MANUAL OF

Pediatric Hematology and *Oncology*

FOURTH EDITION

MANUAL OF
Pediatric Hematology AND *Oncology*

FOURTH EDITION

Philip Lanzkowsky, M.B., Ch.B., M.D.,
Sc.D. (honoris causa), F.R.C.P., D.C.H., F.A.A.P.

Chief Emeritus and Consultant
Division of Pediatric Hematology-Oncology
Chairman, Department of Pediatrics
Chief-of-Staff and Executive Director
Schneider Children's Hospital
New Hyde Park, New York
Vice President, Children's Health Network
North Shore-Long Island Jewish Health System
Professor of Pediatrics
Albert Einstein College of Medicine of Yeshiva University
Bronx, New York

ALISTAIR MacKENZIE LIBRARY

ELSEVIER
ACADEMIC
PRESS

AMSTERDAM • BOSTON • HEIDELBERG • LONDON
NEW YORK • OXFORD • PARIS • SAN DIEGO
SAN FRANCISCO • SINGAPORE • SYDNEY • TOKYO

Elsevier Academic Press
30 Corporate Drive, Suite 400, Burlington, MA 01803, USA
525 B Street, Suite 1900, San Diego, California 92101-4495, USA
84 Theobald's Road, London WC1X 8RR, UK

This book is printed on acid-free paper. ∞

Library of Congress Cataloging-in-Publication Data
Lanzkowsky, Philip, 1932-
    Manual of pediatric hematology and oncology / Philip Lanzkowsky. – 4th ed.
       p. ; cm.
    Includes bibliographical references and index.
    ISBN 0-12-088524-7 (alk. paper)
  1. Pediatric hematology–Handbooks, manuals, etc. 2. Tumors in children–Handbooks, manuals, etc.
    [DNLM: 1. Hematologic Diseases–Child. 2. Hematologic Diseases–Infant. 3. Neoplasms–Child.
4. Neoplasms–Infant. WS 300 L297m 2005] I. Title.
    RJ411.L35 2005
    618.92'15–dc22   2004027550

British Library Cataloguing in Publication Data
A catalogue record for this book is available from the British Library

ISBN: 0-12-088524-7

For all information on all Academic Press publications
visit our Web site at www.academicpress.com

Printed in the United States of America
05 06 07 08 09 9 8 7 6 5 4 3 2 1

Working together to grow
libraries in developing countries

www.elsevier.com | www.bookaid.org | www.sabre.org

ELSEVIER   BOOK AID   Sabre Foundation
            International

In Memory of
my parents—Abe and Lily Lanzkowsky—
who instilled in me
the importance of integrity,
the rewards of industry, and
the primacy of being a mensch

Dedicated to
my devoted and patient wife, Rhona,
who appreciates that the study of medicine
is a lifelong and consuming process

and

to our pride and joy
our children and grandchildren
Shelley and Sergio – Joshua Abraham and Sara Lily Bienstock;
David Roy – Jessica Anne, Brandon Benjamin, and Alex Lanzkowsky;
Leora and Alan – Chloe Hannah, Justin Noah, and Jared Isaac Diamond;
Marc and Lisa Joy – Jacob Tyler and Carly Beatrice Lanzkowsky;
Jonathan and Debra Ann – Hana Julia and Judah Aiden Lanzkowsky

and

to my patients, students, pediatric house staff,
fellows in Pediatric Hematology-Oncology,
and my colleagues,
who have taught me so much over the years

Today he can discover his errors of yesterday
And tomorrow he may obtain new light
On what he thinks himself sure of today

Moses Maimonides

Every care has been taken to ensure that various protocols, drugs, and dosage recommendations are precise and accurate, and that generic and trade names of drugs are correct. However, errors can occur and readers should confirm all dosage schedules against the manufacturer's package information data and standard reference sources. Some dosages and delivery methods may not reflect package insert information, due to clinical experience and current usage.

The reader is referred to Appendix 4, which lists the pharmacologic properties and synonyms of the commonly used chemotherapy agents.

CONTENTS

Contributors / ix

Preface to Fourth Edition / xi

Preface to Third Edition / xiii

Preface to Second Edition / xv

Preface to First Edition / xvii

1. Classification and Diagnosis of Anemia during Childhood / 1

2. Anemia during the Neonatal Period / 12

3. Iron-Deficiency Anemia / 31

4. Megaloblastic Anemia / 47

5. Hematologic Manifestations of Systemic Illness / 71

6. Bone Marrow Failure / 94

7. Hemolytic Anemia / 136

8. Polycythemia / 199

9. Disorders of the White Blood Cells / 209

10. Disorders of Platelets / 250

11. Disorders of Coagulation / 295

   Hemostatic Disorders / 295

   Thrombotic Disorders / 328

12. Lymphadenopathy and Splenomegaly / 363

13. Lymphoproliferative Disorders, Myelodysplastic Syndromes, and Myeloproliferative Disorders / 371

14. Leukemias / 415

15. Hodgkin Disease / 453

16. Non-Hodgkin Lymphoma / 491

17. Central Nervous System Malignancies / 512

18. Neuroblastoma / 530

19. Wilms' Tumor / 548

20. Rhabdomyosarcoma and Other Soft-Tissue Sarcomas / 561

21. Malignant Bone Tumors / 585

22. Histiocytosis Syndromes / 604

23. Retinoblastoma / 630

24. Miscellaneous Tumors / 645

25. Hematopoietic Stem Cell Transplantation / 669

26. Supportive Care and Management of Oncologic Emergencies / 695

27. Evaluation, Investigations and Management of Late Effects of Childhood Cancer / 749

Appendix 1   Hematologic Reference Values / 775

Appendix 2   CD Antigen Designations / 800

Appendix 3   Biological Tumor Markers / 803

Appendix 4   Pharmacologic Properties of the Commonly Used Chemotherapy Agents / 805

Index / 808

CONTRIBUTORS

Steven Arkin, M.D.
Associate Professor of Clinical Pediatrics, Albert Einstein College of Medicine of Yeshiva University, Bronx, New York; Attending, Division of Pediatric Hematology-Oncology, Department of Pediatrics, Schneider Children's Hospital, New Hyde Park, New York

Hemostatic Disorders

Mark Atlas, M.D.
Assistant Professor of Pediatrics, Albert Einstein College of Medicine of Yeshiva University, Bronx, New York; Attending, Division of Pediatric Hematology-Oncology, Department of Pediatrics, Schneider Children's Hospital, New Hyde Park, New York

Thalassemia; Non-Hodgkin Lymphoma; Central Nervous System Malignancies; Rhabdomyosarcoma and Other Soft-Tissue Sarcomas

Banu Aygun, M.D.
Assistant Professor of Pediatrics, Albert Einstein College of Medicine of Yeshiva University, Bronx, New York; Attending, Division of Pediatric Hematology-Oncology, Department of Pediatrics, Schneider Children's Hospital, New Hyde Park, New York

Disorders of Platelets; Lymphadenopathy and Splenomegaly; Gaucher Disease and Niemann–Pick Disease; Malignant Bone Tumors; Supportive Care and Management of Oncologic Emergencies

Debra Friedman, M.D.
Assistant Professor of Pediatrics, University of Washington School of Medicine, Seattle; Attending, Division of Pediatric Hematology-Oncology, Department of Pediatrics, Children's Hospital and Medical Center, Seattle, Washington

Retinoblastoma

Gungor Karayalcin, M.D.
Professor of Pediatrics, Albert Einstein College of Medicine of Yeshiva University, Bronx, New York; Associate Chief, Division of Pediatric Hematology-Oncology, Department of Pediatrics, Schneider Children's Hospital, New Hyde Park, New York

Hematologic Manifestations of Systemic Illness; Sickle Cell Anemia; Thrombotic Disorders; Hodgkin Disease

Philip Lanzkowsky, M.B., Ch.B., M.D., Sc.D. (honoris causa), F.R.C.P., D.C.H., F.A.A.P.
Professor of Pediatrics, Albert Einstein College of Medicine of Yeshiva University, Bronx, New York; Chairman, Department of Pediatrics, Schneider Children's Hospital, New Hyde Park, New York; Emeritus Chief, Division of Pediatric Hematology-Oncology, and Chief of Staff and Executive Director, Schneider Children's Hospital

Classification and Diagnosis of Anemia during Childhood; Anemia during Neonatal Period; Iron-Deficiency Anemia; Megaloblastic Anemia; Thrombotic Disorders; Hodgkin Disease

Jeffrey Lipton, M.D., Ph.D.
Professor of Pediatrics, Albert Einstein College of Medicine of Yeshiva University, Bronx, New York; Chief, Division of Pediatric Hematology-Oncology and Stem Cell Transplantation, Department of Pediatrics, Schneider Children's Hospital, New Hyde Park, New York

Bone Marrow Failure; Histiocytosis Syndromes

Arlene Redner, M.D.
Associate Professor of Clinical Pediatrics, Albert Einstein College of Medicine of Yeshiva University, Bronx, New York; Attending, Division of Pediatric Hematology-Oncology, Department of Pediatrics, Schneider Children's Hospital, New Hyde Park, New York

Leukemias; Wilms' Tumor; Evaluation, Investigations, and Management of Late Effects of Childhood Cancer

Indira Sahdev, M.D.
Associate Professor of Clinical Pediatrics, New York University School of Medicine, New York; Attending, Division of Pediatric Hematology-Oncology, Department of Pediatrics, Schneider Children's Hospital, New Hyde Park, New York

Neuroblastoma; Miscellaneous Tumors; Hematopoietic Stem Cell Transplantation

Ashok Shende, M.D.
Associate Professor of Pediatrics, Albert Einstein College of Medicine of Yeshiva University, Bronx, New York; Attending, Division of Pediatric Hematology-Oncology, Department of Pediatrics, Schneider Children's Hospital, New Hyde Park, New York

Polycythemia; Disorders of the White Blood Cells; Lymphoproliferative Disorders, Myelodysplastic Syndromes, and Myeloproliferative Disorders

PREFACE TO THE FOURTH EDITION

This edition of the *Manual of Pediatric Hematology and Oncology* is the fourth edition and the sixth book written by the author on pediatric hematology and oncology. The first book written by the author 25 years ago was exclusively on pediatric hematology and its companion book, exclusively on pediatric oncology, was written 3 years later. The book reviewers at the time suggested that these two books be combined into a single book on pediatric hematology and oncology and the first edition of the *Manual of Pediatric Hematology and Oncology* was published by the author in 1989.

It is from these origins that this 4th edition arises—the original book written in its entirety by the author, was 456 pages, has more than doubled in size. The basic format and content of the clinical manifestations, diagnosis and differential diagnosis has persisted with little change as originally written by the author. The management and treatment of various diseases have undergone profound changes over time and these aspects of the book have been brought up-to-date by the subspecialists in the various disease entities. The increase in the size of the book is reflective of the advances that have occurred in both hematology and oncology over the past 25 years. Despite the size of the book, the philosophy has remained unchanged over the past quarter century. The author and his contributors have retained this book as a concise manual of personal experiences on the subject over these decades rather than developing a comprehensive tome culled from the literature. Its central theme remains clinical as an immediate reference for the practicing pediatric hematologist-oncologist concerned with the diagnosis and management of hematologic and oncologic diseases. It is extremely useful for students, residents, fellows and pediatric hematologists and oncologists as a basic reference assembling in one place essential knowledge required for clinical practice.

This edition has retained the essential format written and developed decades ago by the author and, with usage over the years, has proven to be highly effective as a concise, practical, up-to-date guide replete with detailed tables, algorithms and flow diagrams for investigation and management of hematologic and oncologic conditions. The tables and flow diagrams have been updated with the latest information and the most recent protocols of treatment, that have received general acceptance and have produced the best results, have been included in the book.

Since the previous edition, some five years ago, there have been considerable advances particularly in the management of oncologic disease in children and these sections of the book have been completely rewritten. In addition, advances in certain areas have required that other sections of the book be updated. There has been extensive revision of certain chapters such as on Disorders of the White Cells, Lymphoproliferative Disorders, Myeloproliferative Disorders and Myelodysplastic Syndromes and Bone Marrow Failure. Because of the extensive advances in thrombosis we have rewritten that entire section contained in the chapter on Disorders of Coagulation to encompass recent advances in that area. The book, like it's previous editions, reflects the practical experience of the author and his colleagues based on half a century of clinical experience. The number of contributors has been expanded but consists essentially of the faculty of the Division of Hematology-Oncology at the

Schneider Children's Hospital, all working together to provide the readers of this manual with a practical guide to the management of the wide spectrum of diseases within the discipline of pediatric hematology-oncology.

I would like to thank Laurie Locastro for her editorial assistance, cover design and for her untiring efforts in the coordination of the various phases of the production of this edition. I also appreciate the efforts of Lawrence Tavnier for his expert typing of parts of the manuscript and would like to thank Elizabeth Dowling and Patricia Mastrolembo for proof reading of the book to ensure its accuracy.

Philip Lanzkowsky, M.B., Ch.B., M.D.,
Sc.D. (honoris causa), F.R.C.P., D.C.H., F.A.A.P.

PREFACE TO THE THIRD EDITION

This edition of the *Manual of Pediatric Hematology and Oncology*, published five years after the second edition, has been written with the original philosophy in mind. It represents the synthesis of experience of four decades of clinical practice in pediatric hematology and oncology and is designed to be of paramount use to the practicing hematologist and oncologist. The book, like its previous editions, contains the most recent information from the literature coupled with the practical experience of the author and his colleagues to provide a guide to the practicing clinician in the investigation and up-to-date treatment of hematologic and oncologic diseases in childhood.

The past five years have seen considerable advances in the management of oncologic diseases in children. Most of the advances have been designed to reduce the immediate and long-term toxicity of therapy without influencing the excellent results that have been achieved in the past. This has been accomplished by reducing dosages, varying the schedules of chemotherapy, and reducing the field and volume of radiation.

The book is designed to be a concise, practical, up-to-date guide and is replete with detailed tables, algorithms, and flow diagrams for investigation and management of hematologic and oncologic conditions. The tables and flow diagrams have been updated with the latest information, and the most recent protocols that have received general acceptance and have produced the best results have been included in the book.

Certain parts of the book have been totally rewritten because our understanding of the pathogenesis of various diseases has been altered in the light of modern biological investigations. Once again, we have included only those basic science advances that have been universally accepted and impinge on clinical practice.

I thank Ms. Christine Grabowski, Ms. Lisa Phelps, Ms. Ellen Healy, and Ms. Patricia Mastrolembo for their untiring efforts in the coordination of the writing and various phases of the development of this edition. Additionally, I acknowledge our fellows, Drs. Banu Aygun, Samuel Bangug, Mahmut Celiker, Naghma Husain, Youssef Khabbaze, Stacey Rifkin-Zenenberg, and Rosa Ana Gonzalez, for their assistance in culling the literature.

I also thank Dr. Bhoomi Mehrotra for reviewing the chapter on bone marrow transplantation, Dr. Lorry Rubin for reviewing the sections of the book dealing with infection, and Dr. Leonard Kahn for reviewing the pathology.

Philip Lanzkowsky, M.B., Ch.B., M.D.,
Sc.D. (honoris causa), F.R.C.P., D.C.H., F.A.A.P.

PREFACE TO THE SECOND EDITION

This edition of the *Manual of Pediatric Hematology and Oncology*, published five years after the first edition, has been written with a similar philosophy in mind. The basic objective of the book is to present useful clinical information from the recent literature in pediatric hematology and oncology and to temper it with experience derived from an active clinical practice.

The manual is designed to be a concise, practical, up-to-date book for practitioners responsible for the care of children with hematologic and oncologic diseases by presenting them with detailed tables and flow diagrams for investigation and clinical management.

Since the publication of the first edition, major advances have occurred, particularly in the management of oncologic diseases in children, including major advances in recombinant human growth factors and bone marrow transplantation. We have included only those basic science advances that have been universally accepted and impinge on clinical practice.

I would like to thank Dr. Raj Pahwa for his contributions on bone marrow transplantation, Drs. Alan Diamond and Leora Lanzkowsky Diamond for their assistance with the neuro-radiology section, and Christine Grabowski and Lisa Phelps for their expert typing of the manuscript and for their untiring assistance in the various phases of the development of this book.

Philip Lanzkowsky, M.B., Ch.B., M.D.,
Sc.D. (honoris causa), F.R.C.P., D.C.H., F.A.A.P.

PREFACE TO THE FIRST EDITION

The *Manual of Pediatric Hematology and Oncology* represents the synthesis of personal experience of three decades of active clinical and research endeavors in pediatric hematology and oncology. The basic orientation and intent of the book is clinical, and the book reflects a uniform systematic approach to the diagnosis and management of hematologic and oncologic diseases in children. The book is designed to cover the entire spectrum of these diseases, and although emphasis is placed on relatively common disorders, rare disorders are included for the sake of completion. Recent developments in hematology-oncology based on pertinent advances in molecular genetics, cytogenetics, immunology, transplantation, and biochemistry are included if the issues have proven value and applicability to clinical practice.

Our aim in writing this manual was to cull pertinent and useful clinical information from the recent literature in pediatric hematology and oncology and to temper it with experience derived from active clinical practice. The result, we hope, is a concise, practical, readable, up-to-date book for practitioners responsible for the care of children with hematologic and oncologic diseases. It is specifically designed for the medical student and practitioner seeking more detailed information on the subject, the pediatric house officer responsible for the care of patients with these disorders, the fellow in pediatric hematology-oncology seeking a systemic approach to these diseases and a guide in preparation for the board examinations, and the practicing pediatric hematologist-oncologist seeking another opinion and approach to the these disorders. As with all brief texts, some dogmatism and "matters of opinion" have been unavoidable in the interests of clarity. The opinions expressed on management are prudent clinical opinions; and although they may not be accepted by all, pediatric hematologists-oncologists will certainly find a consensus. The reader is presented with a consistency of approach and philosophy describing the management of various diseases rather than with different managements derived from various approaches described in the literature. Where there are divergent or currently unresolved views on the investigation or management of a particular disease, we have attempted to state our own opinion and practice so as to provide some guidance rather than to leave the reader perplexed.

The manual is not designed as a tome containing the minutiae of basic physiology, biochemistry, genetics, molecular biology, cellular kinetics, and other esoteric and abstruse detail. These subjects are covered extensively in larger works. Only those basic science advances that impinge on clinical practice have been included here. Each chapter stresses the pathogenesis, pathology, diagnosis, differential diagnosis, investigations, and detailed therapy of hematologic and oncologic diseases seen in children.

I would like to thank Ms. Joan Dowdell and Ms. Helen Witkowski for their expert typing and for their untiring assistance in the various phases of the development of this book.

Philip Lanzkowsky, M.D.,
F.R.C.P., D.C.H., F.A.A.P.

1

CLASSIFICATION AND DIAGNOSIS OF ANEMIA DURING CHILDHOOD

Anemia can be defined as a reduction in hemoglobin concentration, hematocrit, or number of red blood cells per cubic millimeter. The lower limit of the normal range is set at two standard deviations below the mean for age and sex for the normal population.*

When a patient presents with anemia, it is important to establish whether the abnormality is isolated to a single cell line (red blood cells only) or whether it is part of a multiple cell line abnormality (red cells, white cells, and platelets). Abnormalities of two or three cell lines usually indicate one of the following:

- Bone marrow involvement (e.g., aplastic anemia, leukemia) or
- An immunologic disorder [e.g., connective tissue disease or immunoneutropenia, idiopathic thrombocytopenic purpura (ITP) or immune hemolytic anemia singly or in combination] or
- Sequestration of cells (e.g., hypersplenism).

Table 1-1 presents an etiologic classification of anemia and the diagnostic features in each case.

The *blood smear* is very helpful in the diagnosis of anemia. It establishes whether the anemia is hypochromic, microcytic, normocytic, or macrocytic and it also shows specific morphologic abnormalities suggestive of red cell membrane disorders (e.g., spherocytes, stomatocytosis, or elliptocytosis) or hemoglobinopathies (e.g., sickle cell disease, thalassemia).

The mean corpuscular volume (MCV) confirms the findings on the smear with reference to the red cell size, for example, microcytic (<70 fL), macrocytic (>85 fL), or normocytic (72–79 fL). Figure 1-1 delineates diagnosis of anemia by examination of the smear, and Table 1-2 lists the differential diagnostic considerations based on specific red cell morphologic abnormalities. The mean corpuscular hemoglobin (MCH) and mean corpuscular hemoglobin concentration (MCHC) are calculated values and generally of less diagnostic value. The MCH usually parallels the MCV. The MCHC is a measure of cellular hydration status. A high value (>35 g/dL) is characteristic of spherocytosis and a low value is commonly associated with iron deficiency.

The MCV and reticulocyte count are helpful in the differential diagnosis of anemia (Figure 1-2). An elevated reticulocyte count suggests chronic blood loss or hemolysis; a normal or depressed count suggests impaired red cell formation.

---

*Children with cyanotic congenital heart disease, respiratory insufficiency, arteriovenous pulmonary shunts or hemoglobinopathies that alter oxygen affinity can be functionally anemic with hemoglobin levels in the normal range.

Table 1-1. Etiologic Classification and Major Diagnostic Features of Anemia in Children

Etiologic classification	Diagnostic features
I. Impaired red cell formation	
A. Deficiency	
Decreased dietary intake (e.g., excessive milk-iron-deficiency anemia, vegan-vitamin B_{12} deficiency	
Increased demand, e.g., growth (iron) hemolysis (folic acid)	
Decreased absorption	
Specific: intrinsic factor lack (Vitamin B_{12})	
Generalized: malabsorption syndrome (e.g., folic acid, iron)	
Increased loss	
Acute: hemorrhage (iron)	
Chronic: gut bleeding (iron)	
Impairment in red cell formation can result from one of the following deficiencies:	
1. Iron deficiency	Hypochromic, microcytic red cells; low MCV, low MCH, low MCHC, high RDW[a], low serum ferritin, high FEP, guaiac positivity
2. Folate deficiency	Macrocytic red cells, high MCV, high RDW, megaloblastic marrow, low serum and red cell folate
3. Vitamin B_{12} deficiency	Macrocytic red cells, high MCV, high RDW, megaloblastic marrow, low serum B_{12} decreased gastric acidity; Schilling test positive
4. Vitamin C deficiency	Clinical scurvy
5. Protein deficiency	Kwashiorkor
6. Vitamin B_6 deficiency	Hypochromic red cells, sideroblastic bone marrow, high serum ferritin
7. Thyroxine deficiency	Clinical hypothyroidism, low T_4, high TSH
B. Bone marrow failure	
1. Failure of a single cell line	
a. Megakaryocytes[b]	
(1) Amegakaryocytic thrombocytopenic purpura with absent radii (TAR)	Limb abnormalities, thrombocytopenic purpura absent megakaryocytes
b. Red cell precursors	
(1) Congenital red cell aplasia (Diamond–Blackfan anemia)	Absent red cell precursors
(2) Acquired red cell aplasia (transient erythroblasto-penia of childhood)	Absent red cell precursors
c. White cell precursors[b]	
(1) Congenital neutropenia	Neutropenia, recurrent infection

(Continues)

Table 1-1. (*Continued*)

Etiologic classification	Diagnostic features
2. Failure of all cell lines (characterized by pancytopenia and acellular or hypocellular marrow)	
a. Constitutional	
(1) Fanconi anemia	Multiple congenital anomalies, chromosomal breakage
(2) Familial without anomalies	Familial history, no congenital anomalies
(3) Dyskeratosis congenita	Marked mucosal and cutaneous abnormalities
b. Acquired	
(1) Idiopathic	No identifiable cause
(2) Secondary	History of exposure to drugs, radiation, household toxins, infections; associated immunologic disease
3. Infiltration	
a. De novo (e.g., leukemia)	Bone marrow: morphology, cytochemistry, immunologic markers, cytogenetics
b. Secondary (e.g., neuroblastoma, lymphoma)	VMA, skeletal survey, bone marrow
c. Dyshematopoietic anemia (decreased erythropoiesis, decreased iron utilization)	
(1) Infection	Evidence of systemic illness
(2) Renal failure and hepatic disease	BUN and liver function tests
(3) Disseminated malignancy	Clinical evidence
(4) Connective tissue diseases	Rheumatoid arthritis
II. Blood loss	Overt or occult guaiac positive
III. Hemolytic anemia	
A. Corpuscular	Splenomegaly, jaundice
1. Membrane defects (spherocytosis, elliptocytosis)	Morphology, osmotic fragility
2. Enzymatic defects (pyruvate kinase, G6PD)	Autohemolysis, enzyme assays
3. Hemoglobin defects	
a. Heme	
b. Globin	
(1) Qualitative (e.g., sickle cell)	Hb electrophoresis
(2) Quantitative (e.g., thalassemia)	HbF, A_2 content
B. Extracorpuscular	
1. Immune	Coombs' test
a. Isoimmune	
b. Autoimmune	
(1) Idiopathic	Coombs' test, antibody identification

(Continues)

Table 1-1. (*Continued*)

Etiologic classification	Diagnostic features
(2) Secondary Immunologic disorder (e.g., lupus)	Decreased C_3, C_4, CH_{50} positive ANA
One cell line (e.g., red cells)	Anemia: Coombs' positive
Multiple cell line (e.g., white blood cells, platelets)	Neutropenia-immunoneutropenia, thrombocytopenia-ITP
2. Nonimmune (idiopathic, secondary)	

Abbreviations: FEP, free erythrocyte protoporphyrin; G6PD, glucose-6-phosphate dehydrogenase; Hb, hemoglobin; ITP, idiopathic thrombocytopenic purpura; MCH, mean corpuscular hemoglobin; MCHC, mean corpuscular hemoglobin concentration; MCV, mean corpuscular volume; RBC, red blood cell; RDW, red cell distribution width (see definition in footnote a); VMA, vanillylmandelic acid.

[a] RDW = coefficient of variation of the RBC distribution width (normal between 11.5% and 14.5%).

[b] Not associated with anemia.

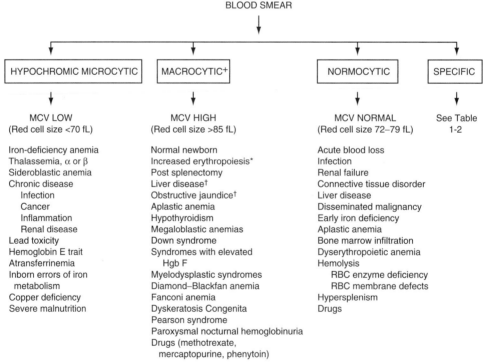

Fig. 1-1. An approach to the diagnosis of anemia by examination of the blood smear.
[+]Spurious macrocytosis (high MCV) may be caused by macroagglutinated red cells (e.g., *Mycoplasma pneumonia* and autoimmune hemolytic anemia).
[*]Increased number of reticulocytes.
[†]On the basis of increased membrane, resulting in an increased membrane/volume ratio. Increased membrane results from exchanges between red cell lipids and altered lipid balance in these conditions.

Table 1-2. Specific Red Cell Morphologic Abnormalities

I. Target cells

Increased surface/volume ratio

Thalassemia

Hemoglobinopathies

Hb AC or CC

Hb SS, SC, S-Thal

Liver disease

Postsplenectomy or hyposplenic states

Severe iron deficiency

Hb E (heterozygote and homozygote)

LCAT deficiency: congenital disorder of lecithin/cholesterol acyltransferase deficiency (corneal opacifications, proteinuria, target cells, moderately severe anemia)

Abetalipoproteinemia

II. Spherocytes

Decreased surface/volume ratio, hyperdense (>MCHC)

Hereditary spherocytosis

ABO incompatibility: antibody-coated fragment of RBC membrane removed

Autoimmune hemolytic anemia: antibody-coated fragment of RBC membrane removed

Microangiopathic hemolytic anemia (MAHA): fragment of RBC lost after impact with abnormal surface

SS disease: fragment of RBC removed in reticuloendothelial system

Hypersplenism

Burns: fragment of damaged RBC removed by spleen

Posttransfusion

Pyruvate kinase deficiency

Water-dilution hemolysis: fragment of damaged RBC removed by spleen

III. Acanthocytes (spur cells)*

Cells with 5–10 spicules of varying length; spicules irregular in space and thickness, with wide bases; appear smaller than normal cells because they assume a spheroid shape

Liver disease

Disseminated intravascular coagulation (and other MAHA)

Postsplenectomy or hyposplenic state

Vitamin E deficiency

Hypothyroidism

Abetalipoproteinemia: rare congenital disorder; 50–100% of cells acanthocytes; associated abnormalities (fat malabsorption, retinitis pigmentosa, neurologic abnormalities)

Malabsorptive states

IV. Echinocytes (burr cells)*

10–30 spicules equal in size and evenly distributed over RBC surface; caused by alteration in extracellular or intracellular environment

Artifact

Renal failure

Dehydration

Liver disease

Pyruvate kinase deficiency

Peptic ulcer disease or gastric carcinoma

Immediately after red cell transfusion

Rare congenital anemias due to decreased intracellular potassium

---

*May be morphologically indistinguishable

(Continues)

Table 1-2. (*Continued*)

V. Pyknocytes*

Distorted, hyperchromic, contracted RBC; can be similar to echinocytes and
acanthocytes

VI. Schistocytes

Helmet, triangular shapes, or small fragments. Caused by fragmentation on impact
with abnormal vascular surface (e.g., fibrin strand, vasculitis, artificial surface in
circulation)

Disseminated intravascular coagulation (DIC)
Severe hemolytic anemia (e.g., G6PD deficiency)
Microangiopathic hemolytic anemia
Hemolytic uremic syndrome
Prosthetic cardiac valve, abnormal cardiac valve, cardiac patch, coarctation of the
aorta
Connective tissue disorder (e.g., SLE)
Kasabach–Merritt syndrome
Purpura fulminans
Renal vein thrombosis
Burns (spheroschistocytes as a result of heat)
Thrombotic thrombocytopenia purpura
Homograft rejection
Uremia, acute tubular necrosis, glomerulonephritis
Malignant hypertension
Systemic amyloidosis
Liver cirrhosis
Disseminated carcinomatosis
Chronic relapsing schistocytic hemolytic anemia

VII. Elliptocytes

Elliptical cells, normochromic; seen normally in less than 1% of RBCs; larger numbers
occasionally seen in a normal patient

Hereditary elliptocytosis
Iron deficiency (increased with severity, hypochromic)
SS disease
Thalassemia major
Severe bacterial infection
SA trait
Leukoerythroblastic reaction
Megaloblastic anemias
Any anemia may occasionally present with up to 10% elliptocytes
Malaria

VIII. Teardrop cells

Shape of drop, usually microcytic, often also hypochromic

Newborn
Thalassemia major
Leukoerythroblastic reaction
Myeloproliferative syndromes

IX. Stomatocytes

Has a slit-like area of central pallor

Normal (in small numbers)
Hereditary stomatocytosis
Artifact
Thalassemia

*May be morphologically indistinguishable

(Continues)

Table 1-2. (*Continued*)

Acute alcoholism
Rh null disease (absence of Rh complex)
Liver disease
Malignancies

X. **Nucleated red blood cells**
Not normal in the peripheral blood beyond the first week of life
Newborn (first 3–4 days)
Intense bone marrow stimulation
Hypoxia (especially postcardiac arrest)
Acute bleeding
Severe hemolytic anemia (e.g., thalassemia, SS hemoglobinopathy)
Congenital infections (e.g., sepsis, congenital syphilis, CMV, rubella)
Postsplenectomy or hyposplenic states: spleen normally removes nucleated RBC
Leukoerythroblastic reaction: seen with extramedullary hematopoiesis and bone
marrow replacement; most commonly leukemia or solid tumor—fungal and
mycobacterial infection may also do this; leukoerythroblastic reaction is also
associated with teardrop red cells, 10,000–20,000 WBC with small to moderate
numbers of metamyelocytes, myelocytes, and promyelocytes; thrombocytosis
with large bizarre platelets
Megaloblastic anemia
Dyserythropoietic anemias

XI. **Blister cells**
Red cell area under membrane, free of hemoglobin, appearing like a blister
G6PD deficiency (during hemolytic episode)
SS disease
Pulmonary emboli

XII. **Basophilic stippling**
Coarse or fine punctate basophilic inclusions that represent aggregates of ribosomal
RNA
Hemolytic anemias (e.g., thalassemia trait)
Iron-deficiency anemia
Lead poisoning
Pyrimidine 5′-nucleotidase deficiency

XIII. **Howell–Jolly bodies**
Small, well-defined, round, densely stained nuclear-remnant inclusions; 1 μm in
diameter; centric in location
Postsplenectomy or hyposplenia
Newborn
Megaloblastic anemias
Dyserythropoietic anemias
A variety of types of anemias (rarely iron-deficiency anemia, hereditary spherocytosis)

XIV. **Cabot's Ring bodies**
Nuclear remnant ring configuration inclusions
Pernicious anemia
Lead toxicity

XV. **Heinz bodies**
Denatured aggregated hemoglobin
Thalassemia
Asplenia
Chronic liver disease
Heinz-body hemolytic anemia

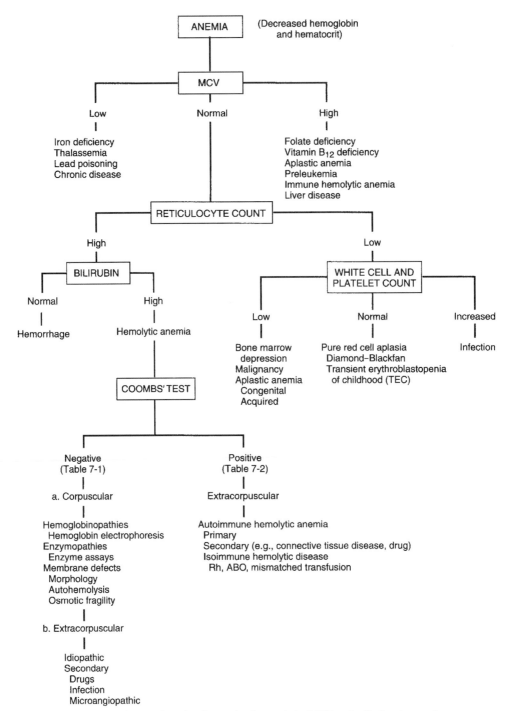

Fig. 1-2. Approach to the diagnosis of anemia by MCV and reticulocyte count.

The reticulocyte count must be adjusted for the level of anemia to obtain the reticulocyte index,* a more accurate reflection of erythropoiesis. In patients with bleeding or hemolysis, the reticulocyte index should be at least 3%, whereas in patients with anemia due to decreased production of red cells, the reticulocyte index is less than 3% and frequently less than 1.5%.

Mean corpuscular volume and red cell distribution width (RDW) indices, available from automated electronic blood-counting equipment, are extremely helpful in defining the morphology and the nature of the anemia and have led to a classification based on these indices (Table 1-3).

In more refractory cases of anemia, bone marrow examination may be indicated. A bone marrow smear should be stained for iron, where indicated, to estimate iron stores and to diagnose the presence of a sideroblastic anemia. Bone marrow examination may indicate a normoblastic, megaloblastic, or sideroblastic morphology. Figure 1-3 presents the causes of each of these findings.

Table 1-4 lists various laboratory studies helpful in the investigation of a patient with anemia. The investigation of anemia entails the following steps:

1. Detailed history and physical examination (see Table 1-1)
2. Complete blood count, to establish whether the anemia is only due to one cell line (e.g., the red cell line only) or is part of a three-cell-line abnormality (abnormality of red cell count, white blood cell count, and platelet count)
3. Determination of the morphologic characteristics of the anemia based on blood smear (Table 1-2) and consideration of the MCV (Figures 1-1 and 1-2) and RDW (Table 1-3) and morphologic consideration of white blood cell and platelet morphology

Table 1-3. Classification of Nature of the Anemia Based on MCV and RDW

	MCV low	MCV normal	MCV high
RDW normal	Microcytic homogeneous	Normocytic homogeneous	Macrocytic homogeneous
	Heterozygous thalassemia Chronic disease	Normal Chronic disease Chronic liver disease Nonanemic hemoglobinopathy (e.g., AS, AC) Chemotherapy Chronic myelocytic leukemia Hemorrhage Hereditary spherocytosis	Aplastic anemia Preleukemia
RDW high	Microcytic heterogeneous	Normocytic heterogeneous	Macrocytic heterogeneous
	Iron deficiency S β-thalassemia Hemoglobin H Red cell fragmentation	Early iron or folate deficiency Mixed deficiencies Hemoglobinopathy (e.g., SS) Myelofibrosis Sideroblastic anemia	Folate deficiency Vitamin B_{12} deficiency Immune hemolytic anemia Cold agglutinins

Abbreviations: MCV, mean corpuscular volume; RDW, red cell distribution width, which is the coefficient of variation of RBC distribution width (normal: 11.5–14.5%).

*Reticulocyte index = reticulocyte count × (patient's hematocrit/normal hematocrit). For example, for a reticulocyte count of 6% and hematocrit of 15%, the reticulocyte index = 6 × (15/45) = 2%.

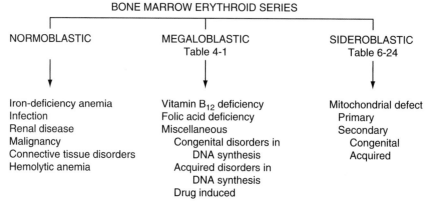

Fig. 1-3. Causes of normoblastic, megaloblastic, and sideroblastic bone marrow morphology.

Table 1-4. Laboratory Studies Often Helpful in the Investigation of a Patient with Anemia

Usual initial studies
  Hemoglobin and hematocrit determination
  Erythrocyte count and red cell indices, including MCV and RDW
  Reticulocyte count
  Study of stained blood smear
  Leukocyte count and differential count
  Platelet count
Suspected iron deficiency
  Free erythrocyte protoporphyrin
  Serum ferritin levels
  Stool for occult blood
  ^{99m}Tc pertechnetate scan for Meckel's diverticulum—if indicated
  Endoscopy (upper and lower bowel)—if indicated
Suspected vitamin B_{12} or folic acid deficiency
  Bone marrow
  Serum vitamin B_{12} level
  Serum folate level
  Gastric analysis after histamine injection
  Vitamin B_{12} absorption test (radioactive cobalt) (Schilling test)
Suspected hemolytic anemia
  Evidence of red cell breakdown
    Blood smear
    Serum bilirubin level
    Urinary urobilinogen
    Hemoglobinuria
    Serum haptoglobin
  Evidence of red cell regeneration
    Reticulocyte count
    Blood smear
    Skeletal radiographs
  Evidence of type of hemolytic anemia: corpuscular
    Membrane
      Blood smear
      Osmotic fragility test
      Autohemolysis test

(Continues)

Table 1-4. (*Continued*)

Hemoglobin
    Sickle test
    Hemoglobin electrophoresis
    Hemoglobin F determination
    Kleihauer–Betke smear
    Heat-stability test
Enzymes
    Enzyme assay
Evidence of type of hemolytic anemia: extracorpuscular
    Immune
        Antiglobulin test
        Acid serum lysis test
        Sucrose lysis test
        Donath–Landsteiner antibody
        ANA
Suspected aplastic anemia or leukemia
    Bone marrow (aspiration and biopsy)—cytochemistry, immunologic markers,
        chromosome analysis
    Skeletal radiographs
Other tests often used especially to diagnose the primary disease
    Viral serology, e.g., HIV
    ANA, complement, CH_{50}
    Blood urea, creatinine, T_4, TSH
    Tissue biopsy (skin, lymph node, liver)

4. Bone marrow aspiration, if required, to examine erythroid, myeloid, and megakaryocytic morphology to determine whether normoblastic, megaloblastic, or sideroblastic erythropoiesis is present and to exclude marrow pathology (e.g., aplastic anemia, leukemia, and benign or malignant infiltration of the bone marrow) (Figure 1-3)
5. Determination of underlying cause of anemia by additional tests (Table 1-4).

SUGGESTED READINGS

Bessman JD, Gilmer PR, Gardner FH. Improved classification of anemias by MCV and RDW. Am J Clin Pathol 1983;80:322.

Blanchette V, Zipursky A. Assessment of anemia in newborn infants. Clin Perinatol 1984;11:489.

Lanzkowsky P. Diagnosis of anemia in the neonatal period and during childhood. In: Pediatric Hematology-Oncology: A Treatise for the Clinician. New York: McGraw-Hill, 1980;3.

2

ANEMIA DURING THE NEONATAL PERIOD

Anemia during the neonatal period is caused by:

- *Hemorrhage:* acute or chronic
- *Hemolysis:* congenital hemolytic anemias or due to isoimmunization, usually associated with indirect hyperbilirubinemia
- *Failure of red cell production:* Diamond–Blackfan anemia (pure red cell aplasia).

Table 2-1 lists the causes of anemia in the newborn.

HEMORRHAGE

Blood loss may occur during the prenatal, intranatal, or postnatal period. Prenatal blood loss may be transplacental, intraplacental, or retroplacental or may be due to a twin-to-twin transfusion.

Prenatal Blood Loss

Transplacental Fetomaternal

In 50% of pregnancies, fetal cells can be demonstrated in the maternal circulation, and in 1% of cases this is of sufficient magnitude to produce anemia in the infant. Transplacental blood loss may be acute or chronic. Table 2-2 lists the characteristics of acute and chronic blood loss in the newborn. Blood loss may be secondary to procedures such as diagnostic amniocentesis or external cephalic version. Fetomaternal hemorrhage is diagnosed by demonstrating fetal red cells by the acid-elution method of staining for fetal hemoglobin (Kleihauer–Betke technique) in the maternal circulation. The optimal timing for demonstrating fetal cells in maternal blood is within 2 hours of delivery and no later than the first 24 hours following delivery.

Intraplacental and Retroplacental

Occasionally, fetal blood accumulates in the substance of the placenta (intraplacental) or retroplacentally, and the infant is born anemic. Intraplacental blood loss from the fetus may occur when there is a tight umbilical cord around the neck or body or when there is delayed cord clamping. Retroplacental bleeding from abruptio placenta is diagnosed by ultrasound or at surgery.

Table 2-1. Causes of Anemia in the Newborn

I. Hemorrhage
- A. Prenatal
    1. Transplacental fetomaternal (spontaneous, traumatic amniocentesis, external cephalic version)
    2. Intraplacental
    3. Retroplacental
    4. Twin-to-twin transfusion
- B. Intranatal
    1. Umbilical cord abnormalities
        a. Rupture of normal cord (unattended labor)
        b. Rupture of varix or aneurysm of cord
        c. Hematomas of cord
        d. Rupture of anomalous aberrant vessels of cord (not protected by Wharton's jelly)
        e. Vasa previa (umbilical cord is presenting part)
        f. Inadequate cord tying
    2. Placental abnormalities
        a. Multilobular placenta (fragile communicating veins to main placenta)
        b. Placenta previa—fetal blood loss predominantly
        c. Abruptio placentae—maternal blood loss predominantly
        d. Accidental incision of placenta during cesarean section
- C. Postnatal
    1. External
        a. Bleeding from umbilicus
        b. Bleeding from gut
        c. Iatrogenic (diagnostic venipuncture, post-exchange transfusion)
    2. Internal
        a. Cephalhematomata
        b. Subaponeurotic hemorrhage
        c. Subdural or subarachnoid hemorrhage
        d. Intracerebral hemorrhage
        e. Intraventricular hemorrhage
        f. Retroperitoneal hemorrhage (may involve adrenals)
        g. Subcapsular hematoma or rupture of liver
        h. Ruptured spleen

II. Hemolytic anemia (see Chapter 7)
- A. Congenital erythrocyte defects
    1. Membrane defects (with characteristic morphology)
        a. Hereditary spherocytosis (pages 143–147)
        b. Hereditary elliptocytosis (pages 147–148)
        c. Hereditary propoikilocytosis (pages 148–149)
        d. Hereditary stomatocytosis (pages 149–150)
        e. Hereditary acanthocytosis (page 150)
        f. Hereditary xerocytosis (pages 150–151)
        g. Infantile pyknocytosis[a]
    2. Hemoglobin defects
        a. α-Thalassemia[b]
        b. γ β-Thalassemia
        c. Unstable hemoglobins (Hb Köln, Hb Zürich[b]) (pages 180–181)
    3. Enzyme defects
        a. Embden–Meyerhof glycolytic pathway
            (1) Pyruvate kinase
            (2) Other enzymes
        b. Hexose-monophosphate shunt
            (1) G6PD (Caucasian and Oriental) with or without drug exposure[b]
            (2) Enzymes concerned with glutathione reduction or synthesis[b]

(Continues)

Table 2-1. (*Continued*)

  B. Acquired erythrocyte defects
    1. Immune
      a. Rh disease, ABO, minor blood groups (M, S, Kell, Duffy, Luther)
    2. Nonimmune
      a. Infections (cytomegalovirus, toxoplasmosis, herpes simplex, rubella, syphilis, bacterial sepsis, e.g., *Escherichia coli*)
      b. Microangiopathic hemolytic anemia with or without disseminated intravascular coagulation: disseminated herpes simplex, coxsackie B infections, gram-negative septicemia, renal vein thrombosis
      c. Toxic exposure (drugs, chemicals) ± G6PD ± prematurity[b]: synthetic vitamin K analogues, maternal thiazide diuretics, antimalarial agents, sulfonamides, naphthalene, aniline-dye marking ink, penicillin
      d. Vitamin E deficiency
      e. Metabolic disease (galactosemia, osteopetrosis)

III. Failure of red cell production
    1. Congenital (Chapter 6)
    Diamond–Blackfan anemia (pure red cell aplasia)
    Dyskeratosis Congenita
    Fanconi anemia
    Congenital dyserythropoietic anemia
    2. Acquired
    Viral infection (hepatitis, HIV, CMV, rubella, syphilis, parvovirus)
    Anemia of prematurity

[a]Not permanent membrane defect but has characteristic morphology.

[b]All of these conditions can be associated with Heinz-body formation and in the past were grouped together as congenital Heinz-body anemia.

Table 2-2. Characteristics of Acute and Chronic Blood Loss in the Newborn

Characteristic	Acute blood loss	Chronic blood loss
Clinical	Acute distress; pallor; shallow, rapid, and often irregular respiration; tachycardia; weak or absent peripheral pulses; low or absent blood pressure; no hepatosplenomegaly	Marked pallor disproportionate to evidence of distress; on occasion signs of congestive heart failure may be present, including hepatomegaly
Venous pressure	Low	Normal or elevated
Laboratory		
Hemoglobin concentration	May be normal initially; then drops quickly during first 24 hours of life	Low at birth
Red cell morphology	Normochromic and macrocytic	Hypochromic and microcytic Anisocytosis and poikilocytosis
Serum iron	Normal at birth	Low at birth
Course	Prompt treatment of anemia and shock necessary to prevent death	Generally uneventful
Treatment	Normal saline bolus or packed red blood cells; if indicated, iron therapy	Iron therapy

From Oski FA, Naiman, JL. Hematologic problems in the newborn. 3rd ed. Philadelphia: Saunders, 1982, with permission.

Twin-to-Twin Transfusion

Significant twin-to-twin transfusion occurs in at least 15% of monochorionic twins. The hemoglobin level differs by 5 g/dL and the hematocrit by 15% or more between individual twins. The donor twin is smaller, pale, may have evidence of oligohydramnios, and may show evidence of shock. The recipient is larger and polycythemic with evidence of polyhydramnios and may show signs of congestive heart failure (Chapter 8).

Intranatal Blood Loss

Hemorrhage may occur during the process of birth as a result of various obstetric accidents, malformations of the umbilical cord or the placenta, or a hemorrhagic diathesis (due to a plasma factor deficiency or thrombocytopenia) (Table 2-1).

Postnatal Blood Loss

Postnatal hemorrhage may occur from a number of sites and may be internal (enclosed) or external. Hemorrhage may be due to:

1. Traumatic deliveries (resulting in intracranial or intra-abdominal hemorrhage)
2. Plasma factor deficiencies (see Chapter 11)
   a. Congenital—hemophilia or other plasma factor deficiencies
   b. Acquired—vitamin K deficiency, disseminated intravascular coagulation
3. Thrombocytopenia (see Chapter 10)
   a. Congenital—Wiskott–Aldrich syndrome, Fanconi anemia
   b. Acquired—isoimmune thrombocytopenia, sepsis.

Clinical and Laboratory Findings

Anemia—pallor, tachycardia, and hypotension (if severe, i.e., ≥20 mL/kg blood loss)
Liver and spleen not enlarged (except in chronic transplacental bleed)
Jaundice absent
Coombs' test negative
Increased reticulocyte count
Polychromatophilia
Nucleated RBCs raised
Fetal cells in maternal blood (in fetomaternal bleed)

Treatment

1. Severely affected
   a. Administer 10–20 mL/kg packed red blood cells (hematocrit usually 50–60%) via an umbilical catheter.
   b. Cross-match blood with the mother. If unavailable, use group O Rh-negative blood or saline boluses (temporarily for shock).
   c. Use partial exchange transfusion with packed red cells for infants in incipient heart failure.
2. Mild anemia due to chronic blood loss
   a. Ferrous sulfate (2 mg elemental iron/kg body weight 3 times a day) for 3 months.

HEMOLYTIC ANEMIA

Hemolytic anemia in the newborn is usually associated with unconjugated hyperbilirubinemia. The hemolytic process is often first detected as a result of the investigation of jaundice during the first week of life. The causes of hemolytic anemia in the newborn are listed in Table 2-1.

Congenital Erythrocyte Defects

Congenital erythrocyte defects involving the red cell membrane, hemoglobin, and enzymes are listed in Table 1-2 and discussed in Chapter 7. Any of these conditions may occur in the newborn and manifest clinically as follows:

Hemolytic anemia (low hemoglobin, reticulocytosis, increased nucleated red cells, morphologic changes)
Unconjugated hyperbilirubinemia
Coombs' test negative.

Infantile Pyknocytosis

Infantile pyknocytosis (see Table 1-2) is characterized by:

1. Hemolytic anemia—Coombs' negative (nonimmune).
2. Distortion of as many as 50% of red blood cells with several to many spiny projections (up to 6% of cells may be distorted in normal infants). Abnormal morphology is extracorpuscular in origin.
3. Disappearance of pyknocytes and hemolysis by the age of 6 months. This is a self-limiting condition.
4. Hepatosplenomegaly.
5. Pyknocytosis may occur in glucose-6-phosphate dehydrogenase (G6PD) deficiency, pyruvate kinase deficiency, vitamin E deficiency, neonatal infections, and hemolysis caused by drugs and toxic agents.

Anemia in the Newborn Associated with Heinz-Body Formation

Red cells of the newborn are highly susceptible to oxidative insult and Heinz-body formation. This may be congenital or acquired and transient.

Congenital

Hemolytic anemia associated with Heinz-body formation occurs in the following conditions:

1. Unstable hemoglobinopathies (e.g., Hb Köln or Hb Zürich)
2. α-Thalassemia, for example, hemoglobin H (β-chain tetrameres)*
3. Deficiency of G6PD, 6-phosphogluconic dehydrogenase, glutathione reductase, glutathione peroxidase.

Acquired

Hemolytic anemia associated with Heinz-body formation occurs transiently in normal full-term infants without red cell enzyme deficiencies if the dose of certain drugs

---

*β-chain hemoglobinopathies such as sickle cell disease or β-thalassemia are generally not apparent until 3–6 months of age when synthesis of the β-globin chain increases, whereas α-chain hemoglobinopathies are evident during fetal life and at birth.

or chemicals is large enough. The following have been associated with toxic Heinz-body formation: synthetic water-soluble vitamin K preparations (Synkayvite), sulfonamides, chloramphenicol, aniline dyes used for marking diapers, and naphthalene used as mothballs.

Diagnosis

1. Demonstrate Heinz bodies on a supravital preparation.
2. Perform specific tests to exclude the various congenital causes of Heinz-body formation mentioned earlier.

Acquired Erythrocyte Defects

Acquired erythrocyte defects may be due to immune (Coombs'-positive) or non-immune (Coombs'-negative) causes. The immune causes are due to blood group incompatibility between the fetus and the mother, for example, Rh (D), ABO, or minor blood group incompatibilities (such as anti-c, Kell, Duffy, Luther, anti-C, and anti-E) causing isoimmunization.

Rh Isoimmunization

Clinical Features

1. Anemia, mild to severe (if severe, associated with hydrops fetalis)
2. Jaundice (indirect hyperbilirubinemia)
   a. Presents during first 24 hours.
   b. May cause kernicterus
      (1) Exchange transfusion should be carried out whenever the bilirubin level in full-term infants rises to, or exceeds, 20 mg/dL.
      (2) Factors that predispose to the development of kernicterus at lower levels of bilirubin, such as prematurity, hypoproteinemia, metabolic acidosis, drugs (sulfonamides, caffeine, sodium benzoate), and hypoglycemia, require exchange transfusions below 20 mg/dL.
   c. Table 2-3 lists the various causes of unconjugated hyperbilirubinemia. Figure 2-1 outlines an approach to the diagnosis of both unconjugated and conjugated hyperbilirubinemia.
3. Hepatosplenomegaly; varies with severity.
4. Petechiae (only in severely affected infants). Hyporegenerative thrombocytopenia and neutropenia may occur during the first week.

Table 2-3. Causes of Unconjugated Hyperbilirubinemia

I. "Physiologic" jaundice: jaundice of hepatic immaturity

II. Hemolytic anemia (see Chapter 7 for more complete list of causes)
   A. Congenital erythrocyte defect
      1. Membrane defects: hereditary spherocytosis, ovalocytosis, stomatocytosis, infantile pyknocytosis
      2. Enzyme defects (nonspherocytic)
         a. Embden–Meyerhof glycolytic pathway (energy potential): pyruvate kinase, triose phosphate isomerase, etc. (pages 152–153)
         b. Hexose monophosphate shunt (reduction potential): G6PD (pages 153–157)
      3. Hemoglobin defects
         Sickle cell hemoglobinopathy[a]

(Continues)

Table 2-3. (*Continued*)

    B. Acquired erythrocyte defect
        1. Immune: allo-immunization (Rh, ABO, Kell, Duffy, Lutheran)
        2. Nonimmune
          a. Infection
            (1) Bacterial: *Escherichia coli*, streptococcal septicemia
            (2) Viral: cytomegalovirus, rubella, herpes simplex
            (3) Protozoal: toxoplasmosis
            (4) Spirochetal: syphilis
          b. Drugs: penicillin
          c. Metabolic: asphyxia, hypoxia, shock, acidosis, vitamin E deficiency in premature infants, hypoglycemia

III. Polycythemia (see Table 8-1 for more complete list of causes)
    A. Placental hypertransfusion
        1. Twin-to-twin transfusion
        2. Maternal–fetal transfusion
        3. Delayed cord clamping
    B. Placental insufficiency
        1. Small for gestational age
        2. Postmaturity
        3. Toxemia of pregnancy
        4. Placenta previa
    C. Endocrinal
        1. Congenital adrenal hyperplasia
        2. Neonatal thyrotoxicosis
        3. Maternal diabetes mellitus
    D. Miscellaneous
        1. Down syndrome
        2. Hyperplastic visceromegaly (Beckwith–Wiedemann syndrome), associated with hypoglycemia

IV. Hematoma
Cephalhematoma, subgaleal, subdural, intraventricular, intracerebral, subcapsular hematoma of liver; bleeding into gut

V. Conjugation defects
    A. Reduction in bilirubin glucuronyl transferase
        1. Severe (type I): Crigler–Najjar (autosomal recessive)
        2. Mild (type II): Crigler–Najjar (autosomal dominant)
        3. Gilbert disease
    B. Inhibitors of bilirubin glucuronyl transferase
        1. Drugs: novobiocin
        2. Breast milk: pregnane-3α, 20β-diol
        3. Familial: transient familial hyperbilirubinemia

VI. Metabolic
Hypothyroidism, maternal diabetes mellitus, galactosemia

VII. Gut obstruction (due to enterohepatic recirculation of bilirubin) (e.g., pyloric stenosis, annular pancreas, duodenal atresia)

VIII. Maternal indirect hyperbilirubinemia (e.g., homozygous sickle cell hemoglobinopathy)

IX. Idiopathic

---

[a]Not usually a cause of jaundice in the newborn because of the predominance of Hgb F (unless associated with concomitant G6PD deficiency).

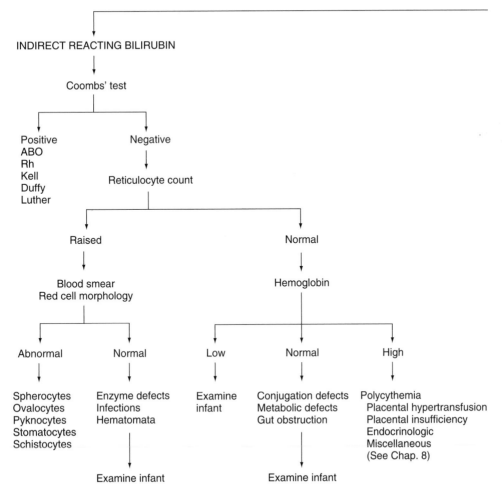

Fig. 2-1. Approach to investigation of jaundice in the newborn.

(Continues)

5. Severe illness with birth of infant with hydrops fetalis, stillbirth, or death *in utero* and delivery of a macerated fetus.
6. Late hyporegenerative anemia with absent reticulocytes. This occurs occasionally during the second to the fifth week and is due to a diminished population of erythroid progenitors (serum concentration of erythropoietin is low and the marrow concentrations of BFU-E and CFU-E are not elevated).

Laboratory Findings

1. Serologic abnormalities (incompatibility between blood group of infant and mother; direct Coombs' test positive in infant; mother's serum has the presence of immune antibodies detected by the indirect Coombs' test)
2. Decreased hemoglobin level, elevated reticulocyte count, smear-increased nucleated red cells, marked polychromasia, and anisocytosis
3. Raised indirect bilirubin level.

Management

Antenatal

Patients should be screened at their first antenatal visit for Rh and non-Rh antibodies. Figure 2-2 shows a schema of the antenatal management of Rh disease. If an

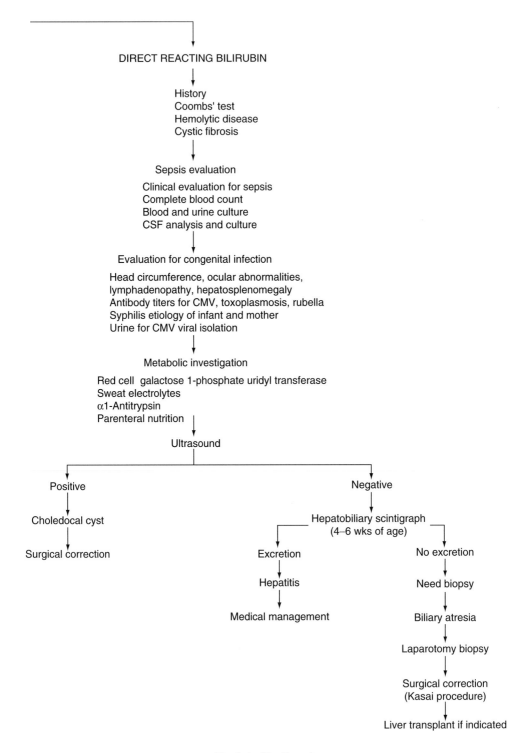

Fig. 2-1. (*Continued*)

immune antibody is detected in the mother's serum, proper management includes the following:

1. Obtain past obstetric history and outcome of previous pregnancies.
2. Determine blood group and conduct indirect Coombs' test (to determine the presence and titer of irregular antibodies). Most irregular antibodies can cause

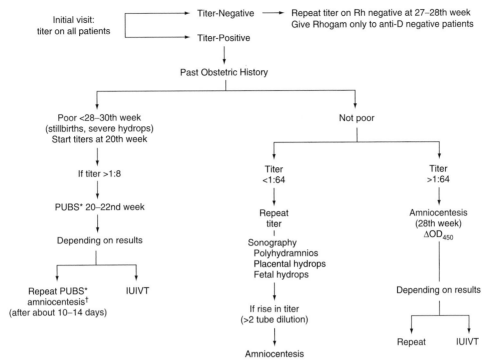

Fig. 2-2. Schema of antenatal management of Rh disease.
Abbreviation: IUIVT, intrauterine intravenous transfusion.
*Percutaneous umbilical vein blood sampling.
[†]Amniotic fluid analysis is less reliable prior to the 26th week of gestation, and PUBS is recommended.

erythroblastosis fetalis; therefore, screening of maternal serum is important. Titers should be determined at various weeks of gestation (Figure 2-2). The frequency depends on the initial or subsequent rise in titers. Theoretically, any blood group antigen (with the exception of Lewis and I, which are not present on fetal erythrocytes) may cause erythroblastosis fetalis. Anti-Le[a], Le[b], M, H, P, S, and I are IgM antibodies and rarely, if ever, cause erythroblastosis fetalis and need not cause concern.

3. Determine zygosity of the father: If the mother is Rh negative and the father is Rh positive, the father's zygosity becomes critical. If he is homozygous, all his future children will be Rh positive. If the father is heterozygous, there is a 50% chance that the fetus will be Rh negative and unaffected. The Rh genotype can be accurately determined by the use of polymerase chain reaction (PCR) of chorionic villus tissue, amniotic cells, and fetal blood when the father is heterozygous or his zygosity is unknown. Mothers with fetuses found to be Rh D negative (dd) can be reassured and further serologic testing and invasive procedures can be avoided. Fetal zygosity can thus be determined by molecular biological means without invading the fetomaternal circulation. It has recently been demonstrated that fetal Rh D genotyping can be performed rapidly on maternal plasma in the second trimester of pregnancy. This is performed by extracting DNA from maternal plasma and analyzing it for the Rh D gene with a fluorescent-based PCR test sensitive enough to detect the Rh D gene in a single cell. The advantage of this test is that neither the mother nor the fetus is exposed to the risks of amniocentesis or chorionic villus sampling.

4. Examination of the amniotic fluid for spectrophotometric analysis of bilirubin. Past obstetric history and antibody titer are indications for serial amniocentesis and spectrophotometric analyses of amniotic fluid to determine the condition of the fetus. Amniotic fluid analysis correlates well with the hemoglobin and hematocrit at birth ($r = 0.9$), but does not predict whether the fetus will require an exchange transfusion after birth. The following are indications for amniocentesis:

   a. History of previous Rh disease severe enough to require an exchange transfusion or to cause stillbirth.

   b. Maternal titer of anti-D, anti-c, or anti-Kell (or other irregular antibodies) of 1:8 to 1:64 or greater by indirect Coombs' test or albumin titration and depending on previous history. An assessment of the optical density difference at 450 μm (ΔOD_{450}) at a given gestational age permits reasonable prediction of the fetal outcome (Figure 2-3). Determination of the appropriate

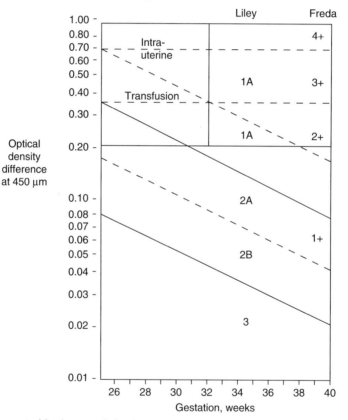

Fig. 2-3. Assessment of fetal prognosis by the methods of Liley and of Freda. Liley's method of prediction: *Zone 1A:* Condition desperate, immediate delivery or intrauterine transfusion required, depending on gestational age. *Zone 1B:* Hemoglobin less than 8 g/dL, delivery or intrauterine transfusion urgent, depending on gestational age. *Zone 2A:* Hemoglobin 8–10 g/dL, delivery at 36–37 weeks. *Zone 2B:* Hemoglobin 11.0–13.9 g/dL, delivery at 37–39 weeks. *Zone 3:* Not anemic, deliver at term. Freda's method of prediction: *Zone 4+:* Fetal death imminent, immediate delivery or intrauterine transfusion, depending on gestational age. *Zone 3+:* Fetus in jeopardy, death within 3 weeks, delivery or intrauterine transfusion as soon as possible, depending on gestational age. *Zone 2+:* Fetal survival for at least 7–10 days, repeat amniocentesis indicated, possible indication for intrauterine transfusion, depending on gestational age. *Zone 1+:* Fetus in no immediate danger. (From Robertson JG. Evaluation of the reported methods of interpreting spectrophotometric tracings of amniotic fluid analysis in Rhesus isoimmunization. Am J Obstet Gynecol 1966;95:120, with permission.)

treatment depends on the ΔOD_{450} of the amniotic fluid, the results of the fetal biophysical profile scoring,* and the assessment of the presence or absence of fetal hydrops (seen on ultrasound) and amniotic phospholipid determinations (lung profile):

Features of lung profile	Immature fetus	Mature fetus
Lecithin/sphingomyelin ratio	<2.0 <45%	>2.0 >50%
Phosphatidylinositol	Absent	Absent
Phosphatidylglycerol	Present (small amounts)	Present (prominent)

If the amniotic fluid ΔOD_{450} indicates a severely affected fetus and phospholipid estimations indicate lung maturity, the infant should be delivered. If the ΔOD_{450} indicates a severely affected fetus and the phospholipid estimations indicate marked immaturity, maternal plasmapheresis and/or intrauterine intravenous transfusion (IUIVT) should be carried out. IUIVT has many advantages over intraperitoneal fetal transfusions and is the procedure of choice. This decision is made in conjunction with the biophysical profile score.

Intensive maternal plasmapheresis antenatally using a continuous-flow cell separator can significantly reduce Rh antibody levels, reduce fetal hemolysis, and improve fetal survival in those mothers carrying highly sensitized Rh-positive fetuses. This procedure together with IUIVT should be carried out when a high antibody titer exists early before a time when the infant can be safely delivered.

If the risk of perinatal death resulting from complications of prematurity is high, then an IUIVT should be carried out. Percutaneously, the umbilical vein is used for blood sampling (PUBS) and venous access and permits a fetal transfusion via the intravascular route (IUIVT). With the availability of high-resolution ultrasound guidance, a fine (20-gauge) needle is inserted directly into the umbilical cord, either at the insertion site into the placenta or into a free loop of cord. This allows the same blood sampling as is available postnatally in the neonate. Temporary paralysis of the fetus with the use of pancuronium bromide (Pavulon) facilitates the procedure, which may be applied to fetuses from 18 weeks' gestation until the gestational age when fetal lung maturity is confirmed. The interval between procedures ranges from 1 to 3 weeks.

The risks of IUIVT include:

Fetal loss (2%)
Premature labor and rupture of membranes
Chorioamnionitis
Fetal bradycardia
Cord hematoma or laceration
Fetomaternal hemorrhage.

The overall survival rate is 88%. Intraperitoneal transfusion can be performed in addition to IUIVT to increase the amount of blood transfused and to extend the interval between transfusions.

Modern neonatal care, including attention to metabolic, nutritional, and ventilatory needs and the use of artificial surfactant insufflation, makes successful earlier delivery possible. The need for IUIVT and intraperitoneal transfusion is rarely, if ever, indicated.

---

*Ultrasound for the assessment of gestational age must be done early in pregnancy. The fetal biophysical profile scoring uses multiple variables: fetal breathing movements, gross body movements, fetal tone, reactive fetal heart rate, and quantitative amniotic fluid volume. This scoring system provides a good short-term assessment of fetal risk for death or damage *in utero*.

Postnatal

Hyperbilirubinemia is the most frequent problem and can be managed by exchange transfusion. Phototherapy is an adjunct rather than the first line of therapy in hyperbilirubinemia due to erythroblastosis fetalis. Postnatal management and criteria for exchange transfusion have changed over the years. We currently use the following management:

1. In hydropic infant at birth:
   a. Adequate ventilation must be established.
   b. Partial exchange transfusion may be necessary to correct severe anemia.
   c. Double-volume exchange transfusion may be required later.
2. A rapid increase in the bilirubin level of greater than 1.0 mg/h and/or a bilirubin level approaching 20 mg/dL at any time during the first few days of life in the full-term infant is an indication for exchange transfusion. In preterm or high-risk infants, exchange transfusion should be carried out at lower levels of bilirubin (e.g., 15 mg/dL).
3. Clinical signs suggesting kernicterus at any time at any bilirubin level are an indication for exchange transfusion.

Prevention of Rh Hemolytic Disease

Rh hemolytic disease can be prevented by the use of Rh immunoglobulin at a dose of 300 μg, which is indicated in the following circumstances:

1. For all Rh-negative, Rh_0 (D^u)-negative mothers who are unimmunized to the Rh factor. In these patients Rh immunoglobulin is given at 28 weeks' gestation and within 72 hours of delivery. Antenatal administration of Rh immunoglobulin is safe for the mother and the fetus
2. For all unimmunized Rh-negative mothers who have undergone spontaneous or induced abortion, particularly beyond the seventh or eighth week of gestation
3. After ruptured tubal pregnancies in unimmunized Rh-negative mothers
4. Following any event during pregnancy that may lead to transplacental hemorrhage, such as external version, amniocentesis, or antepartum hemorrhage in unimmunized Rh-negative women
5. Following tubal ligation or hysterotomy after the birth of an Rh-positive child in unimmunized Rh-negative women
6. Following chorionic villus sampling at 10–12 weeks' gestation. In these patients 50 μg of Rh immunoglobulin should be given.

ABO Isoimmunization

Clinical Features

1. Jaundice (indirect hyperbilirubinemia) usually within first 24 hours; may be of sufficient severity to cause kernicterus
2. Anemia
3. Hepatosplenomegaly.

Table 2-4 lists the clinical and laboratory features of isoimmune hemolysis due to Rh and ABO incompatibility.

Diagnosis

1. Hemoglobin decreased
2. Smear: spherocytosis in 80% of infants, reticulocytosis, marked polychromasia

Table 2-4. Clinical and Laboratory Features of Isoimmune Hemolysis Caused by Rh and ABO Incompatibility

Feature	Rh disease	ABO incompatibility
Clinical evaluation		
Frequency	Unusual	Common
Occurrence in firstborn	5%	40–50%
Predictably severe in subsequent pregnancies	Usually	No
Stillbirth and/or hydrops	Occasional	Rare
Pallor	Marked	Minimal
Jaundice	Marked	Minimal (occasionally marked)
Hepatosplenomegaly	Marked	Minimal
Incidence of late anemia	Common	Uncommon
Laboratory findings		
Blood type, mother	Rh negative	O
Blood type, infant	Rh positive	A or B or AB
Antibody type	Incomplete (7S)	Immune (7S)
Coombs' test, direct	Positive	Usually positive
Coombs' test, indirect	Positive	Usually positive
Hemoglobin level	Very low	Moderately low
Serum bilirubin	Markedly elevated	Variably elevated
Red cell morphology	Nucleated RBCs	Spherocytes
Treatment		
Need for antenatal management	Yes	No
Exchange transfusion		
Frequency	~2:3	~1:10
Donor blood type	Rh-negative group specific, when possible	Rh same as infant group O only

3. Elevated indirect bilirubin level*
4. Demonstration of incompatible blood group
   a. Group O mother may have an infant who is group A or B.
   b. Rarely, mother may be A and baby B or AB or mother may be B and baby A or AB.
5. Direct Coombs' test on infant's red cells usually positive
6. Demonstration of antibody in infant's serum
   a. When free anti-A is present in a group A infant or anti-B is present in a group B infant, ABO hemolytic disease may be presumed. These antibodies can be demonstrated by the indirect Coombs' test in the infant's serum using adult erythrocytes possessing the corresponding A or B antigen. This is proof that the antibody has crossed from the mother's to the baby's circulation.
   b. Antibody can be eluted from the infant's red cells and identified.
7. Demonstration of antibodies in maternal serum. When an infant has signs of hemolytic disease, the mother's serum may show the presence of immune

*In the era of early discharge of newborns, the use of the critical bilirubin level of 4 mg/dL at the sixth hour of life will predict significant hyperbilirubinemia and 6 mg/dL at the sixth hour will predict severe hemolytic disease of the newborn. The reticulocyte count, a positive Coombs' test, and a sibling with neonatal jaundice are additional predictors of significant hyperbilirubinemia and reason for careful surveillance of the newborn.

agglutinins persisting after neutralization with A and B substance and hemolysins.

Treatment

In ABO hemolytic disease, unlike Rh disease, antenatal management or premature delivery is not required. After delivery, management of an infant with ABO hemolytic disease is directed toward controlling the hyperbilirubinemia by frequent determination of unconjugated bilirubin levels, with a view to the need for photo-therapy or exchange transfusion. The principles and methods are the same as those described for Rh hemolytic disease. Group O blood of the same Rh type as that of the infant should be used. Whole blood is used to permit maximum bilirubin removal by albumin.

Late-Onset Anemia in Immune Hemolytic Anemia

Infants not requiring an exchange transfusion for hyperbilirubinemia following immune hemolytic anemia may develop significant anemia during the first 6 weeks of life because of persistent maternal IgG antibodies hemolyzing the infant's red blood cells associated with a reticulocytopenia (antibodies destroy the reticulocytes as well as the red blood cells). For this reason, follow-up hemoglobin levels weekly for 4–6 weeks should be done in those infants.

Nonimmune Hemolytic Anemia

The causes of nonimmune hemolytic anemia are listed in Table 2-1.

Vitamin E Deficiency

Vitamin E is one of several free-radical scavengers that serve as antioxidants to pro-tect cellular components against peroxidative damage. Serum levels of 1.5 mg/dL are adequate; levels greater than 3.0 mg/dL should be avoided because they may be associated with serious morbidity and mortality.

Vitamin E protects double bonds of lipids in the membranes of all tissues, including blood cells. Vitamin E requirements increase with exposure to oxidant stress and increase as dietary polyunsaturated fatty acid (PUFA) content increases. Vitamin E is now supplemented in infant formulas in proportion to their PUFA content in a ratio of E:PUFA > 0.6. The lipoproteins that transport and bind vitamin E are low in neonates.

Clinical Findings

Hemolytic anemia and reticulocytosis
Thrombocytosis
Acanthocytosis
Peripheral edema
Neurologic signs:
  Cerebellar degeneration
  Ataxia
  Peripheral neuropathy.

Hemolytic anemia develops under the following conditions:

Diets high in PUFA supplemented with iron, which is a powerful oxidant
Prematurity
Oxygen administration, a powerful oxidant.

Diagnosis

Peroxide hemolysis test: Red cells are incubated with small amounts of hydrogen peroxide, and the amount of hemolysis is measured.

FAILURE OF RED CELL PRODUCTION

Congenital

The congenital causes that contribute to a failure of red cell production are listed in Table 2-1 and discussed in Chapter 6.

Acquired

Viral Diseases

Viral interference (e.g., CMV, HIV) with fetal hematopoiesis may cause anemia, leukopenia, and thrombocytopenia in the newborn. HIV disease may be associated with a number of hematologic abnormalities (Chapter 5).

ANEMIA OF PREMATURITY

Anemia of prematurity is characterized by reduced bone marrow erythropoietic activity and low serum erythropoietin (EPO) levels. It may be compounded by folic acid, vitamin E, and iron availability and frequent blood sampling.

The low hemoglobin concentration is due to:

- Decreased red cell production (Premature infants have low EPO levels and are less responsive to EPO.)
- Shorter red cell life span
- Increased blood volume with growth.

The nadir of the hemoglobin level is 4–8 weeks and is 7 g/dL.

Treatment

Recombinant human erythropoietin (rHuEPO) corrects anemia of prematurity. The dose is 75–300 units/kg/week subcutaneously for 4 weeks starting at 3–4 weeks of age. This treatment is safe, inexpensive, and effective in reducing the number of transfusions required. It takes about 2 weeks to raise the hemoglobin to a biologically significant degree, which limits its usefulness when a prompt response is needed.

Supplemental oral iron in a dose of at least 2 mg/kg/day is also required to prevent the development of iron deficiency.

The criteria for transfusion of preterm infants vary considerably among different institutions. Table 2-5 gives indications for small-volume red cell transfusions in preterm infants.

PHYSIOLOGIC ANEMIA

In utero, the oxygen saturation of the fetus is 70% (hypoxic levels) and this stimulates erythropoietin, produces a reticulocytosis (3–7%), and increases red cell production causing a high hemoglobin at birth.

Table 2-5. Indications for Small-Volume RBC Transfusions in Preterm Infants

Transfuse well infant at hematocrit ≤20% or ≤25% with low reticulocyte count and tachycardia, tachypnea, poor weight gain, poor suck, or apnea

Transfuse infants at hematocrit ≤30%
  a. If receiving <35% supplemental hood oxygen
  b. If on CPAP or mechanical ventilation with mean airway pressure <6 cm H_2O
  c. If significant apnea (>6/day) and bradycardia are noted while receiving therapeutic doses of methylxanthines
  d. If heart rate >180 beats/min or respiratory rate >80 breaths/min persists for 24 hours
  e. If weight gain <10 g/day is observed over 4 days while receiving ≥100 kcal/kg/day
  f. If undergoing surgery

Transfuse for hematocrit ≤35%
  a. If receiving >35% supplemental hood oxygen
  b. If intubated on CPAP or mechanical ventilation with mean airway pressure >6 cm H_2O

Do not transfuse
  a. To replace blood removed for laboratory tests alone
  b. For low hematocrit value alone

Abbreviation: CPAP, continuous positive airway pressure by nasal or endotracheal route.
Modified from Hume, H. Red blood cell transfusions for preterm infants: the role of evidence-based medicine. Semin Perinatol 1997;21:8–19, with permission.

After birth the oxygen saturation is 95%, EPO is undetectable, and red cell production by day 7 is 10% of the level *in utero*. As a result of this, the hemoglobin level falls to a nadir at 8–12 weeks (physiologic anemia). At this point oxygen delivery is impaired, erythropoietin stimulated, and red cell production increased.

DIAGNOSTIC APPROACH TO ANEMIA IN THE NEWBORN

Figure 2-4 is a flowchart of the investigation of anemia in the newborn and stresses the importance of the Coombs' test, the reticulocyte count, the mean corpuscular volume (MCV), and the blood smear as key investigative tools in elucidating the cause of the anemia. Table 2-6 lists the clinical and laboratory evaluations required in anemia in the newborn.

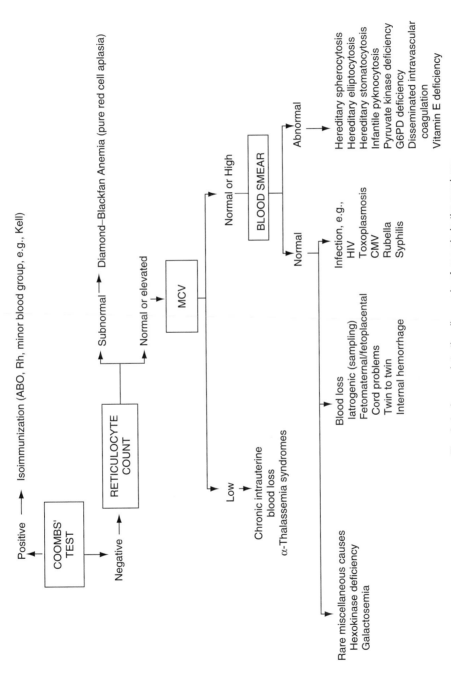

Fig. 2-4. Approach to the diagnosis of anemia in the newborn.

Table 2-6. Clinical and Laboratory Evaluation of Anemia in the Newborn

History
  Obstetrical history
  Family history

Physical examination

Laboratory tests
  Complete blood count
  Reticulocyte count
  Blood smear
  Coombs' test (direct and indirect)
  Blood type of baby and mother
  Bilirubin level
  Kleihauen–Betke test on mother's blood (fetal red cells in maternal blood)
  Studies for neonatal infection
  Ultrasound of abdomen and head
  Red cell enzyme assays (if clinically indicated)
  Bone marrow (if clinically indicated)

SUGGESTED READINGS

Academy of Pediatrics. Provisional Committee for Quality Improvement and Subcommittee on Hyperbilirubinemia. Pediatrics 1994;94:558–65.

Bowman J. The management of hemolytic disease in the fetus and newborn. Semin Perinatol 1997;21:39–44.

Halperin DS, Wacker P, LaCourt G, et al. Effects of recombinant human erythropoietin in infants with the anemia of prematurity: a pilot study. J Pediatr 1990;116:779–96.

Hann IM, Gibson BES, Letsky EA. Fetal and Neonatal Haematology. London: Bailliere Tindall, 1991.

Maier RH, Obladen M, Müller-Hansen I, et al. Early treatment with erythropoietin [beta] ameliorates anemia and reduces transfusion requirements in infants with birth weights below 1000 g. J Pediatr 2002;141:8–15.

Messer J, Haddad J, Donato L, Astruc D, et al. Early treatment of premature infants with recombinant human erythropoietin. Pediatrics 1993;92:519–23.

3

IRON-DEFICIENCY ANEMIA

Iron deficiency is the most common nutritional deficiency in children and is worldwide in distribution. The incidence of iron-deficiency anemia is high in infancy, but it also exists to a lesser extent in schoolchildren and preadolescents. The incidence of iron deficiency is 5.5% in inner-city schoolchildren ranging in age from 5 to 8 years, 2.6% in preadolescents, and 25% in pregnant teenage girls.

PREVALENCE

There is a higher prevalence of iron-deficiency anemia in African-American children than in Caucasian children. Although no socioeconomic group is spared, the incidence of iron-deficiency anemia is inversely proportional to economic status.

Peak prevalence occurs during late infancy and early childhood when the following may occur:

- Rapid growth with exhaustion of gestational iron
- Low levels of dietary iron
- Complicating effect of cow's milk; that is, induced exudative enteropathy due to whole cow's milk ingestion (page 34).

A second peak is seen during adolescence due to rapid growth and suboptimal iron intake. This is amplified in females due to menstrual blood loss.

Table 3-1 lists causes of iron deficiency, and Table 3-2 lists infants at high risk for iron deficiency.

ETIOLOGIC FACTORS

Dietary Requirements

1. One mg/kg/day to a maximum of 15 mg/day (assuming 10% absorption) is required in normal infants.
2. Two mg/kg/day to a maximum of 15 mg/kg/day is required in low-birth-weight infants, infants with low initial hemoglobin values, and those who have experienced significant blood loss.

Table 3-1. Causes of Iron-Deficiency Anemia

I. Deficient intake
Dietary (milk, 0.5–1.5 mg iron/L)

II. Increased demand
Growth (low birth weight, prematurity, low-birth-weight twins or multiple births, adolescence, pregnancy), cyanotic congenital heart disease

III. Blood loss
  A. Perinatal
    1. Placental
       a. Transplacental bleeding into maternal circulation
       b. Retroplacental (e.g., premature placental separation)
       c. Intraplacental
       d. Fetal blood loss at or before birth (e.g., placenta previa)
       e. Fetofetal bleeding in monochorionic twins
       f. Placental abnormalities (Table 2-1)
    2. Umbilicus
       a. Ruptured umbilical cord (e.g., vasa previa) and other umbilical cord abnormalities (Table 2-1)
       b. Inadequate cord tying
       c. Postexchange transfusion
  B. Postnatal
    1. Gastrointestinal tract
       a. Primary iron-deficiency anemia resulting in gut alteration with blood loss aggravating existing iron deficiency: 50% of iron-deficient children have guaiac-positive stools
       b. Hypersensitivity to whole cow's milk ? due to heat-labile protein, resulting in blood loss and exudative enteropathy (leaky gut syndrome) (Table 3-4)
       c. Anatomic gut lesions (e.g., varices, hiatus hernia, ulcer, leiomyomata, ileitis, Meckel's diverticulum, duplication of gut, hereditary telangiectasia, polyps, colitis, hemorrhoids); exudative enteropathy caused by underlying bowel disease (e.g., allergic gastroenteropathy, intestinal lymphangiectasia)
       d. Gastritis from aspirin, adrenocortical steroids, indomethacin, phenylbutazone
       e. Intestinal parasites (e.g., hookworm [*Necator americanus*])
       f. Henoch–Schönlein purpura
    2. Hepatobiliary system: hematobilia
    3. Lung: pulmonary hemosiderosis, Goodpasture syndrome, defective iron mobilization with IgA deficiency
    4. Nose: recurrent epistaxis
    5. Uterus: menstrual loss
    6. Heart: intracardiac myxomata, valvular prostheses or patches
    7. Kidney: microangiopathic hemolytic anemia, hematuria, nephrotic syndrome (urinary loss of transferrin), hemosiderinurias—chronic intravascular hemolysis (e.g., paroxysmal nocturnal hemoglobinuria, paroxysmal cold hemoglobinuria, march hemoglobinuria)
    8. Extracorporeal: hemodialysis, trauma

IV. Impaired absorption
Malabsorption syndrome, celiac disease, severe prolonged diarrhea, postgastrectomy, inflammatory bowel disease, *Helicobacter pylori* infection associated chronic gastritis.

Food Iron Content

A newborn infant is fed predominantly milk. Breast milk and cow's milk contain less than 1.5 mg iron per 1000 calories (0.5–1.5 mg/L). Although cow's milk and breast milk are equally poor in iron, breast-fed infants absorb 49% of the iron, in

Table 3-2. Infants at High Risk for Iron Deficiency

Increased iron needs:
  Low birth weight
  Prematurity
  Multiple gestation
  High growth rate
  Chronic hypoxia—high altitude, cyanotic heart disease
  Low hemoglobin at birth
Blood loss:
  Perinatal bleeding
Dietary factors:
  Early cow's milk intake
  Early solid food intake
  Rate of weight gain greater than average
  Low-iron formula
  Frequent tea intake[a]
  Low vitamin C intake[b]
  Low meat intake
  Breast-feeding >6 months without iron supplements
  Low socioeconomic status (frequent infections)

[a]Tea inhibits iron absorption.
[b]Vitamin C enhances iron absorption.

contrast to the approximately 10% that is absorbed from cow's milk. The bioavailability of iron in breast milk is much greater than in cow's milk.

Table 3-3 lists the iron content of infant foods.

Growth

Growth is particularly rapid during infancy and during puberty. Blood volume and body iron are directly related to body weight throughout life. Each kilogram gain in weight requires an increase of 35–45 mg body iron.

The amount of iron in the newborn is 75 mg/kg. If no iron is present in the diet or if blood loss occurs, the iron stores present at birth will be depleted by 6 months in a full-term infant and by 3–4 months in a premature infant.

The most common cause of iron-deficiency anemia is inadequate intake during the rapidly growing years of infancy and childhood.

Table 3-3. Iron Content of Infant Foods

Food	Iron, mg	Unit
Milk	0.5–1.5	Liter
Eggs	1.2	Each
Cereal, fortified	3.0–5.0	Ounce
Vegetables (starched)		
Yellow	0.1–0.3	Ounce
Green	0.3–0.4	Ounce
Meats (strained)		
Beef, lamb, liver	0.4–2.0	Ounce
Pork, liver, bacon	6.6	Ounce
Fruits (strained)	0.2–0.4	Ounce

Blood Loss

Blood loss, an important cause of iron-deficiency anemia, may be due to prenatal, intranatal, or postnatal causes (see Chapter 2, Table 2-1). Hemorrhage occurring later in infancy and childhood may be either occult or apparent (Table 3-1).

Iron deficiency by itself, irrespective of its cause, may result in occult blood loss from the gut. More than 50% of iron-deficient infants have guaiac-positive stools. This blood loss is due to the effects of iron deficiency on the mucosal lining (e.g., deficiency of iron-containing enzymes in the gut), leading to mucosal blood loss. This sets up a vicious cycle in which iron deficiency results in mucosal change, which leads to blood loss and further aggravates the anemia. The bleeding due to iron deficiency is corrected with iron treatment. In addition to iron deficiency per se causing blood loss, it may also induce an enteropathy, or leaky gut syndrome. In this condition, a number of blood constituents, in addition to red cells, are lost in the gut (Table 3-4).

Cow's milk can result in an exudative enteropathy associated with chronic gastrointestinal (GI) blood loss resulting in iron deficiency. Whole cow's milk should be considered the cause of iron-deficiency anemia under the following clinical circumstances:

1. One quart or more of whole cow's milk consumed per day
2. Iron deficiency accompanied by hypoproteinemia (with or without edema) and hypocupremia (Dietary iron-deficiency anemia unassociated with exudative enteropathy is usually associated with an elevated serum copper level). It is also associated with hypocalcemia, hypotransferrinemia, and low serum immunoglobulins due to the leakage of these substances from the gut.
3. Iron-deficiency anemia unexplained by low birth weight, poor iron intake, or excessively rapid growth
4. Iron-deficiency anemia that recurs after a satisfactory hematologic response following iron therapy
5. Rapidly developing or severe iron-deficiency anemia
6. Suboptimal response to oral iron in iron-deficiency anemia
7. Consistently guaiac-positive stool tests in the absence of gross bleeding and other evidence of organic lesions in the gut
8. Return of GI function and prompt correction of anemia on cessation of cow's milk and substitution by formula.

Blood loss can thus occur as a result of gut involvement due to primary iron-deficiency anemia (Table 3-4) or secondary iron-deficiency anemia as a result of gut abnormalities induced by hypersensitivity to cow's milk, or as a result of demonstrable anatomic lesions of the bowel, for example, Meckel's diverticulum.

Impaired Absorption

Impaired iron absorption due to a generalized malabsorption syndrome is an uncommon cause of iron-deficiency anemia. Because of its effect on the bowel mucosa, severe iron deficiency may induce a secondary malabsorption of iron as well as malabsorption of xylose, fat, and vitamin A (Table 3-4).

Nonhematologic Manifestations

Iron deficiency is a systemic disorder involving multiple systems rather than exclusively a hematologic condition associated with anemia. Table 3-5 lists important iron-containing compounds in the body and their functions, and Table 3-6 lists the tissue effects of iron deficiency.

Table 3-4. Classification of Iron-Deficiency Anemia in Relationship to Gut Involvement

	Primary iron deficiency (dietary, rapid growth)		
	Mild or severe		Severe[a]
Gut changes	None	Leaky gut syndrome	Malabsorption syndrome
Effect	No blood loss	Loss of: Red cells only Loss of: Red cells, Plasma protein, Albumin, Immune globulin, Copper, Calcium	Impaired absorption of iron only Impaired absorption of xylose, fat, lactose, and vitamin A Duodenitis
Result	Iron-deficiency anemia (IDA)	IDA, guaiac-positive IDA, exudative enteropathy	IDA, refractory to oral iron IDA, transient enteropathy
Treatment	Oral iron	Oral iron	IM iron–dextran complex

	Secondary iron deficiency	
	Mild or severe	Severe
Pathogenesis	Cow's milk-induced ? heat-labile protein	Anatomic lesion (e.g., Meckel's diverticulum, polyp, intestinal duplication, peptic ulcer) Blood loss
Effect	Leaky gut syndrome Loss of: Red cells, Plasma protein, Albumin, Immune globulin, Copper, Calcium	
Result	Recurrent IDA, exudative enteropathy	Recurrent IDA
Treatment	Discontinue whole cow's milk; soya milk formula; oral iron	Surgery, specific medical management, iron PO or IM iron dextran

[a]Can occur in severe chronic iron-deficiency anemia from any cause.

Table 3-5. Important Iron-Containing Compounds

Compound	Function
α-Glycerophosphate dehydrogenase	Work capacity
Catalase	RBC peroxide breakdown
Cytochromes	ATP production, protein synthesis, drug metabolism, electron transport
Ferritin	Iron storage
Hemoglobin	Oxygen delivery
Hemosiderin	Iron storage
Mitochondrial dehydrogenase	Electron transport
Monoamine oxidase	Catecholamine metabolism
Myoglobin	Oxygen storage for muscle contraction
Peroxidase	Bacterial killing
Ribonucleotide reductase	Lymphocyte DNA synthesis, tissue growth
Transferrin	Iron transport
Xanthine oxidase	Uric acid metabolism

Table 3-6. Tissue Effects of Iron Deficiency

I. Gastrointestinal tract
   A. Anorexia—common and an early symptom
      1. Increased incidence of low-weight percentiles
      2. Depression of growth
   B. Pica—pagophagia (ice) geophagia (sand)
   C. Atrophic glossitis
   D. Dysphagia
   E. Esophageal webs (Kelly–Paterson syndrome)
   F. Reduced gastric acidity
   G. Leaky gut syndrome
      1. Guaiac-positive stools—isolated
      2. Exudative enteropathy: gastrointestinal loss of protein, albumin, immunoglobulins, copper, calcium, red cells
   H. Malabsorption syndrome
      1. Iron only
      2. Generalized malabsorption: xylose, fat, vitamin A, duodenojejunal mucosal atrophy
   I. Beeturia
   J. Decreased cytochrome oxidase activity and succinic dehydrogenase
   K. Decreased disaccharidases, especially lactase, with abnormal lactose tolerance tests
   L. Increased absorption of cadmium and lead (iron-deficient children have increased lead absorption)
   M. Increased intestinal permeability index

II. Central nervous system
   A. Irritability
   B. Fatigue and decreased activity
   C. Conduct disorders
   D. Lower mental and motor developmental test scores on the Bayley scale that may be long lasting
   E. Decreased attentiveness, shorter attention span
   F. Significantly lower scholastic performance
   G. Reduced cognitive performance
   H. Breath-holding spells
   I. Papilledema

(Continues)

Table 3-6. (*Continued*)

III. **Cardiovascular system**
A. Increase in exercise and recovery heart rate and cardiac output
B. Cardiac hypertrophy
C. Increase in plasma volume
D. Increased minute ventilation values
E. Increased tolerance to digitalis

IV. **Musculoskeletal system**
A. Deficiency of myoglobin and cytochrome C
B. Impaired performance of a brief intense exercise task
C. Decreased physical performance in prolonged endurance work
D. Rapid development of tissue lactic acidosis on exercise and a decrease in mitochondrial α-glycerophosphate oxidase activity
E. Radiographic changes in bone—widening of diploic spaces
F. Adverse effect on fracture healing

V. **Immunologic system**
There is conflicting information as to the effect on the immunologic system of iron-deficiency anemia.
A. Evidence of increased propensity for infection
1. Clinical
a. Reduction of acute illness and improved rate of recovery in iron-replete compared to iron-deficient children
b. Increased frequency of respiratory infection in iron deficiency
2. Laboratory
a. Impaired leukocyte transformation
b. Impaired granulocyte killing and nitroblue tetrazolium (NBT) reduction by granulocytes
c. Decreased myeloperoxidase in leukocytes and small intestine
d. Decreased cutaneous hypersensitivity
e. Increased susceptibility to infection in iron-deficient animals
B. Evidence of decreased propensity for infection
1. Clinical
a. Lower frequency of bacterial infection
b. Increased frequency of infection in iron overload conditions
2. Laboratory
a. Transferrin inhibition of bacterial growth by binding iron so that no free iron is available for growth of microorganisms
b. Enhancement of growth of nonpathogenic bacteria by iron

VI. **Cellular changes**
A. Red cells
1. Ineffective erythropoiesis
2. Decreased red cell survival (normal when injected into asplenic subjects)
3. Increased autohemolysis
4. Increased red cell rigidity
5. Increased susceptibility to sulfhydryl inhibitors
6. Decreased heme production
7. Decreased globin and α-chain synthesis
8. ? Precipitation of α-globin monomers to cell membrane
9. Decreased glutathione peroxidase and catalase activity
a. Inefficient H_2O_2 detoxification
b. Greater susceptibility to H_2O_2 hemolysis
c. Oxidative damage to cell membrane
d. Increased cellular rigidity

(*Continues*)

Table 3-6. (*Continued*)

10. Increased rate of glycolysis-glucose 6-phosphate dehydrogenase, 6-phosphogluconate dehydrogenase, 2,3-diphosphoglycerate (2,3-DPG), and glutathione
11. Increase in NADH-methemoglobin reductase
12. Increase in erythrocyte glutamic oxaloacetic transaminase (EGOT)
13. Increase in free erythrocyte protoporphyrin
14. Impairment of DNA and RNA synthesis in bone marrow cells

B. Other tissues
1. Reduction in heme-containing enzymes (cytochrome C, cytochrome oxidase)
2. Reduction in iron-dependent enzymes (succinic dehydrogenase, aconitase)
3. Reduction in monoamine oxidase (MAO)
4. Increased excretion of urinary norepinephrine
5. Reduction in tyrosine hydroxylase (enzyme converting tyrosine to dihydroxyphenylalanine)
6. Alterations in cellular growth, DNA, RNA, and protein synthesis in animals
7. Persistent deficiency of brain iron following short-term deprivation
8. Reduction in plasma zinc

DIAGNOSIS

Blood

1. *Hemoglobin:* Hemoglobin is below the acceptable level for age (Appendix 1).
2. *Red cell indices:* Lower than normal MCV, MCH, and MCHC for age. Widened red cell distribution width (RDW) in association with a low MCV is one of the best screening tests for iron deficiency.
3. *Blood smear:* Red cells are hypochromic and microcytic with anisocytosis and poikilocytosis, generally occurring only when the hemoglobin level falls below 10 g/dL. Basophilic stippling can also be present but not as frequently as it is present in thalassemia trait. The RDW is high (>14.5%) in iron deficiency and normal in thalassemia (<13%).
4. *Reticulocyte count:* The reticulocyte count is usually normal; however, in severe iron-deficiency anemia associated with bleeding, a reticulocyte count of 3–4% may occur.
5. *Platelet count:* The platelet count varies from thrombocytopenia to thrombocytosis. Thrombocytopenia is more common in severe iron-deficiency anemia; thrombocytosis is present when there is associated bleeding from the gut.
6. *Free erythrocyte protoporphyrin:* The incorporation of iron into protoporphyrin represents the ultimate stage in the biosynthetic pathway of heme. Failure of iron supply will result in an accumulation of free protoporphyrin not incorporated into heme synthesis in the normoblast and the release of erythrocytes into the circulation with high free erythrocyte protoporphyrin (FEP) levels.
   a. The normal FEP level is 15.5 ± 8.3 mg/dL. The upper limit of normal is 40 mg/dL. Table 3-7 gives the causes of elevated levels of FEP and its advantages over transferrin saturation levels as a diagnostic tool.
   b. In both iron deficiency and lead poisoning, the FEP level is elevated. It is much higher in lead poisoning than in iron deficiency. The FEP is normal in α- and β-thalassemia minor. FEP elevation occurs as soon as the body stores of iron are depleted, before microcytic anemia develops. An elevated FEP level, therefore, is an indication for iron therapy even when anemia and microcytosis have not yet developed.
7. *Serum ferritin:* The level of serum ferritin reflects the level of body iron stores; it is quantitative, reproducible, specific, and sensitive and requires only a small

Table 3-7. Causes of Elevated Levels of Free Erythrocyte Protoporphyrin and Advantages of FEP Compared to Transferrin Saturation as a Diagnostic Tool

Causes of raised levels of FEP:
1. Iron-deficiency anemia
2. Conditions with high reticulocyte count[a]
3. Lead poisoning (very high levels)
4. Chronic infection
5. Erythropoietic protoporphyria
6. Acute myelogenous leukemia
7. Rare cases of dyserythropoietic and sideroblastic anemias

Advantages of FEP compared with transferrin saturation:
1. FEP is not subject to daily fluctuations
2. FEP remains elevated during iron treatment (returns to normal after cells with excess FEP are replaced)[b]
3. FEP is not elevated in α- and β-thalassemia

[a]Reticulocytes have a slightly higher concentration of FEP. It occurs in hemolytic anemias (e.g., hemoglobin SS disease).

[b]Useful to know whether a patient who is in the process of receiving iron treatment was iron deficient before commencement of iron therapy.

blood sample. A concentration of less than 12 ng/mL is considered diagnostic of iron deficiency. Normal ferritin levels, however, can exist in iron deficiency when bacterial or parasitic infection, malignancy, or chronic inflammatory conditions coexist because ferritin is an acute-phase reactant. Figure 3-1 depicts the normal range of serum ferritin concentrations at different ages.

8. *Serum iron and iron saturation percentage:* Serum iron estimation as a measure of iron deficiency has serious limitations. It reflects the balance between several factors, including iron absorbed, iron used for hemoglobin synthesis, iron released by red cell destruction, and the size of iron stores. The serum iron concentration represents an equilibrium between the iron entering and leaving the circulation. Serum iron has a wide range of normal, varies significantly with age (see Appendix 1), and is subject to marked circadian changes (as much as 100 µg/dL during the day). The author has abandoned the use of serum iron for the routine diagnosis of iron deficiency (in favor of MCV, RDW, FEP, and serum ferritin) because of the following limitations:
   a. Wide normal variations (age, sex, laboratory methodology)
   b. Time consuming
   c. Subject to error from iron ingestion
   d. Diurnal variation
   e. Falls in mild or transient infection.
9. *Therapeutic trial:* The most reliable criterion of iron-deficiency anemia is the hemoglobin response to an adequate therapeutic trial of oral iron. A reticulocytosis with a peak occurring between the 5th and 10th days followed by a significant rise in hemoglobin level occurs. The absence of these changes implies that iron deficiency is not the cause of the anemia. Iron therapy should then be discontinued and further diagnostic studies implemented. Table 3-8 summarizes the diagnostic tests available for the investigation of iron-deficiency anemia.

Other tests for iron deficiency not in common usage include the following:

1. *Serum transferrin receptor levels (STfR):* This is a sensitive measure of iron deficiency and correlates with hemoglobin and other laboratory parameters of iron

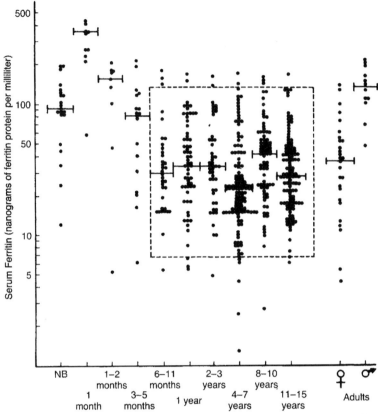

Fig. 3-1. Serum ferritin concentrations during development in the healthy nonanemic newborn, in infants, and in children of various age groups, together with adult male and female values. The median value in each age group is indicated by a horizontal line. The dashed line encloses a square, which includes the 95% confidence levels of the values between the ages of 6 months and 15 years. (From Siimes MA, Addrego JE, Dallman PR. Ferritin in serum: diagnosis of iron deficiency and iron overload in infants and children. Blood 1974;43:581, with permission.)

Note: Normal ferritin levels can occur in iron deficiency in the presence of bacterial or parasitic infection, malignancy, or chronic inflammatory conditions because ferritin is an acute-phase reactant.

status. The STfR is increased in instances of hyperplasia of erythroid precursors such as iron-deficiency anemia and thalassemia and is normal in chronic inflammation. It is therefore of great value in distinguishing iron deficiency from the anemia of chronic disease. It can be measured by a sensitive enzyme-linked immunosorbent assay (ELISA) technique.

2. *Red blood cell zinc protoporphyrin/heme ratio:* When available bone marrow iron is insufficient to support heme synthesis, zinc substitutes for iron in protoporphyrin IX, and the concentration of zinc protoporphyrin relative to heme increases. This test is more sensitive than plasma ferritin level tests, is inexpensive and simple, and is not altered in chronic inflammatory diseases or acute infections.

Differential Diagnosis

Although hypochromic anemia in children is usually due to iron deficiency, it is not necessarily attributable to this condition. A list of the causes of hypochromia is given in Table 3-9. In some of these cases, there is an inability to synthesize hemoglobin normally in spite of adequate iron (e.g., thalassemia, lead poisoning). In unusual or obscure cases of hypochromic anemia, it is necessary to do additional

Table 3-8. Diagnostic Tests for Iron-Deficiency Anemia

1. Blood smear
   a. Hypochromic microcytic red cells, confirmed by RBC indices:
      (1) MCV less than acceptable normal for age (see Appendix 1)
      (2) MCH less than 27.0 pg
      (3) MCHC less than 30%
   b. Wide red cell distribution width (RDW) greater than 14.5%
2. Free erythrocyte protoporphyrin: elevated
3. Serum ferritin: decreased
4. Serum iron and iron binding capacity
   a. Decreased serum iron
   b. Increased iron-binding capacity
   c. Decreased iron saturation (16% or less)
5. Therapeutic responses to oral iron
   a. Reticulocytosis with peak 5–10 days after institution of therapy
   b. Following peak reticulocytosis hemoglobin level rises on average by 0.25–0.4 g/dL/day or hematocrit rises 1%/day
6. Serum transferrin receptor level[a]
7. Red blood cell zinc protoporphyrin/heme ratio[a]
8. Bone marrow[b]
   a. Delayed cytoplasmic maturation
   b. Decreased or absent stainable iron

[a]Rarely required or readily available.
[b]Used only if difficulty is experienced in elucidating cause of anemia.

investigations, such as determination of serum ferritin, serum transferrin receptor levels, hemoglobin electrophoresis, and examination of the bone marrow for stained iron, in order to establish the cause of the hypochromia.

Table 3-10 lists the investigations employed in the differential diagnosis of microcytic anemias and Figure 3-2 depicts a flow chart for the diagnosis of microcytic anemia using MCV and RDW.

Table 3-9. Disorders Associated with Hypochromia

1. Iron deficiency
2. Hemoglobinopathies
   a. Thalassemia (α and β)
   b. Hemoglobin Köln
   c. Hemoglobin Lepore
   d. Hemoglobin H
   e. Hemoglobin E
3. Disorders of heme synthesis caused by a chemical
   a. Lead
   b. Pyrazinamide
   c. Isoniazid
4. Sideroblastic anemias (Table 6-24)
5. Chronic infections or other inflammatory states
6. Malignancy
7. Hereditary orotic aciduria
8. Hypo- or atransferrinemia
   Congenital
   Acquired (e.g., hepatic disorders); malignant disease, protein malnutrition (decreased transferrin synthesis), nephrotic syndrome (urinary transferrin loss)
9. Copper deficiency
10. Inborn error of iron metabolism
    Congenital defect of iron transport to red cells

Table 3-10. Summary of Laboratory

	Ethnic origin	Hb	MCV	MCV in parents	RDW
Iron deficiency	Any	↓	↓	N	↑
β-Thalassemia					
β⁺ trait (heterozygous)	Mediterranean	Slight ↓	↓	One parent ↓	N
β⁰ (homozygous)	Mediterranean	↓	↓	Both parents	N
α-Thalassemia					
Silent carrier (α-thal-2)	Asians, blacks, Mediterranean	N	N	N	N
Trait (α-thal-1)	Asians, blacks, Mediterranean	N or slightly ↓	↓	One parent ↓	N
Hemoglobin H disease		↓	↓		↑
Anemia chronic infection	Any	↓	N	N	N
Sideroblastic	Any	↓	N	N	↑

Abbreviations: Hb, hemoglobin; MCV, mean corpuscular volume; RDW, red cell distribution width; FEP, free erythrocyte protoporphyrin; TIBC, total iron-binding capacity, ↑, abnormally high; ↓, abnormally low; N, normal.

In addition to making a diagnosis of iron-deficiency anemia, its pathogenesis must be established. The history should include conditions resulting in low iron stores at birth, dietary history, and consideration of all factors leading to blood loss. The most common site of bleeding is into the bowel, and the most important investigation is examination of the stool for occult blood. If occult blood is found, its cause should be established by examination of stools for ova, rectal examination, barium enema, upper GI series, ⁹⁹ᵐTc-pertechnetate scan for detection of a Meckel's diverticulum, upper endoscopy, and colonoscopy.

Negative guaiac tests for occult bleeding may occur if bleeding is intermittent; for this reason, occult bleeding should be tested for on at least five occasions when GI bleeding is suspected. The guaiac test is only sensitive enough to pick up more than 5 mL occult blood. Excessive uterine bleeding, epistaxis, renal blood loss (hematuria), and, on rare occasions, bleeding into the lung (idiopathic pulmonary hemosiderosis and Goodpasture syndrome) may all be causes of iron-deficiency anemia. Bleeding into these areas requires specific investigations designed to detect the cause of bleeding.

TREATMENT

Nutritional Counseling

1. Maintain breast-feeding for at least 6 months, if possible.
2. Use an iron-fortified (6–12 mg/L) infant formula until 1 year of age (formula is preferred to whole cow's milk). Restrict milk to 1 pint/day.
3. Use iron-fortified cereal from 6 months to 1 year.

Studies in Microcytic Anemias

FEP	Ferritin	Serum iron	TIBC	Bone marrow iron status	Hb electro-phoresis	Other features
↑	↓	↓	↑	↓	Normal	Dietary deficiency
N	N or ↑	N	N	N	A₂ raised F normal or ↑	Normal examination
↑	↑	↑	↑	↑	F raised (60–90%)	Hepatosplenomegaly Transfusion dependent
N	N	N	N	N	Normal	No hematologic abnormalities
N	N or ↑	N	N	N	Normal	
N	N or ↑	N or ↑	N	↑	Hemoglobin H (2–40%)	Hemolytic anemia of variable severity Inclusion bodies in RBCs
↑	N or ↑	↓	N or ↑	N or ↑	Normal	
N or ↑	N or ↑	N or ↑	N or ↓	↑	Normal	

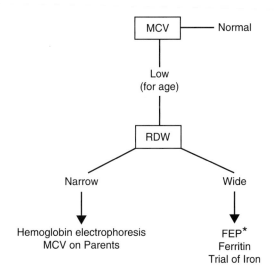

*Also elevated in lead poisoning.
Do serum lead level (if clinically indicated)

Fig. 3-2. Flowchart depicting the diagnosis of microcytic anemia using MCV and RDW.

4. Use evaporated milk or soy-based formula when iron deficiency is due to hypersensitivity to cow's milk.
5. Provide supplemental iron for low-birth-weight infants:
   a. Infants 1.5–2.0 kg: 2 mg/kg/day supplemental iron
   b. Infants 1.0–1.5 kg: 3 mg/kg/day supplemental iron
   c. Infants <1 kg: 4 mg/kg/day supplemental iron. .
6. Facilitators of iron absorption such as vitamin C-rich foods (citrus, tomatoes, and potatoes), meat, fish, and poultry should be included in the diet; inhibitors of iron absorption such as tea, phosphate, and phytates common in vegetarian diets should be eliminated.

Oral Iron Medication

1. *Product:* Ferrous iron (e.g., ferrous gluconate, ferrous ascorbate, ferrous lactate, ferrous succinate, ferrous fumarate, or ferrous glycine sulfate) is effective. Ferric irons and heavily chelated iron should not be used because they are poorly and inefficiently absorbed.
2. *Dose:* 1.5–2.0 mg/kg elemental iron three times daily. Older children: ferrous sulfate (0.2 g) or ferrous gluconate (0.3 g) given three times daily, to provide 100–200 mg elemental iron. In children with GI side effects, iron once every other day may be better tolerated with good effect.
3. *Duration:* 6–8 weeks after hemoglobin level and the red cell indices return to normal.
4. *Response:*
   a. Peak reticulocyte count experienced on days 5–10 following initiation of iron therapy.
   b. Following peak reticulocyte level, hemoglobin rises on average by 0.25–0.4 g/dL/day or hematocrit rises 1%/day during first 7–10 days.
   c. Thereafter, hemoglobin rises more slowly: 0.1–0.15 g/dL/day.
5. *Failure to respond to oral iron:* If patient fails to respond to oral iron, the following reasons should be considered:
   a. Poor compliance (failure or irregular administration of oral iron); administration can be verified by change in stool color to gray-black or by testing stool for iron
   b. Inadequate iron dose
   c. Ineffective iron preparation
   d. Persistent or unrecognized blood loss, with the patient losing iron as fast as it is replaced
   e. Incorrect diagnosis
   f. Coexistent disease that interferes with absorption or utilization of iron (e.g., infection, inflammatory bowel disease, malignant disease, hepatic or renal disease, or concomitant deficiencies of, for instance, vitamin B_{12}, folic acid, thyroid, associated lead poisoning)
   g. Impaired GI absorption (e.g., concurrent administration of large amounts of antacids, which bind iron and histamine-2 blockers).

Parenteral Therapy

Intramuscular

Iron–dextran, a parenteral form of elemental iron, is available for intramuscular use. It is safe, effective, and well tolerated even in infants with a variety of acute illnesses, including acute diarrheal disorders.

Indications

1. Noncompliance with oral administration of iron
2. Severe bowel disease (e.g., inflammatory bowel disease)—use of oral iron might aggravate the underlying disease of the bowel
3. Chronic hemorrhage (e.g., hereditary telangiectasia, menorrhagia, chronic hemoglobinuria from prosthetic heart valves)
4. Acute diarrheal disorder in underprivileged populations with iron-deficiency anemia.

Dose

For intramuscular iron–dextran the following formula is used to raise the hemoglobin level to normal and to replenish iron stores:

$$\frac{\text{Normal hemoglobin} - \text{initial hemoglobin}}{100} \times \text{Blood volume (mL)} \times 3.4 \times 1.5$$

where

Normal hemoglobin is taken from Appendix 1
Blood volume is 80 mL/kg or 40 mL/lb body weight
Multiplication by 3.4 is done to convert grams of hemoglobin into milligrams of iron
The factor of 1.5 provides extra iron to replace depleted tissue stores
Iron–dextran complex provides 50 mg elemental iron/mL.

Side Effects

Staining at the site of intramuscular injection may occur, especially in cases in which the solution is accidentally administered into the superficial tissues. Staining is of a transient type, disappearing after a few weeks or months. The local inflammatory reaction is slight. Nausea and dizziness have been reported in occasional cases. Because of the painful nature of and the skin discoloration that occurs with intramuscular injection, the preferred route for parenteral iron administration is intravenous.

Intravenous

Sodium ferric gluconate (Ferrlecit) or iron(III) hydroxide sucrose complex (Venofer) for intravenous use is effective and has a superior safety profile when compared with intravenous iron–dextran. They are especially useful in anemia associated with renal failure and hemodialysis. Dosage ranges from 1 to 4 mg/kg per week.

Blood Transfusion

A packed red cell transfusion should be given in severe anemia requiring correction more rapidly than is possible with oral iron or parenteral iron or because of the presence of certain complicating factors. This should be reserved for debilitated children with infection, especially when signs of cardiac dysfunction are present and the hemoglobin level is 4 g/dL or less.

Partial Exchange Transfusion

A partial exchange transfusion has been recommended in the management of a severely anemic child under two circumstances:

1. In a surgical emergency, when a final hemoglobin of 9–10 g/dL should be attained to permit safe anesthesia
2. When anemia is associated with congestive heart failure, in which case it is sufficient to raise the hemoglobin to 4–5 g/dL to correct the immediate anoxia.

SUGGESTED READINGS

Ballin A, Berar M, Rubinstein U, et al. Iron state in female adolescents. Am J Dis Child 1992;146:803–5.

Committee on Nutrition. Iron supplementation for infants. Pediatrics 1976;58:765–8.

Dallman PR. Iron deficiency and related nutritional anemias. In: Nathan DG, Oski FA, editors. Hematology of Infancy and Childhood. Philadelphia: WB Saunders, 1987.

Dallman, PR. Progress in the prevention of iron deficiency in infants. Acta Paediatr Scan (Suppl) 1990;365:28–37.

Dallman PR, Reeves JD. Laboratory diagnosis of iron deficiency. In: Steckel A, editor. Iron Nutrition in Infancy and Childhood. New York: Raven Press, 1984;11.

Lanzkowsky P. Iron deficiency anemias: A systemic disease. Trans College Medicine South Africa, July–December, 1982;67–113.

Lanzkowsky P. Iron-deficiency anemia. In: Pediatric Hematology–Oncology: A Treatise for the Clinician. New York: McGraw-Hill, 1980.

Lanzkowsky P. Iron metabolism and iron deficiency anemia. In: Miller DR, Pearson MA, Baehner RL, McMillan CW, editors. Blood Diseases of Infancy and Childhood. 4th ed. St. Louis: CV Mosby, 1978.

Lukens JN. Iron metabolism and iron deficiency anemia. In: Miller DR, Baehner RL, McMillan CW, editors. Blood Diseases of Infancy and Childhood. St. Louis: CV Mosby, 1984.

Oski FA. Iron deficiency in infancy and childhood. N Engl J Med 1993;329:190–3.

4

MEGALOBLASTIC ANEMIA

Megaloblastic anemias are characterized by the presence of megaloblasts in the bone marrow and macrocytes in the blood. In more than 95% of cases, megaloblastic anemia is a result of folate and vitamin B_{12} (cobalamin)* deficiency. Megaloblastic anemia may also result from rare inborn errors of metabolism of folate or vitamin B_{12}. In addition, deficiencies of ascorbic acid, tocopherol, and thiamine may be related to megaloblastic anemia. The causes of megaloblastosis are listed in Table 4-1.

VITAMIN B_{12} DEFICIENCY

Dietary vitamin B_{12} (cobalamin or Cbl), acquired mostly from animal sources, including meat and milk, is absorbed in a series of steps as follows:

- Proteolytic release of Cbl from its associated proteins occurs, and Cbl binds to R-binder proteins made in saliva and the stomach.
- After exposure to pancreatic proteases, Cbl is released from the R proteins.
- Cbl binds to a gastric secretory protein known as intrinsic factor (IF) to form the IF–Cbl complex.
- The IF–Cbl complex is recognized by receptors on ileal mucosal cells.
- Transport occurs across ileal cells in the presence of calcium ions.
- Release into the portal circulation bound to transcobalamin II (TC II), the serum protein that carries newly absorbed Cbl throughout the body, occurs.

Cobalamin is converted into the two required coenzyme forms, adenosylcobalamin (AdoCbl) and methylcobalamin (MeCbl). The cellular metabolism by which the coenzymes are formed involves the following:

- Receptor-mediated binding of the TC II–Cbl complex to the cell surface
- Adsorptive endocytosis of the complex
- Intralysosomal degradation of the TC II
- Release of Cbl into cytoplasm
- Enzyme-mediated reduction of the central cobalt atom
- Cytosolic methylation to form MeCbl or mitochondrial adenosylation to form AdoCbl.

The causes of Cbl deficiency are listed in Table 4-2.

---

*For the purposes of this chapter, vitamin B_{12}, cobalamin, and Cbl are used interchangeably. Vitamin B_{12} contains a metal ion in the form of cobalt and therefore is also known as cobalamin.

Table 4-1. Causes of Megaloblastosis

I. **Vitamin B$_{12}$ (cobalamin) deficiency (Table 4-2)**

II. **Folate deficiency (Table 4-6)**

III. **Miscellaneous**
    A. Congenital disorders in DNA synthesis
        1. Orotic aciduria (uridine responsive)—pyrimidine biosynthesis is interrupted
        2. Thiamine-responsive megaloblastic anemia[a]
        3. Congenital familial megaloblastic anemia requiring massive doses of vitamin B$_{12}$ and folate
        4. Associated with congenital dyserythropoietic anemia (Table 6-5 and Table 6-6)
        5. ? Lesch–Nyhan syndrome (adenine-responsive)—purine nucleotide regeneration is blocked
    B. Acquired defects in DNA synthesis
        1. Liver disease
        2. Sideroblastic anemias (Table 6-24)
        3. Leukemia, especially acute myeloid leukemia (M6) (Chapter 14)
        4. Aplastic anemia (constitutional/acquired)
        5. Refractory megaloblastic anemia
    C. Drug-induced megaloblastosis
        1. Purine analogues (e.g., 6-mercaptopurine, azathioprine, and thioguanine)
        2. Pyrimidine analogues (5-fluorouracil, 6-azauridine)
        3. Inhibitors of ribonucleotide reductase (cytosine arabinoside, hydroxyurea)

[a]Associated in some cases with diabetes and sensorineural hearing impairment and in others with the DID-MOAD syndrome (page 64). There is wide clinical heterogeneity of this rare disorder. Only the anemia is responsive to high doses of thiamine.

Table 4-2. Causes of Vitamin B$_{12}$ Deficiency

I. **Inadequate vitamin B$_{12}$ intake**
    A. Dietary (<2 µg/day): food fads, veganism, malnutrition, poorly controlled PKU diet
    B. Maternal deficiency leading to B$_{12}$ deficiency in breast milk

II. **Defective vitamin B$_{12}$ absorption** (Table 4-3)
    A. Failure to secrete intrinsic factor
        1. Congenital intrinsic factor deficiency (gastric mucosa normal) (OMIM 261000)
            a. Quantitative
            b. Qualitative (biologically inert)[a]
        2. Juvenile pernicious anemia (autoimmune) (gastric atrophy)
        3. Juvenile pernicious anemia (gastric autoantibodies) with autoimmune polyendocrinopathies (OMIM 240300)
        4. Juvenile pernicious anemia with IgA deficiency
        5. Gastric mucosal disease
            a. Corrosives
            b. Gastrectomy (partial/total)
    B. Failure of absorption in small intestine
        1. Specific vitamin B$_{12}$ malabsorption
            a. Abnormal intrinsic factor[a]
            b. Defective cobalamin transport by enterocytes—abnormal ileal uptake (Imerslund–Gräsbeck syndrome) (OMIM 261100)
            c. Ingestion of chelating agents (phytates, EDTA) (binds calcium and interferes with vitamin B$_{12}$ absorption)
        2. Intestinal disease causing generalized malabsorption, including vitamin B$_{12}$ malabsorption:
            a. Intestinal resection (e.g., congenital stenosis, volvulus, trauma)
            b. Crohn's disease

(Continues)

Table 4-2. (*Continued*)

    c. Tuberculosis of terminal ileum
    d. Lymphosarcoma of terminal ileum
    e. Pancreatic insufficiency
    f. Zollinger–Ellison syndrome
    g. Celiac disease, tropical sprue
    h. Other less specific malabsorption syndromes
    i. HIV infection
    j. Long-standing medication that decreases gastric acidity
    k. Neonatal necrotizing enterocolitis
  3. Competition for vitamin B_{12}
    a. Small-bowel bacterial overgrowth (e.g., small-bowel diverticulosis, anastomoses and fistulas, blind loops and pouches, multiple strictures, scleroderma, achlorhydria, gastric trichobezoar)
    b. *Diphyllobothrium latum* (takes up free B_{12} and B_{12} intrinsic factor complex), *Giardia lamblia, Plasmodium falciparum, Strongyloides stercoralis*

III. Defective vitamin B_{12} transport
  A. Congenital TC II deficiency (OMIM 275350)
  B. Transient deficiency of TC II
  C. Partial deficiency of TC I (R-binder deficiency) (OMIM 193090)

IV. Disorders of vitamin B_{12} metabolism
  A. Congenital
    1. Adenosylcobalamin deficiency CblA (OMIM 251100) and CblB diseases (OMIM 251100)
    2. Deficiency of methylmalonyl-CoA mutase (mut°, mut⁻)
    3. Methylcobalamin deficiency CblE (OMIM 236270) and CblG diseases (OMIM 250940)
    4. Combined adenosylcobalamin and methylcobalamin deficiencies: CblC (OMIM 277400), CblD (OMIM 277410), and CblF diseases (OMIM 277380)
  B. Acquired
    1. Liver disease
    2. Protein malnutrition (kwashiorkor, marasmus)
    3. Drugs associated with impaired absorption and/or utilization of vitamin B_{12} (e.g., *p*-aminosalicylic acid, colchicine, neomycin, ethanol, oral contraceptive agents?, metformin)

Abbreviation: OMIM, Online Mendelian Inheritance in Man (Page 50).
[a]Same condition.

Clinical Manifestations

Cbl deficiency is characterized by the following:

- Failure to thrive, anorexia, weakness, glossitis
- Pallor, scleral icterus
- Anemia with high MCV, hypersegmented neutrophils, leukopenia, thrombocytopenia
- Megaloblastic bone marrow
- Elevated urinary and plasma methylmalonic acid and homocysteine
- Muscle hypotonia, tremor, myoclonus.

Nutritional Deficiency

The daily allowance of vitamin B_{12} for children is 2.5 μg/day. The most common cause of Cbl deficiency in infants is dietary deficiency in the mother. Cbl in breast milk parallels that in serum and is deficient when the mother is a vegan or has unrecognized pernicious anemia or has had previous gastric bypass surgery or short-gut syndrome.

Defective Absorption

Table 4-3 lists the features of congenital and acquired defects of vitamin B_{12} absorption.

Food Cobalamin Malabsorption

Some patients suffer from an inability to release cobalamin from the protein-bound state in which it is normally encountered in food. This process requires both an acid pH and peptic activity. Impaired absorption occurs when there is impaired gastric function (e.g., atrophic gastritis, partial gastrectomy). In this condition, there is a low serum cobalamin, mild increase in methylmalonic acid and homocysteine, and a normal Schilling test (see page 67).

Intrinsic Factor Deficiency

Patients with absent or defective intrinsic factor (also known as S-binder) have low serum B_{12}, megaloblastic anemia, developmental delay, and myelopathy. Patients have a mild increase in methylmalonic acid and homocysteine. This autosomal recessive disorder usually appears early in the second year of life, but may be delayed until adolescence or adulthood. The abnormal absorption of cobalamin is corrected by mixing the vitamin with a source of normal intrinsic factor. Some patients have no detectable intrinsic factor, whereas others have intrinsic factor that can be detected immunologically but lacks function. The gene for human intrinsic factor has been cloned and localized to chromosome 11.

Defective Cobalamin Transport by Ileal Enterocyte Receptors for the IF–Cbl Complex (Imerslund–Gräsbeck Syndrome)

Imerslund–Gräsbeck syndrome is an autosomal recessive disorder that usually presents with pallor, weakness, anorexia, failure to thrive, delayed development, recurrent infections, and gastrointestinal symptoms within the first 2 years of life. In many patients, proteinuria of the tubular type is found that is not corrected by systemic cobalamin. Most of the known patients are found in Norway, Finland, and Saudi Arabia and among Sephardic Jews in Israel. In these patients, intrinsic factor level is normal, they do not have antibodies to intrinsic factor, and the intestinal morphology is normal. They have a low serum B_{12} due to a selective defect in cobalamin absorption that is not corrected by treatment with intrinsic factor. They have a mild increase in methylmalonic acid and homocysteine. In some cases the ileal receptor for IF–Cbl complex is absent, whereas in other patients it is present.

There has been a decrease in the number of new cases, suggesting that dietary or other factors may influence the expression of this disease. The locus for Imerslund–Gräsbeck syndrome has been assigned to chromosome 10. Imerslund–Gräsbeck–causing mutations are found in either of two genes encoding the epithelium proteins: cubilin and amnionless (AMN). The gene receptor cubilin P1297L (OMIM 602997)* is a 460-kDa protein that recognizes IF–Cbl and various

---

*The six-digit number is the entry number for the disorder in Online Mendelian Inheritance in Man (OMIM), a continuously updated electronic catalog of human genes and genetic disorders. The online version is accessible through the World Wide Web (http://www.ncbi.nlm.nih.gov/omim/).

Table 4-3. Features of Congenital and Acquired Defects of Vitamin B$_{12}$ Absorption

Condition	Stomach			Schilling test		Serum antibodies		
	Histology	Intrinsic factor[a]	Hydrochloric acid (HCL)	Without IF	With IF	Intrinsic factor	Parietal cell	Associated features
Congenital pernicious anemia	Normal	Absent	Normal	Decreased	Normal	Absent	Absent	None; relative of patient may exhibit defective vitamin B$_{12}$ malabsorption
Juvenile pernicious anemia (autoimmune)	Atrophy	Absent	Achlorhydria	Decreased	Normal	Present (90%)	Present (10%)	Occasional lupus erythematosus, IgA deficiency, moniliasis, endocrinopathy in siblings
Juvenile pernicious anemia with polyendocrinopathies or selective IgA deficiency	Atrophy	Absent	Achlorhydria	Decreased	Normal	Present	Present	Hypothyroidism (chronic autoimmune thyroiditis—Hashimoto thyroiditis) insulin-dependent diabetes mellitus, primary ovarian failure, myasthenia gravis, hypoparathyroidism, Addison disease, moniliasis, or selective IgA deficiency
Enterocyte vitamin B$_{12}$ malabsorption (Imerslund–Gräsbeck)	Normal	Present	Normal	Decreased	Decreased	Absent	Absent	Benign proteinuria, aminoaciduria, no generalized malabsorption[b]
Generalized malabsorption	Normal	Present	Normal	Decreased	Decreased	Absent	Absent	Malabsorption syndrome; history of ileal resection, Crohn disease, lymphoma

[a] Either absent secretion of immunologically recognizable IF or secretes immunologically reactive protein that is inactive physiologically. The latter group includes patients whose IF has reduced affinity for the ileal IF receptor, reduced affinity for cobalamin, or increased susceptibility for proteolysis.

[b] Rare cases have been described of this syndrome associated with generalized malabsorption reversed by vitamin B$_{12}$ administration, and rare cases have been described without proteinuria or aminoaciduria.

51

other proteins to be endocytosed in the intestine and kidney. The exact function of AMN is unknown but mutations affecting either of the two proteins may cause Imerslund–Gräsbeck syndrome.

Table 4-4 lists the inborn errors of cobalamin transport and metabolism.

Defective Transport

Abnormalities of Transcobalamin II (OMIM 275350)

Transcobalamin II is the principal transport system of cobalamin; in its absence, a serious and potentially fatal condition occurs. It presents clinically as follows:

- Age 3–5 weeks
- Autosomal recessive inheritance
- Failure to thrive
- Vomiting and diarrhea
- Progressive pancytopenia
- Megaloblastic bone marrow
- Immunologic deficiency both cellular and humoral
- Neurologic disease (appears years after onset of symptoms)
- Homocystinuria and methylmalonic aciduria
- Normal serum cobalamin levels (most of the cobalamin in serum is bound to transcobalamin I).

Diagnosis

Absence of protein capable of binding radiolabeled cobalamin and migrating with TC II on chromatography or gel electrophoresis, or by immunologic techniques. TC II is synthesized by amniocytes, permitting prenatal diagnosis.

Treatment

1000 μg vitamin B_{12} intramuscularly 1–2 times weekly.

Partial Deficiency of Transcobalamin I (R-Binder Deficiency) (OMIM 193090)

Partial deficiency of transcobalamin I (also known as R-binder or haptocorrin) has been reported. Serum vitamin B_{12} concentrations are persistently low and patients show no signs of vitamin B_{12} deficiency because their TC II–Cbl levels are normal. TC I concentrations range from 25% to 54% of the mean normal concentration.

Clinically this syndrome is characterized by a myelopathy not attributable to other causes, and the etiology of these symptoms remains unclear.

Disorders of Metabolism

Congenital

The conversion of a vitamin to its active coenzyme and subsequent binding to an apoenzyme producing active holoenzyme are fundamental biochemical processes. Therefore, deficient activity of an enzyme can result not only from a defect of the enzyme protein itself, which may involve interaction of a coenzyme with an apoenzyme, but also from a defect in the conversion of the vitamin to a coenzyme.

Once vitamin B_{12} has been taken up into cells, it must be converted to an active coenzyme in order to act as a cocatalyst with vitamin B_{12}-dependent apoenzymes. Two enzymes are known to depend for activity on vitamin B_{12} derivatives:

- Methylmalonyl coenzyme A (CoA) mutase, which requires adenosylcobalamin. Methylmalonyl CoA mutase catalyzes the conversion of methylmalonyl CoA to succinyl CoA. A decreased activity of methylmalonyl CoA mutase is reflected by the excretion of elevated amounts of methylmalonic acid.
- N^5-Methyltetrahydrofolate homocysteine methyltransferase, which requires methylcobalamin. Lack of methylcobalamin leads to deficient activity of N^5-methyltetrahydrofolate homocysteine methyltransferase, with reduced ability to methylate homocysteine, resulting in hyperhomocysteinemia and homocystinuria.

Patients with inborn errors of cobalamin utilization present with methylmalonic acidemia and hyperhomocysteinemia, either alone or in combination. Methylmalonic acidemia occurs as a result of a functional defect in the mitochondrial methylmalonyl CoA mutase or its cofactor adenosylcobalamin. Hyperhomocysteinemia occurs as a result of a functional defect in the cytoplasmic methionine synthase or its cofactor methylcobalamin. The sites of the defects and their frequency are shown in Figure 4-1. Tables 4-4 and 4-5 list the main features of genetic defects in processing cobalamins.

Severe metabolic acidosis, with the accumulation of large amounts of methylmalonic acid in blood, urine, and cerebrospinal fluid, characterizes the methylmalonic acidurias. The incidence is estimated at 1:61,000. All the disorders of Cbl metabolism are inherited as autosomal recessive traits and prenatal diagnosis is possible. Classification has relied on somatic cell complementation studies in cultured fibroblasts. Prenatal detection of fetuses with defects in the complementation groups *cblA*, *cblB*, *cblC*, *cblE*, and *cblF* has been accomplished using cultured amniotic cells and chemical determinations on amniotic fluid or maternal urine. In several cases, *in utero* Cbl therapy has been attempted with apparent success.

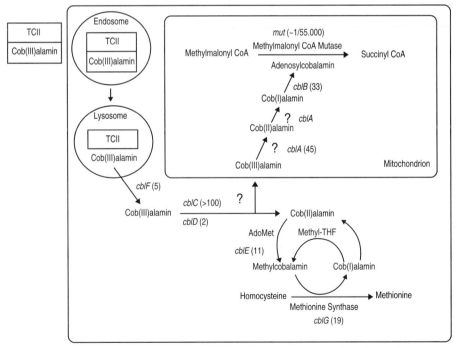

Fig. 4-1. Cobalamin metabolism in cultured mammalian cells and the sites of the known inborn errors of cobalamin metabolism. AdoMet, S-adenosylmethionine; cob(III)alamin, cob(II)alamin, cob(II)alamin represent cobalamin with its cobalt in the 3+, 2+, or 1+ oxidation state; methyl-THF is 5-methyltetrahydrofolate. The incidence or minimum numbers of patients with a given disease are shown in parentheses. (From Rosenblatt DS, Whitehead VM. Cobalamin and folate deficiency: acquired and hereditary disorders in children. Semin Hematol 36:1999, with permission.)

Table 4-4. Autosomal Recessive Inborn Errors of Cobalamin Transport and Metabolism

Condition (OMIM No.)	Defect	Typical clinical manifestations	Typical onset	Laboratory findings	Treatment and response
TC II deficiency (OMIM 275350)	Defective/absent TC II	Failure to thrive, megaloblastic anemia, later neurologic features, and immuno-deficiency	Early infancy 3–5 weeks	Usually normal serum Cbl; elevated serum MMA, homocysteine; absent/defective TC II	High doses of Cbl by injection; good response to treatment if begun early
TC I (R-binder) deficiency (OMIM 193090)	Deficiency/absence of TC I in plasma, saliva, leukocytes	Neurologic symptoms (myelopathy) reported, but unclear if these are related to condition	Unclear if observed symptoms are related to condition	Low serum Cbl, normal TC II-Cbl levels. No increase in MMA or homocysteine.	Cbl therapy does not appear to be of benefit
Defective synthesis of AdoCbl: cblA (OMIM 251100) cblB (OMIM 251110)	Defective synthesis of AdoCbl	Lethargy, failure to thrive, recurrent vomiting, dehydration, hypotonia, ketoacidosis hypoglycemia	First weeks or months of life	Normal serum Cbl, homocysteine, and methionine; elevated MMA, ketones, glycine, ammonia; leukopenia, thrombocytopenia, anemia	Pharmacologic doses of Cbl, dietary protein restriction, oral antibiotics. Treatment response for cblA better than for cblB

Defect	Defective synthesis	Clinical features	Onset	Laboratory findings	Treatment
Defective synthesis of MeCbl: cblE (OMIM 236270) cblG (OMIM 250940)	Defective synthesis of MeCbl	Vomiting, poor feeding, lethargy, severe neurologic dysfunction, megaloblastic anemia	Most in first 2 years of life	Normal serum Cbl and folate; homocystinuria, hypomethioninemia	Pharmacologic doses of Cbl, betaine; good treatment response in some patients treated early
Defective synthesis of AdoCbl and MeCbl: cblC (OMIM 277400) cblD (OMIM 277410) cblF (OMIM 277380)	Impaired synthesis of both AdoCbl and MeCbl	Failure to thrive, developmental delay, neurologic dysfunction, megaloblastic anemia, some cases with retinal findings	Variable from neonatal period to adolescence; majority with neonatal onset	Normal serum Cbl, TC II; methylmalonic aciduria, homocystinuria, hypomethioninemia	Pharmacologic doses of hydroxocobalamin, moderate protein restriction, betaine treatment. Response often not optimum

Abbreviations: TC II, transcobalamin II; OMIM, Online Mendelian Inheritance in Man; Cbl, cobalamin; MMA, methylmalonic acid; TC I, transcobalamin I; AdoCbl, adenosylcobalamin; MeCbl, methylcobalamin.
Modified from Rasmussen SA, Fernhoff PM, Scanlon KS. Vitamin B_{12} deficiency in children and adolescents. J of Pediatrics 2001;138:10–17.

Table 4-5. Main Features of Genetic Defects of Processing of Cobalamins

Defect	Serum B_{12}	Clinical/biochemical
Food cobalamin malabsorption	Low	NA ± anemia, mild ↑ MMA/tHcy
Intrinsic factor deficiency	Low	Anemia, delayed development, mild ↑ MMA/tHcy
Enterocyte cobalamin malabsorption (Imerslund–Gräsbeck)	Low	Anemia, proteinuria, delayed development, mild ↑ MMA/tHcy
Transcobalamin I (R-binder) deficiency	Low	No abnormality, no ↑ MMA/tHcy
Transcobalamin II deficiency	Normal	NA ± anemia, failure to thrive, mild ↑ MMA/tHcy
Intracellular defects of cobalamin	Normal	Severe disease, ↑ MMA/tHcy

Abbreviations: NA, neurologic abnormalities; MMA, methylmalonic acid; tHcy, total homocysteine; ↑, increased.

Adenosylcobalamin Deficiency CblA (OMIM 251100) and CblB (OMIM 251110) Diseases

Deficiencies of adenosylcobalamin synthesis lead to impaired methylmalonyl CoA mutase activity and result in methylmalonic acidemia. Cobalamin-responsive methylmalonic aciduria characterizes both CblA and CblB diseases. Intact cells from both CblA and CblB patients fail to synthesize adenosylcobalamin. However, cell extracts from CblA patients can synthesize adenosylcobalamin when provided with an appropriate reducing system, whereas extracts from CblB patients cannot. The defect in CblA may be related to a deficiency of a mitochondrial nicotinamide adenine dinucleotide phosphate (NADPH)-linked aquacobalamin reductase. The defect in CblB affects adenosyltransferase, which is involved in the final step in adenosylcobalamin synthesis.

This group of patients presents with:

- Life-threatening or fatal ketoacidosis in the first few weeks or months of life
- Hypoglycemia and hyperglycinemia
- Failure to thrive or developmental retardation (may be a consequence of the acidosis and reversed by relief of the ketoacidosis)
- Normal serum cobalamin concentrations.

Both CblA and CblB are autosomal recessive diseases. Studies of these patients have shown that intact cells fail to oxidize propionate normally. Methylmalonyl CoA arises chiefly through the carboxylation of propionate, which in turn derives largely from degradation of valine, isoleucine, methionine, and threonine.

Treatment

Ninety percent of CblA patients respond to therapy with systemic hydroxocobalamin or cyanocobalamin, whereas only 40% of CblB patients respond to this therapy. Only 30% have long-term survival.

Deficiency of Methylmalonyl-CoA Mutase (mut°, mut⁻)

Defects in methylmalonyl CoA mutase apoenzyme formation can occur and result in methylmalonic aciduria, which is accompanied by life-threatening or fatal ketoacidosis, unresponsive to vitamin B_{12}.

Protein feeding induces symptoms rapidly. Symptoms include lethargy, failure to thrive, muscular hypotonia, respiratory distress, and recurrent vomiting and dehydration. Children normally excrete <15–20 ng of methylmalonic acid per gram of creatinine, whereas patients with methylmalonyl CoA mutase deficiency excrete >100 mg up to several grams daily. Patients may have elevated levels of ketones, glycine, and ammonia in the blood and urine. Many also have hypoglycemia, leukopenia, and thrombocytopenia.

Treatment
Treatment involves protein restriction using a formula deficient in valine, isoleucine, methionine, and threonine, with the goal of limiting amino acids that use the propionate pathway. Therapy with carnitine has been advocated for those patients who are carnitine deficient. Lincomycin and metronidazole have been used to reduce enteric propionate production by anaerobic bacteria. These patients do not respond well to vitamin B$_{12}$ therapy. Despite therapy, a number of patients have experienced basal ganglia infarcts, tubulointerstitial nephritis, acute pancreatitis, and cardiomyopathy as complications. Liver transplantation has been attempted.

Cultures of patients' fibroblasts show two classes of mutase deficiency: those having no detectable enzyme activity are designated mut°, whereas those with residual activity, which can be stimulated by high levels of cobalamin, are termed mut⁻. Some mut° cell lines synthesize no detectable protein.

Methylcobalamin Synthesis Deficiency: CblE (OMIM 236270) and CblG (OMIM 250940) Diseases

Abnormalities in methylcobalamin synthesis result in reduced N^5-methyltetrahydrofolate:homocysteine methyltransferase and consequently lead to homocystinuria with hypomethioninemia. Thus, homocystinuria and hypomethioninemia, usually without methylmalonic aciduria, characterize functional methionine synthase deficiency (CblE, CblG), although one CblE patient had transient methylmalonic aciduria. Fibroblasts from CblE and CblG patients show a decreased accumulation of methylcobalamin with a normal accumulation of adenosylcobalamin after incubation with cyanocobalamin. Their fibroblasts show decreased incorporation of labeled methyltetrahydrofolate as well. Cyanocobalamin uptake and binding to both cobalamin-dependent enzymes is normal in CblE fibroblasts and in most CblG fibroblasts.

Clinical findings
- In most patients, illness within the first 2 years of life, but a number of patients have been diagnosed in adulthood
- Megaloblastic anemia
- Various neurologic deficits including developmental delay, cerebral atrophy, EEG abnormalities, nystagmus, hypotonia, hypertonia, seizures, blindness, and ataxia
- Failure to thrive.

Treatment
Hydroxocobalamin is administered systemically, daily at first, then once or twice weekly. Usually this corrects the anemia and the metabolic abnormalities. Betaine supplementation may be helpful to reduce the homocysteine further. The neurologic findings are more difficult to reverse once established, particularly in CblG disease. There has been successful prenatal diagnosis of CblE disease in amniocytes, and the mother with an affected fetus can be treated with twice weekly hydroxocobalamin after the second trimester.

Combined Adenosylcobalamin and Methylcobalamin Deficiency CblC (OMIM 277400), CblD (OMIM 277410), and CblF (OMIM 277380) Diseases

These disorders result in failure of cells to synthesize both methylcobalamin (resulting in homocystinuria and hypomethioninemia) and adenosylcobalamin (resulting in methylmalonic aciduria) and, accordingly, deficient activity of methylmalonyl

CoA mutase and N^5-methyltetrahydrofolate: homocysteine methyltransferase. Fibroblasts from CblC and CblD patients accumulate virtually no adenosylcobalamin or methylcobalamin when incubated with labeled cyanocobalamin. In contrast, fibroblasts from CblF patients accumulate excess cobalamin, but it is all unmetabolized cyanocobalamin, nonprotein bound, and localized to lysosomes. In CblC and CblD, the defect is believed to involve cob(III)alamin* reductase or reductases, whereas in CblF, the defect involves the exit of cobalamin from the lysosome. Partial deficiencies of cyanocobalamin beta-ligand transferase and microsomal cob(III)alamin reductase have been described in CblC and CblD fibroblasts as well.

These patients present in the first year of life with:

- Poor feeding, failure to thrive, and lethargy
- Macrocytosis, hypersegmented neutrophils, thrombocytopenia, and megaloblastic anemia
- Developmental retardation
- Spasticity, delirium, and psychosis (in older children and adolescents)
- Hydrocephalus, cor pulmonale, and hepatic failure, as well as a pigmentary retinopathy with perimacular degeneration
- Methylmalonic acid levels that are lower than in methylmalonyl CoA mutase deficiency, but greater than in defects of cobalamin transport.

In addition, many patients with the onset of symptoms in the first month of life die, whereas those with a later onset have a better prognosis.

CblC, CblD, and CblF diseases can be differentiated using cultured fibroblasts. Failure of uptake of labeled cyanocobalamin distinguishes CblC and CblD from all other *cbl* mutations. There is reduced incorporation of propionate and methyltetrahydrofolate into macromolecules in all three disorders and reduced synthesis of adenosylcobalamin and methylcobalamin. Complementation analysis between an unknown cell line and previously defined groups establishes the specific diagnosis. Prenatal diagnosis has been successfully accomplished in CblC disease using chorionic villus biopsy material and cells.

Treatment
The treatment of CblC disease can be difficult. Daily therapy with oral betaine and twice weekly injections of hydroxocobalamin improve lethargy, irritability, and failure to thrive; reduce methylmalonic aciduria; and return serum methionine and homocysteine concentrations to normal. There has been incomplete reversal of the neurologic and retinal findings. Surviving patients usually have moderate to severe developmental delay, even with good metabolic control.

Acquired

In protein malnutrition (kwashiorkor, marasmus) and liver disease, impaired utilization of vitamin B_{12} has been reported. Certain drugs are associated with impaired absorption or utilization of vitamin B_{12} (see Table 4-2).

FOLIC ACID DEFICIENCY

Folate coenzymes are the central participants in single-carbon transfer reactions. 5,10-Methylene tetrahydrofolate is used unchanged for the synthesis of thymidylate,

---

*In this form of cobalamin, the cobalt atom is trivalent (cob[111]) and must be reduced before it can bind to the respective enzyme.

reduced to 5-methyltetrahydrofolate for the synthesis of methionine, or oxidized to 10-formyltetrahydrofolate for the synthesis of purines.

The causes of folic acid deficiency are listed in Table 4-6.

Acquired Folate Deficiency

Folate deficiency, next to iron deficiency, is one of the most common micronutrient deficiencies worldwide. It is a component of malnutrition and starvation. Women are more frequently affected than men. Folate deficiency is common in mothers, particularly where poverty or malnutrition is prevalent, and dietary supplements are not provided. Folate stores are depleted after 3 months or sooner when the growing fetus and lactation impose increased demands for folate. The major benefit of folate sufficiency for the fetus is the prevention of neural tube defects. This is currently best achieved by administering folate (and cobalamin) to mothers during the periconceptional period.

Table 4-6. Causes of Folic Acid Deficiency

I. Inadequate intake
   A. Poverty, ignorance, faddism
   B. Method of cooking (sustained boiling loses 40% folate)
   C. Goat's-milk feeding (6 µg folate/L)
   D. Malnutrition (marasmus, kwashiorkor)
   E. Special diets for phenylketonuria or maple syrup urine disease
   F. Prematurity
   G. Post–bone marrow transplantation (heat-sterilized food)

II. Defective absorption
   A. Congenital, isolated defect of folate malabsorption[a]
   B. Acquired
      1. Idiopathic steatorrhea
      2. Tropical sprue
      3. Partial or total gastrectomy
      4. Multiple diverticula of small intestine
      5. Jejunal resection
      6. Regional ileitis
      7. Whipple disease
      8. Intestinal lymphoma
      9. Broad-spectrum antibiotics
      10. Drugs associated with impaired absorption and/or utilization of folic acid, e.g., diphenylhydantoin (Dilantin), primidone, barbiturates, oral contraceptive agents, cycloserine, metformin, ethanol, dietary amino acids (glycine, methionine)
      11. Post–bone marrow transplantation (total body irradiation, drugs, intestinal GVH disease)

III. Increased requirements
   A. Rapid growth (e.g., prematurity, pregnancy)
   B. Chronic hemolytic anemia, especially with ineffective erythropoiesis (e.g., thalassemia major)
   C. Dyserythropoietic anemias
   D. Malignant disease (e.g., lymphoma, leukemia)
   E. Hypermetabolic states (e.g., infection, hyperthyroidism)
   F. Extensive skin disease (e.g., dermatitis herpetiformis, psoriasis, exfoliative dermatitis)
   G. Cirrhosis
   H. Post–bone marrow transplantation (bone marrow and epithelial cell regeneration)

(Continues)

Table 4-6. (*Continued*)

IV. Disorders of folic acid metabolism
  A. Congenital[b]
  1. Methylenetetrahydrofolate reductase (MTHFR) deficiency (OMIM 236250)
  2. Glutamate formiminotransferase deficiency (OMIM 229100)
  3. Functional N^5-methyltetrahydrofolate:homocysteine methyltransferase deficiency caused by cblE (OMIM 236270) or cblG (OMIM 250940) disease
  4. Dihydrofolate reductase deficiency (less well established)
  5. Methenyl-tetrahydrofolate cyclohydrolase (less well established)
  6. Primary methyl-tetrahydrofolate: homocysteine methyltransferase deficiency (less well established)
  B. Acquired
  1. Impaired utilization of folate
    a. Folate antagonists (drugs that are dihydrofolate reductase inhibitors, e.g., methotrexate, pyrimethamine, trimethoprim, pentamidine)
    b. Vitamin B_{12} deficiency
    c. Alcoholism
    d. Liver disease (acute and chronic)
    e. Other drugs (IIB10 above)

V. Increased excretion (e.g., chronic dialysis, vitamin B_{12} deficiency, liver disease, heart disease)

Abbreviation: OMIM, Online Mendelian Inheritance in Man (page 50).

[a]Rare disorder. Isolated disorder of folate transport resulting in low CSF folate and mental retardation. The ability to absorb all other nutrients is normal. Defect is overcome by pharmacologic oral doses of folic acid or intramuscular folic acid (Lanzkowsky P, Erlandson, ME, Bezan AI. Isolated defect of folic acid absorption associated with mental retardation and cerebral calcifications, Blood 1969;34:452–65; Am J Med 1970;48:580–3).

[b]These disorders are associated with megaloblastic anemia, mental retardation, disorders in gait, and both peripheral and central nervous system disease.

In addition, low daily folate intake is associated with a twofold increased risk for preterm delivery and low infant birth weight. These findings suggest that maternal folate status may affect birth outcome in ways other than neural tube defects.

Clinical folate deficiency is seldom present at birth. However, rapid growth in the first few weeks of life demands increased folate. There is a need for folate supplements at this time, particularly for premature infants, in doses of 0.05–0.2 mg/day.

Inborn Errors of Folate Transport and Metabolism

Inborn errors include hereditary folate malabsorption, methylene-tetrahydrofolate reductase (MTHFR) deficiency, and glutamate formiminotransferase deficiency. In addition to these rare severe deficiencies, polymorphisms in the MTHFR gene have been implicated with neural defects and vascular thrombosis. Table 4-7 lists the clinical and biochemical features of inherited defects of folate metabolism.

Hereditary Folate Malabsorption (OMIM 229050)

Hereditary folate malabsorption (congenital malabsorption of folate) is due to a rare autosomal recessive trait and is characterized by megaloblastic anemia, chronic or recurrent diarrhea, mouth ulcers, failure to thrive, and usually loss of developmental milestones, seizures, and progressive neurologic deterioration. The most important diagnostic feature is megaloblastic anemia in the first few months of life, associated with low serum, red cell, and cerebrospinal fluid folate levels.

All patients have an abnormality in the absorption of oral folic acid or of reduced folates. They may have an elevated excretion of formiminogiutamic (FIGLU) acid

Table 4-7. Clinical and Biochemical Features of Inherited Defects of Folate Metabolism

Clinical sign	Hereditary folate malabsorption	Methylene-H$_4$ folate reductase deficiency	Glutamate formiminotransferase deficiency	Functional methionine synthase deficiency	
				CblE	CblG
Prevalence	13 cases	>30 cases	13 cases	8 cases	12 cases
Megaloblastic anemia	A	N	N[a]	A	A
Developmental delay	A	A	N[a]	A	A
Seizures	A	A	N[a]	A	A
Speech abnormalities	N	N	A[a]	N	N
Gait abnormalities	N	A	N[a]	N	A[a]
Peripheral neuropathy	N[a]	A	N[a]	N	A[a]
Apnea	N	A	N[a]	N[a]	N
Biochemical findings					
Homocystinuria/homocysteinemia	N	A	N	A	A
Hypomethioninemia	N	A	N	A	A
Formiminoglutamic aciduria	A[a]	N	A	N	N[a]
Folate absorption	A	N	N	N	N
Serum Cbl	N	N	N[a]	N	N
Serum folate	A	A	N[a]	N	N
Red blood cell folate	A	A[a]	N[a]	N	N

(Continues)

Table 4-7. (Continued)

	Hereditary folate malabsorption	Methylene-H$_4$ folate reductase deficiency	Glutamate formiminotransferase deficiency	Functional methionine synthase deficiency	
				CblE	CblG
Defects detectable in cultured fibroblasts					
Whole cells					
CH$_3$H$_4$ folate uptake	N	N	N	A	A
CH$_3$H$_4$ folate content	N	A	N	N	N
CH$_3$B$_{12}$ content	N	N^a	N	A	A
Extracts					
Activity of holoenzyme of methionine synthase	N	N^a	N	N^b	A
Glutamate forminotransferase			Activity undetectable in cultured cells; ? Abnormal in liver and erythrocytes		
Methylene-H$_4$ folate reductase	N	A	N	N	N
Treatment	Folic acid or reduced folates in pharmacologic doses	Folates, betaine, methionine	? Folates	OH-Cbl, folinic acid, betaine	

Abbreviations: N, normal; A, abnormal (i.e., clinical findings or laboratory findings present).

^{a}Exceptions described in some cases.

^{b}Abnormal activity with low concentrations of reducing agent in assay.

From Rosenblatt DS. Inherited disorders of folate transport and metabolism. In: Scriver CR, Beaudet AL, Sly WS, Valle D, editors. The metabolic and molecular bases of inherited disease. 7th ed. New York: McGraw-Hill, 1995, with permission.

and of orotic acid. This disease indicates that there is a specific transport system for folates across both the intestine and the choroid plexus and that this carrier system is coded by a single gene. Even when blood folate levels are increased sufficiently to correct the anemia, folate levels in the cerebrospinal fluid (CSF) remain low. These patients are unable to achieve the normal 3:1 CSF:serum folate ratio. The uptake of folate into other cells is probably not defective, and the uptake of folate into cultured cells is not abnormal.

Oral folic acid in doses of 5–40 mg/day and lower parenteral doses correct the hematologic abnormality, but CSF folate levels remain low. Oral methyltetrahydrofolate and folinic acid can increase CSF folate levels, but only slightly.

In treating these patients, it is essential to maintain levels of folate in the blood and in the cerebrospinal fluid in the range associated with folate sufficiency. Oral doses of folates may be increased to 100 mg or more daily if necessary; if oral therapy is not effective, systemic therapy with reduced folates should be tried. It may be necessary to give intrathecal reduced folates if CSF levels cannot be normalized.

Methylene-Tetrahydrofolate Reductase Deficiency (OMIM 236250)

Clinical Findings

Clinically asymptomatic but biochemically affected individuals have been reported. The condition can present severely in early infancy (first month of life) or much more mildly as late as 16 years of age. Clinical symptoms vary and consist of developmental delay, which is the most common clinical manifestation; motor and gait abnormalities; recurrent strokes; seizures; mental retardation; psychiatric manifestations; microcephaly; and vasculopathy. Megaloblastic anemia is uncommon in patients with this disease because reduced folates are still available for purine and pyrimidine synthesis. MTHFR deficiency results in elevated plasma homocysteine and homocystinuria and decreased plasma methionine levels because levels of methyltetrahydrofolate serve as one of three methyl donors for the conversion of homocysteine to methionine.

Pathologic findings in patients with severe MTHFR deficiency include vascular changes such as thrombosis of both cerebral arteries and veins, dilated cerebral vessels, internal hydrocephalus, microgyria, perivascular changes, demyelination, macrophage infiltration, gliosis, astrocytosis, and subacute combined degeneration of the spinal cord. By interfering with methylation, methionine deficiency may cause demyelination.

Diagnosis

MTHFR deficiency can be diagnosed by measuring enzyme activity in liver, white blood cells, and cultured fibroblasts. In fibroblasts, the specific activity of MTHFR is dependent on the stage of the culture cycle. A rough correlation exists between the degree of enzyme deficiency and clinical severity. The proportion of total folate in fibroblasts that is methyltetrahydrofolate and the extent of labeled formate incorporated into methionine are better indicators of clinical severity.

Prognosis

Prognosis is poor in early-onset severe MTHFR deficiency.

Treatment

MTHFR deficiency is resistant to treatment. Regimens have included folic acid, methyltetrahydrofolate, methionine, pyridoxine, various cobalamins, carnitine, and betaine. Betaine therapy after prenatal diagnosis has resulted in the best outcome to date since it has the theoretical advantage of both lowering homocysteine levels and supplementing methionine levels.

Prenatal diagnosis is possible by enzyme assay in amniocytes, chorionic villus biopsy samples, or cultured chorionic villus cells. The phenotypic heterogeneity in MTHFR deficiency is reflected by genotypic heterogeneity.

Glutamate Formiminotransferase Deficiency (OMIM 229100)

Glutamate formiminotransferase and formiminotetrahydrofolate cyclodeaminase are involved in the transfer of a formimino group to tetrahydrofolate followed by the release of ammonia and the formation of 5,10-methyltetrahydrofolate. These activities are found only in the liver and kidneys and are performed by a single octameric enzyme. It is not clear that glutamate formiminotransferase deficiency is associated with disease, even though FIGLU acid excretion is the one constant finding. Twenty patients have been described, with ages ranging from 3 months to 42 years at diagnosis. Some have been asymptomatic and several patients have macrocytosis and hypersegmentation of neutrophils.

Mild and severe phenotypes have been described. Patients with severe form show mental and physical retardation, abnormal EEG activity, and dilatation of the cerebral ventricles with cortical atrophy. In the mild form, there is no mental retardation but massive excretion of FIGLU acid.

Liver-specific activity ranges from 14% to 54% of control values. It is not possible to confirm the diagnosis using cultured cells because the enzyme is not expressed. There is dispute as to whether the enzyme is expressed in red cells.

Patients may have elevated to normal serum folate levels and elevated FIGLU acid levels in the blood and urine after a histidine load. Plasma amino acid levels are usually normal, but hyperhistidinemia, hyperhistidinuria, and hypomethioninemia have been found. The excretion of hydantoin-5-propionate, the stable oxidation product of the FIGLU precursor, 4-imidazolone-5-propionate, and 4-amino-5-imidazolecarboxamide, an intermediate in purine synthesis, has been seen in some patients.

Autosomal recessive inheritance is the probable means of transmission because there have been affected individuals of both sexes with unaffected parents.

Functional Methionine Synthase Deficiency (OMIM 250940)

Functional methionine synthase deficiency due to the *cblE* and *cblG* mutations is characterized by homocystinuria and defective biosynthesis of methionine. Most patients have presented in the first few months of life with megaloblastic anemia and developmental delay. The distribution of cobalamin derivatives was altered in cultured cells, with decreased levels of methylcobalamin as compared with normal fibroblasts. The *cblE* mutation is associated with low methionine synthase activity when the assay is performed with low levels of thiol, whereas the *cblG* mutation is associated with low activity under all assay conditions. *cblE* and *cblG* represent distinct complementation classes. Both diseases respond to treatment with hydroxocobalamin (OH-cbl).

Other Megaloblastic Anemias

Thiamine-Responsive Anemia in DIDMOAD (Wolfram) Syndrome: Autosomal Recessive Inheritance

Megaloblastic anemia and sideroblastic anemia with ringed sideroblasts may be present. Neutropenia and thrombocytopenia are present. It is accompanied by diabetes insipidus (DI), diabetes mellitus (DM), optic atrophy (OA), and deafness (D) (hence, the term *DIDMOAD*). It is due to a defect in thiamine transport, possibly deficient thiamine pyrophosphokinase activity.

Treatment

Anemia responds to 100 mg thiamine daily but megaloblastic changes persist. Insulin requirements decrease.

Orotic Aciduria

Orotic aciduria is a rare autosomal recessive defect of pyrimidine synthesis with failure to convert orotic acid to uridine and excretion of large amounts of orotic acid in the urine, sometimes with crystals. It is associated with severe megaloblastic anemia, neutropenia, and failure to thrive, and physical and mental retardation are frequently present.

Treatment

Treatment is with oral uridine (1–1.5 g/day). The anemia is refractory to vitamin B_{12} and folic acid.

Lesch–Nyhan Syndrome

In Lesch–Nyhan syndrome, mental retardation, self-mutilation, and choreoathetosis result from impaired synthesis of purines due to lack of hypoxanthine phosphoribosyltransferase. Some patients have megaloblastic anemia.

Treatment

Megaloblastic anemia responds to adenine therapy (1.5 g/day).

CLINICAL FEATURES OF COBALAMIN AND FOLATE DEFICIENCY

1. *Insidious onset*: Pallor, lethargy, fatigability, and anorexia; sore red tongue and glossitis; episodic or continuous diarrhea.
2. *History:* Similarly affected sibling or a sibling who died; maternal vitamin B_{12} deficiency or poor maternal diet.
3. *Vitamin B_{12} deficiency:* All infants show signs of developmental delay, apathy, weakness, irritability, or evidence of neurodevelopmental delay, loss of developmental milestones, particularly motor achievements (head control, sitting, and turning). Athetoid movements, hypotonia, and loss of reflexes occur. In older children signs of subacute dorsolateral degeneration of the spinal cord may occur. The usual symptoms are paresthesias in the hands or feet and difficulty in walking and use of the hands. Symptoms arise because of a peripheral neuropathy (especially paresthesias and numbness) associated with degeneration of posterior and lateral tracts of the spinal cord. Loss of vibration and position sense with an ataxic gait and positive Romberg's sign are features of posterior column and peripheral nerve loss. Spastic paresis may occur, with knee and ankle reflexes increased because of lateral tract loss, but flaccid weakness may also occur when these reflexes are lost but the Babinski sign remains

extensor. MRI findings include increased signals on T_2-weighted images of the spinal cord, brain atrophy, and retarded myelination.

4. Deleterious effect of cobalamin or folate deficiency apart from neurologic complications are increased risk of vascular thrombosis due to hyperhomocysteinemia.

5. Maternal folate deficiency results in neural tube defects, prematurity, fetal growth retardation, and fetal loss.

6. Inborn errors of metabolism of cobalamin and folate result in failure to thrive, neurologic disorders, unexplained anemias, or cytopenias. Plasma levels of methylmalonic acid and homocysteine should be determined in these cases to elucidate the precise diagnosis. Elevation of these levels reflects a functional lack of cobalamin and/or folate by tissues even when plasma vitamin levels are at the lower level of normal.

DIAGNOSIS

The age of presentation may help to focus on the most likely diagnosis (Table 4-8).

1. *Red cell changes:*
   a. *Hemoglobin:* Usually reduced, may be marked.
   b. *Red cell indices:* MCV increased for age and may be raised to levels of 110–140 fL; MCHC normal.
   c. *Red cell distribution width (RDW):* Increased.
   d. *Blood smear:* Many macrocytes* and macro-ovalocytes; marked anisocytosis and poikilocytosis; presence of Cabot rings, Howell–Jolly bodies, and punctate basophilia.
2. *White blood cell count:* Reduced to 1500–4000/mm³; neutrophils show hypersegmentation, that is, nuclei of more than five lobes.
3. *Platelet count:* Moderately reduced to 50,000–180,000/mm³.
4. *Bone marrow:* Megaloblastic appearance.
   a. The cells are large, and the nucleus has an open, stippled, or lacy appearance. The cytoplasm is comparatively more mature than the nucleus, and this dissociation (nuclear-cytoplasmic dissociation) is best seen in the later cells. Orthochromatic cells may be present with nuclei that are still not fully condensed.
   b. Mitoses are frequent and sometimes abnormal[†]; nuclear remnants, Howell–Jolly bodies, bi- and trinucleated cells, and dying cells are evidence of gross dyserythropoiesis.
   c. The metamyelocytes are abnormally large (giant) and have a horseshoe-shaped nucleus.
   d. Hypersegmented polymorphs may be seen, and the megakaryocytes show an increase in nuclear lobes.
5. *Serum vitamin B_{12} level:* Normal values 200–800 pg/mL (levels <80 pg/mL are almost always indicative of vitamin B_{12} deficiency).
6. *Serum and red cell folate levels:* Wide variation in normal range; serum levels less than 3 ng/mL = low, 3–5 ng/mL = borderline, and >5–6 ng/mL = normal. Red cell folate levels 74–640 ng/mL.
7. Urinary excretion of orotic acid to exclude orotic aciduria.

---

*Macrocytosis can be masked by associated iron deficiency and thalassemia.

†Megaloblastic cells exhibit increased frequency of chromosomal abnormalities, especially random breaks, gaps, and centromere spreading. A rare case of nonrandom, transient 7q- has been described in acquired megaloblastic anemia.

Table 4-8. Disorders Giving Rise to Megaloblastic Anemia in Early Life and Their Likely Time of Presentation

Disease	Likely time of presentation (months)		
	2–6	7–24	>24
Folate deficiency			
Inadequate supply			
Prematurity	+		
Dietary (e.g., goat's milk)	+		
Chronic hemolysis			+
Defective absorption			
Celiac disease/sprue			+
Anticonvulsant drugs			+
Congenital	+		
Cobalamin deficiency			
Inadequate supply			
Maternal cobalamin deficiency		+	
Nutritional			+
Defective absorption			
Juvenile pernicious anemia			+
Congenital malabsorption		+	±
Congenital absence of intrinsic factor		+	±
Defective metabolism			
Transcobalamin II deficiency	+		
Inborn errors of cobalamin utilization	+		
Thiamine responsive			+
Orotic aciduria	+		
Lesch–Nyhan syndrome			+

8. *Deoxyuridine suppression test:* This test can discriminate between folate and cobalamin deficiencies.

If vitamin B$_{12}$ deficiency is suspected proceed as follows:

1. Obtain a detailed dietary history and history of previous surgery.
2. Conduct a Schilling urinary excretion test.* This test measures both intrinsic factor availability and intestinal absorption of vitamin B$_{12}$.
3. If the Schilling test is abnormal, repeat with commercial intrinsic factor. If absorption occurs, abnormality is due to lack of intrinsic factor. If no absorption occurs then there is specific ileal vitamin B$_{12}$ malabsorption (Imerslund–Gräsbeck) or transcobalamin II deficiency. When bacterial competition (blind-loop syndrome) is suspected, the test may be repeated after treatment with tetracycline and will often revert to normal.
4. Gastric acidity after histamine stimulation, intrinsic factor content in gastric juice, serum antibodies to intrinsic factor, and parietal cells and gastric biopsy help to establish a precise diagnosis.

---

*The Schilling test is performed by administering 0.5–2.0 µg of radioactive vitamin B$_{12}$ PO. This is followed in 2 hours by an intramuscular injection of 1000 µg nonradioactive vitamin B$_{12}$ to saturate the B$_{12}$-binding proteins and allow the subsequently absorbed oral radioactive vitamin B$_{12}$ to be excreted in the urine. All urine is collected for 24 hours and may be collected for a second 24 hours, especially if renal disease is present. Normal subjects excrete 10–35% of the administered dose; those with severe malabsorption of vitamin B$_{12}$, because of lack of intrinsic factor or intestinal malabsorption, excrete less than 3%.

5. Measure serum holo-transcobalamin II (cobalamin bound to transcobalamin II). In patients with vitamin B_{12} deficiency, holo-translocation II falls below the normal range before total serum cobalamin does.
6. Ileal disease should be investigated by barium studies and small-bowel biopsy.
7. Disorders of vitamin B_{12} metabolism should be excluded by serum and urinary levels of excessive methylmalonic acid and homocysteine as well as by other sophisticated enzymatic assays. In folate deficiency, serum methylmalonic acid is normal whereas homocysteine is increased. Therefore, evaluation of both methylmalonic acid and total homocysteine is helpful in distinguishing between folate and vitamin B_{12} deficiency.
8. Persistent proteinuria is a feature of specific ileal vitamin B_{12} malabsorption.

If folic acid deficiency is suspected, proceed as follows:

1. Detailed dietary and drug history (e.g., antibiotics, anticonvulsants) and gastroenterologic symptoms (e.g., malabsorption, diarrhea, dietary history)
2. Tests for malabsorption:
   a. Oral doses of 5 mg pteroylglutamic acid should yield a plasma level in excess of 100 ng/mL in 1 hour. If there is no rise in plasma level, congenital folate malabsorption should be considered.
   b. A 24-hour stool fat and blood D-xylose test should be done to exclude generalized malabsorption.
3. Upper gastrointestinal barium study and follow-through
4. Upper gut endoscopy and jejunal biopsy
5. Sophisticated enzyme assays to diagnose congenital disorders of folate metabolism.

TREATMENT
Vitamin B_{12} Deficiency

Prevention

In conditions in which there is a risk of developing vitamin B_{12} deficiency (e.g., total gastrectomy, ileal resection), prophylactic vitamin B_{12} should be prescribed.

Active Treatment

Once the diagnosis has been accurately determined, several daily doses of 25–100 µg may be used to initiate therapy as well as potassium supplements.* Alternatively, in view of the ability of the body to store vitamin B_{12} for long periods, maintenance therapy can be started with monthly intramuscular injections in doses between 200 and 1000 µg. Most cases of vitamin B_{12} deficiency require treatment throughout life.

Patients with defects affecting the intestinal absorption of vitamin B_{12} (abnormalities of IF or of ileal uptake) will respond to parenteral B_{12}. This bypasses the defective step completely.

Patients with complete TC II deficiency respond only to large amounts of vitamin B_{12} and the serum cobalamin level must be kept very high. Doses of 1000 µg IM two or three times weekly are required to maintain adequate control.

Patients with methylmalonic aciduria with defects in the synthesis of cobalamin coenzymes are likely to benefit from massive doses of vitamin B_{12}. These children

---

*Hypokalemia has been observed during B_{12} initiation treatment in adults.

may require 1–2 mg vitamin B_{12} parenterally daily. However, not all patients in this group benefit from administration of vitamin B_{12}.

It may be possible to treat vitamin B_{12}-responsive patients *in utero*. Congenital methylmalonic aciduria has been diagnosed *in utero* by measurements of methylmalonate in amniotic fluid or maternal urine.

In vitamin B_{12}-responsive megaloblastic anemia, the reticulocytes begin to increase on the 3rd or 4th day, rise to a maximum on the 6th to 8th day, and fall gradually to normal by about the 20th day. The height of the reticulocyte count is inversely proportional to the degree of anemia. Beginning bone marrow reversal from megaloblastic to normoblastic cells is obvious within 6 hours and is complete in 72 hours. Neurologically, the level of alertness and responsiveness improves within 48 hours and developmental delays may catch up in several months in young infants. Permanent neurologic sequelae often occur. Prompt hematologic responses are also obtained with the use of oral folic acid, but it is contraindicated because it has no effect on neurologic manifestations and may precipitate or accelerate their development.

Folic Acid Deficiency

Successful treatment of patients with folate deficiency involves:

1. Correction of the folate deficiency
2. Treatment of the underlying causative disorder
3. Improvement of the diet to increase folate intake
4. Follow-up evaluations at intervals to monitor the patient's clinical status.

Optimal response occurs in most patients with 100–200 μg folic acid per day. Because the usual commercially available preparations include a tablet (0.3–1.0 mg) and an elixir (1.0 mg/mL), these available preparations are utilized. Before folic acid is given, it is necessary to exclude vitamin B_{12} deficiency.

The clinical and hematologic response to folic acid is prompt. Within 1–2 days, the appetite improves and a sense of well-being returns. There is a fall in serum iron (often to low levels) in 24–48 hours and a rise in reticulocytes in 2–4 days, reaching a peak at 4–7 days, followed by a return of hemoglobin levels to normal in 2–6 weeks. The leukocytes and platelets increase with reticulocytes and the megaloblastic changes in the marrow diminish within 24–48 hours, but large myelocytes, metamyelocytes, and band forms may be present for several days.

Folic acid is usually administered for several months until a new population of red cells has been formed. Folinic acid is reserved for treating the toxic effects of dihydrofolate reductase inhibitors (e.g., methotrexate, pyrimethamine).

It is often possible to correct the cause of the deficiency and thus prevent its recurrence, for example, improved diet, a gluten-free diet in celiac disease, or treatment of an inflammatory disease such as tuberculosis or Crohn's disease. In these cases, there is no need to continue folic acid for life. In other situations, it is advisable to continue the folic acid to prevent recurrence of, for example, chronic hemolytic anemia such as thalassemia or in patients with malabsorption who do not respond to a gluten-free diet.

Cases of hereditary dihydrofolate reductase deficiency respond to *N*-5-formyl tetrahydrofolic acid and not to folic acid.

SUGGESTED READINGS

Carmel R. Beyond megaloblastic anemia: new paradigms of cobalamin and folate deficiency. Semin Hematol 1999;36(1).

Chanarin I. Management of megaloblastic anemia in the very young. Brit J Haematol 1983;53:1–3.

Chanarin I. The Megaloblastic Anemias. 3rd ed. Oxford: Blackwell Scientific Publications, 1990.

Cooper BA, Rosenblatt DS, Whitehead VM. Megaloblastic anemia. In: Hematology of Infancy and Childhood. Philadelphia: WB Saunders, 1993.

Heisel, MA, Siegel SE, Falk RE, et al. Congenital pernicious anemia: report of seven patients with studies of the extended family. J Pediatr 1984;105:564–8.

Lanzkowsky P. The megaloblastic anemias: folate deficiency II. Clinical, pathogenetic and diagnostic considerations in folate deficiency. In: Nathan DG, Oski FA, editors. Hematology of Infancy and Childhood. Philadelphia: WB Saunders, 1987.

Lanzkowsky P. The megaloblastic anemias: vitamin B_{12} (cobalamin) deficiency and other congenital and acquired disorders. Clinical, pathogenetic and diagnostic considerations of vitamin B_{12} (cobalamin) deficiency and other congenital and acquired disorders. In: Nathan DG, Oski FA, editors. Hematology of Infancy and Childhood. Philadelphia: WB Saunders, 1987.

5

HEMATOLOGIC MANIFESTATIONS OF SYSTEMIC ILLNESS

A variety of systemic illnesses including acute and chronic infections, neoplastic diseases, connective tissue disorders, and storage diseases are associated with hematologic manifestations. The hematologic manifestations are the result of the following mechanisms:

1. Bone marrow dysfunction
   a. Anemia or polycythemia
   b. Thrombocytopenia or thrombocytosis
   c. Leukopenia or leukocytosis
2. Hemolysis
3. Immune cytopenias
4. Alterations in hemostasis
   a. Acquired inhibitors to coagulation factors
   b. Acquired von Willebrand disease
   c. Acquired platelet dysfunction
5. Alterations in leukocyte function.

HEMATOLOGIC MANIFESTATIONS OF DISEASES OF VARIOUS ORGANS

Heart

The major hematologic complications of cardiac disease are discussed in the following subsections.

Hemolysis

Hemolysis occurs with prosthetic valves or synthetic patches utilized for correction of cardiac defects (particularly when there is failure of endothelialization). It has the following characteristics:

- Hemolysis is secondary to fragmentation of the red cells as they are damaged against a distorted vascular surface.
- Hemolysis is intravascular and may be associated with hemoglobinemia and hemoglobinuria.

71

- Iron deficiency occurs secondary to the shedding of hemosiderin within renal tubular cells into the urine.
- Thrombocytopenia secondary to platelet adhesion to abnormal surfaces also occurs.
- Autoimmune hemolytic anemia may occasionally occur after cardiac surgery with the placement of foreign material within the vascular system.

Coagulation Abnormalities

- A coagulopathy exists in some patients with cyanotic heart disease. The coagulation abnormalities correlate with the extent of the polycythemia. Hyperviscosity may lead to tissue hypoxemia, which could trigger disseminated intravascular coagulation (DIC).
- Marked derangements in coagulation (such as disseminated intravascular coagulation, thrombocytopenia, thrombosis, and fibrinolysis) can accompany surgery involving cardiopulmonary bypass. Heparinization must be strictly monitored.

Platelet Abnormalities

Quantitative and qualitative platelet abnormalities are associated with cardiac disease:

- Thrombocytopenia occurs secondary to microangiopathic hemolysis associated with prosthetic valves.
- Cyanotic heart disease can produce prolonged bleeding time and abnormal platelet aggregation.

Polycythemia

- The hypoxemia of cyanotic heart disease produces a compensatory elevation in erythropoietin and secondary polycythemia.
- Patients are at increased risk for cerebrovascular accidents secondary to hyperviscosity.

Gastrointestinal Tract

Esophagus

- Iron-deficiency anemia may occur as a manifestation of gastroesophageal reflux.
- Endoscopy may be required in unexplained iron deficiency.

Stomach

- The gastric mucosa is important in both vitamin B_{12} and iron absorption.
- Chronic atrophic gastritis produces iron deficiency. There may be an associated vitamin B_{12} malabsorption.
- Gastric resection may result in iron deficiency or in vitamin B_{12} deficiency due to lack of intrinsic factor.
- Zollinger–Ellison syndrome (increased parietal cell production of hydrochloric acid) may cause iron deficiency through mucosal ulceration.

Small Bowel

- Celiac disease or tropical sprue may cause malabsorption of iron and folate.
- Inflammatory bowel disease may cause iron deficiency from blood loss.

- Eosinophilic gastroenteritis can produce peripheral eosinophilia.
- Diarrheal illnesses of infancy can produce life-threatening methemoglobinemia.

Lower Gastrointestinal Tract

- Ulcerative colitis is often associated with iron-deficiency anemia.
- Peutz–Jeghers syndrome (intestinal polyposis and mucocutaneous pigmentation) predisposes to adenocarcinoma of the colon.
- Hereditary hemorrhagic telangiectasia (Osler–Weber–Rendu disease) may produce iron deficiency, platelet dysfunction, and hemostatic defects.

Pancreas

- Hemorrhagic pancreatitis produces acute normocytic, normochromic anemia. It may also be associated with DIC.
- Shwachman–Diamond syndrome is characterized by congenital exocrine pancreatic insufficiency, metaphyseal bone abnormalities, and neutropenia. There may also be some degree of anemia and thrombocytopenia.
- Cystic fibrosis produces malabsorption of fat-soluble vitamins (e.g., vitamin K) with impaired prothrombin production.
- Pearson syndrome is characterized by exocrine pancreatic insufficiency and severe sideroblastic anemia.

Liver Disease

Anemia

Anemias of diverse etiologies occur in acute and chronic liver disease. Red cells are frequently macrocytic (mean corpuscular volume [MCV] of 100–110 fl). Target cells and acanthocytes (spur cells) are frequently seen. Some of the pathogenetic mechanisms of anemia include:

1. Shortened red cell survival and red cell fragmentation (spur cell anemia) in cirrhosis
2. Hypersplenism with splenic sequestration in the presence of secondary portal hypertension
3. Iron-deficiency anemia secondary to blood loss from esophageal varices in portal hypertension
4. Chronic hemolytic anemia in Wilson's disease secondary to copper accumulation in red cells
5. Aplastic anemia resulting from acute viral hepatitis (particularly hepatitis B) in certain immunologically predisposed hosts
6. Megaloblastic anemia secondary to folate deficiency in malnourished individuals.

Coagulation Abnormalities

The liver is involved in the synthesis of most of the coagulation factors. Liver dysfunction can be associated with either hyper- or hypocoagulable states because both procoagulant and anticoagulant synthesis is impaired.

Factor I (fibrinogen)
Fibrinogen levels are generally normal in liver disease. Low levels may be seen in fulminant acute liver failure.

Factors II, VII, IX, and X (vitamin K–dependent factors)
These factors are reduced in liver disease secondary to impaired synthesis. Factor VII is the most sensitive.

Factor V
Levels generally parallel factors II and X. If there is associated DIC, factor V level is markedly depressed. In cholestatic liver disease, factor V may be markedly elevated as an acute-phase reactant.

Factor VIII
Procoagulant activity is generally normal in liver disease. If there is associated DIC, factor VIII will be markedly depressed.

Plasminogen and antithrombin
Levels are depressed in acute and chronic liver disease. Liver disease results in a hypercoagulable state and may be associated with an increased incidence of DIC.

α_2-Macroglobulin and plasmin
Inhibitor of thrombin α_2-macroglobulin and plasmin is elevated in cirrhosis. Tests for coagulation disturbances prothrombin time (PT) is the most convenient test for monitoring liver function.

Kidneys

Renal disease may affect red cells, white cells, platelets, and coagulation. Severe renal disease with renal insufficiency is frequently associated with chronic anemia (and sometimes pancytopenia). This type of anemia is characterized by:

1. Hemoglobin as low as 4–5 g/dL
2. Normochromic and normocytic red cell morphology unless there is associated microangiopathic hemolytic anemia (as in the hemolytic uremic syndrome), in which case schistocytes and thrombocytopenia are seen
3. Low reticulocyte count
4. Decreased erythroid precursors in bone marrow aspirate.

The following mechanisms are involved in the pathogenesis of this type of anemia:

1. Erythropoietin deficiency is the most important factor (90% of erythropoietin synthesis occurs in the kidney).
2. Shortened red cell survival is secondary to uremic toxins or in hemolytic uremic syndrome (HUS) secondary to microangiopathic hemolysis.
3. Uremia itself inhibits erythropoiesis and in conjunction with decreased erythropoietin levels produces a hypoplastic marrow.
4. Increased blood loss from a hemorrhagic uremic state and into a hemodialysis circuit causes iron deficiency.
5. Dialysis can lead to folic acid deficiency.

Treatment

1. Recombinant human erythropoietin (rHuEPO)*:
   a. Determine the baseline serum erythropoietin and ferritin levels prior to starting rHuEPO therapy. If ferritin is less than 100 ng/mL, give ferrous sulfate 6 mg/kg/day aimed at maintaining a serum ferritin level above 100 ng/mL and a threshold transferrin saturation of 20%.
   b. Start with rHuEPO treatment in a dose of 150 units/kg/day SC three times a week.
   c. Monitor blood pressure closely (increased viscosity produces hypertension in 30% of cases) and perform complete blood count (CBC) weekly.

---

*Thrombosis of vascular access occurs in 10% of cases treated with rHuEPO.

    d. Titrate the dose:
       (1) If no response, increase rHuEPO to 300 units/kg/day SC three times a week.
       (2) If hematocrit (Hct) reaches 40%, stop rHuEPO until Hct is 36% and then restart at 25% dose.
       (3) If Hct increases very rapidly (>4% in 2 weeks), reduce dose by 25%. The potential benefits of rHuEPO are listed in Table 5-1.
2. Folic acid 1 mg/day is recommended because folate is dialyzable.
3. Packed red cell transfusion is rarely required.

Endocrine Glands

Thyroid

Anemia is frequently present in hypothyroidism. It is usually normochromic and normocytic. The anemia is sometimes hypochromic because of associated iron deficiency, and occasionally macrocytic because of vitamin B_{12} deficiency. The bone marrow is usually fatty and hypocellular, and erythropoiesis is usually normoblastic. The finding of a macrocytic anemia and megaloblastic marrow in children with hypothyroidism should raise the possibility of an autoimmune disease with antibodies against parietal cells as well as against the thyroid, leading to vitamin B_{12} deficiency (juvenile pernicious anemia with polyendocrinopathies).

Adrenal Glands

- Androgens stimulate erythropoiesis.
- Conditions of androgen excess such as Cushing syndrome and congenital adrenal hyperplasia can produce secondary polycythemia.
- In Addison disease, some degree of anemia is also present but may be masked by coexisting hemoconcentration. The association between Addison disease and megaloblastic anemia raises the possibility of an inherited autoimmune disease directed against multiple tissues, including parietal cells (juvenile pernicious anemia with polyendocrinopathies).

Lungs

- Hypoxia secondary to pulmonary disease results in secondary polycythemia.
- Idiopathic pulmonary hemosiderosis is a chronic disease characterized by recurrent intra-alveolar microhemorrhages with pulmonary dysfunction, hemoptysis,

Table 5-1. Potential Benefits of Recombinant Human Erythropoietin in Children with Renal Disease

1. Elimination of transfusion dependency, including:
   Decreased risks of transfusion
   Elimination of chronic iron overload
   Reduced sensitization to histocompatibility locus antigen (HLA)—easier to transplant
2. Increased energy and activity levels
3. Better appetite, resulting in better nutrition (dietary potassium and phosphate restrictions must be observed)
4. Improved growth
5. Improved cognition
6. Healthier psychosocial development
7. Improved cardiac function

and hemosiderin-laden macrophages, resulting in iron-deficiency anemia. A precise diagnosis can be established by the presence of siderophages in the gastric aspirate. A lung biopsy may be necessary.

Treatment is controversial and may involve:

- Corticosteroids
- Withdrawal of cow's milk
- Packed red cell transfusions when indicated.

Skin

Mast Cell Disease

Mast cell disease or mastocytosis is associated with abnormal accumulation of mastocytes (closely related to monocytes or macrophages rather than to basophils) that occur in the dermis (cutaneous mastocytosis) or in internal organs (systemic mastocytosis). The systemic form is rare in children. In children, this condition is more common under 2 years of age. It usually presents either as a solitary cutaneous mastocytoma or, more commonly, as urticaria pigmentosa. Involvement beyond the skin is unusual in children; bone lesions are the most common, but bone marrow involvement is rare.

Eczema and Psoriasis

Patients with extensive eczema and psoriasis commonly have a mild anemia. The anemia is usually normochromic and normocytic (anemia of chronic disease).

Dermatitis Herpetiformis

- Macrocytic anemia secondary to malabsorption
- Hyposplenism: Howell–Jolly bodies maybe present on blood smear.

Dyskeratosis Congenita

This disease is characterized by ectodermal dysplasia and aplastic anemia (also see pages 112–114). The aplastic anemia is associated with high MCV, thrombocytopenia, and elevated fetal hemoglobin. This may occur before the onset of the skin manifestations.

Hereditary Hemorrhagic Telangiectasia

This autosomal dominant disorder is associated with bleeding disorder. Easy bruisability, epistaxis, and respiratory and gastrointestinal bleeding may be caused by telangiectatic lesions.

Ehlers–Danlos syndrome
This condition may be associated with platelet dysfunction: reduced aggregation with ADP, epinephrine, and collagen. An unusual sensitivity to aspirin is described in type IV syndrome (see page 291).

CHRONIC ILLNESS

Chronic illnesses such as cancer, connective tissue disease, and chronic infection are associated with anemia. The anemia has the following characteristics:

- Normochromic, normocytic, occasionally microcytic
- Usually mild, characterized by decreased plasma iron and normal or increased reticuloendothelial iron
- Impaired flow of iron from reticuloendothelial cells to the bone marrow
- Decreased sideroblasts in the bone marrow.

Treatment involves treating the underlying illness. Iron is of little value because the iron is cleared by the reticuloendothelial system.

Connective Tissue Diseases

Rheumatoid Arthritis

- Anemia of chronic illness (normocytic, normochromic)
- High incidence of iron deficiency
- Leukocytosis and neutropenia common in exacerbations of juvenile rheumatoid arthritis (JRA)
- Thrombocytosis associated with a high level of interleukin 6 (IL-6) occurs in many patients, although there may be transient episodes of thrombocytopenia

Felty's Syndrome

- Triad of rheumatoid arthritis, splenomegaly, and neutropenia
- Granulocyte colony-stimulating factor (G-CSF) is effective treatment in some cases

Systemic Lupus Erythematosus

- Two types of anemia are common: anemia of chronic illness (normocytic, normochromic) and acquired autoimmune hemolytic anemia (Coombs' positive).
- Neutropenia is common as a result of decreased marrow production and immune mediated destruction.
- Lymphopenia with abnormalities of T-cell function occurs.
- Immune thrombocytopenia occurs.
- A circulating anticoagulant (antiphospholipid antibody) may be present and is associated with thrombosis.

Polyarteritis Nodosa

- Microangiopathic hemolytic anemia, possibly associated with renal disease or hypertensive crises
- Prominent eosinophilia.

Wegener Granulomatosis

This autoimmune disorder is rare in children. Hematologic features include:

- Anemia: normocytic; RBC fragmentation with microangiopathic hemolytic anemia
- Leukocytosis with neutrophilia
- Eosinophilia
- Thrombocytosis.

Kawasaki Syndrome

- Mild normochromic, normocytic anemia with reticulocytopenia
- Leukocytosis with neutrophilia and toxic granulation of neutrophils and vacuoles

- Decreased T-suppressor cells
- High C_3 levels
- Increased cytokines IL-1, IL-6, IL-8, interferon-α, and tumor necrosis factor (TNF)
- Marked thrombocytosis (mean platelet count of 700,000/mm^3)
- DIC.

Henoch–Schönlein Purpura

Henoch–Schönlein purpura (HSP) is called anaphylactoid purpura, which is associated with systemic vasculitis characterized by unique purpuric lesions, transient arthralgias or arthritis (especially affecting knees and ankles), colicky abdominal pain, and nephritis (see page 293).

- Anemia occasionally occurs as a result of GI bleeding or decreased RBC production caused by renal failure.
- Transient decreased F XIII activity may occur.
- Vitamin K deficiency from severe vasculitis-induced intestinal malabsorption has been reported.

Infections

Anemia

- Chronic infection is associated with the anemia of chronic illness.
- Acute infection, particularly viral infection, can produce transient bone marrow aplasia or selective transient erythrocytopenia.
- Parvovirus B19 infection in people with an underlying hemolytic disorder (such as sickle cell disease, hereditary spherocytosis) can produce a rapid fall in hemoglobin and an erythroblastopenic crisis marked by anemia and reticulocytopenia. There may be an associated neutropenia.
- Many viral and bacterial illnesses may be associated with hemolysis.

White Cell Alterations

- Viral infections can produce leukopenia and neutropenia. Neutrophilia with an increased band count and left shift frequently results from bacterial infection.
- Neonates, particularly premature infants, may not develop an increase in white cell count in response to infection.
- Eosinophilia may develop in response to parasitic infections.

Clotting Abnormalities

Severe infections, for example, gram-negative sepsis, can produce DIC.

Thrombocytopenia

Infection can produce thrombocytopenia through decreased marrow production, immune destruction, or DIC.

Viral and Bacterial Illnesses Associated with Marked Hematologic Sequelae

Parvovirus

Parvovirus B19 has a peculiar predilection for rapidly growing cells, particularly red cell precursors in the bone marrow. It has a preference for the red cell precursors because it uses P antigen as a receptor. This viral infection is associated with a transient erythroblastopenic crisis, particularly in individuals with an underlying hemolytic disorder. In addition, it can produce thrombocytopenia, neutropenia, and a hemophagocytic syndrome. In immunocompromised individuals, parvovirus B19 infection can produce prolonged aplasia.

Epstein–Barr Virus

Epstein–Barr virus (EBV) infection is associated with the following hematologic manifestations:

- Atypical lymphocytosis
- Acquired immune hemolytic anemia
- Agranulocytosis
- Aplastic anemia
- Lymphadenopathy and splenomegaly
- Immune thrombocytopenia.

EBV infection also has immunologic and oncologic associations (see Chapter 13):

- X-linked lymphoproliferative syndrome associated with fatal EBV infection, acquired hypogammaglobulinemia, and lymphoma
- Clonal T-cell proliferations
- Hemophagocytic syndrome
- Endemic form of Burkitt's lymphoma in Africa.

Human Immunodeficiency Virus

The main pathophysiology of human immunodeficiency virus (HIV) infection is a constant decline in CD4+ lymphocytes, leading to immune collapse and death. The other bone marrow cell lines also decline in concert with CD4+ cell numbers as HIV disease (acquired immunodeficiency syndrome [AIDS]) progresses.

HIV infection has the hematologic manifestations discussed next.

Thrombocytopenia

Thrombocytopenia occurs in about 40% of patients with AIDS. Initially, the clinical findings resemble those of immune thrombocytopenic purpura (ITP). Some degree of splenomegaly is common and the platelet-associated antibodies are often in the form of immune complexes that may contain antibodies with anti-HIV specificity. Megakaryocytes are normal or increased, and production of platelets is reduced in the bone marrow. Thrombotic thrombocytopenic purpura (TTP) is also associated with HIV disease. This occurs in advanced AIDS.

Anemia and Neutropenia

HIV-infected individuals develop progressive cytopenia as immunosuppression advances. Anemia occurs in approximately 70–80% of patients and neutropenia in 50%. Cytopenias in advanced HIV disease are often of complex etiology and include the following:

- A production defect appears to be most common.
- Antibody and immune complexes associated with red and white cell surfaces may contribute. Up to 40% have erythrocyte-associated antibodies. Specific antibodies against i and U antigens have occasionally been noted. About 70% of patients with AIDS have neutrophil-associated antibodies.

The pathogenesis of the hematologic disorders includes:

- *Infections:* Myelosuppression is frequently caused by involvement of the bone marrow by infecting organisms (e.g., mycobacteria, cytomegalovirus [CMV], parvovirus, fungi, and, rarely, *Pneumocystis carinii*).
- *Neoplasms:* Non-Hodgkin lymphoma (NHL) in AIDS patients is associated with infiltration of the bone marrow in up to 30% of cases. It is particularly prominent in the small noncleaved histologic subtype of NHL.
- *Medications:* Widely used antiviral agents in AIDS patients are myelotoxic; for example, zidovudine (AZT) causes anemia in approximately 29% of patients. Ganciclovir and trimethoprim/sulfamethoxazole or pyrimethamine/sulfadiazine cause neutropenia. In general, bone marrow suppression is related to the dosage and to the stage of HIV disease. Importantly, the other nucleoside analogues of anti-HIV compounds (dideoxycytidine [ddC], dideoxyinosine [ddI], stavudine [d4T], or lamivudine [3TC]) are usually not associated with significant myelotoxicity.
- *Nutrition:* Poor intake is common in advanced HIV disease and is occasionally accompanied by poor absorption. Vitamin B_{12} levels may be significantly decreased in HIV infection although vitamin B_{12} is not effective in treatment. The reduction in serum vitamin B_{12} levels is due to vitamin B_{12} malabsorption and abnormalities in vitamin B_{12}–binding proteins.

Coagulation Abnormalities

The following abnormalities occur:

- Dysregulation of immunoglobulin production may affect the coagulation cascade. The dysregulation of immunoglobulin production may also occasionally result in beneficial effects, as in the resolution of anti–factor VIII antibodies in HIV-infected hemophiliacs.
- Lupus-like anticoagulant (antiphospholipid antibodies) or anticardiolipin antibodies occur in 82% of patients. This is not associated with thrombosis in AIDS patients.
- Thrombosis may occur secondary to protein S deficiency. Low levels of protein S occur in 73% of patients.

Role of Hematopoietic Growth Factors in AIDS

- rHuEPO results in a significant improvement in hematocrit and reduces transfusion requirements while the patient is receiving zidovudine. rHuEPO therapy should be initiated if the erythropoietin threshold is less than 500 IU/L.
- G-CSF in a dose of 5 µg/kg/day SC is the most widely used growth factor in neutropenia.
- Granulocytic-macrophage colony-stimulating factor (GM-CSF) improves neutrophil counts in drug-induced neutropenia. The effects of GM-CSF are seen within 24–48 hours with relatively low doses of GM-CSF (250 µg/m² 3 × week).
- Interleukin-3 (IL-3) given in doses of 0.5–5 mg/kg/day increases neutrophil counts.

Cancers in Children with HIV Infection

Malignancies in children with HIV infection are not as common as those in adults. Table 5-2 lists AIDS-related neoplasms in adults, and Table 5-3 lists AIDS-related neoplasms in children with HIV infection in the order of frequency.

Table 5-2. AIDS-Related Neoplasms in Adults

Kaposi sarcoma
Non-Hodgkin lymphoma
Anogenital cancers
Cervical cancer
   Epithelioid anal cancer
Hodgkin disease
Leiomyosarcoma
Testicular tumors
Conjunctival tumors
Melanoma
Renal tumors
Skin cancer
   Basal cell carcinoma
   Squamous cell carcinoma
Lung cancer
   Adenocarcinoma

Table 5-3. AIDS-Related Neoplasms in Children

Non-Hodgkin lymphoma
   Burkitt lymphoma (B-cell, small noncleaved)
   Immunoblastic lymphoma (B-cell, large cell)
   Central nervous system lymphomas
   Mucosa-associated lymphoid tissue (MALT) type
Leiomyosarcoma and leiomyoma
Kaposi's sarcoma
Leukemias

Non-Hodgkin lymphoma (NHL)

NHL is the most common malignancy secondary to HIV infection in children. It is usually of B-cell origin as in Burkitt (small noncleaved cell) or immunoblastic (large cell) NHL. The mean age of presentation of malignancy in congenitally transmitted disease is 35 months, with a range of 6–62 months. In transfusion-transmitted disease, the latency from the time of HIV seroconversion to the onset of lymphoma is 22–88 months. The CD4 lymphocyte count is less than $50/\text{mm}^3$ at the time of diagnosis of the malignancy.

The presenting manifestations include:

- Fever
- Weight loss
- Extranodal manifestations (e.g., hepatomegaly, jaundice, abdominal distention, bone marrow involvement, or central nervous system [CNS] symptoms).

Some patients will already have had lymphoproliferative diseases such as lymphocytic interstitial pneumonitis or pulmonary lymphoid hyperplasia. These children usually have advanced (stage III or IV) disease at the time of presentation.

Central nervous system lymphomas

Children with CNS lymphomas present with developmental delays or loss of developmental milestones and encephalopathy (dementia, cranial nerve palsies, seizures, or hemiparesis).

The differential diagnosis includes infections such as toxoplasmosis, cryptococcosis, or tuberculosis. Contrast-enhanced computed tomography (CT) studies of the brain show hyperdense mass lesions that are usually multicentric or periventricular. CNS lymphomas in AIDS are fast growing and often have central necrosis and a "rim of enhancement" as in an infectious lesion. A stereotactic biopsy will give a definitive diagnosis.

Treatment of HIV infection–related lymphomas. Treatment consists of standard protocols as described in Chapter 16 on non-Hodgkin lymphoma. Treatment of CNS lymphomas is more difficult. Intrathecal therapy is indicated even for those without evidence of meningeal or mass lesions at diagnosis of NHL. Radiation therapy may be a helpful adjunct for CNS involvement.

The following are more favorable prognostic features in NHL secondary to AIDS:

- CD4 lymphocyte count greater than $100/mm^3$
- Normal serum LDH level
- No prior AIDS-related symptoms
- Good Karnofsky score (80–100).

Proliferative lesions of mucosa-associated lymphoid tissue

Mucosa-associated lymphoid tissue (MALT) shows reactive lymphoid follicles with prominent marginal zones containing centrocyte-like cells, lymphocytic infiltration of the epithelium (lymphoepithelial lesion), and the presence of plasma cells under the surface epithelium. These lesions may be associated with the mucosa of the gastrointestinal tract, Waldeyer ring, salivary glands, respiratory tract, thyroid, and thymus. Proliferative lesions of MALT can be benign or malignant (such as lymphomas).

The proliferative lesions arising from MALT form a spectrum or a continuum extending from reactive to neoplastic lesions. The neoplastic lesions are usually low grade but may progress into high-grade MALT lymphomas (Table 5-4). MALT lymphomas characteristically remain localized, but if dissemination occurs, they are usually confined to the regional lymph nodes and other MALT sites. MALT lesions represent a category of pediatric HIV-associated disease that may arise from a combination of viral etiologies, including HIV, EBV, and CMV.

Treatment of low-grade MALT lymphoma involves:

- *α-Interferon:* 1,000,000 units/m^2 SC three times a week; continue until regression of disease or severe toxicity occurs.
- *Rituxan (monoclonal antibody-anti-CD20):* 375 mg/m^2 IV weekly for 4 weeks; courses may be repeated as clinically indicated.

Table 5-4. Spectrum of Systemic Lymphoproliferation in Children with AIDS

Follicular hyperplasia (lymph nodes, gastrointestinal tract)
Lymphoid follicles/nodular (liver, thymus)
Thymitis and multilocular thymic cyst PLH/LIP complex, typical and atypical
Polyclonal polymorphic B-cell lymphoproliferative disorder
Myoepithelial sialoadenitis
Myoepithelial sialoadenitis with lymphoma
MALT lymphoma (involving lungs, tonsils, and salivary glands)
Non-MALT lymphoma (involving nodal and extranodal sites)

Abbreviations: PLH/LIP, pulmonary lymphoid hyperplasia/lymphoid interstitial pneumonitis; MALT, mucosa-associated lymphoid tissue.

From McClain KL, Joshi VV. Cancer in children with HIV infection. Hematol Oncol Clin North Am 1996;10:1189, with permission.

Some patients may not require any treatment because of the indolent nature of the disease.

Leiomyosarcomas and leiomyomas
Malignant or benign smooth muscle tumors, leiomyosarcoma (LS) and leiomyoma (LM), are the second most common type of tumor in children with HIV infection. The incidence in HIV patients is 4.8% (in non-HIV children, it is 2 per million). The most common sites of presentation are the lungs, spleen, and gastrointestinal tract. Patients with endobronchial LM or LS often have multiple nodules in the pulmonary parenchyma. Bloody diarrhea, abdominal pain, or signs of obstruction may signal intraluminal bowel lesions. These tumors are clearly associated with EBV infection. *In situ* hybridization and quantitative polymerase chain reaction studies of LM and LS demonstrated that high copy numbers of EBV are present in every tumor cell. The EBV receptor (CD21/C3d) is present on tumor tissue at very high concentrations, but is present at lower concentrations in normal smooth muscle or control leiomyomas/leiomyosarcomas that had no EBV DNA in them. In AIDS patients, the EBV receptor may be unregulated, allowing EBV to enter the muscle cells and cause their transformation.

Treatment involves:

- Chemotherapy, including doxorubicin or α-interferon
- Radiotherapy
- Complete surgical resection prior to chemotherapy, where feasible.

Despite surgery and chemotherapy, the disease tends to recur.

Kaposi sarcoma
Kaposi sarcoma (KS) is rare in children and constitutes the third most common malignancy in pediatric AIDS patients; it occurs in 25% of adults with AIDS. KS occurs only in those HIV-infected children who were born to mothers with HIV. The lymphadenopathic form of KS is seen mostly in Haitian and African children and may represent the epidemic form of KS unrelated to AIDS. The cutaneous form is a true indicator of the disease related to AIDS. Visceral involvement has not been pathologically documented in children with AIDS.

Leukemias
Almost all leukemias are of B-cell origin. They represent the fourth most common malignancy in children with AIDS. The clinical presentation and biologic features are similar to those found in non-HIV children.

Treatment involves chemotherapy designed for B-cell leukemias and lymphomas.

Miscellaneous tumors
There is no increase of Hodgkin disease in children with AIDS as compared to adult patients. Children with AIDS rarely develop hepatoblastoma, embryonal rhabdomyosarcoma, fibrosarcoma, and papillary carcinoma of the thyroid. The occurrence of these tumors is probably unrelated to the HIV infection.

Torch Infections

This is a group of congenital infections including toxoplasma, rubella, CMV, herpes simplex virus (HSV), and syphilis. They can all cause neonatal anemia, jaundice, thrombocytopenia, and hepatosplenomegaly.

Bordetella **Pertussis**

This organism causes pertussis (whooping cough). It is invariably associated with marked lymphocytosis (>25,000/mm^3) in early stages of infection.

Acute Infectious Lymphocytosis

Acute infectious lymphocytosis is caused by a coxsackievirus and is a rare benign, self-limiting childhood condition. It is associated with a low-grade fever, diarrhea, and marked lymphocytosis (50,000/mm^3). Lymphocytes are mainly CD4 T cells. The condition resolves in 2–3 weeks without treatment (page 242).

Bartonellosis

Bartonellosis is caused by a gram-negative bacillus *Bartonella bacilliformis* confined to the mountain valleys of the Andes. The vector is a local sand fly. Infection from this organism causes a fatal syndrome of severe hemolytic anemia with fever (Oroya fever). Another species of *Bartonella, B. henselae,* causes "cat scratch fever." It is associated with a regional (following a scratch by a cat) lymphadenitis. Thrombocytopenia may occur in this condition.

Tuberculosis

Tuberculosis is caused by *Mycobacterium tuberculosis*. Hematologic manifestations include leukemoid reaction mimicking CML, monocytosis, and rarely pancytopenia.

Leptospirosis (Weil Disease)

This disease is caused by *Leptospira icterohaemorrhagiae*. A coagulopathy occurs that is complex and can be corrected with vitamin K administration. Thrombocytopenia commonly occurs but DIC is rare.

Parasitic Illnesses Associated with Marked Hematologic Sequelae

Malaria

Acute infections cause anemia which is multifactorial:

- Intracellular parasite metabolism alters negative charges on the RBC membrane, which causes altered permeability with increased osmotic fragility. Spleen removes the damaged RBC or the parasites are "pitted" during the passage from the spleen, which results in microspherocytes of RBC.
- Autoimmune hemolytic anemia may also occur. An IgG antibody is formed against the parasite and resulting immune complex attaches nonspecifically to RBC, complement is activated, and cell destruction occurs. Positive Coombs' test due to IgG is found in 50% of patients with *P. falsiparum* malaria.
- Thrombocytopenia without DIC is common. IgG antimalarial antibody bonds to the platelet-bound malaria antigen, and the IgG platelet parasite complex is removed by the reticulo-endothelial (R-E) system.

Babesiosis

Babesiosis is caused by several species from the genus *Babesia* that colonize erythrocytes. It is a zoonotic disease transmitted by the Ixodes tick. The clinical features are similar to those of malaria and include fever, myalgia, and arthralgia with hepatosplenomegaly and hemolysis.

Leishmaniasis

The protozoal species *Leishmania* causes progressive splenomegaly and pancytopenia (anemia, neutropenia, and thrombocytopenia). The bone marrow usually is hypercellular with hemophagocytosis. Some children may show coagulopathy.

Hookworm

Worldwide hookworm is a major cause of anemia. Two species infest humans:

- *Ancylostoma duodenale* is found in the Mediterranean region, in North Africa, and on the west coast of South America.
- *Necator americanus* is found in most of Africa, Southeast Asia, the Pacific islands, and Australia.

Hookworms penetrate exposed skin, usually the soles of bare feet, and migrate through the circulation to the right side of the heart, then lungs (causing hypereosinophilic syndrome), and through the airway down to the esophagus. They mature in the small intestine and attach their mouth parts to the mucosa. They suck blood with each adult *A. duodenale* consuming about 0.2 mg/day. Heavily infested children may present with profound iron-deficiency anemia, hypoproteinemia, and marked eosinophilia.

Tapeworm

Diphyllobothrium latum is a fish tapeworm. It is acquired by eating uncooked freshwater fish. This worm infestation in the intestine results in vitamin B_{12} deficiency.

Trypanosomiasis

A diagnosis of trypanosomiasis can be made by finding trypanosomes in a blood and bone marrow smear.

LEAD INTOXICATION

One of the most striking hematologic features of lead intoxication is basophilic stippling of RBC (coarse basophilia). It is caused by precipitation of denatured mitochondria secondary to inhibition of pyrimidine-5'-nucleotidase. Lead also produces ring sideroblast in the marrow and is associated with hypochromic microcytic anemia and markedly elevated free erythrocyte protoporphyrin levels.

NUTRITIONAL DISORDERS

Protein-Calorie Malnutrition

Protein deficiency in the presence of adequate carbohydrate caloric intake (kwashiorkor) is associated with mild normochromic, normocytic anemia secondary to reduced RBC production despite normal or increased erythropoietin levels as well as reduced red cell survival. Protein calorie malnutrition is also associated with impaired leukocyte function.

Scurvy

With scurvy, mild anemia is common. There is a bleeding tendency due to loss of vascular integrity, which may result in petechiae or subperiosteal, orbital, or subdural hemorrhages. Hematuria and melena may occur.

Anorexia Nervosa

Anorexia nervosa produces the following hematologic changes in more advanced stages:

- Gelatinous changes of bone marrow, which may become severely hypoplastic
- Mild anemia (macrocytic), neutropenia, and thrombocytopenia
- Predisposition of infection associated with neutropenia
- Irregularly contracted red cells are seen (as in hypothyroidism) secondary to a disturbance in the composition of membrane lipids.

BONE MARROW INFILTRATION

The bone marrow may be infiltrated by nonneoplastic disease (storage disease) or neoplastic disease. In storage disease, a diagnosis is established on the basis of the clinical picture, enzyme assays of white cells or cultured fibroblasts, and bone marrow aspiration revealing the characteristic cells of the disorder. Neoplastic disease may arise *de novo* in the marrow (leukemias) or invade the marrow as metastases from solid tumors (neuroblastoma or rhabdomyosarcoma). Table 5-5 lists the diseases that may infiltrate the marrow.

Gaucher Disease

Gaucher disease is the most common lysosomal storage disease, resulting from deficient activity of β-glucocerebrosidase. It is inherited in an autosomal recessive manner. More than 100 mutations are now known to cause Gaucher disease in the glucocerebrosidase gene. The degree of clinical involvement differs greatly in individual patients, even those with the same genotype and those affected within the same family.

Pathogenesis

Glucocerebrosidase is necessary for the catabolism of glucocerebroside. Deficiency of glucocerebrosidase leads to accumulation of glucocerebroside in the lysosomes of macrophages in tissues of the reticuloendothelial system. Figure 5-1 shows a diagram of the cellular pathophysiology of Gaucher disease. Accumulation in splenic macrophages and in the Kupffer cells of the liver produces hepatosplenomegaly.

Table 5-5. Diseases Invading Bone Marrow

I. Nonneoplastic
   A. Storage diseases
      1. Gaucher disease
      2. Niemann–Pick disease
      3. Cystine storage disease
   B. Marble bone disease (osteopetrosis)
   C. Langerhans cell histiocytosis (Chapter 22)

II. Neoplastic
   A. Primary
      1. Leukemia (Chapter 14)
   B. Secondary
      1. Neuroblastoma (Chapter 18)
      2. Non-Hodgkin lymphoma (Chapter 16)
      3. Hodgkin lymphoma (Chapter 15)
      4. Wilms' tumor (rarely) (Chapter 19)
      5. Retinoblastoma (Chapter 23)
      6. Rhabdomyosarcoma (Chapter 20)

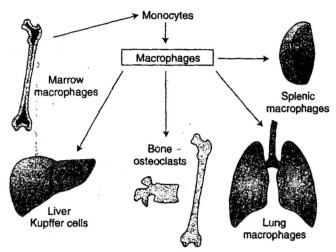

Fig. 5-1. Diagram of the cellular pathophysiology of Gaucher disease. Monocytes are produced in the bone marrow and mature to macrophages in the marrow or in specific sites of distribution as liver Kupffer cells, bone osteoclasts, and lung and tissue macrophages. Once resident, they accumulate glucosylceramide by phagocytosis and become end-stage Gaucher cells. (From Grabowski GA, Leslie N. Lysosomal storage diseases: Perspectives and principles. In: Hoffmann R, Benz EJ, Shattil SJ, Furie B, Cohen HJ, Silberstein LE, McGlave P, editors. Hematology Basic Principles and Practice. 3rd ed. Philadelphia: Lippincott-Raven, 2000, with permission.)

Hypersplenism produces anemia and thrombocytopenia. Glucocerebroside accumulation in the bone marrow results in osteopenia, lytic lesions, pathologic fractures, chronic bone pain, bone infarcts, osteonecrosis, and acute excruciating bone crises.

Gaucher disease is classified into three types based on the presence and degree of neuronal involvement. Table 5-6 outlines the clinical manifestations of the three types of Gaucher disease.

Patients with Type 1 Gaucher disease present with:

- Hepatosplenomegaly (rarely, portal hypertension develops)
- Pancytopenia secondary to hypersplenism and rarely from infiltration of the bone marrow with Gaucher cells
- Bone pain, osteoporosis, pathologic fractures, and bone crises
- Growth delay (Fifty percent of the symptomatic children are at or below the third percentile for height, and another 25% are shorter than expected based on their midparental height.)
- Typical foamy cells in the bone marrow
- Erlenmeyer flask deformity of the distal femora on radiographs
- Decreased glucocerebrosidase activity of white cells
- Characteristic mutations of the glucocerebrosidase gene on chromosome 1 on DNA analysis.

Diagnosis

Glucocerebrosidase assay on leukocytes or cultured skin fibroblasts is the most efficient method of diagnosis. The typical child with type 1 Gaucher's disease will have enzyme activity that is 10–30% of normal.

Further Evaluation

- DNA evaluation for glucocerebrosidase gene abnormalities in patient, parents, and siblings
- Complete blood count

Table 5-6. Clinical Classification of Gaucher Disease

Clinical features	Type 1	Type 2	Type 3a	Type 3b	Type 3c
Onset	Childhood/ adulthood	Infancy	Childhood	Childhood	Childhood
Hepatosplenomegaly	+ to +++	+	+++	+++	+
Hypersplenism	+ to +++	+	+++	+++	+
Bone crises/fractures	+ to +++	—	++	+++	+
Neurodegenerative course	—	+++	++	+	+
Survival	6–80+ years	<2 years	2nd to 4th decade	2nd to 4th decade	2nd to 4th decade
Ethnic predilection	Ashkenazi Jewish	Panethnic	Northern Swedish	Panethnic	Panethnic

Note + to +++; occasionally present to commonly present; – not present

- Serum chemistry with liver function tests
- Acid phosphatase level
- Angiotensin-converting enzyme
- Chitotriosidase
- Liver/spleen volume with magnetic resonance imaging (MRI) or CT radiographs of femora and lateral spine
- MRI of femora
- Bone density of the spine and hips (DEXA)
- Chest radiograph.

Treatment

Enzyme replacement therapy is recommended for the treatment of symptomatic type 1 patients. Recombinant human macrophage-targeted human glucocerebrosidase (imiglucerase, Cerezyme, manufactured by Genzyme, Cambridge, MA) is used for enzyme replacement therapy. The initial dose is 30–60 units/kg IV every 2 weeks. The initial dose must be individualized for each patient based on disease severity and rate of progression. Maintenance dose is 15–60 units/kg IV every 2 weeks. Children who require treatment need to continue therapy indefinitely to maintain their clinical improvement. Prolonged periods off therapy are not appropriate.

Recommendations for monitoring of children with type 1 Gaucher disease receiving and not receiving enzyme replacement therapy are outlined in Table 5-7.

Iron therapy in Gaucher disease patients with anemia is not recommended because Gaucher cells avidly take up iron, which leads to hemochromatosis and decreased iron availability for erythropoiesis.

Response to therapy

The earliest response is an improvement in hematologic parameters. A progressive decrease in liver/spleen size is regarded as a positive response. Skeletal response occurs more slowly (after 2–4 years), along with a decrease in pain and bone crises.

Approximately 5% of patients develop hypersensitivity to enzyme replacement therapy. These reactions respond to interruption of infusion and administration of antihistamine and glucocorticoids. Subsequent reactions can usually be prevented by reducing the initial rate of infusion, so that no more than 10 units/min are administered. These reactions commonly occur during the first 12 months of treatment. For this reason, the first year of treatment should be administered under the direct supervision of a physician. Following 1 year, therapy can be administered at home by

Table 5-7. Recommendations for Monitoring Children with Type 1 Gaucher Disease (Minimal Evaluations Only)

	All patients, baseline	Patients not receiving enzyme therapy		Patients receiving enzyme therapy		
		Every 12 months	Every 12–24 months	Every 3 mo[a]	Every 12 mo[a]	At time of dose change
Hematologic						
Hemoglobin	X	X		X		X
Platelet count	X	X		X		X
Acid phosphatase (total, non-prostatic), Angiotensin converting enzyme, chitotriosidasc[b]	X	X		X		X
Visceral[c]						
Spleen volume (volumetric MRI or CT)	X		X		X	X
Liver volume (volumetric MRI or CT)	X		X		X	X
Skeletal[d]						
MRI (coronal; T1- and T2-weighted) of entire femora[e]	X		X		X	X
Radiograph: AP view of entire femora[e] and lateral view of spine	X		X		X	X
Bone density (DEXA): spine and hips	X		X		Every 12–24 mo	
Quality of life[f]						
Patient reported functional health and well-being	X	X			X	

Abbreviation: DEXA, dual energy x-ray absorptiometry.

[a]For patients who have reached clinical goals and for whom there has been no change in dose, the frequency of monitoring can be decreased to every 12–24 months.

[b]One or more of these markers should be consistently monitored (at least once every 12 months) in conjunction with other clinical assessments of disease activity and response to treatment. Of the three currently recommended biochemical markers, chitotriosidasc activity, when available as a validated procedure from an experienced laboratory, may be the most sensitive indicator of changing disease activity, and is therefore preferred.

[c]Obtain contiguous transaxial 10-mm-thick sections for sum of region of interest.

[d]Additional skeletal assessments that are optional include bone age for patients ≤14 years old. Follow-up is recommended if baseline is abnormal.

[e]Optimally, obtain hips to below knees. As an alternative, obtain hips to distal femur.

[f]Ideally, quality of life should be assessed every 6 months using a standard and valid instrument.

From Charrow J, Anderson HC, Kaplan P, et al. Enzyme replacement therapy and monitoring for children with Type 1 Gaucher disease: Consensus recommendations. J Pediatr 2004;144:112–20, with permission.

home nursing services. The nonneutralizing IgG antibodies that develop in up to 13% of patients are not clinically relevant.

Niemann–Pick Disease

Niemann–Pick disease types A and B result from deficient activity of acid sphingomyelinase, encoded by a gene on chromosome 11. The defect results in accumulation of sphingomyelin in the monocyte-macrophage system. The progressive deposition of sphingomyelin in the central nervous system leads to type A, and in nonneuronal tissues leads to type B. Type C is a neuropathic form that results from the defective cholesterol transport.

Clinical Manifestations

Depending on the type, Niemann–Pick disease has classic signs, including:

- Hepatosplenomegaly
- Cherry red spot in macula
- Psychomotor deterioration
- Reticular pulmonary infiltrates
- Foamy cells in the bone marrow

Table 5-8 lists the clinical features of the different types of Niemann–Pick disease.

Diagnosis

Diagnosis involves examining leukocytes or cultured fibroblasts to determine sphingomyelinase activity.

Table 5-8. Classification of Niemann–Pick Disease

	Type		
	A (acute infantile with CNS involvement)	B (chronic visceral)	C/D (chronic neuropathic)
Age of presentation	3–6 months	Infancy/childhood	Infancy to early adulthood
Inheritance	Autosomal recessive	Autosomal recessive	Autosomal recessive
Ethnicity	Mainly Ashkenazi Jews	Panethnic	Nova Scotia (D)
Neurologic symptoms	Developmental delay Neurologic regression	None	Psychomotor retardation Down-gaze paralysis Ataxia
Hepatosplenomegaly	Present	Present	Present/absent
Cherry red macula	50% of cases	Absent	Absent
Lymphocyte vacuoles	Present	None	Present
Niemann–Pick cells in marrow	Present	Present	Present
Sphingomyelinase activity in tissue	Marked reduction (<10% of controls)	Marked reduction (<10% of controls)	Normal range[a]
Storage product	Sphingomyelin	Sphingomyelin	Sphingomyelin and cholesterol

[a]Deficiency in cultured fibroblasts to esterify exogenous cholesterol.

Treatment

There is no specific treatment for Niemann–Pick disease. Bone marrow transplantation in type B patients has been successful in reducing spleen and liver volumes, the sphingomyelin content in the liver, the Niemann–Pick cells in the bone marrow, and the radiologic infiltration of the lungs.

Splenectomy in Type B patients frequently causes progression of pulmonary disease and should be avoided if possible.

"Foam Cells" in Bone Marrow

Foam cells are seen in the bone marrow in the following conditions:

1. Neimann–Pick disease (types A, B, C, D)
2. Gaucher disease (types 1, 2, 3)
3. G_{m1} gangliosidosis (type 1)
4. G_{m2} gangliosidosis (Sandhoff variant)
5. Lactosyl ceramidosis
6. Sialidosis I
7. Sialidosis II, late infantile type
8. Mucolipidosis II
9. Mucolipidosis III
10. Mucolipidosis IV
11. Fucosidosis
12. Mannosidosis
13. Neuronal ceroid-lipofuscinosis
14. Farber disease
15. Wolman disease
16. Cholesteryl ester storage disease
17. Cerebrotendinous xanthomatosis
18. Chronic hyperlipidemia
19. Chronic corticosteroid therapy
20. Hematologic malignancies (e.g., Hodgkin disease, leukemia, myeloma)
21. Hematologic disease (e.g., aplastic anemia, ITP).

A careful history (including ethnic and family history), physical examination, examination of bone marrow using phase electron microscopy and special stains, and liver biopsy for biochemical analysis (enzyme assays on white blood cells or cultured skin fibroblasts) can assist in making a specific diagnosis of these storage diseases.

Cystinosis

An autosomal recessive defect, cystinosis is associated with generalized deposits of cystine in the tissues. Cystinosis occurs in the first year of life with the following manifestations:

- Thermal instability, polydipsia, polyuria
- Failure to thrive
- Recurrent episodes of vomiting and dehydration
- Dwarfism and rickets often prominent
- Early renal involvement with tubular dysfunction manifesting as a secondary Fanconi syndrome, leading to chronic renal failure.

Diagnosis

- Cystine crystals in the bone marrow
- Elevated cystine levels in leukocytes or fibroblasts.

Infantile Malignant Osteopetrosis (Marble Bone Disease)

Osteopetrosis is a hereditary disorder that may be present in either a severe or a mild form.

Severe Form (Autosomal Recessive)

The marrow space is progressively obliterated by excessive osseous growth. The difficulty in obtaining marrow by aspiration is a diagnostic clue. Radiologic changes are characteristic and diagnostic, consisting of generalized osteosclerosis. The cranial foramina progressively narrow, resulting in blindness due to optic atrophy, deafness, and other cranial nerve lesions.

The hematologic characteristics include the following:

- Progressive pancytopenia due to encroachment on the hematopoietic marrow by the overgrowth of bone
- Compensatory extramedullary hematopoiesis with resultant leukoerythroblastic anemia (circulating normoblasts, tear-drop-shaped poikilocytosis, and early myelocytes), hepatosplenomegaly, and lymphadenopathy
- Bone marrow hypoplasia
- Hemolysis due to splenic sequestration of red cells and perhaps general overactivity of the reticuloendothelial system.

Treatment

Allogeneic stem cell transplantation provides multipotent hematopoietic stem cells, which serve as a source of normal osteoclasts.

Mild Form (Autosomal Dominant)

Pathologic fractures occur in sclerotic bone. Nerve entrapment syndromes may also be present.

Neoplastic Disease

Neoplastic disease can be associated with the following hematologic alterations:

- Hemorrhage
- Nutritional deficiency states
- Dyserythropoietic anemias (including erythroid hypoplasia, sideroblastic anemia, and anemia similar to that seen in chronic inflammation)
- Defect in erythropoietin production
- Hemodilution
- Hemolysis
- Pancytopenia secondary to marrow invasion or to cytotoxic therapy
- Acquired von Willebrand disease as in Wilms' tumor
- Hypercoagulable states as in non-Hodgkin lymphoma
- Coagulopathy as in acute promyelocytic leukemia
- Leukoerythroblastic anemia and marrow
- Infiltration cytotoxic drug therapy.

Marrow infiltration is suspected when leukoerythroblastic anemia develops. This term signifies the presence of myelocytes and normoblasts with anemia, thrombocytopenia, and neutropenia. The explanation of this blood picture is that extramedullary erythropoiesis occurs when the marrow is infiltrated, permitting the escape of early myeloid and erythroid cells into the circulation. Normal blood findings, however, do not exclude marrow infiltration.

Bone marrow examination frequently demonstrates infiltration with tumor cells in the presence of pancytopenia. Because metastatic bone marrow involvement from solid tumors may be patchy, a single aspiration is not diagnostic. At least two aspirates and two biopsies should be performed.

The hematologic alterations associated with malignancy should be managed supportively and should resolve if the underlying neoplasms can be successfully treated.

SUGGESTED READINGS

Charrow J, Anderson HC, Kaplan P, et al. Enzyme replacement therapy and monitoring for children with Type 1 Gaucher disease: consensus recommendations. J Pediatr 2004;144:112–20.

Eschbach J, Abdulhadi M, et al. Recombinant human erythropoietin in anemic subjects with end-stage renal disease: results of phase III multicenter clinical trial. Am Intern Med 1989;111:992.

Grabowski GA, Leslie N. Lysosomal storage diseases: perspectives and principles. In: Hoffmann R, Benz EJ, Shattil SJ, Furie B, Cohen HJ, Silberstein LE, McGlave P, editors. Hematology Basic Principles and Practice. 3rd ed. Philadelphia: Lippincott-Raven, 2000.

Granovsky MO, Mueller BU, Nicholson HS, Rosenberg PS, Rabkin CS. Cancer in human immunodeficiency virus–infected children: a case series from the Children's Cancer Group and the National Cancer Institute. J Clin Oncol 1998;16:1729.

Kolodney EH, Charria-Ortiz G. Storage diseases of the reticuloendothelial system. In: Nathan D, Orkin SH, Ginsburg D, Look AT, editors. Nathan and Oski's Hematology of Infancy and Childhood. 6th ed. Philadelphia: WB Saunders, 2003.

McClain KL, Joshi VV. Cancer in children with HIV infection. Hematol Oncol Clin North Am 1996;10:1189.

McGovern MM, Desnick RJ. Lipidoses. In: Behrman RE, Kliegman RM, Jenson HB, editors. Nelson Textbook of Pediatrics. 17th ed. Philadelphia: WB Saunders, 2004.

Mueller BU, Pizza PA. Cancer in children with primary or secondary immunodeficiencies. J Pediatr 1995;126:1.

Scadden DT. Hematologic disorders and growth factor in HIV infection. Hematol Oncol Clin North Am 1996;10:1149.

Sinai-Trieman L, Salusky I, et al. The use of subcutaneous recombinant erythropoietin in children undergoing continuous cycling peritoneal dialysis. J Pediatr 1989;114:550.

Stockman J, Ezekowitz A. Hematologic manifestations of systemic diseases. In: Nathan D, Orkin S, editors. Nathan and Oski's Hematology of Infancy and Childhood. 5th ed. Philadelphia: WB Saunders, 1998;1841–91.

6

BONE MARROW FAILURE

Bone marrow failure may manifest as an isolated quantitative failure of one cell line, a single cytopenia (e.g., erythroid, myeloid, or megakaryocytic), or as pancytopenia, an acquired or inherited failure of all three cell lines with a hypoplastic or aplastic marrow (Table 6-1) or it may be due to an inherited qualitative failure of the bone marrow (e.g., congenital dyserythropoietic anemia). Bone marrow failure may also be due to invasion of the bone marrow by nonneoplastic (e.g., storage cells) or neoplastic conditions, primary or metastatic.

Table 6-2 lists the inherited bone marrow failure syndromes with their known and presumed genes. The inherited bone marrow failure syndromes had usually been divided into those resulting in pancytopenia (Fanconi anemia and dyskeratosis congenita) and those apparently restricted to a single hematopoietic lineage (Diamond–Blackfan anemia, congenital neutropenia [Kostmann syndrome, cyclic neutropenia, Shwachman Diamond syndrome], congenital amegakaryocytic thrombocytopenia, and thrombocytopenia absent radii [TAR] syndrome). However, it has become evident that most of these "single-cell cytopenias" may manifest abnormalities in other hematopoietic cell lines; for example, in Shwachman Diamond syndrome and congenital amegakaryocytic thrombocytopenia, pancytopenia is fairly common (Table 6-1).

DIAMOND–BLACKFAN ANEMIA (CONGENITAL PURE RED CELL APLASIA)
Pathophysiology

Diamond–Blackfan anemia (DBA) is a rare, pure red cell aplasia predominantly of infancy and childhood resulting from an intrinsic hematopoietic cell defect in which erythroid progenitors and precursors are highly sensitive to death by apoptosis.

Genetics

1. *Dominant inheritance:*
   a. The first DBA gene, *DBA1,* has been cloned and identified as *RPS 19,* a gene that codes for a ribosomal protein, located at chromosome 19q13.2. Studies show that *RPS 19* mutations account for only 20–25% of both sporadic and familial cases. The function of this protein is not fully understood.

Table 6-1. Causes of Single Cell Line Failure and Generalized Bone Marrow Failure

Failure of single cell line (single cytopenia)
Red cells
  Inherited
    Diamond–Blackfan anemia (pure red cell aplasia)
    Congenital dyserythropoietic anemia (CDA)
    Pearson syndrome
  Acquired
    Idiopathic
      Transient erythroblastopenia of childhood (TEC)
    Secondary
      Drugs
      Infection
      Malnutrition
      Thymoma
      Hematologic conditions
        Chronic hemolytic anemia (with associated parvovirus B19 infection)
        Chronic parvovirus B19 infection
White blood cells (Chapter 9)
  Shwachman Diamond syndrome
  Severe congenital neutropenia (Kostmann syndrome)
  Reticular dysgenesis (congenital aleukosis)
Platelets (Chapter 10)
  Congenital amegakaryocytic thrombocytopenia
  Thrombocytopenia absent radii (TAR) syndrome

Failure of all three cell lines (generalized pancytopenia)
Inherited
  Fanconi anemia (associated with chromosomal breakages induced by clastogens, e.g., diepoxybutane [DEB])
  Familial aplastic anemia (not associated with clastogen-induced chromosomal breakages, DEB negative, no abnormal physical stigmata)
  Dyskeratosis congenita
  Shwachman Diamond syndrome (predominantly neutropenia)[a]
  Congenital amegakaryocytic thrombocytopenia (predominantly thrombocytopenia)[a]
  Diamond–Blackfan anemia (predominantly anemia)[a]
  Aplastic anemia with constitutional chromosomal abnormalities
  Dubowitz syndrome (congenital abnormalities, mental retardation, aplastic anemia)
Acquired
  Idiopathic
  Secondary (see Table 6-17)

[a]Can have reduction in other cell lines.

A second gene, *DBA2*, has been localized by linkage analysis to chromosome 8p22-23. This second locus may account for 40–45% of patients.

More than 30% of families are inconsistent for linkage to either 19q or 8p, strongly suggesting further genetic heterogeneity. Approximately 10% of families have more than one clearly affected individual. The vast majority of these cases appear to be of dominant inheritance. Within these pedigrees there exists considerable heterogeneity in the expression of the DBA phenotype.

  b. Laboratory studies used for identification of dominant inheritance in family members of a proband with DBA include hemoglobin level, mean corpuscular volume (MCV), and erythrocyte adenosine deaminase activity. Note, however, that the absence of these markers clearly does not exclude dominant inheritance. By carefully evaluating families, it appears that at least 40–50% of cases of DBA are dominantly inherited.

Table 6-2. Inherited Bone Marrow Failure Syndrome Genes, Known and Presumed

Disorder	Gene	Locus	Genetics	Gene product
Fanconi anemia	FANCA	16q24.3	Autosomal recessive	FANCA
	FANCB	Xp22.31	X-linked recessive	FANCB
	FANCC	9q22.3	Autosomal recessive	FANCC
	FANCD1	13q12.3	Autosomal recessive	BRCA2
	FANCD2	3p25.3	Autosomal recessive	FANCD2
	FANCE	6p21.3	Autosomal recessive	FANCE
	FANCF	11p15	Autosomal recessive	FANCF
	FANCG	9p13	Autosomal recessive	FANCG
	FANCI/J	?/?	Autosomal recessive	?/?
	FANCL	2p16.1	Autosomal recessive	FANCL
Dyskeratosis congenita	DKC1	Xq28	X-linked recessive	Dyskeratin
	hTR (DKC2)	3q	Autosomal dominant	Telomerase RNA
	DKC3	?	Autosomal recessive	?
Shwachman Diamond syndrome	SBDS	7q11	Autosomal recessive	SBDS
Diamond–Blackfan anemia	RPS19 (DBA1)	19q13.2	Autosomal dominant	RPS19
	DBA2	8p23.3-p22	Autosomal dominant	?
	DBA3	?	Autosomal dominant	?
	?	?	?	?
Kostmann syndrome (SCN)	ELA2	19p13.3	Autosomal dominant	Neutrophil elastase
	?	?	Autosomal recessive	?
Amegakaryocytic thrombocytopenia	c-mpl	1p34	Autosomal recessive	Thrombopoietin receptor
Thrombocytopenia absent radii (TAR) syndrome	?	?	Autosomal recessive	?

Abbreviation: SCN, severe congenital neutropenia.

2. *Recessive inheritance:* This is suggested in some instances but has not been confirmed.

To provide meaningful genetic counseling, it is important to perform the previously mentioned laboratory studies to reduce the possibility of missing dominant inheritance in presumed recessive or sporadic cases. It is also important to perform these laboratory studies in potential family stem cell donors to increase the likelihood of detection of a silent phenotype.

Clinical Features

The following clinical features include findings of the DBA Registry (DBAR) of North America.

1. Rare disorder; autosomal dominant and possible autosomal recessive mode of inheritance.
2. The median age at presentation of anemia is 2 months and the median age at diagnosis of DBA is 3 months. More than 90% of the patients present during the first year of life.
3. Platelet and white cell counts are usually normal; thrombocytosis occurs rarely; neutropenia and/or thrombocytopenia may occur. Instances of significant cytopenias including aplastic anemia are emerging.
4. Physical anomalies, excluding short stature, are found in 47% of the patients. Of these, 50% are of the face and head, 38% upper limb and hand, 39% genitourinary, and 30% cardiac. Twenty-one percent of the patients have more than one anomaly.
5. Karyotype generally normal.
6. No hepatosplenomegaly.
7. Malignant potential; DBA has been recognized as a cancer predisposition syndrome. The precise incidence of cancer is unknown. Of the approximately 30 reported cases of malignancy, the most common have been hematopoietic (acute myeloid leukemia [AML], myelodysplastic syndrome [MDS], lymphoma). Osteogenic sarcoma is next most common and cases of breast, colon, and other solid tumors have been reported.

Diagnosis

1. Elevated erythrocyte adenosine deaminase (eADA) activity is found in approximately 85% of patients. Macrocytosis and an elevated fetal hemoglobin are supportive but not diagnostic of DBA. These parameters may be useful in avoiding potential matched related hematopoietic stem cell transplant (HSCT) donors with genotypic DBA and have been helpful in distinguishing DBA from transient erythroblastopenia of childhood (TEC) (Table 6-3).
2. Bone marrow with virtual absence of normoblasts, in some cases with relative increase in proerythroblasts or normal number of proerythroblasts with a maturation arrest; normal myeloid and megakaryocytic series.

Table 6-4 lists the diagnostic criteria for Diamond–Blackfan anemia.

Differential Diagnosis

This condition must be differentiated from:

• *Transient erythroblastopenia of childhood:* Table 6-3 differentiates TEC from DBA. Congenital hypoplastic anemia due to transplacental infection with B19

Table 6-3. Differentiating Transient Erythroblastopenia from Diamond–Blackfan Anemia

Feature	Transient erythroblastopenia	DBA (pure red cell aplasia)
Frequency	Common (? increasing)	Rare (5–10 per 10^6 live births)
Age at diagnosis	6 months–4 years, occasionally older	90%, by 1 year 25%, at birth or within first 2 months
Etiology	Acquired (viral, idiopathic)	Genetic
Familial	No	Yes (in at least 10–20% of cases)
Antecedent history	Viral illness	None
Congenital abnormalities	Absent	Present ~50% cases (heart, kidneys, musculoskeletal system)
Course	Spontaneous recovery in weeks to months	Prolonged, 20% actuarial probability of remission
Transfusion dependence	Not dependent	Transfusion or steroid dependent
MCV (for age)	Normocytic	Macrocytic
Hemoglobin F (for age)	Normal	Elevated
i Antigen	Usually normal	Elevated
Erythrocyte adenosine deaminase activity	Not elevated	Elevated (~85% of cases)
Treatment	Packed cell transfusion, if required	Packed red cell transfusion. Prednisone 2 mg/kg/day and taper to lowest effective dose Stem cell transplantation

Table 6-4. Diagnostic Criteria for Diamond–Blackfan Anemia

Diagnostic criteria:
  Normochromic, usually macrocytic anemia, relative to patient's age and occasionally
    normocytic anemia developing in early childhood
  Reticulocytopenia
  Normocellular marrow with selective paucity of erythroid precursors
  Normal or only slightly decreased granulocyte count
  Normal or slightly increased platelet count
Supportive criteria:
  Typical physical abnormalities
  Increased fetal hemoglobin
  Increased erythrocyte adenosine deaminase (eADA) activity

parvovirus can be differentiated from DBA by performing reverse transcriptase polymerase chain reaction (RT-PCR) for B19 parvovirus on a bone marrow sample. Parvovirus may result in a transient or more chronic red cell failure in a patient with underlying hemolytic anemia or in a patient with underlying immune deficiency, respectively.

- Late hyporegenerative anemia due to Rh or ABO hemolytic disease of the newborn. This may rarely last for a few months and should be considered in the differential diagnosis of DBA.
- Pearson syndrome.

- Thymoma, not described in infancy but has been reported in a 5-year-old.
- Viral infections.
- Medications.

Treatment

1. *Packed red cell transfusion, as required:* Leukocyte-depleted packed red cells reduce the incidence of nonhemolytic, febrile transfusion reactions, as well as the risk of transmission of cytomegalovirus (CMV) and the risk of human leukocyte antigen (HLA) alloimmunization. Patients who have previously been treated with immunosuppressive drugs should receive irradiated blood products. Patients in whom stem cell transplantation is contemplated should receive CMV-negative blood products.

2. *Prednisone:* In a dose of 2–4 mg/kg/day given in 3 or 4 divided doses. Reticulocytosis usually occurs in 1–2 weeks but may take slightly longer. When the hemoglobin level reaches 10.0 g/dL, reduce the dose to the minimum necessary to maintain a reasonable hemoglobin level in order to obtain an effective alternate-day schedule. Any patient who experiences significant steroid-related side effects including growth failure should have steroid medication temporarily discontinued and should be placed on a red cell transfusion regimen. Patients with DBA on low-dose alternate-day therapy of long duration, starting in early infancy, may manifest significant steroid toxicity. Steroid-related side effects have been observed in most patients, with 40%, 12%, and 6.8% manifesting cushingoid features, pathologic fractures, and cataracts, respectively. It is recommended that corticosteroids be withheld for the first year of life to reduce these side effects and to allow for safe and effective immunization.

3. *Hematopoietic stem cell transplantation:* Although somewhat controversial, HLA-matched sibling donor transplantation should be considered for any patient with DBA. Consideration should be given to the fact that 20% of all patients attain remission, balanced by the risk of hematologic malignancy, myelodysplasia, or severe aplastic anemia. A family marrow donor must be tested for the presence of a "silent phenotype." Matched unrelated or incompletely matched related donor transplants have proven to be very risky and should be reserved for patients with leukemia, MDS, severe aplastic anemia, or clinically significant neutropenia or thrombocytopenia.

4. *Alternative therapy:* A number of treatments, including erythropoietin, immunoglobulin, megadose corticosteroids, and androgens, have been utilized in DBA patients with little success. Cyclosporine, interleukin-3 (IL-3), and metoclopramide have resulted in occasional responses in DBA. The toxicity of cyclosporine and the lack of availability of IL-3 exclude their use for most patients. A more extensive trial with metoclopramide is required to determine whether it has a place in the treatment of DBA. These agents should be explored on a case-by-case basis as an alternative to corticosteroids, transfusion, or stem cell transplantation when the risk associated with these proven modalities warrants the treatment.

Prognosis

1. Approximately 80% of DBA patients respond initially to corticosteroid therapy. The remaining 20% require transfusion therapy.

2. Remission may occur actuarially in 20% of patients by age 25, irrespective of their pattern of response to treatment, with 77% remitting during the first decade.

3. The major complication of transfusion is iron overload, the consequences of which include diabetes mellitus, cardiac and hepatic dysfunction, growth failure, and endocrine dysfunction. Iron chelation with deferoxamine is therefore an essential component of a transfusion program. New oral iron chelators are under development; however, the oral chelator deferiprone (L1) has caused significant neutropenia in DBA and should not be used. Many patients, however, find nearly daily subcutaneous chelation therapy onerous and compliance is often poor. Sustained hematologic remissions defined as stable hemoglobin levels without transfusion or steroid requirement for 6 months may occur. Only about half of steroid-responsive patients remain on prednisone for long periods of time. In summary, both chronic corticosteroid therapy and chronic transfusion therapy may lead to a number of significant immediate and long-term complications, supporting a role for HSCT. Survival of patients into adulthood in remission or sustainable on steroids is in the range of 85–100%. Only about 60% of transfusion-dependent patients survive to middle age.

4. HLA-matched-sibling stem cell transplantation patients have long-term survival of about 80%, whereas unrelated or partially matched related transplants yield survivals under 20%. Favorable transplantation outcomes are most likely if the patient is in good health at the time of HSCT without complications of iron overload and allosensitization. Improvements in supportive care, graft versus host disease (GVHD) prophylaxis, and infection control have resulted in a marked decrease in HLA-matched related HSCT transplant-related morbidity and mortality. Sibling HSCT is recommended for young DBA patients, prior to development of significant allosensitization or iron overload, when there is an available HLA-matched related donor.

5. Patients with DBA who become pregnant may develop either an increased requirement for steroid therapy or red cell transfusions due to worsening anemia and should be considered high risk and require appropriate follow-up. This appears to be a hormonally induced problem because oral contraceptives may cause the same problem in patients with DBA.

6. Fetal hydrops secondary to fetal DBA has been reported.

CONGENITAL DYSERYTHROPOIETIC ANEMIAS

The congenital dyserythropoietic anemias (CDAs) are a group of conditions characterized by ineffective erythropoiesis (intramedullary red cell death, i.e., anemia with reticulocytopenia and marrow erythroid hyperplasia) and by specific morphologic abnormalities in the bone marrow consisting of increased numbers of multinucleated red cell precursors. There are 3 major types of CDA (I, II, and III).

Clinical Manifestations

CDA has the following clinical manifestations:

- Chronic mild anemia (red cells have nonspecific abnormalities; basophilic stippling, occasional normoblasts, suboptimal reticulocyte count for degree of anemia in the context of erythroid hyperplasia in marrow), usually presenting in childhood
- Granulopoiesis and thrombopoiesis normal
- Chronic or intermittent mild jaundice
- Splenomegaly
- High plasma iron turnover rate and low iron utilization by erythrocyte (ineffective erythropoiesis) resulting in hemosiderosis

- Red cell survival time shortened
- Progressive iron overload leading to hemosiderosis.

Marrow findings tend to distinguish the three types from one another. Other clinical manifestations of CDA include the following:

- CDA associated with atypical hereditary ovalocytosis
- CDA of neonatal onset (with severe anemia at birth, hepatosplenomegaly, jaundice, syndactyly, and small for gestational age)
- CDA associated with hydrops fetalis and hypoproteinemia.

Table 6-5 lists the clinical features of congenital dyserythropoietic anemia, types I–III. Cases with clinical manifestations that do not fit the classical categories of CDA have been described. Table 6-6 lists the clinical features of so-called types IV–VI. Table 6-7 lists the myeloid/erythroid (M/E) ratios and percentages of erythroblasts showing various dysplastic changes in 10 healthy adults and 12 patients with CDA type I. Table 6-8 lists the diagnostic tests necessary when CDA is suspected. The diagnosis of CDA can only be made after the exclusion of other causes of congenital dyserythropoiesis such as thalassemia syndromes and hereditary sideroblastic anemias. Recently, familial dyserythropoietic anemia with thrombocytopenia has been shown to be associated with mutations in GATA-1.

Treatment

- Splenectomy performed in severely affected patients results in moderate to marked improvement, with CDA type I having the poorest response.

Table 6-5. Clinical and Laboratory Features of Congenital Dyserythropoietic Anemia, Types I–III

Feature	Type I	Type II (HEMPAS)[a]	Type III
Inheritance	Autosomal recessive	Autosomal recessive	Autosomal dominant
Clinical	Hepatosplenomegaly	Hepatosplenomegaly	Hepatosplenomegaly
	Jaundice	Variable jaundice	Hair-on-end
	Some patients respond to α-interferon 2a treatment	Gallstones Hemochromatosis	appearance on skull radiograph Increased prevalence of lymphoproliferative disorders
Gene locus (in some cases)	15q15.1–15.3[b]	20q11.2	15q21–25[b]
Red cell size	Macrocytic	Normo or macrocytic	Macrocytic
Anemia	Mild to moderate Hemoglobin 8–12 g/dL	Moderate Hemoglobin 6–7 g/dL	Mild to moderate Hemoglobin 7–8.5 g/dL
Reticulocytes	1.5%	±2%	2–4%
Smear	Macrocytic: Marked anisocytosis and poikilocytosis; basophilic stippling	Normocytic: Anisocytosis and poikilocytosis; basophilic stippling; "teardrop" cells; irregular contracted cells; occasionally, normoblasts	Macrocytic: Anisocytosis and poikilocytosis; basophilic stippling

(Continues)

Table 6-5. *(Continued)*

Feature	Type I	Type II (HEMPAS)[a]	Type III
Marrow normoblasts	Megaloblastoid: Binucleated, 2–5%; internuclear chromatin bridges, 1–2%	Normoblastic: Bi- and multi-nucleated, 10–50%; binuclearity predominates	Megaloblastic: Multinuclearity (up to 12 nuclei gigantoblasts), 10–50%
Serology:			
Ham test	Negative	Positive	Negative
Anti-i agglutinability	Normal	Strong	Normal
Marrow iron	Scant increase	Increased	Increased
Serum bilirubin and urine urobilinogen	Elevated	Elevated	Elevated

[a]Pathognomonic finding in CDA type II is that the patient's red cells are lysed by approximately 30% of acidified sera from normal individuals, but not from patient's own acidified serum. The red cells contain a specific HEMPAS (hereditary erythroblastic multinuclearity associated with a positive acidified-serum test) antigen; many normal sera contain an IgM that is anti-HEMPAS.

[b]May apply only to a proportion of cases.

Table 6-6. Clinical Features of Congenital Dyserythropoietic Anemia, Types IV–VI

	Type IV	Type V	Type VI
Clinical	Mild to moderate splenomegaly	Spleen palpable in few cases Unconjugated hyperbilirubinemia due to intramedullary destruction of morphologically normal, but functionally abnormal erythroblasts/marrow reticulocytes	Spleen not palpable
Hemoglobin	Very low, transfusion dependent	Normal or near normal	Normal or near normal
MCV	Normal or mildly elevated	Normal or mildly elevated	Very high (119–125) without vitamin B_{12}, folic acid, or other causes of megaloblastic anemia
Erythropoiesis	Normoblastic or mildly to moderately megaloblastic	Normoblastic	Grossly megaloblastic
Nonspecific erythroblast dysplasia	Present	Absent or little	Present

Table 6-7. M/E Ratios and Percentages of Erythroblasts Showing Various Changes in 10 Healthy Adults and 12 Patients with CDA Type I

	Healthy volunteers		CDA type I	
	Mean	Range	Mean	Range
M/E ratio	3.1	2–8.3	0.54	0.20–1.30
Cytoplasmic stippling (%)	0.24	0–0.91	7.10	1.02–15.04
Cytoplasmic vacuolation (%)	0.39	0–0.70		
Intererythroblastic cytoplasmic bridges (%)	2.38	0.72–4.77		
Markedly irregular or karyorrhectic nuclei (%)	0.22	0–0.55	3.00	1.32–5.03
Howell–Jolly bodies (%)	0.18	0–0.39	0.97	0.41–1.58
Binuclearity (%)	0.31	0–0.57	4.87	3.50–7.02
Internuclear chromatin bridges (%)	0	0	1.59	0.60–2.83
Number of erythroblasts assessed per subject	713	548–1022	817	500–1185

From Wickramasinghe SN. Dyserythropoiesis and congenital dyserythropoietic anemias. Br J Haematol 1997;98:785–97, with permission.

Table 6-8. Diagnostic Tests for Congenital Dyserythropoietic Anemia

Complete blood count, including MCV, red cell distribution width (RDW), blood smear examination
Absolute reticulocyte count
Quantitative light and if needed electron microscope analysis of the bone marrow
Serum vitamin B_{12} and red cell folate measurements
Parvovirus B19
Serum bilirubin levels
Hemoglobin (Hb) electrophoresis: Hb A2, Hb F assays
Red cell enzyme assays (pyruvate kinase, glucose-6-phosphate dehydrogenase)
SDS polyacrylamide gel electrophoresis of red cell membranes
Acidified serum lysis test
Sucrose lysis test
Serum ferritin level
Test for urinary hemosiderin
Cytogenetic studies of bone marrow cells
Mutation analysis for known CDA genes
Studies of globin chain synthesis
Studies of globin gene analysis

Abbreviation: SDS, sodium dodecyl sulfate.

- Prophylactic phlebotomy when the hemoglobin level permits and/or deferoxamine (newer oral iron chelators when available) iron chelation should be administered to ameliorate the effects of iron overload.
- Folic acid, 1 mg per week, should be administered. Iron therapy is contraindicated.
- Vitamin E has been used in the treatment of CDA type II, with an apparent improvement in red cell survival and a reduction in serum bilirubin and reticulocyte count.
- Recombinant α-interferon 2a has been used in CDA type I, resulting in an increase in hemoglobin level, a decrease in MCV and red cell distribution width (RDW), a reduction in serum bilirubin and lactic dehydrogenase (LDH) levels,

an improvement in morphology of erythroblasts, and a reduction in ineffective erythropoiesis.
• Successful stem cell transplant has been performed in type I CDA.

TRANSIENT ERYTHROBLASTOPENIA

Transient erythroblastopenia of childhood must be differentiated from Diamond–Blackfan anemia in order to avoid unnecessary corticosteroid use (Table 6-3). TEC has the following features:

1. *Pathophysiology:* The following clinical and laboratory observations have shed light on the basic mechanisms of the pathogenesis of TEC:
   a. *Virus:* There is usually a history of a preceding nonspecific viral illness 1–2 months prior to TEC.
   b. *Erythropoietin levels:* Serum erythropoietin levels are high in keeping with the degree of anemia.
   c. *CFU-E and BFU-E:* Both are decreased in 30–50% of patients, suggesting that the defect might be at the CFU-E and BFU-E levels.
   d. *Serum inhibitors of erythropoiesis:* Immunoglobulin G (IgG) inhibitors of normal progenitor cells have been found in 60–80% of patients with TEC.
   e. *Cellular inhibitors of erythropoiesis:* Inhibitory mononuclear cells have been observed in approximately 25% of patients with TEC.

   On the basis of the preceding observations, it has been speculated that a nonspecific virus is cleared as the host develops IgG antibody. This IgG antibody probably recognizes shared viral and erythroid progenitor epitopes.
2. *Age:* Usually between 6 months and 4 years of age. With more children attending day care programs, younger patients with TEC are being identified.
3. *Sex:* Equal frequency in boys and girls.
4. *Hematologic values:*
   a. Hemoglobin falls to levels ranging from 3 to 8 g/dL.
   b. Reticulocyte count is 0%.
   c. White blood cell and platelet count are usually normal.
      Note, however, that approximately 10% of patients may have significant neutropenia (absolute neutrophil count [ANC], <1000/mm^3) and 5% have thrombocytopenia (platelet count, <100,000/mm^3). (Table 6-3 lists the hematologic characteristics.) An analysis of 50 patients presenting with TEC at our institution revealed a high incidence of neutropenia (64% with an ANC of <1500/mm^3).
5. *Bone marrow:* Absence of red cell precursors, except when the diagnostic bone marrow is performed during early recovery (prior to a reticulocytosis) when variable degrees of erythroid maturation may be observed.
6. *Prognosis:* Spontaneous recovery occurs within weeks to months with the vast majority of patients recovering within 1 month. Recurrent TEC occurs only rarely.
7. *Treatment:* Transfusion of packed red blood cells if there is impending cardiovascular compromise. Because recovery is usually prompt, restraint should be exercised with regard to red cell transfusions.

Other instances of transient red cell failure may occur secondary to:

• *Drugs:* chloramphenicol, penicillin, phenobarbital, and diphenylhydantoin
• *Infections:* viral infections (e.g., mumps, EBV, parvovirus B19, atypical pneumonia) and bacterial sepsis
• *Malnutrition:* kwashiorkor and other disorders

- *Chronic hemolytic anemia:* hereditary spherocytosis, sickle cell anemia, β-thalassemia, and other congenital or acquired hemolytic anemias. The etiologic agent is human parvovirus B19.

APLASTIC ANEMIA

Aplastic anemia is a physiologic and anatomic failure of the bone marrow characterized by a marked decrease or absence of blood-forming elements in the marrow and peripheral pancytopenia (decreased red cells, white blood cells, and platelets). Splenomegaly, hepatomegaly, and lymphadenopathy are not characteristic of this condition. Aplastic anemia may be congenital or acquired.

Figure 6-1 delineates in schematic form an approach to the differential diagnosis of pancytopenia, and Table 6-9 lists the investigations to be carried out in a patient with pancytopenia.

CONGENITAL APLASTIC ANEMIAS

Fanconi Anemia

Fanconi anemia (FA) is a rare (heterozygote frequency in the general population of 1/300; 1/100 in Ashkenazi Jews and South African Afrikaners due to "founder effect") autosomal recessive inherited bone marrow failure syndrome generally associated with multiple congenital anomalies. Very rarely (FANCB) the disease may be transmitted as an X-linked recessive (Table 6-2).

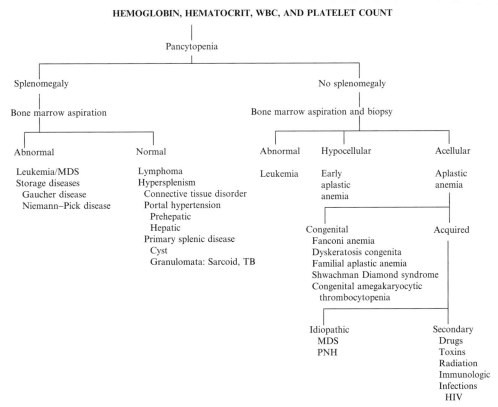

Fig. 6-1. Approach to the differential diagnosis of pancytopenia.

Table 6-9. Investigations in Patients with Pancytopenia

1. Detailed drug history, toxin and radiation exposure, family history of aplastic anemia, physical examination for congenital anomalies
2. Blood count: absolute reticulocyte count, granulocyte count, Hb, Hct, MCV, platelet count
3. ANA and DNA titer, Coombs' test, rheumatoid factor, liver function tests, tuberculin test
4. Viral serology: HIV, EBV, parvovirus, hepatitis A, B, C. PCR for virus when indicated
5. Serum vitamin B$_{12}$, red cell, and serum folate levels
6. Bone marrow aspirate and trephine biopsy (Because of patchiness of bone marrow involvement, biopsy at multiple sites may be required.)
7. Chromosome breakage assay on blood lymphocytes or skin fibroblasts using clastogen stimulation (e.g., diepoxybutane or mitomycin C) to diagnose Fanconi anemia (Skeletal radiographs, renal, cardiac, abdominal ultrasound, chest x-ray to determine congenital anomalies in Fanconi anemia.)
8. Cytogenetic studies on bone marrow to exclude myelodysplastic syndromes
9. Flow cytometric immunophenotypic analysis of erythrocytes for deficiency of GPI-linked surface protein (e.g., CD55/59) to exclude paroxysmal nocturnal hemoglobinuria
10. Diagnostic tests to rule out Shwachman Diamond syndrome (see Chapter 9) such as skeletal radiograph, chest radiograph, pancreatic ultrasound, serum trypsinogen, and isoamylase
11. Mutation analysis for inherited bone marrow failure syndromes when suspected.

Abbreviations: Hb, hemoglobin; Hct, hematocrit; MCV, mean corpuscular volume; HIV, human immunodeficiency virus; EBV, Epstein–Barr virus; PCR, polymerase chain reaction.

Pathophysiology of Fanconi Anemia

Somatic cell hybridization studies have thus far defined 11 FA complementation groups. Of these, nine FA genes have been cloned (Table 6-10). The gene products of these nine genes have been shown to cooperate in a common pathway. Six of the FA proteins (FANCA, C, E, F, G, and L) assemble in a nuclear complex that is required to monobuiquinate and activate FANCD2. Ubiquinated FANCD2 is translocated to a nuclear focus containing BRCA1. Recently FANCD1 has been identified as BRCA2. The exact mechanism of FANCD2 monobuiquitination and the role of FANCD2, BRCA2 (FANCD1), and BCRA1 in DNA repair are yet to be unraveled. Despite the identification of this pathway, the manner in which disruption in this cascade of events results in a faulty DNA-damaged response and genomic instability leading to hematopoietic failure and cancer predisposition remains to be determined.

Fanconi anemia cells are characterized by hypersensitivity to chromosomal breakage as well as hypersensitivity to G$_2$/M cell cycle arrest induced by DNA cross-linking agents. In addition there is sensitivity to oxygen-free radicals and to ionizing radiation.

Clinical Features

1. FA is inherited as an autosomal recessive disorder in over 99% of cases and is the most frequently inherited aplastic anemia. Recently FANCB has been found to be inherited by an X-linked recessive. Of the 11 defined FA complementation groups, with 9 genes cloned thus far (Table 6-10), FANCA is the most common complementation group, representing about 70% of cases. FANCC may have an earlier onset of pancytopenia and shorter survival. However, genotype–phenotype correlation is complex and probably relates as much to the nature of the gene product and other factors as to the specific complementation group.
2. All racial and ethnic groups are affected.
3. Pancytopenia is the usual finding.

Table 6-10. Complementation Groups of Fanconi Anemia

Complementation Group/Gene	Percentage of FA Patients[a]	Locus	Gene Product (M.W. kDa)
FANCA	66%	16q24.3	FANCA (163)
FANCB	<1%	Xp22.31	FANCB (95)
FANCC	9.5%	9q22.3	FANCC (63)
FANCD1	3.3%	13q12.3	BRCA2 (380)
FANCD2	3.3%	3p25.3	FANCD2 (155, 162)
FANCE	2.5%	6p21.3	FANCE (60)
FANCF	2.1%	11p15	FANCF (42)
FANCG	8.7%	9p13	FANCG (68)
FANCI/J	1.6%/1.6%	?/?	?/?
FANCL	<1%	2p16.1	FANCL (43)

[a]Data derived from European Fanconi Anemia Research Programme (1994–2003), Levitus M et al. Heterogeneity in Fanconi anemia: evidence for 2 new genetic subtypes. Blood 2004;103:2498–2503.

a. The median age at hematologic presentation of patients is approximately 7 years. The actuarial risk of developing bone marrow failure is 90% by 40 years of age.

b. Hematologic dysfunction usually presents with macrocytosis, followed by thrombocytopenia, often leading to progressive pancytopenia and severe aplastic anemia (SAA). FA frequently terminates in MDS and/or AML.

c. FA cells are hypersensitive to chromosomal breaks induced by DNA cross-linking agents. This observation is the basis for the commonly used chromosome breakage test for FA. The clastogens diepoxybutane (DEB) and mitomycin C (MMC) are the agents most frequently used *in vitro* to induce chromosome breaks, gaps, rearrangements, quadriradii, and other structural abnormalities. Clastogens also induce cell cycle arrest in G_2/M. The hypersensitivity of FA lymphocytes to G_2/M arrest, detected using cell cycle analysis by flow cytometry either *de novo* or clastogen induced, has more recently been used as a screening tool for FA.

4. Bone marrow examination reveals hypocellularity and fatty replacement consistent with the degree of peripheral pancytopenia. Residual hematopoiesis may reveal dysplastic erythroid (megaloblastoid changes, multinuclearity) and myeloid (abnormal granulation) precursors and abnormal megakaryocytes.

5. Congenital anomalies include increased pigmentation of the skin along with café au lait and hypopigmented areas, short stature (impaired growth hormone secretion), skeletal anomalies (especially involving the thumb, radius, and long bones), male hypogenitalism, microcephaly, abnormalities of the eyes (microphthalmia, strabismus, ptosis, nystagmus) and ears including deafness, hyperreflexia, developmental delay, and renal and cardiac anomalies. Forty percent lack obvious physical abnormalities. There is great clinical heterogeneity even within a genotype (sibling may be phenotypically different).

6. The actuarial risks of developing hematologic (AML/MDS) and nonhematologic (e.g., squamous cell carcinoma of the head and neck, cancer of the breast, kidney, lung, colon, bone, retinoblastoma, and female gynecologic) tumors are 33% and 28%, respectively, by 40 years of age. Androgen-related, usually benign liver neoplasia may also occur. The risk of solid tumors may become even higher as death from aplastic anemia is reduced and as post-HSCT patients survive longer. These data must be considered in the context of HSCT, in particular when the risk of nonhematologic malignancy is likely to increase as a result

of HSCT conditioning regimens and chronic GVHD. Treatment for cancer is generally ineffective.

7. Prenatal diagnosis is possible in amniotic fluid cell cultures and chorionic villus biopsy.

Complications

Table 6-11 describes the complications of malignancy and liver disease associated with Fanconi anemia.

Differential Diagnosis

1. The differential diagnosis of FA generally includes acquired aplastic anemia, congenital amegakaryocytic thrombocytopenia (CAT), TAR syndrome as well as VATER/VACTRL (vertebral anomalies, anal atresia, cardiac anomalies, tracheoesophageal fistula, renal anomalies, limb anomalies) syndromes. FA is easily distinguished from TAR syndrome (Table 6-12). There is an intercalary defect in TAR consisting of absent radii with normal thumbs, whereas in FA the defect is terminal, an abnormal radius always being associated with anomalies of the thumb. FA testing is warranted in any child who presents with hematologic cytopenias, unexplained macrocytosis, aplastic anemia or AML, as well as representative congenital abnormalities or solid tumors typical of FA such as head and neck, esophageal, or gynecologic tumors presenting at an early age (Table 6-13).

2. The critical investigations are aspiration and biopsy of the bone marrow and demonstration in peripheral blood of increased chromosomal fragility or G_2/M arrest induced by clastogens (e.g., DEB, MMC). Complementation group analysis and/or mutation analysis may be helpful after the demonstration of a positive screening test.

Table 6-11. Malignancy and Liver Disease in Fanconi Anemia

	Leukemia	Myelodysplastic syndrome (MDS)	Cancer[a]	Liver disease
Number of patients (%)	84 (9)	32 (3)	47 (5)	37 (4)
Male:female	1.3:1	1.1:1	0.3:1	1.6:1
Age (in years) at diagnosis				
Mean	10	13	13	9
Median	9	12	10	6
Range	0.1–28	1–31	0.1–34	1–48
Percentage ≥16 years old	20	32	31	11
Age (in years) at complication				
Mean	14	17	23	16
Median	14	17	26	13
Range	0.1–29	5–31	0.31–38	3–48
Number without pancytopenia (%)	21 (25)	14 (44)	8 (17)	1 (3)
Number died (%)	40 (48)	20 (63)	18 (38)	1 (3)
Number reported deceased (%)	66 (79)	24 (75)	28 (60)	32 (86)

Note: 150 patients had one or more malignancies; the number of malignancies was 157. MDS cases included seven who developed leukemia.

[a]More recent data describe an actuarial risk of hematologic and non-hematologic cancer of 33% and 28% respectively by 40 years of age.

From Alter BP. Arms and the man or hands and the child: congenital anomalies and hematologic syndromes. J Pediatr Hematol Oncol 1997;19:287–91, with permission.

Table 6-12. Features Differentiating Fanconi Anemia from Amegakaryocytic Thrombocytopenic Purpura (TAR Syndrome)

Feature	Fanconi anemia	TAR
Age at onset of hematologic symptoms	Median of 7 years	Birth to infancy
Low birth weight	~10%	~10%
Stature	Short	Short
Skeletal deformities	66%	100%
Absent radii with fingers and thumbs present	0%	100%
Other hand deformities	~40%	~40%
Lower extremity deformities	~40%	<10%
Cardiovascular anomalies	5–10%	5–10%
Anomalous pigmentation of skin	77%	0%
Hemangiomas	0%	~10%
Mental retardation	17%	7%
Peripheral blood	Pancytopenia Macrocytosis (high MCV)	Thrombocytopenia, eosinophilia, leukemoid reactions, anemia
Bone marrow	Aplastic	Absent or abnormal megakaryocytes, normal myeloid and erythroid precursors
Marrow CFU-GM, CFU-E	Decreased	Normal (decreased CFU-megakaryocytes)
HbF	Increased	Normal
Hexokinase in blood cells	Decreased in some	?
Chromosomal breaks in leukocytes	Present	None
Malignancy	Common	Rare (leukemia only)
Sex ratio (male/female)	~1:1	~1:1
Inheritance pattern	Autosomal recessive	Autosomal recessive
Associated leukemia	Yes	Rare
Prognosis	Poor	Good if patient survives first year when platelet count improves

Modified from Hall JG, Levin J, Kuhn JP, et al. Thrombocytopenia with absent radius (TAR). Medicine (Baltimore) 1969;48:411, with permission.

3. FA somatic mosaics with DEB-positive and DEB-negative (double population) cells belong to distinct groups based on the degree of mosaicism and may present diagnostic problems. Mosaicism leading to a "normal" T cell that is resistant to the less dose-intense HSCT conditioning, used for FA, may result in graft rejection.

Table 6-13 lists the indications for Fanconi anemia screening studies, Table 6-14 lists the laboratory studies required to make the diagnosis of Fanconi anemia, and Table 6-15 lists the initial and follow-up investigations to be performed in a patient with an established diagnosis of Fanconi anemia.

Management

Serial assessment of the bone marrow should be performed to provide evidence of progression and the development or evolution of cytogenetic abnormalities:

Table 6-13. Indications for Fanconi Anemia Screening Studies

All children with unexplained cytopenias

All children with MDS or AML

Patients with classic birth defects suggestive of FA

VATER/VACTRL (vertebral anomalies, anal atresia, cardiac anomalies, tracheoesophageal fistula, renal anomalies, and limb anomalies)

Structural anomalies of the upper extremity and/or genitourinary system

Patients with:

Excessive café au lait spots

Microcephaly

Micro-ophthalmia

Growth failure

Development of squamous cell carcinoma at a young age in esophagus, head, neck, or female genitalia and liver tumors

Patient with leukemia with unusual sensitivity to chemotherapy

Karyotype with spontaneous chromosome breaks

Patients with unexplained macrocytosis and an elevated HbF

Males with unexplained infertility

Table 6-14. Laboratory Studies for Diagnosis of Fanconi Anemia

1. Screening tests:
   a. Demonstration of the presence of increased chromosomal breakage in T-lymphocytes cultured in the presence of DNA cross-linking agents such as mitomycin C (MMC) or diepoxybutane (DEB). DEB test is used more widely.
   b. Flow cytometry study: A flow cytometric technique for the analysis of alkylating agent–treated cells can determine the percentage of cells arrested in G_2M because a characteristic distribution clearly distinguishes FA cells from normal cells.
2. Definitive test:
   a. Mutation analysis (see Table 6-10 for cloned FANC genes)[a]
   b. Western blot for D2-L (long protein formed by ubiquitination of FANC D2[b])
3. Prenatal diagnosis of FA: DEB test can be used in either chorionic villus or amniocentesis-derived samples.
4. Detection of carrier state: In an FA family, if proband has been identified to have a defect in one of the nine cloned genes, molecular testing is available for the extended family members.
   Population-based screening is done only in the at-risk Askenazi Jewish population (FANCC).

Note: Some patients with FA may have two populations of cells exhibiting either a normal or an FA phenotype. Such mosaicism may result in a false-negative chromosome breakage study if the percentage of normal cells is high. The study of fibroblasts are useful in this circumstance.

[a]Done only in specialized laboratories

[b]Currently available only as a research study

- Bone marrow aspiration should be performed for cytology, cytogenetics with FISH analysis for cytogenetic abnormalities that may be predictive of leukemia (e.g., 3q gain, 1q gain, 7q deletion, 5q deletion).
- Bone marrow biopsy should be done for cellularity.

The patient's complete blood counts should be monitored. The degree of cytopenia guides management as follows:

	Mild	Moderate	Severe
Hemoglobin level	≥8.0 gm/dL	<8.0 gm/dL	<8.0 gm/dL
ANC	>1000/mm^3	<1000/mm^3	<500/mm^3
Platelet count	≥50,000/mm^3	<50,000/mm^3	<30,000/mm^3

Table 6-15. Diagnostic Investigations to Be Performed in a Patient with Established Diagnosis of Fanconi Anemia

Endocrine studies for:
  Short stature (growth hormone deficiency)
  Glucose intolerance
  Hypothyroidism
  Pubertal delay
  Evaluation of undescended testes
Imaging studies[a] and evaluation of:
  Orthopedic anomalies
  Genitourinary abnormalities
Hepatic ultrasound every 6 months while taking androgens
Serum chemistries for:
  Liver function
  Kidney function
Hearing test
Monitoring for iron overload for patients on red cell transfusion therapy
  1. Ferritin
  2. Liver enzymes
  3. Liver biopsy
  4. Superconductivity quantum interference device-biosuseptometry (SQUID)
Survey of family members:
  1. To exclude diagnosis of FA in any other family members
  2. To type family members to determine the potential availability of an HLA-matched sibling for future consideration of bone marrow transplant
  3. To provide genetic counseling to parents and patient
Prospective counseling and screening:
  1. Avoid exposure to potential mutagens or carcinogens (e.g., insecticides, organic solvents, hair dye, papillomavirus)
  2. Cancer surveillance:
    a. Examine bone marrow yearly with histologic and cytogenetic studies for evidence of myelodysplasia or leukemia
    b. Yearly head and neck examination over age 7 years
    c. Yearly gynecologic examination beginning at age 16 years
    d. Breast self-examination beginning at age 16 years
Mutation analysis:
  These studies are performed in specialized laboratories only. Mutation analysis may help predict the phenotype as more data become available.

---

[a]Limit exposure to radiation by using appropriate restraint and nonradiologic imaging studies.

When cytopenias are in the mild to moderate range and in the absence of cytogenetic abnormalities, counts should be monitored every 3–4 months and bone marrow aspiration should be performed yearly. Monitoring of blood counts and bone marrow should be increased for mild cytopenia in the presence of cytogenetic abnormalities without frank MDS. With falling (or in some cases rising) counts, surveillance must be increased.

Other management modalities include:

- *Androgen and cytokine therapy:* Androgen therapy (oxymetholone 2–5 mg/kg/day and tapered to the lowest effective dose) and cytokines (granulocyte colony-stimulating factor [G-CSF] or granulocyte-macrophage colony-stimulating factor [GM-CSF]) should be administered when moderate to severe cytopenia is present. Approximately 50% of patients will respond to androgens.
- *Transfusions:* Treatment with packed red blood cells and platelets should be minimized and reserved for patients who fail androgen therapy. Blood products

should be irradiated, leukocyte depleted, and of single donor origin, when possible. Blood relatives should not be used as blood donors until a matched allogeneic related donor transplant is ruled out. Iron status should be monitored at regular intervals to determine the degree of iron overload and the institution of chelation treatment in chronically transfused patients.

- *Allogeneic hematopoietic stem cell transplantation:* HLA typing should be done at diagnosis to facilitate therapeutic planning. Evidence of true MDS (as opposed to benign clonal abnormalities) or evolution to leukemia are clear indications for transplant. The sensitivity of FA patients to traditional transplant conditioning regimens requires the use of lower doses of chemotherapy and radiation therapy (page 677). Before a family member is used as a donor, the donor should be evaluated to exclude a diagnosis of Fanconi anemia.
- *Endocrine follow-up:* Patients should be periodically evaluated. The majority of patients with FA have short stature. Up to 50% of them are deficient in growth hormone. Because of a theoretical association of growth hormone and leukemia, growth hormone should be used with that understanding in patients with FA. Patients should be evaluated for the relatively common findings of hypothyroidism, diabetes mellitus, and reduced fertility.
- *Gene therapy:* This approach is experimental and will only be performed in approved clinical trials.

Prognosis

Current results of matched sibling transplantation prior to development of overt leukemia show a long-term disease-free survival of 80–90%. However, the long-term risks of late sequelae from hematopoietic stem cell transplantation, although not sufficiently understood, probably include an increase in cancer risk. Unrelated donor transplant should be reserved for androgen refractory patients and those with MDS or leukemia.

Dyskeratosis Congenita

Dyskeratosis congenita (DC) is characterized by ectodermal dysplasia and hematopoietic failure. The classic triad of ectodermal dysplasia consists of abnormal skin pigmentation, dystrophic nails, and leukoplakia of mucous membranes. In addition to the classic triad, there are a number of other somatic findings in DC. The most common of these are epiphora (tearing due to obstructed tear ducts), developmental delay, pulmonary disease, short stature, esophageal webs, dental caries, tooth loss, premature gray hair, and hair loss. Other ocular, dental, skeletal, cutaneous, genitourinary, gastrointestinal, and CNS abnormalities have also been reported.

The median age for the onset of mucocutaneous abnormalities is 6–8 years. Nail changes occur first. The median age for the onset of pancytopenia is 10 years. Approximately 50% of patients develop severe aplastic anemia and greater than 90% develop at least a single cytopenia by 40 years of age. The anemia is associated with a high MCV and elevated fetal hemoglobin. In a number of cases, aplastic anemia precedes the onset of abnormal skin, dystrophic nails, or leukoplakia. As with FA it is the nonhematologic manifestations of DC that are of particular concern especially when hematopoietic stem cell transplantation for bone marrow failure is considered.

Pathophysiology

Recent evidence establishes DC to be the result of deficient telomerase activity. Telomerase adds DNA sequence back to the ends of chromosomes that are eroded with each DNA replication. Telomerase activity is found in tissues with rapid turnover such as the basal layer of the epidermis, squamous epithelium of the oral cavity, hematopoietic stem cells and progenitors, and in other tissues affected in DC. The lack of telomerase activity also gives rise to chromosome instability resulting in the high rate of premature cancer observed in these tissues. Epithelial malignancies develop at or beyond the third decade of life. About one in five patients will develop progressive pulmonary disease characterized by fibrosis, resulting in diminished diffusion capacity and/or restrictive lung disease. Of note, type 2 alveolar epithelial cells express telomerase. It is likely that more pulmonary disease would be evident if patients did not succumb earlier to the complications of severe aplastic anemia and cancer.

Genetics

Dyskeratosis congenita is most commonly inherited as an X-linked recessive gene with 86% of patients being male, although some of these represent autosomal dominant or recessive inheritance. The gene responsible for the X-linked form was mapped to Xq28 and subsequently identified as *DKC1*. *DKC1* codes for dyskerin, a nucleolar protein associated with nucleolar RNAs. Dyskerin is also associated with the telomerase complex. This later function appears to be the one involved in the pathophysiology of DC, as the dominant form has recently been mapped to a gene that encodes telomerase RNA (*hTR*). Autosomal recessive forms have been inferred from pedigrees, in particular those described with brother–sister pairs in consanguineous families. All three genetic subtypes have many common features; however, autosomal recessive patients appear to have a more severe phenotype. Affected members within the same family may exhibit wide variability in clinical presentation, suggesting the influence of modifying genes and environmental factors.

Clinical Course

- *Bone marrow failure:* Sixty-seven percent of the deaths are a consequence of bone marrow failure, and 9% die of lung disease with or without HSCT.
- *Malignancy:* Almost 9% of patients develop cancer (MDS, Hodgkin disease, and carcinoma). The degree of predisposition to leukemia is yet to be clearly defined.
- *Immunodeficiency:* Significant progressive immunodeficiency occurs in DC. The vast majority of patients (80%), with or without neutropenia, die from infection, some opportunistic, usually before 30 years of age. Although DC is predominantly a cellular immune defect, it is reasonable to assume that immunodeficiency as well as neutropenia play a significant role in the infectious morbidity and mortality in DC.
- *Outcome:* Median survival of approximately 35 years for both X-linked and autosomal recessive forms of DC. There are too few autosomal dominant cases for such an analysis. The prognosis for patients with DC is poor.

Therapy

Responses to androgens, G-CSF or GM-CSF, as well as erythropoietin and rarely splenectomy, have been documented. However, for the most part these responses have been transient. Immunomodulatory therapy is ineffective. Supportive care with blood products, antibiotics, and antifibrinolytic agents is similar to that used for idiopathic aplastic anemia. Once these measures are required, HSCT should be considered for those patients with an HLA-matched related donor or an acceptable alternative donor and no DC-related contraindications. The results have been poor with failure due predominantly to pulmonary complications. All DC patients are at a high risk of interstitial pulmonary disease when undergoing HSCT. Unfortunately, there have been too few transplant survivors to determine whether an increase in the prevalence of cancer will follow as a consequence of HSCT. An immunoablative rather than a myeloablative approach may reduce the incremental risk of pulmonary toxicity as well as the potential for nonhematologic cancer risk.

Aplastic Anemias with Constitutional Chromosomal Abnormalities

Rare cases of aplastic anemia have been associated with Down syndrome; congenital trisomy-8 mosaicism; familial Robertsonian translocation (13;14); nonfamilial translocation in a male with t(1;20); (p22;q13.3) and cerebellar ataxia; bone marrow monosomy-7 manifesting prior to pancytopenia (familial ataxia–pancytopenia syndrome); and increased spontaneous chromosomal breakage without further increase in breakage with mitomycin C as well as other very rare cases with familial associations.

ACQUIRED APLASTIC ANEMIA
Pathophysiology

The effectiveness of immunosuppressive therapy implies that in many patients with acquired aplastic anemia, bone marrow failure results from an immunologically mediated, tissue-specific, organ-destructive mechanism. The fact that 50% of identical twins with severe aplastic anemia will not engraft with no conditioning after the infusion of syngeneic stem cells supports this notion in at least half the cases. A reasonable theory suggests that exposure to an inciting antigen, cells, and cytokines of the immune system destroys stem cells in the marrow, resulting in pancytopenia. Treatment with immunosuppressive modalities leads to marrow recovery.

Clinical and laboratory studies have suggested that interferon γ (IFN-γ) plays a central role in the pathophysiology of aplastic anemia. *In vitro* studies show that the T cells from aplastic anemia patients secrete IFN-γ and tumor necrosis factor (TNF). Long-term bone marrow cultures (LTBMCs) have shown that IFN-γ and TNF are potent inhibitors of both early and late hematopoietic progenitor cells. Both of these cytokines suppress hematopoiesis by their effects on the mitotic cycle and, more importantly, by the mechanism of cell killing. The mechanism of cell killing involves the pathway of apoptosis (i.e., IFN-γ and TNF unregulate each other's cellular receptors, as well as the Fas receptors in hematopoietic stem cells). Cytotoxic T cells also secrete interleukin-2 (IL-2), which causes polyclonal expansion of the T cells. Activation of the Fas receptor on the hematopoietic stem cell by the Fas ligand present on the lymphocytes leads to apoptosis of the targeted hematopoietic progenitor cells. Additionally, IFN-γ mediates its hematopoietic suppressive activity through interferon regulatory factor 1 (IRF-1), which inhibits the transcription of cellular genes and their entry into the cell cycle. IFN-γ also induces the production of the toxic gas nitric oxide, diffusion of which causes additional toxic effects on the hematopoietic progenitor cells. Direct cell–cell interactions between effective lymphocytes and targeted hematopoietic cells probably also occur.

In vivo observation in aplastic anemia patients supports the following *in vitro* findings:

1. IFN-γ messenger RNA, which is undetectable in normal marrow, is detectable in most patients with aplastic anemia.
2. Hematopoietic cells of patients with aplastic anemia express Fas receptors and, as a result, their marrow contains an increased number of apoptotic cells.
3. An increased number of activated cytotoxic lymphocytes are present in the blood and bone marrow of these patients.

4. Successful treatment with antithymocyte globulin and cyclosporine results in a decrease in the number of these cytotoxic cells.
5. The importance of immunosuppressive therapy was recognized when (a) an unexpected improvement in pancytopenia was observed in aplastic anemia patients following failure of engraftment in allogeneic bone marrow transplantation and (b) the need for immunosuppressive preparative therapy was realized for successful engraftment in about half of hematopoietic stem cells in identical twin bone marrow transplantation performed for aplastic anemia.

Table 6-16 shows an etiologic classification of aplastic anemia, and Table 6-17 lists the various causes of acquired aplastic anemia.

Table 6-16. An Etiologic Classification of Aplastic Anemia

Direct toxicity
  Radiation[a]
  Chemotherapy[a]
  Benzene[a]
  Intermediate metabolites of some common drugs
Immune-mediated causes
  Iatrogenic causes[a]
  Transfusion-associated graft versus host disease[a]
  Eosinophilic fasciitis[a]
  Hepatitis-associated disease[a]
  Pregnancy
  Intermediate metabolites of some common drugs
  Idiopathic aplastic anemia

[a]Indicates relatively well-established mechanism.
From Young NS, Macijewski J. The pathophysiology of acquired aplastic anemia. N Engl J Med 1997;336:1365–72, with permission.

Table 6-17. Causes of Acquired Aplastic Anemia[a]

I. Idiopathic (70% or more of cases)

II. Secondary
  A. Drugs[b]
    1. Predictable, dose dependent, rapidly reversible (affects rapidly dividing maturing hematopoietic cells rather than pluripotent stem cells)
      a. 6-Mercaptopurine
      b. Methotrexate
      c. Cyclophosphamide
      d. Busulfan
      e. Chloramphenicol
    2. Unpredictable, normal doses (defect or damage to pluripotent stem cells)
      a. Antibiotics: chloramphenicol, sulfonamides
      b. Anticonvulsants: mephenytoin (Mesantoin), hydantoin
      c. Antirheumatics: phenylbutazone, gold
      d. Antidiabetics: tolbutamide, chlorpropamide
      e. Antimalarial: quinacrine
  B. Chemicals: insecticides (e.g., DDT, Parathion, Chlordane)
  C. Toxins (e.g., benzene, carbon tetrachloride, glue, toluene)
  D. Irradiation
  E. Infections
    1. Viral hepatitis (hepatitis A, B, and C and non-A, non-B, non-C, and non-G hepatitis)
    2. HIV infection (AIDS)
    3. Infectious mononucleosis (Epstein–Barr virus)

(Continues)

Table 6-17. (*Continued*)

    4. Rubella[c]
    5. Influenza[c]
    6. Parainfluenza[c]
    7. Measles[c]
    8. Mumps[c]
    9. Venezuelan equine encephalitis
    10. Rocky Mountain spotted fever[c]
    11. Cytomegalovirus (in newborn)
    12. Herpes virus (in newborn)
    13. Chronic parvovirus
 F. Immunologic disorders
   Graft versus host reaction in transfused immunologically incompetent subjects
   X-linked lymphoproliferative syndrome (Chapter 13)
 G. Aplastic anemia preceding acute leukemia (hypoplastic preleukemia)
 H. Myelodysplastic syndromes (Chapter 13)
  I. Thymoma
  J. Paroxysmal nocturnal hemoglobinuria
 K. Malnutrition
    1. Kwashiorkor
    2. Marasmus[c]
    3. Anorexia nervosa[c]
 L. Pregnancy

[a]For an etiologic classification of aplastic anemia, see Table 6-16.
[b]Partial listing.
[c]Pancytopenia with temporary marrow hypoplasia.

The immune mechanism plays a central role in the pathophysiology of aplastic anemias caused by a variety of agents. For example:

Antigenetic stimulus (e.g., hepatitis virus, drug causing
idiosyncratic reaction, aberrantly expressed gene and its
protein product in a hematopoietic progenitor cell)

Aberrant cellular protein expression by hematopoietic progenitor (in hepatitis
viral protein expression, in idiosyncratic drug reaction expression of altered
cellular protein due to binding of drug/its products, or in hematopoietic
malignancy expression of genetically altered cellular protein)

Uptake of these aberrant proteins by antigen-presenting cells, which
process them into peptides. These peptides form cellular complexes
with major histocompatibility-complex molecules

Presentation of complexed peptides to naive T cells

Immune response

Destruction of aberrant antigen-expressing hematopoietic progenitor cells

Clinical Findings

Acquired aplastic anemia may be idiopathic or secondary. About 70% of cases are considered idiopathic, without an identifiable cause. The onset of acquired aplastic anemia is usually in retrospect gradual, and the symptoms are related to the pancytopenia:

1. Anemia results in pallor, easy fatigability, weakness, and loss of appetite.
2. Thrombocytopenia leads to petechiae, easy bruising, severe nosebleeds, and bleeding into the gastrointestinal and renal tracts.
3. Leukopenia leads to increased susceptibility to infections and oral ulcerations that respond poorly to antibiotic therapy.
4. Hepatosplenomegaly and lymphadenopathy do not occur; their presence suggests an underlying leukemia.
5. Hyperplastic gingivitis is also a symptom of aplastic anemia.

Laboratory Investigations

1. *Anemia:* Normocytic or macrocytic normochromic.
2. *Reticulocytopenia:* Absolute count more reliable.
3. *Leukopenia:* Granulocytopenia often less than 1500/mm^3.
4. *Thrombocytopenia:* Platelets often less than 30,000/mm^3.
5. *Fetal hemoglobin:* May be slightly to moderately elevated.
6. *Bone marrow:*
   a. Marked depression or absence of hematopoietic cells and replacement by fatty tissue–containing reticulum cells, lymphocytes, plasma cells, and usually tissue mast cells.
   b. Megaloblastic changes and other features indicative of dyserythropoiesis frequently seen in the erythroid precursors present.
   c. Bone marrow biopsy essential for diagnosis to exclude the possibility of poor aspiration technique or poor bone marrow sampling; additionally, rules out granulomas, myelofibrosis, or leukemia.
   d. Chromosomal analysis normal; rules out Fanconi anemia and myelodysplastic syndromes.
   e. Bone marrow cultures for infectious agent and/or DNA; antigen-based evaluation for infectious agent when indicated.
7. *Chromosome breakage assay:* Performed on peripheral blood to rule out Fanconi anemia.
8. *Flow cytometry (CD55/59):* Performed to exclude paroxysmal nocturnal hemoglobinuria.
9. *Physical examination, appropriate laboratory and imaging studies and if warranted mutation analysis:* Performed to rule out other inherited bone marrow failure syndrome (DC, DBA, SDS, CAT)
10. *Liver function chemistries:* Performed to exclude hepatitis.
11. *Renal function chemistries:* Performed to exclude renal disease.
12. *Viral serology testing:* Hepatitis A, B, and C antibody panel; Epstein–Barr virus antibody panel; parvovirus B19 and IgG and IgM antibodies; varicella antibody titer; cytomegalovirus antibody titer, etc.
13. *Quantitative immunoglobulins, C3, C4, and complement.*
14. *Autoimmune disease evaluation:* Antinuclear antibody (ANA), total hemolytic complement (CH50), Coombs' test.
15. *HLA typing:* Patient and family done at the time of diagnosis of severe aplastic anemia to ensure a timely transplant.

16. *Blood group typing:* On the patient.
17. *Clotting profile:* Prothrombin time (PT), activated partial thromboplastin time (APTT), fibrinogen.

Severity

Severe aplastic anemia is defined as a bone marrow cellularity of less than 25% and at least two of the following findings: granulocyte count, $<500/mm^3$ ($<200/mm^3$ in very severe aplastic anemia); platelet count, $<20,000/mm^3$; and reticulocyte count, $<40,000/mm^3$. The definition of mild and moderate aplastic anemia varies among researchers and institutions.

Table 6-18 lists the recommendations for the treatment of moderate and severe aplastic anemia. Table 6-19 lists the favorable and unfavorable prognostic factors in acquired aplastic anemia.

Treatment

Supportive Care

1. Avoid exposure to hazardous drugs and toxins.
2. The risk of serious bleeding and symptomatic anemia must be balanced against the risk of transfusion sensitization and iron overload. Unless symptomatic,

---

Table 6-18. Recommendations for Treatment of Aplastic Anemia

1. Moderate aplastic anemia:
   Observe with close follow-up and supportive care
   If the patient develops:
   a. Severe aplastic anemia
      and/or
   b. Severe thrombocytopenia with significant bleeding
      and/or
   c. Chronic anemia requiring transfusion treatments
      and/or
   d. Serious infections
   Then treat with the same recommended therapy for severe aplastic anemia
2. Severe aplastic anemia:
   Allogeneic bone marrow transplantation when HLA-matched sibling donor available
   In the absence of an HLA-matched sibling marrow donor:
   Treat the patient with ATG, cyclosporine A (CSA), methylprednisolone, and growth factors such as G-CSF or GM-CSF
   If no response or waning of response and recurrence of severe aplastic anemia, a second course of immunosuppressive therapy is not recommended since the use of a second course is controversial. The following is recommended:
   a. HLA-matched (genotypic matched preferred) unrelated bone marrow, peripheral blood or umbilical cord blood transplant if a suitable donor is available. In the absence of availability of such a donor an HLA-mismatched (1 antigen) bone marrow or mismatched (1-2 antigens) umbilical cord transplant is recommended
   b. High-dose cyclophosphamide and cyclosporine therapy without stem cell transplant is carried out in some institutions

---

Notes: Partial response: absence of infections and transfusion dependency and sustained increase in all cell counts as follows: reticulocyte count, $\geq20,000/mm^3$; platelet count, $\geq20,000/mm^3$; absolute neutrophil count, $\geq500/mm^3$. Complete response: Normal counts. Partial response and complete response are considered as responses for the evaluation of the success of immunosuppressive therapy.

Table 6-19. Prognostic Factors in Acquired Aplastic Anemia

Factor	Favorable	Unfavorable
Granulocyte count	>500/mm^3	<500/mm^3 (<200/mm^3 is more unfavorable)
Platelet count	>20.000/mm^3	<20.000/mm^3
Bone marrow	Retained cellular elements	Totally aplastic with <20% hematopoietic cells remaining
Age	Younger	Older
Hemorrhagic manifestations	Absent	Present
Infection	Absent	Present

transfusions of red cells and platelets should be reserved for patients with hemoglobin levels and platelet counts of around 7 g/dL and 10,000/mm^3, respectively. Performance of HSCT as rapidly as is feasible minimizes transfusions in patients undergoing histocompatible HSCT. To avoid sensitization to transplant antigens, there should be no transfusions from blood relatives and transfusions should be restricted, if possible, to single unrelated donors to decrease the likelihood of sensitization to donor antigens. In all patients blood products should be leukocyte depleted to reduce the risk of sensitization and CMV infection. CMV-negative blood products should be used when patients have negative serology for CMV and are potential candidates for HSCT.

Patients receiving chronic red cell transfusion should be followed for evidence of iron overload and chelated appropriately. The use of single donor platelets, when available, is recommended. In females, menses should be suppressed by the use of oral contraceptives. Drugs that impair platelet function, such as aspirin, should be avoided. Intramuscular injections should be given carefully, followed by ice pack application to injection sites.

3. The antifibrinolytic agent epsilon aminocaproic acid (Amicar) can be used to reduce mucosal bleeding in thrombocytopenic patients with good hepatic and renal function. Hematuria is a contraindication to its use. A dose of 100 mg/kg/dose every 6 hours is used. The maximum daily dose is 24 grams. Teeth should be brushed with a cloth or soft toothbrush.

4. Avoid infection. Keep patients out of the hospital as much as possible. Good dental care is important. Rectal temperatures should not be taken, and the rectal areas should be kept clean and free of fissures. If a patient is febrile:

   a. Culture possible sources, including blood, sputum, urine, stool, skin, and sometimes spinal fluid and bone marrow for aerobes, anaerobes, fungi, viruses, and tubercle bacilli.

   b. Patients with fever and neutropenia should be treated with broad-spectrum antibiotic coverage (Chapter 26). The specific therapy depends on the clinical status of the patient, the presence of indwelling vascular access devices, and knowledge of the local flora pending specific culture results and antibiotic sensitivities. In patients who remain febrile 4–7 days in the face of broad antibacterial coverage, antifungal therapy with amphotericin B should be started empirically. Therapy should be continued until the patient is afebrile and cultures are negative or a specific organism is identified. An appropriate course of therapy is administered if an organism is identified. In the presence of perirectal infection, clindamycin or Flagyl should be added for anaerobic coverage.

5. Maintain hemoglobin level. Prior to any transfusion, perform complete blood group typing to minimize the risk of sensitization to minor blood group antigens and to permit identification of antibodies should they subsequently develop.

6. Patients who were previously treated with immunosuppressive therapy should receive irradiated cellular blood products to prevent complications of GVHD. Patients receiving immunosuppressive therapy should also receive *Pneumocystis carinii* prophylaxis with trimethoprim and sulfamethoxazole (Bactrim/Septra). No antibacterial prophylaxis should be administered to afebrile, neutropenic patients.

Patients with mild to moderate aplastic anemia should be observed for spontaneous improvement or complete resolution. The treatment of choice for SAA, for patients who have an HLA-matched related donor, is hematopoietic stem cell transplantation. An increasing number of centers are treating moderate aplastic anemia in a fashion similar to SAA.

Specific Therapy

Hematopoietic Stem Cell Transplantation

As soon as the diagnosis of SAA is suspected in children, HLA typing should be performed where potential donors exist. Patients with related histocompatible donors (complete HLA match or a mismatch at a single HLA-A or -B locus) should have an HSCT as soon as possible (complete investigations to exclude FA, paroxysmal nocturnal hemoglobinuria (PNH), or other inherited bone marrow failure syndromes should be carried out) because the risk of transplant-related morbidity and mortality increases with increasing age, an increasing interval from diagnosis to transplant, multiple transfusions, and the occurrence of serious infections.

Because graft rejection is the major cause of morbidity and mortality in HSCT for SAA, the pretransplantation preparative regimen of cyclophosphamide (Cytoxan) and antithymocyte globulin, ATG (ATGAM/thymoglobulin) with the inclusion of cyclosporin A (CSA [Sandimmune]) in the GVHD prophylaxis regimen is designed to be highly immunosuppressive. Table 6-20 lists the HSCT preparative regime for SAA. Even when an identical twin donor is used, a similar preparatory regimen is recommended. Long-term survival in the range of 90% can be expected with HSCT using histocompatible related donors. The overall risk of unrelated or mismatched related donor transplantation precludes its use as a front-line therapy for SAA at this time. However, as improved HLA typing, preparative regimens, and

Table 6-20. Hematopoietic Stem Cell Transplantation Preparative Regimen for Severe Aplastic Anemia

Day –5	Morning: Cyclophosphamide, 50 mg/kg IV over 1 hour.
	Afternoon: ATG, 30 mg/kg IV. First dose of ATG is given over 8 hours; subsequent doses are given over 4 hours.
This is repeated on Day –4 and Day –3.	
Day –2	Morning: Cyclophosphamide, 50 mg/kg IV over 1 hour.
Day –1	Rest, cyclosporine A, 10 mg/kg/day PO daily adjusted for serum levels.
Day 0	Marrow infusion

Abbreviation: ATG = antithymocyte globulin.
From Vlachos A, Lipton JM. In: Conn's Current Therapy, WB Saunders Company, 2002, with permission.

GVHD prophylaxis are utilized, HSCT will become available to a wider group of patients with SAA.

Immunosuppressive Therapy

Patients unable to undergo HSCT (because no suitable donor is present) should have immunosuppressive therapy based on ATG and CSA, which have become the treatment of choice for these patients. In addition to ATG and CSA corticosteroids, methylprednisolone (Solu-Medrol) or prednisolone (prednisone) is added to prevent serum sickness. GM-CSF (Leukine) or G-CSF (Neupogen) is used to achieve a more rapid increment in the granulocyte count. Short term, the survival using this approach is in the range of 85%.

The regimen of ATG, methylprednisolone, GM-CSF, and CSA treatment for severe aplastic anemia is listed in Table 6-21.

The following criteria are used for exclusion of treatment of patients with immunosuppressive drugs:

1. Serum creatinine, >2 mg%
2. Concurrent pregnancy
3. Sexually active females who refuse contraceptives
4. Patients with concurrent hepatic, renal, cardiac, or metabolic problems of such severity that death is likely to occur within 7–10 days or moribund patients.

Antithymocyte globulin

Test dose. An intradermal ATG test dose should be carried out prior to ATG treatment. The skin test procedure consists of injection of 0.1 mL of a 1:1000 dilution of ATG in 0.9% sodium chloride solution for injection (5 µg equine IgG). A control using 0.9% sodium chloride injection is administered on the contralateral side. Allergy is indicated by erythema greater than 5 mm compared to the saline control, developing

---

Table 6-21. Immunosuppressive Therapy for Severe Aplastic Anemia

1. Antithymocyte globulin: ATGAM antithymocyte globulin (equine) (Pharmacia) 20 mg/kg/day IV once daily, or thymoglobulin (antithymocyte globulin [rabbit], Sang stat) 2.0 mg/kg/day IV once daily days 1 to 8. Diphenhydramine (Benadryl) and Acetominophen (Tylenol) are given as premedication to ATG.
2. Methylprednisolone, 2 mg/kg/day IV days 1 to 8. Divide into 0.5 mg/kg/dose IV every 6 hours.
3. Prednisone taper following an 8-day course of IV methylprednisolone. On days 9 and 10, prednisone, 1.5 mg/kg/day PO to be divided into two equal daily doses. On days 11 and 12, prednisone, 1 mg/kg/day PO to be divided into two equal daily doses. On days 13 and 14, prednisone, 0.5 mg/kg/day PO to be divided into two equal daily doses. On day 15, prednisone, 0.25 mg/kg/day PO to be given in one dose.
4. G-CSF, 5 µg/kg/day, or GM-CSF, 250 µg/m^2/day SC once daily before bedtime starting on day 5. G-CSF or GM-CSF is to be continued until an absolute neutrophil count of > 1000/mm^3 is reached. G-CSF or GM-CSF should then be tapered.
5. CSA, 10 mg/kg/day PO initially starting on day 1. Divide into two equal daily doses. Serum drug levels should be monitored as needed with the first level at 72 hours after initiation of therapy. CSA dose to be adjusted to keep serum trough levels between 100 and 300 ng/mL. CSA should be continued until patient is transfusion independent and GM-CSF has been discontinued; then decrease the dose by 2.0 mg/kg every 2 weeks.

Abbreviations: CSA, cyclosporine (formerly cyclosporin A); GM-CSF, granulocyte-macrophage colony-stimulating factor.

Modified from Vlachos A, Lipton JM. In: Conn's Current Therapy. Philadelphia: WB Saunders, 2002.

within the first hour of the skin test. The patient should also be observed for signs and symptoms of systemic allergic reaction. ATG doses are listed in Table 6-21.

Usual adverse reactions to ATG.

- *Thrombocytopenia:* All patients should receive a daily platelet transfusion on a prophylactic basis to maintain a platelet count of more than 20,000/mm^3 (during administration of ATG). Only irradiated and leukocyte-filtered cellular blood products should be used.
- *Headache, myalgia.*
- *Arthralgia, chills, and fever:* Treatment with an antihistamine and a corticosteroid is indicated.
- *Chemical phlebitis:* A central line (high flow vein) for infusion of ATG should be used and peripheral veins should be avoided.
- *Itching and erythema:* Treatment with an antihistamine with or without cortico-steroids is indicated.
- *Leukopenia.*
- *Serum sickness:* Many patients develop serum sickness approximately 7–10 days following ATG administration. This should be treated by increasing the daily dose of Solu-Medrol until the symptoms abate.

Uncommon adverse reactions to ATG. Dyspnea, chest/back/flank pain, diarrhea, nausea, vomiting, hypertension, herpes simplex infection, stomatitis, laryngospasm, anaphylaxis, tachycardia, edema, localized infection, malaise, seizures, gastrointestinal bleeding/perforation, thrombophlebitis, lymphadenopathy, hepatosplenomegaly, renal function impairment, liver function abnormalities, myocarditis, and congestive heart failure.

CSA preparations

CSA preparations include:

- Neoral oral solution, 100 mg/mL
- Neoral capsule or Sandimmune capsule, 25 mg and 100 mg/capsule.

Oral CSA solution may be mixed with milk, chocolate milk, or orange juice preferably at room temperature. It should be stirred well and drunk at once.

Cyclosporine levels should be performed once a week for the first 2 weeks and then once every 2 weeks for the remainder of the treatment or as necessary to maintain a whole-blood CSA level between 200 and 400 ng/mL. Changes in serum creatinine levels are the principal criteria for dose change. An increase in creatinine level of more than 30% above baseline warrants a reduction in the dose of CSA by 2 mg/kg/day each week until the creatinine level has returned to normal. A serum CSA level of less than 100 ng/mL is evidence of inadequate absorption, and a CSA level above 500 ng/mL is considered an excessive dose. If the CSA level is greater than 500 ng/mL, CSA should be discontinued. Levels should be repeated daily or every other day. When the level returns to 200 ng/mL or less, CSA should be resumed at a 20% reduced dose.

Principal side effects of CSA. Renal dysfunction, tremor, hirsutism, hypertension, and gum hyperplasia.

Uncommon side effects of CSA. Significant hyperkalemia, hyperuricemia, hypomagnesemia, hepatotoxicity, lipemia, central nervous system toxicity, and gynecomastia. An increase of more than 100% in the bilirubin level or of liver enzymes is treated in the same way as an increase of more than 30% in creatinine and warrants a reduction in the dose of CSA by 2 mg/kg/day each week until the bilirubin and/or liver enzymes return to the normal range.

Contraindications to the use of CSA. Hypersensitivity to CSA.

Pharmacokinetic interactions with CSA.

1. *Carbamazepine, phenobarbital, phenytoin, rifampin:* Decreases half-life and blood levels of CSA.
2. *Sulfamethazine/trimethoprim IV:* Decreases serum levels of CSA.
3. *Erythromycin, fluconazole, ketoconazole, nifedipine:* Increases blood levels of CSA.
4. *Imipenem-cilastatin:* Increases blood levels of CSA and central nervous system toxicity.
5. *Methylprednisolone (high dose), prednisolone:* Increases plasma levels of CSA.
6. *Metoclopramide (Reglan):* Increases absorption and increases plasma levels of CSA.

Pharmacologic interactions with CSA.

1. *Aminoglycosides, amphotericin B, nonsteroidal anti-inflammatory drugs, trimethoprim/sulfamethoxazole:* Nephrotoxicity.
2. *Melphalan, quinolones:* Nephrotoxicity.
3. *Methylprednisolone:* Convulsions.
4. *Azathioprine, corticosteroids, cyclophosphamide:* Increases immunosuppression, infections, malignancy.
5. *Verapamil:* Increases immunosuppression.
6. *Digoxin:* Elevates digoxin level with toxicity.
7. *Nondepolarizing muscle relaxants:* Prolongs neuromuscular blockade.

Hematopoietic growth factors

The addition of human recombinant G-CSF or GM-CSF to a regimen of ATG, cyclosporine, and corticosteroids provides improved protection from infectious complications by stimulating granulopoiesis. The regimen we recommend uses GM-CSF and G-CSF interchangeably.

Treatment Choices and Long Term Follow-Up

Although the short-term outcome with immunosuppressive therapy is comparable to that obtained with HLA-matched related HSCT, the decision to choose HSCT for younger patients who have a histocompatible donor is based on the result of long-term follow-up. Although there is some late mortality, due to chronic GVHD and therapy-related cancer, in patients undergoing HSCT for SAA, the survival curves are relatively flat. Improved GVHD prophylaxis and safer preparative regimens should further improve these results. In contrast, the risk of clonal hematopoietic disorders such as MDS, AML, and PNH is unacceptably high relative to both the short- and long-term risks of HSCT. Those undergoing immunomodulation must be closely followed for the development of clonal disorders. In terms of unrelated or poorly matched related donor HSCT, current risks favor the use of immunomodulatory therapy in those patients with SAA who cannot receive a matched related HSCT.

Salvage Therapy

For the patient who fails HSCT, has a partial response (ANC $\geq 500/mm^3$, but still is red cell and platelet transfusion dependent), or relapses following immunomodulatory therapy, management choices include alternative donor HSCT or further immunosuppressive therapy. These choices are under evaluation.

Children and teenagers for whom a fully HLA-matched unrelated donor, determined by high-resolution typing, exists are good candidates for an alternative donor HSCT. A delay in transplantation, along with the associated risk of infection and additional transfusions attendant to a second course of immune therapy, seems unwarranted in this setting. For older patients and those without a good alternative donor, preliminary data suggest that high-dose cyclophosphamide may be more effective than a second course of ATG/CSA/G-CSF. Androgens and alternative cytokines are being evaluated and should be considered experimental.

High-Dose Cyclophosphamide Therapy

Complete remission in severe aplastic anemia after high-dose cyclophosphamide therapy without bone marrow transplantation has been reported. The use of high-dose cyclophosphamide is controversial due to considerable toxicity reported by some investigators. The rationale for the use of high-dose cyclophosphamide is as follows:

1. The majority of patients with severe aplastic anemia lack an HLA-identical sibling for treatment with bone marrow transplantation.
2. Although the majority (80%) of children with severe aplastic anemia benefit from the use of treatment with ATG and cyclosporine, many do not attain completely normal counts and some patients treated successfully with immunosuppressive therapy either relapse or develop late clonal diseases such as paroxysmal nocturnal hemoglobinuria, myelodysplastic syndrome, or acute leukemia.
3. After preparation with cyclophosphamide, most allografts persist indefinitely; however, in several cases, a complete autologous reconstitution of hematopoiesis has occurred.
4. Patients with very severe aplastic anemia (i.e., severe aplastic anemia patients with an absolute neutrophil count of less than 200/mm^3 at diagnosis) respond to immunosuppressive therapy, but have greater morbidity and mortality due to the profound neutropenia.

On this basis, patients with severe aplastic anemia who lack an HLA-identical sibling donor have been treated by some clinicians on high-dose cyclophosphamide as a single course. Table 6-22 lists the high-dose cyclophosphamide therapy regimen for severe aplastic anemia.

Long-Term Sequelae and Outcomes for Severe Aplastic Anemia

Table 6-23 lists the long-term sequelae following treatment of aplastic anemia. Outcomes for both immunosuppressive therapy and HSCT have improved considerably.

1. Survival rates of greater than 80% have been realized with both immunosuppressive therapy or stem cell transplantation. Stem cell transplantation is curative for most patients.

Table 6-22. High-Dose Cyclophosphamide Therapy for Severe Aplastic Anemia

1. Cyclophosphamide,[a] 45 mg/kg/day IV × 4 days
2. Mesna (Mesnex),[a] 360 mg/m^2/dose IV with cyclophosphamide, as a 3-hourly infusion after cyclophosphamide, and as bolus at hours 6, 9, and 12 hours following cyclophosphamide
3. GM-CSF, 250 μg/M^2/day SC starting 24 hours after fourth dose of cyclophosphamide and to continue until absolute neutrophil count >1000/mm^3

Abbreviation: GM-CSF, granulocyte-macrophage colony-stimulating factor.
[a]Not FDA approved for this indication.
From Vlachos A, Lipton JM. In: Conn's Current Therapy. Philadelphia: WB Saunders, 2002, with permission.

Table 6-23. Long-Term Sequelae Following Treatment of Aplastic Anemia[a]

Sequelae	Type of therapy and incidence of complications	
	Immunosuppressive therapy (%)	Bone marrow transplantation (%)
10-Year cumulative cancer incidence	18.8	3.1
10-Year cumulative myelodysplastic syndrome (MDS) incidence	9.6	0.0
10-Year cumulative acute leukemia (AL) incidence	6.6	0.25
10-Year cumulative solid tumor (ST) incidence	2.2	2.9

Conclusion: Survivors of aplastic anemia are at high risk of developing late malignancies. Incidence of MDS and AL is higher in patients treated with immunosuppressive therapies; however, the incidence of ST is the same in both transplantation and immunosuppressive treated patients.

[a]Report of European Bone Marrow Transplantation Working Party on severe aplastic anemia.

2. Immunosuppressive therapy improves hematopoiesis and achieves transfusion independence in the majority of patients, but the time to response is long, hematopoietic response may be partial, and relapses are relatively common.
3. Clonal hematopoietic disorders including PNH, myelodysplasia, and leukemia may develop in up to 10% of patients treated with immunosuppressive therapy (IST). An analysis of 1765 patients with acquired aplastic anemia treated with either sibling transplant ($n = 583$) or IST ($n = 1182$) produced the following results:
   a. Matched sibling donor HSCT is always superior in young patients (<20 years of age) at any neutrophil count.
   b. Immunosuppression is superior in older patients (41–50 years) with a neutrophil count greater than 0.5×10^9/L.
   c. For the 21- to 40-years-of-age group, the differences are less clear.
   d. In all age groups there is a higher percentage of late failures for the immunosuppression-treated patients.
   e. The difference in survival between patients treated with HSCT and immunosuppression is not linear, but increases with time. For the younger group of patients, a 10% advantage in favor of HSCT at 1 year became a 19% advantage at 5 years.
   f. There is a higher risk of late death in patients treated with immunosuppressive therapy due to complications, including relapse and evolution to clonal disorders.

The European Bone Marrow Transplantation Working Party compared the rate of secondary malignancies following HSCT and IST. Forty-two malignancies developed in 860 patients receiving IST, compared to 9 in 748 patients who underwent HSCT. In this study, acute leukemia and myelodysplasia were seen exclusively in IST-treated patients, whereas the incidence of solid tumors was similar in the two groups of patients.

Treatment of Moderate Aplastic Anemia

The natural history of moderate aplastic anemia is uncertain and clinical experience varies widely. For this reason, it is generally thought that these patients should be treated initially with supportive therapy with very close follow-up. Those patients who progress to develop severe aplastic anemia and/or significant and severe thrombocytopenia and bleeding, serious infections, or a chronic red blood transfusion requirement should be treated with the same treatment options as described for severe aplastic anemia.

SIDEROBLASTIC ANEMIAS (MITOCHONDRIAL DISEASES WITH BONE MARROW FAILURE SYNDROMES)

The sideroblastic anemias are a heterogeneous group of mitochondrial disorders characterized by:

- Anemia that may be normocytic, normochromic or microcytic, and hypochromic except in Pearson syndrome, which is characterized by macrocytic anemia probably due to fetal-like erythropoiesis
- Reticulocytopenia
- Ineffective erythropoiesis (i.e., erythroid hyperplasia in bone marrow despite anemia)
- Presence of iron-loaded normoblasts demonstrated as ring sideroblasts (greater than 10% of erythroid precursor) by Pearls' Prussian blue stain (This stain serves as a surrogate technique for electron microscopy or energy dispersive x-ray analysis used for the demonstration of iron-loaded mitochondria in normoblasts.)
- Mild to moderate hemolysis due to peripheral red blood cell destruction of unknown etiology

The sideroblastic anemias can arise from the primary or secondary defects of mitochondria. In congenital sideroblastic anemias, iron rings are predominantly seen in late normoblasts (i.e., orthochromatic and polychromatophilic normoblasts), whereas they are seen in earlier erythroid cells (i.e., basophilic normoblasts) in the acquired form. Table 6-24 shows a classification of the sideroblastic anemias.

Table 6-24. Classification of Sideroblastic Anemias

I. **Primary mitochondrial defects** (i.e., involving 2.7 to 7.767 kb deletional lesion of mitochondrial DNA)
  A. Pearson syndrome (refractory sideroblastic anemia with vacuolization of bone marrow precursors and exocrine pancreatic dysfunction) characterized by:
      Refractory aregenerative macrocytic sideroblastic anemia; thrombocytopenia and neutropenia less significant
      Increased fetal hemoglobin
      Vacuolization of marrow precursors (erythroid and granulocytic series)
      Low birth weight
      Exocrine pancreatic dysfunction
      Hepatic failure, chronic diarrhea
      Severe lactic acidosis
      Diabetes mellitus
      Renal tubular dysfunction
      No reported disease in siblings
  B. Expanded Pearson syndrome:
      Pearson syndrome with Kearns–Sayre syndrome (myopathy, pigmentary retinopathy, cardiac conduction defects, ophthalmoplegia). A mother of a patient with Pearson syndrome has been described to have Kearns–Sayre syndrome.
  C. Wolfram syndrome, also known by the acronym DIDMOAD (diabetes insipidus, diabetes mellitus, optic atrophy, and deafness) (Chapter 4 pages 64–65).

(Continues)

Table 6-24. (*Continued*)

II. **Secondary involvement of mitochondria**
   A. Congenital sideroblastic anemia due to mutations of nuclear DNA
      1. X-linked recessive defect due to point mutation in the gene for erythroid-specific δ-aminolevulinic acid synthase (ALA-S2)
      2. Autosomal dominant sideroblastic anemia
      3. Autosomal recessive sideroblastic anemia
   B. Acquired sideroblastic anemias
      1. Drugs and toxins:
         Chloramphenicol—inhibits mitochondrial protein necessary for normal electron transfer and energy generation
         Isoniazid—inhibits ALA-S
         Cycloserine—inhibits ALA-S
         Lead—inhibits ALA-S, ferrochelatase, δ-aminolevulinic acid dehydratase
         Ethanol—inhibits multiple aspects of mitochondrial function
      2. Sideroblastic anemia of myelodysplastic syndromes:
         In some patients with refractory anemia with ringed sideroblasts (RARS), heteroplastic mutations of mitochondrial DNA affecting subunit 1 of cytochrome C oxidase
      3. Sideroblastic anemias of systemic (rheumatoid arthritis, polyarteritis nodosa), metabolic (pyridoxine responsive anemia), and malignant disorders (leukemia, carcinoma)
      4. Idiopathic sideroblastic anemias
      5. Pyridoxine—responsive anemia

Pathophysiology

Heme biosynthesis involves eight enzymes, four of which are cytoplasmic and four of which are localized in the mitochondria.

There are two distinct types of δ-aminolevulinic acid synthase (ALA-S): ALA-S1 (housekeeping form) occurs in nonerythroid cells and its gene maps on the autosome, and ALA-S2 (erythroid-specific form) occurs in erythroid cells and its gene maps on the X chromosome. Distinct aspects of heme synthesis regulation in nonerythroid and erythroid cells are related to the differences between these two ALA-S enzymes. In nonerythroid cells, the synthesis and activity of ALA-S1 is subject to feedback inhibition by heme, thus making ALA-S1 the rate-limiting enzyme for the heme pathway. In erythroid cells, heme does not inhibit either the activity or the synthesis of ALA-S2, but it does inhibit cellular iron uptake from transferrin without affecting its utilization for heme synthesis.

Table 6-25 shows the distinct features of iron and heme metabolism in erythroid and nonerythroid cells. These differences explain the large amount of heme production by erythroid cells compared to the low amount produced by non-erythroid cells. They also explain the mitochondrial deposition of iron in iron-loaded erythroid precursors.

Sideroblastic anemias result from injury to the mitochondria. Defects attributed to the mitochondrial pathways of heme synthesis result in sideroblastic anemias. Mitochondrial injury results from:

- Defective heme synthesis and the accumulation of iron, especially in erythroid precursors. This iron accumulation causes oxidative damage to the mitochondrial machinery through a Fenton reaction (i.e., the formation of a hydroxyl radical catalyzed by iron and reactive oxygen species damaging mitochondrial DNA by cross-linking DNA strands or by promoting the formation of DNA protein cross links).
- Congenital deletions of mitochondrial DNA.

Table 6-25. Iron and Heme Metabolism: Distinct Features in Erythroid Cells

	Erythroid	Nonerythroid*
Iron		
Iron Source	Exclusivity Tf	Tf + non-Tf Fe
Tf receptors	Differentiation ↑	
	Proliferation ↑	
	Differentiation ↓	
+Fe	Little change	↓↓
Regulation	Transcriptional	Primary mRNA stability
Effect of heme on FE uptake from Tf	Inhibits	No Effect
Fe overload	Mitochondria	Cytosol ferritin (never mitochondria)
Heme	Non Covalent assoc. with globin	Covalent binding to cytochromes
Content	Very high	Trace
Major function	O_2 transport	e^- transport
Control of Synthesis	Fe from Tf	ALA-S
Effect of ALA-S	Translational induction by Fe (IRE in 5' UTR)	Feedback repression by heme (no IRE)
Heme Oxygenase	mRNA↓ during erythroid differentiation	Induced by heme

*"Nonerythroid" cells, in this context, are represented by transformed cells grown in tissue cultures and hepatocytes; it is possible that some specialized cells (eg, macrophages) have other specific iron/heme metabolism characteristics.

Abbreviation: Tf, transferrin; ALA-S, aminolevulinic acid Synthase; IRE, iron-responsive element; 5'UTR, 5' untranslated region.

From Ponka P. Tissue-specific regulation of iron metabolism and heme synthesis: distinct control mechanism in erythroid cells. Blood 1997;89:1-25, with permission.

Toxins or drugs responsible for causing sideroblastic anemia should be eliminated. Oral pyridoxine is used in some patients with either congenital or acquired sideroblastic anemia with partial response.

As a result of mitochondrial damage, there is increased deposition of iron in heme-containing cells (e.g., erythroid cells). Additionally, there is decreased oxidative phosphorylation and decreased adenosine triphosphate (ATP) synthesis in many organs as observed in Pearson syndrome. Figure 6-2 shows a simplified view of the pathophysiologic relationship of various mitochondrial diseases in the context of sideroblastic anemias, bone marrow failure, and/or mitochondrial cytopathies.

Sideroblastic anemia in children is often secondary to defects in the enzymes of the heme biosynthetic pathway, namely, ALA-S deficiency. Impaired production of heme resulting from defects in these enzymes results in mitochondrial iron accumulation, damage to the mitochondrial machinery, and formation of ring sideroblasts. Porphyrias, however, do not display sideroblastic anemia because they are characterized by defects in the cytoplasmic steps of heme synthesis.

Toxins or drugs responsible for causing sideroblastic anemia should be eliminated. Oral pyridoxine is used in some patients with either congenital or acquired sideroblastic anemia with partial response.

Treatment

Treatment of Pearson Syndrome

1. Correction of the metabolic acidosis (e.g., avoidance of fasting, administration of thiamine, riboflavin, carnitine, and coenzyme Q to bypass deleted respiratory enzymes).

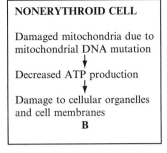

ERYTHROID CELL NORMOBLAST	NONERYTHROID CELL

Involvement of A alone: Sideroblastic anemia without mitochondrial cytopathy
Involvement of B alone: Mitochondrial cytopathies without sideroblastic anemia
Involvement of A and B: Sideroblastic anemias with mitochondrial cytopathies, e.g., Pearson syndrome, Pearson syndrome with Kearns–Sayre syndrome, Wolfram syndrome

Fig. 6-2. Simplified view of pathophysiologic consequences of mitochondrial diseases.

2. Removal of the reactive oxygen radical by the use of ascorbate, vitamin E, or lipoic acid.
3. The diagnosis of anemia occurs between 1 and 6 months in the majority of patients. Patients can be supported with red cell transfusions. G-CSF may be used to support clinically significant neutropenia. If patients do not succumb to metabolic acidosis and organ failure, the majority will improve within the first decade of life.
4. Patients who survive and have resolution of their anemia are at risk of developing Kearns–Sayre syndrome.
5. No experience exists with HSCT or solid organ transplantation.

Note that the efficacy of therapies 1 and 2 listed above is not clear at this time.

PAROXYSMAL NOCTURNAL HEMOGLOBINURIA

PNH is a condition in which hemolytic anemia results from an acquired abnormality of the red blood cell membrane that increases its sensitivity to complement-induced hemolysis.

Pathogenesis

Patients with PNH have a somatic mutation in the *PIG-A* gene (phosphatidylinositol glycan complementation group A). This mutation occurs in primitive hematopoietic stem cells.

A protein product (probably α-1,6N-acetylglucosamine transferase) of the *PIG-A* gene is normally responsible for the transfer of *N*-acetylglucosamine to phosphatidylinositol. In patients with PNH, there is a mutation in the *PIG-A* gene, which results in a decrease in its protein product and leads to a metabolic block in the biosynthesis of the glycolipid (i.e., glycosyl phosphatidylinositol [GPI]) anchor. This anchoring molecule is required for several surface proteins of the hematopoietic cells.

Table 6-26 lists the surface proteins missing on PNH blood cells as a result of a deficiency in the GPI anchor. Thus, the primary defect in PNH resides in the deficient assembly of the GPI anchor and, as a result, all GPI-linked antigens are absent on the surface of PNH cells.

Table 6-26. Surface Proteins Missing on Paroxysmal Nocturnal Hemoglobinuria Blood Cells

Antigen	Expression pattern
Enzymes	
Acetylcholinesterase (AChE)	Red blood cells
Ecto-5-nucleotidase (CD73)	Some B and T lymphocytes
Neutrophil alkaline phosphatase (NAP)	Neutrophils
Adhesion molecules	
Blast-1/CD48	Lymphocytes
Lymphocyte function-associated antigen-3 (LFA-3 or CD58)	All blood cells[a]
Complement regulating surface proteins	
Decay accelerating factor (DAF or CD55)	All blood cells[b]
Homologous restriction factor (HRF or C8bp)	All blood cells[c]
Membrane inhibitor of reactive lysis (MIRL or CD59)	All blood cells
Receptors	
Fcγ receptor III (Fcγ III or CD16)	Neutrophils, NK cells,[d] Macrophages,[d] some T lymphocytes[d]
Monocyte differentiation antigen (CD14)	Monocytes, macrophages, granulocytes
Urokinase-type plasminogen activator receptor (u-PAR)	Monocytes, granulocytes
Blood group antigens	
Comer antigens (DAF)	Red blood cells
Yt antigens (AChE)	Red blood cells
Holley Gregory antigen	Red blood cells
John Milton Hagen antigen (JMH)	Red blood cells, lymphocytes
Dombrock residue	Red blood cells
Neutrophil antigens	
NA1/NA2 (CD16)	Neutrophils
NB1/NB2	Neutrophils
Other surface proteins of unknown functions	
CD52 (CAMPATH)	All blood cells
CD24	B lymphocytes, neutrophils, eosinophils
CD48	
CD66c	
CD67	
JMH-bearing protein	

[a]On lymphocytes expressed in GPI-linked and transmembrane form.

[b]Level of expression on T lymphocytes varies.

[c]Expression of C8bp on human blood cells is controversial (personal communication. Taroh Kinoshita)

[d]Expressed in a transmembrane form.

From Young NS, Bressler M, Casper JT, Liu J. Biology and therapy of aplastic anemia. In: Schacter GP, McArthur TR, editors. Hematology 1996. American Society of Hematology, 1996; with permission; and Ware RE. Autoimmune hemolytic anemia. In: Nathan DG, Orkin SH, Ginsburg D, Look TA, editors. Nathan and Oski's Hematology of Infancy and Childhood. 6th ed. Philadelphia: WB Saunders, 2003, with permission.

Mechanism of Hemolysis and Hemoglobinuria in Paroxysmal Nocturnal Hemoglobinuria

The absence of surface complement-regulatory proteins, namely, CD55 and CD59, allows deposition of complement factors and C3 convertase complexes, which leads to chronic complement-mediated intravascular hemolysis, resulting in hemoglobinuria.

Mechanism of Hypercoagulable State

The mechanism of a hypercoagulable state in PNH is not well understood. Complement deposition on platelets results in vesiculations of their plasma membranes, which leads to increased procoagulant activity of the platelets. The monocytes and granulocytes of PNH cells lack the receptor for the GPI-linked urokinase plasminogen activator and this deficiency may lead to impaired fibrinolysis.

The antithrombin (AT), protein C, and protein S levels are normal in PNH patients.

Mechanism of Defective Hematopoiesis

The mechanism of defective hematopoiesis (macrocytosis with bone marrow erythroid dysplasia) evolving to severe aplastic anemia in some patients is not well understood. However, the following explanations have been considered:

- The initial step is the development of the *PIG-A* mutation. This is followed by a bone marrow insult.
- Resistance of PNH clones to injury by the insulting agents compared with susceptibility of normal hematopoietic stem cells.
- The intrinsic proliferation advantage of PNH stem cells compared with normal hematopoietic stem cells results in selection of abnormal stem cells followed by clonal expansion.
- Suppression of normal hematopoietic stem cells by PNH cells and evolution to MDS or AML

In the preceding list, it is assumed that two populations of stem cells normally reside in bone marrow: (1) a large population of normal stem cells and (2) a minor population of PNH stem cells.

Clinical Manifestations

The three main clinical features of PNH are (1) intravascular hemolysis, (2) bone marrow failure (macrocytosis, pancytopenia to severe aplastic anemia), and (3) the tendency to venous thrombosis. PNH can present as a primary "classic" hemolytic syndrome or it may arise during the course of aplastic anemia (AA) as AA-PNH syndrome. The nature of the pathogenetic link between the two conditions remains unknown. They may be differentiated from each other by the following clinical findings:

Findings	Classic PNH syndrome	Aplastic anemia-PNH syndrome
Hemolysis	Chronic with acute exacerbation.	Hemolysis clinically subtle.
Thrombotic complications	More often present. Acute hemolysis may be preceded by abdominal pain, thought to be due to temporary occlusion of the gastrointestinal veins. Thrombosis of larger abdominal veins may be present.	Occurs less frequently. Bone marrow failure predominantly the picture.
Abnormal erythrocyte or granulocyte CD55/CD59	Positive from the time of diagnosis.	Positive in 20–50% of patients with SAA. May evolve post immunosuppressive therapy.

Many patients have an overlap of the aforementioned findings and do not fit precisely into one of these two groups.

Course of the Disease

The onset of PNH is insidious. There is no familial tendency. Venous thrombosis is more often responsible for death than bone marrow failure in patients with PNH. Spontaneous long-term remission or leukemia transformation may occur in some patients.

Patients with classic PNH may have cytopenia of one or all blood cell lineages and the degree of bone marrow failure may vary from mild to severe. About 15% of patients with aplastic anemia develop overt PNH; however, 35–50% of aplastic anemia patients may have flow cytometric evidence of deficiency of GPI-linked molecules at some stage of their disease as evidence of subclinical PNH.

Complications

Intravascular hemolysis:

Hemoglobinuria (dark urine)
Iron deficiency
Acute renal failure.

Venous thrombosis:

Peripheral veins
Superior and inferior vena cava
Hepatic veins (Budd–Chiari syndrome)
Mesenteric veins
Sagittal sinus
Splenic vein
Abdominal wall veins
Intrathoracic veins.

Defective hematopoiesis:

Pancytopenia
Macrocytosis
Aplastic anemia
Evolution to AML.

Infectious:

Sinopulmonary
Blood borne.

Diagnosis

Table 6-27 lists the laboratory findings in PNH.

Flow Cytometric Analysis of GPI-Linked Molecules

Flow cytometric analysis of blood cells with the use of monoclonal antibodies to GPI-linked surface antigens is a very sensitive method for the diagnosis of PNH and has replaced the Ham test.

All blood cell lineages (i.e., red blood cells, lymphocytes, monocytes, granulocytes) can be analyzed by the flow cytometric technique. Heterogeneous patterns of the phenotypic expressions of various blood cells can be identified with the flow cytometric technique. For example, red blood cell phenotypes can be identified by their CD59 expression:

Table 6-27. Laboratory Findings in Paroxysmal Nocturnal Hemoglobinuria

Nonspecific findings	Cytopenia involving one or more cell lineages
	Macrocytosis, anisocytosis, polychromasia
	Reticulocytosis
	Decreased neutrophil alkaline phosphatase
	Increased level of lactate dehydrogenase
	Decreased haptoglobin
	Hemoglobinuria, hemosiderinuria
	Iron deficiency, folate deficiency
Bone marrow findings	Varies from hyperplastic with predominant erythropoiesis to hypoplastic with little or patchy hematopoiesis
	Hypoplasia or aplasia of one or more hematopoietic lineages
	Increased number of mast cells
Cytogenesis	Usually normal
Specific test for PNH	Flow cytometric analysis glycosyl phosphatidylinositol (GPI)-linked cell surface proteins (CD55/59) on peripheral blood or bone marrow cells.

Adapted from Young NS, Bressler M, Casper JT, Liu J. Biology and therapy of aplastic anemia. In: Schacter GP, McArthur TR, editors. Hematology 1996. American Society of Hematology, 1996; with permission.

PNH type I = Normal expression of CD59
PNH type II = Partially deficient or residual expression of CD59
PNH type III = Complete absence of expression of CD59.

The proportion of the three different phenotypes may vary from patient to patient. Because other blood cell lineages can be analyzed, the transfusion of red blood cells to a patient does not interfere with the diagnosis of PNH.

The percentage of granulocytes with a PNH phenotype is usually higher than the percentage of red cells lacking CD59. Thus, flow cytometric analysis of the granulocytes increases sensitivity in the diagnosis of PNH.

Treatment

Hematopoietic Stem Cell Transplantation

HSCT is the only curative treatment for PNH. If a fully matched family donor is available, then HSCT is the treatment of choice, especially for patients who develop bone marrow failure.

Immunosuppressive Therapy

Therapy with cyclosporine and ATG is indicated in the setting of PNH-associated aplastic anemia. This treatment may lead to improvement in aplastic anemia but not in the hemolysis of PNH.

Use of Hematopoietic Growth Factor

The use of G-CSF, GM-CSF, and erythropoietin may be attempted in the setting of pertinent cytopenia.

Supportive Therapy

Long-term anticoagulant therapy (e.g., with warfarin) is indicated for patients with venous thrombosis. Iron and folate supplements are indicated due to chronic hemoglobinuria accompanied by iron loss and chronic hemolysis with increased erythroid marrow activity requiring supplementation of additional folate. Red blood cell transfusion as needed.

SUGGESTED READINGS

Alter B, Lipton J. Anemia, Fanconi. EMedicine J [serial online]. 2002. Available at http://www.emedicine.com/ped/topic3022.htm.

Bacigalupo A, Brand R, Oneto R, et al. Treatment of acquired severe aplastic anemia: bone marrow transplantation compared with immunosuppressive therapy—the European Group for Blood and Marrow Transplantation Experience. Semin Hematol 2000;37:69–80.

Ball SE. The modern management of severe aplastic anemia. Br J Haematol 2001;110:41–53.

Bridges KR. Sideroblastic anemia: a mitochondrial disorder. J Pediatr Hematol Oncol 1997;19:274–8.

Brodsky RA, Sensenbrenner LL, Jones RJ. Complete remission in severe aplastic anemia after high dose cyclophosphamide without bone marrow transplantation. Blood 1996;87:491–4.

Brown KE, Tisdale J, Barnett J, Dunbar CE, Young NS. Hepatitis associated aplastic anemia. N Engl J Med 1997;336:1059–64.

Camitta B, Thomas ED, Nathan DG, et al. A prospective study of androgens and bone marrow transplantation for treatment of severe aplastic anemia. Blood 1979;53:504–15.

Cherrick I, Karayalcin G, Lanzkowsky P. Transient erythroblastopenia of childhood. Am J Pediatr Hematol Oncol 1994;16:320–4.

Connor JM, Gatherer D, Gray FC, Pirrit LA, Affara NA. Assignment of the gene for dyskeratosis congenita to Xq28. Human Genet 1986;72:348–51.

De Plauque M, Bacigalupo A, Wursch A, Hows JM, et al. Long term follow-up of severe aplastic anemia patients treated with antithymocytic globulin. Br J Haematol 1989;73:121–6.

Dokal I. Dyskeratosis congenita in all its forms (Review). Br J Haematol 2000;110:768–79.

Draptchinskaia N, Gustavsson P, Andersson B, Pettersson M, Willig T-N, et al. The gene encoding ribosomal protein S19 is mutated in Diamond–Blackfan anemia. Nat Genet 1999;21:169–75.

Frickhofen N, Kaltwasser JP, Schrezenmeir H, Raghavachar A, et al. Treatment of aplastic anemia with antilymphocyte globulin and methylprednisolone with or without cyclosporine. N Engl J Med 1991;324:1297–1304.

Gazda H, Lipton JM, Willig T-N, Ball S, et al. Evidence for linkage of familial Diamond–Blackfan anemia to chromosome 8p23.2-23.1 and non-19q non-8p familial disease. Blood 2001;97:2145–50.

Grompe M. FANCD2: a branch-point in DNA damage response? Nat Med 2002;8:555–6.

Hedberg VA, Lipton M. Thrombocytopenia with absent radii. A review of 100 cases. Am J Pediatr Hematol Oncol 1988;10:51–64.

Hillmen P, Lewis SM, Bressler M, Luzzatto L, Dacie JV. Natural history of paroxysmal nocturnal hemoglobinuria. N Engl J Med 1995;333:1253–8.

Joenje H, Patel KJ. The emerging genetic and molecular basis of Fanconi anemia. Nat Rev Genet 2001;2:446–57.

Kerr DS. Protein manifestations of mitochondrial disease: a mini-review. J Pediatr Hematol Oncol 1997;19:279–86.

Koenig JM, Ashton D, DeVore GR, Christensen RD. Late hyporegenerative anemia in Rh-hemolytic disease. J Pediatr 1989;115:315–8.

Kojima S, Horibe K, Inaba J, et al. Long term outcome of acquired aplastic anemia in children: comparison between immunosuppressive therapy and bone marrow transplantation. Br J Haematol 2000;11:321–8.

Lipton JM, Federman N, Khabbaze, Schwartz CL, et al. Osteogenic sarcoma associated with Diamond–Blackfan anemia: a report from the Diamond–Blackfan Anemia Registry. J Pediatr Hematol Oncol 2001;23:39–44.

Nathan DG, Orkin SH. Hematology of Infancy and Childhood. 5th ed. Philadelphia: WB Saunders, 1998.

Perdahl EB, Naprstek BL, Wallace WC, Lipton JM. Erythroid failure in Diamond–Blackfan anemia is characterized by apoptosis. Blood 1994;83:645–50.

Ponka P. Tissue-specific regulation of iron metabolism and heme synthesis: distinct control mechanism in erythroid cells. Blood 1997;89:1–25.

Rosenberg PS, Greene MH, Alter BP. Cancer incidence in persons with Fanconi's anemia. Blood 2003;101:822–826.

Shalev H, Tamary H, Shaft D, Reznitsky P, Zaizov R. Neonatal manifestations of congenital dyserythropoietic anemia type I. J Pediatr 1997;131:95–7.

Socie G, Henry-Amar M, Bacigalupo A, et al. Malignant tumors occurring after treatment of aplastic anemia. European Bone Marrow Transplantation—Severe Aplastic Anemia Working Party. N Engl J Med 1993;329:1152–7.

Vlachos A, Klein GW, Lipton JM. The Diamond–Blackfan Anemia Registry: tool for investigating the epidemiology and biology of Diamond–Blackfan anemia. J Pediatr Hematol Oncol 2001;23:377–82.

Vulliamy T, Marron A, Goldman F, Dearlove A, et al. The RNA component of telomerase is mutated in autosomal dominant dyskeratosis congenita. Nature 2001;413:432–5.

Wickramasinghe SN. Dyserythropoiesis and congenital dyserythropoietic anemias. Br J Haematol 1997;98:785–97.

Young NS, Alter BP. Aplastic Anemia: Acquired and Inherited. Philadelphia: WB Saunders, 1994.

7

HEMOLYTIC ANEMIA

APPROACH TO DIAGNOSIS

An essential feature of hemolytic anemia is a reduction in the normal red cell survival of 120 days. Premature destruction of red cells may result from corpuscular abnormalities (within the red cell corpuscle), that is, abnormalities of membrane, enzymes, or hemoglobin; or from extracorpuscular abnormalities, that is, immune or nonimmune mechanisms. Tables 7-1 and 7-2 list the causes of hemolytic anemia due to corpuscular and extracorpuscular defects, respectively.

The approach to the diagnosis of hemolytic anemia should include:

1. Consideration of the clinical features suggesting hemolytic disease
2. Laboratory demonstration of the presence of a hemolytic process
3. Determination of the precise cause of the hemolytic anemia by special hematologic investigations.

Clinical Features

The following clinical features suggest a hemolytic process:

1. *Ethnic factors:* Incidence of sickle gene carrier in the African-American population (8%), high incidence of thalassemia trait in people of Mediterranean ancestry, and high incidence of glucose-6-phosphate dehydrogenase (G6PD) deficiency among Sephardic Jews
2. *Age factors:* Anemia and jaundice in an Rh-positive infant born to a mother who is Rh negative or a group A or group B infant born to a group O mother (setting for a hemolytic anemia)
3. History of anemia, jaundice, or gallstones in family
4. Persistent or recurrent anemia associated with reticulocytosis
5. Anemia unresponsive to hematinics
6. Intermittent bouts or persistent indirect hyperbilirubinemia
7. Splenomegaly
8. Hemoglobinuria
9. Presence of multiple gallstones
10. Chronic leg ulcers
11. Development of anemia or hemoglobinuria after exposure to certain drugs
12. Cyanosis without cardiorespiratory distress
13. Polycythemia
14. Dark urine due to dipyrroluria.

Table 7-1. Causes of Hemolytic Anemia Due to Corpuscular Defects

I. **Membrane defects**
 A. Primary membrane defects with specific morphologic abnormalities
   1. Hereditary spherocytosis
   2. Hereditary elliptocytosis/pyropoikilocytosis
   3. Hereditary stomatocytosis with:
      a. Increased osmotic fragility (high Na^+, low K^+)
      b. Decreased osmotic fragility (high Na^+, low K^+)
      c. Normal osmotic fragility
      d. Rh_{null}
   4. Congenital hemolytic anemia with dehydrated red cells (high Na^+, low K^+, decreased osmotic fragility)
 B. Secondary membrane defects: abetalipoproteinemia

II. **Enzyme defects**
 A. Energy potential defects (Embden–Meyerhof: anaerobic; ATP-producing pathway deficiencies)
   1. Hexokinase
   2. Glucose phosphate isomerase
   3. Phosphofructokinase
   4. Triosephosphate isomerase
   5. Phosphoglycerate kinase
   6. 2,3-Diphosphoglyceromutase (polycythemia and no hemolysis)
   7. Pyruvate kinase
 B. Reduction potential defects (hexose monophosphate: aerobic; NADPH-producing pathway deficiencies)
   1. G6PD[a]
   2. 6-Phosphogluconate dehydrogenase (6PGD)
   3. Glutathione reductase
   4. Glutathione synthetase
   5. 2,3-Glutamyl-cysteine synthetase
 C. Abnormalities of erythrocyte nucleotide metabolism
   1. Adenosine triphosphatase deficiency
   2. Adenylate kinase deficiency
   3. Pyrimidine 5′-nucleotidase (P5N) deficiency
   4. Adenosine deaminase excess

III. **Hemoglobin defects**
 A. Heme: congenital erythropoietic porphyria
 B. Globin
   1. Qualitative: hemoglobinopathies (e.g., Hb S, C, H, M)
   2. Quantitative: α- and β-thalassemias

IV. **Congenital dyserythropoietic anemias**
 A. Type I
 B. Type II
 C. Type III
 D. Type IV

Abbreviations: ATPase, adenosine triphosphatase; G6PD, glucose-6-phosphate dehydrogenase.

[a]World Health Organization (WHO) classification of G6PD variant: Class I variant: Chronic hemolysis due to severe G6PD deficiency, e.g., G6PD deficiency Harilaou. Class II variant: Intermittent hemolysis in spite of severe G6PD deficiency, e.g., G6PD Mediterranean. Class III variant: Intermittent hemolysis associated usually with drugs/infections and moderate G6PD deficiency, e.g., G6PDA variant. Class IV variant: No hemolysis, no G6PD deficiency, e.g., normal G6PD (B+ variant).

Table 7-2. Causes of Hemolytic Anemia Due to Extracorpuscular Defects

I. Immune
  A. Isoimmune
    1. Hemolytic disease of the newborn
    2. Incompatible blood transfusion
  B. Autoimmune: IgG only; complement only; mixed IgG and complement
    1. Idiopathic
       a. Warm antibody
       b. Cold antibody
       c. Cold–warm hemolysis (Donath–Landsteiner antibody)
    2. Secondary
       a. Infection, viral: infectious mononucleosis—Epstein–Barr virus (EBV),
          cytomegalovirus (CMV), hepatitis, herpes simplex, measles, varicella, influenza
          A, coxsackie virus B, human immunodeficiency virus (HIV); bacterial:
          streptococcal, typhoid fever, *Escherichia coli* septicemia, *Mycoplasma pneumoniae*
          (atypical pneumonia)
       b. Drugs and chemicals: quinine, quinidine, phenacetin, *p*-aminosalicylic acid,
          sodium cephalothin (Keflin), penicillin, tetracycline, rifampin, sulfonamides,
          chlorpromazine, pyradone, dipyrone, insulin; lead
       c. Hematologic disorders: leukemias, lymphomas, lymphoproliferative syndrome,
          associated idiopathic thrombocytopenic purpura (Evans syndrome), paroxysmal
          cold hemoglobinuria, paroxysmal nocturnal hemoglobinuria
       d. Immunopathic disorders: systemic lupus erythematosus, periarteritis nodosa,
          scleroderma, dermatomyositis, rheumatoid arthritis, ulcerative colitis,
          agammaglobulinemia, Wiskott–Aldrich syndrome, dysgammaglobulinemia, IgA
          deficiency, thyroid disorders, giant cell hepatitis, Evans syndrome, autoimmune
          lymphoproliferative syndrome (ALPS), common variable immune deficiency
       e. Tumors: ovarian teratomata, dermoids, thymoma, carcinoma, lymphomas

II. Nonimmune
  A. Idiopathic
  B. Secondary
    1. Infection, viral: infectious mononucleosis, viral hepatitis; bacterial: streptococcal, *E.
       coli* septicemia, *Clostridium perfringens*, *Bartonella bacilliformis*; parasites: malaria,
       histoplasmosis
    2. Drugs and chemicals: phenylhydrazine, vitamin K, benzene, nitrobenzene,
       sulfones, phenacetin, acetinalimide; lead
    3. Hematologic disorders: leukemia, aplastic anemia, megaloblastic anemia,
       hypersplenism, pyknocytosis
    4. Microangiopathic hemolytic anemia: thrombotic thrombocytopenic purpura,
       hemolytic uremic syndrome, chronic relapsing schistocytic hemolytic anemia,
       burns, post cardiac surgery, march hemoglobinuria
    5. Miscellaneous: Wilson disease, erythropoietic porphyria, osteopetrosis,
       hypersplenism

Laboratory Findings

Laboratory findings of hemolytic anemia consist of:

1. Reduced red cell survival and evidence of accelerated hemoglobin catabolism
2. Evidence of increased erythropoiesis.

Accelerated Hemoglobin Catabolism

Accelerated hemoglobin catabolism varies with the type of hemolysis as follows:

- Extravascular hemoglobin catabolism (see Figure 7-1)
- Intravascular hemoglobin catabolism (see Figure 7-2).

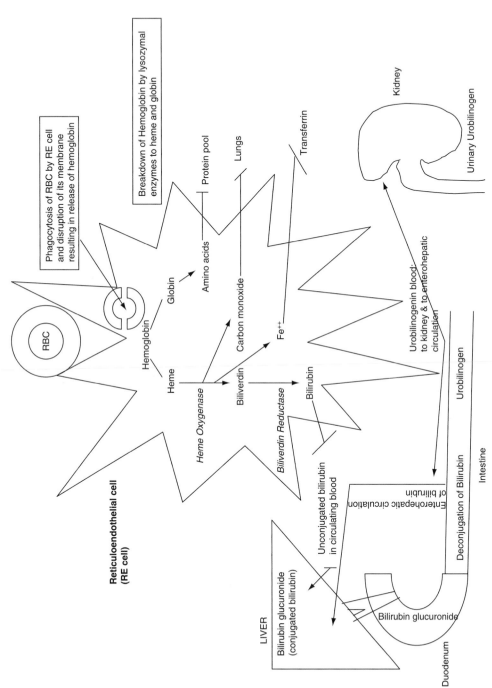

Fig. 7-1. Extravascular hemoglobin catabolism following extravascular destruction of the RBC.

139

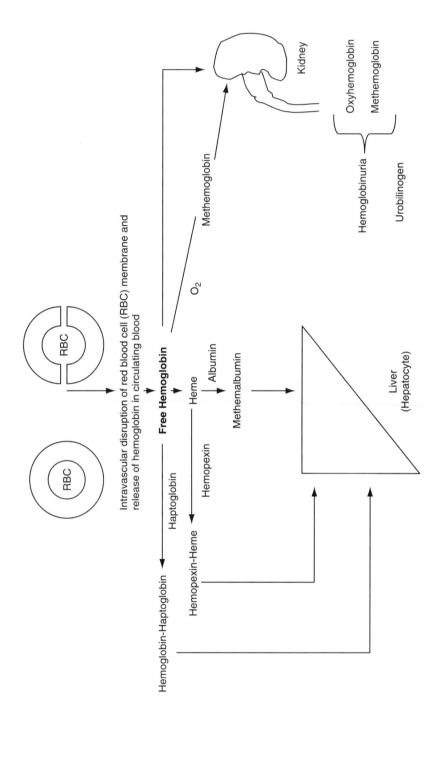

Fig. 7-2. Intravascular hemoglobin catabolism following intravascular hemolysis. Hemoglobin-haptoglobin, hemopexin-heme, and methemalbumin are cleared by hepatocytes. Heme is converted to iron and bilirubin. The common pathway for both extravascular and intravascular hemolysis is the conjugation of bilirubin (bilirubin glucuronide) by the hepatocytes, its excretion in bile, and ultimately formation of the urobilinogen by the bacteria in the gut. Part of urobilinogen enters in enterohepatic circulation and part is excreted by the kidney in urine, and the remainder of urobilinogen is excreted in stool (see Fig. 7-1).

Signs of extravascular hemolysis:

1. Increased unconjugated bilirubin
2. Increased fecal and urinary urobilinogen
3. Increased rate of carbon monoxide production.

Signs of intravascular hemolysis:

1. Raised plasma hemoglobin level (normal value <1 mg hemoglobin/dL plasma, visibly red plasma contains >50 mg hemoglobin/dL plasma)
2. Hemoglobinuria (Table 7-3 lists the causes of hemoglobinuria)
3. Hemosiderinuria (due to sloughing of iron-laden tubular cells into urine)
4. Low or absent plasma haptoglobin (normal level, 128 ± 25 mg/dL)
5. Raised plasma methemalbumin (albumin bound to heme; unlike haptoglobin, albumin does not bind intact hemoglobin)
6. Raised plasma methemoglobin (oxidized free plasma hemoglobin) and raised levels of hemopexin-heme complex in plasma.

Increased Erythropoiesis

Erythropoiesis increases in response to a reduction in hemoglobin and is manifested by:

1. *Reticulocytosis:* Frequently up to 10–20%; rarely, as high as 80%
2. Increased mean corpuscular volume (MCV) due to the presence of reticulocytosis and increased red cell distribution width (RDW) as the hemoglobin level falls
3. Increased normoblasts in peripheral blood
4. *Specific morphologic abnormalities:* Sickle cells, target cells, basophilic stippling, irregularly contracted cells (schistocytes), and spherocytes

---

Table 7-3. Causes of Hemoglobinuria

I. Acute
- A. Mismatched blood transfusions
- B. Drugs and chemicals
  - 1. Regularly causing hemolytic anemia
    - a. Drugs: phenylhydrazine, sulfones (dapsone), phenacetin, acetanilid (large doses)
    - b. Chemicals: nitrobenzene, lead, inadvertent infusion of water
    - c. Toxins: snake and spider bites
  - 2. Occasionally causing hemolytic anemia
    - a. Associated with G6PD deficiency: antimalarials (primaquine, chloroquine), antipyretics (aspirin, phenacetin), sulfonamides (Gantrisin, lederkyn), nitrofurans (Furadantin, Furacin), miscellaneous (naphthalene, vitamin K, British antilewisite [BAL], favism)
    - b. Associated with Hb Zürich: sulfonamides
    - c. Hypersensitivity: quinine, quinidine, *para*-aminosalicylic acid (PAS), phenacetin
- C. Infections
  - 1. Bacterial: *Clostridium perfringens, Bartonella bacilliformis* (Oroya fever)
  - 2. Parasitic: malaria
- D. Burns
- E. Mechanical (e.g., prosthetic valves)

II. Chronic
- A. Paroxysmal cold hemoglobinuria; syphilis; idiopathic
- B. Paroxysmal nocturnal hemoglobinuria
- C. March hemoglobinuria
- D. Cold agglutinin hemolysis

5. *Erythroid hyperplasia of the bone marrow:* Erythroid:myeloid ratio in the marrow increasing from 1:5 to 1:1
6. Increased red cell creatine levels
7. Erythroid hyperplasia in bone marrow
8. Expansion of marrow space in chronic hemolysis resulting in:
    a. Prominence of frontal bones
    b. Broad cheekbones
    c. Widened intratrabecular spaces, hair-on-end appearance of skull radiographs
    d. Biconcave vertebrae with fish-mouth intervertebral spaces
9. Decreased red cell survival demonstrated by ^{51}Cr red cell labeling.

Table 7-4 lists the investigations used to demonstrate the presence of a hemolytic process.

Determination of Cause

Once the presence of a hemolytic process has been established, the precise cause of the hemolytic anemia must be determined. Table 7-5 lists the tests used to establish the cause of hemolytic anemia.

CORPUSCULAR HEMOLYTIC ANEMIAS
Membrane Defects

Hereditary spherocytosis, elliptocytosis, stomatocytosis, acanthocytosis, xerocytosis, and pyropoikilocytosis can be diagnosed on the basis of their characteristic morphologic abnormalities. Spectrin is responsible for maintaining red cell shape and is composed of two subunits, α- and β-spectrin, which are structurally distinct and are encoded by separate genes. A variety of mutations in α- and β-spectrin have been reported. Spectrin regulates the lateral mobility of integral membrane proteins and provides structural support for the lipid bilayer. Disruption of spectrin self-association leads to disorders characterized by abnormally shaped red cells. Enzyme defects and many hemoglobinopathies have nonspecific morphologic abnormalities.

Table 7-4. Tests Used to Demonstrate a Hemolytic Process

Accelerated hemoglobin catabolism
    Serum bilirubin level
    Urinary urobilinogen excretion
    Fecal urobilinogen excretion
    Haptoglobin level
    Plasma hemoglobin level
    Methemoglobin level
    Methemalbumin level
    Carboxyhemoglobin
    Urinalysis for hemoglobinuria and hemosiderinuria
    Blood smear: red cell fragments (schistocytes), spherocytes
    Red cell survival studies: ^{51}Cr, difluorophosphate-32 (^{32}DFP)
Increased erythropoiesis
    Reticulocyte count/reticulocyte index
    Macrocytosis
    Normoblastemia
    Bone marrow examination for erythroid hyperplasia
    Radiography: hair-on-end appearance

Table 7-5. Tests Used to Establish a Specific Cause of Hemolytic Anemia

Corpuscular defects
  Membrane
    Blood smear: spherocytes, ovalocytes, pyknocytes, stomatocytes[a]
    Osmotic fragility (fresh and incubated)[a]
    Autohemolysis[a]
    Cation permeability studies
    Membrane phospholipid composition
    Scanning electron microscopy
  Hemoglobin defects
    Blood smear: sickle cells, target cells (Hb C)[a]
    Sickling test[a]
    Hemoglobin electrophoresis[a]
    Quantitative fetal hemoglobin determination[a]
    Kleihauer–Betke smear[a]
    Heat stability test for unstable hemoglobin
    Oxygen dissociation curves
    Rates of synthesis of polypeptide chain production
    Fingerprinting of hemoglobin
  Enzyme defects
    Heinz-body preparation[a]
    Osmotic fragility[a]
    Autohemolysis test[a]
    Screening test for enzyme deficiencies[a]
    Specific enzyme assays[a]
  Extracorpuscular defects
    Coombs' test: IgG (gamma), C'3 (complement), broad-spectrum (both gamma and
      complement)[a]
    Acidified serum lysis (Ham's) test[a]
    Donath–Landsteiner test[a]
    Flow cytometric analysis of red cells with monoclonal antibodies to GP1-linked surface
      antigens (for PNH)

[a]Tests commonly employed and most useful in establishing a diagnosis.

Hereditary Spherocytosis

Genetics

1. Autosomal dominant inheritance (75% of cases). The severity of anemia and the degree of spherocytosis may not be uniform within an affected family.
2. No family history in 25% of cases. Some show minor laboratory abnormalities, suggesting a carrier (recessive) state. Others are due to a *de novo* mutation.
3. Most common in people of northern European heritage, with an incidence of 1 in 5000.

Pathogenesis

In hereditary spherocytosis (HS), the primary defect is membrane instability due to dysfunction or deficiency of a red cell skeletal protein. A variety of membrane skeletal protein defects have been found in different families. These include:

1. *Ankyrin mutations:* Account for 50–67% of HS. In many patients, both spectrin and ankyrin proteins are deficient. Mutations of ankyrin occur in both dominant and recessive forms of HS. Clinically, the course varies from mild to severe. Red cells are typically spherocytes.

2. α-Spectrin mutations occur in recessive HS and account for less than 5% of HS. Clinical course is severe. Contracted cells, poikilocytes, and spherocytes are seen.
3. β-Spectrin mutations occur in dominant HS and account for 15–20% of HS. Clinical course is mild to moderate. Acanthocytes, spherocytic elliptocytes, and spherocytes are seen.
4. Protein 4.2 mutations occur in the recessive form of HS and account for less than 5% of HS. Clinical course is mild to moderate. Spherocytes, acanthocytes, and ovalocytes are seen.
5. Band 3 mutations occur in the dominant form of HS and account for 15–20% of HS. Clinical course can be mild to moderate. Spherocytes are occasionally mushroom-shaped or pincered cells.

Deficiency of these membrane skeletal proteins in HS results in vertical defect, which causes progressive loss of membrane lipid and surface area. The loss of surface area results in characteristic microspherocytic morphology of HS red cells.
The sequelae are as follows:

1. Sequestration of red cells in the spleen (due to reduced erythrocyte deformability)
2. Depletion of membrane lipid
3. Decrease in membrane surface area relative to volume, resulting in a decrease in surface area-to-volume ratio
4. Tendency to spherocytosis
5. Influx and efflux of sodium increased; cell dehydration
6. Rapid adenosine triphosphate (ATP) utilization and increased glycolysis
7. Premature red cell destruction.

Hematology

1. *Anemia:* Mild to moderate in compensated cases. In erythroblastopenic crisis, hemoglobin may drop to 2–3 g/dL.
2. MCV usually decreased; mean corpuscular hemoglobin concentration (MCHC) raised and RDW elevated.*
3. Reticulocytosis (3–15%).
4. *Blood film:* Microspherocytes[†] (vary in number); hyperdense cells,[‡] polychromasia.
5. Coombs' test negative.
6. Increased red cell osmotic fragility (spherocytes lyse in higher concentrations of saline than normal red cells) occasionally only demonstrated after incubation of blood sample at 37°C for 24 hours. In spite of normal osmotic fragility, increased MCHC or an increase of hyperdense red cells is highly suggestive of HS.
7. Autohemolysis at 24 and 48 hours increased, corrected by the addition of glucose.
8. Survival of ^{51}Cr-labeled cells reduced with increased splenic sequestration.
9. *Marrow:* Normoblastic hyperplasia; increased iron.

---

*The MCHC is only raised in hereditary spherocytosis, hereditary xerocytosis, hereditary pyropoikilocytosis, and cold agglutinin disease. The presence of elevated RDW and MCHC (performed by aperture impedance instruments, e.g., Coulter) makes the likelihood of hereditary spherocytosis very high, because these two tests used together are very specific for hereditary spherocytosis.

[†]The percentage of microspherocytes is the best indicator of the severity of the disease but not a good discriminator of the HS genotype.

[‡]Hyperdense cells are seen in HbSC disease, HbCC disease, and xerocytosis. In HS, hyperdense cells are a poor indicator of disease severity but an effective discriminating feature of the HS phenotype.

Biochemistry

1. Raised bilirubin, mainly indirect reacting
2. Obstructive jaundice with increased direct-reacting bilirubin; may develop due to gallstones, a consequence of increased pigment excretion.

Clinical Features

1. Anemia and jaundice: Severity depends on rate of hemolysis, degree of compensation of anemia by reticulocytosis, and ability of liver to conjugate and excrete indirect hyperbilirubinemia.
2. Splenomegaly.
3. Presents in newborn (50% of cases) with hyperbilirubinemia, reticulocytosis, normoblastosis, spherocytosis, negative Coombs' test, and splenomegaly.
4. Presents before puberty in most patients.
5. Diagnosis sometimes made much later in life by chance.
6. Co-inheritance of HS with hemoglobin S-C disease may increase the risk of splenic sequestration crisis.
7. Co-inheritance of β-thalassemia trait and HS may worsen, improve, or have no effect on the clinical course of HS.
8. Iron deficiency may correct the laboratory values but not the red cell life span in HS patients.
9. HS with other system involvement:
   a. Interstitial deletion of chromosome 8p11.1–8p21.1 causes ankyrin deficiency, psychomotor retardation, and hypogonadism.
   b. HS may be associated with neurologic abnormalities such as cerebellar disturbances, muscle atrophy, and a tabes-like syndrome.

Classification

Table 7-6 lists a classification of hereditary spherocytosis in accordance with clinical severity and indications for splenectomy.

Diagnosis

1. Clinical features and family history
2. Hematologic features.

Complications

1. *Hemolytic crisis:* With more pronounced jaundice due to accelerated hemolysis (may be precipitated by infection)
2. *Erythroblastopenic crisis:* Dramatic fall in hemoglobin level (and reticulocyte count); usually due to maturation arrest and often associated with giant pronormoblasts in the recovery phase; usually associated with parvovirus B19 infection*
3. *Folate deficiency:* Caused by increased red cell turnover; may lead to superimposed megaloblastic anemia. Megaloblastic anemia may mask HS morphology as well as its diagnosis by osmotic fragility

---

*Parvovirus B19 infects developing normoblasts, causing a transient cessation of production. The virus specifically infects CFU-E and prevents their maturation. Giant pronormoblasts are seen in bone marrow. Diagnosis is made by increased IgM antibody titer against parvovirus and PCR for parvovirus on bone marrow.

Table 7-6. Classification of Spherocytosis and Indications for Splenectomy

Classification	Trait	Mild spherocytosis	Moderate spherocytosis	Severe spherocytosis[a]
Hemoglobin (g/dL)	Normal	11–15	8–12	6–8
Reticulocyte count (%)	≤3	3.1–6	≥6	≥10
Bilirubin (mg/dL)	≤1.0	1.0–2.0	≥2.0	≥3.0
Reticulocyte production index	<1.8	1.8–3	>3	
Spectrin per erythrocyte[b] (percentage of normal)	100	80–100	50–80	40–60
Osmotic fragility				
Fresh blood	Normal	Normal to slightly increased	Distinctly increased	Distinctly increased
Incubated blood	Slightly increased	Distinctly increased	Distinctly increased	Distinctly increased
Autohemolysis				
Without glucose (%)	>60	>60	0–80	50
With glucose (%)	<10	≥10	≥10	≥10
Splenectomy	Not necessary	Usually not necessary during childhood and adolescence	Necessary during school age before puberty	Necessary, not before 3 years of age
Symptoms	None	None	Pallor, erythroblastopenic crises, splenomegaly, gallstones	Pallor, erythroblastopenic crises, splenomegaly, gallstones

[a]Value before transfusion.

[b]Normal (mean±SD): 226 ± 54 × 10³ molecules per cell.

From Eber SW, Armburst R, Schröter W. J Pediat 1990;117:409.

4. *Gallstones:* In approximately one-half of untreated patients; increased incidence with age. Occasionally, HS may be masked or improved in obstructive jaundice due to increase in surface area of red cells and formation of targets cells
5. *Hemochromatosis:* Rarely.

Treatment

1. Folic acid supplement (1 mg/day)
2. Leukocyte-depleted packed red cell transfusion for severe erythroblastopenic crisis
3. Splenectomy* for moderate to severe cases. Most patients with less than 80% of normal spectrin content require splenectomy. Splenectomy should be carried out early in severe cases but not before 5 years of age, if possible. The management of the splenectomized patient is detailed in Chapter 26. Although spherocytosis persists postsplenectomy, the red cell life span becomes essentially normal and complications are prevented, especially transient erythroblastopenia and persistent hyperbilirubinemia, which leads to gallstones
4. Ultrasound should be carried out before splenectomy to exclude the presence of gallstones. If present, cholecystectomy is also indicated.

Hereditary Elliptocytosis

Hereditary elliptocytosis (HE) is clinically and genetically a heterogeneous disorder.

Pathogenesis

HE is due to various defects in the skeletal proteins, spectrin, and protein 4.1. The basic membrane defects consist of:

1. Defects of spectrin self-association involving the α-chains
2. Defects of spectrin self-association involving the β-chains
3. Deficiency of protein 4.1
4. Deficiency of glycophorin.

Deficiencies of these skeletal proteins result in decreased horizontal stability and reduced pliability of red blood cells. Thus, a red blood cell is unable to regain its biconcave shape after its distortion in the microcirculation.

The membrane defect results in decreased cellular deformability as a result of increased membrane rigidity, which is a consistent feature in all cases. In addition, cell dehydration is present. In HE, cell fragmentation is the result of the loss of mechanical integrity of the skeleton. The cell remnants contain a full complement of various membrane proteins and represent a true fragmentation process in which microcytic red blood cells with decreased hemoglobin content are generated. In HS, however, continuous loss of the lipid-rich and skeleton-free domains of the membrane during the red cell life span results in spherocytic red cells with near-normal hemoglobin content and the absence of fragmented cells with markedly decreased hemoglobin content.

---

*Laparoscopic splenectomy is safe in children. Although it requires more operative time than open splenectomy, it is superior with regard to postoperative analgesia, smaller abdominal wall scars, duration of hospital stay, and more rapid return to a regular diet and daily activities. It is not known if accessory spleens are readily identified with the laparoscope although the magnification afforded by the laparoscope might be advantageous in some cases.

Genetics

HE is characterized by an autosomal dominant mode of inheritance (with variable penetrance), affecting about 1 in 25,000 of the population. Two types of inheritance occur:

1. Non-Rh-linked, associated with a high incidence of severe anemia in the homozygote
2. Rh-linked, usually associated with a milder disorder.

Clinical Features

1. Varies from patients who are symptom free to severe anemia requiring blood transfusions. The percentage of microcytes best reflects the severity of the disease.
2. About 12% have symptoms indistinguishable from hereditary spherocytosis.
3. The percentage of elliptocytes varies from 50% to 90%. No correlation has been established between the degree of elliptocytosis and the severity of the anemia.
4. HE has been classified into the following clinical subtypes:
   a. Common HE, which is divided into several groups: silent carrier state, mild HE, HE with infantile pyknocytosis
   b. Common HE with chronic hemolysis, which is divided into two groups: HE with dyserythropoiesis and homozygous common HE, which is clinically indistinguishable from hereditary pyropoikilocytosis (see later discussion)
   c. Spherocytic HE, which clinically resembles HS; however, a family member usually has evidence of HE
   d. Southeast Asian ovalocytosis, in which the majority of cells are oval; however, some red cells contain either a longitudinal or transverse ridge.

Laboratory Findings

1. Blood smear: 25–90% of cells elongated oval elliptocytes
2. Osmotic fragility normal or increased
3. Autohemolysis usually normal but may be increased and usually corrected by the addition of glucose or ATP.

Treatment

The indications for transfusion, splenectomy, and prophylactic folic acid are the same as for hereditary spherocytosis.

Hereditary Pyropoikilocytosis

Definition

Hereditary pyropoikilocytosis (HPP) is a congenital hemolytic anemia associated with *in vivo* red cell fragmentation and marked *in vitro* fragmentation of red cells at 45°C. Because of the similarities in the membrane defect in this condition and HE, it is viewed as a subtype of HE.

Genetics and Etiology

1. Homozygous or doubly heterozygous for the spectrin chains (e.g., Sp-$\alpha^{1/74}$ and Sp-$\alpha^{1/46}$). The spectrin chain defects found in HPP are similar to those found in HE.

2. Increased ratio of cholesterol to membrane protein.
3. Decreased cell deformability.

Clinical Features

1. Anemia characterized by extreme anisocytosis and poikilocytosis
   a. Red cell fragments, spherocytes, and budding red cells (the red cells are exquisitely sensitive to temperature and fragment after 10 minutes of incubation time at 45–46°C *in vitro;* heating for 6 hours at 37°C explains *in vivo* formation of fragmented red cells and chronic hemolysis)
   b. Hemoglobin level, 7–9 g/dL
   c. Marked reduction in MCV and elevated MCHC
2. Jaundice
3. Splenomegaly
4. Osmotic fragility and autohemolysis increased
5. Mild HE present in one of the parents or siblings.

Differential Diagnosis

Similar cells are seen in microangiopathic hemolytic anemias, after severe burns or oxidant stress, and in pyruvate kinase deficiency.

Treatment

Patients respond well to splenectomy with a rise in hemoglobin to 12 g/dL. Following splenectomy, hemolysis is decreased but not totally eliminated.

Hereditary Stomatocytosis

Definition and Genetics

The stomatocyte has a linear slit-like area of central pallor rather than a circular area. When suspended in plasma, the cells assume a bowl-shaped form. This hereditary hemolytic anemia of variable severity is characterized by an autosomal dominant mode of inheritance.

Etiology

The cells contain high Na^+ and low K^+ concentrations. The disorder is probably due to a membrane and protein defect. The cells are abnormally rigid and poorly deformable, contributing to their rapid rate of destruction. There are many biochemical variants.

Clinical Features

1. Very variable
2. Jaundice at birth
3. Pallor: marked variability depending on severity of anemia
4. Splenomegaly
5. Hematology
   a. Anemia
   b. Smear, 10–50% stomatocytes
   c. Reticulocytosis
   d. Increased osmotic fragility and autohemolysis.

Differential Diagnosis

Stomatocytosis may occur with thalassemia, some red cell enzyme defects (glutathione peroxidase deficiency, glucose phosphate isomerase deficiency), Rh_{null} red cells, viral infections, lead poisoning, some drugs (e.g., quinidine and chlorpromazine), some malignancies, liver disease, and alcoholism.

Treatment

Splenectomy may be beneficial if hemolysis is severe.

Hereditary Acanthocytosis

Definition

Acanthocytes have thorn-like projections that vary in length and width and are irregularly distributed over the surface of red cells.

Genetics

The mode of inheritance is autosomal recessive.

Clinical Features

1. *Steatorrhea:* Only fat malabsorption
2. *Neurologic symptoms:* Weakness, ataxia and nystagmus, atypical retinitis pigmentosa with macular atrophy, blindness
3. *Anemia:* Mild hemolytic anemia; 70–80% acanthocytes; slight reticulocytosis.

Diagnosis

1. Clinical syndrome
2. Absent β-lipoprotein in plasma
3. Diagnostic findings on small intestine biopsy.

Differential Diagnosis

During the neonatal period, hereditary acanthocytosis may have to be distinguished from the benign nonhereditary disorder of infantile pyknocytosis. Acquired acanthocytosis occurs under the following conditions: renal failure, cirrhosis, microangiopathic hemolytic anemia, hypothyroidism, pyruvate kinase deficiency, and in association with some neoplasms.

Hereditary Xerocytosis

Definition

Hereditary xerocytosis is a familial condition characterized by red cells that appear to be shrunken, with hemoglobin puddled at the periphery or center of the cell. The defect in these cells permits increased permeability of univalent cations Na^+ and K^+. The accompanying cell water loss results in dehydrated red cells. There is an increased proportion of phosphatidylcholine in the membrane.

Genetics

The mode of inheritance of this rare condition is autosomal dominant.

Clinical Features

1. Few symptoms, moderate anemia; red cell morphology, stomatocytic
2. Elevated reticulocytes
3. Splenomegaly and gallstones
4. MCHC elevated, MCV increased
5. Osmotic fragility reduced
6. Increased heat stability (46 and 49°C for 60 minutes).

Treatment

Transfusions are generally not required. The benefit of splenectomy is slight.

Enzyme Defects

There are two major biochemical pathways in the red cell: the Embden–Meyerhof anaerobic pathway (energy potential of the cell) and the hexose monophosphate shunt (reduction potential of the cell). Figure 7-3 illustrates the enzyme reactions in the red cell.

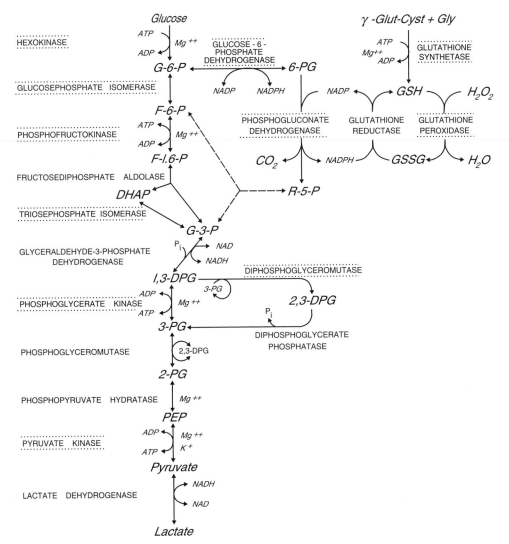

Fig. 7-3. Enzyme reactions of Embden–Meyerhof and hexose monophosphate pathways of metabolism. Documented hereditary deficiency diseases are indicated by enclosing dotted lines.

Pyruvate Kinase Deficiency

Pyruvate kinase (PK) is an enzyme active in the penultimate conversion in the Embden–Meyerhof pathway. Although deficiency is rare, it is the most common enzyme abnormality in the Embden–Meyerhof pathway.

Genetics

1. Autosomal recessive inheritance
2. Significant hemolysis seen in homozygotes
3. Found predominantly in people of northern European origin
4. Deficiency not simply quantitative; probably often reflects the production of PK variants with abnormal characteristics.

Pathogenesis

1. Defective red cell glycolysis with reduced ATP formation
2. Red cells rigid, deformed, and metabolically and physically vulnerable (reticulocytes less vulnerable because of ability to generate ATP by oxidative phosphorylation).

Hematology

1. Features of nonspherocytic hemolytic anemia: macrocytes, oval forms, polychromatophilia, anisocytosis, occasional spherocytes, contracted red cells with multiple projecting spicules, rather like acanthocytes or pyknocytes
2. Erythrocyte PK activity decreased to 5–20% of normal; 2,3-diphosphoglycerate (2,3-DPG) and other glycolytic intermediary metabolites increased (because of two- to threefold increase in 2,3-DPG, there is a shift to the right in P_{50}*)
3. Autohemolysis markedly increased, showing marked correction with ATP but not with glucose.

Clinical Features

1. Variable severity; can cause moderately severe anemia (not drug induced)
2. Usually presents with neonatal jaundice
3. Splenomegaly common but not invariable
4. Late: gallstones, hemosiderosis (from multiple transfusions), bone changes of chronic hemolytic anemia
5. Erythroblastopenic crisis due to parvovirus B19 infection.

Treatment

1. Folic acid supplementation
2. Transfusions as required
3. Splenectomy (if transfusion requirements increase); splenectomy does not arrest hemolysis, but decreases transfusion requirements.

Other Enzyme Deficiencies

1. Hexokinase deficiency, with many variants
2. Glucose phosphate isomerase deficiency

---

*Because of the right shift of P_{50}, patients do not exhibit fatigue and exercise intolerance proportionate to the degree of anemia.

3. Phosphofructokinase deficiency, with variants
4. Aldolase
5. Triosephosphate isomerase deficiency
6. Phosphoglycerate kinase deficiency
7. 2,3-DPG deficiency due to deficiency of diphosphoglycerate mutase
8. Adenosine triphosphatase deficiency
9. Enolase deficiency.

These enzyme deficiencies have the following features:

1. *General hematologic features:*
   a. Autosomal recessive disorders except phosphoglycerate kinase deficiency, which is sex linked
   b. Chronic nonspherocytic hemolytic anemias (CNSHAs) of variable severity
   c. Osmotic fragility and autohemolysis normal or increased
   d. Improvement in anemia after splenectomy
   e. Diagnosed by specific red cell assays
2. *Specific nonhematologic features:*
   a. Phosphofructokinase deficiency associated with type VII glycogen storage disease and myopathy
   b. Triosephosphate isomerase deficiency associated with progressive debilitating neuromuscular disease with generalized spasticity and recurrent infections (some patients have died of sudden cardiac arrest)
   c. Phosphoglycerate kinase deficiency associated with mental retardation and a behavioral disorder.

Note the three exceptions to the general hematologic features listed above: (1) Adenosine deaminase excess (i.e., not an enzyme deficiency) is an autosomal dominant disorder. (2) Pyrimidine 5′-nucleotidase deficiency is characterized by marked basophilic stippling, although the other chronic nonspherocytic hemolytic anemias lack any specific morphologic abnormalities. (3) Deficiency of diphosphoglycerate mutase results in polycythemia.

Glucose-6-Phosphate Dehydrogenase Deficiency

Glucose-6-phosphate dehydrogenase (G6PD) is the first enzyme in the pentose phosphate pathway of glucose metabolism. Deficiency diminishes the reductive energy of the red cell and may result in hemolysis, the severity of which depends on the quantity and type of G6PD and the nature of the hemolytic agent (usually an oxidation mediator that can oxidize NADPH, generated in the pentose phosphate pathway in red cells).

Genetics

1. Sex-linked recessive mode of inheritance by a gene located on the X chromosome (similar to hemophilia).
2. Disease is fully expressed in hemizygous males and homozygous females.
3. Variable intermediate expression is shown by heterozygous females (due to random deletion of X chromosome, according to Lyon hypothesis).
4. As many as 3% of the world's population is affected; most frequent among African Americans and those of Mediterranean origin.

The molecular basis of G6PD deficiency and its clinical implications follow:

1. Deletions of G6PD genes are incompatible with life because it is a housekeeping gene and complete absence of G6PD activity, called hydeletions, will result in death of the embryo.

2. Point mutations are responsible for G6PD deficiencies. They result in:
   a. *Sporadic mutations:* They are not specific to any geographic areas. The same mutation may be encountered in different parts of the world that have no causal (e.g., encountering G6PD Guadalajara in Belfast) relationship with malarial selection. These patients manifest with chronic nonspherocytic hemolytic anemia (CNSHA WHO Class I).
   b. *Polymorphic mutations:* These mutations have resulted from malaria selection; hence, they correlate with specific geographic areas. They are usually WHO Class II or III and not Class I.

The World Health Organization (WHO) classification of G6PD variants on the basis of magnitude of the enzyme deficiency and the severity of hemolysis are shown here:

WHO Class	Variant	Magnitude of enzyme deficiency	Severity of hemolysis
I	Harilaou, Tokyo, Guadalajara, Stonybrook, Minnesota	2% of normal activity	Chronic nonspherocytic hemolytic anemia
II	Mediterranean	3% of normal activity	Intermittent hemolysis
III	A⁻	10–60% of normal activity	Intermittent hemolysis usually associated with infections or drugs
IV	B (Normal)	100% of normal activity	No hemolysis

Pathogenesis

1. Red cell G6PD activity falls rapidly and prematurely as red cells age
2. Decreased glucose metabolism
3. Diminished NADPH/NADP and GSH/GSSG ratios
4. Impaired elimination of oxidants (e.g., H_2O_2)
5. Oxidation of hemoglobin and of sulfhydryl groups in the membrane
6. Red cell integrity impaired, especially on exposure to oxidant drugs and chemicals.

Clinical Features

Episodes of hemolysis may be produced by:

- Drugs (Table 7-7)
- Fava bean (broad bean, *Vicia fava*): ingestion or exposure to pollen from the bean's flower (hence favism)
- Infection (in more susceptible subjects).

1. Drug-induced hemolysis
   a. Typically in African Americans but also in Mediterranean and Canton types
   b. List of drugs (see Table 7-7); occasionally need additional stress of infection or the neonatal state
   c. Acute self-limiting hemolytic anemia with hemoglobinuria
   d. Heinz bodies in circulating red cells
   e. Blister cells, fragmented cells, and spherocytes
   f. Reticulocytosis
   g. Hemoglobin normal between episodes

Table 7-7. Agents Capable of Inducing Hemolysis in G6PD-Deficient Subjects[a]

Clinically significant hemolysis	Usually not clinically significant hemolysis
Analgesics and antipyretics	
Acetanilid	Acetophenetidin (phenacetin)
	Acetylsalicylic acid (large doses)
	Antipyrine[a,b]
	Aminopyrine[b]
	p-Aminosalicylic acid
Antimalarial agents	
Pentaquine	Quinacrine (Atabrine)
Pamaquine	Quinine[b]
Primaquine	Chloroquine[c]
Quinocide	Pyrimethamine (Daraprim)
	Plasmoquine
Sulfonamides	
Sulfanilamide	Sulfadiazine
N-Acetylsulfanilamide	Sulfamerazine
Sulfapyridine	Sulfisoxazole (Gantrisin)[c]
Sulfamethoxypyridazine (Kynex)	Sulfathiazole
Salicylazosulfapyridine (Azulfidine)	Sulfacetamide
Nitrofurans	
Nitrofurazone (Furacin)	
Nitrofurantoin (Furadantin)	
Furaltadone (Altafur)	
Furazolidone (Furoxone)	
Sulfones	
Thiazolsulfone (Promizole)	
Diaminodiphenylsulfone (DDS, dapsone)	Sulfoxone sodium (Diasone)
Miscellaneous	
Naphthalene	
Phenylhydrazine	Menadione
Acetylphenylhydrazine	Dimercaprol (BAL)
Toluidine blue	Methylene blue
Nalidixic acid (NegGram)	Chloramphenicol[b]
Neoarsphenamine (Neosalvarsan)	Probenecid (Benemid)
Infections	Quinidine[b]
Diabetic acidosis	Fava beans[b]

[a]Many other compounds have been tested but are free of hemolytic activity. Penicillin, the tetracyclines, and erythromycin, for example, will not cause hemolysis, and the incidence of allergic reactions in G6PD-deficient persons is not any greater than that observed in others. Any drug, therefore, not included in the list of those known to cause hemolysis may be given.

[b]Hemolysis in Caucasians only.

[c]Mild hemolysis in African Americans, if given in large doses.

2. Favism
   a. Acute life-threatening hemolysis, often leading to acute renal failure caused by ingestion of fava beans
   b. Associated with Mediterranean and Canton varieties
   c. Blood transfusion required

3. Neonatal jaundice
   a. Usually associated with Mediterranean and Canton varieties
   b. Infants may present with pallor, jaundice (can be severe and produce kernicterus*), and dark urine.

Often no exposure to drugs; occasionally exposure to naphthalene (mothballs), aniline dye, marking ink, or a drug. In a majority of neonates, the jaundice is not hemolytic but hepatic in origin.

4. Chronic nonspherocytic hemolytic anemia
   a. Occurs mainly in people of northern European origin
   b. Hematologic picture
      (1) Chronic nonspherocytic anemia
      (2) Reticulocytosis
      (3) Shortened red cell survival
      (4) Increased autohemolysis with only partial correction by glucose
      (5) Slight jaundice
      (6) Mild splenomegaly.

Treatment

1. Avoidance of agents that are deleterious in G6PD deficiency
2. Indication for transfusion of packed red blood cell in children presenting with acute hemolytic anemia:
   a. Hemoglobin (Hb) level below 7 g/dL
   b. Persistent hemoglobinuria and Hb below 9 g/dL
3. Chronic nonspherocytic hemolytic anemia (NSHA):
   a. In patients with severe chronic anemia: transfuse red blood cells to maintain Hb level 8–10 g/dL and iron chelation, when needed
   b. Indications for splenectomy
      (1) Hypersplenism
      (2) Severe chronic anemia
      (3) Splenomegaly causing physical impediment
   c. Genetic counseling and prenatal diagnosis for severe CNSHA if the mother is a heterozygote.

Other Defects of Glutathione Metabolism

Glutathione Reductase

In this autosomal dominant disorder, hemolytic anemia is precipitated by drugs having an oxidant action. Thrombocytopenia has occasionally been reported. Neurologic symptoms occur in some patients.

Glutamyl Cysteine Synthetase

In this autosomal recessive disorder, there is a well-compensated hemolytic anemia.

Glutathione Synthetase

In this autosomal recessive disorder, there is a well-compensated hemolytic anemia, exacerbated by drugs having an oxidant action.

---

*The excessive jaundice is not only due to hemolysis but may be due to reduced glucuronidation of bilirubin caused by defective G6PD activity in the hepatocytes.

Glutathione Peroxidase

In this autosomal recessive disorder, acute hemolytic episodes occur after exposure to drugs having an oxidant action.

HEMOGLOBIN DEFECTS
Sickle Cell Disease

Incidence

Sickle hemoglobin is the most common abnormal hemoglobin found in the United States (approximately 8% of the African-American population has sickle cell trait). The expected incidence of sickle cell disease (SCD) at birth is 1 in 625.

Genetics

1. Sickle cell disease is transmitted as an incomplete autosomal dominant trait.
2. Homozygotes (two abnormal genes) do not synthesize hemoglobin A (HbA); red cells contain 90–100% hemoglobin S (HbS).
3. Heterozygotes (one abnormal gene) have red cells containing 20–40% HbS.
4. HbS arises as a result of spontaneous mutation and deletion of the β-globin gene on chromosome 11, which results in selective advantage against *Plasmodium falciparum* malaria in carriers (balanced polymorphism).
5. α-Thalassemia (frequency of 1–3% in African Americans) may be co-inherited with sickle cell trait or disease. Individuals who have both α-thalassemia and sickle cell anemia are less anemic than those who have sickle cell anemia alone. However, α-thalassemia trait does not appear to prevent frequency or severity of vaso-occlusive complications.

Results of DNA polymorphism linked to the β^s gene suggest that it arose from three independent mutations in tropical Africa:

1. Benin–Central West African haplotype (the most common haplotype)
2. Senegal–African West Coast haplotype
3. Bantu–Central African Republic (CAR) haplotype

The Benin type is also found in Ibadan, Algeria, Sicily, Turkey, Greece, Yemen, and southwest Saudi Arabia. In Caribbean and North American patients of African heritage with SCD, 50–70% of chromosomes are Benin, 15–30% are Bantu-CAR, and 5–15% are Senegal. The Benin and Senegalese patients have higher levels of fetal hemoglobin (HbF) and fewer dense cells compared with Bantu-CAR patients. Patients with Senegal haplotype have the least severe disease, whereas patients with Bantu-CAR haplotype have most severe disease.

Pathophysiology

Figure 7-4 depicts the pathophysiology of sickle cell disease.
A single amino acid substitution (valine for glutamic acid) occurs in the β-polypeptide chain. This simple alteration has the following consequences:

1. Hemoglobin S has a higher net electrical charge than that of hemoglobin A and hence a different electrophoretic mobility.
2. Hemoglobin S in the reduced form (deoxygenated) is less soluble than hemoglobin A. The molecules form rod-like tactoids; these in turn distort the red cell, which takes on the sickle form (Figure 7-4).

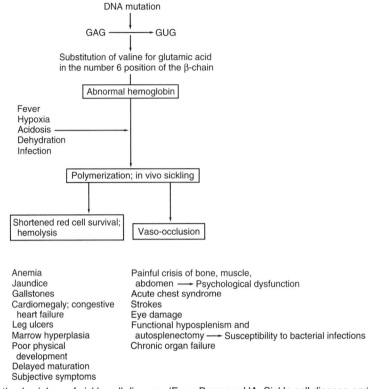

Fig. 7-4. Pathophysiology of sickle cell disease. (From Pearson, HA. Sickle cell disease and its crisis. In: Dickerman JD, Lucey JF, editors. Smith's the Critically Ill Child. Philadelphia: WB Saunders, 1985;229, with permission.)

3. Sickle cells are prematurely destroyed, causing a hemolytic anemia (Figure 7-4).
4. Sickle cells result in increased blood viscosity and impaired blood flow and initiate thrombi.
5. Hemoglobin F effects HbS by decreasing polymer content in cells. The effect of HbF on HbS may have direct and indirect effects on other RBC characteristics (i.e., percentage of HbF affects the RBC adhesive properties in patients with SCD). The higher the HbF concentration in cells, the milder the clinical severity of sickle cell anemia.

Clinical Features

Figure 7-5 displays the clinical problems of sickle cell disease by age.

Hematology

1. *Anemia:* Moderate to severe normochromic, normocytic
2. *Sickle cell preparation:* Reducing agent (e.g., sodium metabisulfite) positive
3. Reticulocytosis
4. Neutrophilia common
5. Platelets often increased
6. *Blood smear:* Sickle cells, increased polychromasia, nucleated red cells, and target cells (Howell–Jolly bodies may indicate hyposplenism)
7. *Erythrocyte sedimentation rate (ESR):* Low (sickle cells fail to form rouleaux)
8. *Hemoglobin electrophoresis:* Hemoglobin S migrates slower than hemoglobin A, giving the diagnostic SS pattern.

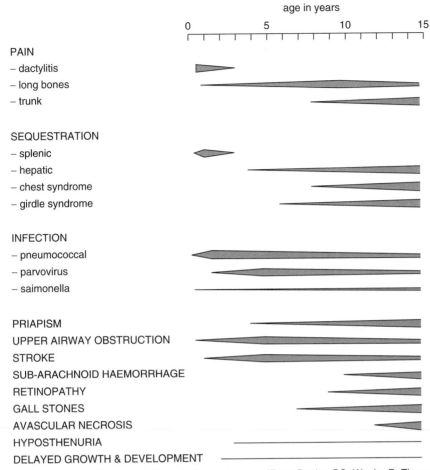

Fig. 7-5. The clinical problems of sickle cell disease by age. (From Davies SC, Wonke B. The management of hemoglobinopathies. In: Hann IM, Gibson ES, guest editors. Bailliere's Clinical Hematology. London: Bailliere Tindall, 1991;361, with permission).

Crises

1. Vaso-occlusive or symptomatic crisis (see Table 7-8)
2. Splenic sequestration crisis:
   a. Uncommon, but may be rapidly fatal
   b. Occurrence between 5 and 24 months of age
   c. Splenomegaly due to pooling of large amounts of blood in the spleen
   d. Abdominal pain of sudden onset accompanied by nausea and vomiting
   e. Hemoglobin level: may drop precipitously, followed by hypovolemic shock and death
3. Erythroblastopenic (aplastic) crisis:
   a. Cessation of red cell production that may persist for 10–14 days with profound drop in hemoglobin (as low as 1 g/dL)
   b. Reticulocyte count and the number of nucleated red cells in the marrow sharply decrease; platelet and white blood cell counts are generally unaffected
   c. May occur in several members of a family and can occur at any age
   d. Almost invariably associated with infection (the most common cause is parvovirus B19, which causes fifth disease in normal people)

Table 7-8. Symptomatology and Clinical Manifestations of Vaso-occlusive Crisis

Symptomatology	Manifestations
Hand–foot syndrome (dactylitis)	Under 5 years of age; painful swelling of the hands and feet
Bone crises	Painful bone crises usually beginning at age 3 or 4 years; must be distinguished from osteomyelitis (Table 7-9)
Abdominal crises (sickle cell girdle syndrome)	Related to sickle cell vaso-occlusion of mesenteric blood supply and infarction in the liver, spleen, or lymph nodes that results in capsular stretching. Table 7-10 lists the differentiation between painful abdominal crisis and acute abdomen.
CNS crises	May include convulsions, meningeal signs, blindness, radiculopathy, vertigo and acute mental syndrome, cerebral infarction. Incidence: 7–29%; mean age of onset: 7.7 years and increased incidence of subarachnoid hemorrhage. Figure 7-6 depicts the investigations and treatment of neurologic deficit
Pulmonary crises (acute chest syndrome)	Presents with chest pain that may be pleuritic, unexplained dyspnea, and fever; differential diagnosis from pneumonia may be difficult (Table 7-11); it may be associated with full-blown sickle cell girdle syndrome
Priapism	Predisposing factors: sexual intercourse, masturbation, infection, and local trauma; impotence in many cases
Hematuria	Painless and usually mild; defect is papillary necrosis
Intrahepatic vaso-occlusive crisis (hepatic sequestration)	Sudden, painful enlargement of liver; massive rise in bilirubin (mostly direct) and liver enzymes; it may occur at any age once the spleen has atrophied and fibrosed

Table 7-9. Differentiation between Bone Infarction and Osteomyelitis

Features	Favoring osteomyelitis	Favoring vaso-occlusion
History	No previous history	Preceding painful crisis
Pain, tenderness, erythema, swelling	Single site	Multiple sites
Fever	Present	Present
Leukocytosis	Elevated band count ($>1000/mm^3$)	Present
ESR	Elevated	Normal to low
α-HBD	Normal	Elevated
Radiograph	Abnormal	Abnormal
Bone scan	Abnormal ^{99m}Tc-diphosphonate	Abnormal ^{99m}Tc-diphosphonate
	Normal ^{99m}Tc-colloid marrow uptake	Decreased ^{99m}Tc-colloid marrow uptake
Blood culture	Positive (*Salmonella, Staphylococcus*)	Negative
Recovery	Only with appropriate antibiotic therapy	Spontaneous

Abbreviation: α-HBD, α-hydroxybutyric dehydrogenase.

    e. Terminates spontaneously usually after about 10 days (recovery occurs with reticulocytosis and nucleated red cells in the blood; reticulocyte count may reach 50–60%, with hemoglobin returning to precrisis level)

    f. Folate supplementation required to prevent development of megaloblastic anemia

Table 7-10. Differentiation between Painful Abdominal Crisis and Acute Abdomen

Features	Painful crisis	Acute abdomen
History of previous episodes	Present	Absent
Abdominal pain and distention	Present	Present
Signs of peritoneal irritation	Absent	Present
Decreased peristalsis	Present	Present
α-HBD	Elevated	Normal
Leukocytosis	Present	Elevated band count (>1000/mm^3)
Response to symptomatic treatment	Present	Absent

Table 7-11. Differentiation between Pneumonia and Pulmonary Infarction

Feature	Favoring pneumonia	Favoring pulmonary infarction
Chest pain, fever, hypoxia	Present	Present
Age	<5 years	>5 years
Associated painful crisis	Absent	May be present
Chills	Present	Absent
Leukocytosis	Elevated band count (>1000/mm^3)	Present
Blister cells on smear	Absent	Present
ESR	Elevated	Low
α-HBD	Normal	Elevated
Chest radiograph	Upper lobe infiltrate	Normal
VQ scan	Normal	Positive
Cultures	Positive blood and sputum or cold agglutinins and *Mycoplasma* titers	Negative

4. Hyperhemolytic crisis:
   a. Very unusual; may ensue in association with certain drugs or acute infections; G6PD deficiency is a possible contributing cause
   b. Patient begins to feel weak, looks paler, and shows more scleral icterus; may have abdominal pain
   c. Hematocrit falls to 15% or less in a few days; reticulocyte count rises; after several days, excessive hemolysis gradually subsides.

Organ dysfunction

Central nervous system

Acute infarction of the brain can result in a stroke, which occurs in approximately 7% of children with SCD. The incidence is 0.7% per year during the first 20 years of life, with the highest rates in children 5–10 years of age. An additional 20% of patients with sickle cell disease have evidence of asymptomatic cerebral infarction on MRI of the brain. These individuals may have significant neuropsychological deficit. The most common underlying lesion is intracranial arterial stenosis or obstruction, usually in the internal carotid, often in the proximal middle cerebral or anterior cerebral arteries. Chronic injury to the endothelium of vessels by sickled red blood cells (SRBCs) results in changes in the intima with proliferation of fibroblasts and smooth muscle; the lumen is narrowed or completely obliterated, which progresses to moyamoya. *Acute* sickling may result in acute cerebral infarction, manifesting as:

Motor disabilities (e.g., hemiparesis, gait dysfunction)
Focal seizures
Speech defects
Deficit in IQ
Cortical atrophy and ventricular dilatation on computed tomography (CT).

In untreated patients, the mortality rate is approximately 20%, with about 70% of patients experiencing a recurrence within 3 years.

Patients at high risk for first stroke include those with a high white cell count and those with a low borderline hematocrit. Note that coexistent α-thalassemia may reduce the risk of a stroke.

Figure 7-6 depicts the investigations and treatment of neurologic deficit in sickle cell disease.

Diagnosis
- *Head CT scan:* May not be positive for infarction within the first 6 hours of the episode.
- *Brain MRI:* May become abnormal in 2–4 hours in about 90% of patients.
- *Magnetic resonance arterial angiography (MRA):* Very useful in the early evaluation of the patient with new symptoms.

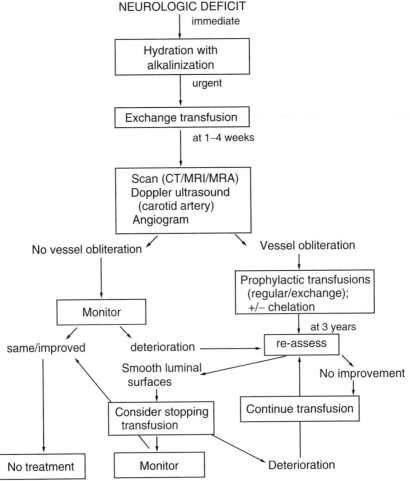

Fig. 7-6. The investigations and treatment of neurologic deficit in sickle cell disease. (Modified from Davies SC, Wonke B. The management of hemoglobinopathies. In: Hann IM, Gibson BES, guest editors. Bailliere's Clinical Hematology. London: Bailliere Tindall, 1991;361.)

- *Transcranial Doppler (TCD) measurement:* TCD measurements record the highest time-averaged mean blood flow velocity in 2-mm increments in the middle cerebral artery, the distal internal carotid artery, the anterior or posterior cerebral arteries, and the basilar artery. The results are categorized as normal (velocity <170 cm/sec); conditional (170–200 cm/sec); and abnormal (>200 cm/sec). It is a noninvasive assessment of brain blood flow identifying children with SCD at high risk for stroke and "asymptomatic" brain disease. TCD can be used as a screening tool in children as young as 2 years of age and should be performed yearly. If the results are conditional (170–200 cm/sec), then the patient should have an examination every 2 months. Patients with abnormal velocities (>200 cm/sec) need to have repeat TCD to ensure that they do not progress to abnormal within 2–8 weeks. In patients with an abnormal TCD, a chronic transfusion regime reduces the risk of stroke by >90%.

Treatment
- *Exchange transfusion:* This limits the amount of acute sickling in poorly perfused areas of the brain. Patients usually show marked improvement in motor function. After initial exchange, a maintenance exchange transfusion program should be carried out (for about 4 years). A regular program designed to keep HbS less than 20% lowers the recurrence rate of stroke to less than 10%.
- *Fetal hemoglobin stimulating agents (e.g., hydroxyurea):* These may prevent further stroke.
- *Nitric oxide (NO):* This is a potent vasodilator. Inhaled NO in SCD patients with acute chest syndrome produces a dramatic improvement in oxygenation.
- *Stem cell transplantation.*

Cardiovascular system
Abnormal cardiac findings are present in most patients and are primarily a result of chronic anemia and the compensatory increased cardiac output.

1. *Cardiomegaly:* Found in most patients. Left ventricular hypertrophy occurs in about 50% of patients. Decreased left ventricular contractility occurs in one third of SCD patients.
2. *Myocardial dysfunction:* Secondary to fibrosis and hemosiderosis.
3. *Heart sounds:* Moderate intensity murmur, blowing in character with wide splitting of second heart sound.
4. *Electrocardiogram (ECG) abnormalities:* Sinus tachycardia; left ventricular hypertrophy; left axis deviation; inverted T waves; sinus arrhythmia.
5. *Radiologic findings:* Cardiac enlargement involving all chambers; prominent pulmonary artery segment.
6. *Echocardiographic findings:* Both left and right ventricular dilatation; increased stroke volume; abnormal septal motion.
7. *Pulmonary hypertension and cor pulmonale:* Usually occurs in older patients and may be related to previous repeated chest syndromes.

Lungs
1. Reduced PaO_2.
2. Reduced PaO_2 saturation.
3. Increased pulmonary shunting.
4. Acute chest syndrome (ACS): This is the most common cause of death and the second most common cause of hospitalization. Distinguishing ACS from infectious and noninfectious causes is often difficult (see Table 7-11). The incidence is about 24 events per 100 patients in young children. The incidence in other sickle cell genotypes is lower (SS > Sβ^0-thalassemia > SC > Sβ^+-thalassemia), and concomitant α-thalassemia does not appear to affect ACS rates. Fetal

hemoglobin (HbF) levels are inversely proportional to the frequency of ACS, and an increase in HbF (10–15%) decreases the incidence of ACS by about 50% in all age groups. This may also explain why patients with the homozygous CAR haplotype have ACS more commonly and severely than do those with either homozygous Benin or Senegal haplotypes.

The incidence of ACS has been shown to be inversely proportional to the degree of anemia and directly proportional to the white blood cell count; increased levels of cytokines and/or white cell adhesion to the endothelium may play a role in this. ACS has a striking association with vaso-occlusive crisis (VOC). About 30% of all ACS events are preceded or accompanied by a pain crisis. About 50% of ACS events are associated with infections. *Streptococcus pneumoniae* is the most common causative organism in ACS in young children. *Mycoplasma* and *Chlamydia* are two common organisms that may be related to severe ACS. Parvovirus infection can also result in ACS not only by direct infection, but also by causing bone marrow necrosis with subsequent pulmonary fat embolism (PFE) syndrome. The frequency of PFE in patients with SCD is not uncommon (15%). It usually follows a VOC. Pulmonary infarction is usually due to obstruction of small or medium-sized vessels and is possibly secondary to occlusion from adhesion of sickled RBCs to endothelial cells.

The treatment for ACS is:

Intravenous (IV) antibiotics.

Hydration with alkalinization (hydration: IV plus oral fluids at one time maintenance are sufficient). Overhydration may result in pulmonary edema because patients with ACS are particularly susceptible.

Pain control: nonsteroidal agents (narcotic sparing effect) and narcotics. Careful monitoring is required to reduce the risk of hypoventilation.

Adrenergic bronchodilators (to improve peak expiratory flow rates).

Oxygen therapy (in hypoxemic patients).

Exchange transfusions (in severe hypoxemia: PaO_2 <70 mmHg in room air); prophylactic transfusions (in recurrent ACS).

Hydroxyurea (in recurrent ACS).

Stem cell transplantation (in recurrent ACS).

5. Pulmonary fibrosis—chronic lung disease: Early identification of progressive lung disease using pulmonary function testing is imperative. Aggressive treatment has little benefit in end-stage lung disease and this should be avoided by prophylactic transfusions.

Kidney
1. Increased renal flow.
2. Increased glomerular filtration rate.
3. Enlargement of kidneys; distortion of collecting system on intravenous pyelogram.
4. Hyposthenuria (urine concentration defect): Hyposthenuria is the first manifestation of sickle cell–induced obliteration of the vasa recta of the renal medulla. Edema in the medullary vasculature is followed by focal scarring, interstitial fibrosis, and destruction of the countercurrent mechanism. Hyposthenuria results in a concentration capacity of more than 400–450 mOsm/kg and an obligatory urinary output as high as 2000 mL/m²/day, causing the patient to be particularly susceptible to dehydration. The increased urine output is associated with *nocturia*, often manifesting as *enuresis*. Treatment of enuresis includes imipramine (adolescents) at a starting dose 25 mg/day, increasing to a maxi-

mum of 100 mg/day; intranasal 1-deamino-8-D-arginine vasopressin (DDAVP) (0.01%): 10–40 µg at bedtime.

5. Hematuria: Papillary necrosis is usually the underlying anatomic defect. Treatment of papillary necrosis is aggressive IV hydration. Frank hematuria usually resolves, although bleeding can be prolonged.
6. Renal tubular acidification defect.
7. Increased urinary sodium loss (may result in hyponatremia).
8. Hyporeninemic hypoaldosteronism and impaired potassium excretion are results of renal vasodilating prostaglandin increase in patients with SCD.
9. Proteinuria: Persistent increasing proteinuria is an indication of glomerular insufficiency, perihilar focal segmental sclerosis, and renal failure. Intraglomerular hypertension with sustained elevations of pressure and flow is the prime etiology of the hemodynamic changes and subsequent proteinuria. If proteinuria persists for more than 4–8 weeks, angiotensin-converting enzyme (ACE) inhibitors (i.e., enalapril) are recommended.
10. Nephrotic syndrome: A 24-hour urine protein of more than 2 g/day, edema, hypoalbuminemia, and hyperlipidemia may indicate progressive renal insufficiency. The efficacy of steroid therapy in the management of nephrotic syndrome in SCD is not clear. Carefully monitored use of diuretics is indicated to control edema.
11. Chronic renal failure—uremia. Renal failure can be managed with peritoneal dialysis, hemodialysis, and transplantation.

Liver and biliary system
1. Chronic hepatomegaly.
2. Liver function tests: Increased serum glutamic-oxaloacetic transaminase (SGOT) and serum glutamic pyruvic transaminase (SGPT).
3. Cholelithiasis (incidence):
   a. 2–4 years: 12%
   b. 15–18 years: 42%

   All patients with SCD should have periodic routine sonographic examinations of the gallbladder. Even if patients have asymptomatic cholelithiasis, laparoscopic cholecystectomy is recommended. Children tolerate elective cholecystectomy well with little morbidity if prepared properly for surgery. Operating during the acute phase, however, carries a significant risk of complications. Persistent *Salmonella* bacteremia is also an indication for elective cholecystectomy in a patient with gallstones.
4. Transfusion-related hepatitis.
5. Intrahepatic crisis: Intrahepatic sickling can result in massive hyperbilirubinemia, elevated liver enzyme values, and a painful syndrome mimicking acute cholecystitis or viral hepatitis. Fulminant hepatic failure, massive cholestasis, hepatic encephalopathy, and shock are rare complications and require exchange transfusion.
6. Hepatic necrosis, portal fibrosis, regenerative nodules, and cirrhosis are common postmortem findings that may be a consequence of recurrent vascular obstruction and repair.

Bones
Skeletal changes in SCD are common because of expansion of the marrow cavity, bone infarcts, or both.

1. Dactylitis: First few years of life. Dactylitis usually is not seen in older children because as the child ages, the sites of hematopoiesis move from a peripheral location such as the fingers and toes to more central locations such as the arms,

legs, ribs, and sternum. Infants with dactylitis often tolerate these episodes very well and may require only acetaminophen or nonsteroidal inflammatory agents (NSAIDs).

2. Avascular necrosis (AVN): The most common cause of AVN of the femoral head is sickle cell disease. The incidence is much higher with coexistent α-thalassemia in patients who have frequent painful crises and in those with the highest hematocrits. The pathophysiology is sludging in marrow sinusoids, marrow necrosis, healing with increased intramedullary pressure, bone resorption, and eventually collapse. About 50% of patients are asymptomatic. Symptomatic patients have significant chronic pain and limited joint mobility. The diagnosis is made radiographically and shows subepiphyseal lucency and widened joint space and flattening or fragmentation and scarring of the epiphysis. On MRI, avascular necrosis of femoral head can be detected before deformities are apparent on radiograph.

   Treatment: Therapy for AVN is largely supportive, with bed rest, NSAIDs, and limitation of movement during the acute painful episode. Transfusion therapy does not seem to delay progression of AVN. Core decompression of the affected hip has been reported to reduce pain and stop progression of the disease. In this procedure, avascularized bone is removed to decompress the area with the potential for subsequent new bone formation. This procedure seems to be beneficial only in the early stages of AVN and before loss of the integrity of the femoral head. AVN of the hip may have its onset in childhood, so thorough musculoskeletal examination with concentration on the hips should be performed at least yearly in children with SCD. This ensures that AVN is detected early when it is in its most treatable form. Total hip replacement may be the only option for severely compromised patients; 30% of replaced hips require surgical revision within 4.5 years, and more than 60% of patients continue to have pain and limited mobility postoperatively. Avascular necrosis of the humeral head is uncommon. Patients are less symptomatic, and arthroplasty is exceedingly rare.

3. Widening of medullary cavity and cortical thinning: Hair-on-end appearance of skull on radiograph.

4. Fish-mouth vertebra sign on radiograph.

Eyes

1. *Retinopathy:* Sickle retinopathy is common in all forms of SCD, but particularly in those patients with hemoglobin SC disease.

   Nonproliferative retinopathy: Occlusion of small blood vessels of the eye and retinal neovascularization are very common (30% as young as 5–7 years of age) and are usually not associated with defects in visual acuity.

   Treatment: Hydroxyurea therapy may slow or prevent further vaso-occlusion. This in turn may have a favorable effect by reducing subsequent neovascularization.

   Proliferative retinopathy: Occlusion of small blood vessels in the peripheral retina may be followed by enlargement of existing capillaries or development of new vessels. Clusters of neovascular tissue "sea fans" grow into vitreous and along the surface of the retina. Sea fans may cause vitreous hemorrhage, which results in transient or prolonged loss of vision. Small hemorrhages resorb, but repeated leaks cause formation of fibrous strands. Shrinkage of these strands can cause retinal detachment.

   Treatment: Photocoagulation may be effective in retinal detachment.

   With proper screening and new methods such as laser surgery most of the complications of retinopathy can be avoided. Annual ophthalmologic examinations including inspection of the retina are indicated for children older than 5 years of age.

2. *Angioid streaks:* These are pigmented striae in the fundus caused by abnormalities in Baruch's membrane due to iron or calcium deposits or both. They usually produce *no* problems for the patient, but occasionally they can lead to neovascularization that can bleed into the macula and decrease vision.

3. *Hyphema:* Blood in the anterior chamber (hyphema) rarely occurs secondary to sickling in the aqueous humor, because of its low pH and PaO_2. Anterior chamber paracentesis may be performed if pressure is increased.

4. *Conjunctivae:* Comma-shaped blood vessels, seemingly disconnected from other vasculature, can be seen in the bulbar conjunctiva of patients with SCD and variants (SS > SC > Sβ-thalassemia). These produce no clinical disability. Their frequency may be related to the number of irreversibly sickled cells in the blood. This abnormality can be identified by using the +40 lens of an ophthalmoscope.

Ears

Twelve percent of patients have high-frequency sensorineural hearing loss. The pathophysiology of the auditory apparatus appears to be sickling in the cochlear vasculature with destruction of hair cells.

Adenotonsillar hypertrophy

Adenotonsillar hypertrophy giving rise to upper airway obstruction can become a problem from the age of 18 months. The marked hypertrophy is compensation for the loss of lymphoid tissue in the spleen. It occurs in at least 18% of patients. In severe cases, this can cause hypoxemia at night with consequent sickling. Early tonsillectomy may be indicated in these patients.

Skin

Cutaneous ulcers of the legs occur over the external or internal malleoli. Leg ulcers usually do not occur in childhood. Ulceration may result from increased venous pressure in the legs caused by the expanded blood volume in the hypertrophied bone marrow. The incidence is higher in patients with low steady-state hemoglobin values or low fetal hemoglobin production.

Treatment

Rest; elevation of the leg
Protection of the ulcer by the application of a soft sponge-rubber doughnut
Debridement and scrupulous hygiene
Iodosorb wound dressing to induce localized proinflammatory cytokines such as tumor necrosis factor (TNF) and interleukin-6 (IL-6)
Low-pressure elastic bandage and above-the-knee elastic stockings to improve venous circulation
Exchange transfusion therapy if ulcers persist despite optimal care
Antistaphylococcal antibiotic treatment if skin colonized with *Staphylococcus aureus*
Oral administration of zinc sulfate (220 mg three times a day) to promote healing of leg ulcers
Split-thickness skin grafts.

Genitourinary-priapism

Priapism is marked by a painful failure of detumescence of the penis. Mean age of priapism in patients with SCD is about 12 years. Priapism usually occurs at early morning hours, probably related to sleep acidosis. The normal slow blood flow pattern in the penis is similar to the blood flow in the spleen and renal medulla. Failure of detumescence is due to venous outflow obstruction or to prolonged smooth muscle relaxation, either singly or in combination. Postpubertal patients tend to have prolonged and recurrent episodes. With repeated episodes, the cavernosa is fibrosed and hyalinized and blood no longer flows. Treatment decisions must be made and implemented promptly within 12 hours, because the time the patient has been in the priapismic state correlates with the presence of irreversible infarction and future dysfunction.

A history should be obtained as to the precise timing of the onset and the state of recurrence. If the shaft of the penis is hard and painful in the area of the cavernosa but the glans is soft and the patient is able to urinate, there is relatively little involvement of the spongiosa. Urinary obstruction is the clinical hallmark, along with engorgement of the glans, of secondary involvement of the corpora spongiosa. An MRI scan of the penis can determine if the obstruction is confined to the corpora cavernosa (bicorporal) or if there is involvement of the spongiosa (tricorporal). Involvement of the spongiosa is indicative of cavernosa infarction.

Treatment:

Hydration
Partial exchange transfusion (most effective within 24 hours from the onset)
Analgesia (i.e., morphine sulfate)
Sedation (i.e., hydroxyzine pamoate [Vistaril])
Oxygen
Sitz bath or hot compresses.

Surgical procedures for acute episodes:

Corporal aspiration and irrigation (repeat, if necessary)
Cavernoglans shunt
Cavernosaphenous shunt.

Surgical procedures for impotence:

Insertion of penile prosthesis.

Prevention of priapism. For recurrent priapism, prophylactic exchange transfusion is very effective. In children (Tanner 1, 2, 3) and adolescents (Tanner 4, 5) who still retain penile function after a major episode of priapism, treatment with hydroxyurea might be considered. Treatment for at least 2 years might allow for healing and should not interfere with normal sexual activity.

Growth and Development

1. Birth weight is normal. However, by 2–6 years of age, the height and weight are significantly delayed. The weight is more affected than the height, and patients with sickle cell anemia and $S\beta^0$-thalassemia experience more delay in growth than patients with HbSC disease and $S\beta^+$-thalassemia. In general, by the end of adolescence, patients with sickle cell disease have caught up with controls in height but not weight. The poor weight gain is likely to represent increased caloric requirements in anemic patients with increased bone marrow activity and cardiovascular compensation. Zinc deficiency may be a cause of poor growth. In these patients, zinc supplementation (dose of 220 mg three times a day) at about 10 years of age should be administered. Growth hormone levels and growth hormone stimulation studies appear to be normal in children who have impaired growth.
2. Delayed sexual maturation: Tanner 5 is not achieved until the median ages of 17.3 and 17.6 years for girls and boys, respectively. In males, decreased fertility with

abnormal sperm motility, morphology and numbers is prominent. Zinc sulfate 220 mg three times a day may be effective for sexual maturity in these patients; females are more responsive than males.

Functional Hyposplenism

1. By 6 months of age, significant splenomegaly is apparent and persists during childhood, after which the spleen undergoes progressive fibrosis (autosplenectomy).
2. Functional reduction of splenic activity precedes autosplenectomy in early life. This is the consequence of altered intrasplenic circulation caused by intrasplenic sickling. It can be temporarily reversed by transfusion of normal red cells. Children with functional hyposplenia are 300–600 times more likely to develop overwhelming pneumococcal and *Haemophilus influenzae* sepsis and meningitis than are normal children; other organisms involved are gramnegative enteric organisms and *Salmonella*. The period of greatest risk of death from severe infection occurs during the first 5 years of life.
3. Functional hyposplenism may be demonstrated by the following:
   a. Presence of Howell–Jolly bodies on blood smear
   b. ^{99m}Tc-gelatin sulfur colloid spleen scan: no uptake of the radioactive colloid by enlarged spleen
   c. Twenty percent (range 12–40%) pitted red cells on interference phase-contrast microscopy (Nomarski optics).

Hemostatic Changes

Almost all of the components of hemostasis are altered, resulting in a hypercoagulable state:

- *Increased platelet activation and secretion:* Increased sickle red blood cell (SRBC) adhesion to endothelium
- *Increased von Willebrand factor (vWF):* Abnormal adherence of SRBCs to endothelium
- *Increased activated factor VII (factor VIIa) and factor X (factor Xa):* Increased thrombin formation
- *Increased factor VIII and fibrinogen*
- *Decreased protein C and protein S:* Increased risk of thrombosis.

Hemostatic changes may explain some of the clinical manifestations of SCD. It is still difficult to prove that these changes are indeed involved in the pathophysiology of vaso-occlusive crisis in SCD.

Therapeutic Approaches to Altering Sickle Red Blood Cell/Endothelial Cell Interaction
- *Hydroxyurea:* May result in reduction of adhesive receptors on SRBCs
- *Nitric oxide:* Inhibits platelet activation, aggregation, and secretion; inhibits SRBC adhesion to the endothelium; reduces HbS polymerization
- *Arginine:* When given orally increases levels of exhaled and plasma nitric oxide (transient effect)
- *Anticoagulants:* (1) Minidose heparin (SC): reduces in-hospital stay; (2) low-intensity coumadin: reduces thrombin generation; and (3) low-molecular-weight heparin (LMWH): has specific activity against factors VIIa and Xa
- *Antiplatelet agents:* (1) Acetylsalicylic acid (ASA): no significant effect on pain crises; and (2) ASA plus dipyridamole: modest benefit.

Diagnosis

1. *In utero:* Sickle cell disease can be diagnosed accurately *in utero* by restriction endonuclease analysis of DNA prepared from fetal fibroblasts (obtained by amniocentesis). Chorionic villus biopsy offers an alternative to amniocentesis. With the advent of PCR amplification of specific DNA sequences, sufficient DNA can be obtained from a very small number of fetal cells, thereby eliminating the necessity of culturing fetal fibroblasts from amniotic fluid. These techniques should be employed before 10 weeks' gestation.
2. *During newborn period:* The diagnosis of sickle cell disease can be established by electrophoresis using:
   a. High-performance liquid chromatography (most commonly used)
   b. Citrate agar with a pH of 6.2, a system that provides distinct separation of hemoglobins S, A, and F
   c. Acid and alkaline electrophoresis
   d. PCR amplification of DNA.
   These tests can be performed on cord blood or on a dried blood specimen blotted on filter paper.
3. *In older children:* Table 7-12 lists the diagnosis and differential diagnosis of various sickle cell syndromes.

Prognosis

The survival time is unpredictable and is related in part to the severity of the disease and its complications (with active management, 85% survive to 20 years of age).

Causes of Death

1. Infection (peak incidence between 1 and 3 years of age)
   a. Sepsis
   b. Meningitis
   Infection is the most common cause of death and is due to splenic dysfunction. The risk of acquiring sepsis or meningitis is greater than 15% in children younger than 5 years, with a mortality rate of 30%.
2. Organ failure
   a. Heart
   b. Liver
   c. Kidney.
3. Thrombosis of vessels supplying vital organs
   a. Lungs: most common cause in adults
   b. Brain: most common cause in adolescents.

Ameliorating Factors

1. Persistent production of HbF into adolescence and adulthood
   a. A level of more than 10% HbF offers protection against stroke and avascular necrosis.
   b. A level of more than 20% HbF offers protection from episodic manifestations such as painful crises or pulmonary complications.
2. Co-inheritance of α-thalassemia, which reduces the levels of hemolysis (higher hemoglobin and lower reticulocyte count)
3. Environmental factors (i.e., socioeconomic status).

Table 7-12. Differential Diagnosis in Sickle Cell Syndromes

Syndrome[a]	Clinical severity	Spleno-megaly	Mean hemoglobin (g/dL)	Mean hematocrit (%)	Mean corpuscular volume (fL)	Reticulocytes (%)	Red cell morphology	Electrophoresis
AS	Asymptomatic	(−)	Normal	Normal	Normal	Normal	Few target cells	35–45% S; 55–60% A; F[b]
SS	Severe	YC (+) OC (−)	7.5	22	85	5–30	Many target cells, ISCs (4+), and NRBCs	80–96% S; 2–20% F[b]
SC	Mild/moderate	(+)	11	33	80	2–6	Many target cells, few ISCs (1+)	50–55% S; 45–50% C; F[b]
S/β-thalassemia	Moderate/severe	(+)	8.5	28	65	3–20	Marked hypochromia and microcytosis; many target cells, ISCs (3+), and NRBCs	50–85% S; 2–30% F[b]; >3.5% A2
S/β+-thalassemia	Mild/moderate	(+)	10	32	72	2–6	Mild microcytosis and hypochromia; many target cells, few ISCs (1+)	50–80% S; 10–30% A; 0–20% F[b], <3.5% A2
SS/α-thalassemia-1	Mild/moderate	(+)	10	27	70	5–10	Mild hypochromia and microcytosis; few ISCs (2+)	80–100% S; 0–20% F[b]
S/HPFH	Asymptomatic	(−)	14	40	85	1–3	Occasional target cells, no ICSs	60–80% S; 15–35% F[c]

Abbreviations: HPFH, high persistent fetal hemoglobin; ISC, irreversible sickle cell; NRBC, nucleated red blood cell; OC, older child; YC, young child (−) absent, (+) present.

[a] All syndromes have positive sickle preparations.

[b] Hemoglobin F distribution; heterogeneous.

[c] Hemoglobin F distribution; homogeneous.

Management

1. *Comprehensive care:* Prevention of complications is as important as treatment. Optimal care is best provided in a comprehensive setting.
2. *Infection:* Because of a marked incidence of bacterial sepsis and meningitis and fatal outcome under 5 years of age, the following management is recommended:

   All children with sickle cell disease should receive oral penicillin prophylaxis starting at 3–4 months of age:

   62.5 mg bid (up to 1 year)

   125 mg bid (1–3 years)

   250 mg bid (3–6 years)

   In patients allergic to penicillin erythromycin ethyl succinate 10 mg/kg orally twice a day should be prescribed.

   All children with SCD should receive a 24-valent pneumococcal vaccine at 2 years of age. Revaccination after 4 years improves the protective levels of antibodies without serious adverse reactions. Conjugate *Haemophilus influenzae* vaccine should be given (three injections at 2-month intervals) between 2 and 6 months of age. Influenza virus vaccine should be given yearly, each fall.

   Early diagnosis of infections requires:

   - Education of the family to identify a child with fever: Families should be instructed to call their physician immediately if their child develops a single temperature greater than 38.5°C (by mouth) or two elevations between 38°C and 38.5°C. The child should be seen immediately by a physician.
   - Proper investigation of the patient to determine the etiology of the fever.
   - Prompt antibiotic coverage.

   Table 7-13 outlines the protocol to manage children under 5 years of age with fever.
3. *Painful crisis:* Most painful crises (mild or mild to moderate) can be treated at home with increased fluid intake and oral analgesics. The level of α-hydroxybutyric dehydrogenase (α-HBD) is of great value in the clinical diagnosis of

---

Table 7-13. Protocol for Patients under 5 Years of Age Presenting with Fever

1. Physical examination
2. Laboratory evaluation

   Blood count, band count, and reticulocyte count

   Blood culture

   Chest radiograph

   Urinalysis, culture, and sensitivity

   Mycoplasma titer

   Stool culture (if diarrhea present)

   Lumbar puncture: performed in all patients under 1 year of age or patients with even minimal signs suggestive of meningitis

   Evaluation for osteomyelitis (see Table 7-9)
3. All patients under age 5 with a documented temperature (by mouth) above 38.5°C should be admitted to the hospital
4. If meningitis not suspected or ruled out, patient is placed on ceftriaxone to cover *S. pneumoniae* and *H. influenzae* at a dose of 75 mg/kg/day; antibiotics continued until blood cultures negative for 72 hours
5. Discharge after 72 hours on oral Ceclor or Augmentin if afebrile, nontoxic, and safe hemoglobin level; during hospitalization, blood and reticulocyte counts ordered a minimum of every other day
6. Reevaluation within 1 week of discharge

From Vishinsky E, Lubin BH. Suggested guidelines for treatment of children with sickle cell anemia. Hematol Oncol Clin North Am 1987;1:483, with permission.

vaso-occlusive crisis. It permits a distinction between true painful crises, infection, and fake symptoms. Table 7-14 lists the values of α-HBD in the steady state, during vaso-occlusive crisis, and during infection. Moderate to severe and severe painful episodes must be treated in the hospital in the following manner:

a. Increased hydration. 1.5 times maintenance fluid (2250 mL/m²/day with DW/50% N sodium bicarbonate (88 mEq/L).
b. Analgesic treatment (see Table 7-15).
c. Partial exchange transfusion for refractory crisis (more than 5 days' duration). The aim is to reduce HbS to less than 40% and keep the hemoglobin

Table 7-14. Serum α-Hydroxybutyric Dehydrogenase in Sickle Cell Disease

	Steady state	Vaso-occlusive crisis	Infection
α-HBD (mU/mL)	305.4±47.0 (255–378)	517.5±86.3 (417–773)	306.6±44.8 (205–375)

Table 7-15. Recommended Initial Dose and Interval of Analgesics Necessary to Obtain Adequate Pain Control in Sickle Cell Disease

	Maximum dose (mg)	Route	Interval	Comments
Severe pain				
Morphine	0.15 mg/kg/dose (max 10 mg)	SC, IM	q3h	Drug of choice
Meperidine	1.5 mg/kg/dose (max 100 mg)	IM	q3h	Increased incidence of seizures; avoid in patients with renal or neurologic disease
Moderate pain				
Oxycodone (Percocet or Percodan)	1–2 tabs/dose (1 tab=5 mg)	PO	q4h	Patients over age 5
Methadone	0.15 mg/kg/dose	PO	q6h	Effective in patients usually requiring parenteral narcotics; NOT FOR ROUTINE USE
Meperidine	1.5 mg/kg/dose (max 100 mg/dose)	PO	q3½h	
Mild pain				
Codeine	0.75 mg/kg/dose	PO	q4h	May be effective up to 6 hours
Aspirin	1.5 g/m²/day divided into 6 doses	PO	q4h	May be given with a narcotic for added analgesia
Acetaminophen	1.5 g/m²/day divided into 6 doses	PO	q4h	May be given with a narcotic for added analgesia
Ibuprofen (Motrin)	300–600 mg	PO	q6h	

Note: The combination of continuous intravenous and oral morphine and patient education reduces hospital stay. Undertreatment of pain leads to repeated hospitalization and conflict between patient and physician. Sickle cell pain should be treated like cancer pain.

From Vichinsky E, Lubin BH. Suggested guidelines for treatment of children with sickle cell anemia. Hematol Oncol Clin North Am 1987;1:483, with permission.

level at 10–12 g/dL because of the risk of increasing whole-blood viscosity, while maintaining a steady blood volume. In children, this is usually achieved by exchanging 1.5 times the total calculated blood volume on three occasions at 6–8 hourly intervals. Total volume exchanged (mL) = 35 × weight (kg). In the author's institution, the procedure is performed as follows: 15 mL/kg packed red cells is transfused; simultaneously, 20 mL/kg whole blood is continuously removed (the procedure lasts from 1 to 2 hours). The entire procedure is repeated on the following day (expected HbS level, <40%).

4. *Splenic sequestration crisis:* Table 7-16 lists the management.
5. *Acute chest syndrome (ACS):* Table 7-17 lists the management.
6. *Transfusion therapy:* Always consider the risk of infection (hepatitis B virus, hepatitis C virus, HIV), iron overload, and alloimmunization. The incidence of alloimmunization is 17.6%: mostly Kell (26%) and Rh (E [24%] and C [16%], respectively) antibodies. Other antibodies also occur in the following order of frequency: Jk^b (10%), Fy^a (6%), M (4%), Le^a (4%), S (3%), Fy^b (3%), e (2%), and Jk^a (2%).

   All children with SCD should have a red cell phenotype identified at diagnosis. This allows determination of the child's red cell antigen phenotype before any transfusion. The patients should receive blood that is leukocyte depleted, sickle cell negative, and phenotypically matched to the patient for the Rh and Kell antigens. These measures decrease the incidence of transfusion reactions and alloimmunization.

   Red cell transfusions or partial exchange transfusions may be used as primary treatments for the following conditions:
   Anemia
   Erythroblastopenic crisis
   Splenic sequestration (see Table 7-16)
   Hyperhemolytic crisis
   Refractory painful crisis
   Acute chest syndrome (see Table 7-17)
   Congestive heart failure
   Priapism
   Chronic leg ulcers
   Cerebrovascular accidents (HbS must be reduced to less than 20% at all times)
   Serious infections (i.e., sepsis, meningitis)
   Pregnancy
   Elective surgical procedures.
7. Recombinant human erythropoietin may ameliorate the anemia of sickle cell disease.

Table 7-18 lists routine health maintenance–related laboratory and special studies in patients with sickle cell disease.

Table 7-16. Management of Splenic Sequestration Crisis

Treatment of acute splenic sequestration crisis
   Transfuse to hemoglobin of 9–10 g/dL
   Partial exchange transfusion if any signs of cardiorespiratory distress
   Prophylactic exchange transfusion program until age 2 to maintain HbS at less than 30%
Indications for surgery
   One major or two minor acute splenic sequestration episodes (age >2 years or patient age <2 years and no evidence of splenic function)

Table 7-17. Management of Acute Chest Syndrome

Investigations
  Chest radiograph
  Blood count, reticulocyte count
  Blood culture, sputum culture (if possible)
  Arterial blood gas in room air
  Mycoplasma titer (acute and follow-up)
  VQ scan
  ECG
  Viral studies
Antibiotic therapy
  IV Ceftriaxone (75 mg/kg/day) started immediately; erythromycin may be added if
    Mycoplasma suspected
  If pleural fluid is contributing to respiratory distress, thoracentesis indicated
  Arterial blood gas closely monitored; oxygen administered if the patient has hypoxia
    (PaO_2, <70 mmHg)
  Partial exchange transfusion should be initiated for any of the following criteria:
    PaO_2, <70 mmHg
    25% drop in baseline PaO_2
    Acute congestive heart failure or acute right heart strain
    Rapidly progressive pneumonia
    Marked dyspnea with tachypnea

From Vichinsky E, Lubin BH with modifications. Suggested guidelines for treatment of children with sickle cell anemia. Hematol Oncol Clin North Am 1987;1:483, with permission.

Table 7-18. Routine Health Maintenance–Related Laboratory and Special Studies in Patients with Sickle Cell Disease

	Starting age	Frequency
Laboratory studies		
Complete blood count	At diagnosis	Yearly
Red cell antigen typing	At diagnosis	—
Liver and renal functions	At diagnosis	Yearly
Urinalysis	1 year	Yearly
Special studies		
Pulmonary function	5 years	Every 3 years
Chest x-ray	5 years	Every 3 years
Eye examinations	5 years	Every 3 years
Transcranial Doppler	2 years	Yearly

Management of Pregnancy

In women with SCD, pregnancy may be associated with serious problems for both the mother and the fetus. Maternal complications may include:

Increase in frequency of vaso-occlusive crises
Acute chest syndrome (specifically in third trimester)
Exaggeration of physiologic anemia
Toxemia
Death.

Because of sickling in the placenta, fetal complications may include:

Spontaneous abortion

Prematurity
Intrauterine growth retardation.

With modern obstetric management, regular prenatal care, and better nutrition, maternal mortality and perinatal death rates have been reduced (1% and 15%, respectively).
The following management is recommended:

- Complete red cell typing of both mother and father should be performed with antibody screening in the mother.
- Iron and folate should be prescribed.
- Early stages of pregnancy should be monitored with serial ultrasonographic studies.
- Transfusions or exchange transfusions* should be immediately initiated for the following indications: (1) mother symptomatic with either VOC or anemia-related problems or (2) any sign of fetal distress or poor growth.

Psychological Support

As for any chronic disease, patients require psychological support. Major problems that occur are:

- Coping with chronic pain
- Inability to keep up with peers
- Fears of premature death
- Delayed sexual maturity
- Increased doubts about self-worth.

These concerns should be addressed openly with appropriate psychological support. Self-help groups for patients and families should be provided

New Treatment Modalities

1. Antisickling therapy:
   Fetal hemoglobin production stimulating agents:
   5-Azacytidine
   Hydroxyurea
   Recombinant human erythropoietin
   Short-chain organic acids
2. Hematopoietic stem cell transplantation.

Hydroxyurea Therapy

Hydroxyurea (HU) is the most commonly used drug for HbF modulatory therapy. HU results in the upregulation of HbF. HbF, within the red cell, interferes with polymerization of HbS, and therefore decreases the propensity of the red cell to sickle. HU also increases red cell hydration and decreases the expression of red cell adhesion molecules, therefore providing additional salutary effects on the red cells. Numerous studies in adults and children have shown the beneficial effect of HU in SCD:

- Reduces number of VOC crises.
- Reduces incidence of ACS.
- Reduces transfusion needs.

---

*Blood transfusion should be carefully selected to be compatible in minor group antigens for which the mother is negative and the father positive. This approach minimizes the risk of maternal sensitization against fetal antigens.

HU is not yet approved by FDA for use in children. Efficiency and safety in children as young as 2 years of age have been as good as adult experience. However, the use of HU in children should be considered investigational, particularly because of concerns regarding potential leukemogenesis, teratogenesis, and adverse effect on growth and development.

Dose

The starting dose of HU is 15 mg/kg/day. It is increased every 6–8 weeks by 5 mg/kg/day until a total dose of 35 mg/kg/day is reached or until a favorable response is obtained or until signs of toxicity appear. Evidence of toxicity includes:

Neutrophil count, <2000/mm^3
Platelets, <80,000/mm^3
Hemoglobin drop, 2 g/dL
Absolute reticulocyte count <80,000/mm^3.

Clinical Response

HbF greater than 20% and a rise in total hemoglobin of 1–2 g/dL.

Follow-Up

The patient should be monitored with a complete blood count and HbF determination by hemoglobin electrophoresis twice monthly. Once a stable and maximum tolerated dose is obtained, the patient can be monitored monthly.

Indications

More than three painful crises in 1 year
Cerebrovascular accident (CVA) with alloimmunization
Recurrent ACS
Chronic leg ulcers that fail conventional therapy
Persistent occurrences of priapism despite standard therapy
Creatinine levels less than or equal to 1.7 mg/dL
Reticulocyte count greater than 150,000/mm^3.

Side Effects

Myelosuppression
Hair loss; skin pigment changes
Gastrointestinal (GI) disturbance
Birth defects (Female patient on hydroxyurea should not become pregnant or should be on birth control because of potential for birth defects.)
Increase in GGTP
Increase in creatinine.

Contraindications

Creatinine level greater than 2.0 mg/dL
Active liver disease.

Hematopoietic Stem Cell Transplantation (HSCT)

Currently HSCT (including umbilical cord blood) is the only curative therapy. The results of transplantation are best when performed in children with a sibling donor who is HLA identical.

The Eligibility criteria for HSCT for SCD:

1. Inclusions:
   - Patients <16 years of age with sickle cell anemia (SCD-SS or SCD-Sβ thalassemia)
   - One or more of the following complications:
     Stroke or CNS event lasting longer than 24 hours
     Impaired neuropsychological function and abnormal MRI scan
     Recurrent ACS or stage 1 or 2 sickle lung disease*
     Recurrent VOC disease
     Sickle nephropathy (GFR 30–50% predicted normal)
     Osteonecrosis of multiple bones.

2. Exclusions:
   - Patients >16 years of age
   - HLA-non-identical donor
   - One or more of the following conditions:
     Lansky performance score <70%
     Acute hepatitis or biopsy evidence of cirrhosis
     Renal impairment (GFR <30% predicted normal)
     Stage 3 or 4 sickle lung disease.*

Approximately 150 patients have undergone HSCT from HLA-identical siblings worldwide. Transplant morbidity is about 5%, and more than 90% patients survive. Approximately 85% survive free from SCD after HSCT. About 10% of patients experience recurrence. Neurologic complications such as seizures may occur after transplantation. Patients who have stable engraftment of donor cells experience no subsequent sickle cell–related events and experience stabilization of preexisting organ damage. There is also splenic function recovery. Linear growth is normal or accelerated after transplantation in the majority of patients.

About 5% of the patients develop clinical grade III acute or extensive graft versus host disease (GVHD; see Chapter 25). The risk of secondary cancers is estimated to be less than 5%.

Recommendations

- Children with SCD who experience significant sickle cell complications should be considered for HSCT.
- HLA typing should be performed on all siblings.
- Families should be counseled about the collection of UCB from prospective siblings.
- For severely affected children who have HLA-identical sibling donors, families should be informed about the benefits, risks, and treatment alternatives regarding HSCT.

Sickle Cell Trait (Heterozygous Form, AS)

The concentration of HbS in red cells is low, and sickling does not occur under normal conditions.

---

*The staging system for chronic lung disease is based on clinical, physiological, and roentgenographical criteria. Stage 1 and 2 are characterized by a mild reduction in lung volumes (vital capacity, total lung capacity) and FEV_1/FVC ratio (defines air flow obstruction). Stage 3 is where hypoxemia is first observed during stable periods, and a severe reduction in lung volumes and flows is seen with associated borderline pulmonary hypertension and fibrosis on chest radiograph. Stage 4 is characterized by severe pulmonary fibrosis and pulmonary hypertension. Patients progress from one stage to the next every 2 to 3 years. Chronic lung disease is a prime contributor to mortality in young adults with sickle cell anemia.

Hematology

1. *Indices:* Usually normal
2. *Blood smears:* Normal with few target cells
3. *Sickle cell preparation:* Reducing agents (e.g., sodium metabisulfite) to induce sickling *in vitro*
4. *Hemoglobin electrophoresis:* AS pattern (HbA, 55–60%; HbS, 35–45%).

Clinical Features

1. Usually asymptomatic
2. Hematuria rarely
3. Infarction rare, occurring during flights in unpressurized aircraft.

Significance

The genetic implications mandate counseling. Table 7-12 lists the differential diagnosis of sickle cell syndromes.

Hemoglobin C

Basic Features and Pathology

1. *Carrier state:* 2% in African Americans
2. *Amino acid substitution (the same codon in the β-chain as in hemoglobin S):* Lysine for glutamic acid
3. *Hemoglobin C tendency to form rhomboidal crystals with increases in osmolality:* Red cell deformability impaired and splenic sequestration increased.

Hemoglobin C Disease (Homozygous CC)

Hematology

1. *Anemia:* Usually mild, hemolytic
2. *Blood smear:* Numerous target cells, as well as some spherocytes (the result of membrane loss in the spleen); a bar of crystalline hemoglobin across cell due to alteration in intracellular hemoglobin is a frequent finding
3. *Hemoglobin electrophoresis:* CC pattern.

Clinical Features

1. Less severe than hemoglobin SS
2. Splenomegaly
3. Dehydration, leading to marked hemolysis and microcirculatory problems.

Hemoglobin C Trait (Heterozygous Form, AC)

Asymptomatic with only genetic significance.

Hemoglobin SC Disease

Combination of hemoglobin S and hemoglobin C.

Hematology

1. *Anemia:* If present, usually mild, hemolytic
2. *Blood smear:* Many target cells; sickle cells occasionally seen

3. *Sickle cell preparations:* Positive
4. *Hemoglobin electrophoresis:* SC pattern (HbS ±50%; HbC, ±50%).

Clinical Features

1. Similar to, but less severe than, sickle cell anemia
2. Severe infarctions on occasion (e.g., during pregnancy or the puerperium); may prove fatal.

Hemoglobin S/Thalassemia

1. Combination of hemoglobin S and β-thalassemia trait
2. Hematology and clinical features vary; severity depends on the amount of normal adult hemoglobin synthesized (0–30%)
3. With no hemoglobin A, disease comparable to sickle cell anemia.

Hemoglobin D and E

These β-chain variants cause relatively little morbidity; the diagnosis is made on hemoglobin electrophoresis.

Unstable Hemoglobins

Unlike the amino acid substitutions in hemoglobin S and hemoglobin C, which affect the polarity of the external surface of the hemoglobin molecule, resulting in polymerization (HbS) or crystallization (HbC), the substitutions in unstable hemoglobins occur within the heme cavity or pocket of the α- or β-polypeptide chain. Substitution in the region of heme attachment causes gross molecular instability.

The hereditary methemoglobinopathies are closely related to the unstable hemoglobins. The substitution in these cases is also in the region of heme attachment, but it results in increased susceptibility to oxidation of heme Fe^{2+} to Fe^{3+} with consequent methemoglobin accumulation and cyanosis rather than hemolysis. There is some overlap between these two disorders, insofar as there is an increase in methemoglobin formation in most types of unstable hemoglobinopathies.

Changes in the oxygen affinity have also been found in some of the unstable hemoglobins and some of the M hemoglobins. An increase in oxygen affinity results in greater tissue anoxia and greater erythropoietin stimulation for a given level of anemia. In at least one hemoglobinopathy, hemoglobin Chesapeake, the only clinical manifestation is mild polycythemia.

Table 7-19 lists the various clinical manifestations that suggest unstable hemoglobinopathies, and Table 7-20 presents laboratory data that suggest unstable hemoglobinopathies.

Table 7-19. Clinical Manifestations of Unstable Hemoglobins

Chronic nonspherocytic hemolytic anemia, varying from mild to severe
Intraerythrocyte inclusions (Heinz bodies) demonstrable by incubation of the cells with brilliant cresyl blue or methyl violet
Urinary dipyrrolic pigment excretion
Drug-induced hemolytic anemia
Methemoglobinemia
Cyanosis
Polycythemia
Chronic hemolytic anemia with normal hemoglobin electrophoresis
Variable response of hemolytic anemia to splenectomy

Table 7-20. Laboratory Data in Unstable Hemoglobinopathies

Chronic hemolytic anemia with normal red cell morphology, red cell enzymes, and hemoglobin electrophoresis
Abnormal heat stability test; tendency to precipitate on heating at 50°C
Presence of Heinz bodies
Raised methemoglobin levels
Dipyrroluria

THALASSEMIAS

Basic Features

Thalassemia syndromes are characterized by varying degrees of ineffective hematopoiesis and increased hemolysis. Clinical syndromes are divided into α- and β-thalassemias, each with varying numbers of their respective globin genes mutated. There is a wide array of genetic defects and a corresponding diversity of clinical syndromes. Most β-thalassemias are due to point mutations in one or both of the two β-globin genes (chromosome 11), which can affect every step in the pathway of β-globin expression from initiation of transcription to messenger RNA synthesis to translation and post translation modification. Figure 7-7 shows the organization of the genes (i.e., ε and γ, which are active in embryonic and fetal life, respectively) and activation of the genes in the locus control region (LCR), which promote transcription of the β-globin gene.

There are four genes for α-globin synthesis (two on each chromosome 16). Most α-thalassemia syndromes are due to deletion of one or more of the α-globin genes rather than to point mutations. Mutations of β-globin genes occur predominantly in children of Mediterranean, Southern, and Southeast Asian ancestry. Those of α-globin are most common in those of Southeast Asian and African ancestry. The main genetic variants are listed as follows.

β-Thalassemia

1. *β⁰-Thalassemia:* No detectable β-chain synthesis due to absent β-chain messenger RNA (mRNA)
2. *β⁺-Thalassemia:* Reduced β-chain synthesis due to reduced or nonfunctional β-chain mRNA
3. *δβ-Thalassemia:* δ- and β-chain genes deleted

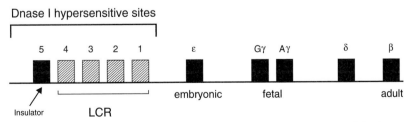

β-globin gene transcription is regulated by activation of the genes of the locus control region (LCR) and repression of the early genes

Fig. 7-7. The structure of the human β-globin locus in chromosome 11. (From Nathan D, Orkin S, editors. Nathan and Oski's Hematology of Infancy and Childhood. 5th ed. Philadelphia: WB Saunders, 1998;817, with permission.)

4. *Eβ-Thalassemia:* Hemoglobin E (lysine → glutamic acid at 26) and β-chain genes deletion

5. *Hb Lepore:* A fusion globin due to unequal crossover of the β- and δ-globin genes (the globin is produced at a low level because it is under δ-globin regulation).

α-Thalassemia

1. *Silent carrier α-thalassemia:* Deletion of one α-globin gene
2. *α-Thalassemia trait:* Deletion of two α-globin genes
3. *Hb Constant Spring:* Abnormal α-chain variant produced in very small amounts, thereby mimicking deficiency of the gene
4. *HbH disease:* Deletion of 3 α-globin genes, resulting in significant reduction of α-chain synthesis
5. *Hydrops fetalis:* Deletion of all 4 α-globin genes; no normal adult or fetal hemoglobin production.

In many populations, α- and β-thalassemia and structural hemoglobin variants (hemoglobinopathies) exist together, resulting in a wide spectrum of clinical disorders. Tables 7-21 and 7-22 list some features of the heterozygous and homozygous or doubly heterozygous states, respectively, of β-thalassemia and its variants. Table 7-23 lists the α-thalassemia syndromes.

β-Thalassemia: Homozygous or Doubly Heterozygous Forms (Major and Intermedia)

Pathogenesis

1. Variable reduction of β-chain synthesis ($β^0$, $β^+$, and variants)
2. Relative α-globin chain excess resulting in intracellular precipitation of insoluble α-chains
3. Increased but ineffective erythropoiesis with many red cell precursors prematurely destroyed; related to α-chain excess
4. Shortened red cell life span; variable splenic sequestration.

Table 7-21. Heterozygous States of β-Thalassemia and Variants

Type	HbA_2	HbF
$β^+$-Thalassemia	Increased	Normal to slightly increased
$β^0$-Thalassemia	Increased	Normal to slightly increased
δβ-Thalassemia	Normal	Increased (2–10%)
HPFH	Normal	Increased (10–40%)

Table 7-22. Homozygous or Doubly Heterozygous States of β-Thalassemia and Variants

Type	Anemia	δ-Globin chain	β-Globin chain	β-Globin mRNA	Gene mutation
β-Thalassemia	Severe	Present	Decreased	Decreased	Point mutations or deletions
$β^0$-Thalassemia	Severe	Present	Absent	Absent or abnormal	Point mutations or deletions
δβ-Thalassemia	Mild	Absent	Absent	Absent	Deletion mutation
HPFH	None	Absent	Absent	Absent	Point mutations or deletions

Table 7-23. α-Thalassemia Syndromes*

Syndrome	Genetics	Number of α-genes deleted	Newborn Hb Barts (γ_4) (%)	α/β synthesis ratio	Comments
Silent carrier of α-thalassemia	Heterozygous silent carrier	1	1–2	0.8–0.9	No anemia; no microcytosis; detectable by genetic interaction (i.e., two silent carriers can produce a child with α-thalassemia trait; a silent carrier and a person with α-thalassemia trait can produce a child with Hb H disease); also detectable by molecular studies
α-Thalassemia trait	Heterozygous α-thalassemia trait OR Homozygous silent carrier OR Homozygous Hb Constant Spring	2	3–10	0.7–0.8	Microcytosis; hypochromia; mild anemia
Hemoglobin H disease	Heterozygous α-thalassemia trait/ silent carrier OR α-thalassemia trait/Constant Spring	3	25	0.3–0.6	Hemolytic anemia of variable severity; relatively little ineffective erythropoiesis; no transfusion requirement; Hb H ($\beta4$) present
Hydrops fetalis	Homozygous α-thalassemia trait Hb Barts (γ_4)	4	80–100	0	Death *in utero* or shortly after birth

*This may be associated with a syndrome known as α-Thalassemia X-linked mental retardation syndrome characterized by hemoglobin H inclusions (β-globin tetramers), distinctive cranial features, genital anomalies, developmental delay with hypotonia and mental retardation.

Sequelae

1. Hyperplastic marrow (bone marrow expansion with cortical thinning and bony abnormalities)
2. Increased iron absorption and iron overload (especially with repeated blood transfusion), resulting in
   a. Fibrosis/cirrhosis of the liver
   b. Endocrine disturbances (e.g., diabetes mellitus, hypothyroidism, hypogonadism, hypoparathyroidism, hypopituitarism)
   c. Skin hyperpigmentation
   d. Cardiac hemochromatosis manifesting as pericarditis, arrhythmias, cardiomegaly, pericarditis, and ultimately, cardiac failure
3. Hypersplenism
   a. Plasma volume expansion
   b. Shortened red cell life (of autologous and donor cells)
   c. Leukopenia
   d. Thrombocytopenia.

Hematology

1. Anemia: Hypochromic, microcytic
2. Reticulocytosis
3. Leukopenia and thrombocytopenia (may develop with hypersplenism)
4. Blood smear: Target cells and nucleated red cells, extreme anisocytosis, contracted red cells, polychromasia, punctate basophilia, circulating normoblasts
5. ^{51}Cr-labeled red cell life span reduced (but the ineffective erythropoiesis is more important in the production of anemia)
6. Hemoglobin F raised; hemoglobin A2 increased
7. Bone marrow: May be megaloblastic (due to folate depletion); erythroid hyperplasia
8. Osmotic fragility: Decreased
9. Serum ferritin: Raised.

Biochemistry

1. Raised bilirubin (chiefly indirect)
2. Evidence of liver dysfunction (late, as cirrhosis develops)
3. Evidence of endocrine abnormalities, for example, diabetes (typically late), hypogonadism (low estrogen and testosterone).

Clinical Features

Because of the variability in the severity of the fundamental defect, there is a spectrum of clinical severity (major to intermedia) that considerably influences management. β-Thalassemia intermedia is defined as homozygous or doubly heterogeneous thalassemia, which is generally not transfusion dependent. Clinical manifestations include:

1. Failure to thrive in early childhood
2. Anemia
3. Jaundice, usually slight; gallstones
4. Hepatosplenomegaly, which may be massive; hypersplenism
5. Abnormal facies, prominence of malar eminences, frontal bossing, depression of bridge of the nose, and exposure of upper central teeth
   a. Skull radiographs showing hair-on-end appearance due to widening of diploic spaces

    b. Fractures due to marrow expansion and abnormal bone structure

    c. Generalized skeletal osteoporosis

6. Growth retardation, delayed puberty, primary amenorrhea in females, and other endocrine disturbances secondary to chronic anemia and iron overload
7. Leg ulcers
8. Skin bronzing

If untreated, 80% of patients die in the first decade of life. With current management, the life expectancy has dramatically increased. Patients now reach the fifth decade of life and are expected to live well beyond.

Complications

Complications develop as a result of:

- Chronic anemia in patients who are undertransfused or in untransfused thalassemia intermedia patients
- Chronic transfusion with resultant hemosiderosis and hemochromatosis
- Poor compliance with chelation therapy (generally).

Even in carefully managed patients, the following complications may develop:

- Endocrine disturbances (e.g., growth retardation, pituitary failure with impaired gonadotropins, hypogonadism, insulin-dependent diabetes mellitus, adrenal insufficiency, hypothyroidism, hypoparathyroidism)
- Cirrhosis of the liver and liver failure
- Cardiac failure due to myocardial iron overload (often associated with arrhythmias and pericarditis)
- Extramedullary hematopoiesis, resulting in bony deformities
- Marked osteoporosis is nearly uniformly present by the time patients reach adolescence. The causes of this include medullary expansion, deficiency of estrogen and testosterone, nutritional deficiency, and desferrioxamine toxicity. Manifestations include rickets, scoliosis, spinal deformities, nerve compression, fractures, and severe osteoporosis. Osteoporosis can be delayed by the early institution of chelation in childhood and sex hormone replacement early in adolescence.

Causes of Death

1. Congestive heart failure
2. Arrhythmia
3. Sepsis secondary to increased susceptibility to infection post-splenectomy
4. Multiple organ failure due to hemochromatosis.

Management

Hypertransfusion Protocol

The hypertransfusion protocol is used to maintain a pretransfusion hemoglobin between 10.5 and 11.0 g/dL at all times using 15 cc/kg leukocyte-depleted cross-matched packed red cells. Post-transfusion hemoglobin falls roughly 1 gram per week, necessitating transfusions every 3–4 weeks. Transfusion therapy should be started when a diagnosis is made and the hemoglobin level falls below 7 g/dL. Hypertransfusion results in:

1. Maximizing growth and development
2. Minimizing extramedullary hematopoiesis and decreasing facial and skeletal abnormalities

3. Reducing excessive iron absorption from gut
4. Retarding the development of splenomegaly and hypersplenism by reducing the number of red cells containing α-chain precipitates that reach the spleen
5. Reducing and/or delaying the onset of complications (e.g., cardiac).

Chelation Therapy

The objectives of chelation therapy are:

1. To bind free extracellular iron
2. To remove excess intracellular iron
3. To attain a negative iron balance (i.e., iron excretion > iron input).

Iron overload results from:

1. Ongoing transfusion therapy
2. Increased gut absorption of iron
3. Chronic hemolysis.

Chelation using desferrioxamine (Desferal) is recommended as follows:

1. Chelation should be instituted when the ferritin level is greater than 1000 ng/mL and adequate iron is excreted into the urine with the desferrioxamine challenge.
2. The desferrioxamine challenge is performed as follows:
   a. A 24-hour urine collection is started.
   b. Desferrioxamine 40 mg/kg is infused IV over 8 hours, starting at the beginning of the collection.
   c. The urine collection continues for 16 more hours, and the urine is assayed for total iron content.
   d. If the 24-hour urinary iron excretion is greater than or equal to 50% of the daily iron overload, the patient is ready for chelation.
   e. Daily iron load is calculated using roughly 1 mg iron/1 mL packed red blood cells (PRBCs). For example, if a patient receives 210 cc PRBCs every 21 days, the daily iron load is 10 mg. If the patient excretes 5 mg iron with the 24-hour challenge, chelation should be started.
3. Desferrioxamine, 40–60 mg/kg/day, is infused subcutaneously over 8–10 hours nightly via a portable electronic pump 4–6 nights per week, depending on iron overload.
4. In selected cases, with severe iron overload, desferrioxamine is administered IV in a high dose, maximum 10 g/day. This may be done immediately post-transfusion to bind transiently increased free serum iron.
5. The aim is to maintain the serum ferritin level close to 1000 ng/mL. The ferritin level should be monitored every 3–6 months.

The complications of desferrioxamine administration include:

Swelling at infusion site
Local reactions: pruritus, rash, and hyperemia (add hydrocortisone 2 mg/mL to the desferrioxamine solution)
Anaphylactoid reactions (treat by desensitization)
Toxic effects on the eye; cataracts, reduction of visual fields and visual acuity, and night blindness; occurs with prolonged or high-dose therapy or if desferrioxamine is used without sufficient iron overload
Hearing impairment with prolonged or high-dose therapy, typically without sufficient iron overload

Metaphyseal dysplasias

Desferrioxamine toxicity exacerbated when there is insufficient excretable iron relative to the amount of desferrioxamine given.

Splenectomy

1. Splenectomy reduces the transfusion requirements in patients with hypersplenism. It is usually performed in adolescents when transfusion requirements have increased secondary to hypersplenism.
2. Two weeks prior to splenectomy, a polyvalent pneumococcal and meningococcal vaccine should be given. If the patient has not received a *Haemophilus influenzae* vaccine, this should also be given. Following splenectomy, prophylactic penicillin 250 mg bid is given to reduce the risk of overwhelming postsplenectomy infection. Management of the febrile splenectomized patient is detailed in Chapter 26.
3. Indications for splenectomy include:
   a. Persistent increase in blood transfusion requirements by 50% or more over initial needs for more than 6 months
   b. Annual packed cell transfusion requirements in excess of 250 mL/kg/year in the face of uncontrolled iron overload (ferritin greater than 1500 ng/mL or increased hepatic iron concentration)
   c. Evidence of severe leukopenia and/or thrombocytopenia.

Supportive Care

1. Folic acid is not necessary in hypertransfused patients; 1 mg daily orally is given to patients on low transfusion regimens.
2. Hepatitis B vaccination should be given to all patients.
3. Appropriate inotropic, antihypertensive, and antiarrhythmic drugs should be administered when indicated for cardiac dysfunction.
4. Endocrine intervention (i.e., thyroxine, growth hormone, estrogen, testosterone) should be implemented when indicated.
5. Cholecystectomy should be performed if gallstones are present.
6. Patients with high viral loads of hepatitis C that are not spontaneously decreasing should be treated with PEG-interferon and ribavirin. Ribavirin increases hemolysis and transfusion requirements typically increase during therapy.
7. HIV-positive patients should be treated with the appropriate antiviral medications.
8. Genetic counseling and antenatal diagnosis (when indicated) should be carried out using chorionic villus sampling or amniocentesis.
9. Management of osteoporosis includes:
   a. Periodic screening and prevention through early hormonal replacement.
   b. Yearly screening of adolescents with bone densitometry and gonadal hormone evaluation.
   c. Early in adolescence, patients should receive estrogen/progesterone or testosterone replacement to prevent gonadal insufficiency–induced bone loss, which may result in a decreased adult height due to fusion of the epiphyses. The possible increased risk of breast cancer with hormonal replacement therapy should be explained to female patients.
   d. Two new agents are available to treat osteoporosis: (1) Calcitonin prevents trabecular bone loss by inhibiting osteoclastic activity. Parenteral and intranasal preparations are available. Miacalcin is the intranasal preparation. The dose is 1 spray into alternating nostrils daily. Miacalcin should be

taken with calcium carbonate 1500 mg daily and vitamin D 400 units daily. (2) Bisphosphonates (alendronate sodium) also inhibit osteoclast-mediated bone resorption. The usual dose of Fosamax is 10 mg orally taken daily with a full glass of water 30 minutes before breakfast.

Follow-up of patients with thalassemia includes:

Monthly: Measure the pretransfusion hemoglobin.

Every 3 months: Measure height and weight; measure ferritin; perform complete blood chemistry, including liver function tests.

Every 6 months: Complete physical examination and dental examination.

Every year: Evaluate growth and development; evaluate iron balance; complete evaluation of cardiac function (echocardiograph, ECG, Holter monitor as indicated); endocrine function (TFTs, PTH, FSH/LH, testosterone/estradiol, IGF-1, fasting cortisol); visual and auditory acuity; viral serologies (HAV, HBV panel, HCV [or if HCV+, quantitative HCV RNA PCR], HIV); bone densitometry; ongoing psychosocial support.

Every 1–2 years: Evaluation of tissue iron burden: SQUID (superconducting quantum interference device) measurement of liver iron; T_2-star measurement of cardiac iron (in select patients with cardiac disease); liver biopsy for iron concentration and histology.

Future Directions

Ongoing research to investigate better therapies for thalassemia patients is critical. The National Institutes of Health recently established the Thalassemia Clinical Research Network to facilitate clinical research trials in thalassemia.

Alternative Methods of Chelation

Nightly subcutaneous administration of desferrioxamine is time consuming and interferes in many ways with the lifestyle of the patient. For this reason, compliance is often suboptimal and patients develop hemochromatosis.

Clinical testing of a number of oral chelating compounds is under way. Deferiprone (L1) in a dose of 75 mg/kg/day is currently being used in Europe and is undergoing further clinical trials for FDA approval. Controversy exists at present about its potential toxicity, including idiosyncratic neutropenia, arthropathy, and possible adverse redistribution of iron. Many studies find deferiprone clinically useful without an unduly high risk of causing neutropenia. Preliminary data indicate that it may be particularly useful in reducing cardiac iron overload either as a single agent or in combination with desferrioxamine. ICL-670, a tri-dentate oral chelator, appears clinically effective in early trials. With a relatively long half-life, early results indicate that it may be equally as effective as desferrioxamine. A direct comparison trial must be completed to prove this and to study long-term efficacy and toxicity.

Pharmacologic Upgrading of Fetal Hemoglobin Synthesis

High levels of HbF ameliorate the symptoms of β-thalassemia by increasing the hemoglobin concentration of the thalassemic red cells and decreasing the accumulation of unmatched α-chains, which cause ineffective erythropoiesis. Hydroxyurea has been demonstrated to increase HbF production and mean hemoglobin levels in patients with thalassemia intermedia or Eβ-thalassemia, decreasing or eliminating the need for transfusion. Additionally, there are reports of a few β-thalassemia major patients who became transfusion free using hydroxyurea. Butyric acid analogues and erythropoietin as well as further testing with hydroxyurea are avenues of further investigation. Although these agents can decrease transfusion dependence, they have serious side effects, including neutropenia, increased susceptibility to infection, and possible oncogenicity.

Hematopoietic Stem Cell Transplantation

1. Stem cell transplantation from an HLA-identical sibling is a curative mode of therapy.
2. The greater the degree of hepatomegaly, hemosiderosis, and portal fibrosis of the liver prior to transplant, the worse the outcome.
3. Stem cell transplantation is a controversial mode of therapy because its risks must be weighed against the fact that patients who are least symptomatic have the best transplant results.

The following information is available about transplantation:

Results are better among patients less than 3 years of age who have received few transfusions and are without significant complications.

GVHD occurs less frequently in younger patients.

The refinement of methods of preparation for transplantation has brought about a drastic reduction in morbidity and mortality.

Gene Therapy

Research is under way on methods of inserting a normal β-globin gene into mammalian cells. Ultimately, the aim is to insert the gene into stem cells and utilize these for stem cell transplant.

Management of the Acutely Ill Thalassemic Patient

Acute illness requiring urgent treatment occurs secondary to:

- Sepsis, usually with encapsulated organisms
- Cardiomyopathy secondary to myocardial iron overload
- Endocrine crises such as diabetic ketoacidosis.

Prevention of these crises should be the primary treatment. Preventive measures include:

- Management of the splenectomized patient as outlined in Chapter 26
- Adequate chelation to prevent secondary hemochromatosis
- Routine monitoring of cardiac and endocrine function.

If a patient presents with signs of shock, the following measures should be instituted:

1. Determine hemoglobin, electrolyte, calcium, and glucose levels; perform urinalysis.
2. Obtain blood cultures.
3. Distinguish between cardiogenic shock and septic shock because the management of each differs. To distinguish between the two, obtain an ECG; echocardiograph, looking at left ventricular contractility; and central venous pressure (CVP).
4. If the patient is in cardiogenic shock, management includes diuretics, inotropic support, and careful monitoring of CVP and cardiac output. Management also includes desferrioxamine chelation as a continuous intravenous infusion at a dose of 15 mg/kg/h. (Once cardiac iron toxicity has reached the point of cardiac failure, it is extremely difficult to reverse; however, approximately 50% of patients will survive if aggressive chelation and cardiac management are insti-

tuted.) If Deferiprone is available, it may be added to desferrioxamine to further increase iron excretion.

5. If the patient is in septic shock, management consists of:
   Blood cultures, at least two peripheral sites
   Broad-spectrum antibiotics IV (e.g., third-generation cephalosporin and an aminoglycoside)
   Fluid boluses of 10 cc/kg normal saline to restore blood pressure
   Pressors such as dopamine, as indicated
   Coagulation studies to evaluate for disseminated intravascular coagulation (DIC)
   CVP monitoring to guide fluid management
   Arterial blood gas and chest radiograph.
6. If the patient is in diabetic ketoacidosis, manage the ketoacidosis in the usual manner with careful monitoring of cardiac function when the patient is being vigorously hydrated.

β-Thalassemia Intermedia

Although patients are homozygous or doubly heterozygous, the resultant anemia is milder than in thalassemia major.

Clinical Features

1. Patients generally do not require transfusions and maintain a hemoglobin between 7 and 10 g/dL.
2. Marked medullary expansion, hepatosplenomegaly, growth retardation, facial anomalies, and hyperbilirubinemia occur if patients are not adequately transfused.
3. Patients are most healthy if management is as vigorous as that for thalassemia major.

Management

1. Folic acid 1 mg/day PO should be administered.
2. Meats, particularly those rich in iron (e.g., liver and beef), and iron-supplemented cereals should be avoided. A cup of tea with every meal will reduce the absorption of nonheme iron.
3. Chelation therapy is required at an older age than in thalassemia major because patients have received fewer transfusions. It should be started when the serum ferritin level has risen to more than 1000 ng/mL and the desferrioxamine challenge produces sufficient urine iron excretion.
4. Transfusions generally are not required except during periods of erythroblastopenia (aplastic crises) or during acute infection. If hemoglobin falls below 7 g/dL, transfusion therapy should be initiated. Thalassemia intermedia patients who are inadequately transfused show the most extreme bony abnormalities (worse than adequately transfused thalassemia major patients).
5. Splenectomy may be required.
6. Cardiac and endocrine evaluation and bone densitometry should be performed as in thalassemia major.

β-Thalassemia Minor or Trait (Heterozygous β⁰ or β+)

Clinical Features

1. Asymptomatic (physical examination is normal)
   a. Discovered on routine blood test: slightly reduced hemoglobin, basophilic stippling, low MCV, normal RDW.

b. Discovered in family investigation or family history of heterozygous or homozygous β-thalassemia.

c. Confirmed with hemoglobin electrophoresis, demonstrating slightly decreased hemoglobin A (90–95% typically), increased hemoglobin A_2 (>4%); hemoglobin F mildly elevated in 50% of cases.

2. Thalassemia trait of unusual severity. There are cases of β-thalassemia trait of unusual severity secondary to the co-inheritance of α-gene duplication with increased α-globin synthesis, thereby increasing α- and β-chain imbalance.

α-Thalassemias

The major syndromes resulting from decreased α-chain synthesis are listed in Table 7-23. α-Thalassemia may present as silent carrier, thalassemia trait, hemoglobin H disease, or hydrops fetalis. Hemoglobin H disease is clinically milder than homozygous β-thalassemia and does not require a hypertransfusion protocol. Hydrops fetalis is not compatible with life and presents with intrauterine or neonatal death, though some babies have survived with fetal packed red blood cell transfusions when antenatal diagnosis was made. These patients should continue on hypertransfusion regimens and be treated as if they had β-thalassemia major, or treated with allogeneic stem cell transplant.

Differential Diagnosis

The differential diagnosis of the thalassemia syndromes and other microcytic anemias is listed in Table 3-10.

EXTRACORPUSCULAR HEMOLYTIC ANEMIAS

The causes of hemolytic anemia due to extracorpuscular defects are listed in Table 7-2; they may be immune or nonimmune.

Immune Hemolytic Anemia

Immune hemolytic anemia can be either isoimmune or autoimmune. Isoimmune hemolytic anemia results from a mismatched blood transfusion or from hemolytic disease in the newborn. In autoimmune hemolytic anemia (AIHA), shortened red cell survival is caused by the action of immunoglobulins, with or without the participation of complement on the red cell membrane. The red cell autoantibodies may be of the warm type, the cold type, or the cold–warm Donath–Landsteiner type. Complement participation is usually confined to the IgM type of antibody; only rarely is it associated with IgG. AIHA may be idiopathic or secondary to a number of conditions listed in Table 7-2.

Warm Autoimmune Hemolytic Anemia

Antibodies of the IgG class are most commonly responsible for AIHA in children. The antigen to which the IgG antibody is directed is one of the Rh erythrocyte antigens in more than 70% of cases. This antibody usually has its maximal activity at 37°C, and the resultant hemolysis is called warm antibody-induced hemolytic anemia. Rarely, warm reacting IgM antibodies may be responsible for hemolytic anemia. As in all patients with AIHA, erythrocyte survival is generally proportional to the amount of antibody on the erythrocyte surface.

Clinical Features

1. Severe, life-threatening condition
2. Sudden onset of pallor, jaundice, dark urine
3. Splenomegaly
4. Laboratory findings
   a. Hemoglobin level: very low
   b. Reticulocytosis: common
   c. Smear: prominent spherocytes, polychromasia, macrocytes, autoagglutination
   d. Neutropenia and thrombocytopenia (occasionally)
   e. Increased osmotic fragility and autohemolysis proportional to spherocytes
   f. Direct Coombs' test: positive
   g. Hyperbilirubinemia
   h. Haptoglobin level: markedly decreased
   i. Hemoglobinuria, increased urinary urobilinogen.

Management

Because this is a life-threatening condition, the following must be monitored carefully:

1. Hemoglobin level (q4h)
2. Reticulocyte count (daily)
3. Splenic size (daily)
4. Hemoglobinuria (daily)
5. Haptoglobin level (weekly)
6. Coombs' test (weekly).

Treatment

Blood Transfusion

1. If a specific antibody is identified, a compatible donor may be selected. The antibody usually behaves as a panagglutinin, and no totally compatible blood can be found.
2. Washed packed red cells should be used from donors whose erythrocytes show the least agglutination in the patient's serum.
3. The volume of transfused blood should only be of sufficient quantity to relieve any cardiopulmonary embarrassment from the anemia.
4. In our experience, the use of such poorly matched blood is made relatively safe by biologic cross-matching, transfusing of relatively small volumes of blood at any given time, and concomitant use of high-dose corticosteroid therapy.

Corticosteroid Therapy

1. Hydrocortisone 8–40 mg/kg/day IV in divided doses (q8h) or prednisone 2–10 mg/kg/day PO is administered.
2. High-dose corticosteroid therapy should be maintained for several days. Thereafter, corticosteroid therapy in the form of prednisone should be slowly tapered off over a 3- to 4-week period.
   a. The dose of prednisone should be tailored to maintain the hemoglobin at a reasonable level; when the hemoglobin stabilizes, the corticosteroids should be discontinued.

b. Lack of response for 21 days should be considered a steroid failure and other modalities should be considered.

Intravenous Gammaglobulin

Intravenous gammaglobulin (IVGG) in a dose of 5 g/kg, a much larger dose than used in idiopathic thrombocytopenic purpura or autoimmune neutropenia, may be effective.

Splenectomy

1. Splenectomy may be beneficial in some patients.
2. Splenectomy is indicated if the hemolytic process continues to be brisk despite high-dose corticosteroid therapy and IVGG for 3–4 weeks and the necessity of frequent packed red cell transfusions to maintain a reasonable hemoglobin level.
3. The results of splenectomy are unpredictable, but it is usually beneficial.

Cytotoxic Agents

1. Antimetabolites: azathioprine, 6-mercaptopurine, and thioguanine
2. Alkylating agents: chlorambucil and cyclophosphamide
3. Mitotic inhibitors: vincristine and vinblastine.

These agents have been used with variable success, but their use has not been completely evaluated, nor do any studies indicate preference in the use of cytotoxic agents. This type of therapy should be used only in patients refractory to steroids and splenectomy.

Plasmapheresis

Plasmapheresis has been successful in slowing the rate of hemolysis in patients with severe IgG-induced immune hemolytic anemia. The effect is short lived if antibody production is ongoing, and success is limited, possibly because more than half of the IgG is extravascular and the plasma contains only small amounts of the antibody; most of the antibody is on the red cell surface. Plasmapheresis has been more effective in IgM-induced hemolytic anemia.

Immunosuppressive Therapy

Cyclosporine A, an immunosuppressive agent that has been used extensively in the treatment of rejection in organ transplantation and more recently in autoimmune diseases and aplastic anemia, may have a role in the treatment of immune-mediated hemolysis, although prospective trials have not been completed. The potential role of monoclonal antibodies (anti-Fc antibodies) in the treatment of immune-mediated hemolysis has yet to be fully evaluated.

Hormonal Therapy

There has been recent success with danazol (synthetic androgen), which has a masculinizing effect. Danazol's early effect appears to be due to decreased expression of macrophage Fc-receptor activity and danazol may become an alternative to corticosteroid therapy in some patients with IgG-induced immune hemolytic anemia. The effect of these agents in IgM-induced hemolysis is untested.

Giant Cell Hepatitis and Coombs-Positive Autoimmune Hemolytic Anemia

This is a specific rare entity of unknown etiology, although an autoimmune component has been suggested because of the association of Coombs-positive AIHA and response to immunosuppression.

Clinical Findings

Age: 6–24 months, occasionally older age
Fever
Pallor
Jaundice (progressing to cirrhosis and liver failure)
Firm hepatomegaly and splenomegaly
Associated convulsions
Prognosis: Poor.

Laboratory Findings

Direct Coombs' test: mixed (IgG and complement); no evidence of other autoimmunity
Hemolytic anemia
Liver function abnormality: high direct bilirubin, transaminase, and serum globulin values; prolonged prothrombin time
Liver histology: marked lobular fibrosis, extensive necrosis with central-portal bridging, and giant cell transformation.

Treatment

The use of corticosteroids in combination with immunosuppressive therapy (e.g., azathioprine) has met with some success. Vincristine, α-interferon, and intravenous immunoglobulin have also been used.

Cold Autoimmune Hemolytic Anemia

IgM antibodies are found less often in association with hemolysis in the pediatric age group. Most IgM autoantibodies that cause immune hemolytic anemia in humans are cold agglutinins, and cold hemagglutinin disease is almost always caused by an IgM antibody. The destruction of red blood cells is usually triggered by cold exposure. Cold hemagglutinin disease usually occurs during *Mycoplasma pneumoniae* infection. It may also occur with other infections, such as infectious mononucleosis, cytomegalovirus, and mumps. Cold hemagglutinin disease or IgM-induced hemolysis is usually due to reaction with antigens of the I/i system. Anti-I is characteristic of *M. pneumoniae*–associated hemolysis and anti-i cold agglutinins are usually found in infectious mononucleosis. *M. pneumoniae* adherence to the red cell membrane appears to be mediated by sialic acid–containing receptors, associated with terminal galactose residues of the I antigen. The association of the infecting organism with the red blood cell may alter the antigenic structure of red blood cell membrane antigen, rendering it immunogenic. IgM antibody is usually polyclonal and immunologically heterogeneous.

Clinical Features

This disease may be idiopathic but is more frequently seen in conjunction with infections such as *M. pneumoniae* (atypical pneumonia) and less commonly with lymphoproliferative disorders. The hematologic features in cold autoimmune hemolytic anemia are similar to those in warm autoimmune hemolytic anemia but less marked.

Treatment

Treatment consists of control of the underlying disorder. Transfusions may be necessary; again, identification of compatible blood may prove difficult. Warming the blood to 37°C during administration by means of a heating coil or water bath is indicated to avoid further temperature activation of the antibody. Efficient in-line blood warmers (McGaw Water Bath; Fenwall Dry Heat Warmer) are designed to deliver blood at 37°C to the patient. Unmonitored or uncontrolled heating of blood is extremely dangerous and should not be attempted. Red cells heated too long are rapidly destroyed *in vivo* and can be lethal to the patient.

If the anemia is severe, a trial of cytotoxic drug therapy is appropriate. Alkylating agents such as cyclophosphamide and chlorambucil may be capable of lowering the titer of cold agglutinins and, less commonly, reducing the degree of hemolysis. Treatment with corticosteroids or splenectomy is generally not effective. Plasmapheresis is a valuable approach to reducing the level of cold agglutinins. If the blood is obtained at 37°C, with the patient's arm warmed by hot pads, the warm unit can be separated quickly by centrifugation and the red cells returned to the patient through an efficient in-line blood warmer.

Donath–Landsteiner Cold Hemolysin

This is an unusual IgG antibody with anti-P specificity, originally described in cases of syphilis. This antibody, although uncommon, is most frequently found in children with viral infections. Hemolysis in this syndrome is most commonly intravascular as a result of the unusual complement-activating efficiency of this IgG antibody. Hemolysis, which is usually mild, may occasionally be severe but resolves as the infection clears.

Nonimmune Hemolytic Anemia

This group of conditions is due to extracorpuscular causes of hemolytic anemia in which the antiglobulin (Coombs') test is negative. The various causes are listed in Table 7-2. Those conditions caused by various infections, drugs, and underlying hematologic disease respond to treatment of the underlying condition, as well as the necessary acute supportive care.

Microangiopathic Hemolytic Anemia

Microangiopathic hemolytic anemia (MAHA) is a result of diverse causes that have in common a relatively uniform hematologic picture and in general a common pathogenesis. Table 7-24 lists the various causes of MAHA.

Diagnosis

The blood smear is characterized by the presence of burr erythrocytes, schistocytes, helmet cells, and microspherocytes. This occurs in association with evidence of hemolysis and usually, but not invariably, thrombocytopenia. The severity of both

Table 7-24. Causes of Microangiopathic Hemolytic Anemia

Renal disease
  Hemolytic uremic syndrome
  Renal vein thrombosis
  Renal transplant rejection
  Radiation nephritis
  Chronic renal failure
Cardiac conditions
  Malignant hypertension
  Coarctation of aorta
  Severe valvular heart disease
  Subacute bacterial endocarditis of aortic valve
  Intracardiac prosthesis
Liver disease
  Severe hepatocellular disease
Infections
  Disseminated herpes infection
  Meningococcal septicemia
  Cerebral falciparum malaria
Hematologic
  Thrombotic thrombocytopenic purpura (hereditary or secondary) (Chapter 10)
Miscellaneous
  Severe burns
  Giant hemangioma
  Disseminated intravascular coagulation of any causation; sometimes accompanied by consumption of circulating coagulation factors (consumption coagulopathy)

the anemia and the thrombocytopenia, as well as the degree of compensatory erythroid response, varies greatly. Intravascular hemolysis occurs in all forms; plasma hemoglobin levels may be elevated, haptoglobin absent, hemosiderinuria present, and urinary iron excretion increased in the more chronic forms.

Elevated serum fibrin degradation products in some cases of MAHA may represent evidence of associated DIC. The thrombocytopenia is due to consumption of platelets in the microthrombi and is an example of excessive platelet destruction rather than a failure of production. The marrow, therefore, shows normal numbers of megakaryocytes together with erythroid hyperplasia. Acute forms of MAHA are sometimes accompanied by disseminated intravascular coagulation (DIC).

Hypersplenism

Whether splenic enlargement is caused by infection or is secondary to such diseases as thalassemia, portal hypertension, or storage diseases, a shortened red cell survival with excessive sequestration can be demonstrated in many patients with clinical splenomegaly. Typically, hypersplenism is accompanied by moderate neutropenia and thrombocytopenia with active erythropoiesis, myelopoiesis, and thrombopoiesis in the marrow. Splenectomy is followed by the return to normal of the blood values.

SUGGESTED READINGS

General

Becker P, Lux S. Disorders of the red cell membrane. In: Nathan D, Oski F, editors. Hematology of Infancy and Childhood. Philadelphia: WB Saunders, 1993.

Dacie J. The Haemolytic Anaemias 3. The Auto-Immune Haemolytic Anaemias. 3rd ed. Edinburgh: Churchill Livingstone. 1992.

Lanzkowsky P. Hemolytic anemia. In: Pediatric Hematology Oncology: A Treatise for the Clinician. New York: McGraw-Hill, 1980.

Luzzatto L. G6PD deficiency and hemolytic anemia. In: Nathan DG, Oski FA, editors. Hematology of Infancy and Childhood. Philadelphia: WB Saunders, 1993.

Mentzer W. Pyruvate kinase deficiency and disorders of glycolysis. In: Nathan DG, Oski FA, editors. Hematology of Infancy and Childhood. Philadelphia: WB Saunders, 1987.

Mentzer W, editor. Clinics in Haematology: Enzymopathies. Philadelphia: WB Saunders, 1981;10.

Nathan D, Orkin S. Nathan and Oski's Hematology of Infancy and Childhood. 5th ed. Philadelphia: WB Saunders, 1998:811–87.

Schreiber A, Gill F. Autoimmune hemolytic anemia. In: Nathan DG, Oski FA, editors. Hematology of Infancy and Childhood. Philadelphia: WB Saunders, 1987.

Sickle Cell

Adekile AD, Tuli M, Haider MZ, et al. Influence of α-thalassemia trait on spleen function in sickle cell anemia patients with high HbF. Am J Hematol 1996;36:184–9.

Bernaudin F, Soullet G, Vannier JP, et al. Bone marrow transplantation in 14 children with severe sickle cell disease: the French experience. GEGMO Bone Marrow Transplantation 1993;12:118.

Bounga JC, Mouélé R, Préhu C, et al. Glucose-6-phosphate dehydrogenase deficiency and homozygous sickle cell disease in Congo. Hum Hered 1998;48:192–7.

Driscoll MC, Hurlet A, Berman B, et al. Stroke risk in sibling pairs with sickle cell disease. Am J Hum Genet 1999;65:A201.

Ferrone F, Nagel, RL. Polymer structure and polymerization of deoxyhemoglobin S. In: Steinberg MH, Forget BG, Higgs DR, et al., editors. Disorders of Hemoglobin: Genetics, Pathophysiology, Clinical Management. Cambridge, UK: Cambridge University Press, 2001.

Ferster A, Vermylen C, Cornu G, et al. Hydroxyurea for treatment of severe sickle cell anemia: pediatric clinical trial. Blood 1996;88:1960.

Garner C, Tatu T, Reittie JE, et al. Genetic influences on F cells and other hematologic variables: a twin heritability study. Blood 2000;95:342–6.

Gore L, Lane P, Quinones RR, Giller RH. Successful cord blood stem cell transplantation for sickle cell anemia from an HLA-identical sibling. Blood 1997;90:388b.

Nagel RL. Severity, pathobiology, epistatic effects, and genetic markers in sickle cell anemia. Semin Hematol 1991;28:180–201.

Noguchi CT, Rodgers GP, Serjeant G, et al. Levels of fetal hemoglobin necessary for treatment of sickle cell disease. N Engl J Med 1988;318:96–9.

Powars DR. Dr. Sickle cell anemia: βˢ-gene-cluster haplotypes as prognostic indicators of vital organ failure. Semin Hematol 1991;28:202–8.

Powars DR. βˢ-gene-cluster haplotypes in sickle cell anemia. Clinical and hematologic features. Hematol Oncol Clin North Am 1991;5:475–93.

Rogers Z. Hydroxyurea therapy for diverse pediatric population with sickle cell disease. Semin Hematol 1997;34:42.

Steinberg MH. Compound heterozygous and other sickle hemoglobinopathies. In: Steinberg MH, Forget BG, Higgs DR, et al., editors. Disorders of Hemoglobin: Genetics, Pathophysiology, Clinical Management. Cambridge, UK: Cambridge University Press, 2001.

Vermylen C, Cornu G. Hematopoietic stem cell transplant for sickle cell anemia. Curr Opin Hematol 1997;4:377.

Weiss M, Blobel G. Nuclear factors that regulate erythropoiesis. In: Steinberg MH, Forget BG, Higgs DR, et al., editors. Disorders of Hemoglobin: Genetics, Pathophysiology, Clinical Management. Cambridge, UK: Cambridge University Press, 2001.

Thalassemia

Anderson LJ, Wonke B, Prescott E, et al. Comparison of effects of oral deferiprone and subcutaneous desferrioxamine on myocardial iron concentrations and ventricular function in beta-thalassemia. Lancet 2002;360:516–20.

Anderson LJ, Holden S, Davis B, et al. Cardiovascular T_2-star (T_2*) magnetic resonance for the early diagnosis of myocardial iron overload. Eur Heart J 2001;22:2171–9.

Angelucci E, Brittenham GM, McLaren C, et al. Hepatic iron concentration and total body iron stores in thalassemia major. N Engl J Med 2000;343:327–31.

Chui DHK, Fucharoen S, Chan V. Hemoglobin H disease: not necessarily a benign disorder. Blood 2003;101:791–800.

Cohen A. Cooley's anemia seventh symposium. Ann NY Acad Sci 1998;850.

Cunningham M, Macklin E, Neufeld E, Cohen A. Complications of β-thalassemia major in North America. Blood 2004;104:34–9.

Lawson SE, Roberts IA, Amrolia P, Dokal I, Szydlo R, Darbyshire PJ. Bone marrow transplantation for beta-thalassaemia major: the UK experience in two paediatric centres. Br J Haematol 2003;120(2):289–95.

Lowrey C, Nienhuis A. Brief report: treatment with azacytidine of patients with end-stage beta-thalassemia. N Engl J Med 1993;329(12):845–8.

Lucarelli G, Galimberti M, Pochi P, et al. Marrow transplantation in patients with thalassemia responsive to iron chelation therapy. N Engl J Med 1993;29:840–4.

Olivieri N. The β-thalassemias. N Engl J Med 1999; 341(2):99–109.

Orkin SH, Nathan, DG. The Thalassemias. In: Nathan D, Oski F, editors. Hematology of Infancy and Childhood. 6th ed. Philadelphia: WB Saunders, 2003.

8

POLYCYTHEMIA

POLYCYTHEMIA IN THE NEWBORN

Definition

A venous hematocrit reading of more than 65% or a venous hemoglobin concentration in excess of 22.0 g/dL any time during the first week of life should be considered evidence of polycythemia. Capillary blood samples should not be relied on for the diagnosis of polycythemia because they are significantly higher than venous hemoglobin or venous hematocrit and vary with the temperature of the extremity from where the sample is taken. Hematocrit values determined on a microcentrifuge include a small amount of trapped plasma and have a higher value than hematocrit values determined from automated analyzers.

A patient with a very high hematocrit should not have blood drawn into commercially available tubes, because the ratio of anticoagulant to blood is inappropriate. To adjust the anticoagulant for a known hematocrit, the proper amount of 3.2% sodium citrate (as indicated in the following table) should be added to the test tube making a total volume (blood and citrate) of 5 or 10 mL.

Hematocrit %	Anticoagulant required (mL)	
	In 5 mL	In 10 mL
55	0.40	0.80
60	0.38	0.75
63	0.35	0.70
65	0.33	0.65

Incidence

The incidence is 0.4–4.0% of all births. Incidence of neonatal polycythemia is higher at high altitudes than at sea level.

Etiology

The causes of neonatal polycythemia are listed in Table 8-1.

Symptoms

Symptoms are a consequence of the increase in blood viscosity. Hematocrit up to 65% has a linear correlation with viscosity, and beyond 65% it has an exponential

Table 8-1. Causes of Neonatal Polycythemia

I. Intrauterine hypoxia
- A. Placental insufficiency
  1. Small-for-gestational age (intrauterine growth factor)
  2. Dysmaturity
  3. Postmaturity
  4. Placenta previa
  5. Maternal hypertension syndromes (toxemia of pregnancy)
- B. Severe maternal cyanotic heart disease
- C. Maternal smoking

II. Hypertransfusion
- A. Twin-to-twin transfusion
- B. Maternal to fetal transfusion
- C. Placental-cord transfusion (delayed cord clamping, cord stripping, third stage of labor underwater at body temperature, holding baby below mother with cord attached)

III. Endocrine causes
- A. Congenital adrenal hyperplasia
- B. Neonatal thyrotoxicosis
- C. Congenital hypothyroidism
- D. Maternal diabetes mellitus

IV. Miscellaneous
- A. Chromosomal abnormalities
  1. Trisomy 13
  2. Trisomy 18
  3. Trisomy 21 (Down syndrome)
- B. Beckwith–Wiedemann syndrome (hyperplastic visceromegaly)
- C. Oligohydramnios
- D. Maternal use of propranolol
- E. High-altitude conditions
- F. High oxygen affinity hemoglobinopathies (Table 8-4)

relationship. Viscosity depends on a number of factors (Table 8-2). Table 8-3 lists the symptoms, signs, and complications of neonatal polycythemia. Some of the symptoms may result from an underlying cause such as intrauterine hypoxia, maternal diabetes, or placental insufficiency.

Table 8-2. Factors Increasing Viscosity

1. Hematocrit >60%
2. Larger mean cell volume (MCV)
3. Decreased deformability of fetal erythrocytes
4. Plasma protein levels especially high fibrinogen
5. Decreased flow rate—vessel diameter and endothelial integrity, e.g., increased levels of erythropoietin, in addition to inducing erythrocytosis, may induce other effects such as:
   a. Hematocrit-independent, vasoconstriction-dependent hypertension
   b. Upregulation of tissue renin
   c. Increased endothelin production
   d. Stimulation of endothelial and vascular smooth muscle proliferation
   e. Change in vascular tissue prostaglandin production
   f. Stimulation of angiogenesis.

Laboratory Findings

When polycythemia is due to maternofetal transfusion, the following laboratory findings may be present:

1. Increased quantities of immunoglobulin (IgA and IgM) in the infant's serum
2. Reduction in fetal hemoglobin to less than 60%
3. The presence of red cells bearing maternal blood group antigens in the baby's circulation and, if the infant is a male, the presence of XX cells of maternal origin in the baby's circulation.

Table 8-3. Symptoms, Signs, and Complications of Neonatal Polycythemia

Clinical

"Feeding problems" (60%)
Lethargy
Hypotonia
Weak suck
Difficult to arouse
Tremulousness
Easily startled
Hepatomegaly
Vomiting
Tachypnea
Tachycardia
Cardiomegaly
Plethora
Cyanosis
Jaundice

Laboratory

Venous hemoglobin >22 g/dL
Venous hematocrit >65%
Thrombocytopenia
Reticulocytosis
Normoblastemia
Increased blood viscosity (normal 12.1 cP ± 3.9)
Presence of IgM or IgA in serum
Unconjugated hyperbilirubinemia
Hypoglycemia (12–40%)
Hypocalcemia (1–11%)
Hypomagnesemia
EEG abnormal
ECG abnormal
Chest radiograph
   Increased vascularity
   Pleural fluid
   Hyperaeration
   Alveolar infiltrates
   Cardiomegaly

Complications

Transient tachypnea of newborn
Respiratory distress
Congestive heart failure
Convulsions
Intracranial hemorrhage
Peripheral gangrene
Priapism
Necrotizing enterocolitis
Ileus
Acute renal failure
Testicular infarction
Disseminated intravascular coagulation

When polycythemia is due to intrauterine hypoxia it is usually accompanied by an increase in the nucleated red blood cells (nRBCs) in the blood during the early neonatal period. The mean value of nRBCs in the first few hours of life in a healthy full-term neonate is 500 nRBCs/mm^3 or 0–10 nRBCs/100 white blood cells (WBCs). A value of greater than 1000 nRBCs/mm^3 or 10–20 nRBCs/100 WBCs is considered abnormal. The other hematologic indices of fetal hypoxia include higher absolute lymphocyte counts and lower platelet counts in comparison with normal full-term neonates without hypoxia during fetal life.

Treatment

Because instruments to measure viscosity are not clinically available, neonatal hyperviscosity is diagnosed by a combination of symptoms and an abnormally high hematocrit.

Treatment should be reserved for infants with respiratory, cardiac, or central nervous system (CNS) symptoms and a venous hematocrit of 65–69% or an asymptomatic infant with a venous hematocrit of >70%. All polycythemic infants, however, should be carefully monitored for evidence of hypoglycemia, hypocalcemia, and hyperbilirubinemia. Treatment should be designed to reduce the venous hematocrit to approximately 50–55%. This can be accomplished by a partial exchange transfusion, using 5% human albumin, Ringer's lactate, or normal saline. It is better to avoid the use of fresh frozen plasma because it may contain infectious agents. Normal saline or Ringer's lactate solutions have the advantages that they are easily available and equally effective. However, it is important to take into account the patient's renal status and serum sodium level when a decision is made to use albumin, Ringer's lactate, or normal saline to avoid sodium overload. Partial exchange has a favorable effect on cerebral blood flow velocity in newborn infants with polycythemia because it reduces the hematocrit while maintaining blood volume.

The following formula is employed to approximate the volume of exchange required to reduce the hematocrit reading to the desired level:

$$\text{Volume of exchange (mL)} = \text{Blood volume (mL)} \times \frac{\text{Observed Hct} - \text{Desired Hct}}{\text{Observed Hct}}$$

Partial exchange transfusion has been shown to increase capillary perfusion, cerebral blood flow, and cardiac function and to reduce the risk of tissue damage caused by ischemia in various organs, resulting from severe slowing in the microcirculation due to a high hematocrit and low shear rates. However, there is little evidence that the long-term outcome of infants is improved by the procedure.

POLYCYTHEMIA IN CHILDHOOD

The term *polycythemia* applies to an increase in circulating red cell mass to above the normal upper limits of 30 mL/kg body weight (excluding hemoconcentration due to dehydration). For practical purposes, this means a hemoglobin level higher than 17 g/dL or a hematocrit level of 50% or more during childhood.

Figure 8-1 depicts the pathogenesis of polycythemia, and Table 8-4 classifies various causes of polycythemia.

Primary polycythemia results from congenital ([germline] erythropoietin receptor mutation) or acquired ([somatic] polycythemia vera) mutations that make erythroid progenitor cells exquisitely sensitive to circulating cytokines, resulting in increased red cell mass. *Secondary polycythemia*, on the other hand, results from the action of an excessive amount of circulating cytokines on the normal responsive erythroid progenitor cells. The cytokine usually is erythropoietin. However, in some clinical con-

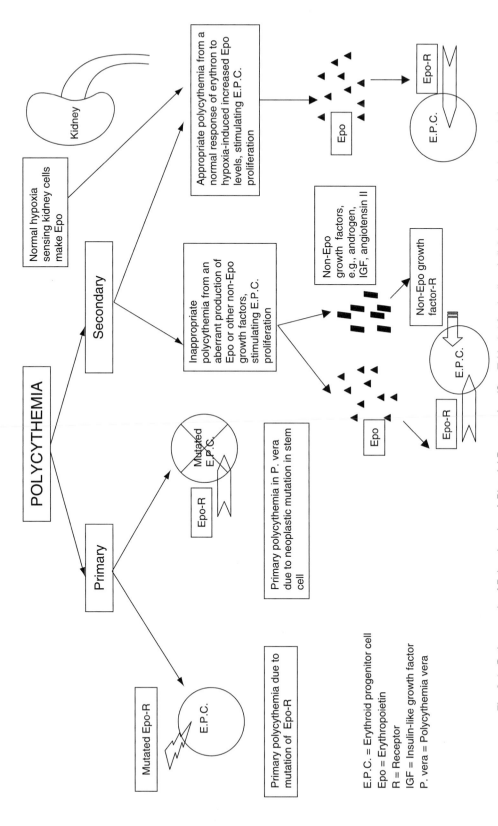

Fig. 8-1. Pathogenesis of Polycythemia – A Pictorial Presentation (See Table 8-4 for the list of clinical causes of polycythemia)

Table 8-4. Classification of Polycythemia

I. **Relative polycythemia** (hemoconcentration, dehydration)

II. **Primary polycythemia** (results from somatic or germline mutations of erythroid
progenitor cells that make them exquisitely sensitive to erythropoietin or other cytokines)
    A. Polycythemia vera (results from somatic mutation)
    B. Erythropoietin receptor mutation (results from germline mutation)

III. **Secondary polycythemia**
    A. Insufficient oxygen delivery (also known as *appropriate* polycythemia because it
results from a normal response of erythron to hypoxia)
        1. Physiologic
            a. Fetal life
            b. Low environmental O_2 (high altitude)
        2. Pathologic
            a. Impaired ventilation: pulmonary disease, obesity
            b. Pulmonary arteriovenous fistula
            c. Congenital heart disease with left-to-right shunt (e.g., tetralogy of Fallot,
Eisenmenger syndrome)
            d. Abnormal hemoglobins (reduced P_{50} in whole blood)
                (1) Methemoglobin (congenital and acquired)
                (2) Carboxyhemoglobin
                (3) Sulfhemoglobin
                (4) High oxygen affinity hemoglobinopathies[a] (hemoglobin
Chesapeake, Ranier, Yakima, Osler, Tsurumai, Kempsey, and
Ypsilanti)
                (5) 2,3-DPG mutase deficiency in red cells resulting in 2-3
bisphosphoglycerate (BPG) deficiency.
    B. Increase in erythropoietin (also known as *inappropriate* polycythemia because it
results from an aberrant production of erythropoietin or other growth factors)
        1. Endogenous
            a. Renal: Wilms' tumor,[b] hypernephroma, renal ischemia, e.g., renal
vascular disorder, congenital polycystic kidney, benign renal lesions
(cysts, hydronephrosis).
Post-transplant erythrocytosis (occurs in 10–15% of renal graft
recipients). Contributing factors include persistence of erythropoietin
secretion from the recipients's diseased and ischemic kidney, and
secretion of angiotensin II, androgen, and insulin-like growth factor.
            b. Adrenal: pheochromocytoma, Cushing syndrome, congenital adrenal
hyperplasia, adrenal adenoma with primary aldosteronism
            c. Liver: hepatoma, focal nodular hyperplasia,[c] hepatocellular carcinoma,
hepatic hemangioma, Budd-Chiari syndrome (some of these patients
may have overt or latent myeloproliferative disorder)
            d. Cerebellum: hemangioblastoma, hemangioma, meningioma
            e. Uterus: leiomyoma, leiomyosarcoma
        2. Exogenous
            a. Administration of testosterone and related steroids
            b. Administration of growth hormone
    C. Polycythemia with characteristics of both primary and secondary polycythemias
            a. Chuvashian polycythemia
            b. Non-Chuvashian polycythemias

IV. **Neonatal polycythemia**

---

[a]Some of these are electrophoretically silent and require hemoglobin oxygen association kinetics for diagnosis.
[b]Associated with male gender, low clinical stage, and usually >16 years of age. May occur with a normal
serum erythropoietin.
[c]Histologically stains positively for erythropoietin by immunohistochemistry.

ditions, nonerythropoietin growth factors (e.g., angiotensin II, androgens, and insulin-like growth factor I in recipients of renal graft during the post-transplant period) may also play a role in inducing erythrocytosis.

Combined Characteristics of Primary and Secondary Polycythemias

Recently, various molecular polycythemic lesions have been described. These include von Hippel–Lindau mutations, erythropoietin receptor mutations, globin mutations, and bisphosphoglycerate deficiency in decreasing order of frequency.

Von Hippel–Lindau Mutations Causing Polycythemia

- *Chuvashian* polycythemia (familial benign polycythemia):* Autosomal recessive inheritance mutation of von Hippel–Lindau gene results in defective hypoxic sensing by kidney cells and increased production of erythropoietin. Some patients may have a normal level of erythropoietin. However, their erythroid progenitors are hypersensitive to the normal levels of erythropoietin.

  Clinical manifestations include varicose veins, thrombotic and hemorrhagic complications, strokes, increased levels of vascular endothelial growth factor and plasminogen activator inhibitor-1 but they do not develop von Hippel–Lindau syndrome and its complications (hemangioblastomas, pheochromocytoma, or renal cell carcinoma) and vice versa; patients with von Hippel–Lindau syndrome do not manifest erythrocytosis.

- *Non-Chuvashian polycythemias:* Several patients of other than Chuvash ethnicity have been found to have polycythemia resulting from mutations at various regions of the von Hippel–Lindau gene. These mutations may be heterozygous or homozygous.

Table 8-5 compares the clinical manifestations of polycythemia vera, primary familial and congenital polycythemia and Chuvashian polycythemia. Table 8-6 lists the criteria for a diagnosis of polycythemia vera.

Treatment

1. *Erythrocytosis:* Partial exchange transfusions (phlebotomy) to maintain hemoglobin levels of 16–17 g/dL (i.e., less than 20 g/dL) are the mainstay of treatment for erythrocytosis. The underlying cause, if known, should be treated.
2. *Polycythemia secondary to high oxygen affinity hemoglobin or deficiency of bisphosphoglycerate:* Phlebotomy is usually not beneficial in the treatment of polycythemia secondary to high oxygen affinity hemoglobins or those conditions resulting from deficiency of bisphosphoglycerate, because they cause a decrease in exercise tolerance.
3. *Post-transplant erythrocytosis in renal graft recipients:* These patients respond to drugs that cause inactivation of the renin-angiotensin system (e.g., captopril, enalapril, losartan, lisinopril, and fosinopril). Patients unable to tolerate angiotensin-converting enzyme inhibitors can be treated with an angiotensin II AT1 receptor antagonist, losartan. Theophylline, a nonselective adenosine receptor antagonist in low dose, has been found effective in suppression of erythropoiesis.
4. *Congenital erythropoietin-dependent erythrocytosis:* Successful treatment of congenital erythropoietin-dependent erythrocytosis, clinically similar to Chuvashian polycythemia, has been reported with the use of theophylline.

---

*The Chuvash Republic is located on the west bank of the Volga River in the central part of European Russia. The first reports of congenital polycythemia in Chuvashia appeared in the 1970s (Blood 1997;89:2148–54).

Table 8-5. Clinical Manifestations of Polycythemia Vera (PV), Primary Familial and Congenital Polycythemia (PFCP), and Chuvashian Polycythemia (CP)

Clinical entities	Polycythemia vera (PV)	Primary familial and congenital polycythemia (PFCP)	Chuvashian polycythemia (CP)
Frequency	Rare	Unknown	Unknown
Inheritance	None	Dominant	Recessive
Underlying cause	None	Erythropoietin receptor mutation is found only in 12%	Functional deficiency of VHL
Symptoms of polycythemia (e.g., headache, dizziness, lethargy, blurred vision)	Present	Usually diagnosed on routine blood count	Present
Signs	Plethora, splenomegaly	Plethora, no splenomegaly	Plethora, no splenomegaly, varicosities of peripheral veins
Erythropoietin level	Undetectable	Normal or low	Increased but high or normal in sporadic non-CP
Course	Thrombosis or hemorrhage (other myelo-proliferative disorders)	Benign	Thrombosis or hemorrhage
Diagnosis		Molecular analysis for truncation of cytosolic portion of ER and *in vitro* hypersensitivity to EPO	Molecular analysis of VHL protein gene levels of VEGF and PAI-1
Treatment	Phlebotomy, α-IFN, ASA, HU, Anagrelide	Phlebotomy	Phlebotomy

VHL, von Hippel–Lindau; VEGR, vascular endothelial growth factor; PAI-1, plasminogen activator inhibitor; α-IFN, α interferon; ASA, aspirin; HU, hydroxyurea; ER, Erythropoietin receptor; EPO, Erythropoietin.

Theophylline results in the reduction of serum levels of erythropoietin and transferrin receptor, leading to decrease in hemoglobin levels.

5. *Polycythemia vera:* In *low-risk patients,* defined as:
   - Asymptomatic individuals under 40 years of age
   - Platelet count <1.0 million/mm^3
   - No comorbidities
   - No history of thrombosis.

   If the hematocrit is effectively controlled by phlebotomy there is no need for cytoreduction. Low-dose aspirin is also beneficial.

   In *high-risk patients,* defined as:

   - Patients 60 years of age or older or
   - Symptomatic patients or

Table 8-6. Criteria for Diagnosis of Polycythemia Vera[a]

Category A
1. Increased red cell volume (male $\geq$36 mL/kg; female $\geq$32 mL/kg)
2. Arterial oxygen saturation $\geq$92%
3. Splenomegaly

Category B
1. Thrombocytosis (>400,000 cells/mm³)
2. Leukocytosis (>12,000 cells/mm³)
3. Increased leukocyte alkaline phosphatase
4. Increased vitamin B_{12} (>900 pg/mL) or unsaturated B_{12}-binding capacity (>2200 pg/mL)

   For diagnosis patient must have:

       A1 + A2 + A3

      OR

       A1 + A2 + any 2 from category B

[a]Increased expression of m-RNA of a receptor PRV-1 (polycythemia rubra vera-1) in granulocytes, but not in their progenitors, is a useful diagnostic marker that distinguishes polycythemia vera from secondary erythrocytosis. Polycythemia vera patients express significantly high amount of PRV-1. Quantitative RT-PCR assay for PRV-1 has high sensitivity and specificity.

(Adapted from Berlin NI (1975): Diagnosis and classification of the polycythemias. Semin Hematol 12:339, with permission.)

- Patients with platelet counts >1.0 million/mm³ or
- Patients with comorbidities or
- Patients with a history of thrombosis.

In these cases cytoreductive therapy, preferably with α-interferon rather than hydroxyurea, in young patients is utilized. Anagrelide is also useful to decrease platelet counts. An induction dose of Anagrelide in children of 0.5 mg twice daily, followed by a maintenance dose of 0.5–1.0 mg twice a day, adjusted to maintain a platelet count within the normal range, is employed. The dosage is adjusted to the lowest effective dosage required to reduce and maintain the platelet count below 600,000/mm³, and ideally to maintain it in the normal range.

In *intermediate-risk patients*, defined as:

- 40–60 years of age and
- Platelet count of 600,000/mm³ to 1.0 million/mm³.

These patients are treated with phlebotomy and Anagrelide.

SUGGESTED READINGS

Cazzola M, Guarnone R, et al. Congenital erythropoietin-dependent erythrocytosis responsive to theophylline treatment. Blood 1998;91:360.

Ebert BL, Bunn HF. Regulation of the erythropoietin gene. Blood 1999;94:1864.

Fisher JW. Erythropoietin: physiology and pharmacology update. Exp Biol Med 2003;228:1–14.

Gilbert HS. Modern treatment strategies in polycythemia vera. Semin Hematol 2003;40:26–9.

Hermansen MC. Nucleated red blood cells in the fetus and newborn. Arch Dis Child Fetal Neonatal Ed 2001;84:F211–5.

Linndemann R, Haga P. Evaluation and treatment of polycythemia in the neonate. In: Editor: Christensen, RD. Hematologic Problems of the Neonate. Philadelphia: WB Saunders, 2000.

Prchal JT. Classification and molecular biology of polycythemias (erythrocytoses) and thrombocytosis. Hematol Oncol Clin North Am 2003;17:1151–8.

Prchal JT, Sokol L. "Benign erythrocytosis" and other familial and congenital polycythemias. Eur J Haematol 1996;57:263–8.

Sergeyeva A, Gordeuk VR, et al. Congenital polycythemia in Chuvashia. Blood 1997;89:2148.

Vlahakos DV, et al. Posttransplant erythrocytosis. Kidney Int 2003;63:1187–94.

Werner EJ. Neonatal polycythemia and hyperviscosity. Clin Perinatol 1995;22:693.

9

DISORDERS OF WHITE BLOOD CELLS

The total white blood cell count and the differential count are valuable guides in the diagnosis, treatment, and prognosis of various childhood illnesses.

LEUKOCYTES

Table 9-1 lists the causes of leukocytosis. The normal leukocyte counts and the absolute counts of different classes of leukocytes vary with age in children, and their ranges are listed in Appendix Table A1-15. Leukocytosis may be acute or chronic and may result from an increase in one or more specific classes of leukocytes.

Table 9-2 lists the causes of monocytosis and monocytopenia, Table 9-3 the causes of basophilia, and Table 9-4 the causes of neutrophilia. Eosinophils and lymphocytes are discussed later in this chapter.

For the purposes of quantitative interpretation, it is important to calculate the absolute count of each class of white blood cell (WBC) rather than the relative percentage count. If nucleated red blood cells (nRBCs) are present, the total WBC count includes the total nucleated cell count (TNCC). Under these circumstances the true total WBC count is calculated by subtracting the absolute nRBC count from the TNCC. This correction is generally required in the hemolytic anemias.

Blood smear examination of the white cell morphology is important in the diagnosis of various causes of leukocytosis; for example, in severe infections or other toxic states, the neutrophils may contain fine deeply basophilic granules (toxic granulation) or larger basophilic cytoplasmic masses (Döhle bodies); vacuolization of neutrophils may also occur. Döhle bodies are also found in pregnancy, burns, cancer, May Hegglin anomaly, and many other conditions. Infants and children have a tendency to release immature granulocytes into the circulation, and the WBC count may reach very high levels (>50,000/mm³). This is called a leukemoid reaction. The shift to the left may be so marked as to suggest myeloid leukemia. Table 9-5 lists the distinguishing features of leukemoid reaction and true leukemia.

Leukopenia

Leukopenia exists when the total WBC count is less than 4000/mm³. Leukopenia may result from a decrease in one or more specific classes of leukocytes. The causes of neutropenia are listed in Table 9-6, lymphopenia in Table 9-14, and monocytopenia in Table 9-2. Leukopenia can result from a number of conditions. However,

Table 9-1. Causes of Leukocytosis

Physiologic
  Newborn (maximal 38,000/mm^3)
  Strenuous exercise
Emotional disorders; fear, agitation
Ovulation, labor, pregnancy
Acute infections
  Bacterial, viral, fungal, protozoal, spirochetal
Metabolic causes
  Diabetic coma
  Acidosis
  Anoxia
  Azotemia
  Thyroid storm
  Acute gout
  Burns
  Seizures
Drugs
  Steroids
  Epinephrine
  Endotoxin
  Lithium
  Serotonin, histamine, heparin, acetylcholine
Poisoning
  Lead, mercury, camphor
Acute hemorrhage
Malignant neoplasms
  Carcinoma
  Sarcoma
  Lymphoma
Connective tissue diseases
  Rheumatic fever
  Rheumatoid arthritis
  Inflammatory bowel disease
Hematologic diseases
  Splenectomy, functional asplenia
  Leukemia and myeloproliferative
    disorders
  Hemolytic anemia
    Transfusion reaction
  Megaloblastic anemia during
    therapy

Table 9-2. Causes of Monocytosis and Monocytopenia

Monocytosis
  Hematologic disorders
    Leukemia
    Acute myelogenous leukemia
    Chronic myelogenous leukemia
    Lymphoma (Hodgkin and non-Hodgkin)
    Chronic neutropenia
    Histiocytic medullary reticulosis
  Connective tissue disorders
    Systemic lupus erythematosus
    Rheumatoid arthritis
    Myositis
  Granulomatous diseases
    Inflammatory bowel disease
    Sarcoidosis
  Infections
    Subacute bacterial endocarditis
    Tuberculosis
    Syphilis
    Rocky Mountain spotted fever
    Kala-azar
  Malignant disease (usually carcinomas)
  Miscellaneous disorders
    Postsplenectomy state
    Tetrachloroethane poisoning
    Lipidoses (e.g., Niemann–Pick disease)

Monocytopenia
  Glucocorticoid administration
  Infections associated with endotoxemia

Table 9-3. Causes of Basophilia

Hypersensitivity reactions
  Drug and food hypersensitivity
  Urticaria
Inflammation and infection
  Ulcerative colitis
  Rheumatoid arthritis
  Influenza
  Chickenpox
  Smallpox
  Tuberculosis
Myeloproliferative diseases
  Chronic myeloid leukemia
Myeloid metaplasia

Table 9-4. Causes of Neutrophilia

Increased production
Clonal disease
  Myeloproliferative disorders
    Chronic myelogenous leukemia
    Chronic neutrophilic leukemia
  Juvenile myelomonocytic leukemia
  Transient myeloproliferative disorder of Down syndrome
Hereditary
  Autosomal dominant form of hereditary neutrophilia
  Familial cold urticaria
Reactive
  Chronic infection
  Chronic inflammation
    Juvenile rheumatoid arthritis
    Inflammatory bowel disease
    Kawasaki disease
  Hodgkin disease
  Drugs: lithium, G-CSF, GM-CSF, chronic use of corticosteroids
  Leukemoid reaction
  Chronic idiopathic neutrophilia

Increased mobilization from marrow storage pool
Drugs: Corticosteroids, G-CSF
Stress
Acute infection
Hypoxia

Decreased margination
Exercise
Epinephrine

Decreased egress from circulation
Leukocyte adhesion deficiency (LAD)
  LAD type I: deficiency of CD 11/CD 18 integrins on leukocytes
  LAD type II: absence of neutrophil sialyl Lewis X structures
Asplenia

Modified from Dinaur MC. The phagocyte system and disorders of granulopoiesis and granulocyte function. In: Nathan and Oski's Hematology of Infancy and Childhood. 5th ed. Philadelphia: WB Saunders, 1998, with permission.

Table 9-5. Features of Leukemoid Reaction and Leukemia

Feature	Leukemoid reaction	Leukemia
Clinical	Evidence of infection	Hepatosplenomegaly Lymphadenopathy
Hematologic	No anemia No thrombocytopenia	Anemia Thrombocytopenia
Bone marrow	Normal, hypercellular	Blasts Decreased megakaryocytes Decreased erythroid precursors
Leukocyte alkaline phosphatase	High	Absent

Table 9-6. Causes of Neutropenia

I. **Decreased production**
  A. Congenital
    1. Neutropenia in various ethnic groups[a]
    2. Hereditary
      a. Severe congenital neutropenia: sporadic (most common) or autosomal dominant or Kostmann disease—autosomal recessive
      b. Familial benign chronic neutropenia—autosomal dominant
    3. Chronic benign neutropenia[b]
    4. Reticular dysgenesis
    5. Cyclic neutropenia
    6. Neutropenia associated with agammaglobulinemia and dysgammaglobulinemia
    7. Neutropenia associated with abnormal cellular immunity in cartilage-hair hypoplasia
    8. Neutropenia associated with pancreatic insufficiency [Shwachman–Diamond syndrome (see page 221) and Pearson syndrome (see page 126); (Chapter 6; Table 6-24)]
    9. Neutropenia associated with hyperimmunoglobulin M syndrome
    10. Neutropenia associated with metabolic disease
      a. Glycogen storage disease (type IB)
      b. Idiopathic hyperglycinemia
      c. Isovaleric acidemia
      d. Methylmalonic acidemia
      e. Propionic acidemia
      f. Thiamine-responsive anemia in DIDMOAD syndrome (see pages 64–65)
      g. Barth syndrome[c] (see page 223)
    11. Bone marrow aplasia
      a. Fanconi anemia
      b. Familial congenital aplastic anemia without anomalies
      c. Dyskeratosis congenita (see pages 112–114) (Chapter 6)
    12. Bone marrow infiltration: osteopetrosis, cystinosis, Gaucher disease, Niemann–Pick disease
  B. Acquired
    1. Acute
      a. Acute transient neutropenia
      b. Viral infection (e.g., HIV, EBV, hepatitis A and B, respiratory syncytial virus, measles, rubella, varicella)
      c. Bacterial infection (e.g., typhoid, paratyphoid, tuberculosis, brucellosis)
      d. Rickettsial infection

(Continues)

Table 9-6. (*Continued*)

2. Chronic
   a. Bone marrow aplasia
      (1) Idiopathic
      (2) Secondary: drugs, chemicals, irradiation, infection, immune reaction, malnutrition, copper deficiency, vitamin B_{12} deficiency, folate deficiency
   b. Bone marrow infiltration, neoplastic
      (1) Primary: leukemia
      (2) Secondary: neuroblastoma, lymphoma, rhabdomyosarcoma

II. **Failure to release mature neutrophils from the bone marrow (myelokathexis)**
    (ineffective myelopoiesis)
    Cortisone stimulation test (Table 9-8)

III. **Increased margination of neutrophils (pseudoneutropenia)**
     Epinephrine stimulation test (Table 9-8)

IV. **Increased destruction**
    A. Immune
       1. Drug induced (e.g., anticonvulsants)
       2. Alloimmune (isoimmune)
          a. Maternofetal
          b. Multitransfusion
       3. Autoimmune neutropenia
          a. Idiopathic[a]
          b. Secondary: systemic lupus erythematosus, lymphoma, leukemia, rheumatoid arthritis, HIV infection (in 20–44% of AIDS patients), infectious mononucleosis, associated with autoimmune thrombocytopenia and/or autoimmune hemolytic anemia
    B. Nonimmune
       1. Infections
       2. Hypersplenism

[a]Chronic, mild with a benign course.
[b]Probably same condition as idiopathic autoimmune neutropenia.
[c]Rare genetic disorder consisting of neutropenia, cardiomyopathy, muscle weakness, failure to thrive and growth retardation.

isolated leukopenia resulting from a decrease in all classes of leukocytes is observed uncommonly.

Neutropenia

Neutropenia is defined as a decrease in the absolute neutrophil count (ANC). The ANC is calculated by multiplying the total WBC count by the percentage of segmented neutrophils and bands. Neutropenia is defined as an ANC of less than $1000/mm^3$ in infants between 2 weeks and 1 year of age and less than $1500/mm^3$ beyond 1 year of age.

Severity and duration of neutropenia correlate with susceptibility to developing various types of bacterial infections. Severity of neutropenia is graded according to ANC as follows:

Severe neutropenia: ANC less than $500/mm^3$
Moderate neutropenia: ANC $500–1000/mm^3$
Mild neutropenia: ANC $1000–1500/mm^3$.

Neutropenic patients are usually infected with their own endogenous bacterial flora that reside in the mouth, oropharynx, gastrointestinal tract, and skin. For this reason, the frequency of gram-negative bacterial infections and *Staphylococcus aureus* infections is high in these patients. Neutropenia alone does not, per se, predispose them to parasitic, viral, or fungal infections.

Benign ethnic neutropenia is observed in a variety of populations including Africans, West Indians, Yemenite and Ethiopian Jews, Beduin Arabs, and Jordanians. In these groups an ANC as low as 1000/mm³ may be considered normal.

Clinical Features

Severe neutropenia has the following common clinical manifestations:

1. High fever, chills, severe prostration, and irritability
2. Extensive necrotic and ulcerative lesions: oropharyngeal and nasal tissues, skin, gastrointestinal (GI) tract, vagina, and uterus
3. Gram-negative septicemia.

The risk of infection is inversely proportional to the ANC. When the ANC falls below 1000/mm³, stomatitis, gingivitis, and cellulitis dominate the clinical picture. More severe infections occur when the ANC is below 500/mm³ with perirectal abscesses, pneumonia, and sepsis being common.

Granulocyte colony-stimulating factor (G-CSF) produces a sustained neutrophil recovery in patients with severe chronic neutropenia, reduces the incidence and severity of infection, and improves the quality of life. The drug is tolerated well and adverse effects are transient and mild. Neutropenia can be transient (<8 weeks) or chronic (>8 weeks). Table 9-6 lists the causes of neutropenia, and Figure 9-1 shows an approach to the diagnosis of neutropenia.

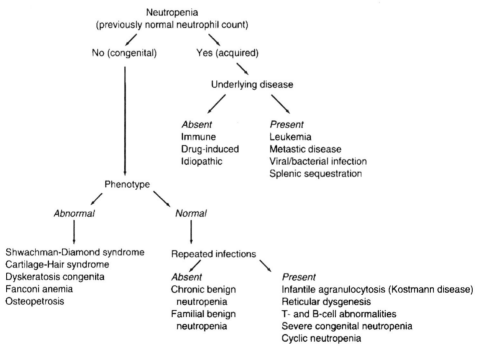

Fig. 9-1. Approach to diagnosis of neutropenia. (From Roskos RR, Boxer LA. Clinical disorders of neutropenia. Pediatr Rev 1991;12:208–12, with permission.)

DECREASED POLYMORPHONUCLEAR LEUKOCYTE PRODUCTION

Table 9-7 summarizes the features of some of the congenital neutropenias.

Severe Congenital Neutropenia and Kostmann Disease

Epidemiology

Severe congenital neutropenia (SCN) includes a heterogeneous group of disorders with different patterns of inheritance. Kostmann disease follows an autosomal recessive pattern of inheritance. Its underlying genetic defect is unknown. Other SCN may follow autosomal dominant or sporadic patterns of inheritance; in this group of patients, most of them have diverse mutations in the neutrophil elastase gene (*ELA-2*). These mutations affect only one allele. The majority of patients present with a sporadic pattern, because autosomal dominant inheritance is relatively more lethal. Some patients may exhibit germline mosaicism.

Incidence

The incidence of SCN is 2 per million population.

Clinical Manifestations

During the first year of life, omphalitis, otitis media, upper respiratory tract infections, pneumonitis, skin abscesses, and liver abscesses occur commonly with positive cultures for staphylococci, streptococci, *Pseudomonas*, *Peptostreptococcus*, and fungi. Splenomegaly may be present. Other manifestations include the following:

- *Blood counts:* ANC less than 200/mm^3, mild anemia, thrombocytosis, moderate eosinophilia, and marked monocytosis are present in the blood counts.
- *Bone marrow:* Bone marrow examination shows maturation arrest of myelopoiesis at the promyelocyte or myelocyte stage with marked paucity of mature neutrophils. There is an increase in monocytes, eosinophils, macrophages, and plasma cells.
- *Pathogenesis: In vitro* studies show a reduced number of formation of granulocyte-macrophage colonies in SCN patients. There is also a reduced number of CD34+/Kit+/G-CSFR+ myeloid progenitor cells in the bone marrow.
- *Neutrophil elastase gene (ELA-2) mutations:* It has been hypothesized that mutations of *ELA-2* in SCN result in a high rate of premature apoptosis in neutrophil precursors, which results in decreased myelopoiesis. Neutrophil elastase is a serine protease localized in the granules of neutrophils and monocytes. A mutant enzyme has a dominant negative effect on the normal wild-type elastase. This explains the defective proteolysis in the SCN neutrophils even though half of the normal amount of the elastase is present in the neutrophils of these patients. The gene responsible for the autosomal recessive form of SCN in the original cases described by Kostmann is still unknown.

Cytogenetic Evaluation

Initial cytogenetic studies of bone marrow at diagnosis are normal. However, during the course of the disease, clonal abnormalities may emerge, 50% of which are monosomy 7. Because 12% of patients with SCN develop myelodysplastic syndrome (MDS) and/or acute myelogenous leukemia (AML), it is important to perform

Table 9-7. Clinical and Hematologic Features of Some Congenital Neutropenias

Feature	Severe congenital neutropenia (SCN) and Kostmann disease (KD)	Familial benign neutropenia	Chronic benign neutropenia[a]	Reticular dysgenesis[b]
Inheritance	Autosomal recessive (KD) Autosomal dominant or sporadic (SCN)	Dominant	Not hereditary	Not hereditary
Severity	Severe illness Life-threatening pyogenic infections in first months of life	Variable; benign to severe infections	Benign	Severe, fatal thymic dysplasia Lymphoid hypoplasia
Clinical findings	Skin infection Aphthous ulcers Septicemia Meningitis Peritonitis Lung abscess Lymphadenopathy Splenomegaly (20%)	Less troublesome infection to severe infection	Paronychia Gingivitis Impetigo: mild infections, localized	Severe bacterial and viral infection Neonatal death

Hematologic findings	Anemia Neutropenia, <200/mm^3 Monocytosis Eosinophilia Risk of leukemia	Neutropenia, usually <300/mm^3 Monocytosis	No anemia Absent mature PMN Some band forms Monocytosis	Neutropenia Lymphopenia
Marrow findings	↑ Promyelocytes Absent MM, B, PMN ↑ Monocytes ↑ Eosinophils ↑ Plasma cells	↓ MM, B, PMN "Maturation arrest"	Absent PMN Normal myeloid cells to band stage; lymphocytes increased	Absent myeloid and absent lymphoid cells Normal thrombopoiesis and erythropoiesis
Treatment	Antibiotics Supportive measures G-CSF Stem cell transplantation	No therapy G-CSF, if indicated	Antibiotics, as indicated G-CSF, if indicated	Stem cell transplantation

Abbreviations: B, bands; MM, metamyelocytes; PMN, polymorphonuclear leukocytes; G-CSF, granulocyte colony-stimulating factor.

[a]Most of these cases are autoimmune in origin and pathogenesis, even though antineutrophil antibodies may not always be demonstrated. This condition is probably the same as idiopathic autoimmune neutropenia (see pages 224–225).

[b]Failure of stem cells committed to myeloid and lymphoid development.

periodic bone marrow examinations for morphology and cytogenetic studies in the follow-up of these patients.

G-CSF Receptor in SCN

G-CSF receptor is normal in patients with SCN. However, patients with SCN are predisposed to develop acquired (somatic) mutations of the cytoplasmic domain of the G-CSF receptor. There is a good correlation between the development of leukemia/MDS and the acquisition of G-CSF receptor mutations in patients with SCN. The time interval between these two events varies considerably.

Treatment

The dose of G-CSF employed is 5.0 µg/kg/day. Response occurs 7–10 days from the start of treatment with an increase in ANC to greater than $1000/mm^3$. More than 95% of patients with SCN respond to G-CSF. After beginning the G-CSF dose of 5.0 µg/kg/day, the dose should be adjusted at 1- to 2-week intervals until the lowest effective dose is achieved.

Patients who require greater than a 100 µg/kg/day dose of G-CSF should be considered as candidates for hematopoietic stem cell transplantation (HSCT). The other indications for HSCT in SCN include emergence of MDS/AML or refractoriness to G-CSF treatment. However, some experts favor the treatment with HSCT for all patients with SCN who have an HLA-matched sibling donor available.

Complications associated with the use of G-CSF include bone pain, splenomegaly, hepatomegaly, thrombocytopenia, osteopenia/osteoporosis, Henoch-Schönlein purpura type of immune-complex-induced vasculitis of the skin, and/or glomerulonephritis. The leading cause of death in SCN is from MDS/leukemia.

Chronic Benign Neutropenia

1. This is the most common form of neutropenia in infants under 4 years of age. The rate of infection decreases with age.
2. Ninety percent of cases occur before 14 months of age.
3. The clinical course is variable, ranging from benign to life threatening. Patients with an ANC greater than $400/mm^3$ do not have a higher incidence of infection than normal children. Day-to-day variations occur in the white cell counts.

Laboratory Findings

The ANC is usually less than $500/mm^3$. The bone marrow shows myeloid hyperplasia with a reduction in mature neutrophil precursors (maturation arrest).

Treatment

Treatment includes supportive care, antibiotics, and G-CSF, if indicated.

Cyclic Neutropenia

1. Rare disorder; presents in infancy or childhood; usually benign, but 10% die from overwhelming infection.
2. Autosomal dominant mode of inheritance in some patients and sporadic in others.
3. Genetic and molecular studies by linkage analysis have localized the genetic defect to chromosome 19p13.3. Gene sequencing revealed mutations in the gene

for neutrophil elastase (*ELA-2*), a serine protease synthesized during the promyelocyte/myelocyte stage. It has been speculated that neutropenia results from activation of the apoptotic pathway by mutant forms of *ELA-2*.

4. Marked neutropenia (ANC less than 500/mm^3, usually less than 200/mm^3) at regular intervals, usually every 21 days, persisting for 3–6 days. ANC then increases to the lower limit of normal, about 2000/mm^3, and remains approximately at this level until the next neutropenic period. Cycles may vary from 14 to 40 days.

5. Infections: Coincident with neutropenia, patient manifests the following clinical signs:
   Fever
   Ulceration of oral, vaginal, or rectal mucous membranes
   Gingivitis, stomatitis
   Furunculosis, cellulitis
   Perirectal abscess
   Cervical lymphadenopathy
   Fatal Clostridial bacteremia from gastrointestinal tract ulcers
   Other infections (e.g., mastoiditis, pneumonia, adenitis).

6. Hematology
   Monocytosis during neutropenic nadir
   Neutrophil granulocytes affected
   Oscillations in reticulocyte and platelet counts in most patients and fluctuations of eosinophil and lymphocyte counts in some patients
   Bone marrow—absent late myeloid precursors before development of neutropenia, but during the neutropenic phases, marrow shows myeloid hyperplasia.

7. Therapy includes antibiotic therapy (as indicated). Prophylactic therapy with G-CSF is recommended to all patients with cyclic neutropenia to prevent the severe dental complications and also to prevent development of life-threatening infections. G-CSF is started in a dose of 5.0 µg/kg/day and then the dose of G-CSF is adjusted at 1- to 2-week intervals until the lowest effective dose is achieved. It may be administered daily or on alternate days.

   Granulocytic-macrophage colony-stimulating factor (GM-CSF) is used less frequently for long-term treatment because of its side effects. It is less effective than G-CSF in elevating the ANC but is effective in reducing the nadir in cyclic neutropenia.

Patients with cyclic neutropenia are not predisposed to develop malignancies.

Neutropenia Associated with X-Linked Agammaglobulinemia

1. Inherited as X-linked recessive trait; caused by mutations in the gene encoding a tyrosine kinase known as Bruton's or B-cell tyrosine kinase (BTK).

2. Severe decrease in serum IgG, IgA, and IgM levels and marked decrease in B lymphocytes, but normal T-cell function.

3. BTK gene is also expressed in myeloid cells and its product participates in signal transduction for myeloid maturation.

4. Patients with neutropenia are more prone to develop fungal or *Pneumocystis carinii* infections.

5. Neutropenia is observed only when rapid production of these cells is required.

6. A short course of G-CSF with antibiotic may be used, when needed, although no evidence-based data are available.

Neutropenia Associated with Autosomal Recessive Agammaglobulinemia

Autosomal recessive agammaglobulinemia due to mutations of the gene encoding for μ heavy chain is also associated with neutropenia and absent B cells. A short course of G-CSF may be used, when needed, although no evidence-based data are available.

Neutropenia Associated with Abnormal Cellular Immunity in Cartilage–Hair Hypoplasia

This condition is characterized by:

1. Autosomal recessive mode of inheritance; found in Amish and Finnish population
2. Short-limbed dwarfism
3. Fine hair
4. Moderate to severe neutropenia and increased susceptibility to infection
5. Lymphopenia, macrocytic anemia
6. Impaired cellular immune function due to impaired T-cell function caused by mutations in the *RMRP* gene, which encodes the RNA component of a ribonuclear protein ribonuclease; diminished delayed skin hypersensitivity and rejection of skin allograft.

Treatment

Treatment includes allogeneic stem cell transplantation. There are no reports of the use of G-CSF in this disorder.

Neutropenia Associated with Common Variable Immunodeficiency

Common variable immunodeficiency (CVID) is used to describe patients with hypogammaglobulinemia of undetermined origin. The IgG level is low but IgM and IgA levels vary. *In vitro* response of B cells to pokeweed mitogen to produce immunoglobulin is impaired in patients whose B cells fail to differentiate into mature cells.

Clinical Manifestations

CVID usually becomes manifest in patients between 20 and 30 years of age and only occasionally in childhood. Most patients manifest recurrent infections of the sinopulmonary tract. They are also prone to develop noncaseating granulomas of the skin, gut, and other organs. These patients are predisposed to develop autoimmune disorders such as immune thrombocytopenic purpura (ITP), systemic lupus erythematosus (SLE), and thyroiditis.

Treatment

Neutropenia in CVID is explained on an autoimmune basis. Patients respond to G-CSF treatment, IV immunoglobulin, and antibiotics.

Myelokathexis and WHIM Syndrome

Inheritance is autosomal dominant. Patients display **W**arts, **H**ypogammaglobulinemia, **I**nfections, and **M**yelokathexis, hence, the term **WHIM** syndrome.

Hematologic Findings

- Moderate to severe neutropenia. Neutrophils and eosinophils contain vacuoles, prominent granules, and nuclear hypersegmentation with pyknotic nuclei connected to each other by thin filaments. Normal morphology of lymphocytes, monocytes, and basophils. Neutrophil function is usually normal.
- Bone marrow shows granulocytic hyperplasia and neutrophils with similar degenerative changes as in the blood, that is, congenital dysmyelopoietic neutropenia. Ineffective myelopoiesis due to increased apoptosis of neutrophils in bone marrow because of decreased expression of antiapoptotic factor *bcl-x*.

Treatment

Prompt response to G-CSF or GM-CSF. Immunoglobulin levels return to normal after treatment with G-CSF.

Selective IgA Deficiency and Neutropenia

Selective IgA deficiency may be associated with neutropenia that is autoimmune in nature. It is not known if the use of G-SCF is effective in this condition.

Dubowitz Syndrome

This condition is characterized by dysmorphic facies, mental retardation, microcephaly, growth retardation, eczema, association with recurrent neutropenia, and low IgG and IgA with elevated IgM levels. The mode of inheritance is autosomal recessive.

Neutropenia Associated with Pancreatic Insufficiency (Shwachman–Diamond Syndrome) (SDS)

This condition is characterized by:

1. Autosomal recessive mode of inheritance. It is a rare multiorgan disease.
2. Metaphyseal chondrodysplasia
   a. Dwarfism
   b. Impaired gait due to hip dysplasia.
3. Abnormal hematopoiesis: Abnormal bone marrow stroma with its reduced ability to support hematopoiesis, increased expression of Fas on hematopoietic progenitor cells resulting in increased apoptosis, and stem cell abnormality characterized by decreased growth potential of CFU-GM and CFU-E on culture.
   a. Neutropenia: 200–400 cells/mm^3; cyclic pattern (occasionally)
   b. Myeloid hypoplasia
   c. Recurrent bacterial infection (e.g., otitis media, pneumonia).
4. Polymorphonuclear motility defect due to impairment of the cellular cytoskeleton or microtubular function.
5. Pancreatic exocrine insufficiency
   a. Diarrhea, steatorrhea
   b. Failure to thrive, growth failure.
6. Increased frequency of myocardial necrosis.

Diagnosis

- Fecal fat (72 hours)
- Pancreatic function tests (duodenal intubation to demonstrate absence of trypsin, amylase, and lipase)
- Low serum trypsinogen levels in young patients (may improve with age)

- Congenital lipomatosis of the pancreas revealed on pancreatic CAT scan imaging to identify gross fatty changes, especially in the body of the pancreas and ductal ectasia and calcification
- Normal sweat electrolyte test.

Genetics

The gene for SDS has been mapped to a single locus at the chromosome 7 centromere and hypothetically it may be involved in the development of pancreas, hematopoiesis, and chondrogenesis. Chromosome 7 abnormalities such as deletions of the long arm, isochromosome 7, and loss of chromosome 7 occur in the majority of patients with SDS who develop myelodysplasia. It is unclear if this somatic mutation in the marrow stem cells results because of the congenital mutations in the SDS locus.

Hematologic Complications

- Anemia.
- Thrombocytopenia (9% have platelet counts less than $50,000/mm^3$); the development of thrombocytopenia may signal conversion to aplastic anemia or myelodysplasia.
- Aplastic anemia.
- AML; incidence increases with age, starting at about 10 years of age.
- Myelodysplasia; incidence increases with age, starting at about 10 years of age.

The overall incidence of AML and myelodysplasia is about 16%. Both are resistant to chemotherapy and only respond to allogeneic stem cell transplantation.

Treatment

- Pancreatic enzymes.
- GCSF.
- GM-CSF.
- Allogeneic HSCT. Indications and optimum timing for transplantation are unclear. Most of the patients have been transplanted for the treatment of myelodysplasia, AML, or severe pancytopenia. The following contribute to unsatisfactory results of HSCT: hepatic and cardiac toxicity, preexisting infections, poor nutritional status, marrow stromal defect not corrected by HSCT, presence of MDS/AML, and excessive sensitivity of critical organs to radiation therapy and/or chemotherapy.

Neutropenia Associated with Hyperimmunoglobulin M Syndrome

Immunodeficiency with hyper-IgM may be caused by one of the following molecular genetic defects:

1. X-linked recessive trait, caused by mutations in the gene for the CD40 ligand, a molecule on T cells that binds to its receptor CD40 on B cells, to induce immunoglobulin class switching from production of IgM to IgG and IgA.
2. X-linked recessive form of the hyper-IgM syndrome caused by a mutation in IκB kinase γ subunit/NF-κB essential modulator (NEMO) and associated with hypohidrotic ectodermal dysplasia (conical teeth, inadequate sweating, and poor antibody production to polysaccharide antigens).
3. An autosomal recessive form of hyper-IgM syndrome caused by a defect in the gene for activation-induced cytidine deaminase. This enzyme is needed for Ig class switch, recombination, and somatic hypermutation.

The mechanism of neutropenia is a decreased interaction between T cells and bone marrow stromal cells, resulting in reduced production of G-CSF.

Clinical Manifestations

- Severe recurrent pyogenic bacterial infections
- Infections by opportunistic organisms including *Pneumocystis carinii*, histoplasmosis, cryptosporidium, and *Toxoplasma*
- Neutropenia, transient, cyclic (10%), or chronic (50% of cases)
- Coombs' positive autoimmune hemolytic anemia
- Lymphoid hyperplasia
- Low serum immunoglobulin A (IgA), IgE, and IgG; elevated IgM
- Number of circulating B cells are normal or increased and T cells are normal.

Treatment

IV immunoglobulin and G-CSF (mainstay of therapy); also HSCT.

Neutropenia Associated with Metabolic Diseases

The presenting clinical features in neutropenia associated with metabolic diseases (Table 9-6) are lethargy, vomiting, ketosis, and dehydration during the neonatal period, failure to thrive, and growth retardation. The marrow is hypoplastic in these conditions, with decreased numbers of myeloid precursors. Idiopathic hyperglycinemia and methylmalonic acidemia also have associated thrombocytopenia.

In glycogen storage disease type IB, there is impairment of glucose-6-phosphate-translocase, an enzyme necessary for the transport of glucose-6-phosphate from the cytoplasm to the endoplasmic reticulum, the site where glucose-6-phosphate is hydrolyzed to glucose and inorganic phosphate by an enzyme glucose-6-phosphatase. As a result of the low availability of glucose, these patients develop hypoglycemia, defective chemotaxis, and recurrent infections. The mechanism of neutropenia is not known in this disease. The bone marrow is hypercellular with abundant neutrophils.

Barth syndrome is characterized by cardiomyopathy, neutropenia, skeletal myopathy, growth retardation, low creatinine levels, mitochondrial abnormalities, and organic aciduria. It is a sex-linked recessive disorder. It results from mutations in the gene *G4.5*, a member of a tafazzin family protein.

Bone Marrow Disease

Bone marrow aplasia, whether congenital (Fanconi anemia, dyskeratosis congenita) or acquired (idiopathic or secondary), or bone marrow infiltration, whether nonneoplastic (e.g., storage diseases such as Gaucher disease or Niemann–Pick disease, osteopetrosis, and cystinosis) or neoplastic (e.g., leukemia and neuroblastoma), may present with neutropenia as a component of the pancytopenia of the disorder.

INCREASED DESTRUCTION OR DISORDERS OF DISTRIBUTION OF POLYMORPHONUCLEAR LEUKOCYTES

Immunoneutropenia

Drug-Induced Neutropenia

Drug-induced neutropenia may be due to:

1. Idiosyncratic suppression of myeloid production affecting a few exposed persons; for example, antibiotics (novobiocin, methicillin), sulfonamides, antidiabetics

(tolbutamide, chlorpropamide), antithyroids (propylthiouracil, methimazole), antihistamines, and antihypertensives (chlorothiazides, Aldomet)

2. Regularly occurring dose-dependent myeloid suppression from cytotoxic drugs or antimetabolites; for example, 6-mercaptopurine, methotrexate, and nitrogen mustard
3. Destruction of white cells produced by the marrow due to differences in individual ability to metabolize a drug; for example, phenothiazine and thiouracil
4. Drug-haptene disease, in which antibodies to the drug–leukocyte complex are produced, resulting in demonstrable *in vitro* leukoagglutinins; for example, amidopyrine-related drugs (dipyrone, phenylbutazone), sulfapyridine, mercurial diuretics, and chlorpropamide.

Neonatal Neutropenia

Immunoneutropenias may be alloimmune (isoimmune), with immunization to foreign antigens on the fetal leukocytes similar to Rh isoimmunization, or autoimmune, in infants born to mothers with neutropenia who have antileukocyte antibodies (e.g., a mother who has SLE).

Alloimmune Neonatal Neutropenia

In alloimmune neonatal neutropenia, alloantibodies are frequently directed to the neutrophil-specific NA antigen system, of which there are two alleles: NA1 and NA2.

Clinical Features

- Infants may be asymptomatic or they may have infections (e.g., pyoderma, omphalitis, pneumonia).
- Neutropenia usually resolves at 2 months of age.
- Bone marrow is hypercellular with an increase in neutrophil precursors and a paucity of mature neutrophils.

Treatment

Antibiotics, as indicated; IVIG, G-CSF.

Autoimmune Neutropenia

Autoimmune neutropenia can be primary or secondary.

Primary Autoimmune Neutropenia

Primary autoimmune neutropenia is probably the same entity as idiopathic chronic benign neutropenia of infancy and childhood.

Neutropenia may result from antibodies against leukocytes on an idiopathic basis. It is analogous to autoimmune hemolytic anemia or autoimmune thrombocytopenia. Neutrophil antibodies may adversely affect the function of neutrophils, producing qualitative defects in the neutrophils and amplifying the risk of infection associated with neutropenia. Neutrophil autoantibodies may also affect myeloid precursor cells. When this occurs, it can produce profound neutropenia. The disease is characterized by the following:

1. Age: 3–30 months; median age, 8 months; has occurred as early as 1 month of age. Occasionally, it may be congenital.

2. It is nonfamilial.
3. Physical examination: normal; occasionally, slight splenomegaly.
4. Benign infections of skin and upper respiratory tract, as well as otitis media in 90% of cases; not life threatening; responsive to standard antibiotics.

Diagnosis

1. Neutrophil counts range from 0 to 1000 cells/mm^3. Monocytosis is common.
2. The bone marrow may be normal or may show evidence of myeloid hyperplasia with marked reduction in segmented neutrophils due to their destruction by antibodies.
3. Epinephrine or hydrocortisone administration results in the rise of neutrophil counts.
4. Antineutrophil antibodies are not always present, and screening has to be repeated for antibody detection. Immunoassay is more sensitive than leukoagglutination testing for diagnosing immune neutropenia. In most patients the autoantibody is auto-anti-NA1, and some have auto-anti-NA2.

Prognosis
Spontaneous recovery within a few months to a few years. The median age at recovery is 30 months (range of 7–73 months). In 95% of cases, recovery occurs by 4 years of age.

Treatment
In patients with severe neutropenia and severe or recurrent infections:

- Appropriate antibiotics for acute infections or prophylactic antibiotics such as trimethoprim/sulfamethoxazole
- Prednisone 2 mg/kg orally for 1 month; about 75% response rate
- Intravenous immunoglobulin (IVIG) 1 g/kg/day for 3–5 days until absolute neutrophil count is greater than 1000/mm^3; about 50% response rate
- High-dose IV immunoglobulin 3 g/kg/day for 3–5 days
- Concomitant administration of intravenous immunoglobulin and high-dose Solu-Medrol or prednisone to produce a synergistic effect
- Recombinant human granulocytic-macrophage colony-stimulating factor (rHuGM-CSF) or G-CSF to treat patients with active infections; almost 100% response rate (G-CSF in a dose of 5 µg/kg/day SC is given until the absolute neutrophil count is greater than 5000/mm^3). IV IG or G-CSF are preferred for the treatments of infections in these patients.

Secondary Autoimmune Neutropenia

Secondary autoimmune neutropenia is more common in adults than in children. Associated diseases include Evans syndrome, autoimmune hemolytic anemia, autoimmune thrombocytopenia, thyroiditis, insulin-dependent diabetes mellitus, and combined immune deficiency. Autoantibody specificity is Pan-FcR γIIIb.

Treatment
Treat the associated condition and use G-CSF.

Nonimmune Neutropenia

Pseudoneutropenia

In this condition, a normal neutrophil population may be shifted toward the marginating compartment, leaving fewer cells in the circulating compartment. The WBC count measures only the circulating cells and not the marginating pool; therefore, this represents a pseudoneutropenia. The bone marrow is normal in appearance. The neutrophils function normally, and the leukocyte changes are usually found incidentally on blood count. Marginating neutrophils may be uncovered by the injection of epinephrine.

Ineffective Myelopoiesis

This condition is a chronic neutropenia with the ability to respond with a neutrophil leukocytosis at times of infection. Marrow examination shows a shift to the right among the granulocytic series, the predominant cells resembling degenerating polymorphs with dense pyknotic chromatin. The fundamental defect appears to be intramedullary death of the neutrophils (or ineffective myelopoiesis). Corticosteroids and splenectomy do not influence the course of the disease.

Infections

Viral infections and certain bacterial infections, such as typhoid fever, paratyphoid fever, and rickettsial disease, may be associated with neutropenia. Staphylococcal or pneumococcal infections associated with neutropenia indicate a grave prognosis.

Hypersplenism

Hypersplenism causes peripheral sequestration not only of red cells and platelets but of granulocytes as well. The marrow in such cases shows myeloid hyperplasia with normal maturation to the polymorph stage. Splenomegaly from any cause (e.g., thalassemia, storage diseases, portal hypertension, lymphomas) may produce hypersplenism. Occasionally, splenomegaly and neutropenia of unknown cause (primary splenic neutropenia) occur in which the hematologic abnormality can be cured by splenectomy.

Investigations in Neutropenia

Table 9-8 lists the investigations required in patients with neutropenia.

Management of Neutropenia

Table 9-9 lists the management required in the care of neutropenic patients.

DISORDERS OF LEUKOCYTE FUNCTION

Table 9-10 classifies the diseases of leukocyte dysfunction and lists the investigations to be carried out in patients with leukocyte dysfunction.

Leukocyte Adhesion Disorders

Leukocyte Adhesion Deficiency Type I

Leukocyte adhesion deficiency (LAD) type I is characterized by a deficiency of glycoprotein CD 11b, which forms the α-subunit of the Mac-1 β_2-integrin (CD 11b/CD18) on the cell surface of the neutrophils. Intercellular molecule 1 (ICAM-1) expressed on the vascular endothelium serves as a ligand to Mac-1 for the neutrophil adhesion. Because of the mutation and the absence of Mac-1, neutrophils in LAD type I are not

Table 9-8. Investigations of Patients with Neutropenia[a]

1. History of drug ingestion, toxin exposure
2. Physical examination—nature of infectious lesions, growth and development, presence of anomalies
3. Familial: absolute granulocyte count in family members
4. Blood count: platelet count, absolute granulocyte count, and reticulocyte count; absolute granulocyte count 3 times per week for 2 months (to exclude cyclic neutropenia)
5. Bone marrow
   a. Maturation characteristics of myeloid series; ? reduction in mature granulocytes
   b. Maturation and number of megakaryocytes and erythroid precursors
   c. Karyotype (to identify myelodysplasia or acute myelocytic leukemia)
   d. Electron microscopy (subcellular morphology, congenital dysgranulopoiesis)
6. Presence of leukoagglutinins
   a. Serum antibodies directed against granulocytes
7. Estimate of marginating granulocyte reserve pool
   a. Epinephrine stimulation tests (0.1 mL 1:1000 epinephrine SC)
      (1) Absolute granulocyte counts at 5, 10, 15, and 30 minutes
      (2) Normal: double base count
8. Estimate of bone marrow granulocyte reserve pool
   a. Cortisone stimulation tests (5 mg/kg IV)
      (1) Absolute granulocyte counts hourly for 6 hours
      (2) Normal: increase of more than 2000 neutrophils/mm^3
   b. Typhoid stimulation tests (0.5-mL vaccine SC)
      (1) Absolute granulocyte count at 3, 6, 12, and 24 hours
      (2) Normal: threefold to fourfold increase
9. Rebuck skin window (to assess leukocyte migration and chemotaxis)
   Normal: at 3 hours, neutrophils; at 6 hours, mixed neutrophils and monocytes; at 24 hours, monocytes
10. Immunologic tests:
    a. Immune globulins (IgA, IgG, IgM, IgE)
    b. Cellular immunity (skin-test activity, purified protein derivative [PPD], T- and B-cell evaluation; suppressor T-cell assay)
    c. Antinuclear antibodies, C_3, C_4, CH_{50}
11. Evidence of metabolic disease
    a. Plasma and urine amino acid screening
    b. Serum vitamin B_{12}, folic acid, and copper
12. Evidence of pancreatic disease
    Exocrine pancreatic function: stool fat, pancreatic enzyme assays, CT scan of pancreas for pancreatic lipomatosis, serum levels of trypsinogen and isoamylase
13. Chromosomal analysis (Fanconi anemia)
14. Radiographic bone survey (cartilage–hair hypoplasia, Shwachman–Diamond syndrome, Fanconi anemia)
15. Serum muramidase (ineffective myelopoiesis)
16. Colony-forming unit (CFU) assays (adequacy of myeloid-committed stem cell compartment)
17. Colony-stimulating activity (CSA) assay (inhibition of CSA effect or production)
18. Flow cytometric analysis (paroxysmal nocturnal hemoglobinuria)
19. Bone density studies (14% of patients with chronic neutropenia show nonclinical osteoporosis or osteopenia)
20. Neutrophil elastase (ELA-2) mutation gene analysis

[a]Absolute granulocyte count less than 1500/mm^3.

Table 9-9. Management of Neutropenic Patient[a]

1. Admit to hospital for persistent fever over 101°F.
2. Obtain appropriate cultures (blood, throat, urine, infected area) and sensitivity.
3. Administer parenteral antibiotics (Chapter 26)
    a. If an organism is isolated, 10–14 days' intravenous treatment is required.
    b. If no organism is isolated, antibiotic is continued until afebrile or neutropenia is resolved.
4. Place on reverse isolation to prevent superinfection with antibiotic-resistant organisms.
5. Observe strict hand-washing procedures.
6. Wash skin carefully with a Povidine-containing solution before all skin puncture procedures.
7. Minimize manipulation of skin, oral mucosa, perineum, and rectum; rectal temperatures and enemas are contraindicated.
8. Treat mouth ulcerations and gingivitis with appropriate systemic antibiotics if secondary bacterial infection is found and 3% hydrogen peroxide–1% alum mouthwash, which usually produces symptomatic relief.
9. Administer recombinant human G-CSF (rHu-GCSF)[b] for treatment of Kostmann disease (severe congenital agranulocytosis), Shwachman–Diamond syndrome, other congenital neutropenias, and severe neutropenia following chemotherapy (the starting dose is 5 μg/kg SC with dose modification according to the patient's absolute neutrophil count).

[a]Neutrophil count less than 500 cells/mm^3.

[b]G-CSF specifically stimulates myeloid progenitor cells in the bone marrow and enhances neutrophil production and function.

Table 9-10. Classification and Investigation of Diseases of Leukocyte Dysfunction

Function	Disease	Investigations
Motility and migration Chemotaxis	Leukocyte adhesion deficiency Lazy-leukocyte syndrome Syndrome of elevated IgE, eczema, and recurrent infection	All tests below may be abnormal Rebuck skin window: at 3 hours, neutrophils; at 6 hours, mixed neutrophils and monocytes; at 24 hours, monocytes
Opsonization	Complement deficiency Specific bacterial antibody deficiency	Serum complement levels Immunoglobulin levels Specific bacterial antibody levels
Bacterial killing	Chédiak–Higashi syndrome Myeloperoxidase deficiency Chronic granulomatous disease (CGD) Job's disease Leukocyte glutathione peroxidase deficiency Glucose-6-phosphate dehydrogenase (G6PD) deficiency	Morphologic tests Chédiak–Higashi giant granules Peroxidase stain Bacterial test Killing of catalase-positive (*Staphylococcus aureus*) and catalase-negative (streptococcal) bacteria Metabolic tests Nitroblue tetrazolium (NBT) reduction test[a] Glucose 1–^{14}C oxidation with phagocytosis Oxygen consumption during phagocytosis H_2O_2-dependent ^{14}C-formate oxidation with phagocytosis Iodine-125 fixation during phagocytosis[b]

[a]Impaired in CGD due to nicotinamide adenine dinucleotide phosphate (NADPH) oxidase deficiency, deficiency of glutathione reductase of G6PD. Normal in myeloperoxidase deficiency.

[b]Impaired in CGD and in myeloperoxidase deficiency.

able to attach to the endothelium and undergo transendothelial migration. Additionally, their ability for chemotaxis, phagocytosis, degranulation, and respiratory burst activity is also impaired. Survival of neutrophils is prolonged in LAD type I.

Clinical Features

- Rare autosomal recessive disorder
- Persistent neutrophilia and lack of pus formation
- Frequent skin and periodontal infection
- Omphalitis, delayed umbilical cord separation (normal mean age of cord separation: 7–15 days)
- Perirectal abscess
- Sepsis
- Necrotizing enterocolitis
- Pneumonia
- Sinusitis
- Infecting organisms: *Staphylococcus aureus, Pseudomonas aeruginosa, Proteus, Escherichia coli, Klebsiella, Candida albicans,* and *Aspergillus.*

Diagnosis

1. Flow cytometry for assessment of expression of CD 11b or CD 18 on neutrophil cell surfaces with the use of specific monoclonal antibodies
2. *In vitro* functional assays of neutrophil adhesion, chemotaxis, and phagocytosis.

Treatment

For mild and moderate disease: oral hygiene with antimicrobial mouthwash, for example, chlorhexidine gluconate, prophylactic use of trimethoprim/sulfamethoxazole (co-trimoxazole), and aggressive treatment of infections. For severe cases, HSCT is recommended.

Leukocyte Adhesion Deficiency Type II

Extremely rare condition caused by the absence of neutrophil sialyl Lewis X structure. Patients have rare Bombay (hh) red cell phenotype. Compared with LAD type I, these patients suffer from less serious types of infections. They are unable to form pus in spite of leukocytosis of $30,000–150,000/mm^3$.

Lazy-Leukocyte Syndrome

An altered membrane microfilamentous protein structure or function leads to rigidity and impaired mobility of the neutrophils, causing difficulty in their entering and exiting the circulation.

The disease is characterized by:

1. Poor polymorphonuclear leukocyte response to bacterial pyrogen injection, indicating impaired marrow release of polymorphs
2. Recurrent stomatitis, otitis, gingivitis, and low-grade fever, frequently staphylococcal aureus infections
3. Low or normal absolute granulocyte counts with normal phagocytic and bactericidal activity in the polymorphs
4. Normal bone marrow findings

5. Defective recruitment of polymorphs to skin windows, recruitment of mono-cytes normal.

Syndrome of Elevated Immunoglobulin E, Eczema, and Recurrent Infection (Job Syndrome)

Clinical Manifestations

- Chronic eczema, delay in shedding primary teeth, hyperextensible joints, scolio-sis, osteopenia, and tendency to fractures, growth retardation, and coarse facies
- Recurrent severe staphylococcal abscesses
- Recurrent cutaneous, pulmonary, and joint abscesses
- Chronic candidiasis of mucosa and nails.

Laboratory Findings

- Very high serum IgE level (greater than 2500 IU/mL)
- Defect in T lymphocytes that results in reduced production of IFN-γ and tumor necrosis factor
- Molecular basis of hyper IgE syndrome unknown
- Striking defect in neutrophil granulocyte chemotactic responsiveness; neutrophil migration, phagocytosis, and bactericidal activity normal.

Treatment

- Prophylactic antibiotics: trimethoprim/sulfamethoxazole or dicloxacillin
- rhIFN-γ: 50 μg/m^2 subcutaneously three times per week; however, evidence-based data for its efficacy are not available.

Localized Juvenile Periodontitis/Localized Aggressive Periodontitis in Children

Localized juvenile periodontitis (LJP) is characterized by severe alveolar bone loss localized to the first molars and incisors. It is frequently associated with the presence of the bacterium *Actinobacillus actinomycetemcomitans*. Age of onset is usually at puberty.

Its etiology is defective neutrophil chemotaxis in the majority of patients. This defect is attributed to neutrophil chemotactic inhibitors. Phagocytosis is also abnor-mal in many of these patients. Unstimulated neutrophils from these patients show reduced Lewis X, sialyl Lewis X, and L-selectin expression.

Treatment

- Deep subgingival scaling and root planning
- Adjunctive systemic use of antibiotics: simultaneous use of metronidazole and amoxicillin or amoxicillin with clavulanic acid (Augmentin)
- Local delivery of antibiotics: Not much information is available. However, the use of doxycycline or minocycline, in local delivery formulation, may be consid-ered in eliminating infection with *A. actinomycetemcomitans*.

Chédiak–Higashi Syndrome

This syndrome is characterized by:

1. Autosomal recessive syndrome with repeated pyogenic infections; mean age at death, 6 years

2. Photophobia, pale optic fundi, nystagmus, partial oculocutaneous albinism, and excessive sweating
3. Hepatosplenomegaly, generalized lymphadenopathy
4. Hematologic features:
   a. Anemia, neutropenia, and thrombocytopenia.
   b. Giant refractile peroxidase-positive granules (1–4 μm) are present in the neutrophils, eosinophils, basophils, and platelets. They stain greenish gray.
   c. Granules fail to discharge lysosomal enzymes into the phagocytic vacuole, leading to increased susceptibility to infection.
   d. A defect in chemotaxis and neutropenia contributes further to lower bacterial resistance.
   e. Platelets are deficient in dense bodies and may contain the giant granules.
5. An accelerated phase occurs in 85% of cases. It is characterized by infiltration of the central nervous system and peripheral nerves, liver, spleen, and other organs by histiocytes and atypical lymphocytes. A lymphoma-like picture with fever, jaundice, hepatosplenomegaly, lymphadenopathy, bleeding tendency, and pancytopenia develops.

Treatment

1. Ascorbic acid (20 mg/kg/day) may normalize the chemotactic defect and bactericidal function.
2. Antibiotics. Prophylactic antibiotics include trimethoprim/sulfamethoxazole. Therapeutic use of antibiotics is recommended to treat infections.
3. Vincristine and corticosteroids may induce temporary remissions when used in accelerated phase.
4. Allogeneic HSCT is potentially curative.

Chronic Granulomatous Disease

Pathogenesis

In chronic granulomatous disease (CGD), neutrophils show normal phagocytosis but defective killing of microorganisms as a result of markedly deficient or absent superoxide production due to inherited mutations of polypeptides of reduced nicotinamide adenine dinucleotide phosphate (NADPH) oxidase (also known as respiratory burst oxidase) in phagocytes. Superoxide is a precursor of microbicidal oxidants such as hydrogen peroxide and hypochlorous acid.

Table 9-11 lists the reactions of the respiratory burst pathway. Organisms that make their own catalase are more often responsible for severe infections in these patients. These organisms are able to convert their own hydrogen peroxide to water, thus making it unavailable to the phagocyte for the microbicidal purpose. As a consequence, the ingested bacteria or fungi remain viable in the phagocytes and are protected from host humoral immunity and from antibiotics, which fail to penetrate the cell. The mobility of the phagocytes leads to generalized seeding of the reticuloendothelial system with live microorganisms. This results in the formation of generalized chronic granulomatous lesions, characterized by recurrent suppurative infection with bacteria of low virulence (e.g., *Staphylococcus aureus, Staphylococcus epidermidis, Aerobacter aerogenes,* and *Serratia marcescens*), *Burkholderia (Pseudomonas) capacia* and *Salmonella,* or infection with mycotic organisms (e.g., *Aspergillus*). *S. aureus* is the most frequently isolated organism. However, the most common causes of death are pneumonia and/or sepsis due to *Aspergillus* or *B. capacia.*

Table 9-11. Reactions of Respiratory Burst Pathway in a Neutrophil (Activated for Phagocytosis)

1. Assembly of respiratory oxidase, also known as NADPH oxidase, a multisubunit enzyme complex consisting of four essential phagocyte oxidase (PHOX) polypeptides: gp91^{PHOX}, p22^{PHOX}, p47^{PHOX}, and p67^{PHOX}. NADPH oxidase catalyzes the transfer of an electron from NADPH to molecular oxygen as a result of which superoxide (O$_2^-$) is formed.
$$NADPH + 2O_2 \xleftarrow{\text{NADPH oxidase}} NADP + H^+ + 2O_2$$
2. Conversion of superoxide to hydrogen peroxide (H$_2$O$_2$) by superoxide dismutase or spontaneously and also formation of hydroxyl radical (OH).
3. Hypochlorous acid (HOCL) formation: $H_2O_2 \xrightarrow{\text{Myeloperoxidase}} HOCl$.
4. Conversion of hydrogen peroxide to water by glutathione peroxidase:
GSH (reduced glutathione) + H$_2$O$_2$ $\xrightarrow{\text{glutathione peroxidase}}$ GSSG (oxidized glutathione) + H$_2$O.
5. Hydrogen peroxide is also converted to water by catalase.
6. Restoration of GSH by conversion of GSSG by glutathione reductase:
$$NADPH + GSSG \xrightarrow{\text{glutathione reductase}} GSH + NADP$$
7. Generation of NADPH through G6PD (glucose-6-phosphate dehydrogenase) reaction.

Genetics

CGD results from mutations in any of the four genes encoding essential subunits of the NADPH oxidase. A genetic classification of CGD according to the component of NADPH oxidase affected follows:

Component affected	Gene locus	Inheritance	Frequency (% of cases)
gp91^{phox*}	Xp21.1	X-linked	65
p22^{phox*}	16q24	Autosomal recessive	7
p47^{phox*}	7q11.23	Autosomal recessive	23
p67^{phox*}	1q25	Autosomal recessive	5

Note: pHOx, phagocyte oxidase.

Clinical Features

1. Incidence: between 1/200,000 and 1/250,000 live births.
2. First symptoms may manifest in infancy or childhood.
3. Lymphadenopathy (nodes suppurative and drain pus) and hepatosplenomegaly.
4. Recurrent suppurative infections: pneumonitis, subcutaneous abscesses, impetiginous rashes, and osteomyelitis (often small bones of the hands and feet).
5. Urologic problems (e.g., granulomatous ureteral or urethral strictures, bladder granulomas, and urinary tract infections) in 38% of cases.
6. Gastrointestinal problems: colitis, enteritis, granulomatous obstruction of gastric outlet.
7. Hematologic features:
   a. Appropriate neutrophil leukocytosis.
   b. Anemia due to infection.
   c. McLeod syndrome (i.e., mild hemolytic anemia, acanthocytosis, decreased expression of Kell antigen due to defect in K$_x$ antigen on red cells); this occurs in rare patients with large deletions of Xp 21.1 gene.
   d. Hypergammaglobulinemia.
8. Noninfectious complications: noninfectious granulomata resulting in colitis, granulomatous cystitis, and urethritis, cutaneous granulomata, pericarditis,

and recurrent gastrointestinal strictures occur in patients with CGD as a result of a failure of phagocytes to clear both exogenous and endogenous debris.

Diagnosis

A nitroblue tetrazolium (NBT) dye test can be used to establish a diagnosis.

Treatment

1. The use of prophylactic antibiotics and antifungal agents:
   Antibacterial: trimethoprim/sulfamethoxazole (co-trimoxazole) Dose: 5 mg/kg/day, once a day orally based on trimethoprim component, or dicloxacillin for patients allergic to sulfa.
   Antifungal antibiotic: itraconazole: 3–5 mg/kg/day once a day orally.
2. The use of rhIFN-γ (interferon-γ) in a dose of 50 mcg/m² SC three times a week. Beneficial effect of interferon-γ is probably related to increased synthesis of nitric oxide (NO) through the NO synthase pathway. NO causes nitration of bacteria. Interferon-γ may also stimulate other nonoxidative microbicidal pathways. It also increases superoxide production in phagocytes. Interferon-γ as prophylaxis has been recommended only in patients with significant infections despite appropriate oral agents, or as an adjunct to the treatment of deep-seated infections. Oral antibiotic prophylaxis appears to be adequate in most of the patients.
3. Granulocyte transfusions to provide short-term relief at times of crisis.
4. Steroids should be used cautiously to treat granulomatous disease in the gastrointestinal or urinary tract.
5. Allogeneic stem cell transplantation is rarely used to treat CGD. It may be indicated in patients with severe disease. Trials are being conducted using a nonmyeloablative regimen. Identification of patients with poor outcome still remains unknown.

Prognosis

With the use of prophylactic antibiotics and recombinant human interferon-γ (rhIFN-γ) the prognosis of CGD has improved remarkably in the past two decades.

Myeloperoxidase Deficiency

Myeloperoxidase participates in the halogenation reaction in the neutrophils and is useful in killing bacteria phagocytosed by the neutrophils. This condition has the following characteristics:

1. Rare
2. Autosomal recessive inheritance
3. Less severe than chronic granulomatous disease
4. Normal NBT test and glucose metabolism
5. Abnormal iodination, cytochemical peroxidase staining, and bactericidal tests
6. Infections generally mild, but with more susceptibility for candida infections, which need to be treated aggressively.

Glutathione Synthetase Deficiency

1. Autosomal recessive
2. Relatively benign disorder

3. Intermittent neutropenia
4. Severe metabolic acidosis as a result of increased levels of 5-oxoproline, a metabolite formed during the biochemical steps of glutathione synthesis
5. Hemolysis induced by oxidant stress
6. Treatment:
    a. Correction of acidosis
    b. Use of vitamin E, 400 units per day, to treat hemolysis and infections
    c. Antibiotic therapy for infections
7. Respiratory burst is normal in neutrophils, and phagocytosis abnormal only in patients with severe deficiency of glutathione synthetase.

Glutathione Reductase Deficiency

1. Autosomal recessive
2. Accumulation of H_2O_2 in neutrophils
3. Hemolysis induced by oxidant stress
4. Frequency of infections not increased
5. Avoid use of oxidant foods and drugs.

Glucose-6-Phosphate Dehydrogenase Deficiency in Leukocytes

In some cases of Caucasian glucose-6-phosphate dehydrogenase (G6PD) deficiency, the enzyme is severely depressed (less than 5% of normal) in the neutrophil. As a result the conversion of NADP to NADPH is decreased, leading to decreased respiratory burst and abnormal NBT test. Persistent and eventually fatal bacterial infection occurs because of the inability of the leukocytes to generate H_2O_2. Clinical manifestations are similar to CGD. Hemolytic anemia may occur.

Treatment

1. Aggressive treatment of infections
2. Avoidance of oxidant drugs and foods
3. Red cell transfusions for anemia.

Neutrophil Production and Destruction in Newborn Infants

Neutrophil production: Using soluble Fc receptor III (sFcR III) as a surrogate marker for estimation of total neutrophil mass, it has been shown that newborn infants born before 32 weeks of gestation have 20% of the adult neutrophil mass. Normal levels of neutrophil mass are attained at 4 weeks of age in premature neonates. However, full-term neonates have neutrophil stores within the normal adult range.

Neutrophil Function in the Newborn

- *Chemotaxis:* Decreased in newborn infants. Normal chemotactic ability is attained at 2 weeks of age in term and preterm neonates.
- *Vascular rolling of neutrophils:* Also decreased due to decreased expression of L-selectin on the neutrophil cell membrane.
- *Vascular endothelial adhesion:* Also decreased due to decreased expression of β_2-integrin Mac-1 on the neutrophil cell membrane in neonates.
- *Dynamics of change of shape:* Newborn neutrophils are rigid because of impaired ability to form polymers of actin (P-actin) and reduced formation of microtubules.

- *Phagocytosis:* Neutrophils of term neonates have a normal ability for phagocytosis of gram-positive and gram-negative bacteria. However, their ability for phagocytosis of candida is abnormal up to 2 weeks of age. Preterm neonates have abnormal bacterial phagocytosis. However, when treated with therapeutic doses of intravenous gamma globulin G (IV IG) the neutrophils are able to ingest bacteria normally.
- *Respiratory burst:* Respiratory burst in term neonates is normal under normal conditions. In contrast, it is less active under the conditions of stress and sepsis. For this reason, neonates are more susceptible to overwhelming infections with group B streptococci, *Staphylococcus epidermis, S. aureus,* and *E. coli.* Respiratory burst performance of neutrophils in preterm neonates remains abnormal for more than 2 months of age. In term neonates, the generation of superoxide and hydrogen peroxide is increased, but because the levels of lactoferrin and myeloperoxidase are low, there is truncation of the later respiratory burst activity, resulting in abnormal bacterial killing.

Therapeutic Implications

G-CSF or GM-CSF may be helpful in term and preterm neonates during sepsis. The prophylactic use of G-CSF is more effective in preterm infants. The use of IVIgG to improve opsonization and phagocytosis has been disappointing.

Neonatal Preeclampsia-Associated Neutropenia

Neonatal preeclampsia-associated neutropenia occurs in low-birth-weight neonates with a maternal history of pregnancy-induced hypertension. Treatment includes the prophylactic use of G-CSF.

EOSINOPHILS

Table 9-12 lists the nonclonal (reactive) causes of eosinophilia, and Figure 9-2 shows the nonclonal (reactive) and clonal causes of eosinophilia.

Table 9-12. Nonclonal (Reactive) Causes of Eosinophilia

Allergic disorders
  Asthma, hay fever, urticaria, drug hypersensitivity
Immunologic disorders
  Omenn syndrome (severe combined immunodeficiency and eosinophilia)
Skin disorders
  Eczema, scabies, erythema toxicum, dermatitis herpetiformis, angioneurotic edema, pemphigus
Parasitic infestation
  Helminthic: *Ascaris lumbricoides,*[a] trichinosis, echinococcosis, visceral larva migrans,[a,b] hookworm,[a] strongyloidiasis,[a] filariasis[a]
  Protozoal: malaria, pneumocystis, toxoplasmosis
Hematologic disorders
  Hodgkin disease, postsplenectomy state, eosinophilic leukemoid reaction, congenital immune deficiency syndromes, Fanconi anemia, thrombocytopenia with absent radii, Kostmann disease, infectious mononucleosis, familial reticuloendotheliosis
Familial eosinophilia
Irradiation
Pulmonary eosinophilia
  Eosinophilic pneumonitis (Loeffler syndrome), pulmonary eosinophilia with asthma, tropical eosinophilia

(Continues)

Table 9-12. (*Continued*)

Gastrointestinal disorders
  Eosinophilic gastroenteritis, milk precipitin disease, ulcerative colitis, protein-losing
    enteropathy, regional enteritis, allergic granulomatosis
Miscellaneous
  Idiopathic hypereosinophilic syndrome,[b] periarteritis nodosa, metastatic neoplasm,
    cirrhosis, peritoneal dialysis, chronic renal disease, Goodpasture syndrome, sarcoidosis,
    thymic disorders, hypoxia
Idiopathic

[a]Helminth infestations associated with eosinophilia and pulmonary infiltrates.

[b]Conditions associated with striking eosinophilia. Leukocyte counts of 30,000–100,000/mm³ are characteristic, with 50–90% of leukocytes being eosinophils. In all other conditions, the white blood cell count is normal or only slightly elevated, and eosinophils make up 10–40% of the leukocyte count.

Eosinophilia

Normal mean eosinophil count in the circulating blood is $400/mm^3$. Normally, most of the eosinophils reside in the connective tissue located in the immediate proximity of the epithelial lining of the gut, respiratory tract, and urogenital tract. Their number and activation increase as a response to antigens, especially when these antigens are deposited in the above tissues. A response is characterized by an immediate hypersensitivity reaction, mediated by IgE or delayed hypersensitivity reaction, mediated by T lymphocytes.

Severity of eosinophilia is graded according to the presence of their absolute number in the circulating blood as follows:

Mild eosinophilia: $400–1500/mm^3$
Moderate eosinophilia: $1500–5000/mm^3$
Severe eosinophilia: greater than $5000/mm^3$.

Figure 9-3 illustrates mechanisms of eosinophil production, activation, and migration in the tissues. Following activation, the eosinophil expresses its effector function, which includes the release of highly toxic granule proteins and other mediators of inflammation.

Finally, eosinophils undergo apoptosis or necrosis and are ingested by professional macrophages. Engulfment of apoptotic eosinophils prevents spillage of the eosinophil tissue-toxic contents. It also results in release of anti-inflammatory cytokines such as transforming growth factor β, interleukin-10, and prostaglandin E2 by macrophages. In contrast to this, when eosinophils undergo necrosis, the tissue-toxic contents of eosinophils, such as major basic protein, lipids, cationic proteins, and neurotoxins, are released. Ingestion of necrotic eosinophils by macrophages results in release of proinflammatory cytokines, for example, thromboxane B_2 and GM-CSF.

For this reason, in treatment of eosinophilic diseases, the use of the drugs that induce eosinophil apoptosis (e.g., corticosteroids, cyclosporin, and theophylline) is desirable, rather than the drugs that induce eosinophil necrosis.

Figure 9-2 shows the causes of eosinophilia.

Idiopathic Hypereosinophilic Syndrome

Idiopathic hypereosinophilic syndrome (HES) includes a heterogeneous group of disorders defined by:

1. A persistent eosinophilia of $>1500/mm^3$ for longer than 6 months
2. Absence of evidence of known causes of eosinophilia despite a comprehensive workup for such causes

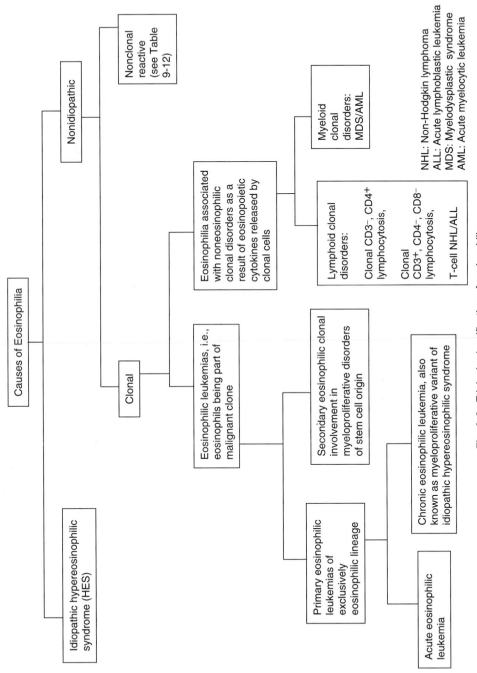

Fig. 9-2. Etiologic classification of eosinophilia.

Causes of Eosinophilia

Idiopathic hypereosinophilic syndrome (HES)

Nonidiopathic

Clonal

Nonclonal reactive (see Table 9-12)

Eosinophilic leukemias, i.e., eosinophils being part of malignant clone

Eosinophilia associated with noneosinophilic clonal disorders as a result of eosinopoietic cytokines released by clonal cells

Primary eosinophilic leukemias of exclusively eosinophilic lineage

Secondary eosinophilic clonal involvement in myeloproliferative disorders of stem cell origin

Lymphoid clonal disorders:

Clonal CD3$^-$, CD4$^+$ lymphocytosis,

Clonal CD3$^+$, CD4$^-$, CD8$^-$ lymphocytosis,

T-cell NHL/ALL

Myeloid clonal disorders: MDS/AML

Acute eosinophilic leukemia

Chronic eosinophilic leukemia, also known as myeloproliferative variant of idiopathic hypereosinophilic syndrome

NHL: Non-Hodgkin lymphoma
ALL: Acute lymphoblastic leukemia
MDS: Myelodysplastic syndrome
AML: Acute myelocytic leukemia

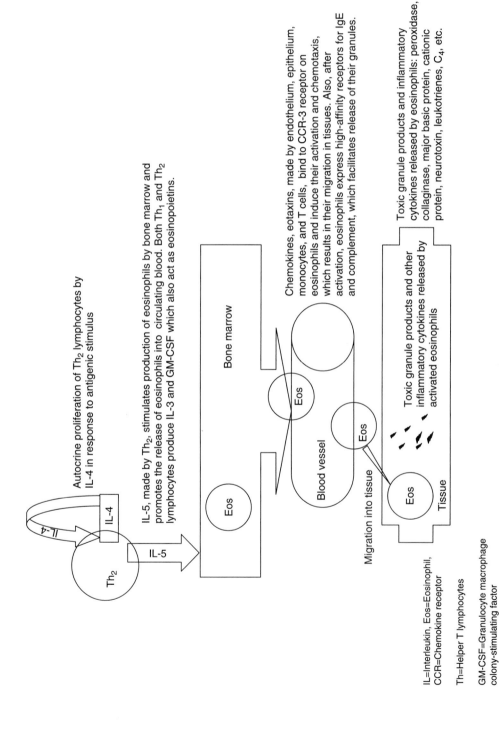

Autocrine proliferation of Th$_2$ lymphocytes by IL-4 in response to antigenic stimulus

IL-5, made by Th$_2$, stimulates production of eosinophils by bone marrow and promotes the release of eosinophils into circulating blood. Both Th$_1$ and Th$_2$ lymphocytes produce IL-3 and GM-CSF which also act as eosinopoietins.

Chemokines, eotaxins, made by endothelium, epithelium, monocytes, and T cells, bind to CCR-3 receptor on eosinophils and induce their activation and chemotaxis, which results in their migration in tissues. Also, after activation, eosinophils express high-affinity receptors for IgE and complement, which facilitates release of their granules.

Toxic granule products and inflammatory cytokines released by eosinophils: peroxidase, collaginase, major basic protein, cationic protein, neurotoxin, leukotrienes, C$_4$, etc.

Toxic granule products and other inflammatory cytokines released by activated eosinophils

Bone marrow

Blood vessel

Migration into tissue

Tissue

Eos

Th$_2$

IL-4

IL-5

IL=Interleukin, Eos=Eosinophil, CCR=Chemokine receptor

Th=Helper T lymphocytes

GM-CSF=Granulocyte macrophage colony-stimulating factor

Fig. 9-3. Mechanism of eosinophil production in bone marrow, release in circulation, and migration in tissue.

3. Signs and symptoms of organ involvement directly attributable to eosinophilia, including hepatomegaly, splenomegaly, heart disease, diffuse or focal central nervous system (CNS) abnormalities, pulmonary fibrosis, fever, weight loss, or anemia (i.e., evidence of end organ damage with histologic demonstration of tissue infiltration by eosinophils or objective evidence of clinical pathology in any organ system associated with eosinophilia and not clearly attributable to another cause).

Epidemiology

HES most commonly occurs between the ages of 20 and 40 years with a male to female ratio of 4:1. Clinical manifestations of HES in the pediatric age group are similar to HES in adult patients. In children HES may be associated with trisomy 8 or trisomy 21.

Clinical Presentation

The disease generally has a gradual onset. The chief complaints include anorexia, fatigue, weight loss, recurrent abdominal pain, fever, night sweats, persistent non-productive cough, chest pain, pruritus, skin rash, and congestive heart failure.

Organ Involvement

Cardiovascular Disease

HES-associated heart disease evolves through three stages:

1. Early acute phase, associated with degranulating eosinophils in the heart muscle (5–6 weeks into eosinophilia)
2. Subacute thrombotic stage (10 months into eosinophilia)
3. Chronic stage of fibrosis (24 months into eosinophilia). Cardiac disease involves both ventricles and can cause incompetence of mitral and tricuspid valves.

Coagulation System

Eosinophilia can cause a hypercoagulable state, the etiology of which is unclear. Eosinophil major basic proteins inactivate thrombomodulin, resulting in the unavailability of activated protein C. Intracardiac thrombus, deep-venous thrombosis, dural sinovenous thrombosis, and/or arterial thrombosis can occur.

Nervous System Complications

- Encephalopathy (altered behavior and cognitive function)
- Thrombotic strokes
- Peripheral neuropathies including mononeuritis multiplex, symmetrical sensorimotor neuropathy, and radiculopathy
- Retinal hemorrhages.

Gastrointestinal Complications

- Hepatomegaly due to eosinophilic infiltration of the liver results in liver function abnormalities.
- Enteropathy due to blunting of the villi and cellular infiltration in the lamina propria results in diarrhea and fat malabsorption.
- Eosinophilic infiltration of colon results in colitis.

Spleen

Splenomegaly with disruption of its architecture can occur.

Dermatologic Manifestations

The most common lesions include pruritic papules and nodules, urticarial plaques, and angioedema. Vesiculobullous lesions, generalized erythroderma, and aquagenic pruritus occur in some patients. Digital necrosis may result from vasculitis and microthrombi.

Pulmonary Complications

Nocturnal cough, fever, and diaphoresis can occur due to accumulation of eosinophils in the lungs. Pulmonary fibrosis can also occur.

Treatment

Table 9-13 lists the treatment of idiopathic HES.

Non-idiopathic Eosinophilia

Eosinophilia, for which a cause is ascertained, can be clonal or reactive.

Primary Clonal Eosinophilic Disorders

The primary clonal eosinophilic disorders include eosinophilic leukemias of exclusively eosinophilic lineage, for example, acute eosinophilic leukemia and chronic eosinophilic leukemia (also known as myeloproliferative variant of idiopathic hypereosinophilic syndrome). The following karyotypic abnormalities associated with chronic eosinophilic leukemia have been reported: The majority of patients have t (5 ; 12) (q33 : p 13). Sporadic patients have trisomy 8, i (17q), t (5 ;12) (q 31: q13), t (1; 5) (q 23: q 33), t (2; 5) (p 13: q 35), t (5; 9) (q 32: q33), t (5 ; 16) (q 33 : p 13), trisomy 10, 17q+, 15q–, –7,t (7; 12) (q11: p11), or t (4;16) (q11 or 12: p13).

HES with FIP1L1-PDGFRA fusion gene

A special variant of HES with a fusion gene *FIP1L1-PDGFRA* occurring as a result of interstitial deletion on chromosome 4q12 has recently been described. The fusion gene makes an activated tyrosine kinase, which results in a myeloproliferative variant of HES. It is characterized by increased levels of tryptase, increased atypical mast cells in bone marrow, and tissue fibrosis (myelofibrosis, endomyocardial fibrosis, pulmonary fibrosis). They respond well to imatinib mesylate treatment, which targets the fusion tyrosine kinase. Some patients with the *FIP1L1-PDGFRA* fusion gene may not have the classic characteristics of a myeloproliferative variant of HES and also respond well to imatinib. Some patients with HES may not have the *FIP1L1-PDGFRA* fusion gene and still respond to imatinib.

Secondary Clonal Eosinophilic Disorders

Secondary clonal involvement of eosinophil lineage can occur in myeloproliferative disorders of stem cell origin, for example, Ph¹-positive chronic myeloid leukemia. Eosinophilia is observed less commonly in polycythemia vera, myelofibrosis, and essential thrombocythemia.

Noneosinophilic Clonal Disorders

In noneosinophilic clonal disorders, clonal cells release eosinopoietic cytokines and, thus, are associated with eosinophilia. These noneosinophilic clonal disorders

Table 9-13. Treatment of Eosinophilia

Treatment of reactive or nonclonal eosinophilia: Treat the underlying cause, e.g., treatment of parasitic infections with appropriate antiparasitic drugs

Treatment of clonal disease: Myeloid clonal disease: Treat with appropriate chemotherapy ± hematopoietic stem cell transplantation.

Lymphoid malignancies: Treat with appropriate chemotherapy.

CD3–, CD4+ Lymphoid clonal disease with high levels of IL-5, usually associated with dermatologic manifestations: Treat with cyclosporine A, glucocorticoids or 2CDA.

CD3+, CD4–, CD8– Lymphoid clonal induced eosinophilia with high levels of IL-5 and usually associated with dermatologic manifestations: Treat with glucocorticoids, cyclosporine A.

Treatment of HES caused by interstitial deletion of 4q12 resulting in a fusion gene *FIP1L1-PDGFRA*: Imatinib mesylate, adult dose: 400 mg day. Pediatric dose: not established.

Treatment of idiopathic HES: Glucocorticoids, hydroxyurea, α-interferon, vincristine, thioguanine, or etoposide. Use these agents sequentially and if the response is unsatisfactory then treat with imatinib mesylate at doses of 100–200 mg/day (of interest is that patients with normal serum interleukin-5 values respond to imatinib, but not the ones with high values). During acute life-threatening presentation of HES, high-dose 10–20 mg/kg of Solu-Medrol (methylprednisolone) may be required but usually 1–2 mg/kg of prednisone may be sufficient.

Treatment with allogeneic hematopoietic stem cell transplantation is reserved for patients with HES refractory to above-mentioned therapies.

Treatment of patients with idiopathic HES but without organ involvement: None. Treatment is not necessary, but continuous periodic monitoring for organ involvement and emergence of clonality is warranted. Also, continue search for rare reactive causes of eosinophilia.

The following eosinophilic disorders with single-organ involvement may progress into HES:

Eosinophilic gastroenteritis

Gleich syndrome (episodic eosinophilia with angioedema)

Loeffler syndrome

Schulman syndrome (eosinophilic fascitis)

Well syndrome (eosinophilic cellulitis)

Parasitic infections with eosinophilia.

Note: Doses of some of the drugs: thioguanine, 40–60 mg/m^2/day orally. Vincristine, 1.5 mg/m^2/week IV. Etoposide, 60–100 mg/m^2/day for 3–5 days IV every 3–6 weeks. Hydroxyurea, 10–20 mg/kg/day orally. Cyclosporine 6 mg/kg/day orally (trough level, 100–200 µg/L). α-Interferon, 5×10^6 units/m^2/day SC or IM.

may be lymphoid or myeloid in their clonality. Lymphoid clonal disorders associated with eosinophilia include dermatologic patients with abnormal clones of T cells producing interleukin-5, patients with acute lymphoblastic leukemia, and T-lymphoblastic lymphoma. Myeloid clonal disorders associated with eosinophilia include myelodysplastic syndromes, acute myeloid leukemia with chromosome 16 abnormality, the 8p myeloproliferative syndrome, myelodysplastic syndromes, and systemic mastocytosis. The following cytogenetic abnormalities associated with acute myeloid leukemia with eosinophilia have been reported: inv (16) (p13: q22), t(16:16)(p 13: q22), t(5; 16) (q33:q22), and monosomy 7.

Reactive or nonclonal eosinophilic conditions are listed in Table 9-12.

Eosinophilia during the Newborn Period

A mild eosinophilia with eosinophil count greater than 700/mm^3 is observed in 75% of growing preterm infants. It is present in the second or third week of life and persists for several days or sometimes for weeks. Eosinophilia of prematurity is considered to be benign although it could be associated with a higher incidence of sepsis, especially with gram-negative bacteria.

A complete absence of eosinophils is observed in neonates who fare poorly and subsequently die.

Familial Eosinophilia

Familial eosinophilia is an autosomal dominant disorder. A genome-wide search showed evidence of linkage on chromosome 5q31-33 between markers D55642 and D55816. Some of the affected members are found to have high WBC counts, lower RBC counts, intermittent thrombocytopenia, cellular infiltration with mast cells in the liver and bone marrow, or involvement of the heart and nervous system. The levels of IL-3, IL-5, and GM-CSF are normal.

Figure 9-4 shows the diagnostic studies for evaluation of eosinophilia, and Table 9-13 lists the treatment of conditions that cause eosinophilia.

LYMPHOCYTES

Table 9-14 lists the causes of lymphocytosis and lymphopenia.

Acute Infectious Lymphocytosis

This disorder can be characterized by:

1. Discovery on routine blood count. It is caused by a Coxsackie virus.
2. Mild complaints: vomiting, diarrhea, upper respiratory tract infection, abdominal pain, slight or absent fever; symptoms of short duration.
3. No enlargement of liver, spleen, or lymph nodes.
4. Hematologic findings:
   a. WBC counts varying from 40,000 to 100,000/mm³
   b. Absolute increase in lymphocytes, with a lymphocyte predominance of more than 70%
   c. No anemia or thrombocytopenia.
5. No evidence of Epstein–Barr virus (EBV) infection.
6. Condition to be differentiated from acute leukemia, infectious mononucleosis, and lymphocytosis accompanying certain infections, particularly pertussis.
7. Prognosis excellent and no treatment required.

INFECTIOUS MONONUCLEOSIS

Infectious mononucleosis is an acute infectious disease caused by EBV. This common disease occurs in epidemic form in children of all ages but is rare in infants under 6 months of age. Infectious mononucleosis is usually a benign, self-limited disease; occasionally, it is associated with severe and fatal complications. Table 9-15 lists the frequency of various signs and symptoms of infectious mononucleosis, and Table 9-16 lists the laboratory and diagnostic findings.

Differential Diagnosis

Mononucleosis-like syndromes are common in infants and children and are generally due to EBV infection. The heterophil-negative EBV-negative mononucleosis-like syndrome is due to the following agents:

1. Cytomegalovirus
2. *Toxoplasma gondii*

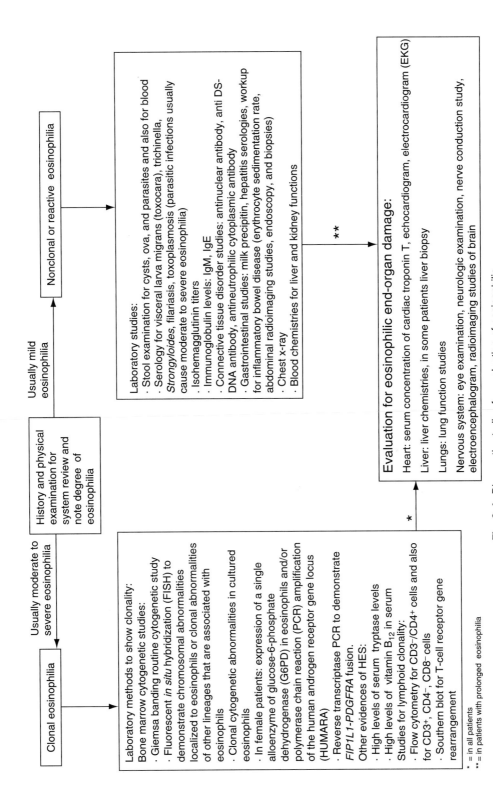

Fig. 9-4. Diagnostic studies for evaluation of eosinophilia.

243

Table 9-14. Causes of Lymphocytosis and Lymphopenia

I. Lymphocytosis
- A. Physiologic: 4 months–4 years
- B. Infections
  - 1. Acute
    - a. Moderate lymphocytosis: measles, rubella, varicella, mumps, roseola infantum, brucellosis, typhoid, paratyphoid, autoimmune diseases, granulomatous diseases, postimmunization states, drug reactions, graft rejection
    - b. Marked lymphocytosis: acute infectious lymphocytosis, infectious mononucleosis, cytomegalovirus infection, toxoplasmosis, pertussis
  - 2. Chronic
    Tuberculosis, syphilis
- C. Leukemia: acute lymphoblastic leukemia

II. Lymphopenia
Sex-linked agammaglobulinemia

III. Alymphocytosis
Swiss-type agammaglobulinemia

3. Drugs (para-aminosalicylic acid, Dilantin, sulfone)
4. Other agents (adenovirus, herpes simplex, rubella).

Leukemia and lymphomas must always be considered and can be excluded by a bone marrow examination, if sufficient doubt exists about the diagnosis. See Table 9-17 for a list of the causes of atypical lymphocytosis.

Table 9-15. Approximate Frequency of Various Signs and Symptoms in Infectious Mononucleosis

Symptom or sign	Percentage
Adenopathy[a]	100
Malaise and fatigue	90–100
Fever	89–95
Sweats	80–95
Sore throat, dysphagia	80–95
Pharyngitis[b]	65–85
Anorexia	50–80
Nausea	50–70
Splenomegaly	50–60
Headache	40–70
Chills	40–60
Bradycardia	35–50
Cough	30–50
Periorbital edema	25–40
Palatal enanthem	25–35
Liver or splenic tenderness	15–30
Myalgia	12–30
Hepatomegaly	15–25
Rhinitis	10–25
Ocular muscle pain	10–20
Chest pain	5–20
Jaundice	5–10
Arthralgia	5–10

(Continues)

Table 9-15. (*Continued*)

Symptom or sign	Percentage
Diarrhea or soft stools	5–10
Photophobia	5–10
Skin rash[c]	3–6
Conjunctivitis	<5
Abdominal pain	<5
Gingivitis	<3
Pneumonitis	<3
Epistaxis	<3

[a]Chiefly cervical (posterior cervical); commonly axillary, epitrochlear, and inguinal nodes, but any nodes may be involved. Rarely, mediastinal nodes are enlarged.

[b]Tonsils may be covered with membrane resembling diphtheria.

[c]Rash may be scarlatiniform, morbilliform, vesicular, maculopapular, and salmon colored. When ampicillin is given, rash occurs in 75–100% of patients.

Complications

Numerous and bizarre complications have been described in infectious mononucleosis, as listed in Table 9-18.

Treatment

1. Acetaminophen, in a dose of 10–15 mg/kg, is usually sufficient as an analgesic and antipyretic agent.
2. Corticosteroids are indicated in the following clinical situations:
   a. Severe pharyngitis with dysphagia and potential airway obstruction
   b. Acute and severe hemolytic anemia
   c. Severe life-threatening complications
   d. Rapidly progressive thrombocytopenic purpura
   e. Left upper quadrant abdominal pain with subcapsular splenic hemorrhage (not rupture).

Prednisone 1–2 mg/kg is typically given under these circumstances. Corticosteroids are not without harmful side effects and should be used only for the treatment of disabling disease; the course of corticosteroids should be short.

Table 9-16. Laboratory Findings in Infectious Mononucleosis

1. Increase in atypical lymphocytes (seen in other conditions; Table 9-17). 25% or more of leukocytes during second or third week are Downey type I, II, and III cells[a]
2. Leukocyte count usually elevated, but may be normal or low. Neutropenia, slight thrombocytopenia
3. EBV-specific antibodies. Acute or recent primary infection is indicated by the following:
   a. Presence of viral capsid antigen (VCA)-specific IgM antibodies
   b. High titers of VCA-specific IgG antibodies (1:320 or greater)
   c. Detection of anti–early antigen (EA) (1:10 or greater)
   d. Absence of anti-Epstein–Barr nuclear antigen (EBNA) (see Figure 9-5 for antibody responses during EBV-induced infectious mononucleosis)
4. Heterophile antibody test positive (4 or 5 days after onset)
   a. Sheep red cell agglutinins also develop during serum sickness, in other disease entities (infectious hepatitis, rubella, tuberculosis, leukemia, and Hodgkin disease), and in normal persons.

(Continues)

Table 9-16. (*Continued*)

b. In the latter conditions, the antibodies exist in a low titer and can be differentiated from those in infectious mononucleosis by absorption tests with guinea pig kidney and beef red cells as follows:

	Titer after absorption	
	Guinea pig kidney	Beef red cells
Infectious mononucleosis	Present	Absent
Normal serum	Absent	Present
Serum sickness	Absent	Present

5. Monospot test
   a. 96–99% reliable in older children and adults; however, detects disease in only less than 50% of children under 4 years of age
   b. Can detect heterophile titers as low as 1:56
6. Evidence of hepatic dysfunction in 75% of cases
7. Occasionally false-positive Venereal Disease Research Laboratory (VDRL), antinuclear antibody (ANA), and febrile agglutination reactions
8. Abnormalities of immune system

*These cells vary markedly in size and shape and are T lymphocytes. The cytoplasm is vacuolated, with a foamy appearance, and the periphery of the cytoplasm is characteristically indented and deformed by the surrounding erythrocytes. The nucleus is round, bean shaped, or lobulated, with no nucleolus (Downey type I monocytoid cells). Some lymphocytes have deep blue-staining cytoplasm and nuclei that appear immature (Downey type II plasmacytoid cells); some may have nucleoli (Downey type III blastoid cells).

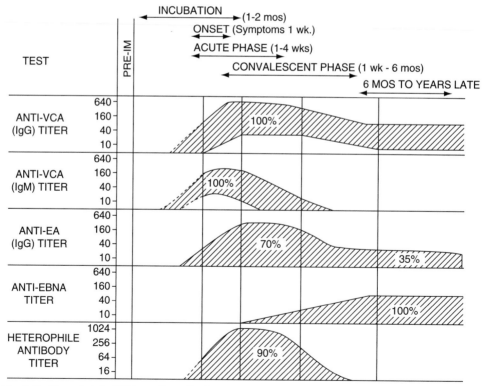

Fig. 9-5. Characteristic EBV-specific antibody responses during EBV-induced infectious mononucleosis. (Adapted from Henle G, Henle W, Horowitz CA. Epstein–Barr virus specific diagnostic tests in infectious mononucleosis. Hum Pathol 1974;5:551, with permission.)

Table 9-17. Causes of Atypical Lymphocytosis

I. Less than 20%
 A. Infections
  1. Bacterial: brucellosis, tuberculosis
  2. Viral: mumps, varicella, rubeola, rubella, atypical pneumonia, herpes simplex, herpes zoster, roseola infantum
  3. Protozoal: toxoplasmosis
  4. Rickettsial: rickettsialpox
  5. Spirochetal: congenital syphilis, tertiary syphilis
 B. Radiation
 C. Miscellaneous
  1. Hematologic: Langerhans cell histiocytosis, leukemia, lymphoma, agranulocytosis
  2. Other: lead intoxication, stress

II. More than 20%
 A. Infectious mononucleosis
 B. Infectious hepatitis
 C. Post-transfusion syndrome
 D. Cytomegalovirus syndrome
 E. Drug hypersensitivity: *p*-aminosalicylic acid (PAS), phenytoin (Dilantin), mephenytoin (Mesantoin), organic arsenicals

Table 9-18. Complications of Infectious Mononucleosis

Neurologic[a]: Bell palsy, cerebellar syndrome, meningoencephalitis, Guillain–Barré syndrome, myelitis, peripheral neuritis, radiculoneuritis, convulsions, coma
Cardiac: myocarditis, pericarditis
Respiratory: laryngeal obstruction, peritonsillar abscess, respiratory obstruction, pleural effusion, pneumonitis
Hematologic: acquired hemolytic anemia (usually Coombs' positive), immunopathic thrombocytopenic purpura, neutropenia, pancytopenia, aplastic anemia, eosinophilia, splenic rupture
Oncologic: nasopharyngeal carcinoma, Burkitt lymphoma, Hodgkin disease, lymphoproliferative disease, nasal T cell/natural killer cell lymphoma, lymphomatoid granulomatosis, angioimmunoblastic lymphadenopathy, central nervous system lymphoma in immunocompromised host, smooth muscle tumors in transplant patients, gastric carcinoma, peripheral T cell lymphoma with virus-associated hemophagocytic syndrome (see Chapter 13)
In HIV patients with AIDS: oral hairy leukoplakia, lymphoid interstitial pneumonitis, non-Hodgkin lymphoma
Renal: nephritis, nephrotic syndrome, hematuria, hemoglobinuria, proteinuria
Hepatic: jaundice, hepatic dysfunction, hepatic necrosis, Reye syndrome
Gastrointestinal: protein-losing enteropathy, melena, pancreatitis
Genitourinary: orchitis, azoospermia, endocervicitis
Ocular: eyelid edema, conjunctivitis, papilledema, uveitis, nystagmus, diplopia, retro-orbital pain, scotomata

[a]May precede, follow, or occur simultaneously with acute phase of disease. Brain, meninges, spinal cord, and cranial and peripheral nerves may be involved separately or in combination, producing bizarre neurologic signs and symptoms.

CHRONIC INFECTIOUS MONONUCLEOSIS

This term is used for patients who have the following clinical syndrome:

1. Chronic and relapsing illness and fatigue, myalgia, adenopathy, hepatospleno-megaly, mild pharyngitis, and intermittent fever
2. Absence of known predisposing cause or chronic illness

3. Anemia, neutropenia, lymphocytopenia, or lymphocytosis, thrombocytopenia, polyclonal hypergammaglobulinemia may be present.

To diagnose this condition, the following criteria must be met and the symptoms must be present for more than 1 year:

1. Elevated IgG antibody titers to viral capsid antigen (VCA) greater than 5120, VCA IgA positive. Early antigen diffuse (EAD) IgG greater than 640, EAD IgA positive. Early antigen restricted (EAR) IgG greater than 640 or detection of genomes in affected tissues, EBNA1 low or negative—an indicator of recent EBV infection
2. Detection of EBV genome in affected tissues.
3. Oligoclonal or monoclonal EBV-infected lymphocyte population may be of T- or B-cell lineage. Occasionally, there may be hemophagocytic lymphohistiocytosis (HLH).

Therapy

Symptomatic patients with active EBV infection are treated. Treatments are similar to those used for EVB-virus infected immunodeficient patients:

1. Antiviral drugs: acyclovir, ganciclovir, adenosine arabinoside
2. Intravenous immunoglobulin
3. Chemotherapy: etoposide, dexamethasone for patients with EBV associated hemophagocytic syndrome.
4. Anti-CD20 (Rituximab) antibody infusion in patients with B-cell proliferation.

SUGGESTED READINGS

Bernini, JC. Diagnosis and management of chronic neutropenia during childhood. Pediatr Clin North Am 1996;43:773–86.

Brito-Babapulle, F. The eosinophilias, including the idiopathic hypereosinophilic syndrome. Br J Haematol 2003;121:203–23.

Bux J, Mueller-Eckhardt C. Autoimmune neutropenia. Semin Hematol 1992;29:45–53.

Boxer L, Dale DC. Neutropenia: causes and consequences. Semin Hematol 2002; 39: 75–81.

Carr, R. Neutrophil production and function in newborn infants. Br J Haematol 2000;110:18–28.

Cartron J, Tchernia G, Cleton J, Damay M, Cheron G, Farrokhi P, Badoual J. Alloimmune neonatal neutropenia. Am J Pediatr Hematol Oncol 1991;13:21–25.

Cottle TE, Fier CJ, Donadieu J, Kinsey SE. Risk and benefit of treatment of severe neutropenia with granulocyte colony-stimulating factor. Semin Hematol 2002; 39: 134–140.

Dale, DC. Guest editor. Severe Chronic Neutropenia, Seminars in Hematology, 2002; 29, 73–133. Philadelphia: WB Saunders.

Dinauer, MC. The phagocyte system and disorders of granulopoiesis and granulocyte function. In: Nathan DG, Orkin SH, Ginsburg D, Look AT, editors. Hematology of Infancy and Childhood. 6th ed. Philadelphia: WB Saunders, 2003.

Horwitz M, Li F, et al. Leukemia in severe congenital neutropenia: Defective proteolysis suggests new pathways to malignancy and opportunities for therapy. Cancer Investigation 2003;21:579–87.

Jonsson OG, Buchanan GR. Chronic neutropenia during childhood: A 13-year experience in a single institution. Am J Dis Child 1991;145:232–5.

Karlsson S. Treatment of genetic defects in hematopoietic cell function by gene transfer. Blood 1991;78:2481–92.

Klion AO, Robyn J, et al. Molecular remission and reversal of myelofibrosis in response to imatinib mesylate treatment in patients with the myeloproliferative variant of hypereosinophilic syndrome. Blood 2004;103:473–76.

Lalezari P, Khorshidi M, Petrosova M. Autoimmune neutropenia of infancy. J Pediatr 1986;109:764.

Shastri KA, Logue GL. Autoimmune neutropenia. Blood 1993;81:1984–95.

Sullivan JL. Hematologic consequences of Epstein–Barr virus infection. Hematol Oncol Clin North Am 1987;1:397.

Vlachos A, Lipton JM. Hematopoietic stem cell transplantation for inherited bone marrow failure syndromes. In: Mehta P, editor. Pediatric Stem Cell Transplantation. Boston: Jones and Bartlett Publishers, 2004.

Yang K, Hill H. Neutrophil function disorders: pathophysiology, prevention, and therapy. J Pediatr 1991;119:343–54.

10

DISORDERS OF PLATELETS

Platelets are an important component in the first phase of hemostasis—platelet plug formation (Chapter 11). When platelets are reduced in number or defective in function, bleeding may occur. Table 10-1 lists the causes of thrombocytopenia based on platelet size, and Table 10-2 lists the causes of thrombocytopenia according to pathophysiology. Bleeding due to platelet disorders typically involves skin and mucous membranes, including petechiae, purpura, ecchymosis, epistaxis, hematuria, menorrhagia, and gastrointestinal hemorrhage. Intracranial hemorrhage rarely occurs.

The characteristics of platelets are as follows:

- *Size:* 1–4 µm (younger platelets are larger)
- *Mean platelet volume (MPV):* 8.9 ± 1.5 µm^3
- *Number:* 150,000–400,000/mm^3
- *Distribution:* one third in the spleen; two thirds in the bloodstream
- *Life span:* 7–10 days.

IMMUNE THROMBOCYTOPENIA

The most frequent cause of thrombocytopenia is immune-mediated platelet destruction due to autoantibodies, drug-dependent antibodies, or alloantibodies.

Immune (Idiopathic) Thrombocytopenic Purpura

Immune thrombocytopenic purpura (ITP) is a syndrome characterized by:

1. Thrombocytopenia (platelet count less than 100,000/mm^3)
2. Shortened platelet survival
3. Presence of antiplatelet antibody in the plasma
4. Increased megakaryocytes in the bone marrow.

This condition may be acute, chronic, or recurrent. In the *acute form,* the platelet count returns to normal (>150,000/mm^3) within 6 months after diagnosis, and relapse does not occur. In the *chronic form,* the platelet count remains low beyond 6 months. In the *recurrent form,* the platelet count decreases after having returned to normal levels. In adults, the chronic form is more common, whereas in children, the acute form is more common. The clinical features of acute and chronic ITP are listed in Table 10-3.

Table 10-1. Platelet Diseases Based on Platelet Size

Macrothrombocytes (MPV raised)
ITP or any condition with increased platelet turnover (e.g., DIC)
Bernard–Soulier syndrome
May Hegglin anomaly and other MYH-9–related diseases (Table 10-14)
Swiss cheese platelet syndrome
Montreal platelet syndrome
Gray platelet syndrome
Various mucopolysaccharidoses

Normal size (MPV normal)
Conditions in which marrow is hypocellular or infiltrated with malignant disease

Microthrombocytes (MPV decreased)
Wiskott–Aldrich syndrome
TAR syndrome
Some storage pool diseases
Iron-deficiency anemia

Abbreviations: MPV, mean platelet volume (as determined by automated electronic counters); normal, 8.9 ± 1.5 μm^3; ITP, idiopathic thrombocytopenic purpura; DIC, disseminated intravascular coagulation; MYH-9, non-muscle myosin heavy chain 9 gene; TAR, thrombocytopenic absent radii.

Table 10-2. Pathophysiological Classification of Thrombocytopenic States

I. **Increased platelet destruction** (normal or increased megakaryocytes in the marrow—megakaryocytic thrombocytopenia)
   A. Immune thrombocytopenias
      1. Idiopathic
         a. Immune (idiopathic) thrombocytopenic purpura
      2. Secondary
         a. Infection induced (e.g., viral—HIV, CMV, EBV, varicella, rubella, rubeola, mumps, measles, pertussis, hepatitis, parvovirus B19; bacterial—tuberculosis, typhoid)
         b. Drug induced (see Table 10-4)
         c. Post-transfusion purpura
         d. Autoimmune hemolytic anemia (Evans syndrome)
         e. Systemic lupus erythematosus
         f. Hyperthyroidism
         g. Lymphoproliferative disorders
      3. Neonatal immune thrombocytopenias
         a. Neonatal autoimmune thrombocytopenia
         b. Neonatal alloimmune thrombocytopenia
         c. Erythroblastosis fetalis–Rh incompatibility
   B. Nonimmune thrombocytopenias
      1. Due to platelet consumption
         a. Microangiopathic hemolytic anemia: HUS, TTP, HSCT-associated microangiopathy
         b. Disseminated intravascular coagulation
         c. Virus-associated hemophagocytic syndrome
         d. Kasabach–Merritt syndrome (giant hemangioma)
         e. Cyanotic heart disease
      2. Due to platelet destruction
         a. Drugs (e.g., ristocetin, protamine sulfate, bleomycin)
         b. Infections

(Continues)

Table 10-2. (*Continued*)

    c. Cardiac (e.g., prosthetic heart valves, repair of intracardiac defects, left ventricular outflow obstruction)

    d. Malignant hypertension

II. Disorders of platelet distribution or pooling

    A. Hypersplenism (e.g., portal hypertension, Gaucher disease, cyanotic congenital heart disease, neoplasm, infection)

    B. Hypothermia

III. Decreased platelet production—deficient thrombopoiesis (decreased or absent megakaryocytes in the marrow—amegakaryocytic thrombocytopenia)

    A. Hypoplasia or suppression of megakaryocytes[a]

       1. Drugs (e.g., chlorothiazides, estrogenic hormones, ethanol, tolbutamide)

       2. Constitutional

         a. Thrombocytopenia absent radii—TAR syndrome

         b. Congenital amegakaryocytic thrombocytopenia

         c. Amegakaryocytic thrombocytopenia with radio-ulnar synostosis

         d. Thrombocytopenia agenesis of corpus callosum syndrome

         e. Paris-Trousseau syndrome

         f. Rubella syndrome

         g. Trisomy 13, 18

       3. Ineffective thrombopoiesis

         a. Megaloblastic anemias (folate and vitamin B_{12} deficiencies)

         b. Severe iron-deficiency anemia

         c. Certain familial thrombocytopenias

         d. Paroxysmal nocturnal hemoglobinuria

       4. Disorders of control mechanism

         a. Thrombopoietin deficiency

         b. Tidal platelet dysgenesis

         c. Cyclic thrombocytopenias

       5. Metabolic disorders

         a. Methylmalonic acidemia

         b. Ketotic glycinemia

         c. Holocarboxylase synthetase deficiency

         d. Isovaleric acidemia

         e. Idiopathic hyperglycinemia

         f. Infants born to hypothyroid mothers

       6. Hereditary platelet disorders[b]

         a. Bernard–Soulier syndrome

         b. May Hegglin anomaly and other MYH-9 gene–related disorders (Table 10-14)

         c. Wiskott–Aldrich syndrome

         d. Pure sex-linked thrombocytopenia

         e. Mediterranean thrombocytopenia

       7. Acquired aplastic disorders

         a. Idiopathic

         b. Drug induced (e.g., dose related: antineoplastic agents; benzene, organic and inorganic arsenicals, Mesantoin, Tridione, antithyroids, antidiabetics, antihistamines, phenylbutazone, insecticides, gold compounds; idiosyncrasy: chloramphenicol)

         c. Radiation induced

         d. Viral infections (e.g., hepatitis, HIV, EBV)

    B. Marrow infiltrative processes

       1. Benign

         a. Osteopetrosis

         b. Storage diseases

(Continues)

Table 10-2. (*Continued*)

2. Malignant
   a. *De novo*—leukemias, myelofibrosis, Langerhans cell histiocytosis, histiocytic medullary reticulosis
   b. Secondary—lymphomas, neuroblastoma, other solid tumor metastases

IV. Pseudothrombocytopenia
   A. Platelet activation during blood collection
   B. Undercounting of megathrombocytes
   C. *In vitro* agglutination of platelets due to EDTA
   D. Monoclonal antibodies that bind to platelet glycoprotein receptors such as abciximab, eptifibatide, tirofiban

[a]A bone marrow biopsy, in addition to marrow aspiration, should always be carried out to avoid sampling errors and to establish the presence of a decreased number of megakaryocytes in the marrow.

[b]These conditions are associated with normal or increased bone marrow megakaryocytes.

Abbreviations: HUS: hemolytic-uremic syndrome, TTP: thrombotic thrombocytopenic purpura, HSCT: hematopoietic stem cell transplant.

Table 10-3. Features of Acute and Chronic ITP

Feature	Acute	Chronic
Age	Children 2–6 years of age	Adults
Sex distribution	Equal	Female/male 3:1
Seasonal predilection	Springtime	None
Preceding infection	~80%	Unusual
Associated autoimmune conditions (e.g., SLE)	Uncommon	More common
Onset	Acute	Insidious
Platelet count	<20,000/mm^3	40,000–80,000/mm^3
Eosinophilia and lymphocytosis	Common	Rare
IgA levels	Normal	Lower than normal
Duration	Usually 2–6 weeks	Months to years
Prognosis	Spontaneous remission in 80% of cases	Fluctuating chronic course

Incidence

The true incidence of ITP is unknown because the disease is often transient. The estimated incidence is about 1 in 10,000 children per year.

Pathogenesis

Figure 10-1 shows the possible pathophysiology of immune thrombocytopenia.

Platelet Antibodies

ITP is caused by autoantibodies against platelet membrane glycoproteins such as GP IIb/IIIa, GP Ib/IX, GP Ia/IIa, GP V, and GP IV. These antibodies are detected by the antigen capture method either on the platelets or in the plasma of patients with ITP. However, even with newly developed techniques, 20% of ITP patients do not have any detectable antibodies. Therefore, ITP is still a clinical diagnosis and platelet antibody tests remain unreliable to confirm or exclude the diagnosis.

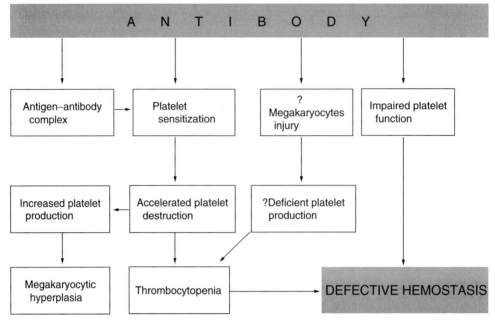

Fig. 10-1. Possible pathophysiology of immune thrombocytopenia.

Platelet Survival

Platelet survival is greatly shortened. Chromium-51 (^{51}Cr) labeled platelets have a life span of a few minutes to 1–4 hours.

Clinical Features

1. *Age:* The greatest frequency of occurrence is between ages 2 and 8 years. Infants less than 2 years old (infantile ITP) have the following clinical features:
   a. Higher male/female ratio
   b. Less frequent occurrence of infection before ITP
   c. Less frequent occurrence of chronic ITP
   d. Poor response to treatment
   e. More severe clinical course.
2. *Sex:* Both sexes are equally affected.
3. *Predisposing factors:* A history of preceding infection, usually viral, is noted within the preceding 3 weeks in 50–80% of cases. Nonspecific upper respiratory infections are the most common cause in postinfectious cases. In about 20% of cases, a specific infection can be identified, such as rubella, measles, varicella, pertussis, mumps, infectious mononucleosis, cytomegalovirus, hepatitis A, B, C, parvovirus or bacterial infection. ITP may also be due to smallpox or live measles vaccination.

Symptoms

Petechiae, purpura, ecchymoses, and mucous membrane bleeding are the symptoms associated with ITP. Figure 10-2 outlines a clinical approach based on platelet count and bleeding time.

Skin

Ecchymoses or purpura are usually found on the anterior surface of the lower extremities and over bony prominences, such as the ribs, scapula, shoulders, legs,

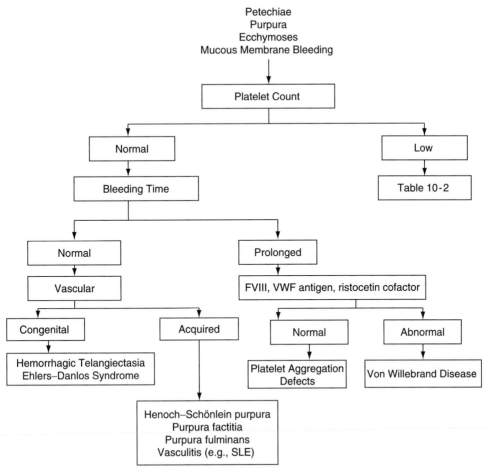

Fig. 10-2. Clinical approach to petechiae, purpura, and mucous membrane bleeding based on platelet count and bleeding time. A few patients with Ehlers-Danlos syndrome have prolonged bleeding time and abnormal platelet aggregation.

and pubic area. Symptoms are mild in 50% of cases, with few bruises on the legs or trunk.

Mucous Membranes

Petechiae may be found in the subconjunctival, buccal mucosa, soft palate, and skin. Bleeding from the nose, gums, mucous membranes, gastrointestinal tract, or kidneys is not uncommon, especially at the onset of disease. Menorrhagia may occur and may be severe. Hematemesis and melena are infrequent.

Internal Organs

Bleeding may occur into the following organs:

1. Central nervous system: a serious complication, usually preceded by headache and dizziness and acute bleeding manifestations elsewhere
2. Retinal hemorrhage
3. Middle ear: uncommon; leads to hearing impairment
4. Deep muscle hematomata and hemarthrosis: rare; characteristic of plasma coagulation factor disorders; seen after intramuscular injection or significant trauma.

Signs

With the exception of hemorrhagic manifestations, the physical examination is not significant. Pallor is usually absent unless there has been significant bleeding. The tip of the spleen is palpable in fewer than 10% of patients. The finding of splenomegaly suggests the probability of leukemia, systemic lupus erythematosus (SLE), infectious mononucleosis, or hypersplenism. Cervical lymphadenopathy is not present unless the precipitating factor is a viral illness.

Laboratory Findings

1. *Platelet count:*
   a. Always less than 150,000/mm^3.
   b. Often less than 20,000/mm^3 in patients with severe generalized hemorrhagic manifestations.
   c. MPV increased (on automated counting equipment); normal MPV, 8.9±1.5 μm^3. (Table 10-1 lists the platelet diseases according to platelet size.)
2. *Blood smear:* Thrombocytopenia determined by automated analyzer must be confirmed by an examination of the peripheral smear to exclude the diagnosis of pseudothrombocytopenia, presence of megathrombocytes, and other hematologic conditions.
   a. Blood smear normal, apart from thrombocytopenia (if active infection, increased neutrophils, lymphocytes, or atypical mononuclear cells may be present).
   b. Anemia present only in proportion to amount of blood loss.
3. *Bone marrow:*
   a. Increased megakaryocytes, often immature and with absence of budding
   b. Normal erythroid and myeloid cells
   c. Increased eosinophils occasionally seen
   d. Erythroid hyperplasia if significant blood loss.
   (Marrow findings are diagnostic of ITP *only* when consistent with the clinical state and presence of a low platelet count and when other causes of secondary thrombocytopenia are excluded. The main purpose of performing a bone marrow examination is to exclude other hematologic disorders, e.g., leukemia.)
4. *Coagulation profile:*
   a. Bleeding time—usually abnormal
   b. Prothrombin time (PT), activated partial thromboplastin time (APTT), and fibrinogen level—normal.

Investigations in Patients with Purpura

- Complete blood count (CBC), including blood smear (careful examination of red cell and white cell morphology) and platelet count.
- Bone marrow aspiration (BMA): BMA is not necessary in a clinically and hematologically typical case of ITP. It is very unlikely (<0.1%) for acute leukemia to present with isolated thrombocytopenia and an otherwise normal CBC. Therefore, if the presentation is typical for ITP, the CBC is normal other than thrombocytopenia (including the white and red cell morphology), and there is no hepatosplenomegaly or lymphadenopathy, bone marrow examination is not required, irrespective of therapy. If the patient has atypical features, or is not responding to therapy, a bone marrow examination should be performed.
- Antinuclear antibody (ANA), and anti-ds-DNA as clinically indicated.
- Blood type, Coombs' test as clinically indicated.

- PT, APTT, fibrinogen level, and split products of fibrinogen (SPF) as clinically indicated.
- Liver function tests with blood urea nitrogen (BUN) and creatinine as clinically indicated.
- Monospot test and/or Epstein–Barr virus (EBV), human immunodeficiency virus (HIV), parvovirus titers as clinically indicated.
- Exclusion of secondary causes of thrombocytopenia.

Diagnosis

Criteria for the diagnosis are as follows:

1. *Clinical examination:* purpura with an otherwise essentially normal physical examination, with no significant splenomegaly and no lymphadenopathy
2. *Platelet count and blood smears:* thrombocytopenia only, with no evidence of red cell or white blood cell abnormalities
3. *Bone marrow:* normal to increased number of megakaryocytes with normal myeloid and erythroid elements
4. Exclusion of secondary causes of thrombocytopenia, such as hypersplenism, microangiopathic hemolytic anemia, disseminated intravascular coagulation (DIC), drug-induced thrombocytopenia (Table 10-4), SLE, infections such as EBV, HIV, and parvovirus.

Table 10-4. Drugs Proved or Suspected to Induce Drug-Dependent Antibody-Mediated Immune Thrombocytopenia

Anti-inflammatory
  Acetaminophen
  Acetylsalicylic acid
  Diclofenac
  Ibuprofen
  Indomethacin
  Meclofenamate
  Mefenamic acid
  Naproxen
  Oxyphenbutazone
  Phenylbutazone
  Piroxicam
  Sodium-p-amino salicylic acid
  Sulfasalzine
  Sulindac
  Tolmetin

Antibiotics
  Antituberculous drugs
    Ethambutol
    Isoniazid
    Para-aminosalicylic acid (PAS)
    Rifampin
    Streptomycin
  Penicillin group
    Ampicillin
    Methicillin
    Penicillin
    Mezlocillin
    Piperacillin

Cephalosporin
  Cefamandole
  Cefotetan
  Ceftazidime
  Cephalothin
Sulfonamides
  Sulfamethoxazole
  Sulfamethoxypyridazine
  Sulfisoxazole
Other antibiotics
  Amphotericin B
  Ciprofloxacin
  Clarithromycin
  Fluconazole
  Gentamicin
  Indinavir
  Nalidixic acid
  Novobiocin
  Pentamidine
  Sodium Stibogluconate
  Stibophen
  Suramin
  Vancomycin

Antineoplastic
  Actinomycin-D
  Aminoglutethimide
  Tamoxifen

(Continues)

Table 10-4. (*Continued*)

Anticonvulsants, sedatives, and antidepressants	H2-antagonists
Amitriptyline	Cimetidine
Carbamazepine	Ranitidine
Desipramine	**Cinchona alkaloids**
Diazepam	Quinidine
Doxepin	Quinine
Haloperidol	**Miscellaneous**
Imipramine	Antazoline
Lithium	Chlorpheniramine
Mianserin	Chlorpropamide
Phenytoin	Danazol
Valproic acid	Desferrioxamine
	Diethylstilbestrol
Cardiac and antihypertensive drugs	Etretinate
Acetazolamide	Glibenclamide
Amiodarone	Gold salts
Alprenolol	Heparin
Captopril	Interferon-α
Chlorothiazide	Iodinated contrast agents
Chlorthalidone	Isotretinoin
Digoxin	Minoxidil
Digitoxin	Levamisole
Furosemide	Lidocaine
Hydrochlorothiazide	Morphine
α-methyldopa	Papaverine
Oxprenolol	Ticlopidine
Procainamide	**Foods**
Spironolactone	Beans

Intracranial Hemorrhage in ITP

Table 10-5 lists the clinical manifestations of intracranial hemorrhage (ICH) in ITP.

Treatment

No treatment is required when the platelet count is greater than 20,000/mm^3 and the patient is asymptomatic or has mild bruising but no evidence of mucous membrane bleeding. Competitive contact sports should be avoided. Depo-Provera or any other long-acting progesterone is useful in suspending menstruation for several months, to prevent excessive menorrhagia in menstruating females. Aspirin, nonsteroidal anti-inflammatory agents, and any other drugs that interfere with platelet function should not be given.

Treatment is indicated for children with platelet counts less than 20,000/mm^3 and significant mucous membrane bleeding, and those with platelet counts less than 10,000/mm^3 and minor purpura. The treatment choices are steroids, IVIG, or anti-D. Their mechanisms of action are listed on Table 10-6.

Steroid Therapy

1. Rationale:
   a. Inhibits phagocytosis of antibody-coated platelets in the spleen and prolongs platelet survival.

Table 10-5. Clinical Manifestations of Intracranial Hemorrhage (ICH) in ITP

Incidence:	0.1–0.5%
Age:	13 months–16 years
Platelet count:	<10,000/mm³ in 73% of cases; 10–20,000/mm³ in 25% of cases; >20,000/mm³ in 2% of cases
Interval between diagnosis of ITP and ICH:	<4 weeks (51% of cases) 4 weeks–9 years (49% of cases) Mean 27 weeks

Presence of identifiable risk factors in 45% of cases of ICH include:
- Head injuries (29%)
- Aspirin treatment (5%)
- AV malformation (17%)
- Mucocutaneous hemorrhage (49%)

Site of ICH
- Intracerebral (77% of cases)—87% supratentorial; 13% posterior fossa
- Subdural hematoma (23% of cases)

Prior treatment
- 50% had prior treatment with steroids and/or IVIG

Survival
- 54% survive—most without permanent damage

Table 10-6. Mechanism of Action of Corticosteroids, IVGG, and Anti-D

Effect	Corticosteroids	IVGG	Anti-D
Improving capillary resistance	+	−	−
Reticuloendothelial blockade	±	+	+
Platelet antibody binding	+	±	−
Altered Fc R binding	+	+	±
T-cell suppression	+	+	−
Immunoglobulin synthesis	D	D	N/D
Cytokine production	D	D	N

Abbreviations: D, decreased; N, normal.

b. Improves capillary resistance and thereby improves platelet economy.
c. Inhibits platelet antibody production.
2. Dose and duration:
a. A course of prednisone, 2 mg/kg/day (maximum 60 mg/day), is given in divided doses. Prednisone is reduced in a stepwise fashion at 5- to 7-day intervals, irrespective of the platelet count, and is stopped at the end of 21–28 days, regardless of the response. A shorter course of prednisone at 4 mg/kg/day for 4 days has also been used with success.
b. In severe cases, methylprednisolone (Solu-Medrol) 30 mg/kg/day (500 mg/m²/day; maximum 1 g/day) for 3 days produces a more rapid response than steroids in conventional doses.
c. Prolonged use of steroids in ITP is undesirable. Large doses or prolonged steroid usage may perpetuate the thrombocytopenia and depress platelet production. It also leads to side effects including weight gain, cushingoid facies, fluid retention, acne, hyperglycemia, hypertension, mood swings, pseudotumor cerebri, cataracts, growth retardation, and avascular necrosis.

High-Dose Intravenous Gammaglobulin

1. Mechanisms of action for high-dose intravenous gammaglobulin (IVGG) include:
   a. Reticuloendothelial Fc-receptor blockade
   b. Activation of inhibitory pathways
   c. Decrease in autoantibody synthesis.
2. Indications in acute ITP:
   a. Neonatal symptomatic immune thrombocytopenia and infants less than 2 years of age who are generally more refractory to steroid treatment
   b. Alternative therapy to corticosteroid therapy but is much more expensive, has significant side effects, is not significantly clinically better than steroid therapy to justify expense and side effects of its use.
3. Dosage:
   a. Acute ITP: a total dose of 2 g/kg body weight given as follows:
      (1) 0.4 g/kg IVGG per day for 5 days OR
      (2) 1 g/kg per day for 2 days.
          Lower doses of 800 mg/kg/day as a single dose or 250 mg/kg/day for 2 days have been used with success.
   b. Chronic ITP:
      (1) Initial IVGG dose of 1 g/kg body weight daily for 2 days, followed by periodic single infusions (0.4–1 g/kg depending on response) to maintain platelet count at a safe level (>20,000/mm^3)
      (2) Alternate-day corticosteroids is useful adjunctive therapy when IVGG is used.
4. Response:
   a. Acute ITP: 80% respond initially
      More rapid increase in platelet counts compared to steroid treatment.
5. IVGG toxicity:
   a. Anaphylaxis in IgA-deficient patients because of preexisting IgA antibodies that react with small amounts of IgA present in commercially available gammaglobulin.
   b. Postinfusion headache in 20% of patients; transient and possibly severe (in severe cases, administer postinfusion dexamethasone 0.15–0.3 mg/kg IV). Severe headache in ITP may suggest the presence of intracranial hemorrhage and if clinically indicated may require a CT scan.
   c. Fever and chills in 1–3% of patients; prophylactic acetaminophen (10–15 mg/kg, 4 hourly, as required) and diphenhydramine (1 mg/kg, 6–8 hourly, as required) to reduce the incidence and severity.
   d. Coombs-positive hemolytic anemia because of the presence of blood group antibodies (anti-A, anti-B, and anti-D) present in IVGG.
   e. Hepatitis C virus (HCV) infection reported in patients receiving IVGG; however, no reports of HIV infection with any licensed preparation in the United States has been described.

Anti-D Therapy

Anti-D is a plasma-derived gamma immune globulin containing a high titer of antibodies to Rh antigens of the red blood cells (RBC) for IV injection. WinRho SDF (Nabi, Boca Raton, FL, USA) has been licensed in the United States, Canada, and Ireland.

Infusion of IV anti-D immunoglobulin to Rh-positive individuals causes a transient hemolytic anemia in the recipient. The mechanism for the beneficial effect of anti-D in ITP is blockade of the Fc receptors of reticuloendothelial cells with antibody-coated autologous red blood cells (Table 10-6). Because the Fc receptors are blocked with antibody-coated RBCs, the receptors are not available to antibody-coated platelets in ITP. The increase in platelet count occurs after 48 hours; therefore, this therapy is not appropriate for emergency treatment. Patients who have not undergone splenectomy are more likely to respond to IV anti-D than are splenectomized patients.

Prerequisite for use
The patient must be Rh positive for this mode of therapy to be beneficial.

Dose
Anti-D 50–75 µg/kg IV infusion over a 3- to 5-minute period. The hemoglobin level should be checked approximately 1 week later, but no sooner than 3–4 days. If the hemoglobin level decrease is 1 g/dL or less, the dose can be increased up to 70–80 µg/kg dose. Repeat anti-Rh D treatment at 3- to 8-week intervals, maintaining a platelet count of more than 20,000/mm^3.

Viral safety
No cases of viral transmission have been reported in patients receiving WinRho, anti-D.

Adverse drug reactions
Fever
Chills
Headache
Drop in hemoglobin and hematocrit attributed to anti-D-related hemolysis.

   These symptoms are directly attributable to anti-D-related hemolysis and a positive Coombs reaction.

Hypersensitivity reactions
Acute anaphylactic reaction is a remote possibility. IgE-mediated and immune complex reactions have been reported with the use of anti-D. No reactions to anti-D have been reported in IgA-deficient patients.

Hemolysis
In four clinical studies with a mean dose of 50 µg/kg WinRho, the mean decrease of hemoglobin was 1.7 g/dL (range, 0.4–6.1 g/dL). Hemolysis is usually extravascular. A few cases of intravascular hemolysis resulting in renal impairment have been reported.

Results
This is a safe, convenient, inexpensive, and effective therapy for chronic ITP. It is more effective in children than in adults.

Rituximab

Rituximab is a humanized mouse monoclonal antibody against the B-cell surface antigen CD-20. It is used for the treatment of non-Hodgkin lymphoma and causes B-cell lysis. The rationale for its use in ITP is to eliminate autoreactive B cells.

Dose
375 mg/m^2 IV weekly for 4 weeks.

Adverse drug reactions

- Fever, chills
- Headache, dizziness
- Nausea, vomiting
- Hypotension, sinus tachycardia

- Mucocutaneous reactions including Stevens-Johnson syndrome, lichenoid dermatitis, vesiculobullous dermatitis, and toxic epidermal necrolysis
- Immunosuppression.

The following drugs, while effective, are rarely necessary or employed in ITP.

Vinca alkaloids
Vincristine
Vinblastine
Danazol
Cyclophosphamide
Azathioprine
Cyclosporine
α-Interferon 2b
Dapsone
Colchicine
Epsilon-aminocaproic acid
Recombinant factor VIIa.

Plasmapheresis

In patients who manifest thrombocytopenia and life-threatening bleeding despite medical intervention and splenectomy, protein A column treatment of plasma and reinfusion can be used for rapid removal of platelet antibodies. By accelerating the clearance of circulating antiplatelet factors, this may be useful in patients with severe ITP.

Platelet Transfusions

Platelet transfusions are indicated when there are neurologic signs suggestive of intracranial bleeding, signs of internal bleeding, or if an emergency surgery is indicated. Although platelet survival is short, a platelet transfusion may have a temporary beneficial hemostatic effect. Fear of prolonging the duration of ITP by enhancing sensitization is theoretical.

Splenectomy

Indications
Splenectomy is indicated for severe acute ITP with acute life-threatening bleeding, which is nonresponsive to medical treatment. Splenectomy is also indicated for chronic purpura with bleeding symptoms or platelet count persistently below 30,000/mm³, which is nonresponsive to medical treatment for several years. In very active patients subject to frequent trauma, earlier splenectomy may be indicated. Because of the hazards of overwhelming postsplenectomy infection (OPSI), the procedure should be undertaken only when clearly indicated. Indications for splenectomy are rare because of judicious use of steroids and IVGG. It is rarely necessary to perform a splenectomy before 2 years after diagnosis because the thrombocytopenia is generally well tolerated and easily controlled. Spontaneous recovery may occur after 4 or 5 years and, therefore, a very conservative approach to splenectomy in ITP should be adopted. Laparoscopic splenectomy appears to be preferable to open splenectomy in experienced hands.

Preparation for splenectomy
Corticosteroids, IVIG, or anti-D can be used to raise the platelet count perioperatively. If active bleeding is occurring just prior to surgery, platelet transfusion may be

required before surgery as well as methylprednisolone 500 mg/m^2/day IV. If the patient undergoing splenectomy has adrenal suppression following previous corticosteroid administration, corticosteroids at full dosage should be administered the day before, the day of, and for a few days after surgery. Patients should be immunized with pneumococcal and meningococcal vaccines preferably 2 weeks prior to splenectomy. They should also receive *Haemophilus influenzae b* vaccine if they have not received it before. Because the protection provided by the vaccines is incomplete, daily prophylaxis with penicillin 250 mg twice daily is recommended. All febrile episodes should be carefully assessed, and patients should be empirically treated with parenteral antibiotics pending blood culture results.

Prognosis
Up to 70% of patients have a complete and long-lasting recovery after splenectomy. Response to steroids and IVGG is a good indication of the likelihood of response to splenectomy (about 80–90%). Forty percent of patients with persistent thrombocytopenia after splenectomy have an accessory spleen.

Treatment of Children with Life-Threatening Hemorrhage

1. Platelet transfusion
2. methylprednisolone 500 mg/m^2 IV per day for 3 days
3. IVGG 2 g/kg
4. Emergency splenectomy.

These measures can be used singly or in combination, depending on the severity and response to treatment. Patients refractory to these measures may benefit from vincristine sulfate 2 mg/m^2 IV and protein A column treatment of plasma and reinfusion of the plasma.

Prognosis

1. Excellent; 50% recover usually within 1 month and 70–80% recover within 6 months.
2. Spontaneous remission after 1 year is uncommon, although may occur even after several years.
3. When a demonstrable underlying cause of ITP exists, the prognosis is related to cause.
4. Age older than 10 years, insidious onset, and female gender are associated with the development of chronic ITP.
5. Of all chronic patients, 50–60% eventually stabilize without any therapy and without recourse to splenectomy.

SECONDARY THROMBOCYTOPENIC PURPURA

Thrombocytopenia may be idiopathic or secondary to known causative agents. This latter group can be further subdivided into those disorders associated with normal or increased megakaryocytes and those associated with decreased or absent megakaryocytes (Table 10-2).

Human Immunodeficiency Virus Thrombocytopenia

Thrombocytopenia is a relatively frequent complication of HIV-1 infection. Thrombocytopenia is seen in 3–8% of seropositive individuals and 30–45% of patients with fully developed acquired immunodeficiency syndrome (AIDS). During the initial phases of HIV infection, thrombocytopenia may be the only manifestation of HIV infection and is immunologically mediated (HIV-ITP). However, patients with late-stage HIV-1 infection (AIDS) have anemia, leukopenia, and thrombocytopenia due to direct marrow suppression by the virus.

Other factors contributing to thrombocytopenia are other infections (e.g., *Pneumocystis carinii* pneumonia, *Mycobacterium avium*, cytomegalovirus [CMV]), myelosuppressive drugs, chronic DIC, and severe malnutrition.

Treatment

In addition to steroids, anti-D, and IVIG, dapsone, vincristine, zidovudine, didanosine, and splenectomy have been used to treat HIV-related thrombocytopenia.

Autoimmune Disorders

Thrombocytopenia is often associated with a variety of autoimmune disorders:

1. *Systemic lupus erythematosus (SLE):* Thrombocytopenia occurs in 15–25% of patients with SLE as a result of peripheral destruction of platelets. Treatment: corticosteroids, IVGG, immunosuppressive agents (e.g., azathioprine, cyclophosphamide), and vinca alkaloids. Splenectomy should be reserved for refractory cases and/or life-threatening hemorrhage.
2. *Autoimmune lymphoproliferative syndrome (ALPS):* This syndrome is characterized by massive lymphadenopathy, hepatosplenomegaly, hypergammaglobulinemia, and autoimmune cytopenias including ITP. The pathogenesis is inherited defects in FAS and other genes that regulate lymphocyte apoptosis. The treatment is steroids.
3. *Antiphospholipid antibody syndrome:* Antiphospholipid antibodies enhance platelet activation. These patients have recurrent arterial or venous thrombi. The treatment is steroids and/or immunosuppressive agents.
4. *Evans syndrome:* Evans syndrome is the combination of autoimmune hemolytic anemia and thrombocytopenia and/or neutropenia. These patients have a poor response to steroids, IVIG, or splenectomy.
5. *Other autoimmune processes:* Hodgkin disease, non-Hodgkin lymphoma, juvenile rheumatoid arthritis, dermatomyositis, Graves' disease, Hashimoto thyroiditis, myasthenia gravis, inflammatory bowel disease, sarcoidosis, and protein losing enteropathy may be associated with autoimmune thrombocytopenia.

Heparin-Induced Thrombocytopenia

Heparin-induced thrombocytopenia (HIT) is defined by a fall in the platelet count to less than $150,000/mm^3$, or a decrease in the platelet count by 50% in patients with preexisting thrombocytopenia. It is due to an autoantibody directed against heparin in association with platelet factor 4. This antibody binds to and activates the Fc receptor on the platelet surface leading to platelet activation. HIT occurs 5 or more days after starting heparin, if the patient has not received heparin before. In patients with previous exposure, it can develop within 48 hours. In patients with suspected HIT, heparin should be discontinued immediately. Alternative anticoagulation therapy (discussed on pages 354-355) should be utilized. If the patient has arterial or venous thrombosis, low-molecular-weight heparin (LMWH) or warfarin should not be used. There is a high risk of cross-reactivity between LMWH and heparin-dependent antibody. Warfarin can lead to skin necrosis or worsening of thrombosis.

Drug-Induced Thrombocytopenia

Drugs can cause thrombocytopenia by two different mechanisms: marrow depression and increased platelet destruction. A marrow examination will distinguish between thrombocytopenia caused by toxic depression, in which the megakaryocytes are scanty or absent, and thrombocytopenia resulting from peripheral destruction, in which the megakaryocytes are normal or increased in number.

Marrow Depression

Drugs can be classified as those that produce a dose-related marrow depression, such as cytotoxic drugs (e.g., 6-mercaptopurine, methotrexate, cyclophosphamide), and those that have an idiosyncratic effect (e.g., chloramphenicol).

Increased Platelet Destruction

Increased platelet destruction is mediated by the binding of the Fab terminus of IgG to a complex of drug (or a drug metabolite) and a platelet membrane component (GP Ib/IX or GP IIb/IIIa). The Fc portions of the IgG molecules interact with the Fc receptors on phagocytic cells of the reticuloendothelial system.

These patients usually present with sudden onset of bleeding 1–2 weeks after starting the drug and have severe thrombocytopenia. The platelet count begins to rise within a few days after discontinuing the drug. A high index of clinical suspicion is required to make the diagnosis. The sensitivity of *in vitro* assays is relatively low. Treatment is IVIG or steroids.

Table 10-4 lists the drugs proved or suspected to induce drug-dependent antibody-mediated immune thrombocytopenia.

Microangiopathic Hemolytic Anemia

Thrombocytopenia is a typical component of microangiopathic hemolytic anemia. Some of these conditions are associated with DIC.

Disseminated Intravascular Coagulation

Thrombocytopenia is seen in several syndromes associated with DIC, including purpura fulminans, overwhelming sepsis, and giant hemangioma. In an unusual case of thrombocytopenia, the PT, PTT, fibrinogen, and fibrin split products should be determined as screening tests to exclude DIC as the cause of the thrombocytopenia.

Hemolytic Uremic Syndrome

Hemolytic uremic syndrome (HUS) is associated with acute hemolytic anemia, thrombocytopenia, and renal failure in infants and young children (between 6 months and 5 years of age).

Etiology and Pathogenesis

Shigella toxins produced by *Escherichia coli* O157:H7 and *Shigella dysenteriae* type I have been associated with the pathogenesis of HUS and thrombotic thrombocytopenic purpura (TTP). *Shigella* toxins may exert a direct effect on platelets, increasing their likelihood of clumping and the toxins may have a local effect on endothelial cells, causing thrombus formation.

Increased platelet consumption may result from a generalized increase in platelet activation. Aggregates of platelets may then become trapped in the small blood vessels, resulting in damage to circulating erythrocytes and a microangiopathic hemolytic anemia.

Clinical Features

- An infection, either mild or severe, associated with gastrointestinal symptoms, including vomiting and bloody diarrhea, precedes the development of HUS.
- The onset of oliguria associated with hypertension may lead to renal failure within days of the initial illness.
- Children between the ages of 4 months and 2 years are typically affected. It is less common in older children. It can give a picture very similar to TTP.

Laboratory Findings

- Thrombocytopenia
- Microangiopathic hemolytic anemia
- Reduced large multimers of von Willebrand factor (consumed during *in vivo* platelet aggregation)
- Decreased immunoglobulins in some patients
- Depleted prostaglandin I2 (PGI2) in some patients.

Treatment

- Aggressive management of renal failure with fluid restriction and peritoneal dialysis, when indicated.
- Correction of anemia with red cell transfusion.
- Life-threatening bleeding due to thrombocytopenia is uncommon. Platelet transfusions can worsen thrombotic complications of the illness and should not be given to a patient with HUS.

Thrombotic Thrombocytopenic Purpura

TTP, or Moschowitz syndrome, is a rare multisystem disease. It can be acute (acquired) or chronic (inherited). It may be secondary to an underlying disease (Table 10-7). Estimated annual incidence is 1–4 in 1,000,000. It is more common in women than in men (3:2). Although it occurs in children, the peak incidence is

Table 10-7. Clinical Classification and Causes of Thrombotic Thrombocytopenic Purpura Syndrome

Idiopathic
  Acute (acquired)
  Chronic (inherited)
Secondary
  Pregnancy, postpartum
  Autoimmune disorders
  Neoplastic disorders
  Infection
  Bacterial endocarditis
  Drug induced
  Stem cell transplantation
  Miscellaneous

at 30–40 years of age. Thrombotic thrombocytopenic purpura can develop secondary to bacterial or viral infections, pregnancy, autoimmune disorders, malignancy, stem cell transplantation, or drugs (ticlopidine, clopidogrel, quinine, mitomycin C, cyclosporine, and tacrolimus).

TTP can be classified as follows:

- *Chronic hereditary TTP:* Unusually large multimers of von Willebrand factor (UL-vWF) bind to platelet GP Ib/IX and GP IIb/IIIa complexes efficiently and induce platelet aggregation. These UL-vWF multimers are synthesized by endothelial cells and processed into multimers of normal size through the action of a vWF-cleaving metalloproteinase, *ADAMTS13* (*a d*isintegrin-like *a*nd *m*etalloprotease with *t*hrombospondin type 1 repeat). In chronic relapsing TTP, mutations in the *ADAMTS13* gene result in markedly decreased protease activity and the accumulation of very large size vWF multimers in the plasma that are responsible for the initiation and propagation of intravascular coagulopathy observed in TTP. Thirteen percent of patients with TTP have severe *ADAMTS13* deficiency. The presenting features, clinical outcome, and response to treatment do not correlate with severity of the *ADAMTS13* deficiency. Severe deficiency does not detect all patients with TTP. Therefore, the diagnosis of TTP is still a clinical diagnosis.
- Hereditary TTP also occurs in another genetic disease characterized by abnormalities of complement factor H that normally regulates the alternative pathway of complement activation. Factor H binds to complement (C3b) and regulates the activity of the alternate pathway. Mutations of the HF gene results in mutated factor H. As a result of this mutation, complement deposition and damage to the renal endothelial cells occur and it may cause local release of vWF and microangiopathy.
- *Sporadic TTP:* In sporadic TTP, gene mutations may be less severe or there may be polymorphisms.
- *Acute acquired TTP:* This has been attributed to an autoantibody and is best termed *autoimmune TTP* because of the presence of *ADAMT13* IgG inhibitors.
- *Secondary TTP:* See Table 10-7.

Clinical and Laboratory Features

The spectrum of systemic involvement varies from patient to patient and from time to time and may be acute, chronic, or relapsing.

Constitutional/nonspecific:

Fever
Headache
Malaise
Nausea/vomiting
Abdominal pain
Chest pain
Arthralgia/myalgia.

Hematologic and laboratory findings:

Microangiopathic hemolytic anemia (blood smear reveals polychromasia, basophilic stippling, schistocytes, microspherocytes, and nucleated red blood cells)
Thrombocytopenia
DIC
Purpura
Pallor
Jaundice

Abnormally elevated factor VIII:vWF antigen in plasma
Reduced haptoglobin level
Presence (usually) of hemoglobinuria and hemosiderinuria
Increased unconjugated bilirubin
Increased lactate dehydrogenase levels (sensitive index of response to therapy or
    development of relapse).

Organ damage:

Fluctuating neurologic signs and symptoms
Progressive renal failure (occurs in 25% of chronic patients).

Pathology

The hallmark of TTP is the widespread presence of segmental hyaline microthrombi
in the microvasculature. These hyaline deposits originate in the subendothelium,
focally occlude vascular lumina, and are composed of compacted platelet debris,
p-aminosalicylic acid (PAS)-positive endothelial fibrils, vWF, and variable amounts
of fibrin. The hyaline occlusions of TTP are most consistently visible in lymph node
biopsies and sections of spleen.

Diagnosis

The histopathologic diagnosis of TTP is often difficult. Skin and muscle biopsies
yield a low percentage of positive findings (32%). Gingival biopsies are diagnostic in
about 50% of cases.

Treatment

- Exchange plasmapheresis provides remission in 50–80% of patients. This
  removes platelet-aggregating substances (e.g., unusually large vWF multimers,
  autoantibodies, and other cofactors).
- Fresh frozen plasma (FFP) infusion provides the vWF-cleaving metalloproteinase.
- Dextran, steroids, vincristine, cyclophosphamide, azathioprine, cyclosporin A,
  IVGG, staphylococcal protein A columns, splenectomy, and antiplatelet agents
  (e.g., acetylsalicylic acid [ASA], dipyridamole) have not been systematically
  evaluated. Splenectomy provides 50% improvement in chronic refractory cases.
- Rituximab, 375 mg/m^2 weekly for 2–8 weeks, has been successful where other
  measures have failed. (Rituximab increases the *ADAMTS13* level and decreases
  the inhibitor level to *ADAMTS13* if it exists). Plasma exchange, if deemed clinically necessary, should be postponed as long as possible after rituximab administration.

Cyanotic Congenital Heart Disease

Thrombocytopenia frequently occurs in children with severe cyanotic congenital
heart disease, usually when the hematocrit levels are more than 65% and when the
arterial oxygen saturation is less than 65%. This may be due to margination of
platelets in the small blood vessels, which may occur in the presence of a high hematocrit level. Thrombocytopenia can occasionally be cyclic, occurring at intervals of
10–25 days. During periods of thrombocytopenia, there are high thrombopoietin levels in the plasma; when platelet counts are normal, thrombopoietin levels are low.

Cyanotic congenital heart disease may be associated with prolonged bleeding
time in spite of normal platelet counts, which is related to an impairment in platelet

aggregation by adenosine diphosphate (ADP), norepinephrine, and collagen. This impairment is correlated with the severity of hypoxia. Affected children usually experience little bleeding during corrective surgery, which, if successful, results in an improved platelet count.

Hypersplenism

A variety of conditions characterized by splenomegaly are associated with thrombocytopenia, presumably resulting from the sequestration or destruction of platelets by the enlarged spleen. This is usually associated with neutropenia and anemia. Megakaryocytes are plentiful in the marrow. Hypersplenism occurs in patients who have splenomegaly, irrespective of cause.

Thrombopoietin Deficiency

Thrombopoietin deficiency is a rare congenital cause of chronic thrombocytopenia with numerous immature megakaryocytes in the bone marrow. Infusion of normal plasma and plasma from patients with ITP is followed by a rise in the platelet count to normal, with apparent maturation of the megakaryocytes.

NEONATAL THROMBOCYTOPENIA

Neonates with severe thrombocytopenia may have bleeding that leads to lifelong residual defects (e.g., intracranial hemorrhage) or death. The incidence of neonatal thrombocytopenia (cord blood platelet count <50,000/mm^3) is 0.3% and that of severe neonatal thrombocytopenia (platelet count <20,000/mm^3) is 0.04%. Most infants who have thrombocytopenia appear ill, are premature, and have other disorders that contribute to the thrombocytopenia, including bacteremia and DIC. In these sick infants, the incidence of thrombocytopenia is as high as 15% and it is most severe several days after delivery.

Table 10-8 lists the causes of neonatal thrombocytopenia, and Figure 10-3 shows an approach to the diagnosis of thrombocytopenia in the infant.

Table 10-8. Causes of Neonatal Thrombocytopenia

I. **Normal or increased megakaryocytes in the marrow (megakaryocytic thrombocytopenia)**
  A. Immune disorders
   1. Autoimmune (passive transfer of platelet antibody) (NITP)
     a. Maternal ITP
     b. Maternal drug-induced thrombocytopenia
     c. SLE
   2. Alloimmune (NATP)
     a. Isolated platelet group incompatibility
     b. Associated with blood group incompatibility
  B. Infection
   1. Bacterial: gram-negative and gram-positive septicemia, listeriosis
   2. Viral: cytomegalovirus, rubella, herpes simplex, coxsackievirus
   3. Protozoal: toxoplasmosis
   4. Spirochetal: syphilis
  C. Drugs
   1. Immune: drug–hapten disease (e.g., quinine, quinidine, sedormid)
   2. Nonimmune: thiazide, tolbutamide (given to mother)

(Continues)

Table 10-8. (*Continued*)

  D. Disseminated intravascular coagulation
    1. Prenatal causes
        a. Preeclampsia and eclampsia
        b. Abruptio placentae
        c. Dead twin fetus
        d. Amniotic fluid embolism
    2. Intranatal causes
        a. Breech delivery
        b. Fetal distress
    3. Postnatal causes
        a. Infections
        b. Hypoxia and acidosis
        c. Respiratory distress syndrome
        d. Renal vein thrombosis
        e. Indwelling catheters
        f. Giant hemangioma
  E. Inherited thrombocytopenia
    1. Sex-linked
        a. Pure
        b. Wiskott–Aldrich syndrome[a]
    2. Autosomal
        a. Pure (dominant or recessive)
        b. Bernard-Soulier syndrome
        c. May Hegglin anomaly

II. Decreased or absent megakaryocytes in the marrow (amegakaryocytic thrombocytopenia)
  A. Isolated megakaryocytic hypoplasia (Table 10-9)
    1. Thrombocytopenia absent radii (TAR syndrome)
    2. Congenital megakaryocytic hypoplasia without anomalies
    3. Congenital hypoplastic thrombocytopenia with microcephaly
    4. Rubella syndrome[b]
    5. Congenital hypoplastic thrombocytopenia associated with trisomy syndromes
    6. Thrombocytopenia agenesis of corpus callosum
    7. Fanconi anemia
    8. Hoyeraal–Hreidarsson syndrome
    9. Amegakaryocytic thrombocytopenia with radio-ulnar synostosis (ATRUS)
    10. Dyskeratosis congenita (DC)
  B. Generalized bone marrow disorders
    1. Bone marrow aplasia
        a. Fanconi anemia
        b. Pancytopenia without congenital anomalies
        c. Osteopetrosis
    2. Bone marrow infiltration
        a. Congenital leukemia
        b. Langerhans cell histiocytosis
        c. Congenital neuroblastoma
  C. Metabolic causes
    1. Associated with acidosis and ketosis
        a. Hyperglycinemia
        b. Methylmalonic acidemia
        c. Isovaleric acidemia
        d. Propionic acidemia
    2. Other
        a. Maternal hyperthyroidism[c]

[a]Decreased production and poor survival of small defective platelets.
[b]Decreased megakaryocytes but not confirmed at autopsy. ? Error in sampling.
[c]Pathogenesis not determined.

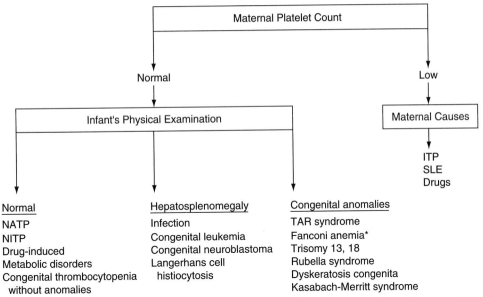

Fig. 10-3. Diagnostic approach to infant with thrombocytopenia. *Thrombocytopenia usually occurs at 4–6 years of age in Fanconi anemia.

Normal or Increased Megakaryocytes in the Marrow: Megakaryocytic Thrombocytopenia

Neonatal Idiopathic (Autoimmune) Purpura: Passive Transfer of Platelet Antibody from Mother

Pregnant women with ITP are at a 50% risk for delivering thrombocytopenic infants, whether or not the mother is thrombocytopenic during pregnancy or at the time of delivery. This results from the transplacental passage of maternal IgG autoantibodies into the fetal circulation, with destruction of fetal platelets. Although self-limiting, neonatal ITP (NITP) may last for several weeks. Infants with severe thrombocytopenia (platelet counts <50,000/mm^3) have a 1% risk for intracranial hemorrhage (ICH). The risk of severe neonatal thrombocytopenia appears higher if the mother has had a previously affected fetus. True maternal ITP must be distinguished from "gestational" thrombocytopenia. This is a common disorder, in which maternal thrombocytopenia is not severe (platelet counts ≥100,000/mm^3) and infants are not at risk for thrombocytopenia.

Patients identified by the following criteria should be managed by a high-risk obstetric team:

- History of a previously affected infant
- Mother splenectomized for ITP
- Mother with thrombocytopenia (<100,000/mm^3) in the current pregnancy.

Treatment

The best approach to managing delivery in women with ITP remains controversial. There is no generally accepted noninvasive methods to identify neonates at risk. Percutaneous umbilical blood sampling and fetal scalp sampling are associated with risks. The benefits of cesarean section have not been proven to reduce the occurrence of intracranial hemorrhage.

1. Prenatal:
   a. IVGG therapy, 1 g/kg/day administered weekly, is recommended for pregnant women who have a platelet count of <30,000/mm³ or bleeding during the third trimester. The role of IVGG therapy administered to the pregnant subject with ITP for the sole benefit of the fetus is more controversial.
   b. The fetal platelet count may be determined by percutaneous umbilical vessel or scalp vein sampling.
   c. Cesarean section is recommended when the fetal platelet count is less than 50,000/mm³.
2. Postnatal:
   a. IVGG therapy, 1 g/kg/day for 2 days for platelet counts less than 50,000/mm³, is the treatment of choice for affected infants. A platelet count greater than 50,000/mm³ and a platelet count at least twice the pretreatment value 48 hours after completion of the IVGG infusion are indicators of a good response to therapy.
   b. Ultrasound of the head should be performed to exclude the presence of intracranial hemorrhage and should be repeated at 1 month of age to identify hydrocephalus and/or intracranial bleeding as early as possible.
   c. Corticosteroids are administered in the form of prednisone or methylprednisolone IV in a dose of 1–3 mg/kg/day. Corticosteroids should be reserved for those infants who are unresponsive or poorly responsive to IVGG therapy or for those in whom significant clinical bleeding is present (in these, combined therapy with IVGG should be considered).
   d. Exchange transfusion is not always beneficial.
   e. Random-donor platelet infusions are generally ineffective in infants with autoimmune thrombocytopenia.
   f. In emergency situations (e.g., ICH), combination therapy with high-dose IVGG, corticosteroids, and random-donor platelets should be administered.

The nadir of the platelet count in infants with ITP often occurs a few days after delivery. It is, therefore, important that serial counts be obtained during the period of greatest risk for severe thrombocytopenia, the first week of life. The response to IVGG alone is 70% and to corticosteroids is 80%.

Neonatal Isoimmune (Alloimmune) Thrombocytopenic Purpura

Neonatal isoimmune (alloimmune) thrombocytopenic purpura (NATP) should be suspected in thrombocytopenic infants born to mothers with a normal platelet count, particularly if infants of successive pregnancies are affected. Immunization arises from fetomaternal passage of platelets in which there is incompatibility of fetal and maternal platelet antigens. The pathophysiology is similar to Rh disease. A number of platelet antigens have been implicated in NATP. The platelet antigenic system most commonly associated with NATP has been designated human platelet antigen (HPA-1a) or Pl^{A1}. Because these antibodies can interfere with normal platelet aggregation, a qualitative defect may be present in those platelets that are not yet destroyed by the antibody. This functional platelet defect may explain why the incidence of serious bleeding is higher in infants with NATP than in NITP infants.

Clinical Features

1. The incidence is 1–2 in 10,000. In 50% of cases, first-born offspring are affected, suggesting that antigenic exposure can occur during the early course of pregnancy (unlike Rh incompatibility, which occurs primarily at the time of delivery).

2. This type of neonatal thrombocytopenia accounts for most of the cases of fetal morbidity and mortality. Hemorrhagic manifestations are variable but tend to be more severe than in the passive transfer of a platelet antibody across the placenta (NITP).

3. Generalized petechiae may appear within minutes of birth and be followed by ecchymosis and even cephalhematomata. Intracranial hemorrhage can occur *in utero* and be detected on ultrasonography during apparently uncomplicated pregnancies. Death *in utero* may occur.

4. Bleeding from the umbilicus, skin puncture site, or gastrointestinal or renal tract may also occur.

5. Megakaryocytes are present in normal or increased numbers in the marrow. Reduced numbers of megakaryocytes indicate direct interaction of the antibody with these cells in certain instances.

6. Early jaundice occurs in 20% of cases.

Diagnosis

Laboratory confirmation is difficult* but important with reference to future pregnancies. A diagnosis of NATP is often inferential. The usual criteria include:

1. Congenital thrombocytopenia
2. Normal maternal platelet count and negative history of maternal ITP
3. No evidence of systemic disease, infection, malignancy, or hemangioma
4. Recovery of platelet count within 2–3 weeks
5. Increased megakaryocytes in bone marrow aspiration; however, a reduced number has been noted in a few instances.

Treatment

Active treatment of the infant

Treatment involves administering a maternal platelet concentrate suspended in normal plasma (mother's platelets lack the antigen responsible for isoimmunization). Maternal platelets should be (1) washed with normal plasma to remove antibodies more completely and (2) irradiated to eliminate the risk of graft versus host disease. In this way, platelets compatible with residual neonatal platelet antibody will be infused.

1. If the mother's platelets are not available, HPA-1a-negative platelets may be available from the blood bank. While antigen-negative platelets are being obtained and prepared for transfusion, random-donor platelets should be utilized for immediate therapy in infants with active bleeding. Random donor platelets are unlikely to be as effective as maternal platelets because

---

*The mother's and father's platelets should be typed for HPA1a and for other known alloantigens, if possible. A number of assays are utilized by platelet immunology laboratories, including fluorescence-activated flow cytometry, platelet suspension immunofluorescence, radioimmunoassays, antigen capture techniques such as monoclonal antibody immobilization of platelet antigens (MAIPA), immunoblotting, platelet lysis, and complement fixation. The mother's and infant's serum or plasma should be screened for the presence of antiplatelet antibody. The antibodies responsible for platelet destruction in NATP usually do not fix complement. Antibodies are usually absent from the newborn's plasma but often are found in high titer in the mother's. The most informative antibody assays are those that can detect platelet alloantibodies even in the presence of human leukocyte antigen (anti-HLA) antibodies. Maternal plasma should be studied with paternal or neonatal platelets as targets; maternal (antigen-negative) platelets and paternal plasma are appropriate negative controls. With some assay systems it may be possible to detect alloimmunization even if the precise antigen incompatibility is not known.

98% of the population has HPA1a-positive platelets. However, a transient increase in the platelet count may still occur with a half-life ranging from 1 to 24 hours.

2. IVGG in a dose of 1 g/kg daily for 1–3 days until the platelet count is between 50,000 and 100,000/mm³. After IVGG, the platelet count usually becomes normal within 1 week.
3. Corticosteroids, which reduce platelet destruction and increase vascular integrity, are also recommended.
4. Ultrasound of the newborn's brain should be carried out during the acute phase to detect intracranial hemorrhage. Careful follow-up of these infants is necessary for early detection of the presence of hydrocephalus, which may require shunting.

Antenatal management

Subsequent pregnancies of a mother who has had one infant with NATP are at high risk for recurrence and nearly all subsequent infants with antigen-positive platelets will be thrombocytopenic. The severity of antenatal and perinatal hemorrhage tends to increase in later pregnancies. The family should be advised of the risk of recurrence at the time the first infant is diagnosed. Antiplatelet antibody titers during pregnancy cannot be used to predict whether an individual fetus will be affected.

It is not possible to anticipate the first case of isoimmune purpura in a given family. However, once an index case has occurred, every effort should be made to obtain a determination of the platelet genotypes of the parents. For example, if the father is homozygous HPA1a positive and the mother a sensitized homozygous HPA1a negative, all subsequent infants will be heterozygous HPA1a positive and are likely to be affected. When this is known, the following maternal management is appropriate:

1. Determine fetal platelet count and allotype using blood obtained from percutaneous umbilical blood sampling after about 20 weeks' gestation.
2. Perform frequent ultrasound examination; however, fetal intracranial hemorrhage may not always be detected by ultrasound.
3. Administer prenatal IVGG therapy to the mother. IVGG 1 g/kg may be given weekly from midgestation until birth.
4. Recommend cesarean section for all pregnancies at risk for NATP.
5. Have washed maternal platelet concentrates available for immediate administration to the infant after birth.

Prognosis

The risk of intracranial hemorrhage is 15%.

Thrombocytopenia Associated with Erythroblastosis Fetalis or Exchange Transfusion

Severe cases of erythroblastosis frequently show petechiae and purpura in the first few hours after birth. This may be due to an isoimmune mechanism, or, when associated with hyperbilirubinemia, it may be an effect of bilirubin toxicity on platelet survival.

Thrombocytopenia may also occur following exchange transfusion because of the paucity of platelets in stored blood or from the shorter survival time of transfused platelets. The thrombocytopenia is transient.

Infection

Thrombocytopenia may occur in any form of sepsis (see Table 10-8). These infants are sick and have jaundice, pallor, purpura, and hepatosplenomegaly. The blood picture shows hemolytic anemia with increased normoblasts, reticulocytosis, and thrombocytopenia. Bone marrow biopsy usually shows normal numbers of megakaryocytes; however, in some cases, bone marrow aspiration has been reported as showing reduced numbers of megakaryocytes. The latter finding suggests that the paucity of megakaryocytes may be related to technical difficulties of marrow aspiration in this age group, although, in some cases, it may be a true finding and mirror the bone marrow biopsy findings.

The mechanism for thrombocytopenia includes the following:

1. Hypoplasia of megakaryocytes
2. Decreased platelet production
3. Increased platelet destruction due to splenomegaly and reticuloendothelial hyperactivity
4. DIC.

Therapy is directed toward the underlying infection.

Drug-Induced Thrombocytopenia in the Mother

Neonatal thrombocytopenia may be associated with drug-induced thrombocytopenia in the mother. In this situation, drug-hapten disease is responsible for both maternal and fetal disease (see Table 10-4). Thiazide diuretics have been incriminated as causing neonatal thrombocytopenia, but the mechanism appears to be different, because the maternal platelet count is normal and no antibodies have been demonstrated.

Disseminated Intravascular Coagulation

A number of conditions in the newborn may trigger DIC in which platelets along with other coagulation factors are consumed during the clotting process (Table 10-8).

Giant Hemangioma

Giant hemangioma coupled with thrombocytopenia probably represents a form of localized intravascular coagulation. The association of thrombocytopenic purpura with giant hemangioma is referred to as the Kasabach–Merritt syndrome. Platelet trapping has been demonstrated in giant hemangiomas, accompanied, in some instances, by evidence of the consumption of coagulation factors and an increase in fibrin degradation products.

Treatment

1. Transfusions of platelets and other coagulation factors have only transient effects but may hasten involution of the hemangioma. These modalities may be required because of active bleeding due to thrombocytopenia.
2. Corticosteroid therapy has little immediate effect, but may bring about involution of the hemangioma, especially in very young infants. However, tumor regression is probably a consequence of vascular thrombosis and infarction.
3. External compression of the hemangioma by firm bandaging, when possible, may reduce blood flow and platelet trapping.
4. Surgical excision, when possible, has corrected the thrombocytopenia.
5. Radiation therapy to reduce the size of the hemangioma should be considered when the hemorrhagic manifestations are severe.
6. Interferon α-2a has been shown to be effective. It inhibits angiogenesis, in part by inhibiting the proliferation of endothelial cells, smooth muscle cells, and fibroblasts that have been stimulated by fibroblast growth factor (FGF),

decreasing collagen production and increasing endothelial prostacyclin production.

Inherited Thrombocytopenia

Sex-Linked Thrombocytopenias

Thrombocytopenia with a sex-linked pattern of inheritance has been reported in a number of families. The presence of a normal number of megakaryocytes in the bone marrow suggests that the thrombocytopenia is a result of shortened platelet survival due to an intrinsic platelet defect. The response to steroids is poor. A complete response to splenectomy has occurred in some patients.

X-linked anemia with severe thrombocytopenia, due to defects in the *GATA-1* gene, has been reported. Bone marrow shows many large megakaryocytes with nuclei pushed to the side and unorganized granular content.

Wiskott–Aldrich Syndrome

The Wiskott–Aldrich is an X-linked syndrome consisting of eczema, recurrent infections, and thrombocytopenia. The gene involved is on the short arm of the X chromosome. It has been cloned and designated WASp.

Infants are ill from the first few months of life and die in early childhood. Bleeding is frequently ushered in by melena during the neonatal period, later followed by purpura. Thrombocytopenia is associated with a shortened platelet survival time caused by an intrinsic platelet defect, as well as impaired platelet production. The clinical course is punctuated by recurrent pyogenic infections, including otitis media, pneumonia, and skin infections. There is also lowered resistance to nonbacterial infections, including herpes simplex and *Pneumocystis carinii* pneumonia.

Hematologic findings
1. Thrombocytopenia (platelet count, about 30,000/mm^3); microthrombocytes; low mean platelet volume (MPV)
2. Anemia (due to blood loss)
3. Leukocytosis (due to infection)
4. Normal or increased megakaryocytes
5. Absent isohemagglutinins, reduced IgM, and normal or elevated IgG and IgA
6. Defective cell-mediated immunity in some cases.

Treatment
1. Platelet transfusion: for hemorrhagic episodes
2. Corticosteroids: for eczema; no effect on the thrombocytopenia
3. Splenectomy: reserved only for very severe cases because of high risk of overwhelming infection following splenectomy
4. Hematopoietic stem cell transplantation.

Autosomal Thrombocytopenias

This heterogeneous group of rare disorders includes both dominant and recessive forms of pure thrombocytopenia and the autosomal dominant May Hegglin anomaly.

In the pure form, families with both dominant and recessive modes of inheritance occur. Bone marrow examination usually demonstrates normal numbers of megakaryocytes. Autologous platelet survival studies indicate a shortened life span, pointing to an intrinsic platelet defect.

The *May Hegglin anomaly* consists of:

1. Autosomal dominant inheritance
2. Thrombocytopenia, variable degree
3. Giant platelets; normal platelet function and platelet survival
4. Döhle bodies in the cytoplasm of the granulocytes
5. Normal megakaryocytes
6. Most patients asymptomatic, with only a few showing hemorrhagic manifestations; no sign of bleeding in newborns
7. May Hegglin, Fetchner, Sebastian, and Epstein syndromes all map to the same region on the long arm of chromosome 22 (see Table 10-14 later in the chapter).

Familial platelet deficiency/AML is dominantly inherited. Thrombocytopenia is mild (100,000/mm^3). Some families have a severe storage pool defect. There is a 30% risk of developing AML and other cancers.

Patients with *Paris-Trousseau syndrome* exhibit mild thrombocytopenia with a subpopulation of platelets containing giant α-granules. Bone marrow examination shows expansion of immature megakaryocytic progenitors with normal erythroid and granulocytic series. Some patients have trigonocephaly, facial dysmorphism, cardiac defects, syndactyly, and psychomotor retardation in addition to platelet defects. This constellation of findings is called *Jacobsen syndrome.*

Decreased or Absent Megakaryocytes in the Marrow

Amegakaryocytic Thrombocytopenia

A variety of syndromes have been described that have in common a primary impairment of platelet production as the major cause of thrombocytopenia. Bone marrow examination usually reveals decreased numbers of megakaryocytes. This may be isolated megakaryocytic hypoplasia or part of a generalized bone marrow disease, such as aplasia of the marrow or infiltration of the marrow by nonneoplastic or neoplastic disease. Characteristics of congenital thrombocytopenic syndromes are listed in Table 10-9.

Congenital Amegakaryocytic Thrombocytopenia without Anomalies

Isolated thrombocytopenia and megakaryocytic hypoplasia without any congenital anomalies has been reported. Patients present at a median age of 7 days. Of a series of 26 patients, 11 developed aplastic anemia at a median age of 3 years. One patient developed AML and one developed MDS. The median survival was 6 years. This is an autosomal recessive disorder due to a homozygous or compound heterozygous mutation of c-pml. Patients with complete loss of c-pml function have more severe thrombocytopenia and more rapid progression to pancytopenia. The only curative treatment has been hematopoietic stem cell transplantation.

Congenital Amegakaryocytic Thrombocytopenia with Bilateral Absence of Radii (TAR Syndrome)

Clinical Features

1. Inheritance is not clearly autosomal recessive. Autosomal dominant with incomplete penetrance has been postulated.
2. Bilateral absence of the radii manifests as a shortening of the forearms and flexion at the elbows; occasionally, other limb abnormalities, such as phocomelia and radial deviation of the wrist, are present. Thumbs are functional.
3. Other congenital anomalies are occasionally present, such as deformity of the digits, micrognathia, dislocation of the hip, and congenital heart disease.

Table 10-9. Characteristics of Congenital Thrombocytopenic Syndromes

Clinical features	TACC	TAR	ATRUS	FA	AMT	HH (DC)	WAS	BS	MH	Trisomy 13, 18, 21
Agenesis of corpus callosum	+	—	—	—	—	—	—	—	—	—
Hypoplasia of cerebellar vermis	+	—	—	—	—	+	—	—	—	+
Low birth weight	+	+	—	+	+	+	—	—	—	+
Growth delay	+	+	—	+	—	+	—	—	—	+
Dysmorphic face	+	+	—	±	+	+	—	—	—	+
Developmental delay	+	—	—	±	+	+	—	—	—	±
Thrombocytopenia	+	+	+	+	+	+	+	+	+	+
Platelet size	N	N	N	N	N	N	↓	↑	↑	N
Pancytopenia	—	—	+	+	±	+	—	—	—	—
Immunodeficiency	—	—	—	—	—	—	+	—	—	—
Megakaryocytes, bone marrow	N/↓	↓	↓	↓	↓	↓	N/↑	N/↑	N/↑	N
Skeletal deformities										
Radial x-ray	—	+	+	±	—	—	—	—	—	—
Clinodactyly/syndactyly	±	—	—	±	—	—	—	—	—	±
Enamel hypoplasia	±	—	—	—	—	—	—	—	—	—
Cardiac defects	±	±	—	±	±	—	—	—	—	±
Renal malformations	±	—	—	±	±	—	—	—	—	±
Cutaneous abnormalities	—	—	—	+	—	+[a]	+	—	—	—
Karyotypic abnormalities	—	—	—	—	—	—	—	—	—	+
Chromosome breaks	—	—	—	+	—	—	—	—	—	—

Abbreviations: TACC, thrombocytopenia agenesis of corpus callosum; TAR, thrombocytopenia absent radii; ATRUS, amegakaryocytic thrombocytopenia with radio-ulnar synostosis; FA, Fanconi anemia; AMT, amegakaryocytic thrombocytopenia; HH, Hoyeraal-Hreidarsson syndrome; DC, dyskeratosis congenita; WAS, Wiskott–Aldrich syndrome; BS, Bernard-Soulier syndrome; MH, May Hegglin anomaly; N, normal; ↑, increased; ↓, decreased; +, present; ±, present occasionally; —, absent.

[a] Present at a mean age of 9 years.

4. Purpura is present in the first few days of life or may be delayed for weeks. Hemorrhagic manifestations range from a few petechiae to severe and even fatal intracranial hemorrhage.

Hematologic Findings

1. The platelet counts usually range from 10,000 to 30,000/mm^3.
2. The leukemoid blood picture frequently shows a total white blood cell count as high as 140,000/mm^3.
3. The bone marrow examination reveals myeloid hyperplasia and an almost total absence of megakaryocytes.

Prognosis

1. If patients survive beyond the first year, the platelet count stabilizes and the prognosis is much better.
2. The condition is rarely premalignant with the development of acute leukemia.

Treatment

1. Transfusion of red cells for anemia and transfusion of platelet concentrates for severe bleeding are required for the thrombocytopenia.
2. Corticosteroids and splenectomy offer no constant benefit.
3. Allogeneic stem cell transplantation may be required for severe symptomatic patients.

Amegakaryocytic Thrombocytopenia with Radio-Ulnar Synostosis

Patients with amegakaryocytic thrombocytopenia with radio-ulnar synostosis (ATRUS) present with severe normocytic thrombocytopenia at birth. Bone marrow shows absence of megakaryocytes. These patients have skeletal abnormalities such as radio-ulnar synostosis, clinodactyly, and shallow acetabula. Some patients subsequently develop hypoplastic anemia and pancytopenia.

Congenital Hypoplastic Thrombocytopenia with Microcephaly

Three infants with this syndrome have been reported. The absence of other stigmata and the persistence of the thrombocytopenia beyond the first year of life excluded rubella syndrome as the basis for this association.

Thrombocytopenia Agenesis of Corpus Callosum Syndrome

Three female patients have been reported with thrombocytopenia, agenesis of corpus callosum, low birth weight, growth delay, and dysmorphic facial features.

Thrombocytopenia in Rubella Syndrome

Congenital cardiac defects, cataracts, deafness, thrombocytopenic purpura, jaundice, hepatosplenomegaly, and bone lesions occur. The platelet count is usually low, ranging from 10,000 to 50,000/mm^3. Anemia with increased reticulocytosis and nucleated red cells has been observed and suggests a marrow response to widespread purpura or an associated hemolytic process. Bone marrow examinations reveal a decreased number of megakaryocytes.

Thrombocytopenia Associated with Trisomy Syndromes

Children with trisomy 13, trisomy 18, and trisomy 21 have been described with congenital hypoplastic thrombocytopenia.

Generalized Bone Marrow Disorders

Bone Marrow Aplasia

All causes of constitutional aplastic anemia may present with thrombocytopenia in the newborn (see Chapter 6).

Bone Marrow Infiltration

Benign disease (e.g., Gaucher disease, Niemann–Pick disease, osteopetrosis; Chapter 5) and malignant disease (e.g., congenital leukemia; Chapter 14) can present with neonatal thrombocytopenia.

Metabolic Causes

Hyperglycinemia with ketosis and the closely related metabolic disorder of *methylmalonic acidemia* may cause periodic thrombocytopenia, as well as neutropenia, during infancy. Infants with these metabolic disorders present with lethargy, vomiting, and ketosis during the neonatal period. A similar disorder, *isovaleric acidemia,* is associated with a generalized marrow hypoplasia causing thrombocytopenia and neutropenia. Neonatal thrombocytopenic purpura has been reported in infants born to *hyperthyroid mothers.* The mechanism has not been defined.

CYTOKINES IN THE TREATMENT OF THROMBOCYTOPENIA

Cytokines that stimulate platelet production may act on early, uncommitted progenitors promoting commitment along the megakaryocytic (MK) lineage or may promote survival so that this commitment can occur without a direct influence. Cytokines with potential activity on platelet production currently available for clinical testing include the following: interleukin-3 (IL-3), stem cell factor (SCF), IL-6, IL-11, and thrombopoietin (TPO). IL-11 and TPO have been used in clinical trials to ameliorate chemotherapy-induced thrombocytopenia. However, they have significant side effects and are not routinely used. Trials regarding use of cytokines in treatment of thrombocytopenia are ongoing.

THROMBOCYTOSIS

Thrombocytosis is a platelet count that is more than two standard deviations above the mean. Most thrombocytosis seen in children is secondary to inflammation. Iron-deficiency anemia, major trauma, or surgery are also associated with thrombocytosis. In reactive thrombocytosis, therapy to decrease platelet count is not indicated. Because one third of the platelets are sequestered in the spleen, individuals with functional asplenia or postsplenectomy have elevated platelet counts. Postsplenectomy thrombocytosis with counts in excess of $1,000,000/mm^3$ is common during the immediate postsplenectomy period. Thromboembolism from this cause is rare in children. ASA, 80 mg every other day, should be given to postsplenectomy patients with marked thrombocytosis to prevent the formation of platelet thrombi. Automated platelet counts may be spuriously elevated due to microspherocytes, red cell and leukocyte fragments, bacteria, and Pappenheimer bodies. Table 10-10 lists the conditions associated with thrombocytosis.

Essential Thrombocythemia

Essential thrombocythemia (ET) is rare in infants and children. It is a clonal myeloproliferative disorder characterized by increased platelets without any attributable cause. The course of ET in young patients is more benign than in adults; however, thrombotic (in 30% of cases) and hemorrhagic complications (usually minor) do occur. The diagnostic criteria of ET are as follows:

1. Platelet count: >600,000/mm^3
2. Hemoglobin: ≤13 g/dL
3. Normal red cell mass (males, <36 mL/kg; females, <32 mL/kg)
4. Normal stainable iron in bone marrow
5. Absence of collagen fibrosis of bone marrow
6. Absence of Philadelphia chromosome, including by molecular analysis
7. Abnormal platelet function tests
8. No known cause for reactive thrombocytosis.

Table 10-11 lists the diagnostic features of ET and details its differentiation from reactive thrombocytosis.

Table 10-10. Conditions Associated with Thrombocytosis in Infants and Children

Hereditary	Carcinoma of colon, lung
Asplenia	Hepatoblastoma
Myeloproliferative disorder in Down	Neuroblastoma
syndrome	Myelodysplastic states
Nutritional	5q-syndrome
Iron deficiency (chronic blood loss)	Sideroblastic anemia
Vitamin E deficiency	Traumatic
Megaloblastic anemia	Surgery
Metabolic	Fractures
Hyperadrenalism	Hemorrhage
Immune	Miscellaneous
Graft versus host reaction	Splenectomy
Nephrotic syndrome	Caffey disease
Infectious	Inflammatory bowel disease
Viral (e.g., CMV)	Rheumatoid arthritis
Bacterial	Polyarteritis nodosa
Mycobacterial	Pulmonary embolism
Fungal	Thrombophlebitis
Drug response	Cerebrovascular accident
Vinca alkaloids	Sarcoidosis
Citrovorum factor	Kawasaki disease
Corticosteroid therapy	Acute blood loss
Epinephrine	Hemolytic anemia
Neoplastic	Exercise
Chronic myeloid leukemia	Acute rheumatic fever
Polycythemia vera	Ankylosing spondylitis
Essential thrombocythemia	Spurious
Histiocytosis	Idiopathic
Lymphoma, Hodgkin disease	

Table 10-11. Differentiation of Essential Thrombocythemia and Reactive Thrombocytosis

	Reactive thrombocytosis	Essential thrombocythemia
Clinical and laboratory features		
Thromboembolism and hemorrhage	Uncommon	Common (in adults)[a]
Duration	Often transitory	Usually persistent
Splenomegaly	Usually absent	Present in 80% of cases
Platelet count	Usually <1,000,000/mm^3	Usually >1,000,000/mm^3
Bleeding time	Usually normal	Often prolonged
Platelet morphology and function	Usually normal	Often abnormal
Leukocyte count	Usually normal	Increased in 90% of cases
Thrombokinetic features		
Total megakaryocyte mass	Slightly increased	Greatly increased
Megakaryocyte number	Increased	Increased
Megakaryocyte volume	Decreased	Decreased
Platelet turnover or production rate	Increased	Increased
Total platelet mass	Increased	Increased
Platelet survival	Normal	Normal to slightly decreased

[a]Rare in younger children.

Modified from Bithell TC. Thrombocytosis. In: Wintrobe's Clinical Hematology. 9th ed. Philadelphia: Lea & Febiger, 1993;1391, with permission.

Treatment

Asymptomatic children may not need to be treated. When treatment is required the following drugs can be utilized:

1. Antiplatelet agents:
   a. ASA: 80–160 mg PO once daily
   b. Dipyridamole: 3–6 mg/kg/day PO in 3 divided doses
2. Platelet-lowering drugs:
   a. Hydroxyurea: 20–30 mg/kg PO once daily, until platelet count is between 300,000 and 600,000/mm^3; maintenance therapy is necessary to sustain remission with dosage adjustment.
   b. Anagrelide hydrochloride (Anagralin; Roberts Pharmaceuticals, Eatontown, NJ, USA). Dose is 1 mg PO daily until platelet count is between 300,000 and 600,000/mm^3; maintenance therapy is necessary to sustain remission with dosage adjustment. *Toxicity:* headache, 30%; tachycardia, 27%; fluid retention, 24%; dizziness, 15%; arrhythmias, <10%. *Indications:* The thrombotic risk of asymptomatic children with ET with no history of thrombosis may not significantly differ from that of the general population. Therefore, treatment may not be necessary in this subgroup.
   c. Interferon α-2a: The safety and efficacy in children under 18 years of age have not been established.

QUALITATIVE PLATELET DISORDERS

Qualitative platelet disorders may result from either congenital or acquired conditions. All are characterized by a prolonged bleeding time and a bleeding tendency based on faulty platelet plug formation in the face of normal platelet numbers. The clinical findings are petechiae, purpura, and mucosal bleeding.

Congenital

Table 10-12 lists the congenital disorders causing defective platelet function. Table 10-13 lists the differential laboratory features in inherited disorders of platelet function. Table 11-22 (Chapter 11) lists the genetic transmission and primary and alternative treatment of hereditary disorders of platelet function.

Defects in Platelet Receptor–Agonist Interaction

1. *Selective impairment in platelet responsiveness to adrenaline:* The interaction of platelets with adrenaline in *in vitro* aggregation tests is mediated by α_2-adrenergic

---

Table 10-12. Classification of Congenital Platelet Function Disorders

Defects in platelet–agonist interaction (receptor defects)
  Selective adrenaline defect
  Selective collagen defect
  Selective thromboxane A_2 defect
  Selective ADP defect
Defects in platelet–vessel wall interaction (disorders of adhesion)
  von Willebrand's disease (deficiency or defect in plasma VWF)
  Bernard–Soulier syndrome (deficiency or defect in GPIb)
Defects in platelet–platelet interaction (disorders of aggregation)
  Congenital afibrinogenemia
  Glanzmann thrombasthenia (deficiency or defect in GPIIb/IIIa)
Disorders of platelet secretion
  Storage pool deficiency
    δ-Storage pool deficiency
      Hermansky–Pudlak syndrome
      Chédiak–Higashi syndrome
    α-Storage pool deficiency (gray platelet syndrome)
    $\alpha\delta$-Storage pool deficiency
    May Hegglin anomaly and MYH9-related disease
  Abnormalities in arachidonic acid pathway
    Impaired liberation of arachidonic acid
    Cyclooxygenase deficiency
    Thromboxane synthetase deficiency
    Altered nucleotide metabolism
    Glycogen storage disease
    Fructose-1,6-diphosphonate deficiency
  Primary secretion defect with normal granule stores and normal thromboxane synthesis
    Defects in calcium mobilization
    Defects in phosphatidylinositol metabolism
    Defects in myosin phosphorylation
  Disorders of platelet–coagulant protein interaction
    Defect in factor Va–Xa interaction on platelets
Platelet factor 3 deficiency (Alport syndrome)
Vascular or connective tissue defect
  Ehlers–Danlos syndrome
  Pseudoxanthoma elasticum
  Marfan syndrome
  Osteogenesis imperfecta
  Hereditary hemorrhagic telangiectasia (Osler–Weber–Rendu disease)

Table 10-13. Laboratory Findings in Inherited Platelet Function Disorders

	Glanzmann thrombasthenia	Storage pool deficiency[a]	Collagen receptor defect	Release defect[b]	Bernard–Soulier syndrome	Von Willebrand disease
Platelet count	Normal	Normal	Normal	Normal	Decreased	Normal
Platelet size	Normal	Microplatelets	Normal	Normal	"Giant platelets"	Normal
Bleeding time	Prolonged	Variable	Variable	Variable	Prolonged	Prolonged
Platelet aggregation						
ADP	Absent	No second wave	Normal	No second wave	Normal	Normal
Arachidonic acid	Absent	Variable	Absent	Decreased	Normal	Normal
Collagen	Absent	Decreased	Normal	Absent	Normal	Normal
Ristocetin (1.5 mg/ml)	Normal	Normal	Normal	Normal	Absent	Variable[c]
Ristocetin (0.5 mg/ml)	Absent	Decreased	Absent	Absent	Normal	Variable[c]
Storage nucleotide pool	Normal	Decreased	Normal	Normal	Normal	Normal
Others	HPA1a absent; GP IIb and IIIa deficient	Dense bodies reduced; ATP/ADP ratio increased	GP Ia and IIa deficient	Cyclooxygenase; thromboxane synthetase or TxA₂ receptor deficient	GP Ib deficiency	Decreased FVIII, VWF antigen, and ristocetin cofactor

[a]In Hermansky–Pudlak, Chédiak–Higashi, and Wiskott–Aldrich syndromes.
[b]Classically occurs with acetylsalicylic acid and other drugs affecting arachidonic acid and prostaglandin pathway.
[c]Types I and II, decreased; Type IIb increased; Type III absent.

receptors and results in several responses, including the exposure of fibrinogen receptors, an increase in intracellular ionized calcium, the inhibition of adenylate cyclase activity, and platelet aggregation. Some patients have impaired aggregation and secretion responses only to adrenaline, associated with a decrease in the number of platelet α_2-adrenergic receptors, with a history of easy bruising and minimally prolonged bleeding times. On the other hand, platelets of 10% of apparently normal people may fail to aggregate in response to adrenaline. The clinical significance of this finding is unclear.

2. *Selective impairment in platelet responsiveness to collagen:* Patients have a bleeding disorder characterized by platelets that are selectively unresponsive to collagen. The platelets are deficient in platelet membrane glycoprotein GP Ia and thrombospondin.
3. *Selective impairment in platelet responsiveness to thromboxane A_2:* Patients have selective impairment in responses to thromboxane A_2.
4. *Selective impairment in platelet responsiveness to ADP:* Platelets show diminished response to ADP and decreased number of binding sites for ADP analogs.

Defects in Platelet Vessel–Wall Interaction (Table 10-12)

1. *Von Willebrand disease:* See Chapter 11.
2. *Bernard–Soulier syndrome:* Patients have a prolonged bleeding time and large platelets on a blood smear. The platelet count is variable. The disorder is transmitted as an autosomal recessive disorder. Affected patients experience purpura, epistaxis, gingival bleeding, menorrhagia, gastrointestinal hemorrhage, and hematuria. Bleeding into joints or muscles does not occur.

The primary defect is a deficiency in platelet membrane glycoprotein GP Ib. The α-chain of GP Ib contains a specific receptor for vWF, and platelets deficient in this glycoprotein fail to bind to vWF in the subendothelial matrix and, therefore, do not adhere to damaged blood vessels under conditions of flow. Platelets aggregate normally in the presence of ADP, collagen, and adrenaline; exhibit reduced aggregation responses to low concentrations of thrombin; and fail to agglutinate in the presence of autologous plasma and the negatively charged antibiotic ristocetin. Treatment is platelet transfusions, DDAVP, and activated factor VII.

Defects in Platelet–Platelet Interaction (Table 10-12)

Glanzmann Thrombasthenia

This is an autosomal recessive bleeding disorder characterized by the following:

1. Normal platelet count and morphology
2. Prolonged bleeding time
3. Absent or diminished clot retraction
4. Defective platelet aggregation
5. Repeated mucocutaneous bleeding.

The biochemical defect is a reduction or functional abnormality in the platelet membrane glycoprotein, GP IIb/IIIa, which mediates aggregation of activated platelets by binding the adhesive proteins fibrinogen, vWF, and fibronectin. Thrombasthenic platelets fail to aggregate in response to physiologic agonists such as ADP, thrombin, and adrenaline; they do agglutinate in the presence of ristocetin. Thrombasthenic platelets attach normally to damaged subendothelium but fail to spread normally and do not form platelet aggregates. Treatment is platelet transfusions. Patients may become refractory to transfusions and may require activated factor VII.

Disorders of Platelet Secretion (Table 10-12)

Storage pool disease (SPD) includes patients with deficiencies of dense granules (δSPD), α-granules (α-SPD), or both types of granules (αδ-SPD).

δ-Storage Pool Deficiency

The total adenosine triphosphate (ATP) and adenosine diphosphate (ADP) platelet granule content in patients with δ-SPD is decreased as are other dense granule contents, including calcium, pyrophosphate, and serotonin. Patients have a mild to moderate bleeding disorder. In platelet aggregation studies, the second wave of aggregation with ADP and adrenaline is absent, and the aggregation response to collagen is either markedly impaired or absent. The response to arachidonic acid is variable. Platelet SPD has been reported in patients with prolonged bleeding times and normal platelet aggregation tests. The disorder has also been reported in association with α-granule deficiency and with other inherited disorders such as Hermansky–Pudlak syndrome (HPS), Chédiak–Higashi syndrome (CHS), Wiskott–Aldrich syndrome (WAS), and TAR syndrome.

Hermansky–Pudlak syndrome
The HPS-1 gene is located on the long arm of chromosome 10. Patients have oculocutaneous albinism, photophobia, rotatory nystagmus, loss of visual acuity, ceroid-like material accumulation in reticuloendothelial cells, and mild to moderate hemorrhagic diathesis. Dense bodies are reduced or virtually absent. Platelets contain very low levels of serotonin, adenine nucleotides, and Ca^{2+}. As a result, platelets do not secrete adequate amounts of these messengers and fail to develop secondary waves of aggregation when exposed to concentrations of ADP, adrenaline, and thrombin that cause irreversible clumping of normal cells. The cause of death is pulmonary fibrosis.

Chédiak–Higashi syndrome
The Chédiak–Higashi gene is located on the long arm of chromosome 1. Patients have partial albinism. Leukocytes, lymphocytes, monocytes, and platelets have large intracytoplasmic granules. Immune dysfunction leads to overwhelming infections or lymphoproliferative disease.

α-Granule Storage Pool Deficiency

The term *gray platelet* describes the morphologic appearance of platelets in Romanovsky-stained peripheral blood smears prepared from patients with a deficiency of α-granules. Platelets from these patients contain absent or markedly reduced α-granule proteins: PF4, vWF, fibronectin, and factor V. Affected patients have mild thrombocytopenia, prolonged bleeding times, and a lifelong bleeding diathesis. The most consistent laboratory abnormality has been impairment in thrombin-mediated aggregation and secretion; aggregation responses to collagen and ADP are variable. Electron microscopy studies reveal the virtual absence of α-granules.

Quebec platelet disorder (factor V Quebec)
Quebec platelet disorder (QPD) is an autosomal dominant condition with mild thrombocytopenia, increased megakaryocytes, defective epinephrine-induced platelet aggregation, and decreased concentration of granule proteins. There is increased storage of urokinase-type plasminogen activator (u-PA). The u-PA generates plasmin, causing degradation of platelet fibrinogen and other α-granule proteins important for hemostasis. Measurements of platelet u-PA and α-granule

fibrinogen degradation products allow accurate diagnosis. The granules appear morphologically normal. These patients have mucocutaneous bleeding and some have joint bleeds and bleeding 12 hours or more after trauma. These clinical manifestations are consistent with the abnormalities of QPD, because it is not only a disorder of platelet function with abnormalities of aggregation but also a disorder of fibrin clot formation and fibrinolysis. The bleeding is unresponsive to platelet transfusions.

May Hegglin Anomaly

The May Hegglin anomaly is characterized by the presence of giant platelets, thrombocytopenia, and Döhle bodies in the leukocytes. Platelets may contain giant granules. Some patients with this disorder have platelet function abnormalities. The disorder is inherited in an autosomal dominant fashion and the majority of affected individuals does not have a significant bleeding disorder. Recently a family of macrothrombocytopenias has been linked to non-muscle myosin heavy-chain 9 gene (*MYH9*), which encodes non-muscle myosin heavy chain IIA. These disorders, including May Hegglin anomaly, Alport, Sebastian, Epstein, and Fechtner syndromes have been named MYH9-related disease. Non-muscle myosin heavy-chain IIA is expressed in the platelets, kidney, leukocytes, and cochlea. As a result, these patients have a combination of mild thrombocytopenia, leukocyte inclusions, nephritis, sensorineural deafness and cataracts (Table 10-14).

Miscellaneous platelet function abnormalities have also been reported in WAS, TAR syndrome, hexokinase deficiency and glucose-6-phosphatase deficiency (type I glycogen storage disease).

Abnormalities in Platelet Arachidonic Acid Pathways (Table 10-12)

Impaired Liberation of Arachidonic Acid

A major response of platelets during activation is the release of arachidonic acid from membrane-bound phospholipids and its subsequent oxygenation to thromboxane A_2. Thromboxane A_2 forms an important positive feedback that enhances platelet activation.

Cyclooxygenase and Thromboxane Synthetase Deficiency

Defects in thromboxane A_2 due to deficiencies of cyclooxygenase and thromboxane synthetase have been reported.

Table 10-14. Clinical and Morphologic Features of the Five Autosomal Dominant Macrothrombocytopenias

| | Clinical Feature[a] | | | | |
Disorder	Thrombocy-topenia	Leukocyte inclusions	Nephritis	High-tone sensorineural deafness	Cataracts
May Hegglin anomaly	+	+	—	—	—
Sebastian syndrome	+	+	—	—	—
Epstein syndrome	+	—	+	+	—
Fechtner syndrome	+	+	+	+	+
Alport syndrome	+	—	+	+	+

[a]+, present; —, absent.

Platelet Secretion Defects with Normal Granule Stores and Normal Thromboxane Synthesis (Table 10-12)

Several studies have identified patients with a mild bleeding diathesis whose platelets have normal granule stores and normal thromboxane A_2 synthesis during stimulation. This category also includes patients with behavioral attention deficit disorder or minimal brain damage syndrome and easy bruising. Many affected patients have abnormalities in the aggregation and secretion responses to weak agonists (ADP, adrenaline) but not to relatively stronger agonists such as arachidonic acid or higher concentrations of collagen.

Defects in Ca^{2+} Mobilization

A number of key platelet processes are Ca^{2+} dependent (e.g., liberation of arachidonic acid and phosphorylation of myosin light chain). Patients with deficient Ca^{2+} mobilization have been reported.

Deficiency of Platelet Procoagulant Activity (Table 10-12)

Platelets contain several coagulation factors in their granules and provide negatively charged lipid surfaces on which a number of key coagulation enzymatic reactions proceed. Platelet factor 3 reflects the contribution of platelets to the interaction of factors Xa, Va, and Ca^{2+} in prothrombin activation. In Scott syndrome, platelets have a decreased number of factor Xa binding sites. Bleeding time, platelet aggregation, and secretion are normal. The patients have a shortened PT as a result of reduced prothrombin consumption.

Acquired

Table 10-15 lists the acquired disorders that cause defective platelet function.

Drug Ingestion

Acetylsalicylic acid (ASA) has been shown to impair platelet aggregation *in vivo* and *in vitro* by inhibiting the release of ADP. Accompanying the impaired aggregation is prolongation of the bleeding time. As low a dose as 300 mg may permanently affect the cohort of platelets circulating at the time so that the defect can be detected in decreasing severity over a period of 4–7 days after exposure. This is related to the normal platelet life span.

The practical importance of ASA-induced platelet dysfunction is apparent in the following clinical situations:

1. The relationship between ASA ingestion and excessive post-tonsillectomy bleeding
2. The occurrence of purpura in children after ingestion of ASA
3. The finding of prolonged bleeding time in investigating children with suspected hemostatic defects
4. The risk of mislabeling cases as mild von Willebrand disease because of ASA ingestion prior to testing.

Table 10-16 lists other commonly used drugs that have been implicated in platelet dysfunction.

Platelet aggregation may be impaired in the newborn following maternal drug therapy. For this reason, a history of drug ingestion is an essential part of the investigation of hemorrhagic states in the newborn period.

Table 10-15. Acquired Disorders Causing Defective Platelet Function

I. **Vascular or connective tissue defects**
 A. Scurvy
 B. Amyloidosis

II. **Adhesion defects**
 A. Acquired von Willebrand disease
 B. Renal failure
 C. Drugs: dipyridamole

III. **Platelet aggregation defects**
 A. Fibrin or fibrinogen split products: DIC, liver disease
 B. Macromolecules: paraproteins, dextran
 C. Drugs: penicillin, semisynthetic penicillins, cephalosporins

IV. **Release reaction defects**
 A. Storage pool deficiency
  1. α-Granules: cardiopulmonary bypass
  2. Dense granules: ITP, SLE
  3. Drugs: reserpine, tricyclic antidepressants, phenothiazines
 B. Defective release
  1. Platelet dyspoiesis: myelodysplastic syndromes, acute leukemias, myeloproliferative syndromes
  2. Drugs: aspirin, other nonsteroidal anti-inflammatory agents, furosemide, nitrofurantoin
  3. Ethanol
 C. Altered nucleotide metabolism
  1. Drugs: phosphodiesterase inhibitors or stimulators of adenylcyclase

V. **Other defects**
 A. Drugs: heparin, sympathetic blockers, clofibrate, antihistamines
 B. Infection: viral
 C. Hypothyroidism

Renal Failure

A generalized hemorrhagic state is known to occur in advanced renal failure. Thrombocytopenia is present in a minority of patients, and reduced platelet adhesiveness to glass and defective ADP-induced platelet factor 3 activation occur.

Liver Disease

In addition to a deficiency of coagulation factors of the prothrombin complex in liver disease, an abnormality of platelet function has been described. Platelet aggregation by ADP and thrombin is significantly delayed in patients with cirrhosis and prolonged thrombin time. This is due to the known inhibition of platelet function by fibrinogen degradation products, resulting from excessive fibrinolysis occurring in advanced liver disease.

Management of Defects in Platelet Function

The management of defects in platelet function consists of the following steps:

1. Remove the cause of platelet dysfunction (e.g., drugs).
2. Treat the underlying disorder (e.g., steroids in immune-mediated dysfunction).

Table 10-16. Drugs Implicated in Platelet Dysfunction

Antibiotics
Ampicillin[a]
Carbenicillin[a]
Furadantin[a]
Gentamycin[a]
Keflin[a]
Moxalactam[a]
Nafcillin[a]
Piperacillin[a]
Quinacrin[b]

Anti-inflammatory drugs
Acetylsalicylic acid[b]
Colchicine[c]
Ibuprofen[b]
Indomethacin[b]
Naprosyn[b]
Phenylbutazone[b]

Anesthetics
Cocaine[a]
Nupercaine[a]
Procaine[a]
Xylocaine[a]

Cardiovascular/respiratory
Aminophylline[d]
Dicumarol[e]
Dipyridamole[d]
Heparin[e]
Hydralazine[b]
Nitroglycerin[f]

Papaverine[e]
Propranolol[a]
Reserpine[a]
Theophyllin[d]
Verapamil[b]

Diuretics
Acetazolamide[e]
Ethacrynic acid[e]
Furosemide[b]

Psychiatric drugs
Eventyl[a]
Elavil[a]
Norpramin[a]
Sinequan[a]
Stelazine[a]
Tofranil[a]

Others
Alcohol[a]
Benedryl[a]
Caffeine[d]
Cyclosporine[a,b]
Dextran[a]
Glycerol guaiacolate[e]
Hydrocortisone[b]
Methylprednisolone[b]
Phenergan[a]
Tocopherol[b]
Vinblastine[c]
Vincristine[c]

[a]Interference with membrane receptors.
[b]Interference with prostaglandin synthesis.
[c]Interference with thrombostatin.
[d]Interference with phosphodiesterase.
[e]Unknown mechanism of action.
[f]Interference with platelet cyclic adenosine monophosphate (AMP).

3. Use platelet transfusions during hemorrhagic episodes or major surgery.
4. Administer DDAVP or cryoprecipitate—may shorten bleeding time in some patients with:
   a. Renal failure
   b. Inherited or acquired defects in release reaction
   c. Inherited or acquired von Willebrand disease.
5. Administer ε-aminocaproic acid (EACA)—may have some benefit in mucosal hemorrhage (oral, nasal, and gastrointestinal tract); the dose is 50 mg/kg orally every 6 hours for 7 days. EACA is contraindicated in the management of bleeding in the urinary tract.
6. Administer activated factor VII.

INHERITED VASCULAR AND CONNECTIVE TISSUE DISORDERS

Ehlers–Danlos Syndrome

Ehlers–Danlos syndrome is an uncommon disorder of connective tissues characterized by hyperextensible skin, hypermobile joints, fragile tissues, and a bleeding tendency, mainly subcutaneous hematoma. Affected individuals may present with easy bruising, bleeding from gums after dental extraction, gastrointestinal bleeding, and hemarthroses. Rupture of major arteries may occur in type IV (ecchymotic) Ehlers–Danlos syndrome. This disorder is associated with decreased levels of type III collagen, which predominates in blood vessels and the gastrointestinal tract.

Pseudoxanthoma Elasticum

This is a rare disorder of elastic tissues that is inherited as an autosomal trait. Severely affected individuals present with spontaneous hemorrhage resulting from defective vessels, and bleeding may occur into the skin, eyes, kidney, joints, uterus, and gastrointestinal tract. Fatal outcome is usually due to subarachnoid and gastrointestinal hemorrhage.

Marfan Syndrome

Marfan syndrome is characterized by skeletal abnormalities, cardiovascular abnormalities, and dislocation of the lens. The syndrome is transmitted as an autosomal-dominant trait. Affected individuals experience easy bruising and may bleed excessively during surgery.

Osteogenesis Imperfecta

The defect is transmitted as an autosomal dominant trait and is associated with brittle bones. Patients may present with a bleeding disorder characterized by bruising, epistaxis, hemoptysis, and intracranial hemorrhage. The basic abnormality seems to be a defect in the amino acid composition of collagen fibers.

Hereditary Hemorrhagic Telangiectasia

Hereditary hemorrhagic telangiectasia (*Osler–Weber–Rendu disease*) is the most common of the inherited vascular disorders. The disease is inherited as an autosomal dominant trait and bleeding occurs from vascular lesions on the skin or mucous membranes. Lesions consist of dilated arterioles and capillaries lined by a thin endothelial layer. They are typical in appearance (1–3 mm in diameter, flat, round, and red or violet in color), and they blanch on pressure. Histology of the abnormal vessels shows a deficiency of supporting elastic fibers. Typical lesions occur most often on the nasal mucosa, lips, oral mucosa, tongue, face, hands, gastrointestinal tract, and, rarely, in the respiratory, gynecological, and urinary tracts. Epistaxis is usually the most common symptomatology.

LABORATORY EVALUATION OF PLATELETS AND PLATELET FUNCTION

The following tests are useful in determining platelet number and function.

Examination of Blood Smear

A disproportionate number (>15%) of platelets larger than 2.5 μm^3 in diameter suggests increased platelet turnover. The large platelets represent a younger population. The mean platelet volume using automatic electronic counters is raised (normal, 8.9±1.5 fL). This indicates peripheral platelet destruction rather than impairment of platelet formation. Table 10-1 lists the various platelet diseases based on platelet size.

Bleeding Time

The Milke template method (a modification of the Ivy method) is the most sensitive in general use. The normal bleeding time in children is less than 9 minutes. The bleeding time is prolonged when platelet counts are less than approximately 100,000/mm³ or when platelet adhesion or aggregation is abnormal (e.g., von Willebrand disease, acquired or congenital platelet function abnormalities).

Closure Time

The platelet function analyzer (PFA-100®; Dade Behring, Deerfield, IL, USA) was developed as a rapid, quantitative, *in vitro* test of platelet function at high shear rates. Citrated whole blood is aspirated through a 150-μm-diameter aperture in a membrane coated with collagen and epinephrine or adenosine 5′-diphosphate. This stimulates a high shear condition and results in the vWF-dependent attachment, activation, and aggregation of platelets, resulting in a closure time that is dependent on occlusion of the aperture by a stable platelet plug. Closure time is superior to the bleeding time for most cases of von Willebrand disease, aspirin effect, and for some causes of platelet dysfunction, giving a very high negative predictive value. Because of the dependence on blood flow, test results can be influenced by the sample's hematocrit. Hematocrit of 25–50% and a platelet count of 100,000/mm³ are required for optimal results.

Platelet Aggregation in Platelet-Rich Plasma

Aggregating agents such as ADP, thrombin, and epinephrine induce platelet aggregation and/or cause platelets to release endogenous ADP. Platelet aggregation may be observed with a platelet aggregometer, which is a photo-optical instrument connected to a recording chart. Platelet-rich plasma, which is turbid, is stirred in a cuvette, and the transmittance of light through the sample, relative to a platelet-poor plasma blank, is recorded. When an aggregating agent is added, the formation of increasingly large platelet aggregates is accompanied by a clearing in the platelet-rich plasma, thereby increasing light transmittance through the sample. The light received through the sample is converted through the electronic signals, amplified, and recorded on chart paper.

1. A biphasic aggregation response, that is, a primary and a secondary wave of aggregation, is induced by low concentrations of ADP.
2. Epinephrine also produces a biphasic response.
3. Collagen induces only a single wave of aggregation, which corresponds to the release reaction of platelets.
4. Thrombin induces both a primary and a secondary wave of aggregation.
5. Ristocetin induces a biphasic aggregation response. Because aggregation with ristocetin may be reduced or absent in von Willebrand disease, ristocetin may be used in the quantitative assay of von Willebrand factor.

6. Arachidonic acid causes rapid secondary (irreversible) aggregation. Nonsteroidal anti-inflammatory drugs (NSAIDs), such as indomethacin and aspirin, are potent inhibitors of aggregation induced by arachidonic acid.

Aspirin, aspirin-containing compounds, and other NSAIDs will inhibit platelet aggregation by interfering with the release reaction of the platelet. Therefore, a secondary wave of aggregation will not be produced. Aggregation curves may show either a disaggregation after the primary wave occurs or an absence or reduction of aggregation, which occurs when collagen is the aggregating agent. There are many disorders in which platelet aggregation will be abnormal, either decreased or increased.

Platelet Aggregation in Whole Blood

A platelet aggregation study may be performed on whole blood using an impedance aggregometer (Lumi aggregometer). This technique gives information on the kinetics of aggregate formation, and a simultaneous assessment of secretory exocytosis is possible by measuring the ATP released from dense bodies using the firefly luciferen–luciferase system. This method makes it possible to quickly detect patients who require further study for possible platelet function disorders such as cyclooxygenase deficiency, storage pool defect, thrombasthenia, and von Willebrand disease. The results obtained with this electrical impedance instrument do not differ from those obtained with the conventional optical method. However, it is now possible to recognize a platelet function defect within 30 minutes of obtaining a 5-mL sample of citrated whole blood. Further, platelets of unusual size or density are not lost to testing through centrifugation.

A number of other tests have been utilized to investigate platelet function and may be required in an individual case:

- Platelet retention and adhesiveness
- Platelet factor 3
- Adenosine diphosphate release
- Capillary fragility
- Clot retraction
- Platelet electrophoresis
- Antiplatelet antibodies
- Platelet survival.

NONTHROMBOCYTOPENIC PURPURA

Anaphylactoid Purpura

Henoch–Schönlein purpura is nonthrombocytopenic vascular purpura. The purpuric eruption differs considerably from that due to thrombocytopenia in that lesions are maculopapular, initially resembling urticaria because of edema and perivascular infiltration and later becoming erythematous, with central areas of hemorrhage that finally fade to brown because of denaturation of the extravasated hemoglobin. The rash appears on the buttocks and on the extensor surfaces of the arms and lower legs. Accompanying the rash are joint or gastrointestinal symptoms, localized areas of edema, and renal damage. Initial hematuria occurs in about one third of patients. The platelet count, bleeding time, and tests for hemostasis are normal. A positive tourniquet test is found in 25% of patients. Treatment is symptomatic. When severe abdominal pain is present, steroid therapy is beneficial.

Infections

Any infections may present with nonthrombocytopenic purpura, including acute bacterial endocarditis, meningococcal septicemia, coxsackievirus, and echovirus infections, rubella, and atypical measles.

Drugs

Diffuse, benign, and self-limiting purpura has been described after exposure to certain drugs (e.g., sulfonamide).

Purpura Factitia

Although it is rare, purpura factitia may present a problem in diagnosis. It is self-inflicted purpura, is usually linear, and is always on accessible parts of the body. It is more common in females than in males and frequently indicates deep-seated psychopathology. All hematologic tests are normal.

SUGGESTED READINGS

Bianch V, Robles R, Alberio L, et al. Von Willebrand factor-cleaving protease (ADAMTS13) in thrombocytopenic disorders: a severely deficient activity is specific for thrombotic thrombocytopenic purpura. Blood 2002;100:710–3.

Blanchette VS, Price V. Childhood chronic immune thrombocytopenic purpura: unresolved issues. J Pediatr Hematol Oncol 2003;25:S28–33.

Bolton-Maggs PHB. Idiopathic thrombocytopenic purpura. Arch Dis Child 2000;83:220–2.

Bussell JB, Skupski DW, MacFarland JG. Fetal alloimmune thrombocytopenia: concensus and controversy. The Journal of Maternal-Fetal Medicine 1996;5:281–292.

Cines DB, Blanchette VS. Medical progress: immune thrombocytopenic purpura. New Engl J Med 2002;346(13):995–1008.

Fetal alloimmune thrombocytopenia: consensus and controversy. J Maternal-Fetal Med 1996;5:281–92.

George JN, Woolf SH, Raskob GE, et al. Idiopathic thrombocytopenic purpura: a practice guideline developed by the explicit methods for the American Society of Hematology. Blood 1996;88(1):3–40.

Heath KE, Campos-Barros A, Toren A, et al. Nonmuscle myosin heavy chain IIA mutations define a spectrum of autosomal dominant thrombocytopenias: May-Hegglin anomaly and Fechtner, Sebastian, Epstein and Alport-like syndromes. Am J Hum Genet 2001;69:1033–1045.

Nonmuscle myosin heavy chain IIA mutations define a spectrum of autosomal dominant thrombocytopenias: May-Hegglin anomaly and Fechtner, Sebastian, Epstein, and Alport-like syndromes. Am J Hum Genet 2001;69:1033–45.

Vesely SK, George JN, Lammie B, et al. ADAMTS13 activity in thrombotic thrombocytopenic purpura-hemolytic uremic syndrome: relation to presenting features and clinical outcomes in a prospective cohort of 142 patients. Blood 2003;102(1):60–8.

Wilson DB. Acquired platelet defects. In: Nathan DG, Orkin SH, Ginsburg D, Look AT, editors. Nathan and Oski's hematology of Infancy and Childhood. 6th ed. Philadelphia: W.B. Saunders, 2003.

11

DISORDERS OF COAGULATION

HEMOSTATIC DISORDERS

Physiology of Hemostasis

As a result of injury to the blood vessel endothelium, three events take place simultaneously:

1. Vasoconstriction (vascular phase)
2. Platelet plug formation (primary hemostatic mechanism—platelet phase)
3. Fibrin thrombus formation (initiation, amplification, and propagation phases).

Relevant Components of Hemostasis

Endothelial cells secrete substances that repel platelets (prostaglandin I2 [PGI2], and nitric oxide), initiate coagulation (collagen, fibronectin), promote platelet adhesion (von Willebrand's factor [vWF]), platelet aggregation (adenosine diphosphate [ADP] and fibrin dissolution (tissue plasminogen activator), catalyze the inhibition of thrombin (heparin and thrombomodulin), and inhibit the initiation of fibrin dissolution (tissue plasminogen activator inhibitor).

Participation of platelets in hemostasis is a fundamental component of the physiologic process of coagulation. Platelet interactions in coagulation are initiated by adhesion to areas of vascular injury. Subsequent activation of platelets results in release of ADP, serotonin, and calcium from "dense bodies" and fibrinogen, vWF, factor V, HMW kininogen, fibronectin, α_1-antitrypsin, β-thromboglobulin, platelet factor 4 (PF4), and platelet-derived growth factor from α-granules. Platelets provide surfaces for the assembly of coagulation factors (e.g.,VIIIa/Ca^{2+}/IXa and Va/Ca^{2+}/Xa complexes). The platelets aggregate and increase the mass of the hemostatic plug. They also mediate blood vessel constriction (by releasing serotonin) and neutralize heparin.

All of the plasma coagulation factors are produced in the liver; factor VIII is also produced by endothelial cells. Table 11-1 lists the half-life and plasma levels of the coagulation factors. Factors II, VII, IX, and X are vitamin K dependent and require vitamin K in order to undergo post-translational gamma carboxylation. These vitamin K–dependent factors circulate in zymogen form, are activated on platelet phospholipid surfaces, and upon activation have serine protease activity. The plasma coagulation factors work in an interdependent manner to generate thrombin (factor IIa) from prothrombin (factor II); thrombin then digests fibrinogen to form fibrin monomers. Fibrin monomers polymerize and establish a network. By incorporating

Table 11-1. Half-Life and Plasma Levels of Coagulation Factors

Factors	Common name	Biologic half-life (h)	Plasma concentration (nM)	Plasma levels (units/dL)
I	Fibrinogen	90	8800	200–400[b]
II	Prothrombin[a]	60	1400	50–150
III	Tissue thromboplastin	N/A		0
V	Proaccelerin, labile factor	12–36	20	50–150
VII	Proconvertin,[a] stable factor	6–8	10	50–150
VIII	Antihemophilic factor	8–12	0.7	50–150
IX	Christmas factor[a]	12–24	90	50–150
X	Stuart factor[a]	32–58	170	50–150
XI	Plasma thromboplastin antecedent	48–72	30	50–150
XII	Hageman factor	48–52	375	50–150
XIII	Fibrin-stabilizing factor	72–120	70	50–150
High-molecular-weight kininogen	Fitzgerald factor	136	6000	—
Prekallikrein	Fletcher factor	N/A	450	—

[a]Vitamin K–dependent.
[b]In mg/dL.

into the hemostatic plug, thrombin becomes inactivated. Thrombin plays a central bioregulatory role, promoting platelet aggregation and release reactions and generating a biofeedback-positive loop to form more thrombin at a faster rate. Thrombin activates factor XIII, which in turn cross-links the fibrin network. Thrombin and thrombin complexed to thrombomodulin also activate thrombin activatable fibrinolysis inhibitor (TAFI), a procarboxypeptidase found in plasma that attenuates fibrinolysis of the clot. The three components of hemostasis (blood vessels, platelets, and plasma coagulation factors) do not function independently but are integrated.

Primary Hemostatic Mechanism (Platelet Phase)

This mechanism leads to the formation of a reversible aggregate of platelets: a temporary hemostatic plug (Figure 11-1). Endothelial injury exposes von Willebrand factor and collagen from the subendothelial matrix to flowing blood and shear forces. Plasma vWF binds to the exposed collagen, uncoils its structure, and, in synergy with collagen, supports the adhesion of platelets. Initially the vWF interacts with the GPIb platelet receptor, tethering the platelets. Because the platelet collagen receptors GPVI and $\alpha_2\beta_1$ bind to collagen, the platelets adhere and become activated with a resulting release of platelet alpha and dense granule contents. Platelet activation results in a conformational change in the α11bβ3 receptor, activating it and enhancing its avidity for von Willebrand factor, for vessel wall ligands, and for fibrinogen. The enhanced avidity for von Willebrand factor and fibrinogen mediates platelet-to-platelet interactions, which eventually lead to platelet plug formation.

Fibrin Thrombus Formation

The fibrin thrombus formation component of hemostasis occurs in three overlapping phases: initiation, amplification, and propagation (Figure 11-2). The *initiation phase* begins with cell-based expression of tissue factor (TF) at the site of endothe-

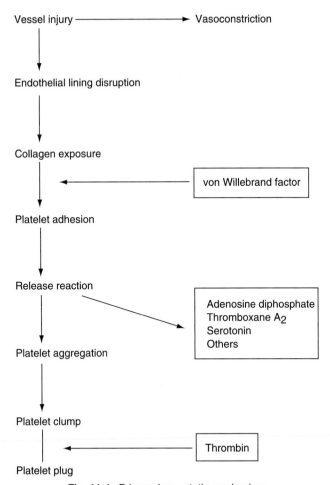

Vessel injury ─────────────────→ Vasoconstriction

Endothelial lining disruption

Collagen exposure

← von Willebrand factor

Platelet adhesion

Release reaction

Adenosine diphosphate
Thromboxane A$_2$
Serotonin
Others

Platelet aggregation

Platelet clump

← Thrombin

Platelet plug

Fig. 11-1. Primary hemostatic mechanism.

lial injury. Factor VII binds to the exposed TF and is rapidly activated. The factor VIIa/TF complex in turn generates factor Xa (FXa) and factor IXa (FIXa). FXa can activate factor V (FV), which complexes with FXa and generates small amounts of thrombin. During the *amplification phase*, the procoagulant stimulus is transferred to the surface of platelets at the site of injury. The small amounts of thrombin enhance platelet adhesion, fully activate the platelets, and activate factors V, VIII, and XI. In the *propagation phase*, the "tenase" complex of FIXa-FVIIIa is assembled on the platelet surface and efficiently generates FXa. Similarly the "prothrombinase" complex of FXa-FVa is assembled on the platelet surface and efficiently generates thrombin.

Unlike FXa generated from TF-FVIIa interactions, FXa complexed to FV is protected from inactivation by tissue factor pathway inhibitor, ensuring adequate thrombin generation. The resulting procoagulant, thrombin, activates factor XIII and cleaves fibrinopeptides (FPs) A and B from fibrinogen. The residual peptide chains aggregate by means of loose hydrogen bonds to form fibrin monomers. Under the influence of FXIIIa, fibrin monomers are converted into fibrin polymers, forming a stable fibrin clot. In the presence of thrombin, the mass of loosely aggregated intact platelets is transformed into a densely packed mass that is bound together by strands of fibrin to form a definitive hemostatic barrier against the loss of blood.

I. Initiation

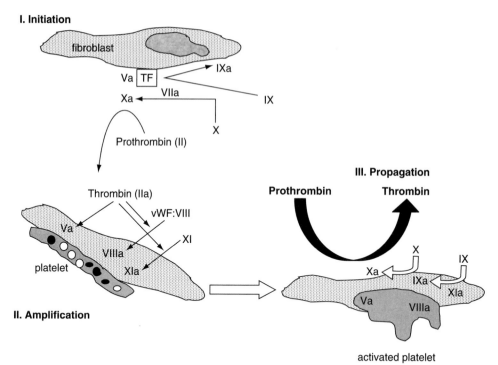

Fig. 11-2. A cell-based model of coagulation. The three phases of coagulation occur on different cell surfaces: initiation on the tissue-factor bearing cell; amplification on the platelet as it becomes activated; and propagation on the activated platelet surface. (Adapted from Hoffman MH, Monroe DM. A cell-based model of hemostasis. Thromb Haemost 2001;85:958–65, with permission.)

Fibrinolysis

The fibrinolytic system provides a mechanism for removal of physiologically deposited fibrin. Clot lysis is brought about by the action of plasmin on fibrin. Fibrinolytic events are shown in Figure 11-3. Plasminogen from circulating plasma is laid down with fibrin during the formation of thrombin. Plasminogen is primarily synthesized in the liver and circulates in two forms, one with an NH_2-terminal glutamic acid residue (glu-plasminogen) and a second form with an NH_2-terminal lysine, valine, or methionine residue (lys-plasminogen). Glu-plasminogen can be converted to lys-plasminogen by limited proteolytic degradation. Lys-plasminogen has a higher affinity for fibrin and cellular receptors and is also more readily activated to plasmin than glu-plasminogen. Both forms of plasminogen bind to fibrin through specific lysine-binding sites. These lysine binding sites also mediate the interaction of plasminogen with its inhibitor, α_2-antiplasmin (α_2AP). Thrombin activated fibrinolysis inhibitor–mediated removal of C-terminal lysine and arginine residues will prevent high-affinity plasminogen binding and will attenuate fibrinolysis. Plasminogen is converted to its enzymatically active form, plasmin, by several activators. These activators are widely distributed in body tissues and fluids. Tissue plasminogen activator (t-PA) is the principal intravascular activator of plasminogen. t-PA is a serine protease that binds to fibrin through lysine-binding sites. When t-PA is bound to fibrin, its plasmin generation efficiency increases markedly. Urokinase-type plasminogen activator (u-PA), a second physiologic activator of plasminogen, is present in urine and activates plasminogen to plasmin equally well in the absence and in the presence of fibrin. Plasmin splits fibrin and fibrinogen into fibrin-degradation products:

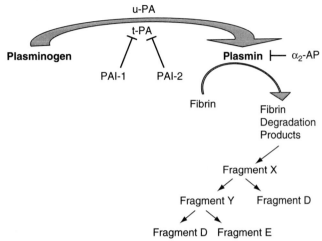

Fig. 11-3. The fibrinolytic pathway. Plasminogen is converted enzymatically to plasmin by t-PA or by u-PA. Plasmin cleaves fibrin and fibrinogen into fibrin degradation products. Major inhibitors of the fibrinolytic pathway are depicted. PAI-1 and PAI-2 inhibit t-PA. Plasmin activity is inhibited by α_2-AP. Abbreviations: t-PA, tissue plasminogen activator; u-PA, urokinase; PAI-1, plasminogen activator inhibitor 1; PAI-2, plasminogen activator inhibitor 2; α_2-AP, α_2 antiplasmin. ⊢ = inhibition.

Fragment X (molecular weight [MW]: 270,000)
Fragment Y (MW: 155,000)
Fragment D (MW: 90,000)
Fragment E (MW: 50,000).

Properties attributed to the various fibrin split products include heparin-like effects, inhibition of platelet adhesion and aggregation, potentiation of the hypotensive effect of bradykinin and chemotactic properties (monocytes and neutrophils). Increased fibrinolysis is usually a reaction to intravascular coagulation (secondary fibrinolysis) rather than the initial event (primary fibrinolysis).

The action of plasmin is negatively regulated by several inhibitors (shown in Table 11-2). These include α_2-antiplasmin and α_2-macroglobulin. Plasminogen activator is in turn regulated by two inhibitors, plasminogen activator inhibitor 1 (PAI-1) and plasminogen activator inhibitor 2 (PAI-2). PAI-1 is the more physiologically important of these inhibitors (Figure 11-3).

Natural Inhibitors of Coagulation

In addition to the physiologic role of fibrinolysis, other inhibitors play critical roles in the control of hemostasis. Table 11-2 lists the plasma fibrinolytic components and hemostatic inhibitors and their principal substrates. All members of this group have overlapping roles in the control of coagulation and fibrinolysis. Major antiproteases of this group of inhibitors include antithrombin, $\alpha2$-antiplasmin, α_2-macroglobulin, the inhibitor of the activated first component of complement (C1 inhibitor), and α_1-antitrypsin.

Antithrombin (AT) neutralizes the procoagulants thrombin, factor IXa, Xa, and XIa (Figure 11-4). When bound to circulating heparin or heparan sulfate on endothelial cells, AT undergoes a conformational change with a dramatic increase in this activity. Tissue factor pathway inhibitor (TFP1) is responsible for inactivation of the FXa/FVIIa/tissue factor complex.

The vitamin K–dependent zymogen, protein C, and its cofactor, protein S, which is also a vitamin K protein, play an important role in the control of hemostasis by

Table 11-2. Plasma Fibrinolytic Components and Hemostatic Inhibitors

	Biologic half-life	Proteases inhibited	Concentration in plasma (mg/dL)
Fibrinolytic components			
Plasminogen[a]	48 h	—	10–15
Plasminogen activators			
Tissue	3–4 min	—	—
Urokinase	9–16 min	—	—
Plasminogen activator inhibitor[a]	—	Plasminogen activator, XIIa	60–200[b]
Inhibitors			
Antithrombin[a] (heparin cofactor)	17–76 h	XIIa, XIa, IXa, Xa, thrombin, kallikrein, plasmin	10–14 104–121[b]
α_2-Plasmin inhibitor[a] (antiplasmin)	30 h	XIIa, XIa, kallikrein, plasmin, thrombin	6–8 80–120[b]
α_2-Macroglobulin[a]	—	XIIa, XIa, thrombin, kallikrein, plasmin	190–310
C1 Inhibitor[a]	—	XIIa, kallikrein	20–25
α_1-Antitrypsin[a]	—	Thrombin, XIa, kallikrein	245–325
Thrombin activatable inhibitor of fibrinolysis (TAFI)			20–400[c]
Tissue factor pathway inhibitor	—	Factor VIIa/tissue factor complex	Endothelial bound
Protein C[a]	6 h	Va, VIIIa, plasminogen activator inhibitor	0.4–0.6 71–109[b]
Protein S	60 h	Va, VIIIa	95–125[b]
Protein C inhibitor[a]	—	Protein Ca	0.5

[a]Enzymatic activity: serine protease.
[b]Activity in plasma (%).
[c]Activity expressed as nM/L.

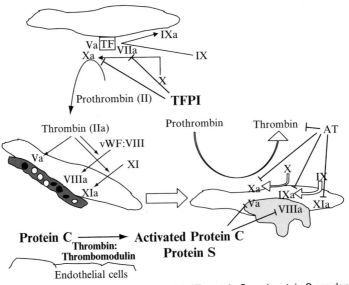

Fig. 11-4. Major inhibitory proteins of coagulation. TFPI, AT, protein C, and protein S are depicted with their target coagulation factor substrates. Abbreviations: TFPI, tissue factor pathway inhibitor; AT, antithrombin. ⊢ = inhibition.

inhibiting activated factors V and VIII (Figure 11-4). Binding of thrombin to thrombomodulin on endothelial cells of small blood vessels neutralizes the procoagulant activities of thrombin and activates protein C. Protein C binds to a specific receptor, and the binding augments the activation of protein C by thrombin. Activated protein C inactivates factors Va and VIIIa in a reaction that is greatly accelerated by the presence of free protein S and phospholipids, thereby inhibiting the generation of thrombin. Free protein S itself has anticoagulant effects: It inhibits the prothrombinase complex (factor Xa, factor Va, and phospholipid), which converts prothrombin to thrombin and inhibits the complex of factor IXa, factor VIIIa, and phospholipid, which converts factor X to factor Xa.

Hemostasis in the Newborn

Table 11-3 lists the hemostatic values in healthy preterm and term infants.

Plasma Factors

In comparison with hemostatic mechanisms in older children and adults, that of the newborn infants is not uniformly developed. In newborns plasminogen levels are only 50% of adult values and α_2AP levels are 80% of adult values, whereas PAI-1 and t-PA levels are significantly increased over adult values. The increased plasma levels of t-PA and PAI-1 in newborns on day 1 of life are in marked contrast to values from cord blood, in which concentrations of these two proteins are significantly lower than in adults. Newborns also have decreased activity of anticoagulant factors, especially antithrombin, protein C, and protein S. In addition the following other physiologic differences are present in normal newborn infants:

Blood vessels:

Capillary fragility is increased.
Prostacyclin production is increased.

Table 11-3. Hemostatic Values in Healthy Preterm and Term Infants

	Normal adults/ children	Preterm infant (28–32 weeks)	Preterm infant (33–36 weeks)	Term infant
PT (s)	10.8–13.9	14.6–16.9	10.6–16.2	10.1–15.9
APTT (s)	26.6–40.3	80–168	27.5–79.4	31.3–54.3
Fibrinogen (mg/dL)	95–425	160–346	150–310	150–280
II (%)	100[a]	16–46	20–47	30–60
V (%)	100[a]	45–118	50–120	56–138
VII (%)	100[a]	24–50	26–55	40–73
VIII (%)	100[a]	75–105	130–150	154–180
vWF Ag (%)	100[a]	82–224	147–224	67–178
vWF (%)	100[a]	83–223	78–210	50–200
IX (%)	100[a]	17–27	10–30	20–38
X (%)	100[a]	20–56	24–60	30–54
XI (%)	100[a]	12–28	20–36	20–64
XII (%)	100[a]	9–35	10–36	16–72
XIII (%)	100[a]	—	35–127	30–122
PK (%)	100[a]	14–38	20–46	16–56
HMW-K (%)	100[a]	20–36	40–62	50–78

Abbreviations: PK, prekallikrein; HMW-K, high-molecular-weight kininogen.
[a]Expressed as a percentage of activity in pooled control plasma.

Platelets:

1. Platelet adhesion is increased due to increased vWF and increased high-molecular-weight (HMW) vWF multimers.
2. Platelet aggregation abnormalities:
   a. Epinephrine-induced aggregation is decreased due to decreased platelet receptors for epinephrine.
   b. Ristocetin-induced aggregation is increased due to increased vWF and increased HMW vWF multimers.
3. Platelet activation is increased, as evidenced by elevated levels of thromboxane A_2, β thromboglobulin, and PF4.

Bleeding Time

The bleeding time is normal because of increased platelet–vessel wall interactions due to increased vWF and HMW vWF, a high hematocrit, and the large red blood cell size.

DETECTION OF HEMOSTATIC DEFECTS

Evaluation of a patient for a hemostatic defect generally entails the following:

1. Detailed history:
   - Symptoms: epistaxis, gingival bleeding, easy bruising, menorrhagia, hematuria, neonatal bleeding, gastrointestinal bleeding, hemarthrosis, prolonged bleeding after lacerations.
   - Response to hemostatic challenge: circumcision, surgery, phlebotomy, immunization/intramuscular injection, suture placement/removal.
   - Underlying medical conditions: known associations with hemostatic defects (liver disease, renal failure, vitamin K deficiency).
   - Medications: antiplatelet drugs (nonsteroidal anti-inflammatory drugs), anticoagulants (warfarin, heparin, low-molecular-weight heparin), antimetabolites (L-asparaginase).
   - Family history: symptoms, response to hemostatic challenge (siblings, parents, aunts, uncles, grandparents).
2. Complete physical examination:
   - Signs consistent with past coagulopathy: petechiae, ecchymoses, hematomas, synovitis/joint effusion, arthropathy, muscle atrophy.
3. Laboratory evaluation (Tables 11-1, 11-2, 11-3, and 11-4):
   Initial screening tests:
   - Complete blood count (CBC): quantitative assessment of platelets.
     Assessments of platelet function:
   - Bleeding time: prolonged with impaired platelet function, platelet counts reduced below 80,000–100,000/mm^3 or impaired vascular integrity.
   - Platelet function analyzer (PFA 100): assesses flow through a membrane; membrane closure time is measured in response to ADP and to epinephrine. Often prolonged with impaired platelet function (see page 292).
     Coagulation factor screening tests (from a laboratory perspective the coagulation system is divided into the intrinsic pathway, the extrinsic pathway, and the common pathway. Such a division, though not relevant for *in vivo* hemostasis, is useful for conceptualizing *in vitro* laboratory testing; Figure 11-5):
   - Prothrombin time (PT) assay (assesses the extrinsic system): utilizes tissue thromboplastin and calcium chloride to initiate the formation of thrombin via the extrinsic pathway.

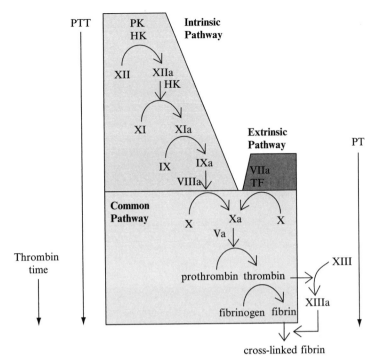

Fig. 11-5. A conceptualization of commonly used screening tests of coagulation and the coagulation parameters they measure. PTT, partial thromboplastin time; PT, prothrombin time.

- Partial thromboplastin time (PTT) assay (assesses the intrinsic system): utilizes a phospholipid reagent, a particulate activator (e.g., ellagic acid, kaolin, silica, soy extract), and calcium chloride to start the enzyme reaction that leads to the formation of thrombin via the intrinsic pathway.

  Common confirmatory coagulation assays:

  Fibrinogen: quantitative measurement of fibrinogen, useful when both the PT and the PTT are prolonged.

  Thrombin time: prolonged when fibrinogen is reduced or abnormal, in the presence of inhibitors (fibrin degradation products, D dimers), and in the presence of thrombin-inhibiting drugs. Useful when both the PT and PTT are prolonged.

  Mixing studies (performed to evaluate a prolonged PT or PTT): the respective assay is performed following addition of normal plasma to patient plasma. Normalization indicates a clotting factor deficiency that was corrected by addition of normal plasma. Continued prolongation indicates presence of a coagulation inhibitor. Such inhibitors may be physiologically relevant or only of *in vitro* significance.

  Clotting factor activity assays: performed to identify clotting factor deficiencies if mixing studies normalize. FXII, FXI, FIX, and FVIII assays are useful if the PTT normalizes in mixing studies. The FVII assay is useful if the PT normalizes in mixing studies. FX, FV, FII, and fibrinogen assays are useful if both PT and PTT normalize in mixing studies. (*Note:* Factor XIII deficiency does not result in prolongation of the PT or PTT.)

  von Willebrand antigen: quantitative assay for von Willebrand factor, useful when bleeding time or PFA-100 closure time is prolonged or when von Willebrand disease is suspected.

Table 11-4. Coagulation Tests and Normal Values

Test	Normal value
Platelet function	
Template bleeding time (min)	<9
Platelet retention (%)	40–90
Platelet aggregation	
Platelet factor 3 availability	
Prothrombin consumption (s)	>25
Clot retraction	Starts at hour 1; completes at hour 24
Clot solubility[a]	
Intrinsic system	
Activated partial thromboplastin time (s)	25–35
Extrinsic system	
Prothrombin time (s)	10–12
Stypven time[b]	
Factor assays	See Tables 11-1 and 11-3
Thrombin time(s)[c]	<24
Reptilase time (s)[c]	<25
Fibrinolytic system	
Staphylococcal clumping (μg/ml)[d]	<9
Thrombo-Wellcotest (μg/ml)[d]	<10
D-Dimer Wellcotest[d]	No latex agglutination

[a]Screening test for factor XIII. Normally clot remains intact after 30 minutes in 1% monochloroacetic acid or 5M urea.
[b]Russell's viper venom test: screening test for factor VII.
[c]Screening test for dysfibrinogenemia, hypofibrinogenemia, and afibrinogenemia.
[d]Split products of fibrinogen.

von Willebrand factor (ristocetin cofactor activity): functional/qualitative assay for von Willebrand factor, useful when the bleeding time or PFA-100 closure time is prolonged or when von Willebrand disease is suspected.

Platelet aggregation studies: a qualitative assessment of platelet function, useful when the bleeding time or PFA-100 closure time is prolonged.

Urea clot lysis assay: useful screen for FXIII deficiency. In the absence of fibrin cross linkage by FXIII, a clot will degrade with incubation in 5 M urea.

Preoperative Evaluation of Hemostasis

1. History (the most important element of the evaluation)
   a. If negative: no coagulation tests are indicated; only a CBC.
   b. If positive or unreliable, the following tests should be performed: CBC, bleeding time, PT, PTT, and fibrinogen.
2. Abnormal tests require further investigation (Figure 11-6).

ACQUIRED COAGULATION FACTOR DISORDERS
Vitamin K Deficiency

The normal full-term infant is born with levels of factors II, VII, IX, and X that are low by adult standards (Table 11-3). The coagulation factors fall even lower over the first few days of life, reaching their nadir on about the third day. This is due to the low body stores of vitamin K at birth. As little as 25 μg vitamin K can prevent this fall in activity of the vitamin K–dependent clotting factors. The vitamin K content of

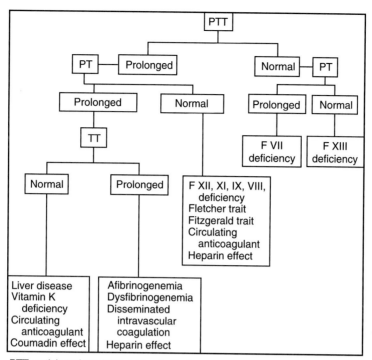

PTT, activitated partial thromboplastin time
PT, prothrombin time
TT, thrombin time

Fig. 11-6. Coagulation tests and interpretation.

cow's milk is about 6 μg/dL and that of breast milk 1.5 μg/dL. It is a combination of low initial stores and subsequent poor intake of vitamin K that occasionally produces an aggravation of the coagulation defect causing primary hemorrhagic disease of the newborn. Vitamin K deficiency results in hemorrhagic disease between the second and fourth days of life and is manifested by gastrointestinal hemorrhage, hemorrhage from the umbilicus, or internal hemorrhage. Bleeding attributable to this cause is responsive to parenteral vitamin K therapy; for this reason, parenteral vitamin K is routinely administered to newborns.

In premature infants of low birth weight, both the vitamin K stores and the level of coagulation factors are even lower than in term infants. The response to vitamin K is slow and inconstant, suggesting that the immature liver has reduced synthetic capability.

Maternal ingestion of certain drugs may result in neonatal hypoprothrombinemia and reduction in factors VII, IX, and X. These drugs include oral anticoagulants and anticonvulsants (phenytoin, primidone, and phenobarbital).

Table 11-5 lists the conditions associated with deficiency of vitamin K–dependent factors in the newborn and in the older child, and Table 11-6 lists the laboratory findings in vitamin K deficiency in relationship to the findings in liver disease and disseminated intravascular disease (DIC).

Hepatic Dysfunction

Any transient inability of the newborn's liver to synthesize necessary coagulation factors, even in the presence of vitamin K, can result in hemorrhagic disease that is nonresponsive to vitamin K therapy. Hepatic dysfunction as a result of immaturity, infection, hypoxia, or underperfusion of the liver can all result in transient inability

Table 11-5. Conditions Associated with Deficiency of Vitamin K–Dependent Factors

Normal newborn (normal by 3 months of age), prematurity
    Vitamin K responsive
    Vitamin K nonresponsive (caused by immaturity, infection, hypoxia, hepatic
       underperfusion)
Dietary
    Cow's milk: 6 µg/L
    Human milk: 1.5 µg/L
Altered bacterial colonization
    Vomiting
    Severe diarrhea malabsorption syndromes
       Celiac disease
       Cystic fibrosis
       Biliary atresia
       Obstruction of gastrointestinal tract
       Antibiotics (including antibiotics in breast milk)
Hepatocellular disease
    Acute
       Reye syndrome
       Acute hepatitis
    Chronic
       Cirrhosis
       Wilson disease
Drugs
    Coumarins

Table 11-6. Laboratory Findings in Vitamin K Deficiency, Liver Disease, and Disseminated Intravascular Coagulation

Component	Vitamin K deficiency	Liver disease	DIC
Red cell morphology	Normal	Target cells	Fragmented cells, burr cells, helmet cells, schistocytes
PTT	Prolonged	Prolonged	Prolonged
PT	Prolonged	Prolonged	Prolonged
Fibrin split products	Normal	Normal or slightly increased	Markedly increased
Platelets	Normal	Normal	Reduced
Factors decreased	II, VII, IX, X	I, II, V, VII, IX, X, XI	Assays are of limited utility

Abbreviations: DIC, disseminated intravascular coagulation; PT, prothrombin time; PTT, partial thromboplastin time.

of the liver to synthesize coagulation factors. This is more prominent in small premature infants. The sites of bleeding in these cases are usually pulmonary and intracerebral with a high mortality. Other causes of hepatocellular dysfunction, affecting patients of all ages, are also listed in Table 11-5. In liver disease vitamin K–dependent factors, factor V, factor XI, and fibrinogen are usually decreased; fibrin split products may be elevated due to impaired clearance (Table 11-6). In contrast, factor VIII levels are usually normal. There is no response to vitamin K. There is usually a clinical response to clotting factor replacement therapy, using fresh frozen plasma and cryoprecipitate (replacement guidelines are the same as those outlined in Table 11-7).

Table 11-7. Treatment of Disseminated Intravascular Coagulation and Purpura Fulminans

Treatment of the underlying disorder
    Treatment of infections with appropriate anti-infectives (antibiotics, antiviral drugs, antifungal drugs)
    Correction of electrolyte imbalances, acidosis, and shock
    Appropriate antineoplastic therapy
    Removal of triggering stimulus
Replacement therapy as indicated
    Platelet concentrates (1 unit/10 kg)
    Cryoprecipitate (50–100 mg/kg fibrinogen)[a]
    Fresh frozen plasma (10–15 mL/kg, initially; may need 5 mL/kg q6h)
Intravenous heparinization[b]
Intravenous direct thrombin inhibitors
Antiplatelet drugs
Antithrombin concentrate
Activated protein C concentrate

[a]One bag of cryoprecipitate contains about 200 mg fibrinogen.
[b]See Heparin Therapy section.

Disseminated Intravascular Coagulation

Disseminated intravascular coagulation is characterized by the intravascular consumption of platelets and plasma clotting factors. Widespread coagulation within the vasculature results in the deposition of fibrin thrombi and the production of a hemorrhagic state when the rapid utilization of platelets and clotting factors results in levels inadequate to maintain hemostasis. The accumulation of fibrin in the microcirculation leads to mechanical injury to the red cells, resulting in erythrocyte fragmentation and microangiopathic hemolytic anemia.

Widespread activation of the coagulation cascade rapidly results in the depletion of many clotting factors as fibrinogen is converted to fibrin throughout the body. Two important mechanisms take place:

1. The generation of thrombin results in intravascular coagulation and rapidly falling platelet count, fibrinogen, and FV, FVIII, and FXIII levels. Paradoxically, *in vitro* bioassays for these factors may be elevated owing to generalized activation of the coagulation system.
2. Concurrently, plasminogen is converted to its enzymatic form (plasmin) by t-PA. Plasmin digests fibrinogen and fibrin (secondary fibrinolysis) into fibrin split products (FSPs), resulting in clot lysis.

Diagnosis of DIC relies on the presence of a well-defined clinical situation associated with a thrombohemorrhagic disorder. The following test results are the most useful and reliable in the diagnostic and therapeutic evaluation of fulminant DIC:

Increased PT and activated partial thromboplastin time (APTT)
Decreased fibrinogen
Decreased platelet count
Fibrin degradation (elevated fibrin degradation products, elevated D dimers)
Presence of fragmented red blood cells (e.g., schistocytes, triangle cells, helmet cells, burr cells)
Increased PF4 (platelet factor 4)
Increased FPA (fibrinopeptide A)
Decreased FV, FVIII, FXIII (useful if levels are decreased).

The typical diagnostic findings of DIC are listed in Table 11-6. Disease states associated with DIC are listed in Table 11-8. Generally available treatment options for treatment of DIC are shown in Table 11-7.

In children the following conditions may be associated with low-grade DIC:

Kasabach–Merritt syndrome
Chronic inflammatory disorders
Arteriovenous fistulae
Vascular prosthesis
Glomerulonephritis.

Low-grade DIC has the potential to accelerate into fulminant DIC. The following laboratory findings are useful in the diagnosis of low-grade DIC:

Presence of fragmented red blood cells
Usually normal or mildly decreased platelet count
Normal or mildly increased PT/APTT
Normal or mildly decreased fibrinogen
Usually increased FSPs
Usually increased PF4
Usually increased FPA levels.

Table 11-8. Disease States Associated with Disseminated Intravascular Coagulation

Causative factors	Clinical situation
Tissue injury	Trauma/crush injuries
	Head injury
	Major surgery
	Heat stroke
	Burns
	Venoms
	Malignancy
	Obstetrical accidents
	Amniotic fluid embolism
	Placental abruption
	Stillborn fetus
	Abortion
	Fat embolism
Endothelial cell injury	Infection (bacterial, viral, protozoal)
AND/OR	Immune complexes
Abnormal vascular surfaces	Eclampsia
	Postpartum renal failure
	Oral contraceptives
	Cardiopulmonary bypass
	Giant hemangioma
	Vascular aneurysm
	Cirrhosis
	Malignancy
	Respiratory distress syndrome
Platelet, leukocyte, or red cell injury	Incompatible blood transfusion
	Infection
	Allograft rejection
	Hemolytic syndromes
	Drug hypersensitivity
	Malignancy

Treatment of low-grade DIC involves treatment of the underlying disease responsible for triggering low-grade DIC and antiplatelet therapy:

Aspirin (5–10 mg/kg/day)
Dipyridamole (3–5 mg/kg/day).

ISOLATED COAGULATION FACTOR DISORDERS

Table 11-9 lists the genetics, prevalence, coagulation studies, and symptoms of inherited coagulation factor disorders. Treatment for the rare coagulation factor deficiencies is shown in Table 11-10.

Hemophilia A and B

The most common coagulation disorders are hemophilia A and B. Hemophilia A is an X-linked recessive bleeding disorder attributable to decreased blood levels of functional procoagulant factor VIII (FVIII, VIII:C, antihemophilic factor). Hemophilia B is also an X-linked recessive disorder and is indistinguishable from hemophilia A with respect to its clinical manifestations. In hemophilia B, the defect is a decreased level of functional procoagulant factor IX (FIX, IX:C, plasma thromboplastin component, or Christmas factor). The incidence of hemophilia is probably 1 per 6,000 live male births. Factor VIII deficiency accounts for 80–85% of cases of

Table 11-9. Genetics, Prevalence, Coagulation Studies, and Symptoms of Inherited Coagulation Factor Deficiencies

Factor deficiency	Genetics	Est. Prevalence	BT	APTT	PT	Associated with bleeding episodes
Afibrinogenemia	AR	1:1 million	N	P	P	++
Dysfibrinogenemia	AR		N	N/P	P	+/−
II	AR	1:2 million	N	P	P	++
V (parahemophilia)	AR	1:1 million	N	P	P	++
VII	AR	1:500,000	N	N	P	+
VIII (hemophilia A)	XLR	1:10,000	N	P	N	+++
von Willebrand disease		1:1,000				
Type 1	AD		N/P	N/P	N	+
Type 2	AD		P	N/P	N	++
Type 3	AR		P	P	N	++
IX (hemophilia B)	XLR	1:60,000	N	P	N	+++
X	AR	1:1 million	N	P	P	++
XI (hemophilia C)	AR	1:1 million	N[a]	P	N	+
XII	AD		N	P	N	−
XIII	AR	1:1 million	N	N	N	+[c]
Prekallikrein (Fletcher trait)	AD		N	P[b]	N	−
HMW kininogen (Fitzgerald trait)	AR		N	P	N	−
Passovoy	AR		N	P	N	+/−

Abbreviations: AD, autosomal dominant; APTT, activated partial thromboplastin time; AR, autosomal recessive; BT, bleeding time; N, normal; P, prolonged; PT, prothrombin time; XLR, X-linked recessive.

[a]Prolonged when associated with platelet dysfunction.
[b]Shortened with prolonged exposure to kaolin.
[c]Umbilical stump bleeding; clot soluble in 5 M urea or 1% monochloracetic acid.

Table 11-10. Treatment of Rare Coagulation Factor Deficiencies[a]

Factor deficiency	Half-life (h)	Percentage increase in plasma concentration after 1 unit/kg IV	Percentage required for hemostasis	Percentage required for minor trauma	Percentage required for surgery and major trauma
Afibrinogenemia	56–82	1–1.5[a]	80[a]	150[a]	200[b]
II	45–60	1	20–30	30	50
V	36	1.5	10–15	10–15	25
VII	5	1	10–15	10–15	20
VWD[c]	24–48	1.5[d]	10	20–30	50
X	24–60	1	10–15	10–15	25
XI	48	1	30	30	>45
XIII	168–240	1	2–3	15	25

[a]see table 11-15 for factor VIII and factor IX deficiency treatment guidelines
[b]In mg/dl.
[c]vWD, von Willebrand's disease.
[d]calculated in units of VWF: Rcof activity

hemophilia, with factor IX deficiency accounting for the remainder. Both types occur with similar incidence among all races and in all parts of the world.

Hemophilia A Carrier Detection

Excessive lyonization may result in reduced FVIII levels in female carriers of hemophilia; hence, a reduced FVIII level can have utility in diagnosing the carrier state.

Direct gene mutation analysis: The FVIII common intron 22 inversion, resulting from an intrachromosomal recombination, is identifiable in 45% of severe hemophilia A patients. For the remaining 55% of severe hemophilia A patients as well as all mild and moderate hemophilia A patients, the molecular defects can usually be detected by efficient screening of all 26 FVIII exons and splice junctions. Therefore, direct gene mutation analysis is the most accurate test for carrier detection and prenatal diagnosis for severe hemophilia A. For rare patients in whom a precise mutation cannot be identified, intragenetic and extragenetic linkage analysis of DNA polymorphisms can be useful with up to 99.9% precision (when an affected male patient and his related family members are available).

When definitive diagnosis of the carrier state cannot be made, determination of the FVIII/vWF:Ag ratio (<1.0) can be used to detect 80% of hemophilia A carriers with 95% accuracy. Use of this methodology requires careful standardization of the laboratory performing the testing.

Hemophilia B Carrier Detection

Hemophilia B carriers have a wide range of FIX levels but, in a subset of cases, can be detected by the measurement of reduced plasma factor IX activity (in 60–70% of cases).

Direct gene mutation analysis: The factor IX gene is located centromeric to the factor VIII gene in the terminus of the long arm of the X chromosome. There is no linkage between the FVIII and FIX genes. The 34-kb FIX coding sequence comprises eight exons and encodes a 461-amino-acid precursor protein that is approximately one-third the size of the factor VIII cDNA. Because of the smaller gene size, FIX mutations can be identified in nearly all patients. Direct FIX mutation testing is available through DNA diagnostic laboratories, with linkage analysis used in those cases where the responsible mutation cannot be identified.

Prenatal Diagnosis

Prenatal diagnosis of hemophilia can be performed by either chorionic villus sampling (CVS) at 10–12 weeks' gestation or by amniocentesis after 15 weeks' gestation. If DNA analysis is not available or if a woman's carrier status cannot be determined, fetal blood sampling can be performed at 18–20 weeks' gestation for direct fetal factor VIII plasma activity level measurement. The normal fetus at 18–20 weeks' gestation has a very low FIX level, which an expert laboratory can distinguish from the virtual absence of FIX in a fetus with severe hemophilia B.

Maternal–fetal combined complication rates for amniocentesis and CVS are 0.5–1.0% and 1.0–2.0%, respectively. Fetal blood sampling is less available; the fetal loss rate for these procedures ranges from 1 to 6%.

Clinical Course of Hemophilia

Hemophilia should be suspected when unusual bleeding is encountered in a male patient. Clinical presentations of hemophilia A and hemophilia B are indistinguishable. The frequency and severity of bleeding in hemophilia are usually related to the plasma levels of factor VIII or IX (Table 11-11), although some genetic modifiers of hemophilia severity have been identified. The median age for first bleeding episode is 10 months, corresponding to the age at which the infant becomes mobile. Table 11-12 shows the common sites of hemorrhage in hemophilia. The incidence of severity and clinical manifestations of hemophilia are listed in Table 11-13.

Treatment (Factor Replacement Therapy)

Factor replacement therapy is the mainstay of hemophilia treatment. The degree of factor correction required to achieve hemostasis is largely determined by the site and nature of the particular bleeding episode. Commercially available products for replacement therapy are listed in Table 11-14. Commercially available FVIII products include high-purity recombinant preparations, highly purified plasma-derived concentrates (monoclonal/immunoaffinity purified), and intermediate-purity plasma-derived preparations. Available FIX products include recombinant FIX and plasma-derived high-purity FIX concentrate (coagulation FIX concentrate). Prothrombin complex concentrates, formerly a mainstay of hemophilia B treatment, are not utilized because of the risk of thrombotic complications associated with intensive treatment. Source plasma for all plasma-derived factor concentrates undergoes donor screening and nucleic acid testing for a variety of viral pathogens. In addition

Table 11-11. Relationship of Factor Levels to Severity of Clinical Manifestations of Hemophilia A and B

Type	Percentage factor VIII/IX	Type of hemorrhage
Severe	<1	Spontaneous; hemarthroses and deep soft tissue hemorrhages
Moderate	1–5	Gross bleeding following mild to moderate trauma; some hemarthrosis; seldom spontaneous hemorrhage
Mild	5–25	Severe hemorrhage only following moderate to severe trauma or surgery
High-risk carrier females	Variable	Gynecologic and obstetric hemorrhage common, other symptoms depend on plasma factor level.

Table 11-12. Common Sites of Hemorrhage in Hemophilia

Hemarthrosis
Intramuscular hematoma
Hematuria
Mucous membrane hemorrhage
  Mouth
  Dental
  Epistaxis
  Gastrointestinal
High-risk hemorrhage
  Central nervous system
    Intracranial
    Intraspinal
  Retropharyngeal
  Retroperitoneal
  Hemorrhage causing compartment syndrome/nerve compression
    Femoral (iliopsoas muscle)
    Sciatic (buttock)
    Tibial (calf muscle)
    Perineal (anterior compartment of leg)
    Median and ulnar nerve (flexor muscles of forearm)

all plasma-derived and many recombinant factor concentrates undergo a viral inactivation treatment, typically with solvent detergent, wet or dry heat treatment, pasteurization, or nanofiltration. Factor concentrates are preferred over fresh frozen plasma or cryoprecipitate because the plasma-derived concentrates undergo viral inactivation treatment in addition to donor screening. Recombinant factor concentrates are widely accepted as the treatment of choice for previously untreated patients, minimally treated patients, and patients who have not had transfusion-associated infections.

Strategies for hemophilia care include on-demand treatment of acute bleeding episodes or, for severe hemophilia patients, prophylactic administration of clotting factor concentrate to maintain trough factor levels >1% augmented with on-demand

Table 11-13. Incidence of Severity and Clinical Manifestations of Hemophilia

Severity	Severe	Moderate	Mild
Incidence			
Hemophilia A	70%	15%	15%
Hemophilia B	50%	30%	20%
Bleeding manifestations			
Age of onset	≤1 year	1–2 years	2 years–adult
Neonatal hemorrhages			
Following circumcision	Common	Common	None
Intracranial	Occasionally	Rare	Rare
Muscle/joint hemorrhage	Spontaneous	Following minor trauma	Following trauma
CNS hemorrhage	High risk	Moderate risk	Rare[a]
Postsurgical hemorrhage	Common	Common	Rare[a]
Oral hemorrhage[b]	Common	Common	Rare[a]

[a]FVIII, >25; FIX, >15.
[b]Following trauma or tooth extraction.

Table 11-14. Commercially Available Coagulation Factor Concentrates

Class	Product	Purity	Procedure	Primary use
FVIII plasma derived	Koate-DVI (Bayer Corp)	Intermediate purity	SD/Dry heat	Hemophilia A
	Humate P (ZLB Behring)	Intermediate purity	P	Hemophilia A/von Willebrand
	Alphanate SD-HT (Grifols Corp)	High purity	SD/Dry heat	Hemophilia A/von Willebrand
	Hemofil M (Baxter Bioscience)	Ultra high purity	SD	Hemophilia A
	Monoclate P (ZLB Behring)	Ultra high purity	P	Hemophilia A
	Monarch M (American Red Cross)	Ultra high purity	SD	Hemophilia A
FVIII recombinant	Recombinate (Baxter Bioscience)	Ultra high purity	None	Hemophilia A
	Helixate (ZLB Behring)	Ultra high purity	SD	Hemophilia A
	ReFacto (Wyeth)	Ultra high purity	SD	Hemophilia A
	Kogenate FS (Bayer Corp)	Ultra high purity	SD	Hemophilia A
	Advate (Baxter Bioscience)	Ultra high purity	SD	Hemophilia A
Prothrombin complex	Profilnine SD (Grifols Corp)	Intermediate	SD	Hemophilia B
	Bebulin VH (Baxter Bioscience)	Intermediate	Vapor heat	Hemophilia B
FIX coagulation concentrate				
Plasma derived	Alphanine SD-VF (Grifols Corp)	High	SD/Nanofiltration	Hemophilia B
Plasma derived	Mononine (ZLB Behring)	High	SD/Ultrafiltration	Hemophilia B
Recombinant	BeneFIX (Wyeth)	High	Nanofiltration	Hemophilia B
Activated prothrombin complex concentrate	FEIBA VH (Baxter Bioscience)	N/A	Vapor heat	Inhibitor bypass therapy
	NovoSeven (NovoNordisk)	N/A	None	Inhibitor bypass therapy, FVII deficiency
Specialty items	Hyate C (Ipsen)	N/A	None	For FVIII inhibitor treatment
	Proplex T (Baxter Bioscience)	Intermediate	Dry heat	FVII replacement (3.5 U FVII/U FIX)

Notes: Purity (international units/mg protein before albumin is added); intermediate <100, high >100, ultra high >1,000; SD, solvent detergent; P, pasteurization; N/A, not applicable.

313

treatment of breakthrough bleeding episodes. The latter strategy pharmacologically converts the severe hemophilia phenotype to a moderate phenotype with an attendant reduction in frequency of bleeding episodes. Nonrandomized studies suggest a markedly reduced incidence of hemophilic arthropathy when prophylaxis is instituted prior to onset of recurrent joint bleeds. This benefit must be balanced with the need for frequent prophylactic infusions (3–4 times/week for FVIII, 2 times/week for FIX), venous access considerations, potential requirements for central venous access devices, increased cost of treatment, and the occasional patient who has a very mild clinical course. Table 11-15 provides generally accepted guidelines for treatment of most types of hemophiliac bleeding. When a bleeding episode is suspected, hemostatic treatment should be rendered first and then diagnostic evaluation(s) may be performed.

Ancillary Therapy

DDAVP

In hemophilia A patients 1-deamino-8-D-arginine vasopressin (DDAVP) increases plasma FVIII levels 2.5- to 6-fold. It is commonly used to treat selected hemorrhagic episodes in mild hemophilia A patients. When used intravenously the dose is 0.3 µg/kg administered in 25–50 mL normal saline over 15–20 minutes. Its peak effect is observed in 30–60 minutes. Subcutaneous DDAVP is as effective as intravenous DDAVP, facilitating treatment of very young patients with limited venous access.

Concentrated intranasal DDAVP (Stimate), available as a 1.5-mg/mL preparation, has approximately two thirds the effect of intravenous DDAVP. Care should be exercised to avoid inadvertent dispensing of the dilute intranasal DDAVP commonly used for treatment of diabetes insipidus. The peak effect of intranasal Stimate is observed 60–90 minutes after administration.

Recommended dosage for use of intranasal Stimate

Body weight <50 kg: 150 µg (one metered dose)
Body weight >50 kg: 300 µg (two metered doses).

Recommendations during the administration of DDAVP are:

1. Mild fluid restriction; avoidance of oral and IV fluid containing low concentration of electrolytes
2. Monitoring of urinary output and daily weights may be useful to track fluid retention.

Responses to DDAVP vary from patient to patient, but in a given patient are reasonably consistent on different occasions. Therefore, a test dose of DDAVP should be administered at the time of diagnosis or in advance of an invasive procedure to assess the magnitude of the patient's response. DDAVP administration may be repeated at 24-hour intervals according to the severity and nature of the bleeding. Administration of DDAVP at shorter intervals results in a progressive tachyphylaxis over a period of 4–5 days.

Side effects of DDAVP

Asymptomatic facial flushing
Thrombosis (a rarely reported complication)
Hyponatremia, more common in very young patients, in patients receiving repeated doses of DDAVP or large volumes of oral or intravenous fluid; hyponatremic seizures have been reported in children under 2 years of age.

Table 11-15. Treatment of Bleeding Episodes

Type of hemorrhage	Hemostatic factor level	Hemophilia A	Hemophilia B	Comment/adjuncts
Hemarthrosis	30–50% minimum	FVIII 20–40 U/kg q12–24h as needed; if joint still painful after 24 h, treat for further 2 days	FIX 30–40 U/kg q24h as needed; if joint still painful after 24 h, treat for further 2 days	Rest, immobilization, cold compress, elevation.
Muscle	40–50% minimum, for iliopsoas or compartment syndrome, 100%, then 50–100% × 2–4 days	20–40 U/kg q12–24h as needed For iliopsoas or compartment syndrome, initial dose is 50 U/kg	40–60 U/kg q24h as needed For iliopsoas or compartment syndrome, initial dose is 60–80 U/kg	Calf/forearm bleeds can be limb threatening. Significant blood loss can occur with femoral-retroperitoneal bleed.
Oral mucosa	Initially 50%, then EACA at 50 mg/kg q6h × 7 days usually suffices	25 U/kg	50 U/kg	Antifibrinolytic therapy is critical. Do not use with PCC or APCC.
Epistaxis	Initially 30–40%, use of EACA 50 mg/kg q6h until healing occurs may be helpful	15–20 U/kg	30–40 U/kg	Local measures: pressure, packing.
Gastrointestinal	Initially 100%, then 50% until healing occurs	FVIII 50 U/kg, then 25 U/kg q12h	FIX 100 U/kg, then 50 U/kg q day	Lesion is usually found, endoscopy is recommended, antifibrinolytic therapy may be helpful.

(Continues)

Table 11-15. (Continued)

Type of hemorrhage	Hemostatic factor level	Hemophilia A	Hemophilia B	Comment/adjuncts
Hematuria	Painless hematuria can be treated with complete bed rest and vigorous hydration for 48 hrs. For pain or persistent hematuria 100%	FVIII 50 units/kg; if not resolved, 30–40 U/kg q day until resolved	FIX 80–100 units/kg; if not resolved, then 30–40 U/kg q day until resolved	Evaluate for stones or urinary tract infection. Lesion may not be found. Prednisone 1–2 mg/kg/d × 5–7 days may be helpful. Avoid antifibrinolytics.
Central nervous system	Initially 100%, then 50–100% for 14 days	50 U/kg, then 25 U/kg q12h	80–100 U/kg, then 50 U/kg q24h	Treat presumptively before evaluating, hospitalize. Lumbar puncture requires prophylactic factor coverage.
Retroperitoneal retropharyngeal	Initially 80–100%, then 50–100% until complete resolution	FVIII 50 units/kg, then 25 U/kg q12h until resolved	FIX 100 U/kg, then 50 U/kg q24h until resolved	Hospitalize.
Trauma or surgery	Initially 100%, then 50% until wound healing is complete	50 U/kg, then 25 U/kg q12h	100 U/kg, then 50 U/kg q24h	Evaluate for inhibitor prior to elective surgery.

Notes: Antifibrinolytic, EACA; epsilon-aminocaproic acid (AMICAR); syrup, 1250 mg/5 mL; tablet, 500 mg.

Antifibrinolytic Therapy

Antifibrinolytic drugs inhibit fibrinolysis by preventing activation of the proenzyme plasminogen to plasmin. This intervention is useful for preventing clot degradation in areas rich in fibrinolytic activity including the oral cavity, the nasal cavity, and the female reproductive tract. Approved antifibrinolytic drugs are:

Epsilon aminocaproic acid (EACA; Amicar): orally; dose is 50–100 mg/kg every 6 hours (maximum, 24 grams total dose per day). Gastrointestinal symptoms may occur at higher doses; therefore, the preferred starting dose is 50 mg/kg. The drug is available as 500-mg tabs or as a flavored syrup (250 mg/mL).

Tranexamic acid (Cyklokapron): 20–25 mg/kg (maximum, 1.5 g) orally or 10 mg/kg (maximum, 1.0 g) intravenously every 8 hours. The oral form, a 500-mg tablet, is not currently available in the United States.

Antifibrinolytic therapy should not be utilized in patients with urinary tract bleeding because of the potential for intrarenal clot formation.

To treat spontaneous oral hemorrhage or to prevent bleeding from dental procedures in pediatric patients with hemophilia, either drug is begun in conjunction with DDAVP or factor replacement therapy and continued for up to 7 days or until mucosal healing is complete. Antifibrinolytic drugs also have efficacy as an adjunct treatment for epistaxis and for menorrhagia. Antifibrinolytic drugs are safe to use in hemophilia B patients receiving coagulation factor IX concentrates but should not be used contemporaneously with prothrombin-complex concentrates (PCCs) because of the thrombotic potential of these concentrates. Initiation of oral antifibrinolytic drug therapy 4–6 hours after the last dose of PCC appears to be well tolerated.

Management of Inhibitors in Hemophilia

Approximately 30% of patients with hemophilia A develop neutralizing alloantibodies (inhibitors) directed against factor VIII. Inhibitors are a major cause of morbidity and mortality in hemophilia. Risk factors for inhibitors include the presence of the common inversion mutation, large deletions of the FVIII gene, African American ethnicity, and a hemophiliac sibling with an inhibitor. Inhibitors are quantitated using the Bethesda assay. Low-responder inhibitors have titers ≤5 Bethesda units (BU) and do not exhibit anamnesis upon repeated exposure to FVIII.

Approximately half of patients with inhibitors will be low responders, and of these, approximately half will have transient inhibitors. Hemophilia A patients with low-responder inhibitors can generally be treated with factor VIII concentrate, albeit at an increased dosing intensity because of reduced *in vivo* recovery and shortened half-life of the FVIII. High-responder inhibitors have titers >5 BU and, although the titer may decay in the absence of FVIII exposure, these patients will display an anamnestic rise in titer upon rechallenge with FVIII. The clinical approach is different for high and low responders (Table 11-16).

Low Responders

For serious limb or life-threatening bleeding, a bolus infusion of 100 units/kg factor VIII is administered; repeat doses of 100 units/kg are administered at 12-hour intervals or, alternatively, the level is maintained with a continuous infusion of 8–10 units/kg/h. A factor VIII assay should be obtained 1 hour after the bolus infusion and trough or steady-state FVIII levels should be followed at least daily thereafter.

For routine joint and muscle hemorrhages, patients can usually be managed with an infusion of 100 units/kg FVIII with follow-up infusions of 100 units/kg FVIII every 12 hours as clinically indicated. During prolonged treatment in FVIII *in vivo*

Table 11-16. Recommendations for Replacement Therapy for Treatment of Bleeding in Patients with Factor VIII Inhibitors

Type of patient	Type of bleed	Recommended treatment
Low responder[a] (<5 BU)	Minor or major bleed	Factor VIII infusions using adequate amounts of factor VIII to achieve a circulating hemostatic level
High responder[b] with low inhibitor level (<5 BU)	Minor/major bleed	PCC, aPCC, or TVIIa infusions
	Life-threatening bleed	Factor VIII infusions until anamnestic response occurs, then aPCC or rVII[a] infusions
High responder with high inhibitor level (>5 BU)	Minor bleed	PCC, aPCC, or TVIIa infusions
	Major bleed	PCC, aPCC, or TVIIa infusions
Porcine FVIII concentrate[c] if porcine inhibitor titer is <20 BU

Abbreviations: BU, Bethesda units; PCC, prothrombin complex concentrates; aPCC, Activated PCC, e.g., Autoplex (Hyland) and FEIBA (factor VIII inhibitor bypassing activity). Nonactivated PCC, e.g., Konyne (Cutter) and Proplex (Hyland). rVIIa, Recombinant activated FVII.
[a]Rise of inhibitor titer is slow to factor VIII challenge.
[b]Rise of inhibitor titer is rapid to factor VIII challenge.
[c]Hyate:C.

recovery and half-life may transiently improve as inhibitor antibody is adsorbed by the FVIII.

High Responders

In high-responder inhibitor patients with limb or life-threatening bleeding, if the inhibitor titer is <20 BU, a high-dose continuous infusion of factor VIII may saturate the antibody, permitting a therapeutic FVIII level. An initial dose of 200 units/kg can be administered with factor VIII levels determined 1 hour after the initiation of the continuous infusion of 40 units/kg-hr.

If a factor VIII level is not attainable or the antibody level is greater than 20 BU, then bypassing agents to initiate hemostasis independent of FVIII should be employed, such as treatment with PCC, aPCC, rFVIIa, or recombinant porcine FVIII (if available) should be employed.

In high responder patients treatment of most bleeding episodes is based on use of bypassing agents to initiate hemostasis independent of FVIII. Available treatments include:

Prothrombin complex concentrate
PCC products can be used to treat routine joint and muscle hemorrhage in hemophilia A patients with inhibitors. They result in the activation of factor X (Xa) or factor II (IIa) with the subsequent formation of the fibrin clot. The initial dose is 75 units/kg of factor IX. Approximately 50% of patients with inhibitors respond to PCCs. If there is no response after two or three infusions given every 12 hours for 1–2 days, an alternative therapy should be employed. If multiple doses are administered, the patient should be monitored for the development of DIC or even myocardial infarction. The simultaneous use of antifibrinolytic therapy (i.e., Amicar) should be avoided to prevent development of thrombosis. Oral antifibrinolytic drug therapy 4–6 hours after the last dose of PCC, however, appears to be well tolerated.

Activated prothrombin complex concentrate (FEIBA)
Activated prothrombin complex concentrate (aPCC) products have increased amounts of activated factor VII (VIIa), factor X (Xa), and thrombin and are effective

in patients even with high titer inhibitors (>50 BU). The initial dose of 75 units/kg can be repeated in 8–12 hours.

Approximately 75% of patients with inhibitors respond to aPCC infusions. For some patients trace amounts of FVIII in aPCC products may cause anamnesis of the inhibitor titer. If multiple doses are administered, the patient should be monitored for the development of DIC or even myocardial infarction. The simultaneous use of antifibrinolytic therapy (i.e., Amicar) should be avoided. Oral antifibrinolytic drug therapy 4–6 hours after the last dose of a PCC, however, appears to be well tolerated.

Recombinant factor VIIa (NovoSeven)

Recombinant activated factor VII (rFVIIa) concentrate can be administered to achieve hemostasis in patients with high-titer inhibitors. The usual dose is 90 µg/kg rFVIIa repeated every 2 hours for 2–3 infusions. The subsequent frequency of infusion and duration of therapy must then be individualized, based on the clinical response and severity of bleeding. Early initiation of hemostatic treatment with rFVIIa produces response rates on the order of 90%. Treatment failures with conventional doses of rFVIIa may respond to higher doses. The incidence of thrombotic complications with this product has been low and anamnesis of the inhibitor does not occur.

Porcine factor VIII concentrate (Hyate C)

Most FVIII inhibitors have notably less affinity for porcine FVIII; therefore, patients who have an antihuman FVIII titer less than 50 BU may respond to porcine FVIII concentrate. Porcine FVIII is able to effect hemostasis in the hemophilia A patient but is less efficiently neutralized by FVIII inhibitors. Measurement of a porcine FVIII inhibitor titer can be helpful in predicting clinical response. The recommended starting dose is 100–150 units/kg, and the response is measured using a standard factor VIII assay. Premedication with Benadryl, acetaminophen, and hydrocortisone is recommended to minimize allergic reactions. Thrombocytopenia has also been reported with porcine FVIII use. Production of porcine plasma-derived FVIII has been recently discontinued. A recombinant porcine FVIII preparation is now entering clinical trials.

Plasmapheresis with Immunoadsorption

When bleeding persists despite active treatment, extracorporeal plasmapheresis (4-liter exchange) over staphylococcal A columns may rapidly reduce the inhibitor titer by adsorbing out offending inhibitory IgG antibodies. This approach is cumbersome and may produce significant fever and hypotension due to the release of staphylococcal A protein from the solid-phase matrix of the chromatographic column. However, it can be life saving in desperate situations and its efficacy can be enhanced by concomitant replacement therapy with FVIII containing concentrates. Availability of staphylococcal protein A columns for immunoadsorption is quite limited.

Immune-Tolerance Induction

Immune-tolerance induction (ITI) intervention is typically reserved for patients with high-responder inhibitors and involves frequent administration of FVIII concentrate over many months to years to induce immune tolerance to exogenous FVIII. Objectives of ITI are an undetectable inhibitor titer, restoring the ability to treat bleeds with FVIII concentrates and restoration of normal *in vivo* FVIII recovery and half-life. A variety of regimens have been used for ITT (Table 11-17), including daily high-dose FVIII (100-Units/kg twice-daily regimen) with or without immunomodulatory therapy, daily intermediate dose FVIII (50–100 Units/kg/day), and alternate-day low dose FVIII (25 IUnits/kg). Immune tolerance is eventually achieved in 60–75% of patients. Until tolerance is successfully attained, episodic bleeds require

Table 11-17. Selected Immune Tolerance Induction Regimens for Hemophilia-Associated Inhibitors

Protocol	FVIII dose	Other agents	% Success rate (number of patients in trial)	Inhibitor elimination time range in months
High dose				
Bonn[1] (Brackman et al.)	100–150 IU/kg twice daily	APCC as required	100 (60)	
Malmo[2] (Berntorp/ Nilsson et al.)	Maintain FVIII>0.40 U/mL	Cyclophosphamide; dose is 12–15 mg/kg IV daily for 2 days followed by 2–3 mg/kg orally given daily for 8–10 days IV lg; dose is 0.4 g/kg daily for 5 days Immunoadsorption	63 (16)	1–2
Intermediate dose				
Kasper/Ewing[3]	50–100 IU/kg daily	Oral prednisone PRN	79 (12)	1–10
Unuvar et al.[4]	50–100 IU/kg daily (induction phase) 25 IU/kg daily (reduction phase)		75 (14)	0–8
Low dose				
Dutch[5] (Mauser-Bunschoten)	25 IU/kg alternate days		87 (24)	2–28

References

1. Oldenburg J, Schwaab R, Brackmann HH. Induction of immune tolerance in haemophilia A inhibitor patients by the "Bonn Protocol": predictive parameter for therapy duration and outcome. Vox Sanguinis 1999;77(Suppl 1):49–54.

2. Freiburghaus C, Berntorp E, Ekman M, et al. Tolerance induction using the Malmo treatment model 1982–1995. Haemophilia 1999;5:32–9.

3. Ewing NP, Sanders NL, Dietrich SL, et al. Induction of immune tolerance to factor VIII in hemophilia A patients with inhibitors. JAMA 1988;259:65–8.

4. Unuvar A, Warrier I, and Lusher JM. Immune tolerance induction in the treatment of paediatric haemophilia A patients with factor VIII inhibitors. Haemophilia 2000;6:150–7.

5. van Leeuwen EF, Mauser-Bunschoten EP, van Dijken PJ. Disappearance of factor VIII:C antibodies in patients with haemophilia A upon frequent administration of factor VIII in intermediate or low dose. Br J Haematol 1986;64,291–7.

alternate treatment, typically with bypassing agents. A low historical peak inhibitor titer, a low inhibitor titer at initiation of ITI, and a low maximum inhibitor titer during ITI all favor success. Success rates may also be higher in young patients and in patients treated on higher dose regimens. Cost and venous access are added obstacles to successfully completing immune tolerance.

Treatment of Factor IX Inhibitors

The frequency of inhibitory antibodies to factor IX is much lower than the frequency seen with factor VIII. The bypassing agents aPCC and rFVIIa have hemostatic efficacy in hemophilia B patients with inhibitors. Their use and dosages are the same as for the treatment of hemophilia A patients with inhibitors. Immune tolerance induction has been successful in some hemophilia B patients with inhibitors. However, many hemophilia B patients, typically those with a history of anaphylaxis to FIX concentrates, develop nephrotic syndrome in response to the frequent high-dose infusions of coagulation FIX concentrates, necessitating termination of the ITI effort.

Spontaneously Acquired Inhibitory Antibodies to Coagulation Factors

Spontaneous autoantibodies to factors VIII and IX and other coagulation factors may arise in nonhemophilia patients in a variety of other clinical conditions.

Acquired Hemophilia A

Autoantibodies (acquired inhibitors) may occur in nonhemophiliacs, resulting in acquired hemophilia A. These develop mainly in adults, more frequently in elderly subjects and in postpartum patients. Associated settings include pregnancy, immune diseases, and hematologic neoplasms (CLL, lymphoma). Symptoms are hemorrhage, typically into soft tissues and mucous membranes with occasional cerebral hemorrhage. Diagnosis is based on history (hemorrhage in the absence of prior patient or family history), prolonged PTT with failure to correct on mixing studies, reduced FVIII level, and the presence of an anti-FVIII inhibitor on Bethesda assay. Affinity of acquired inhibitors for FVIII differs from that of inhibitors (alloantibodies) associated with hemophilia A, resulting in complex kinetics and often incomplete inactivation of FVIII.

Treatment options for minor bleeding episodes in patients with low-titer autoantibodies include augmentation of endogenous FVIII using DDAVP or FVIII concentrates. For more severe bleeding associated with high-titer autoantibodies, hemostatic treatment options include porcine FVIII (if inhibitor titer against porcine FVIII is low), or bypassing agents as used for hemophilia A inhibitors (text above and Table 11-16). Plasmapheresis with or without a staphylococcal A column can be used to transiently lower the inhibitor titer, permitting effective FVIII replacement therapy. Immunosuppression-immunomodulation has been shown to be effective in eliminating autoantibodies. Treatment modalities alone or in combination include high-dose IVIG infusion (400 mg/kg/day for 5 days), prednisone (1 mg/kg/day as a single agent), cyclophosphamide (2 mg/kg/day), or other agents (vincristine, azathioprine, etc.). Cyclosporine A and rituximab are other agents reported to be effective in elimination of autoantibodies. Responses to any individual regimen is variable, requiring individualization of therapy.

Acquired Antibodies to Other Coagulation Factors

Acquired autoantibodies (inhibitors) to factor V are very rare. Some patients may have major hemorrhage (patients with antibodies that also bind to platelet factor V); others may not bleed, even at the time of major surgery. Available treatments for acute hemostasis include platelet transfusion (the factor V contained within the platelet α-granule may be locally protected from the inhibitor) and the use of bypassing agents.

Autoantibodies (inhibitors) to other factors (including prothrombin or factor XI) may occur, most commonly in the setting of systemic lupus erythematosus (SLE) (either isolated or in addition to the lupus anticoagulant) or hematologic malignancy. Some patients, usually those with a profound decrease in prothrombin concentration, may have hemorrhagic symptoms. Acute hemostatic treatment strategies include infusion of fresh frozen plasma or prothrombin complex concentrates. Inhibitor elimination strategies, as for other acquired inhibitors, include the use of plasmapheresis, glucocorticoids, and/or immunosuppression.

Autoantibodies to factor XI are very rare in children. They have been reported following viral infections and are usually transient. Glucocorticoid therapy may be efficacious in their elimination.

Lupus Anticoagulant

See pages 340–341 in the section on thrombotic disorders.

von Willebrand Disease

Von Willebrand disease (vWD) is an autosomally inherited congenital bleeding disorder caused by a deficiency (type 1), dysfunction (type 2), or complete absence (type 3) of von Willebrand factor. vWF has two functions:

1. It plays an integral role in mediating adherence of platelets at sites of endothelial damage, promoting formation of the platelet plug (Figure 11-1).
2. It binds and transports FVIII, protecting it from degradation by plasma proteases.

vWF is a large multimeric glycoprotein that is synthesized in megakaryocytes and endothelial cells as pre-pro-vWF. Sequential cleavage releases mature vWF, which undergoes multimerization and is stored in specific cellular storage granules such as the Weibel–Palade body in endothelial cells and the α-granule in platelets. It is present in normal amounts in plasma, and levels can be significantly increased by administering drugs such as desmopressin (DDAVP) that induce the release of vWF from storage sites into plasma. Deficiency of vWF results in mucocutaneous bleeding and prolonged oozing following trauma or surgery. vWD is the most common hereditary bleeding disorder, with biochemical evidence present in 1–2% of the population and biochemical evidence combined with a bleeding history of 0.1% of the population. Differences between vWD and hemophilia are displayed in Table 11-18. Table 11-19 shows the current classification of vWD, and Figure 11-7 shows the structure of vWF and indicates the location of mutations giving rise to variants of vWD.

Treatment of vWD

Recommended treatment of vWD is indicated in Table 11-20.

Type 1 vWD

This is the most common form of the disorder and is characterized by a mild to moderate decrease in the plasma levels of vWF. Plasma vWF from these individuals has a normal structure. Levels of ristocetin cofactor activity (R:Co or vWF activity) and vWF antigen tend to be decreased in parallel. DDAVP can be used to manage most hemostatic problems in patients with type I vWD. DDAVP treatment generally normalizes FVIII, vWF, and the bleeding time. The standard dose may be repeated daily as necessary. Response to DDAVP should be assessed for each individual patient.

Type 2A vWD

This variant is associated with decreased platelet-dependent vWF function and a lack of large HMW multimers in plasma and platelets. In some patients with type 2A

Table 11-18. Differences between von Willebrand Disease and Hemophilia A

	von Willebrand disease	Hemophilia A
Symptoms	Bruising and epistaxis	Joint bleeding
	Menorrhagia or mucosal bleeding	Muscle bleeding
Sexual distribution	Males = females	Males
Frequency	1:200 to 1:500	1:6000 males
Abnormal protein	vWF	Factor VIII
Molecular weight	$0.6–20 \times 10^6$ Da	280 kDa
Function	Platelet adhesion	Clotting cofactor
Site of synthesis	Endothelial cell or megakaryocytes	
Chromosome	Chromosome 12	X chromosome
Inhibitor frequency	Rare	14–25% of patients
Laboratory tests		
History	Abnormal	Abnormal
Bleeding time	Often abnormal	Usually normal
PTT	Normal or prolonged	Prolonged
Factor VIII	Borderline or decreased	Decreased or absent
vWF Ag	Decreased or absent	Normal or increased
vWF R:Co	Decreased or abnormal	Normal or increased
vWF multimers	Normal or abnormal	Normal

From Montgomery RR, Gill JC, Scott JP. Hemophilia and von Willebrand disease. In: Nathan D, Orkin S, editors. Nathan and Oski's Hematology of Infancy and Childhood. 5th ed. Philadelphia: WB Saunders, 1998:1631–75, with permission.

Abbreviations: vWF Ag = von Willebrand Factor antigen; R: Co = Ristocetin cofactor activity.

vWD, abnormalities have been localized to the A2 domain of vWF (Figure 11-7) and specific gene defects have been described. DDAVP treatment usually increases the FVIII level in type 2A, and the bleeding time may improve in some patients. DDAVP may suffice to control some types of bleeding in patients with this variant. Other patients will require treatment with clotting factor concentrates containing both FVIII and vWF. Use of cryoprecipitate for vWF replacement therapy should not be utilized because this product does not undergo viral inactivation treatment.

Type 2B vWD

This variant is a rare form of vWD characterized by dominant gain in function mutations in the A1 domain of the vWF gene. The HMW multimers bind spontaneously to platelets and are continuously removed from circulation. There may be mild thrombocytopenia due to spontaneous agglutination of the platelets. *In vitro*, this variant is characterized by a reduced threshold for aggregation of platelets on exposure to the antibiotic ristocetin. DDAVP is contraindicated in type 2B vWD because of transient thrombocytopenia resulting from release and clearance of abnormal vWF. Clotting factor concentrates containing both FVIII and vWF are the mainstay of treatment for this vWD variant.

Type 2N vWD

Type 2N vWD is a result of an abnormal vWF molecule that does not bind factor VIII (Figure 11-7). The unbound factor VIII is rapidly cleared from circulation, resulting in reduction of plasma factor VIII as compared with the level of vWF. Some of these patients may be misdiagnosed as having hemophilia A. It appears that the phenotype is expressed only in the presence of a second allele that carries type 1 vWD (compound heterozygous) or in the rare situation of recessive inheritance. In type 2N

Table 11-19. Variants of von Willebrand Disease

	Type 1	Type 2A	Type 2B	Type 2N	Type 2M	Type 3	Platelet type
Genetic transmission	AD	AD	AD	AR	AD	AR	AD
Frequency (%)	70–80	10–12	3–5	1–2	1–2	1–3	0–3
Bleeding time	N	N/prolonged	N/prolonged	N	N/prolonged	Prolonged	Prolonged
Platelet count	N	N	N/decreased	N	N	N	Decreased
FVIII	Decreased	N	Normal	Markedly decreased	Normal	Absent	N
vWF: Ag	Decreased	Decreased	N/decreased	Decreased	N	Absent	N/decreased
R:Co (vWF activity)	Decreased	Decreased	N/decreased	Decreased	Decreased	Absent	N/decreased
RIPA	N/decreased	Decreased	N	Normal	Decreased	Absent	N
RIPA-low dose	Absent	Absent	Increased	Absent	Absent	Absent	N
Multimeric structure	N	Absence of large multimers from plasma and platelets	Reduced large multimers from plasma	N	N	Absent	Reduced large multimers
Response to DDAVP							
FVIII, vWFAg, R:Co	Increases	Increases	Increases	Increases	Increases	NR	Increases
BT	N	Shortens	NR/shortens[a]	N	Shortens	NR	NR

Abbreviations: AD, autosomal dominant; N, normal; vWF: Ag, von Willebrand factor antigen (FVIII-related antigen); RIPA, ristocetin-induced platelet aggregation; RIPA-LD, low-dose RIPA; NR, no response.

[a]Causes platelet aggregation.

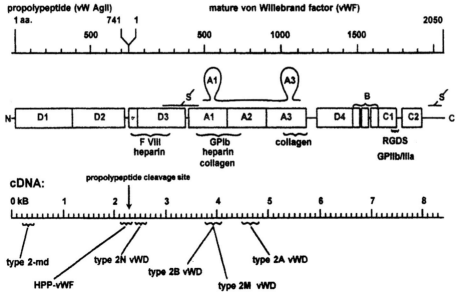

Fig. 11-7. Protein structure of vWF and its large propolypeptide, von Willebrand antigen II (vW AgII). Domains of the vWF molecule have high degrees of similarity, and various protein interactions have been localized to specific regions such as the interaction with platelet glycoprotein Ib or glycoprotein IIb/IIIa. This latter site may be related to an Arg-Gly-Asp-Ser (RGDS) sequence located in the C1 domain. The lower portion of this figure represents the clusters of complementary DNA mutations that cause some of the variants of von Willebrand disease, including types 2A, 2B, 2M, and 2N, as well as the less common variants that prevent propolypeptide cleavage (hereditary persistence of pro-vWF [HPP-vWF]) or a variant that prevents N-terminal multimerization (type 2-md). (From Montgomery RR, Gill JC, Scott JP. Hemophilia and von Willebrand disease. In: Nathan DG, Orkin SH, editors. Nathan and Oski's Hematology of Infancy and Childhood. 5th ed. Philadelphia: WB Saunders, 1998;1631–75, with permission.)

vWD FVIII levels increase following DDAVP infusion but the released FVIII circulates only for a short time because of impaired binding to vWF. For the same reason the half-life of infused high-purity factor VIII is markedly shortened. For major bleeding or surgery, the recommended treatment is a factor VIII concentrate containing high levels of vWF.

Type 2M vWD

Type 2M vWD results from an abnormal binding site on vWF for platelet GP Ib, resulting in reduced ristocetin cofactor (R:Co) activity (functional defect). In this variant multimers of all sizes are present. The vWF protein is released by DDAVP so that patients heterozygous for this variant may respond clinically to standard doses of DDAVP. For homozygotes the vWF released by DDAVP is defective and a poor clinical response occurs. Major bleeding episodes or surgery should be managed with vWF replacement therapy.

Type 3 vWD

This vWD variant occurs in patients with homozygous or doubly heterozygous null mutations or deletions. The clinical phenotype is a severe bleeding disorder with major deficits in both primary and secondary hemostasis. The plasma level of FVIII and vWF is virtually undetectable. Patients are unresponsive to DDAVP (no releasable vWF stores) and require episodic treatment with vWF containing FVIII concentrates. Alloantibodies that inactivate von Willebrand factor develop in 10–15%

Table 11-20. Recommended Treatment in von Willebrand Disease

	Type 1	Type 2A	Type 2B	Type 2N	Type 2M	Type 3	Platelet-type pseudo-vWD
Severe hemorrhages; major surgical procedures	DDAVP	FVIII:vWF concentrates	FVIII:vWF concentrates	FVIII:vWF concentrates	FVIII:vWF concentrates	FVIII:vWF concentrates	Platelet transfusion
Mild hemorrhages; minor surgical procedures	DDAVP	FVIII:vWF concentrates (may respond to DDAVP)	FVIII:vWF concentrates	FVIII:vWF concentrates (may respond to DDAVP)	FVIII:vWF concentrates (may respond to DDAVP)	FVIII:vWF concentrates	Platelet transfusion
Oral surgical procedures	DDAVP and EACA	FVIII:vWF concentrates and EACA	FVIII:vWF concentrates and EACA	FVIII:vWF concentrates and EACA	FVIII:vWF concentrates and EACA	FVIII:vWF concentrates and EACA	Platelet transfusion and EACA

Abbreviations: DDAVP, desmopressin; EACA, amicar; factor VIII: vWF concentrates; see Table 11-14.

of patients with type 3 disease who have received multiple transfusions. Administration of FVIII concentrates containing vWF to these patients is contraindicated because life-threatening anaphylactic reactions may result. In this setting, administration of recombinant FVIII, which is devoid of vWF, can raise FVIII levels to hemostatic levels. In the absence of vWF the half-life of the infused FVIII will be short (1–2 hours) and administration of high doses, at short intervals or by continuous infusion, will be required. Administration of rFVIIa at a dose of 90 µg/kg every 2 hours has produced hemostasis for some of these patients.

Platelet-Type Pseudo–von Willebrand Disease

Platelet-type pseudo-vWD is due to a gain of function mutation defect in the platelet GP Ib receptor. This platelet disorder has a phenotype similar to type 2B vWD. Excessive binding of vWF to platelet GP Ib receptor causes platelet activation and vWF removal from the circulation, plasma concentrations of vWF are reduced, and platelet aggregation is increased. Bleeding in this disorder should be treated with platelet transfusions.

Acquired von Willebrand Disease

Acquired vWD may present as a marked reduction in levels of von Willebrand antigen in a person who does not have a lifelong bleeding disorder. The onset has been associated with a variety of conditions including Wilms' tumor, other neoplasms, autoimmune diseases (e.g., SLE), myeloproliferative disease, lymphoproliferative disorders, use of various drugs, as well as in individuals with angiodysplastic lesions. Proposed mechanisms include specific autoantibodies, adsorption onto malignant cell clones, and depletion in conditions of high vascular shear force. Therapeutic interventions are directed at controlling acute bleeding episodes, treating the underlying disorder in the hope of correcting the abnormalities of vWF, and effecting antibody elimination. DDAVP infusion is the initial treatment of choice for achieving hemostasis; plasma-derived FVIII/vWF concentrates are the second choice. In either case clearance of the von Willebrand factor will be accelerated and levels must be monitored. IVIG, plasmapheresis, and/or immunosuppressive drugs may be useful for eliminating antibody.

Rare Coagulation Factor Deficiencies

Table 11-21 lists the treatment of rare coagulation deficiencies.

HEREDITARY DISORDERS OF PLATELET FUNCTION

Qualitative disorders of platelet function (see Chapter 10) usually manifest with mucocutaneous bleeding. Symptoms include petechiae, ecchymoses, epistaxis, menorrhagia, gastrointestinal bleeding, and abnormal bleeding in association with injury or trauma. Physical examination may reveal associated abnormalities such as nystagmus and oculocutaneous albinism in Hermansky–Pudlack syndrome or eczema in Wiskott–Aldrich syndrome. Laboratory evaluation includes morphologic inspection of the blood smear for platelet size, inclusions, and the presence of a gray or washed-out appearance. Assessment of platelet function by bleeding time, platelet aggregation studies, or PFA-100 closure time will usually be abnormal. Definitive diagnosis of suspected disorders will often require additional studies available only at reference laboratories (e.g., flow cytometry enumeration of receptors, electron

Table 11-21. Treatment of Rare Coagulation Factor Deficiencies[a]

Factor deficiency	Half-life (h)	Percentage increase in plasma concentration after 1 unit/kg IV	Percentage required for hemostasis	Percentage required for minor trauma	Percentage required for surgery and major trauma
Afibrinogenemia	56–82	1–1.5[a]	80[a]	150[a]	200[b]
II	45–60	1	20–30	30	50
V	36	1.5	10–15	10–15	25
VII	5	1	10–15	10–15	20
vWD[c]	24–48	1.5[d]	10	20–30	50
X	24–60	1	10–15	10–15	25
XI	48	1	30	30	>45
XIII	168–240	1	2–3	15	25

[a]See Table 11-15 for factor VIII and factor IX deficiency treatment guidelines.
[b]in mg/dL.
[c]vWD, von Willebrand disease.
[d]Calculated in units of vWF:Rcof activity.

microscopy). Physiologically these disorders may be divided into those caused by abnormal platelet receptors and those with defects in granule content or storage pool release.

Table 11-22 lists the genetic transmission and recommended treatment for these hereditary disorders of platelet function. In some of these disorders, hemostasis will be improved by administration of DDAVP as in von Willebrand disease. Platelet transfusion is often necessary for hemostasis in those disorders not responsive to DDAVP. Leuko-depleted single-donor platelets, HLA matched if available, are preferred in these patients to reduce the risk of platelet allosensitization. Isoantibodies against the platelet proteins absent from the patient are common in these disorders and may render patients refractory to platelet transfusion. Administration of rFVIIa 90 µg/kg can effect hemostasis in some patients not responsive to platelet transfusion. For nonresponders, higher doses may be hemostatic. Antifibrinolytic agents are a useful adjunct in patients with these disorders.

THROMBOTIC DISORDERS

Mechanisms of Thrombosis in Inherited Thrombophilia

In inherited thrombophilias, impaired neutralization of thrombin or a failure to control the generation of thrombin causes thrombosis. There is a malfunction in a system of natural anticoagulants that maintain the fluidity of the blood. Decreases in antithrombin III activity impair the neutralization of thrombin and reduced activity of protein C or protein S diminishes the control of thrombin generation. Both of these mechanisms increase susceptibility to thrombosis (Figure 11-8).

The control of thrombin generation is also compromised by mutations in the gene for factor V or prothrombin. The Arg506Gln substitution in factor V Leiden involves the first of three sites on factor Va that are cleaved by activated protein C. This mutation slows down the proteolytic inactivation of factor Va, which in turn leads to the augmented generation of thrombin. Moreover, the mutant factor V has diminished cofactor activity in the inactivation of factor VIIIa by activated protein C. Both these abnormalities in factor V cause the *in vitro* phenomenon of

Table 11-22. Hereditary Disorders of Platelet Function

Disorder	Transmission/ frequency	Defect	Primary treatment	Alternative treatment
Disorders of receptors				
Glanzmann thrombasthenia	Autosomal recessive, rare	GP IIb/IIIa complex	Platelet transfusion	rFVIIa in instances of platelet alloim-munization
Bernard–Soulier syndrome	Autosomal recessive, Rare	GP Ib/V/IX complex	Platelet transfusion	rFVIIa in instances of platelet alloim-munization
Defects in granule content, storage pool deficiency				
Gray platelet syndrome	Rare	Absent alpha granules	DDAVP (treatment rarely required)	Platelet transfusion for nonresponders
Chédiak–Higashi syndrome	Autosomal recessive, rare	Abnormal granules	DDAVP	Platelet transfusion for nonresponders
Wiskott–Aldrich syndrome	X-linked recessive	WAS protein. Primarily a quantitative defect, storage pool deficiency may also be present	DDAVP for qualitative defect	Platelet transfusion for thrombo-cytopenia
Hermansky–Pudlak syndrome	Autosomal recessive	Absent dense granules	DDAVP	Platelet transfusion for nonresponders
Storage pool release defects	Variable	Impaired secondary wave of aggregation	DDAVP	Platelet transfusion for nonresponders

resistance to activated protein C, resulting in the failure of activated protein C to prolong the activated partial thromboplastin time. For unknown reasons, the G20210A mutation in the 3 untranslated region of the prothrombin gene is associated with an increased level of plasma prothrombin, an effect that promotes the generation of thrombin and impairs the inactivation of factor Va by activated protein C. The mechanisms by which increased levels of factor VIII, factor IX, factor XI, fibrinogen, and homocysteine enhance venous thrombosis are incompletely understood.

Table 11-23 lists the clinical manifestations of a hypercoagulable state, and laboratory findings in hypercoagulable states are listed in Table 11-24.

Venous Thrombosis

Venous thrombotic events develop under conditions of slow blood flow. It may occur by way of activation of the coagulation system with or without vascular dam-

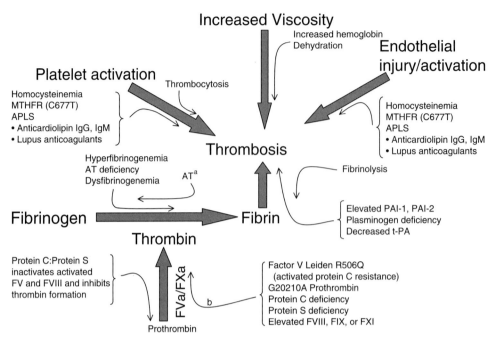

Fig. 11-8. Natural inhibitors of coagulation and the effect(s) of pro-thrombotic states. (a) Leads to neutralization of thrombin. (b) Decreased neutralization or increased generation of thrombin.

age. Venous thrombi are composed of large amounts of fibrin containing numerous erythrocytes, platelets, and leukocytes (red thrombus). The incidence of a venous thrombotic event in children is estimated to be between 0.7 and 1.9 per 100,000 children. Venous thrombosis usually produces significant obstruction to blood flow. The most serious consequence is embolization from a deep-vein thrombosis resulting in pulmonary embolism. Table 11-25 lists the predisposing causes of venous thrombo-

Table 11-23. Clinical Manifestations of Hypercoagulable States

Family history of thrombosis
Recurrent spontaneous thromboses
Thrombosis in unusual sites
Thrombosis at an early age
Resistance to anticoagulant therapy
Coumarin necrosis syndrome
Recurrent spontaneous abortions
Thrombosis during pregnancy/oral contraceptives
Migratory superficial thrombophlebitis
Antiphospholipid syndrome
Autoimmune disorders
   Inflammatory bowel disease
   Systemic lupus erythematosus
   Behçet disease
Malignancy
Nephrotic syndrome
Infections
   Varicella
   HIV
   Suppurative thrombophlebitis

Table 11-24. Laboratory Findings in Hypercoagulable States

Primary hemostasis
Thrombocytosis
Platelet aggregation
  Hyperaggregation
  Spontaneous aggregation
  Circulating platelet aggregates
Increased platelet adhesiveness
Elevated levels of β-thromboglobulin, vWF, and PF4
Short platelet life span

Secondary hemostasis
Shortened PT/PTT
Elevated coagulation factors (i.e., I, II, V, VII, VIII, IX, X, XI)
Reduced antithrombin, heparin cofactor II, plasminogen, tissue plasminogen activator, protein C, protein S, FXII, prekallikrein
Factor V Leiden/APC resistance
Prothrombin gene mutation (G20210A)
Elevated α-2-antiplasmin, α-2-macroglobulin, plasminogen activator inhibitor
Increased lipoprotein (a)
Thrombomodulin deficiency
Presence of fibrinopeptide A (FPA)
Increased fibrin degradation products
Short fibrinogen life span
Dysfibrinogenemia
Homocysteinemia
Presence of lupus anticoagulants
Presence of anticardiolipin antibodies

Table 11-25. Predisposing Factors for Venous Thrombosis

Acquired[a]
Age
Trauma
Venipuncture
Intravenous catheters
Surgery
Thermal injury
Immune complexes
Infections (HIV, varicella, suppurative thrombophlebitis)
Severe dehydration
Shock
Prolonged immobilization
Cancer
L-Asparaginase therapy, prednisone
Oral contraceptives or hormone replacement therapy
Cyanotic heart disease
Pregnancy and the puerperium
Nephrotic syndrome
Liver disease
Neonatal asphyxia
Infant of a diabetic mother
Antiphospholipid syndrome
  Primary
  Secondary
    Systemic lupus erythematosus
    Rheumatoid arthritis

(Continues)

Table 11-25. (Continued)

Resistance to activated protein C not due to factor V Leiden
Systemic lupus erythematosus
　Anticardiolipin antibodies
　Lupus anticoagulants
Hyperviscosity syndromes
　Myeloproliferative disorders
　Polycythemia vera
　Chronic myelogenous leukemia
　Essential thrombocythemia
　Paroxysmal nocturnal hemoglobinuria
Hyperleukocytosis (acute leukemias)
Dysproteinemias
　Multiple myeloma
　Waldenstrom macroglobulinemia
　Cryoglobulinemia
Sickle cell disease
Infusion of concentrated vitamin K–dependent (II, VII, IX, and X) factors

Congenital/inherited[b]
R506Q mutation in the factor V gene [(factor V Leiden)—activated protein C resistance]
G20210A mutation in the prothrombin (factor II) gene
Homozygous C677T mutation in the methylenetetrahydrofolate reductase gene (C677T MTHFR)
Antithrombin (AT) deficiency
Protein C deficiency
Protein S deficiency
Plasminogen deficiency
Reduced levels of tissue thromboplastin activator (t-PA)
Dysfibrinogenemia
FXII (Hageman factor) deficiency
Prekallikrein deficiency
Heparin cofactor II (HC-II) deficiency
Hyperhomocysteinemia (due to C677T MTHFR or folate or vitamin B_{12} deficiency)
Homozygous homocystinuria
Increased levels of factor VIII, factor IX, factor XI, or fibrinogen
Increased thrombin activatable fibrinolysis inhibitor (TAFI)

[a]In inherited thrombophilia these acquired factors increase the risk of venous thrombosis.

[b]The first thrombotic event may occur at an early age in patients who have more than one thrombophilia or who are homozygous for factor V Leiden or the G20210A prothrombin gene mutation or asymptomatic heterozygotes who are relatives of patients with inherited thrombophilia who have had venous thrombosis. The combination of hyperhomocysteinemia with either factor V Leiden or G20210A prothrombin gene mutation significantly increase the risk of venous thrombosis. Recurrent thrombosis is more common in those with more than one thrombophilia.

sis. The detection of venous thrombosis and diagnosis of pulmonary embolism are given in Tables 11-26 and 11-27, respectively.

Newborns are at a high risk for a venous thrombotic event because of decreased activity of anticoagulant factors, specifically antithrombin, protein C, and protein S. Fibrinolytic activity in the newborn period is also decreased by lower serum plasminogen levels. Renal, caval, portal, and hepatic venous system thrombosis are well-known complications of peripartum asphyxia, sepsis, dehydration, and maternal diabetes. The estimated annual incidence of venous thrombotic events is about 0.5 per 10,000 newborns. However, the majority of venous thrombotic events within the first year of life are associated with central venous access devices.

Table 11-26. Detection of Venous Thrombosis

Clinical assessment:
  Symptoms and signs of deep-venous thrombosis
  Presence or absence of an alternative diagnosis
  Presence and number of predisposing factors for venous thrombotic event (Table 11-25)
Venous ultrasound
Impedance plethysmography
D-dimer blood testing:
  High sensitivity and negative predictive value for deep-venous thrombosis
Venogram

Table 11-27. Diagnosis of Pulmonary Embolism

Clinical assessment—typical signs and symptoms
Ventilation-perfusion lung scanning; accuracy is about 80–90%
Pulmonary angiography:
  The gold standard for the diagnosis of pulmonary emboli
Risk factors;
  Recent surgery
  Immobilization (>3 days' bed rest)
  Previous deep-venous thrombosis or pulmonary emboli
  Lower extremity plaster cast
  Lower extremity paralysis
  Strong family history for deep vein thrombosis/pulmonary emboli
  Cancer
  Postpartum

The treatment of venous thrombotic events is given in Table 11-28.

Arterial Thrombosis

Arterial thrombosis initially occurs under conditions of rapid blood flow and often is the result of a process that damages the vessel wall. The thrombus is composed of tightly coherent platelets that contain small amounts of fibrin and few erythrocytes and leukocytes (white thrombus). The most serious consequence of arterial thrombosis is vascular occlusion. Arterial thrombotic events occur in a number of congenital and acquired diseases (Table 11-29).

Cardiac Catheterization

The most common cause of an arterial thrombotic event in children is the use of cardiac vascular catheters. Without prophylactic anticoagulation, the incidence of an

Table 11-28. Treatment of Venous Thrombotic Events and Thromboembolism

Treatment	Indications
Anticoagulant therapy	Majority of patients with a venous thrombotic event (see anticoagulant therapy)
Thrombolytic therapy	Massive pulmonary embolism with hemodynamic compromise; patients with extensive iliofemoral thrombosis (see thrombolytic therapy)
Intracaval filter	Pulmonary embolism despite adequate anticoagulant therapy
Pulmonary embolectomy	Massive pulmonary embolism despite thrombolytic therapy

Table 11-29. Predisposing Causes of Arterial Thrombosis

Acquired
  Catheterization
    Cardiac
    Umbilical artery
    Renal artery—kidney transplantation
    Hepatic artery—liver transplantation
  Vascular
    Injury
    Infections
    Periarteritis nodosa
    Systemic lupus erythematosus (SLE)
    Kawasaki disease
    Hemolytic uremic syndrome (HUS)
    Thrombotic thrombocytopenic purpura (TTP)
  Cardiac
    Blalock–Taussig shunts
    Fontan operation
    Endovascular stents
    Cyanotic congenital heart disease
    Primary endocardial fibroelastosis
    Enlarged left atrium with arterial fibrillation
    Hypertension
    Myocarditis
  Hematologic/Hemostatic
    Elevated levels of LP(a)
    Elevated PAI-1
    Reduced t-PA
    Elevated level of fibrinogen
    Antiphospholipid syndrome (APLS)
    Chronic disseminated intravascular coagulation (DIC)
    Elevated levels of fibrin degradation products (D-dimers)
    Hyperhomocysteinemia
    Hypereosinophilic syndrome
    Myeloproliferative disorders (MDS)
    Polycythemia vera (PV)
    Chronic myelogenous leukemia (CML)
    Essential thrombocythemia (ET)
    Paroxysomal nocturnal hemoglobinuria (PNH)
    Hyperleukocytosis (acute leukemia)
    Sickle cell disease
    Hemoglobin SC disease
    Thrombotic thrombocytopenic purpura (TTP)
    Activated protein C concentrate administration
  Other
    Shock
    Nephrotic syndrome
    Diabetes mellitus
    Hyperlipidemia
    Hypercholesterolemia
    Cigarette smoking
    Elevated CRP
    Malignancy
    Obesity
    Physical inactivity

(Continues)

Table 11-29. (*Continued*)

Congenital/inherited

R506Q mutation in the factor V gene [(factor V Leiden)—activated protein C resistance]

G20210A mutation in the prothrombin (factor II) gene

Homozygous C677T mutation in the methylenetetrahydrofolate reductase gene (C677T MTHFR)

Antithrombin (AT) deficiency

Protein C deficiency

Protein S deficiency

Marfan syndrome

Familial hypercholesterolemia

Mitral valve prolapse

Abbreviations: Lp(a), lipoprotein a; PAI-1, plasminogen activator inhibitor-1; t-PA, tissue thromboplasminogen activator; CRP, C-reactive protein

arterial thrombotic event from femoral artery catheterization is about 40%. Anticoagulation with heparin (100–150 U/kg) reduces the incidence of arterial thrombotic events to 8%.

Cardiac Procedures

Blalock-Taussig Shunts

The short length and very high flow in these shunts may result in arterial thrombosis. The incidence varies from 1 to 17%. For anticoagulant management, see page 361.

Fontan Operation

In this procedure the incidence of an arterial thrombotic event ranges from 3 to 19%. Arterial thrombotic events may occur anytime following the surgery and it is the major cause of early and late morbidity and mortality. For anticoagulant management, see pages 360–361.

Endovascular Stents

These stents are used increasingly to manage some patients with congenital heart disease (e.g., pulmonary artery stenosis, pulmonary vein stenosis, coarctation of aorta). Therapeutic doses of heparin are given at the time of stent insertion, followed by aspirin therapy (5 mg/kg/day).

Umbilical Artery Catheterization

Incidence of an arterial thrombotic event from an umbilical arterial catheter is markedly reduced by a low dose continuous heparin infusion (3 to 5 unit/h).

Renal Artery Thrombosis

Renal arterial thrombosis is commonly associated with kidney transplant. The incidence is about 0.2–3.5% in children. Prophylactic administration of low-molecular-weight heparin (LMWH) 0.4 mg/kg twice daily for 21 days is effective anticoagulant therapy.

Hepatic Artery Thrombosis

Hepatic artery thrombosis is a very serious complication of liver transplantation. It usually occurs within 2 weeks. The reported incidence in children can be as high as

42%. The detection of a hepatic artery thrombosis includes Doppler, angiography, and CT of the liver. The prophylactic use of LMWH and aspirin is controversial. The mortality from hepatic artery thrombosis may be as high as 70% in children. Anticoagulant therapy alone is not effective in hepatic artery thrombosis. Surgical intervention and retransplantation usually are necessary. Thrombolytic therapy has been successful in about 20% of children.

Kawasaki Disease

The acute phase of Kawasaki disease may be associated with arteritis, arterial aneurysms, valvulitis, and myocarditis. The incidence of coronary artery aneurysm, stenosis, or thrombosis is about 25% without initial treatment. There is strong evidence that early use of IV gammaglobulin and aspirin can reduce the coronary artery involvement of Kawasaki disease.

Antiphospholipid Antibody Syndrome

Antiphospholipid antibody syndrome (APLS) may result in an arterial thrombotic event including stroke in children. The lupus anticoagulants and APLS are discussed on pages 338–343.

Specific Risk Factors

Homocysteine

Homocysteine is a sulfur-containing amino acid formed during the metabolism of methionine, an amino acid derived from dietary protein. When excess methionine is present, homocysteine is linked with serine to form cystathionine in a reaction catalyzed by *cystathionine β-synthetase*, a vitamin B_6–dependent enzyme. Otherwise homocysteine acquires a methyl group from N^5-methylhydrofolate in a reaction catalyzed by the vitamin B_{12}–dependent enzyme *methionine synthetase*.

Hyperhomocysteinemia, a risk factor for venous thrombosis, can be caused by genetic disorders affecting the trans-sulfuration or remethylation pathways of homocysteine metabolism, or by folic acid deficiency, vitamin B_{12} deficiency, vitamin B_6 deficiency, renal failure, hypothyroidism, increasing age, and smoking. A rare example of excessive hyperhomocysteinemia is homozygous homocystinuria due to cystathionine β-synthetase deficiency; 50% of affected patients present with venous or arterial thrombosis by the age of 29 years. Homozygosity for the C677T mutation in the methylenetetrahydrofolate reductase gene is a cause of mild hyperhomocysteinemia.

It has been shown that excess homocysteine has the following effects:

- Toxic on the endothelium.
- Promotes thrombosis by platelet activation.
- Causes oxidation of LDL cholesterol.
- Increases levels of von Willebrand factor and thrombomodulin.
- Increases smooth muscle proliferation.

The mean total homocysteine levels in the newborn in various studies are 5.84, 7.4, and 7.8 μmol/L. Daily folic acid (2.5 mg), vitamin B_6 (50 mg), and vitamin B_{12} (1 mg) lower plasma homocysteine levels.

Lipoprotein (a)

Lipoprotein (a), [Lp(a)], is a distinct serum lipoprotein composed of a low-density lipid particle with disulfide links along a polypeptide chain (*apolipoprotein a*). Lp(a) regulates fibrinolysis by competing with plasminogen. Elevated levels of Lp(a) are associated with coronary artery disease and represents an independent risk factor for spontaneous stroke and venous thrombosis in childhood.

Fibrinogen

High levels of fibrinogen are associated with cardiovascular events in both men and women. Individuals with high fibrinogen concentrations have a risk of cardiovascular disease about 2.3 times higher than individuals with lower levels. Cigarette smoking substantially increases fibrinogen levels, a relationship that is both dose-dependent and reversible.

Fibrin Degradation Products (D-Dimers)

The breakdown of cross-linked fibrin yields a number of degradation products, most notably D-dimers. Elevated levels of D-dimers are associated with thrombosis. Low levels of D-dimers are useful for excluding a diagnosis of acute thrombosis. D-dimers are a sensitive marker for fibrin turnover that allow recognition of covert coagulation. Alternately, it may indicate preclinical atherosclerosis, because levels are elevated for years before arterial thrombosis occurs.

Tissue Plasminogen Activator

This fibrinolytic protein is synthesized and secreted in the vascular endothelium and has a very short half-life. Individuals with reduced levels of t-PA are associated with higher risk for coronary artery disease. Low-dose aspirin therapy may reduce coronary artery disease in these individuals.

Plasminogen Activator Inhibitor 1

PAI-1 is an antifibrinolytic protein and is synthesized and secreted in the vascular endothelium. Individuals with elevated levels of PAI-1 antigen are prone to recurrent episodes of spontaneous thrombosis and coronary artery disease. Aspirin therapy may have a beneficial effect in individuals with elevated PAI-1 antigen.

C-Reactive Protein

C-reactive protein (CRP) is a typical acute-phase reactant. In response to acute injury, infection, or other stimuli, serum levels of CRP increase several-fold. It is produced in the liver, regulated primarily via interleukin-6 production by activated leukocytes and fibroblast and endothelial cells. Inflammation plays an essential role in plaque rupture and atherosclerosis. CRP may act as an indirect marker for preclinical atherosclerosis.

General Risk Factors

Cigarette Smoking

Smokers have a twofold increase of developing coronary artery disease and a 50% increased risk of dying from it. Smoking interacts in synergistic fashion with hypercholesterolemia, hypertension, and oral contraceptives.

Cholesterol

The precise mechanism by which LDL cholesterol increases the risk of coronary artery disease and stroke is not known. Lipid parameters other than total cholesterol and LDL cholesterol may be useful predictors of coronary artery disease or may aid in tailoring lipid-lowering therapy. Studies show that for every 1 mg/dL decrease in HDL cholesterol, there is a corresponding 3–4% increase in coronary artery disease.

Hypertension

Studies showed that a 7-mmHg increase from the baseline in diastolic blood pressure is associated with a 27% increase in risk of coronary artery disease and a 42% increase in stroke.

Pregnancy

Venous thrombosis occurs in 60% of women with antithrombin deficiency and in 20% with a deficiency of either protein C or S.

Diabetes

Among people with diabetes, atherosclerotic complications are a major cause of morbidity and mortality. Coronary artery disease is the cause of death in 69% of individuals with diabetes.

Obesity

Obesity early in life is a strong predictor of later cardiovascular disease. Observational studies have demonstrated increased risk of coronary artery disease mortality and morbidity among obese individuals.

Physical Inactivity

Physical inactivity is second only to hypercholesterolemia as a contributing cause of coronary artery disease.

Antiphospholipid Syndrome

Antiphospholipid syndrome (APLS) includes:

Lupus anticoagulant (LA) detected by prolonged APTT
Anticardiolipin antibodies (ACLAs) detected by immunoassays
    Anticardiolipin antibody IgA*
    Anticardiolipin antibody IgG
    Anticardiolipin antibody IgM
Subgroups of antiphospholipid antibodies (APLA) detected by immunoassays
    Anti-beta-2-glycoprotein-I (β-2-GPI) (IgA, IgG, IgM)*
    Anti-phosphatidylserine (IgG, IgA, IgM)*
    Anti-phosphatidylethanolamine (IgG, IgA, IgM)*
    Anti-phosphatidylcholine (IgG, IgA, IgM)*
    Anti-phosphatidylinositol (IgG, IgA, IgM)*
    Anti-annexin-V*

Antiphospholipid antibodies (APLA) are found in 1–5% of young healthy subjects and these increase in prevalence with increasing age. Among patients with SLE, the

---

*These APLAs are not included in the laboratory diagnosis of APLS (see Table 11-30).

prevalence is 12–30% for ACLA and 15–34% for LA. Many patients have laboratory evidence of APLA without clinical consequences.

The APLAs may promote thrombosis by:

Antibody-induced activation of endothelial cells and the secretion of cytokines
Platelet activation
Impaired activation of protein C, annexin V, and tissue factors
Inhibition of β2-GPI (thought to act as a natural anticoagulant)
Impaired fibrinolytic activity
Antibody against endothelial cells.

APLS is the most common acquired condition associated with venous and/or arterial thrombotic events. The thrombotic events associated with APLS include deep-vein thrombosis, pulmonary embolus, coronary artery thrombosis, stroke, transient ischemic attacks, retinal vascular thrombosis, and placental vascular thrombosis (leading to recurrent-miscarriage syndrome). Virtually any organ can be involved and the range of disorders observed within any one organ span a diverse spectrum. The effects of APLS depends on two factors:

1. Nature and size of the vessel affected
2. Acuteness or chronicity of the thrombotic process.

Venous thrombosis, especially deep-venous thrombosis of the legs, is the most common manifestation of the antiphospholipid syndrome. Up to half of these patients have pulmonary emboli. Arterial thromboses are less common than venous thromboses and most frequently manifest with features consistent with ischemia or infarction. The severity of presentation relates to the acuteness and extent of occlusion. The brain is the most common site, with strokes and transient ischemic attacks accounting for almost 50% of arterial occlusions. Coronary occlusions account for an additional 23%; the remaining 27% involve diverse vessels, including subclavian, renal, retinal, and pedal arteries.

In patients with APLS there is an increased rate of heart valve abnormalities, mainly valve masses or thickening that affects primarily the mitral valve. Up to 63% of patients with the antiphospholipid syndrome reveal at least one valvular abnormality on echocardiography. Emboli, especially from mitral-valve or aortic-valve vegetations, can lead to cerebral events. Not all arterial episodes of ischemia or infarction are thrombotic in origin.

Acute involvement at the level of the capillaries, arterioles, or venules may result in a clinical picture resembling hemolytic uremic syndrome and thrombotic thrombocytopenic purpura as well as other thrombotic microangiopathies. Thrombotic microangiopathy may also occur as a more chronic process, resulting in slow, progressive loss of organ function, the underlying reason for which may only be determined by biopsy. Thus, organ involvement in patients with the antiphospholipid syndrome can present in a spectrum from rapidly progressive to clinically silent and indolent. Depending on the size of the vessels affected, organ failure has two predominant causes, thrombotic microangiopathy and ischemia secondary to thromboembolic events.

Other prominent manifestations of the antiphospholipid syndrome include thrombocytopenia, hemolytic anemia, and livedo reticularis. Although renal manifestations are a very common feature of SLE, they have only recently been recognized as part of the antiphospholipid syndrome.

Histopathologic features of APLS consist of:

- Thrombotic microangiopathy
- Ischemia secondary to arterial thromboses or emboli
- Peripheral embolization from venous, arterial, or intracardiac sources.

Table 11-30 shows the criteria for diagnosis of APLS.

Table 11-30. International Consensus Statement on Preliminary Criteria for the Diagnosis of the Antiphospholipid Syndrome[a]

Clinical criteria
Vascular thrombosis
  One or more clinical episodes of arterial, venous, or small-vessel thrombosis, occurring within any tissue or organ
Complications of pregnancy
  One or more unexplained deaths of morphologically normal fetuses at or after the 10th week of gestation; or
  One or more premature births of morphologically normal neonates at or before the 34th week of gestation; or
  Three or more unexplained consecutive spontaneous abortions before the 10th week of gestation

Laboratory criteria[b]
Anticardiolipin antibodies
  Anticardiolipin IgG or IgM antibodies present at moderate or high levels in the blood on two or more occasions at least 6 weeks apart[c]
Lupus anticoagulant antibodies
  Lupus anticoagulant antibodies detected in the blood on two or more occasions at least 6 weeks apart

[a]A diagnosis of definite antiphospholipid syndrome requires the presence of at least one of the clinical criteria and at least one of the laboratory criteria. No limits are placed on the interval between the clinical event and the positive laboratory findings.

[b]The following antiphospholipid antibodies are not included in the laboratory criteria: anticardiolipin IgA antibodies, anti-β_2-glycoprotein I antibodies, and antiphospholipid antibodies directed against phospholipids other than cardiolipin (e.g., phosphatidylserine and phosphatidylethanolamine) or against phospholipid–binding proteins other than cardiolipin-bound β_2-glycoprotein I (e.g., prothrombin, annexin V, protein C, or protein S).

[c]The threshold used to distinguish moderate or high levels of anticardiolipin antibodies from low levels has not been standardized. Many laboratories use 15 or 20 international "phospholipid" units as the threshold separating low from moderate levels of anticardiolipin antibodies or as the 99th percentile of anticardiolipin levels within a normal population.

From Levine JS, Branch W, Rauch J. The antiphospholipid syndrome. N Engl J Med 2002;346:752–63, with permission.

Lupus Anticoagulant and Thrombosis

The so-called "lupus anticoagulant antibody" (LA) was first described in patients with SLE who presented with prolonged APTT. The term is actually a misnomer because only few patients with SLE have LA and the inhibitor is not an anticoagulant. Despite the name, LA antibodies are associated with thromboembolic events rather than clinical bleeding. Approximately 10% of patients with SLE have LA. LA is occasionally found in patients with immune thrombocytopenic purpura (ITP) in whom SLE subsequently develops. Human leukocyte antigen (HLA) HLA-DR antigens (DR7 and DRW35) may play a role in the development of LA in some individuals.

Thromboembolism occurs in about 10% of patients with SLE; however, in patients with SLE and LA the occurrence of thromboembolism is up to 50%. The LA is estimated to account for approximately 6–8% of thrombosis in otherwise healthy individuals. Primary LA thrombosis syndrome consists of patients with LA and thrombosis but who have no secondary underlying disease such as SLE or other autoimmune disorders, malignancy, infection, inflammation, or ingestion of drugs inducing the LA. It is fivefold more common than the secondary type associated with an underlying disease.

Lupus anticoagulant may be associated with the following conditions:

HIV infections
Intercurrent viral infections
Malignancy
Systemic antibiotic therapy
Certain medications (e.g., chlorpromazine, Dilantin, α-interferon, Fansidar, pro-
    cainamide, phenothiazines, phenytoin hydralazine, quinidine, quinine)
Cocaine use
SLE
"Lupus-like" chronic autoimmune disorders
Arterial or venous thrombotic events with no apparent underlying cause
Women with recurrent fetal wastage.

The LA is an acquired circulating immunoglobulin (usually IgG, sometimes IgM or IgA), which binds to negatively charged phospholipid components of factors Xa and Va, phospholipid, and calcium. This circulating anticoagulant is detected by a prolongation of phospholipid-dependent clotting tests such as APTT that do not correct to normal when mixed with normal plasma. More specific tests include a dilute tissue thromboplastin inhibition test, platelet neutralization procedure, dilute Russell viper venom test (DRVVT), or antiphospholipid antibodies by enzyme-linked immunosorbent assay (ELISA). To exclude the presence of LA, two or more assays that are sensitive to these antibodies must be negative.

Because this antibody does not usually cause a bleeding disorder, the primary reason to diagnose it is to avoid intensive workup and therapy prior to surgical procedures. If an antibody is identified in a young child during an acute viral illness, testing should be repeated in several months in order to document its disappearance.

Despite the frequent concordance between LA and either anticardiolipin or anti-B_2-glycoprotein 1 antibodies, these antibodies are not identical. In general, LAs are more specific for APLS whereas ACLAs are more sensitive.

Anticardiolipin Antibodies

Table 11-31 lists the syndromes associated with antiphospholipid antibodies.

Anticardiolipin antibodies (ACLAs) are generally IgG, IgA, and IgM anticardiolipin idiotypes. These antibodies are found in both SLE and non-SLE patients. The ACLAs are associated with venous and arterial thrombotic events. ACLA IgG, IgA, and IgM, and antibodies β-2-GP-1, phosphatidylserine, phosphatidylinositol, phosphatidylcholine, phosphatidylethanolamine, phosphatidylglycerol, or annexin-V are independent risk factors for thrombosis of all types (types I–V). Although there is an association between the LA and ACLAs and an association between LAs and the aforementioned syndromes, LAs, ACLAs, and antibodies to β-2-GP-I, phosphatidylserine, phosphatidylinositol, phosphatidylcholine, phosphatidylethanolamine, phosphatidylglycerol, or annexin-V are separate entities. Most individuals with ACLAs do not have a LA, and most with the LA do not have ACLAs.

ACLAs and Venous or Arterial Thrombosis

ACLAs are associated with many types of venous thrombosis, including deep vein thrombosis (DVT) of the upper and lower extremities, intracranial veins, inferior and superior vena cava, hepatic vein (Budd–Chiari syndrome), portal vein, renal vein, and retinal veins. Arterial thrombotic sites associated with ACLAs include coronary arteries, carotid arteries, cerebral arteries, retinal arteries, subclavian or axillary artery (aortic arch syndrome), brachial arteries, mesenteric arteries, peripheral (extremity) arteries, and both proximal and distal aorta.

Table 11-31. Syndromes of Thrombosis Associated with Antiphospholipid Antibodies

Type I syndrome
Deep-venous thrombosis with or without pulmonary embolus

Type II syndrome
Coronary artery thrombosis
Peripheral artery thrombosis
Aortic thrombosis
Carotid artery thrombosis

Type III syndrome
Retinal artery thrombosis
Retinal vein thrombosis
Cerebrovascular thrombosis
Transient ischemic attacks

Type IV syndrome
Mixtures of types I, II, and III
Type IV patients are rare

Type V (fetal wastage) syndrome
Placental vascular thrombosis
Fetal wastage common in first trimester
Fetal wastage can occur in second and third trimesters
Maternal thrombocytopenia (uncommon)

Type VI syndrome
Antiphospholipid antibody with no apparent clinical manifestations

Modified from Bick RL. Antiphospholipid thrombosis syndromes. Hematol Oncol Clin North Am 2003 17:115–47, with permission.

ACLAs and Cardiac Disease

In patients with high ACLA levels who have coronary artery bypass surgery, there is about a 33% chance of late graft occlusion. More than 20% of young survivors of myocardial infarction have high ACLAs. In those surviving, 60% having these antibodies may experience a later thromboembolic event. ACLAs also are associated with cardiac valvular abnormalities.

ACLAs and Cutaneous Manifestations

ACLAs are associated with livido reticularis. This cutaneous finding is associated with recurrent arterial and venous thromboses, valvular abnormalities, and cerebrovascular thromboses with concomitant essential hypertension. Other cutaneous manifestations include a syndrome of recurrent DVT, necrotizing purpura, and stasis ulcers of the ankles. Other common cutaneous manifestations include livdo vasculitis or reticularis, unfading acral microlivido, peripheral gangrene, necrotizing purpura, hemorrhage (ecchymosis and hematoma formation), and crusted ulcers about the nail beds.

ACLAs and Central Nervous System Manifestations

ACLAs associated with central nervous system (CNS) manifestations include transient ischemic attacks (TIAs), stroke, arterial and venous retinal occlusive disease, cerebral arterial and venous thrombosis, migraine headaches, Guillain–Barré syndrome, chorea, seizures, and optic neuritis. The CNS manifestations of SLE are commonly, but not always, associated with positive antiphospholipid antibodies. Although it is clear that patients with lupus with antiphospholipid antibodies may experience cerebrovascular thromboses, cerebral ischemia, and infarction, these events occur more commonly in patients with the primary anticardiolipin antibody thrombosis syndrome with no underlying autoimmune disease. Multiple cerebral infarctions in patients with antiphospholipid antibodies may result in dementia.

ACLAs and Fetal Wastage Syndrome

These antibodies are associated with high incidence of recurrent miscarriage. Characteristics of this syndrome are:

- Frequent abortions in the first trimester due to placental thrombosis or vasculitis
- Recurrent fetal loss in the second and third trimesters, due to thrombosis or vasculitis
- Premature delivery due to pregnancy-associated hypertensive disease and placental insufficiency
- Maternal thrombocytopenia.

In these individuals there is the presence of high-level IgG ACLAs. This syndrome has been treated successfully by the institution of heparin plus low-dose aspirin. LMWH may be substituted for standard heparin. Women with ACLAs have an approximately 50–75% chance of fetal loss, and successful anticoagulant therapy can increase the chances of normal-term delivery to approximately 97%.

Treatment

Recommended antithrombotic regimens for syndromes of thrombosis associated with APLAs are listed in Table 11-32.

Hereditary Thrombotic Disorders

Inherited thrombophilia* should be suspected when:

- Patient has recurrent or life-threatening venous thromboembolism
- Family history of venous thrombosis
- Is younger than 45 years of age
- No apparent risk factors for thrombosis
- History of multiple abortions, stillbirths, or both.

Factor V Leiden

In Caucasians, factor V Leiden (activated protein C [APC] resistance) is the single most common inherited disorder predisposing to thrombosis. It results from a single G-to-A point mutation at nucleotide 1691 within the factor V gene; arginine is replaced by glutamine at position (R506Q), rendering activated factor V relatively resistant to inactivation by protein C. Approximately 95% of patients with activated protein C resistance test positively for factor V Leiden mutation. The remaining 5%

---

*In thrombophilia multiple gene defects often coexist with the clinical penetrance of the syndrome being the end result of the number of gene defects present in an individual. This has been shown for patients with inherited deficiencies of antithrombin, protein C, or protein S whose risk of developing thrombotic manifestations is enhanced when there is coexistence of factor V Leiden.

Table 11-32. Recommended Antithrombotic Regimens for Syndromes of Thrombosis Associated with Antiphospholipid Antibodies

Type I syndrome
Acute treatment with heparin/LMWH followed by long-term[a] administration of LMWH

Type II syndrome
Acute treatment with heparin/LMWH followed by long-term administration of LMWH

Type III syndrome
  Cerebrovascular
    Long-term administration of subcutaneous LMWH
  Retinal
    Long-term[a] self-administration of subcutaneous porcine heparin/LMWH

Type IV syndrome
  Therapy depends on types and sites of thrombosis

Type V (fetal wastage) syndrome
  Low-dose aspirin before conception and add fixed, low-dose LMWH every 12 hours
    immediately after conception[b]

Type VI syndrome
  No indications for antithrombotic therapy

See Table 11-31 for a description of the various syndromes.
Abbreviation: LMWH, low-molecular-weight heparin.
[a]Antithrombotic therapy should not be stopped unless the ACLA has been absent for 4–6 months.
[b]In women with prior thromboembolism, higher doses of heparin are recommended for full anticoagulation.
Modified from Bick RL. Antiphospholipid thrombosis syndromes. Hematol Oncol Clin North Am 2003;17:115–7, with permission.

of cases are attributable to oral contraceptive usage, presence of a lupus anticoagulant, or other rare mutations in the factor V gene.

The HR_2 haplotype of the factor V gene causes resistance to APC and increases the risk of venous thrombosis when co-inherited with factor V Leiden. There is also a rare mutation in the second of the three sites in factor Va that activated protein C cleaves (Arg306Thr). Additional causes of resistance to APC, probably genetic but as yet unidentified, also increase the risk of venous thrombosis.

Three to 8% of Caucasians carry the factor V Leiden mutation and approximately 0.1% are homozygotes. In contrast this mutation is relatively uncommon in African and Asian populations with a prevalence of <1.0% (heterozygotes). Children with homozygous and heterozygous factor V Leiden usually have their first thrombotic event following puberty with an estimated annual incidence of 0.28%. Heterozygous factor V Leiden increases the risk of thrombosis 5- to 10-fold, whereas homozygous individuals have an 80-fold increased risk. APC resistance even in heterozygotes is a significant risk factor for thrombosis because >20% of patients presenting with a thrombotic event exhibit APC resistance. Forty-two percent of patients who sustain a first venous thrombotic event before 25 years of age and 21% of those between 54 and 70 years of age have APC resistance.

Both heterozygous and homozygous cases of factor V Leiden mutation have increased risk for either venous or arterial thrombosis throughout life but usually are asymptomatic in youth unless associated with other acquired or genetic prothrombotic conditions, including central venous catheters, trauma, surgery, cancer, pregnancy, oral contraceptives, deficient protein C, deficient protein S, or homocysteinemia.

Factor V Leiden mutation has been associated with cerebral infarction and with venous thrombosis in children.

Diagnosis

APTT-based assay (a screening test) can be used to obtain a diagnosis of APC resistance. Patients positive for APC resistance in the clotting assay should undergo genetic testing for factor V Leiden mutation by analyzing genomic DNA in peripheral blood mononuclear cells. This can be readily accomplished by amplifying a DNA fragment containing the factor V mutation site by polymerase chain reaction (PCR).

Prothrombin G20210A Mutation (FII G 20210 A)

The genetic defect is at nucleotide position 20210 in the prothrombin gene. The mutation results in abnormally high prothrombin levels and contributes to thrombotic risk by promoting increased thrombin generation. Prothrombin gene mutation is the second most common inherited thrombotic defect. The frequency of this mutation is about 2–3% in the Caucasian population and 4–5% in Mediterranean populations. The homozygous state is extremely rare. Homozygotes for the prothrombin G200210A mutation have less severe clinical presentations than homozygotes for antithrombin, protein C, and protein S deficiencies. The individual with this genetic defect usually presents with thrombotic episodes in adulthood. The diagnosis of this defect can be made by PCR testing.

Antithrombin (AT) Deficiency

AT functions by forming a complex with the activated clotting factors thrombin, Xa, IXa, and XIa. The relatively slow formation of this complex is greatly accelerated in the presence of heparin or cell-surface heparin sulfate. The incidence of AT deficiency is about 0.2–0.5%. Congenital AT deficiency is a heterozygous disorder; homozygous deficiency, probably incompatible with life, has not been reported.

Two major types of AT deficiency have been described. Type I AT deficiency (low activity and low antigen level) is a quantitative defect caused by a mutation resulting in both decreased synthesis and functional activity of AT, whereas type II AT deficiency is a qualitative defect characterized by decreased AT activity and normal antigenic levels.

Thrombotic complications of AT deficiency usually occur in the second decade of life. However, few pediatric cases with venous thrombotic events have been reported with heterozygous AT deficiency. In affected individuals AT levels are about 40–60% (normal range, 80–120%). The risk of developing thrombotic complications depends on the particular subtype of AT deficiency and on other coexisting inherited or acquired risk factors. In children with heterozygous AT deficiency the relative risk of developing thrombotic episodes is increased 10-fold.

Treatment

AT deficiency is usually treated with oral warfarin-type anticoagulants (Coumadin) to decrease the level of vitamin K–dependent procoagulants so that they are in balance with the level of AT. Heparin requires binding with AT to anticoagulate blood and, for this reason, heparin administration is usually ineffective in AT deficiency states. Because the administration of warfarin may take several days to decrease the vitamin K–dependent factors, acute thrombotic episodes are usually managed with AT replacement therapy, using either fresh frozen plasma or recombinant AT concentrates. Patients are initially treated with approximately 50 units/kg AT, which will increase the baseline level of AT by approximately 50%. AT levels should be maintained at 80% or higher. In patients with severe recurrent thrombosis who cannot be managed with oral anticoagulants, therapeutic or prophylactic replacement therapy can be monitored with AT concentrates.

5,10-Methylenetetrahydrofolate Reductase Mutation

In this condition there is a cytosine to thymine mutation at nucleotide 677 (C677T) of the 5,10-methylenetetrahydrofolate reductase (*MTHFR*) gene. This mutation is a risk factor for stroke in children, venous thrombosis in the young, and coronary artery disease in adults. *MTHFR* is essential for the remethylation of homocysteine to methionine and homozygosity for mutation of *MTHFR* is associated with hyperhomocysteinemia. Hyperhomocysteinemia is a common risk factor for deep-venous thrombosis and increases the risk for DVT in patients with factor V Leiden. The mechanisms whereby excess homocysteine may be a risk factor in thrombosis are listed on page 336.

Protein C Deficiency

Protein C (PC) is a vitamin K–dependent plasma glycoprotein which when activated functions as an anticoagulant by inactivating factors Va and VIIIa. PC activity is enhanced by another vitamin K–dependent inhibitory cofactor, protein S.

PC deficiency is inherited in an autosomal dominant manner and is subdivided into two types. Type I PC deficiency (low activity and low antigen level) is a quantitative deficiency with decreased plasma concentration and functional activity to approximately 50% of normal. Type II PC deficiency (low activity and normal antigen level) is less common and is characterized by a qualitative decrease in functional activity, despite normal levels of PC antigen. Plasma levels of PC below 50% (normal range: 70–110%) are associated with the risk of thrombotic complications.

The population prevalence of heterozygous PC deficiency is estimated at 0.2%. The clinical manifestation of heterozygous PC deficiency is primarily venous thrombotic episodes during the second decade of life or young adulthood. Heterozygous deficiency of PC is not a significant problem during the neonatal period, but homozygous deficiency or compound heterozygous individuals with protein C deficiency may cause a fatal thrombotic disorder. It may present with neonatal purpura fulminans, DIC, progressive skin necrosis with microvascular thrombosis, and thrombosis of the renal veins, mesenteric veins, and dural venous sinuses. Several of the neonates with homozygous deficiency have been subsequently found to be blind.

Treatment

Initially, affected neonates are treated for several months with replacement therapy with fresh frozen plasma (5–10 mL/kg q12h); later, they can usually be managed with long-term oral warfarin or protein C replacement (fresh frozen plasma or prothrombin complex concentrate).

Heterozygous PC deficiency is also one of the major causes of warfarin-induced skin necrosis. Because the half-life of PC is extremely short (2–8 hours), warfarin decreases PC more rapidly than factors IX, X, and prothrombin, resulting in a hemostatic imbalance with resultant microvascular thrombosis. Warfarin-induced skin necrosis is most likely to occur in these patients when loading doses of warfarin are used. This complication can usually be avoided by using low doses of warfarin.

Protein S Deficiency

Protein S deficiency is inherited in an autosomal dominant manner and has a prevalence of 1:33,000. Protein S (PS) is also a vitamin K–dependent anticoagulant that circulates in the plasma in two forms: a free active form (40%) and an inactive form bound to C4b-free binding protein (60%). PS functions as a cofactor to PC by enhancing its activity against factors Va and VIIIa. Free PS levels (normal range: 44–92%) correlate clinically with thrombotic episodes. PS deficiency is classified into three subtypes according to a quantitative defect (type I) (low activity and low antigen level) or a qualitative defect (type II) (low activity and normal antigen level) in which PS activity is reduced as follows:

	Total PS	Free PS	PS Function
Type I	↓	↓	↓
Type IIa	N	↓	↓
Type IIb	N	N	↓

The clinical presentation of protein S deficiency is indistinguishable from that of protein C deficiency. Heterozygous PS deficiency manifests in adulthood as either venous or arterial thrombotic events. Only a few cases with heterozygous protein S deficiency have been reported with thrombotic episodes during childhood. A small number of newborns with either homozygous or compound heterozygous PS deficiency have been reported. These infants, like those with homozygous PC deficiency, may present with purpura fulminans.

Treatment

The acute episodes are usually treated with standard anticoagulation therapy with heparin, followed by oral warfarin administration for 3–6 months. Recurrent thrombosis or a life-threatening thromboembolic event in a patient with PS deficiency is usually managed with long-term oral anticoagulation. Asymptomatic patients are not usually treated but need prophylaxis for high-risk procedures, such as surgery. Pregnancy may be accompanied with a reduction in free PS. Oral contraceptives will also result in a reduction of PS and may precipitate thrombosis in a patient with heterozygous PS deficiency.

Dysfibrinogenemia

Approximately 45 different dysfibrinogenemias that predispose to thrombotic events have been described, with the majority due to single-point mutations. Dysfibrinogenemias are usually inherited as an autosomal recessive condition. Dysfibrinogenemia is a very rare condition: it is estimated to occur in 0.8% of adults presenting with thrombotic episodes. Impaired binding of thrombin to an abnormal fibrin and defective fibrinolysis occurs. Tissue plasminogen activator and plasminogen activation on the abnormal fibrin have been implicated in the development of thrombosis. Congenital dysfibrinogenemias may also be associated with abnormal interactions with platelets and defective calcium binding. Although dysfibrinogenemias are more often associated with bleeding, thrombosis occurs in 20% of cases. The clinical presentation is variable, consisting of venous thrombosis, pulmonary embolism, and arterial occlusion. Some cases of dysfibrinogenemia may have an associated bleeding diathesis. Although it is very rare, intracranial hemorrhage is the most common cause of death in these patients. Homozygosity for dysfibrinogenemia is very rare and associated with juvenile arterial stroke, thrombotic abdominal aortic occlusions, and postoperative thrombotic episodes. Fibrinogen infusions may precipitate the thrombotic events. Slightly decreased fibrinogen levels with prolonged thrombin time (TT) may be indicative of dysfibrinogenemia.

Heparin Cofactor II Deficiency

Heparin cofactor II (HC-II) deficiency is inherited as an autosomal dominant trait. Clinical manifestations of HC-II deficiency are arterial and venous thrombotic events. HC-II deficiency seems to be a rare cause of unexplained thrombotic events.

Hereditary Defects of the Fibrinolytic System

Type I Dysplasminogenemia

Homozygous deficiency of type I dysplasminogenemia clinically manifests as pseudomembranous conjunctivitis, hydrocephalus, obstructive airway disorder, and abnormal wound healing secondary to failure to remove fibrin deposits in various organs. Replacement therapy with plasminogen corrects these defects by allowing the lysis of fibrin deposits. Infants with homozygous deficiency do not seem to have a higher incidence of thrombotic events.

Type II Dysplasminogenemia

Type II dysplasminogenemia is inherited as a mutation at various loci in the plasminogen molecule leading to functional abnormalities and failure of plasminogen activation. Type II defect is associated with increased incidence of thrombotic events.

Tissue Plasminogen Activator Deficiency

There are several families reported with t-PA deficiency with failure to release fibrinolytic activity following venous thrombotic events.

Plasminogen Activator Inhibitor Deficiency

These polymorphic variations of human PAI-1 gene have been reported where specific alleles may be associated with decreased PAI-1 levels. PAI-1 genotype abnormality may represent a risk factor for venous thrombotic events in the setting of PS deficiency.

Prophylaxis in Relatives of Patients with Thrombophilia

First-degree relatives of index patients who are asymptomatic should be advised of the risk of venous thrombosis. Primary prophylaxis in these persons includes the administration of LMWH in high-risk conditions, such as during surgery, trauma, immobilization, and the 6-week postpartum period; maintenance of normal weight and homocysteine levels; and avoidance of contraceptives and hormone replacement therapy. Women with antithrombin deficiency, combined thrombophilia, or homozygosity for factor V Leiden or the G20210A mutation in the prothrombin gene should be treated throughout pregnancy and for 6 weeks postpartum with LMWH.

Thrombotic Disorders in Newborns

Congenital

Newborns comprise the largest group of children developing thrombotic events. Childhood stroke appears to be a diverse condition with many potential risk factors. Inherited thrombophilia is a multiple-gene disorder in which the likelihood of developing thrombotic episodes increases with the number of genetic risk factors present in a subject. The "thrombophilia burden"* is found to be increased in children with stroke.

Acquired

Systemic Venous Thromboembolic Disorders

Incidence of symptomatic venous thrombotic events in newborns (exclusive of CNS) is 0.24 per 10,000. Neonatal thrombotic events including CNS events are 0.51 per 10,000 births with 50% being venous thrombotic events and the other 50% arterial thrombotic events.

The incidence of *sinovenous thrombosis* is 0.7 per 100,000 children per year. The following factors predispose a newborn to sinovenous thrombosis:

- During birth, the normal molding and overlapping of cranial sutures may damage the cerebral sinus structures and provoke sinovenous thrombosis
- Asphyxia
- Dehydration
- Sepsis and meningitis.

The CT scan alone could miss a diagnosis of sinovenous thrombosis. Magnetic resonance imaging (MRI) scanning with venography is the most sensitive and specific test. Doppler flow ultrasound may demonstrate absent or decreased flow within sinovenous channels.

The use of anticoagulants in neonates is controversial and probably not indicated.

Central Venous Catheter–Related Thrombosis

More than 80% of venous thrombotic events are secondary to the use of central venous catheters. Thrombotic events result from damage to vessel walls, disrupted blood flow, infusion of substances in total parenteral nutrition that damage endothelial cells, and thrombogenic catheter materials.

Umbilical venous catheters
Major clinical symptoms of umbilical arterial catheter-related thrombotic events occur in about 3% of infants. Loss of patency due to umbilical arterial catheter–related thrombotic events occur in 13–73% without unfractionated heparin being administered and in 0–13% with unfractionated heparin.

Central venous catheters
Central venous catheters are the most common risk factor for venous thrombotic events in newborns. Right atrial thrombosis commonly occurs in newborns with central venous catheters. Right atrial thrombosis may result in cardiac failure, persistent sepsis, and fatal pulmonary emboli.

Renal Vein Thrombosis

Renal vein thrombosis is the most common non-catheter-related venous thrombotic event in newborns. The incidence is about 10% of all venous thrombotic events. Almost 80% present within the first week of life. Renal vein thrombosis may occur bilaterally in 24% of newborns. The risks of renal vein thrombosis include perinatal

---

*The concomitant presence or any combination of APLA, factor V Leiden, FIIG20210A mutation, AT deficiency, PC deficiency, PS deficiency, or Lp(a). A full thrombophilia workup should be carried out in newborn infants with unexplained prenatal or neonatal cerebral infarction especially if there is a family history of venous thrombosis, early stroke, or heart disease.

asphyxia, shock, polycythemia, cyanotic congenital heart disease, maternal diabetes, and sepsis, which result in reduced renal flow, hyperviscosity, hyperosmolality, and hypercoagulability. Diagnostic ultrasonography is the radiographic test of choice.

Systemic Arterial Thromboembolic Disorders

Arterial ischemic stroke
The incidence of arterial ischemic stroke in newborns is 93 per 100,000 live births. A primary risk factor is identifiable in about 70% of affected newborns. Systemic risk factors include:

- Iatrogenic secondary to indwelling arterial catheters. This is usually related to catheter material, duration of placement, diameter, length, solution infused, and arterial site.
- Cardiac disease.
- Perinatal complications (trauma, hypoxia-ischemia, maternal cocaine abuse).
- Dehydration.
- Congenital thrombophilia (i.e., PC and PS deficiencies, antithrombin deficiency, FII G20210A, MTHFR C 677T, factor V Leiden, elevated Lp[a], maternal APLAs).

Diagnostic radiographic studies include CT scan, MRI, MRA, and less frequently conventional angiogram. Cranial ultrasound has a limited role in arterial ischemic stroke.

Use of anticoagulants is controversial and thrombolytic therapy is rarely indicated.

The risk factors for perinatal stroke are listed in Table 11-33. More than one risk factor is identified in many cases. Diagnosis and treatment of thrombotic events are shown in Table 11-34.

Table 11-33. Risk Factors for Perinatal Stroke

Cardiac disorders
  Congenital heart disease
  Patent ductus arteriosus
  Pulmonary valve atresia

Hematologic disorders
  Polycythemia
  Disseminated intravascular coagulopathy
  Factor V Leiden mutation
  Protein S deficiency
  Protein C deficiency
  Prothrombin mutation
  High homocysteine level
  High lipoprotein (a) level
  Factor VII

Infectious disorders
  CNS infection
  Systemic infection

Maternal disorders
  Autoimmune disorders
  Coagulation disorders
  Anticardiolipin antibodies
  Twin-to-twin transfusion syndrome
  In utero cocaine exposure
  Infection

(Continues)

Table 11-33. (*Continued*)

Placental disorders
    Placental thrombosis
    Placental abruption
    Placental infection (chorioamnionitis)
    Fetomaternal hemorrhage

Vasculopathy
    Vascular maldevelopment

Trauma and catheterization
    Central venous catheters, umbilical venous catheters

Birth asphyxia

Dehydration

Extracorporeal membrane oxygenation

Table 11-34. Diagnosis and Treatment of Neonatal Thromboembolism

Thrombosis	Diagnosis	Treatment
Systemic venous thrombotic events	VG/US	LMWH/UFH/TT[a]
Pulmonary emboli	V/Q scan	LMWH/UFH
Central venous catheter–related thromboembolic event	VG/US	LMWH/UFH/TT[a]
Right atrial thrombosis	ECHO	LMWH/UFH
Umbilical venous catheter	VG	LMWH/UFH
Renal vein thrombosis	US	LMWH/UFH indicated if thrombosis extends to IVC or renal failure
Umbilical arterial catheter	AG	LMWH/UFH prophylaxis: UFH 0.25 unit/mL
Peripheral arterial thrombotic event	AG	LMWH/UFH prophylaxis: UFH 1 unit/mL

Abbreviations: VG, venogram; US, ultrasonogram; LMWH, low-molecular-weight heparin; UFH, unfractionated heparin; TT, thrombolytic therapy; ECHO, echocardiogram; V/Q scan, ventilation perfusion scan; IVC, inferior vena cava; AG, arteriogram.
[a]Recommended only if potential loss of life, organ, or limb.

Antithrombotic Agents

Heparin Therapy

Heparin mediates its activities through catalysis of the natural inhibitor AT. The activities of heparin are considered anticoagulant and antithrombotic. The antithrombotic activities of heparin are influenced by plasma concentration of AT. In the presence of heparin, thrombin generation is decreased in young children compared to adults. Clearance of heparin is also faster in the young. For this reason the optimal dosing of heparin is different in children from adults. In pediatric patients APTT values correctly predict heparin therapy only 70% of the time. The following dosage schedule is utilized for heparinization:

- Loading dose: 75 units/kg IV over 10 minutes
- Initial maintenance dose:
  ≤1 year of age: 28 units/kg/h
  >1 year of age: 20 units/kg/h
- Repeat APTT 4 hours after administration of the heparin loading dose and monitor heparin dose to maintain an APTT at 2.5 times normal for the reference laboratory as follows:

APTT times of normal	Bolus (units/kg)	Dose change (units/kg/hour) (increase or decrease of bolus dose)	Intervals of testing APTT (hours)
<2	50	20% increase	4
2	—	10% increase	4
>2	—	No change	4
2.5	—	No change	24
>2.5[a]	—	10% decrease	4
>3[b]	—	20% decrease	4

Note: Heparin solution at concentrations of 80 units/mL for children 10 kg or less or 40 units/mL for children greater than 10 kg.
[a]Hold the dose 30 minutes.
[b]Hold the dose 1 hour.

- When the patient's APTT achieves a therapeutic level, repeat APTT, CBC with platelet count daily.
- The heparin level should be monitored during the first 48 hours. Heparin level should be 0.2–0.4 units/mL.
- The heparin level is expected to be 0.35–0.70 units/mL by an *anti-factor Xa* assay.
- When heparin is interrupted for more than 1 hour, reestablish the heparin maintenance infusion at the previous rate until the APTT result is available. After that, administer heparin in accordance with the APTT results.
- When the platelet count is 100,000/mm³ or less, consider discontinuing heparin therapy and instituting alternative therapy, because the risk of heparin-induced thrombocytopenia is greater after 5 days of therapy.

Duration of heparin therapy

- Deep-venous thrombosis: A minimum of 5–7 days; maintenance warfarin therapy can be instituted on day 1 or 2 of heparin therapy.
- Pulmonary embolus: 7–14 days; start warfarin therapy on day 5.
- Neonates may be treated for 10–14 days without warfarin.

Avoid acetylsalicylic acid (ASA; aspirin) or other antiplatelet drugs during heparin therapy when possible.

Heparin antidote

- If heparin needs to be discontinued, termination of the heparin infusion will be sufficient (because of the rapid clearance of heparin).
- If an immediate effect is required, protamine sulfate administration may be indicated.
- Following administration of IV protamine sulfate, neutralization occurs within 5 minutes.

The dose of protamine sulfate required to neutralize heparin is as follows:

Last dose of heparin	Protamine dose[a] (per 100 mg heparin)
<30 minutes	1 mg
30 minutes	0.5 mg
1 hour	0.75 mg
>1 hour	0.375 mg
>2 hours	0.25 mg

[a]Maximum dose of protamine sulfate, 50 mg, to be administered in a concentration of 10 mg/mL at a rate not to exceed 5 mg/min. If administered faster, it may cause cardiovascular collapse. Patients with known hypersensitivity reactions to fish and those who have received protamine-containing insulin or previous protamine therapy may be at risk for hypersensitivity reactions to protamine sulfate. Repeat APTT 15 minutes after the administration of protamine sulfate.

Low-Molecular-Weight Heparin

The anticoagulant activities of low-molecular-weight heparin (LMWH) are also mediated by catalysis of the natural inhibitor AT. LMWHs preferentially inhibit factor Xa over thrombin due to the decreased capacity to bind both AT and thrombin simultaneously for thrombin inhibition. Preparations used for children are enoxaparin (Lovenox; Rhone-Poulenc) and reviparin (Cloverine, Knoll Pharma). Young infants have an accelerated clearance of LMWH compared to older children.

Indications for Low-Molecular-Weight Heparin Therapy

- Neonates
- Patients requiring anticoagulation and deemed to be at increased risk for hemorrhage
- Patients in whom venous access for administration and monitoring of standard heparin therapy is difficult.

Dose (Enoxaparin) [Lovenox, Aventis]

Age (months)	Treatment[a] (dose)	Prophylactic (dose)
<2	1.5 mg/kg every 12 h SC	0.75 mg/kg every 12 h SC
>2	1.0 mg/kg every 12 h SC	0.5 mg/kg every 12 h SC

Abbreviation: SC, subcutaneously.
[a]Maximum dose, 2.0 mg/kg every 12 h.

Monitoring of Low-Molecular-Weight Heparin Therapy

- Prior to the initiation of LMWH therapy, a complete blood count, including platelet count, PT, and APTT, should be determined.
- Aspirin or other antiplatelet drugs should be avoided during the therapy.
- Intramuscular injections and arterial punctures should be avoided during the therapy.
- If the platelet count drops to 100,000/mm^3 or less, heparin-induced thrombocytopenia (HIT) must be ruled out; it rarely occurs with LMWH therapy.
- The pretreatment anti-factor Xa level should be determined; thereafter, weekly monitoring should be sufficient 4–6 hours after the SC administration of LMWH.

The therapeutic anti-factor Xa level is 0.5–1.0 units/mL and the prophylactic anti-factor Xa level is 0.1–0.3 units/mL.

- For long-term LMWH therapy, bone densitometry studies should be performed at baseline and then at 6-month intervals to assess for possible osteoporosis.

Duration of Low-Molecular-Weight Heparin Therapy

- LMWH is usually administered up to 3 months without warfarin.
- Extensive thrombus or pulmonary embolus. LMWH for 7–14 days should be administered and warfarin should be started on day 5.
- Newborns may be treated for 10–14 days with LMWH alone.

Adjusting Low-Molecular-Weight Heparin Dose

The dose of LMWH can be adjusted according to the anti–factor X^a level achieved:

Anti–factor Xa level (units/mL)[a]	Dose
<0.35	25% increase
<0.5	10% increase
0.5–1.0	No change
>1.0	20% decrease
>1.5	30% decrease
>2.0	Hold for 24 hours

[a]Repeat anti–factor X level 4 hours post next dose until 0.5–1.0 units/mL, then once weekly at 4 hours post dose.

Antidote for Low-Molecular-Weight Heparin

- Termination of LMWH is usually sufficient.
- When an immediate effect is required, 1 mg protamine per 100 units (1 mg) of LMWH may be given.
- The protamine should be administered intravenously over a 10-minute period. A rapid infusion of protamine may cause hypotension.

Heparin-Induced Thrombocytopenia

Heparin-induced thrombocytopenia (HIT) is an uncommon complication of heparin therapy, and can cause significant morbidity and mortality. The incidence is about 3% in adult patients receiving unfractionated heparin. The incidence in pediatric patients is unknown. It usually begins 5–15 days after commencing heparin therapy (median 10 days) but can occur earlier in patients with prior exposure to heparin. An abrupt decrease of platelet count or a decrease of platelet count by half in 1–2 days should raise suspicion of heparin-induced thrombocytopenia. Any type of heparin including LMWH should be discontinued. Discontinuation of heparin will result in the platelet count returning to normal. In the setting of HIT associated with thrombotic events, heparin must be discontinued and alternative anticoagulation therapy must be initiated until the antibody complex causing HIT is cleared. Alternative intravenous anticoagulation therapy may include the following:

Argatroban

- No loading dose.
- Maintenance dose: Begin at 2 µg/kg/min continuous IV infusion (maximum 10 µg/kg/min).

- Monitor with aPTT beginning 2 hours after the start of therapy; target aPTT = 1.5- to 3-fold greater than the pretreatment value and <100 seconds.
- Excretion: hepatic, reduce dose in patients with hepatic insufficiency.
- Clinical data for use in patients under age 18 are extremely limited.

Lepirudin (recombinant hirudin)

- Loading dose 0.4 mg/kg (up to 44 mg) as an IV bolus.
- Maintenance dose: 0.15 mg/kg/h (up to 16.5 mg/h).
- Monitor with aPTT beginning 4 hours after start of infusion. Adjust infusion for a target aPTT between 1.5- and 2.5-fold greater than the preinfusion value. Recheck aPTT 4 hours after any dosage changes. *APTT >2.5 × original value:* stop infusion for 2 hours, resume at 5% of prior dose. *APTT <1.5 × original value:* increase infusion rate by 20%. Antibodies may develop in up to 40% of patients affecting pharmacokinetics; aPTT monitoring must be ongoing.
- Excretion: renal, reduce for patients with renal insufficiency.
- Clinical data for use in patients under age 18 is extremely limited. Dosing requirements in neonates and newborns may be markedly reduced.

Orgaran (heparan sulfate) (danaparoid sodium)

- Loading dose: 30 units/kg.
- Maintenance dose: 1.2–2.0 units/kg/h.
- Anti-factor Xa activity can be monitored immediately following the bolus dose and every 4 hours until a steady state is reached and then daily to maintain a therapeutic range of 0.4–0.8 units/mL.
- Orgaran is contraindicated in patients with severely impaired renal function.

Ancrod (Russell pit viper venom)

- Ancrod cleaves fibrinopeptide A from fibrinogen.
- Loading dose: 1–2 units/kg intravenous or subcutaneous infusion over 6–24 hours.
- Maintenance dose: 1–2 units/kg every 24 hours (intravenous or subcutaneous infusion) with the dose adjusted to achieve plasma fibrinogen levels of 0.2–1 mg/mL.
- Fresh frozen plasma or anti-ancrod antibody can be used to reverse ancrod's effect.

Warfarin Therapy

Warfarin (4-hydroxycumarin) (Coumadin; Bristol-Myers, Squibb) competitively inhibits vitamin K, an essential cofactor for the post-transitional carboxylation of glutamic acid residues on factors II, VII, IX, and X. Coumadin is the trade name for the most commonly available warfarin preparation.

A loading dose of 0.2 mg/kg by mouth as a single daily dose (maximum initial dose, 10 mg) should be employed when the International Normalized Ratio (INR) is less than 1.3. When it is greater than 1.3, reduce the loading dose to 0.1 mg/kg. For a patient with Fontan procedure or liver dysfunction, the daily dose should be reduced by 50%.

The subsequent dose is age dependent (infants having the highest—0.32 mg/kg—and teenagers the lowest—0.09 mg/kg) and based on the INR response (see the following table). Before the INR was adopted, the prothrombin time (PT) test was used for many years to control oral anticoagulant therapy. The variability of different thromboplastin reagents and instruments used in the performance of the PT made the transferability of results among laboratories difficult and impeded the development of universal guidelines for patient therapy.

Warfarin Daily Loading Doses (Approximately 3–5 Days)

INR[a]	Warfarin loading doses
1.1–1.3	Repeat initial loading dose
1.4–1.9	50% of initial loading dose
2.0–3.0	50% of initial loading dose
3.1–3.5	25% of initial loading dose
>3.5	Hold until INR <3.5, then restart at 50% less than previous dose

[a]The International Normalized Ratio (INR) provides a standardized scale for monitoring patients who are receiving oral anticoagulant therapy. The INR is effectively the PT ratio on which the patient would have been measured had the test been made using the primary World Health Organization International Reference Preparation (IRP). The INR is calculated by use of the International Sensitivity Index (ISI), which is established by the manufacturer for each lot of thromboplastin reagent using a specific instrument: INR = (Patient PT/Normal PT) ^{ISI}.

Warfarin Maintenance Doses for Long-Term Therapy

INR	Warfarin dose
1.1–1.4	Increase dose by 20%
1.5–1.9	Increase dose by 10%
2.0–3.0	No change
3.1–3.5	Decrease dose by 10%
>3.5	Hold until INR <3.5, then restart at 20% less than previous dose

- The warfarin loading period is approximately 3–5 days for most patients before a stable maintenance phase is achieved.
- Warfarin should be started on day 1 or day 2 of heparin therapy. Heparin should be continued for a minimum of 5 days' duration. When the INR is greater than 2.0 for 2 consecutive days and at least 5 days of heparin are completed, heparin can be discontinued.
- For extensive DVT with or without pulmonary emboli, warfarin should be started on day 5 of heparin therapy.
- The INR should be maintained between 2.0 and 3.0 for the vast majority of patients. Children with mechanical heart valves require an INR between 2.5 and 3.5.
- Once the patient has two INRs between 2.0 and 3.0 (or 2.5–3.5 for mechanical valves) obtained weekly, the INR determinations could be carried out every 2 weeks. If INR remains stable, then the INR could be determined once monthly.
- The INR should be monitored a minimum of once monthly.
- If the patient is receiving total parenteral nutrition, vitamin K should be removed from the amino acid solution before warfarin therapy begins.
- If the patient is receiving other medications (i.e., antibiotics, which can affect warfarin), the loading dose may require adjustment.
- The INR should be obtained 5–7 days after initiating a new dose. The maintenance guidelines should be employed for making changes in dosage.
- Children with mechanical heart valves or repeated thromboembolic complications should receive warfarin indefinitely.
- Children with uncomplicated DVT and pulmonary emboli should receive warfarin for a minimum of 3 months.
- Children with a thrombotic event and a persistent, significant, underlying predisposing factor (e.g., continued presence of a central venous catheter, per-

sistence of an antiphospholipid antibody) may be placed on low-dose warfarin (0.1 mg/kg) following 3 months of treatment with full-dose warfarin until the predisposing factor is no longer present.

- Vitamin K is the antidote for warfarin. The patient may also be given fresh frozen plasma or prothrombin complex concentrate infusions to reverse the effects of warfarin. If there is no active bleeding, vitamin K_1 0.5–2 mg SC can be given. If there is active bleeding, vitamin K_1 0.5–2 mg SC (not IM) plus FFP 20 cc/kg IV can be given. If bleeding is significant and life threatening, vitamin K_1 5 mg IV (by slow infusion over 10–20 minutes because of the risk of anaphylactic shock) and prothrombin complex concentrates 50 units/kg IV can be given.
- If low-risk procedures have to be carried out, INR should be reduced to 1.5 or less prior to the procedures. Warfarin should be discontinued 72 hours prior to any high-risk surgery.
- Where surgical procedures have to be carried out and where the risk of thrombosis is high and anticoagulant therapy cannot be reversed for even a short period of time, the following may be considered:
  Discontinue warfarin 72 hours prior to surgery.
  Initiate heparin infusion therapy without a bolus at appropriate dose for age.
  If the INR is more than 1.5 at 12 hours prior to surgery, low-dose vitamin K_1 0.5 mg SC should be given and the INR should be determined approximately 6 hours later.
  Intravenous heparin infusion should be discontinued approximately 6 hours prior to surgery. Preoperative PT and APTT should be within normal limits.
  Heparin should be resumed 8 hours following surgery.
  If the patient develops any signs of bleeding, heparin infusion should be immediately discontinued.
  Oral warfarin should be resumed on the second day post surgery.
  Heparin infusion should be discontinued when a therapeutic INR is reached.
- Where the risk of thrombosis is low and there is no thrombotic event for several weeks, warfarin should be discontinued 72 hours prior to surgery. Warfarin maintenance should be initiated on the day following surgery.
- Both diet and coadministration of certain drugs can have a marked effect on the magnitude of warfarin action (see Table 11-35).

Antiplatelet Therapy

The two most commonly used antiplatelet agents for children are aspirin and dipyridamole. Aspirin acetylates the enzyme cyclooxygenase and thereby interferes with the production of thromboxane A_2 and platelet aggregation. Dipyridamole interferes with platelet function by increasing the cellular concentration of adenosine 3,5-monophosphate (cyclic AMP). This latter effect is mediated by inhibition of cyclic nucleotide phosphodiesterase and/or by blockade of uptake of adenosine, which acts at A_2, receptors for adenosine to stimulate platelet adenylcyclase.

Antiplatelet agents are used in the following conditions:

Cardiac disorders (mechanical prosthetic heart valves, Blalock-Taussig shunts, endovascular shunts)
Cardiovascular events
Kawasaki disease.

Dosage

Aspirin: 5–10 mg/kg/day
Dipyridamole (3–5 mg/kg/day).

Table 11-35. Effect of Drugs on Warfarin Response

**Medications that potentiate
  the effect of warfarin**
Acetaminophen
Acetohexamide
Allopurinol
Androgenic and anabolic steroids
α-Methyldopa
Antibiotics that disrupt intestinal flora
    (tetracyclines, streptomycin
    erythromycin, kanamycin, nalidixic acid,
    neomycin)
Cephaloridine
Chloramphenicol
Chlorpromazine
Chlorpropamide
Chloral hydrate
Cimetidine
Clofibrate
Diazoxide
Disulfiram
Ethacrynic acid
Glucagon
Guanethidine indomethacin
Isoniazid
Mefenamic acid
Methimazole
Methotrexate
Methylphenidate
Nalidixic acid
Nortriptyline
Oxyphenbutazone

p-Aminosalicyclic acid
Paromomycin
Phenylbutazone
Phenytoin
Phenyramidol
Propylthiouracil
Quinidine
Salicylate
Sulfinpyrazone
Sulfonamides
Thyroid hormone
Tolbutamide

**Medications that reduce
  the effect of warfarin**
Antipyrine
Barbiturates
Carbamazepine
Chlorthalidone
Cholestyramine
Digitalis
Ethanol
Ethchlorvynol
Glutethimide
Griseofulvin
Haloperidol
Oral contraceptives
Phenobarbital
Prednisone
All vitamin preparations
    containing vitamin K

Thrombolytic Therapy

In contrast to the anticoagulants heparin and warfarin, which function to prevent fibrin clot formation, the thrombolytic agents act to dissolve established thrombus by converting endogenous plasminogen to plasmin, which can lyse existing thrombus. Thrombolytic therapy should be considered for arterial thrombi using tissue plasminogen activator, urokinase, or streptokinase.

Tissue Plasminogen Activator

A t-PA infusion should be given at a rate of 0.5 mg/kg/h IV for 6 hours.

- Heparin should be given (20 units/kg/h) during t-PA infusion if the patient is not already on heparin.
- Following 6 hours of t-PA infusion and if there is no response to treatment, the plasminogen level should be determined. If the plasminogen level is low, fresh frozen plasma (FFP) 20 cc/kg IV q8h should be administered. A repeat infusion of t-PA may be considered.

Urokinase

Urokinase (UK) should be administered in a loading dose of 4000 units/kg over 10 minutes, followed by 4000 units/kg/h for 6 hours.

- Heparin should be given (20 units/kg/h) during UK infusion if the patient is not already on heparin.
- Following 6 hours of UK infusion and if there is no response to treatment, the plasminogen level should be determined. If the plasminogen level is low, FFP 20 cc/kg IV q8h should be administered. A repeat infusion of UK may be considered.
- Streptokinase can be administered when t-PA and UK are not available.

Streptokinase

Streptokinase (SK) should not be administered if it was used previously or if the plasminogen level is low (i.e., newborns). The loading dose consists of 4000 units/kg (maximum 250,000 units) over 10 minutes, followed by 2000 units/kg/h for 6 hours.

- Heparin should be given (20 units/kg/h) during SK infusion if the patient is not already on heparin.
- If there is no response to treatment, the plasminogen level should be determined. If the plasminogen level is low, FFP 20 cc/kg IV q8h should be given. UK or t-PA should be utilized (not SK) for further thrombolytic therapy.
- Patients must be premedicated with Tylenol and Benadryl before SK (repeat every 4–6 hours).
- Patients should not receive more than one course of SK because of the potential for allergic reactions. An anaphylactic reaction can occur in 1–2% of patients receiving SK. In the event of an anaphylactic reaction, discontinue SK immediately and administer epinephrine, steroids, and antihistamines.

Monitoring Response of Thrombolytic Therapy

- Obtain the PT and APTT every 6 hours.
- Determine the fibrinogen level and/or fibrin/fibrinogen degradation products (FDPs) or D-dimer, every 6 hours.
- Determine the plasminogen level at the end of the 6-hour infusion if there is no response or prior to proceeding to another course of therapy.
- The fibrinogen concentration may decrease by at least 20–50%; and the fibrinogen concentration must be maintained at approximately 100 mg/dL by cryoprecipitate infusions (1 unit/5 kg).
- When the fibrinogen concentration is less than 100 mg/dL and the patient is still receiving infusion of SK, UK, or t-PA, the dose of the thrombolytic agent should be decreased by 25%.
- The platelet count should be maintained at $100,000/m^3$ or higher.
- Six hours following thrombolytic therapy, heparin therapy may be sufficient for 24 hours before reinstituting thrombolytic therapy. There may be ongoing thrombolysis even in the absence of continued administration of the thrombolytic agent.

Complications of Thrombolytic Therapy

Minor bleeding may occur in up to 50% of patients (i.e., oozing from a wound or puncture site). Supportive care and application of local pressure may be sufficient.

When severe bleeding occurs, the infusion of the thrombolytic agent should be terminated, and cryoprecipitate should be administered (usual dose of 1 unit/5 kg).

When life-threatening bleeding occurs, the infusion of the thrombolytic agent should be terminated. The fibrinolytic process can be reversed by infusing Amicar 100 mg/kg (maximum, 5 g) bolus, then 30 mg/kg/h (maximum, 1.25 g/h) until bleeding stops (maximum, 18 g/m²/day). Protamine sulfate may be required to reverse the heparin effect.

The following table lists the management of blocked central venous catheters (CVCs) using t-PA:

Weight	Single-lumen CVC	Double-lumen CVC	Subcutaneous CVC (Mediport)
<10 kg	0.5 mg t-PA diluted in 0.9% NaCl to volume required to fill line.	0.5 mg t-PA diluted in 0.9% NaCl per lumen to fill volume of line. Treat one lumen at a time.	0.5 mg t-PA diluted with 0.9% NaCl to 3 mL.
>10 kg	1.0 mg t-PA in 1.0 mL 0.9% NaCl. Use amount required to fill volume of line, to maximum of 2 mL (2 mg t-PA).	1.0 mg t-PA in 1.0 mL 0.9% NACl. Use amount required to fill volume of line, to a maximum of 2 mL (2 mg t-PA per lumen). Treat one lumen at a time.	2.0 mg t-PA diluted with 0.9% NaCl to 3 mL.

Antithrombotic Therapy in Special Conditions

Valve Replacement

Mechanical Valve Replacement

Heparin

- Heparinization starting at 48 hours postoperatively.
- See heparin dose (pages 351–353).
- Heparin should be stopped for 2 hours before intracardiac lines are removed.
- Chest tube removal or insertion is not a contraindication for heparin.

Warfarin

- Warfarin begins with oral intake and is continued indefinitely.
- See warfarin dose schedule (pages 355–357).
- Aim for an INR of 2.5–3.5.

Aortic Valve Replacement

- Low-dose ASA begins with oral intake (3–5 mg/kg/day) and is continued for 3 months.

Mitral and Tricuspid Valve Replacement

- Atrial fibrillation or has proven intra-atrial thrombus, treatment as per mechanical valve replacement (INR of 2.5–3.5).
- If normal sinus rhythm, anticoagulation will be with warfarin for 3 months (INR of 2.0–3.0), and low-dose ASA (3–5 mg/kg/day), indefinitely.

Pulmonary Valve Replacement

- Currently no treatment.

Fontan Procedure

Heparin

- No heparin loading dose.
- Low-dose heparin infusion of 10 units/kg/h starting 48 hours postoperatively.

- Heparin is stopped for 2 hours before intracardiac lines are removed.
- Chest tube removal or insertion is not a contraindication for heparin.

Warfarin

- Warfarin begins with oral intake and is continued for 3 months.
- Patients after a Fontan procedure are very sensitive to oral anticoagulants. Loading doses of warfarin should be decreased.
- Warfarin dosing should be adjusted according to the warfarin protocol (INR of dose 2.0–3.0).

Aspirin

- Low-dose ASA (3–5 mg/kg/day) starts with oral intake and continues indefinitely.

Blalock-Taussig Shunts

Heparin

- Loading dose of heparin: 75 units/kg over 10 minutes starts immediately postoperative.
- Maintenance dose: 28 units/kg/h ($\leq$1 year old), 20 units/kg/h (>1 year old).

Aspirin

- Low-dose ASA (3–5 mg/kg/day) starts with oral intake and continues indefinitely.

Acute Arterial Infarct

Heparin

- Loading dose of heparin followed by maintenance dose (see heparin dose, pages 351–353).

Warfarin

- Warfarin therapy for a minimum of 3 months (see warfarin dose, page 355–357).

Aspirin

- Low-dose ASA (3–5 mg/kg/day) begins with oral intake and is continued for 3 months.

Idiopathic Arterial Infarct

- Low-dose ASA (3–5 mg/kg/day) for a minimum of 3 months.

Arterial Infarct with Moyamoya Syndrome

- Anticoagulation with heparin or LMWH for 5 days.
- Low-dose ASA (3.5 mg/kg/day) starts at diagnosis and continues indefinitely.

Transient Ischemic Attacks

- Anticoagulation with heparin or LMWH for 5 days.
- Low-dose ASA (3–5 mg/kg/day) starts at diagnosis and continues indefinitely.

Acute Stroke without Hemorrhage

- Anticoagulation with heparin or LMWH for 5 days.
- Subsequent anticoagulation will be according to the underlying etiology.

Sinovenous Thrombosis

- Anticoagulation with heparin or LMWH 10–14 days in newborns. In infants or older children, heparin or LMWH for 5 days followed by warfarin for 3 months (for dosage see heparin nomogram, LMWH dose adjustment schedule, and warfarin dose adjustment schedule).

SUGGESTED READINGS
Hemostatic Disorders

Andrew M, Vegh P, Johnston M, Bowker J, Ofosu F, Mitchell L. Maturation of the hemostatic system during childhood. Blood 1992;80:1998–2005.

Bick R. Disseminated intravascular coagulation: objective criteria for clinical and laboratory diagnosis and assessment of therapeutic response. Clin Appl Thrombosis Hemostasis 1995;1:3–23.

Di Paola J, Nugent D, Young G. Current therapy for rare factor deficiencies. Haemophilia 2001;7 Suppl:16–22.

The diagnosis and management of factor VIII and IX inhibitors: A guideline from the UK Haemophilia Centre Doctor's Organization (UKHCDO). Br J Haematol 2000;111:78–90.

Hemophilia of Georgia. Protocols for the treatment of hemophilia and von Willebrand disease. Hemophilia 2000;6 Suppl 1:84–93.

Hoffman M, Monroe III DM. A cell-based model of hemostasis. Thrombosis Haemostasis 2001;85:958–65.

Hoyer LL. Hemophilia A. N Engl J Med 1994;330:38–47.

Mannucci P. Treatment of Von Willebrand disease. N Engl J Med 2004;351:683–94.

Mannucci PM. Desmopressin: a nontransfusional form of treatment for congenital and acquired bleeding disorders. Blood 1988;72:1449–55.

Thrombotic Disorders

Baker Jr WF. Thrombolytic therapy clinical application. Hematol Oncol Clin North Am 2003;17:283–311.

Bick RL. Antiphospholipid thrombosis syndrome. Hematol Oncol Clin North Am 2003;17:115–47.

Bick RL. Prothrombin G 20210A mutation, heparin cofactor II, protein C and protein S defects. Hematol Oncol Clin North Am 2003;17:9–36.

Crowter MA, Kelton JG. Congenital thrombophilic states associated with venous thrombosis. A qualitative overview and proposed classification system. Ann Intern Med 2003;138:128–34.

Hoppe C, Matsunaga A. Pediatric thrombosis. Pediatr Clin North Am 2002; 49:1257–83.

Kwann HC, Nabhan C. Hereditary and acquired defects in the fibrinolytic system associated with thrombosis. Hematol Oncol Clin North Am 2003;17:103–14.

Levine JS, Branch W, Rauch J. Antiphospholipid syndrome. New Engl J Med 2002;346:752–63.

Meinardi JR, Middeldorp S, De Kam PJ, et al. The incidence of recurrent venous thromboembolism in carriers of factor V Leiden is related to concomitant thrombophilic disorders. Brit J Haematol 2002;116:625–33.

Selighsohn U, Lubertsky A. Genetic susceptibility to venous thrombosis. N Engl J Med 2001;344:1222–31.

Whiteman T, Hassouna H I. Hypercoagulable states. Hematol Oncol Clin North Am 2000;14:355–77.

12

LYMPHADENOPATHY
AND SPLENOMEGALY

Lymphadenopathy and splenomegaly are common findings in children. Both benign and malignant processes can produce these findings, and it is important to distinguish between the two so that appropriate management can be undertaken.

LYMPHADENOPATHY

Enlarged lymph nodes are commonly found in children. Lymphadenopathy might be caused by proliferation of cells intrinsic to the node, such as lymphocytes, plasma cells, monocytes, or histiocytes, or by infiltration of cells extrinsic to the node, such as neutrophils and malignant cells. In most instances, lymphadenopathy represents transient proliferative responses to local or generalized infections. Reactive hyperplasia, defined as a polyclonal proliferation of one or more cell types, is the most frequent diagnosis in pediatric lymph node biopsies.

Lymphadenopathy is also a presenting sign of malignancies such as leukemia, lymphoma, or neuroblastoma, and it is important to be able to differentiate benign from malignant lymphadenopathy.

Lymphadenopathy in the head and neck region must be differentiated from several congenital malformations (Table 12-1).

Systematic palpation of the lymph nodes is important and should include examination of the occipital, posterior auricular, preauricular, tonsillar, submandibular, submental, upper anterior cervical, lower anterior cervical, posterior upper and lower cervical, supraclavicular, infraclavicular, axillary, epitrochlear, and popliteal lymph nodes. Many children have small palpable nodes in the cervical, axillary, and inguinal regions that are usually benign in nature. However, adenopathy in the supraclavicular regions is usually pathologic.

When nodes of significant size are palpated, radiography of the chest should be carried out to determine whether there is an associated mediastinal or hilar lymphadenopathy. The latter may require computed tomography (CT) of the chest. When a malignant disease is suspected, abdominal sonography and CT are required to determine whether retroperitoneal lymph nodes are present. When a child presents with lymphadenopathy, management is based on the following factors.

Table 12-1. Differential Diagnosis of Cervical Lymphadenopathy

Cystic hygroma
Branchial cleft anomalies, branchial cysts
Thyroglossal duct cysts
Epidermoid cysts
Neonatal torticollis
Lateral process of lower cervical vertebra may be misdiagnosed as supraclavicular node.

History

This involves the duration of the lymphadenopathy; fever; recent upper respiratory tract infection; sore throat; skin lesions or abrasions, or other infections in the lymphatic region drained by the enlarged lymph nodes; immunizations; medications; previous cat scratches, rodent bites, or tick bites; arthralgia; sexual history; transfusion history; travel history; and consumption of unpasteurized milk. Significant weight loss, night sweats, or other systemic symptoms should also be recorded as part of the patient's history.

Location

Enlargement of tonsillar and inguinal lymph nodes is most likely secondary to localized infection; enlargement of supraclavicular and axillary lymph nodes is more likely to be of a serious nature. Enlargement of the left supraclavicular node, in particular, should suggest a malignant disease (e.g., malignant lymphoma or rhabdomyosarcoma) arising in the abdomen and spreading via the thoracic duct to the left supraclavicular area. Enlargement of the right supraclavicular node indicates thoracic lesions because this node drains the superior areas of the lungs and mediastinum. Palpable supraclavicular nodes are an indication for a thorough search for intrathoracic or intraabdominal pathology.

Size

Nodes in excess of 2.5 cm should be regarded as pathologic. In addition, nodes that increase in size over time are significant.

Character

Malignant nodes are generally firm, rubbery, and matted. They are usually not tender or erythematous. Occasionally, a rapidly growing malignant node may be tender. Nodes due to infection or inflammation are generally warm, tender, and fluctuant. If infection is considered to be the cause of the adenopathy, it is reasonable to perform a 2-week trial of antibiotic therapy. Failure to produce a reduction in the size of the lymph node within this period is an indication for careful observation. If the size, location, and character of the node suggest malignant disease, the node should be biopsied.

Lymphadenopathy is either localized (one region affected) or generalized (two or more noncontiguous lymph node regions involved). Although localized lymphadenopathy is generally due to local infection in the region drained by the particular lymph nodes, it may also be due to malignant disease, such as Hodgkin disease or neuroblastoma. Lymphadenopathy may initially be localized and subsequently become generalized. Table 12-2 outlines the causes of lymphadenopathy.

Table 12-2. Causes of Lymphadenopathy

I. Nonspecific reactive hyperplasia (polyclonal)

II. Infection
   A. Bacterial:
   Staphylococcus, streptococcus, anaerobes, tuberculosis, atypical mycobacteria, bartonella henselae, brucellosis, salmonella typhi, diphtheria, C. trachomatis (lymphogranuloma venereum), calymmatobacterium granulomatis, francisella tularensis
   B. Viral:
   Epstein-Barr virus, cytomegalovirus, adenovirus, respiratory syncytial virus, influenza, coxsackie virus, rubella, rubeola, varicella, HIV, herpes simplex II
   C. Protozoal:
   Toxoplasmosis, malaria, trypanosomiasis
   D. Pirochetal:
   Syphilis, rickettsia typhi (murine typhus)
   E. Fungal:
   Coccidioidomycosis (valley fever), histoplasmosis, cryptococcus, aspergillosis
   F. Postvaccination: Smallpox, live attenuated measles, DPT, Salk vaccine, typhoid fever

III. Connective tissue disorders
   A. Rheumatoid arthritis
   B. Systemic lupus erythematosus

IV. Hypersensitivity states
   A. Serum sickness
   B. Drug reaction (e.g., Dilantin, mephenytoin, pyrimethamine, phenylbutazone, allopurinol, isoniazid, antileprosy and antithyroid medications)

V. Lymphoproliferative disorders (Chap. 13)
   A. Angioimmunoblastic lymphadenopathy with dysproteinemia
   B. X-linked lymphoproliferative syndrome
   C. Lymphomatoid granulomatosis
   D. Sinus histiocytosis with massive lymphadenopathy (Rosai–Dorfman disease)
   E. Castleman disease (benign giant lymph node hyperplasia, angiofollicular lymph node hyperplasia)
   F. Autoimmune lymphoproliferative syndrome (ALPS) (Canale-Smith syndrome)
   G. Post-transplant lymphoproliferative disorder (PTLD)

VI. Neoplastic diseases
   A. Hodgkin and non-Hodgkin lymphomas
   B. Leukemia
   C. Metastatic disease from solid tumors: neuroblastoma, nasopharyngeal carcinoma, Rhabdomyosarcoma, thyroid cancer
   D. Histiocytosis
      1. Langerhans cell histiocytosis
      2. Familial hemophagocytic lymphohistiocytosis
      3. Macrophage activation syndrome
      4. Malignant histiocytosis

VII. Storage diseases
   A. Niemann–Pick disease
   B. Gaucher disease
   C. Cystinosis

VIII. Immunodeficiency states
   A. Chronic granulomatous disease
   B. Leukocyte adhesion deficiency
   C. Primary dysgammaglobulinemia with lymphadenopathy

Continued

Table 12-2. Causes of Lymphadenopathy—Cont'd

IX. Miscellaneous causes
   A. Kawasaki disease (mucocutaneous lymph node syndrome)
   B. Kikuchi-Fujimoto disease[a]
   C. Sarcoidosis
   D. Beryllium exposure
   E. Hyperthyroidism

[a]A benign form of necrotising apoptotic lymphadenitis of unknown cause. It is rarely associated with systemic lupus erythematosis and can mimic lymphoma.

The following investigations should be carried out to elucidate the cause of either localized or generalized lymphadenopathy:

1. Thorough history of infection, contact with rodents or cats, and systemic complaints.
2. Careful examination of the lymphadenopathy including size, consistency, mobility, warmth, tenderness, erythema, fluctuation, and location. All the lymph node–bearing areas as outlined above should be carefully examined.
3. Physical examination for evidence of hematologic disease, such as hepatosplenomegaly and petechiae.
4. Blood count and erythrocyte sedimentation rate (ESR).
5. Skin testing for tuberculosis.
6. Bacteriologic culture of regional lesions (e.g., throat).
7. Specific serologic tests for Epstein–Barr virus (EBV), *Bartonella henselae*, toxoplasmosis, cytomegalovirus (CMV), and human immunodeficiency virus (HIV).
8. Chest radiograph and CT scan (if necessary); abdominal sonogram and CT, if indicated.
9. EKG and echocardiogram if Kawasaki disease is suspected.
10. Lymph node aspiration and culture; helpful in isolating the causative organism and deciding on an appropriate antibiotic when infection is the cause of the lymphadenopathy.
11. Fine-needle aspiration; may yield a definite or preliminary cytologic diagnosis and occasionally obviate the need for lymph node biopsy; it provides limited material in the event flow cytometry is required, and negative results cannot rule out a malignancy because the sample may be inadequate.
12. Bone marrow examination if leukemia or lymphoma is suspected.
13. Lymph node biopsy if:
    Initial physical examination and history suggest malignancy.
    Laboratory testing is inconclusive and lymph node size is greater than 2.5 cm.
    Lymph node persists or enlarges.
    Appropriate antibiotics fail to shrink node within 2 weeks.

When lymph node biopsy is performed, the results can be maximized when the following precautions are observed:

1. Upper cervical and inguinal areas should be avoided; lower cervical and axillary nodes are more likely to give reliable information.
2. The largest node should be biopsied, not the most accessible one. The oncologist should select the node to be biopsied in consultation with the surgeon.
3. The node should be removed intact with the capsule, not piecemeal.
4. The lymph node should be sent to the pathologist in sufficient tissue culture medium to prevent the tissue from drying out. The node must not be left in

strong light, where it will be subject to heat, and it should not be wrapped in dry gauze, which may produce a drying artifact. Fresh and frozen samples should be set aside for additional studies.

When biopsy is performed, the following studies should be done:

1. Gram stain and culture (bacterial including mycobacterial, viral, and fungal)
2. Light microscopy
3. Immunohistochemical stains (to differentiate tumor types)
4. Flow cytometry (to differentiate cell types in leukemia and lymphoma; e.g., T cell, B cell, pre–B cell)
5. Gene rearrangement studies for the T-cell receptor and the immunoglobulin gene to determine monoclonality in leukemia or lymphoma
6. Electron microscopy.

Once the cause of the lymphadenopathy is ascertained, appropriate management can be undertaken.

SPLENOMEGALY

The tip of the spleen is frequently palpable in otherwise normal infants and young children. It is usually palpable in premature infants and in about 30% of full-term infants. It may normally be felt in children up to 3 or 4 years of age. At an older age, the spleen tip is generally not palpable below the costal margin, and a palpable spleen usually indicates splenic enlargement two to three times its normal size.

Visceroptosis

In children, a palpable spleen may occasionally be due to visceroptosis rather than true splenomegaly. This distinction is important to make so that extensive investigations for the cause of splenomegaly are not undertaken unnecessarily. Visceroptosis may result from congenital or acquired defects in the supporting mechanism responsible for maintaining the spleen in the correct position. The visceroptosed spleen may be felt anywhere from the upper abdomen to the pelvis and may undergo torsion. When the spleen is felt in the upper abdomen, it can easily be pushed under the left costal margin. This finding is helpful in diagnosing visceroptosis and in differentiating it from true splenomegaly.

In addition to this finding, an abdominal radiograph in the upright position may reveal intestinal gas bubbles between the left dome of the diaphragm and the spleen. This sign may be helpful in suggesting the diagnosis. Splenic scans with ^{99m}Tc-sulfur colloid and CT are helpful in defining the position of the spleen more precisely.

Splenomegaly

The significance of splenomegaly depends on the underlying disease. Splenomegaly can be caused by diseases that result in hyperplasia of the lymphoid and reticuloendothelial systems (e.g., infections, connective tissue disorders), infiltrative disorders (e.g., Gaucher disease, leukemia, lymphoma), hematologic disorders (e.g., thalassemia, hereditary spherocytosis), and conditions that cause distention of the sinusoids whenever there is increased pressure in the portal or splenic veins (portal hypertension). Table 12-3 lists the various causes of splenomegaly.

Table 12-3. Causes of Splenomegaly

I. Infectious splenomegaly (due to antigenic stimulation with hyperplasia of the reticuloendothelial and lymphoid systems)
  A. Bacterial: acute and chronic systemic infection, subacute bacterial endocarditis, abscesses, typhoid fever, miliary tuberculosis, tularemia, plague
  B. Viral: infectious mononucleosis (Epstein–Barr virus), cytomegalovirus, HIV, hepatitis A, B, C
  C. Spirochetal: syphilis, lyme disease, leptospirosis
  D. Rickettsial: Rocky Mountain spotted fever, Q fever, typhus
  E. Protozoal: malaria, babesiosis, toxoplasmosis, toxocara canis, toxocara cati, leishmaniasis, schistosomiasis, trypanosomiasis
  F. Fungal: disseminated candidiasis, histoplasmosis, coccidioidomycosis, South American blastomycosis

II. Hematologic disorders
  A. Hemolytic anemias, such as thalassemia, splenic sequestration crisis in sickle cell disease, hereditary spherocytosis
  B. Extramedullary hematopoiesis as in osteopetrosis and myelofibrosis
  C. Myeloproliferative disorders (e.g., polycythemia vera, essential thrombocythemia)

III. Infiltrative splenomegaly
  A. Nonmalignant
    1. Langerhans cell histiocytosis
    2. Storage diseases such as Gaucher disease, Niemann–Pick disease, GM-1 gangliosidosis, glycogen storage disease type IV, Tangier disease, Wolman disease, mucopolysaccharidoses, hyperchylomicronemia types I and IV, amyloidosis, and sarcoidosis
  B. Malignant
    1. Leukemia
    2. Lymphoma: Hodgkin and non-Hodgkin

IV. Congestive splenomegaly
  A. Intrahepatic (portal hypertension): cirrhosis of the liver (e.g., neonatal hepatitis, α_1-antitrypsin deficiency, Wilson disease, cystic fibrosis)
  B. Prehepatic or portal vein obstruction (e.g., thrombosis, vascular malformations)

V. Immunologic diseases
  A. Serum sickness, graft-versus-host disease
  B. Connective tissue disorders (e.g., systemic lupus erythematosus, rheumatoid arthritis—Felty syndrome, mixed connective tissue disorder, Sjögren syndrome, macrophage activation syndrome, systemic mastocytosis)
  C. Common variable immunodeficiency
  D. Autoimmune lymphoproliferative syndrome (ALPS) (Canale–Smith syndrome)

VI. Primary splenic disorders
  A. Cysts
  B. Benign tumors (e.g., hemangioma, lymphangioma)
  C. Hemorrhage in spleen (e.g., subcapsular hematoma)
  D. Partial torsion of splenic pedicle leading to congestive splenomegaly, cyst, and abscess formation

Diagnostic Approach to Splenomegaly

Detailed History

1. Fever or rigors indicative of infection (e.g., subacute bacterial endocarditis [SBE], infectious mononucleosis, malaria)
2. Neonatal omphalitis, umbilical venous catheterization (inferior vena cava or portal vein thrombosis)
3. Jaundice (evidence of liver disease)
4. Abnormal bleeding or bruising (hematologic malignancy)
5. Family history of hemolytic anemia (e.g., hereditary spherocytosis or thalassemia major)
6. Travel to endemic areas (e.g., malaria)
7. Trauma (splenic hematoma).

Physical Examination

1. Size of spleen (measured in centimeters below costal margin); consistency, tenderness, audible rub
2. Hepatomegaly
3. Lymphadenopathy
4. Fever
5. Ecchymoses, purpura, petechiae
6. Stigmata of liver disease such as jaundice, spider angiomata, or caput medusa
7. Stigmata of rheumatoid arthritis or systemic lupus erythematosus (SLE)
8. Osler nodes, Janeway lesions, splinter hemorrhages, fundal hemorrhages (SBE)
9. Cardiac murmurs.

Laboratory Investigations

The extent to which the following investigations are undertaken must be guided by clinical judgment. It is not necessary to perform all the evaluations. If the child appears well, and the index of suspicion is low, it is reasonable to do no further investigations and reexamine the child in 1–2 weeks. If the splenomegaly persists, further workup should be done.

1. *Blood count:* Red cell indices, reticulocyte count, platelet count, differential white blood cell count, and blood film (which may demonstrate evidence of hematologic malignancy, hemolytic disorders, viral and protozoal infections)
2. *Evaluation for infection:* Blood culture and viral studies (CMV, EBV panel, HIV, toxoplasmosis, smear for malaria, tuberculin test)
3. *Evaluation for evidence of hemolytic disease:* Blood count, reticulocyte count, blood smear, haptoglobin level, serum bilirubin, urinary urobilinogen, Coombs' test, osmotic fragility, autohemolysis, and red cell enzyme assays, if indicated
4. *Evaluation for liver disease:* Liver function tests, α_1-antitrypsin deficiency, serum copper, ceruloplasmin (to exclude Wilson disease), and liver biopsy (if indicated)
5. *Evaluation for portal hypertension:* Ultrasound and Doppler of portal venous system and endoscopy (if indicated to exclude esophageal varices)
6. *Evaluation for connective tissue disease:* ESR, C3, C4, CH_{50}, antinuclear antibody (ANA), rheumatoid factor, urinalysis, blood urea nitrogen (BUN), and serum creatinine
7. *Evaluation for infiltrative disease (benign and malignant):*
   a. Bone marrow aspiration and biopsy, looking for blasts, Langerhans cell histiocytes, or storage cells
   b. Enzyme assay for Gaucher disease

8. *Lymph node biopsy:* If there is significant lymphadenopathy, lymph node biopsy may provide the diagnosis
9. *Imaging studies:*
    a. CT scan
    b. Magnetic resonance imaging (MRI)
    c. Liver–spleen scans with ^{99m}Tc-sulfur colloid
10. *Biopsy:* If less invasive studies have failed to provide the diagnosis, it may be necessary to perform a splenectomy or a partial splenectomy. Biopsy and splenic aspiration are rarely performed because there is a significant risk of bleeding. Biopsy material must be processed for cultures and Gram stain, as well as for histology, flow cytometry, histochemical stains, electron microscopy, and gene rearrangement studies. Once the etiology of the splenomegaly is ascertained, further management for the underlying disorder can be instituted.

SUGGESTED READINGS

French J, Camitta BM. The Spleen. In: Behrman R, Kliegman RM, Jenson HB, editors. Nelson Textbook of Pediatrics. 17th ed. New York: Elsevier, 2004.

Leung AKC, Robson WLM. Childhood cervical lymphadenopathy. J Pediatr Health Care 2004;18:3–7.

Link MP, Donaldson SS. The lymphomas and lymphadenopathy. In: Nathan and Oski's Hematology of Infancy and childhood. 6th ed. Philadelphia: WB Saunders, 2003.

Shurin SB. The Spleen and its disorders. In: Hoffman R, Benz EJ, Shattil SJ, Furie B, Cohen HJ, Silberstein LE, editors. Hematology: Basic Principles and Practice. 3rd ed. London: Churchill Livingstone, 2000.

Twist CJ, Link MP. Assessment of lymphadenopathy in children. Pediatr Clin North Am 2002;49:1009–25.

13

LYMPHOPROLIFERATIVE DISORDERS, MYELODYSPLASTIC SYNDROMES, AND MYELOPROLIFERATIVE DISORDERS

LYMPHOPROLIFERATIVE DISORDERS

Lymphoproliferative disorders manifest with uncontrolled hyperplasia of lymphoid tissues (lymph nodes, spleen, bone marrow, liver). They are a heterogeneous group of diseases that range from reactive polyclonal hyperplasia (immunologic disorders) to true monoclonal (malignant) diseases.

Angioimmunoblastic Lymphadenopathy with Dysproteinemia

Manifestations of the clinicopathological syndrome of angioimmunoblastic lymphadenopathy with dysproteinemia (AILD) include:

- Generalized lymphadenopathy (80%)
- Hepatosplenomegaly (70%)
- Fever (70%), malaise, weight loss, polyarthralgia
- Quantitative changes in serum proteins (polyclonal hypergammaglobulinemia, 70%); hypocomplementemia
- Autoantibodies; circulating immune complexes, anti–smooth muscle antibody
- Rashes
- Pulmonary infiltrates, pleural effusions
- Thrombocytopenia
- Hemolytic anemia (often Coombs' positive).

Diagnosis

The lymph node shows architectural effacement, absence of germinal center, and arborization of postcapillary venules and a polymorphous infiltrate that includes immunoblasts and plasma cells. There is also genotypic evidence of T-cell monoclonality. Immunoblasts are CD4 positive. Lymph node cytogenetic studies have shown nonrandom abnormalities, including +3, 14q+, and del(8) (p21). This provides strong evidence of monoclonality.

Prognosis

Spontaneous regression occurs in some cases. Many cases evolve into peripheral T-cell lymphoma and some cases into immunoblastic lymphoma or Hodgkin disease. Death usually results from overwhelming infections. The median survival is 1.5 years.

Treatment of AILD-Type Lymphoma

Chemotherapy: Adriamycin-containing regimens such as CHOP (see Table 13-6 later in this chapter) have been used. Recently, fludarabine has been used successfully in some patients with AILD-type lymphoma.

Small Lymphocytic Infiltrates of the Orbit and Conjunctiva (Ocular Adnexal Lymphoid Proliferation, Pseudolymphoma, Benign Lymphoma, Atypical Lymphocytic Infiltrates)

Lymphocytic infiltrates of the orbit and conjunctiva may be divided into three histologic groups:

1. Monomorphous infiltrates of clearly atypical lymphocytes
2. Infiltrates composed of small lymphocytes with minimal or no cytologic atypia
3. Benign inflammatory pseudotumor or reactive follicular hyperplasia.

On the basis of immunophenotypic criteria, they can be divided into two classes:

1. Infiltrates with monotypic immunoglobulin expression
2. Infiltrates with polytypic immunoglobulin expression.

For the localized small lymphocytic infiltrates, monotypic (monoclonal) immunoglobulin expression confers a 50% risk of dissemination. The initial immunophenotypic (mono- or polyclonal) and molecular studies of various histologic groups fail to correlate with the eventual outcome of these cases because the initial polyclonal tumors may become monoclonal.

All patients presenting with small lymphocyte infiltrates of the orbit and conjunctiva should have a systemic evaluation with serum chemistries, blood counts, and appropriate imaging studies at initial diagnosis and every 6 months for 5 years thereafter.

For localized disease, local radiotherapy is commonly used, regardless of histologic grading.

Angiocentric Immunolymphoproliferative Disorders

These are a collection of entities classified as peripheral T-cell disorders and include lymphomatoid granulomatosis, midline granuloma, and postmalignancy angiocentric immunolymphoproliferative lymphoma.

There are three grades of angiocentric immunolymphoproliferative (AIL) disorders:

Grade I—polymorphic infiltrates with minimal necrosis, few large atypical lymphoid cells, and small lymphocytes lacking nuclear irregularities

Grade II—cytologic atypia of small lymphocytes, scattered large atypical lymphoid cells, and intermediate amount of necrosis

Grade III—lymphoma, either diffuse, mixed, large cell, or immunoblastic, with prominent necrosis.

The cellular origin of AIL lymphoma remains uncertain because of the following findings:

1. Immunophenotype of T cells (CD2+, CD3+, CD4±, CD5±, CD7±)
2. Absence of clonal rearrangements of T-cell receptors
3. Expression of natural killer (NK) cell antigens (CD16+, CD56+, CD57+).

AIL lymphoma has recently been postulated to be a clonal process induced by Epstein–Barr virus (EBV) infection of T lymphocytes.

Clinical Features

Lymphomatoid Granulomatosis

This is a systemic disease characterized by the following:

The lungs are typically involved, presenting with cough, dyspnea, and chest pain. It may be discovered incidentally in asymptomatic patients on a chest radiograph, which shows bilateral nodules, consolidation, or diffuse bilateral reticulonodular infiltrates. There may be mediastinal and hilar lymphadenopathy and pleural effusion.

Purplish skin nodules may undergo spontaneous central necrosis and ulceration.

The kidneys, central nervous system (CNS), skeletal muscles, nasopharynx, or peripheral nerve may also be involved.

Midline Lethal Granuloma

This presents with a progressive necrotizing and destructive process involving the upper airways. There may or may not be a tumor mass. The most common sites of the disease are the nasal fossa, nasal septum, nasopharynx, palate, and adjacent soft tissue or bony structures. There is often a history of long-standing sinusitis with purulent and foul-smelling nasal discharge.

Postmalignancy Angiocentric Immunolymphoproliferative Lymphoma

This rarely occurs in children. Five of the seven childhood cases had acute lymphoblastic leukemia (ALL) previously. The interval between the remission of ALL to the diagnosis of AIL lymphoma ranges from 1 month to 4–5 years. The prognosis is poor.

Treatment

An intensive regimen containing cyclophosphamide and prednisone may improve the chances of survival.

Castleman Disease (Angiofollicular Lymph Node Hyperplasia, Benign Giant Lymph Node Hyperplasia, Angiomatous Lymphoid Hamartoma)

Castleman disease is characterized by an accumulation of nonneoplastic lymphoid tissue interspersed with plasma cells and blood vessels. Vascular hyperplasia has been attributed to a humoral vasoproliferative factor. Table 13-1 shows the relationship between the hyaline vascular (solitary lymph node) and plasma cell (multiple lymph node) histologic types and clinical features in Castleman disease.

The production of interleukin-6 (IL-6) by B cells in the germinal centers of hyperplastic lymph nodes in Castleman disease plays a central role in inducing the variety

Table 13-1. Relationship between Histologic Types and Clinical Features in Castleman Disease

Histologic type (frequency)	Disease sites	Symptoms
Hyaline vascular type (80%)	Solitary lymph node 1.5–16 cm; two thirds in mediastinum; sometimes other sites such as peripheral lymph nodes, abdomen, and pelvis	Asymptomatic; pressure effects referable to the location of the mass may be present
Plasma cell variety (20%)	Involves multiple lymph nodes; involves extranodal sites; splenomegaly present	Associated with systemic symptoms such as fever, sweats, arthralgia, rashes, growth retardation, peripheral neuropathy, nephrotic syndrome Laboratory data: hypergammaglobulinemia, microcytic anemia, raised ESR, amyloidosis; plasma cell proliferation usually polyclonal; increased IL-6 production

of symptoms in this disease. In localized disease, human herpes virus 8 (HHV-8) DNA sequences have been detected in CD19 B cells. In multicentric disease, HHV-8 sequences have been detected in CD19 B cells and CD2 T cells.

Clinical Features

Localized disease
Presents with a mediastinal mass or mediastinal lymphadenopathy.

Multicentric disease
Systemic symptoms: malaise, weakness, fever, weight loss, night sweats, anorexia, or nausea
Physical findings: peripheral lymphadenopathy, may be involvement of abdominal or/and mediastinal lymph nodes; hepatosplenomegaly; edema and/or effusions; central and/or peripheral neurologic manifestations.

Prognosis

Localized disease: excellent
Multicentric disease: poor. Many patients with multicentric disease develop hypergammaglobulinemia. A minority with multicentric disease progress rapidly and develop hemolytic anemia and fatal intercurrent infection. Some develop non-Hodgkin lymphoma or Kaposi sarcoma.

Treatment

Localized disease: surgical resection with or without local radiation
Multicentric disease: glucocorticoids alone or with vincristine; vincristine; monoclonal antibodies; anti-IL-6 or anti-IL-6 receptor antibody. There is limited experience with chemotherapy. Alkylating agents alone or in combination with other agents have been used. Patients' tolerance to intense chemotherapy is poor.

Epstein–Barr Virus–Associated Lymphoproliferative Disorders in Immunocompromised Individuals

EBV is a gamma herpes virus, a subfamily distinguished by its limited tissue tropism and latency. EBV enters via the oropharyngeal route and infects resting B lymphocytes through the interaction between the EBV viral envelope glycoprotein (gp350/220) and the C3d complement receptor (CD21). Infected B cells induce the immunologic response of both virus-specific and virus-nonspecific T cells during primary infection, which leads to regression of a majority of infected B cells. However, the virus persists in its latent state lifelong, by its continued presence in a small number of B cells, which express latent membrane protein 2A (LMP 2A) and small EBV encoded RNA 1 and 2 (EBERs 1 and 2). See the following listing of the functions of EBV latent antigens.

Functions of EBV Latent Antigens

EBV antigen	Function
LMP 1	Prevents apoptosis (through NF-κB and MAPK, induction of antiapoptotic proteins AP-1, bcl-2) and immortalization of B cells, increase in tumor invasiveness (by induction of matrix metalloproteinase).
LMP 2A	Inhibits lysis of B cells.
Lytic antigens	vIL-10 and BHRF1 facilitate lysis of cells and induce survival and proliferation of nearby latently infected B cells.
EBNA 1	Maintains and replicates the EBV episome in latency.
EBNA 2	Has an immortalizing function.

Abbreviations: MAPK, mitogen-activated protein kinase; NF-κB, nuclear factor κB; vIL-10, viral homolog of cellular interleukin-10; BHRF1, viral homolog of cellular bcl-2; bcl-2, B cell lymphoma protein.

EBV Antigens Associated with the Lytic Cycle

Early antigen (EA)
Viral capsid antigen (VCA).

During acute infectious mononucleosis (AIM), humoral responses are directed against both lytic and latent proteins. IgM antibodies to cellular proteins and heterophile antigens are also present during AIM.

Detectable levels of IgG antibodies to VCA and EBNA 1 persist through lifetime.

In conjunction with humoral response, the CD4 and CD8 T cell-mediated responses also play an important role in controlling the EBV infection by identifying and destroying latently infected cells.

Cellular Responses in the Control of EBV Infection

The lymphocytosis during AIM consists of activated CD4 and CD8 T lymphocytes. They are specific for EBV lytic and latent proteins.

Cell	Reactivity (function)
CD8+, CD4+ T cells	Directed toward latent phase proteins: EBNA 3, EBNA 4, LMP 1, EBNA 6
NK (natural killer cells)	Lysis of virus containing cells during lytic phase

Reasons for persistence of latency in EBV infection include:

- Paucity of production of neutralizing antibodies to the gp 350/220 component of the viral glycoprotein, a ligand for interaction with C3d on B cells

- Absence of cytotoxic T lymphocyte (CTL) response to EBNA 1, which is primarily responsible for replication and maintenance of viral genome during host cell division.

A state of balance between the control of EBV infection in the latent state and the host's immune response is achieved in a healthy host after control of the AIM phase. However, this state of balance is offset if the host is immunocompromised. Under this situation, the EBV can proliferate and can cause chronic active EBV infection (CAEBV), hemophagocytic lymphohistiocytosis (HLH), lymphoproliferative disorders (LPDs), lymphomas, and other rare complications.

Figure 13-1 shows latency types and corresponding patterns of gene expression observed in different diseases.

The following immunodeficiencies are associated with the development of LPDs:

1. Inherited immunodeficiencies:
   Ataxia telangiectasia
   Wiscott–Aldrich syndrome
   Common variable immunodeficiency
   Severe combined immunodeficiency (SCID)
   Antibody deficiency syndromes such as hypergammaglobulinemia, hyper IgM
     syndrome, X-linked agammaglobulinemia, IgA and IgG subclass deficiency
   Bloom syndrome
   Chédiak–Higashi syndrome.
   Biological factors of significance involved in the pathogenesis of LPDs in this
     population are:
   a. EBV, which causes B-cell proliferation

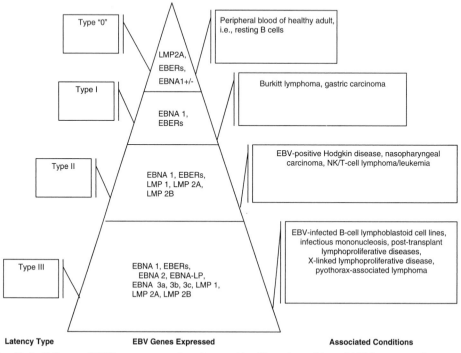

Fig. 13-1. Patterns of EBV gene expression observed in different conditions. LMP, latent membrane protein; EBNA, Epstein–Barr virus nuclear antigen; EBNA-LP, EBNA-leader protein; EBERs, Epstein–Barr-encoded RNAs. (Modified from Swaminathan S. Molecular biology of Epstein–Barr virus and Kaposi's sarcoma associated herpes virus. Semin Hematol 2003;40:107–15; and Tsuchiya S. Diagnosis of Epstein–Barr-associated diseases. Crit Rev Oncol Hematol 2002;44:227–38.)

  b. Imbalanced production of cytokines (e.g., predominance of interleukin-4 [IL-4] and interleukin-6 [IL-6] activates B cells, i.e., humoral arm of immune system)

  c. Genetic defects resulting in ineffective or aberrant rearrangement of T-cell receptor and immunoglobulin genes

 2. Iatrogenically induced immunodeficiencies:

  a. *Organ transplant recipients:* Long-term treatment with immunosuppressive drugs such as cyclosporine and FK-506 increases the risk of infections with EBV. EBV status of the organ transplant recipient plays a significant role. If the patient is EBV seronegative and the donor is seropositive, then the risk of developing clinical infectious mononucleosis followed frequently by LPD increases remarkably. For this reason, post-transplant LPD (PT-LPD) in children differs from that in adults both in frequency and in presentation. The incidence is six times higher in children and it is more likely to present with clinical features of fulminating infectious mononucleosis. Many children have not been previously exposed to EBV and, thus, are more likely to develop a primary EBV infection. PT-LPDs after solid organ transplantation are of B-cell origin and are associated with EBV infection in most patients. A few cases of T-cell PT-LPDs have been reported.

  b. *Hematopoietic stem cell transplant (HSCT) recipients:* HSCT differs in the following respects. The patient receives a new immune system from a donor who is either a full histocompatibility locus antigen (HLA) match or a partial HLA match. The patient's immune system is ablated prior to HSCT. HSCT may require T-cell depletion of the donor's bone marrow.

   The complete recovery of the donor's immune system is delayed by the use of cyclosporine, methotrexate, prednisone, and FK-506, which are used to prevent rejection of graft and graft versus host disease (GVHD). It takes about 6 months to 2 years for immunologic recovery to occur. LPD after HSCT is also associated with EBV-infected B cells. The incidence of LPD in standard matched HSCT is low, but it is 6–12% in HLA-mismatched HSCT due to an increased use of T-cell depletion of the donor's marrow (relative risk factor = 12.3). Also, the use of antithymocyte globulin (ATG) in a preparative regimen increases the risk of PT-LPD (relative risk factor = 3.1). However, depletion of both T and B cells from the graft are associated with a lower incidence of PT-LPD (relative risk factor = 2), since, by removing B cells, it depletes the graft of latent virus creating a balance between latent virus and cellular T cell immunity. If HSCT is performed for immunodeficiency a relative risk factor for post HSCT LPD is 2.5–3.8.

Table 13-2 shows a classification of PT-LPDs.

The frequency of organ involvement with PT-LPDs varies with the type of transplant. For example, liver involvement is 50% in HSCT recipients; lungs 54% in heart transplant recipients and 38% in HSCT recipients; CNS 24% in renal transplant recipients; and kidneys 24% in HSCT recipients and 33% in liver transplant recipients.

Table 13-3 lists the World Health Organization (WHO) classification of PT-LPDs.

Diagnosis of Post-Transplant Lymphoproliferative Disorders

 1. Physical examination: Table 13-4 shows the common sites of involvement in B-cell PT-LPDs.

 2. Biopsy of the appropriate presenting site for histologic studies of immune phenotyping, cytogenetics, molecular analysis, and the examination of EBV genomes in the lymphoid cells (i.e., *in situ* hybridization, Southern blot, polymerase

Table 13-2. Classification of Post-Transplant Lymphoproliferative Disorders

1. Plasmacytic hyperplasia
   Commonly arise in the oropharynx or lymph nodes
   Nearly always polyclonal
   Usually contains multiple clones of EBV
   No oncogenes and tumor suppressor gene alterations
2. Polymorphic B-cell hyperplasia and polymorphic B-cell lymphoma
   Can involve lymph nodes or extranodal sites
   Nearly always monoclonal
   Usually contain a single clone of EBV
   No oncogenes or tumor suppressor gene alterations
3. Immunoblastic lymphoma or multiple myeloma
   Present with widely disseminated disease
   Always monoclonal
   Contains a single clone of EBV
   Contains alterations of one or more oncogenes or tumor suppressor genes (N-*ras*, p53, c-*myc*)

From Magrath IT, Shad AT, Sandlund JT. Lymphoproliferative disorders in immunocompromised individuals. In: Magrath IT, editor. The Non-Hodgkin Lymphoma. 2nd ed. London: Arnold, 1997:955–74, with permission.

Table 13-3. WHO Classification of Post-Transplant Lymphoproliferative Disorders

Early lesions
　Reactive plasmacytic hyperplasia
　Infectious mononucleosis type
PTLD, polymorphic
　Polyclonal (rare)
　Monoclonal
PTLD, monomorphic (classify according to lymphoma classification)
　B-cell lymphomas
　　Diffuse large-cell lymphoma (immunoblastic, centroblastic, anaplastic)
　　Burkitt/Burkitt-like lymphoma
　　Plasma cell myeloma
　T-cell lymphomas
　　Peripheral T-cell lymphoma, not otherwise categorized
　　Other types (hepatosplenic, gamma/delta, T-cell natural killer)
Other types, rare
　Hodgkin disease–like lesions (associated with methotrexate therapy)
　Plasmacytoma-like lesions

From Harris NL, Jaffe ES, Diebold, J, Flandrin G, et al. World Health Organization classification of neoplastic diseases of the hematopoietic and lymphoid tissues: report of the Clinical Advisory Committee Meeting—Airlie House, Virginia, November 1997; J Clin Oncol 1999;17:3835–49.

chain reaction [PCR], terminal repeat probes for clonality). Also, immunostaining of tissues for EBV encoded RNAs (EBVERs) and EBV antigens (proteins) is required for a diagnosis of EBV LPD.

3. Complete blood count.
4. Kidney and liver chemistries, lactic dehydrogenase (LDH).
5. EBV serology (PT-LPD patients have very high anti-VCA titers but lack anti-EBNA antibodies; however, this is not always a consistent finding).
6. A real-time quantitative PCR (qPCR) for EBV-DNA in serum or plasma.
7. A real-time qPCR for EBV-DNA copies in serum or plasma can be used for preemptive diagnosis of post-hematopoietic stem cell PTLD and post–solid organ transplant PTLD.

**Table 13-4. Common Sites of Involvement
in B-Cell Post-Transplant
Lymphoproliferative Disorders**

Site	Percentage of patients
Lymph nodes	59
Liver	31
Lung	29
Kidney	25
Bone marrow	25
Small intestine	22
Spleen	21
Central nervous system	19
Large intestine	14
Tonsils	10
Adrenals	9
Skin/soft tissue	7
Blood	6
Heart	5
Salivary glands	4

From Magrath IT, Shad AT, Sandlund JT. Lymphoproliferative disorders in immunocompromised individuals. In: Magrath IT, editor. The Non-Hodgkin Lymphoma. 2nd ed. London: Arnold, 1997:955–74, with permission.

Table 13-5 shows the comparison of characteristics of LPDs in post–solid organ transplantation (SOT) patients and post-HSCT patients.

Treatment

The indications for treatment of LPD with chemotherapy are:

1. Patient in whom all other measures to control LPD have failed and patient has widespread LPD
2. Patient who has developed monoclonal LPD.

Treatment of B-Cell Lymphoproliferative Disease in Immunosuppressed Patients

General

The following treatment strategy is employed in all patients:

1. Reduction or withdrawal of immunosuppressive therapy (including prednisone and other drugs such as cyclosporine A, azathioprine, and tacrolimus) is attempted as first-line treatment. However, this can aggravate GVHD in HSCT patients and cause graft rejection in organ transplant patients.
2. High-dose acyclovir (500 mg/m² every 8 hours with standard adjustment for impaired renal function) and intravenous immunoglobulin (IVIG): 500 mg/kg/day once a week for 2–4 weeks. Antiviral agents, acyclovir or ganciclovir, may be effective as a preemptive measure.

These measures are usually not effective in HSCT patients because the regenerating donor's immune system cannot provide enough immunity to eradicate EBV-infected B cells. In SOT patients, regression of LPD has been observed in 23–86% of patients with these measures.

For a localized LPD, surgery or local radiation may be helpful.

Table 13-5. Comparison of Lymphoproliferative Disorders: Post–Solid Organ Transplantation and Post–Hematopoietic Stem Cell Transplantation

Characteristic	LPD post-solid organ transplantation	LPD post-hematopoietic stem cell transplantation
Immune system	Patient's own, i.e., organ recipient's own	Replaced by donor's
Immunosuppressive therapy	Lifelong	About 6 months post-transplant, or as long as graft versus host disease persists
Onset of LPD	Highest incidence: 6–12 months after transplant	Highest incidence: 6–12 months after transplant
EBV association	Early-onset LPD: always associated with EBV Late-onset LPD: multifactorial, many patients being EBV negative	Almost always EBV associated
Cellular origin of LPD	LPD arises in patient's, i.e., organ recipient's, own lymphocytes	LPD arises in HSCT donor's lymphocytes; however, sometimes it may arise from blood transfusions
Incidence	EBV status of recipient: Seronegative 15.8% Seropositive 5.4% Organ transplant: Kidney 1.2–9% Liver 6.8–13% Thoracic organ 3.8–11.7% Heart 5–15% Lung 10–20% Intestinal/multivisceral 31% Type of immunosuppression Antithymocyte globulin (ATG) 11.4%	Cumulative incidence 1% at 10 years Mismatched 1% Mismatched and T-cell depletion 1–8% Unrelated 1.5% Unrelated and T-cell depletion 5–29% Unrelated and Campath depletion 1.3%
Treatment	Preemptive therapy Intravenous immunoglobulin infusion Acyclovir or ganciclovir Infusion of patient's (organ recipient's) own EBV-specific cytotoxic T cells (CTL) Infusion of anti-CD20 antibody (rituximab) Therapeutic Same as preemptive plus chemotherapy	Preemptive therapy Intravenous immunoglobulin infusion Acyclovir or ganciclovir Infusion of donor's EBV-specific cytotoxic T cells Infusion of anti-CD20 antibody (rituximab) Therapeutic Same as preemptive plus chemotherapy

Specific

1. Inherited immunodeficiency syndromes:
   Polyclonal or monoclonal with no lymphoma-specific genetic abnormalities:
   a. Localized LPD
      Radiation (low dose)/surgery*
   b. Generalized
      Interferon (see below)
      Anti-B-cell monoclonal antibodies (see below)
      Chemotherapy (Table 13-6) if no response or if LPD is rapidly progressive or recurrent
      Monoclonal with a lymphoma-specific genetic abnormality[†]:
      Chemotherapy[‡] (Table 13-6)
2. Post-SOT:
   Polyclonal or monoclonal with no lymphoma-specific genetic abnormalities:
   Reduce dose of immunosuppressive drugs if possible
   a. Localized LPD
      Radiation/surgery
   b. Generalized LPD
      (1) Interferon:
         Interferon-α (IFN-α). Dose: 3×10^6 units/m^2 (i.e., 3 million units/m^2) once a day subcutaneously for 3 weeks. If there is a response continue for 6 months. IFN-α stimulates NK cells. It also inhibits proliferation of EBV-infected B cells.
      (2) Anti-B-cell monoclonal antibodies:
         a. Humanized anti-CD21 and anti-CD24, although effective in treatment of post–organ transplant LPD, are not commercially available.
         b. Humanized anti-CD20 monoclonal antibody (rituximab) is commercially available. It is administered at a dose of 375 mg/m^2 once a week for 4 weeks after reducing the dose of immunosuppressive drugs. Complete remission rates of 50–65% have been reported. However, it should be used cautiously since it may increase the risk of graft rejection, especially when a reduction in immunosuppressive therapy is attempted at the same time.
            A second course of anti-CD20 may be given for the relapsed patients.
         c. Preemptive therapy with one infusion of 375 mg/m^2 of rituximab in recipients of T-cell-depleted allo-HSCT who develop reactivation of EBV (1000 or more genome-equivalent [geq]/mL) results in a significant reduction of LPD and prevention of LPD-related mortality. Reduction in EBV DNA to less than 50 geq/mL is considered effective therapy.
      (3) Adoptive immunotherapy: Infusion of patient's own EBV-specific cytotoxic T-cells (CTL) has been tried in a few patients with an 80% rate of normalization of EBV DNA viral load.
      (4) Other therapies:
         a. Anti-IL-6 antibody treatment: IL-6 induces proliferation and maturation of EBV-infected B-cells. Anti-IL-6 antibody has been tried in a few patients with some success.
         b. Vaccination of EBV-seronegative recipients before undergoing transplantation.

---

*Avoid radiation therapy in patients with chromosomal instability/DNA repair defect diseases (e.g., ataxia telangiectasia).

[†]Any B-cell malignancy.

[‡]Use smaller doses of chemotherapy agents for patients with chromosomal instability/DNA repair defect diseases (e.g., ataxia telangiectasia).

Chemotherapy: If no response, rapidly progressive, or recurrent.

Monoclonal with a lymphoma-specific genetic abnormality: Table 13-6 lists the treatment regimen with cyclophosphamide, doxorubicin, vincristine, and prednisone (CHOP regimen) used for post-transplant lymphoproliferative disorder.

3. Post-HSCT:

    Interferon (see above)

    Anti-B-cell monoclonal antibodies (see above)

    Donor leukocyte infusions:

    a. Use of unmanipulated donor's T cells
        (1) Without transduction of donor's T cells with a suicide gene that can be turned on in case of worsening of GVHD.
        (2) Transduced donor's T cells with a suicide gene, herpes simplex virus thymidine kinase (HSV-tk), which can be activated by ganciclovir therapy in the event of worsening of GVHD.
    b. Use of selectively *ex vivo* expanded EBV-specific donor's cytotoxic T cells (CTLs).

    Chemotherapy (Table 13-6): If no response or recurrence (see above).

    Monoclonal with a lymphoma specific genetic abnormality: Chemotherapy (Table 13-6).

X-Linked Lymphoproliferative Syndrome

X-linked lymphoproliferative syndrome (XLP) is an X-linked recessive disorder. The pathogenesis is a defect in the regulation of T-cell-mediated immune response, which is induced by EBV. It is unknown why this occurs with EBV and not other viruses in this condition.

Recently, clinical manifestations of XLP such as dysgammaglobulinemia, aplastic anemia, and LPD have been described in the absence of EBV infection.

Pathophysiology

Familial XLP results from mutations in the *SH2D1A* (also known as *SAP*) gene, which makes SAP protein (SLAM-associated protein), which is also known as SH2D1A protein. Normally, in activated T cells and NK cells, SAP levels increase. SAP interacts with SLAM (signaling lymphocyte activation molecule family), a molecule expressed on T-cell surface, B-cell surface, and dendritic cell surface. In T cells,

Table 13-6. Treatment of Post-Transplantation Lymphoproliferative Disorder with Cyclophosphamide, Doxorubicin, Vincristine, Prednisone (CHOP)[a]

Cyclophosphamide	750 mg/m^2 intravenous on day 1 of each cycle
Doxorubicin	50 mg/m^2 intravenous on day 1 of each cycle
Vincristine	1.4 mg/m^2 intravenous (with maximum dose 2 mg) on day 1 of each cycle
Prednisone	100 mg/m^2/day orally (with maximum dose 100 mg) per day on days 1 through 5

Treatment cycles are repeated every 21 days or following hematopoietic recovery. Patients who experience complete remission after four cycles are treated with two additional cycles of chemotherapy. Patients are maintained on reduced cyclosporine level indefinitely.

[a]This same regime (CHOP) can also be utilized for treatment of angioimmunoblastic lymphadenopathy with dysproteinemia (AILD)-type lymphoma.

SAP regulates T-cell receptor (TCR)–induced interferon γ (IFN-γ). In NK cells, SAP binds to 2B4 and NTB-A (which also belong to SLAM family receptors) and activates NK–cell–induced cytotoxicity.

In XLP, various types of *SAP* (*SH2D1A*) gene mutations have been described including deletion, nonsense, missense, and splice site mutations. As a result of this, SAP protein may be absent or truncated or may contain altered amino acid residue at highly conserved sites.

No correlation has been found between genotypes and phenotypes or in the outcomes of these patients. It has been postulated that the mutation of SAP protein in XLP causes defective helper and cytotoxic T cell function. In contrast to familial XLP, no mutations of SAP occur in sporadic XLP.

Clinical Manifestations

Fulminant infectious mononucleosis (frequency 58%; survival 4%). It is characterized by infiltration of various organs with polyclonal B and T cells, production of inflammatory cytokines, and necrosis of liver, bone marrow, lymph nodes, and spleen caused by the invading cytotoxic T-cell and uncontrolled killer cell activity. Death is generally attributable to liver failure with hepatic encephalopathy or bone marrow failure with fatal hemorrhage in the lungs, brain, or gastrointestinal tract and occurs within 1 month of onset of symptoms.

Secondary dysgammaglobulinemia (frequency 30%; survival 55%).

B-cell lymphoproliferative disease including malignant lymphoma (extranodal non-Hodgkin lymphoma) (frequency 25%; survival 35%).

Aplastic anemia

Virus-associated hemophagocytic syndrome. Patients usually die within 1 month of onset of symptoms.

Vasculitis and pulmonary lymphomatoid granulomatosis.

In the same patient, several sequential phenotypes of the disease may manifest over time. This phenotypic variation most often includes dysgammaglobulinemia, malignant lymphoma, and marrow aplasia.

Patients with the XLP syndrome reveal many humoral and cellular immunologic defects, which include the following:

- Selective impaired immunity to EBV but normal immune responses to other herpes viruses
- Uncontrolled TH1 responses (with high levels of IFN-γ in some patients)
- Inverted CD4/CD8 ratio (due to increase in CD8+ cells)
- Dysgammaglobulinemia: low IgG, high IgM, and high IgA
- Defective NK-cell activity
- Decreased T-cell regression assay
- Failure to switch from IgM to IgG class response after secondary challenge with OX174 and diminished mitogen-induced transformation of lymphocytes
- Unchanged lymphocyte-mediated antibody-dependent cellular cytotoxicity.

Table 13-7 lists the diagnostic criteria for XLP.

Treatment

1. Prevention of EBV infection: Prophylactic use of intravenous immunoglobulin (IVIG) has been used without much success. High-dose IVIG 600 mg/kg per month, however, has been effective in some patients.
2. Treatment of acute EBV infection in XLP patients: High-dose IVIG and/or acyclovir are ineffective.

Table 13-7. Diagnostic Criteria for X-Linked Lymphoproliferative Syndrome

Definitive Diagnosis of XLP

Male patient with lymphoma or Hodgkin disease, fatal EBV infection, immunodeficiency, aplastic anemia, or lymphohistiocytic disorder and at least one of the following: (1) mutations in SH2D1A, (2) absent SH2D1A RNA on Northern blot analysis of lymphocytes, and (3) absent SH2D1A protein in lymphocytes.

Probable Diagnosis of XLP

Male patient experiencing death, lymphoma or Hodgkin disease, immunodeficiency, aplastic anemia, or lymphohistiocytic disorder following acute EBV infection and maternal cousins, uncles, or nephews with a history of similar diagnoses following acute EBV infection.

XLP Phenotype

Male patient experiencing death, lymphoma or Hodgkin disease, immunodeficiency disorder, aplastic anemia or lymphohistiocytic disorder following acute EBV infection and who have normal expression of SH2D1A.

Abbreviation: EBV, Epstein–Barr virus.

From: Ochs HD, Nelson DL, Stiehm ER. Other well-defined immunodeficiency syndromes (Contributor: Sullivan, JL). In: Immunologic Disorders in Infants and Children. 5th ed. Philadelphia, WB Saunders, 2004, with permission.

3. Treatment of virus-associated hemophagocytosis: Etoposide and cyclosporine A are effective. Etoposide decreases macrophage activity and cyclosporine A decreases T cell activity. HLH (2004) protocol may be used (see Chapter 22, Histiocytosis Syndromes, page 622).
4. Treatment of aplastic anemia: Etoposide and cyclosporine A are effective.
5. Treatment of lymphoma: Standard therapy for lymphoma is used, that is, chemotherapy and radiation therapy where indicated.

Allogeneic HSCT is the only curative therapy for XLP syndrome. Prognosis: 70% of patients with XLP die before 10 years of age.

Autoimmune Lymphoproliferative Syndrome (Canale–Smith Syndrome)

Autoimmune lymphoproliferative syndrome (ALPS) is characterized by:

- Chronic splenomegaly—can result in hypersplenism.
- Lymphadenopathy—usually involves cervical and axillary lymph nodes; may undergo waxing and waning of the severity of enlargement; other peripheral and intracavitary lymph nodes may also be enlarged; lymph nodes histologically benign. Significant reduction in lymph node size occurs during certain viral and bacterial infections.
- Expansion of α/β, CD3+, CD4–, CD8– T cells, known as double-negative T cells (α/β-DNT cells).
- Hepatomegaly—also attributed to accumulation of excessive number of lymphocytes and occasionally to autoimmune hepatitis.
- Urticarial rash—with pruritus and immune vasculitis.

Hematologic Findings

- Anemia—due to autoimmune hemolytic anemia (AIHA) or hypersplenism
- Dyserythropoiesis
- Neutropenia—due to autoimmune antibodies

- Thrombocytopenia due to immunologic thrombocytopenic purpura (ITP) or hypersplenism causing platelet pooling and sequestration
- Eosinophilia
- Hypersplenism.

Immunologic Findings

- Renal insufficiency—due to glomerulonephritis attributed to immune deposition of antigen–antibody complexes
- Autoimmune hepatitis
- Uveitis, iridocyclitis
- Other autoantibody production—antiphospholipid, anticardiolipin, and antinuclear antibodies
- Hypergammaglobulinemia—due to defective apoptosis of B cells accompanied by hyper-IgG, hyper-IgA, high, normal, or decreased IgM and elevated IgE levels
- Elevated interleukin-10 (IL-10) levels in plasma due to its increased production by α/β-DNT cells and monocytes; IL-10 levels correlate with disease expression in ALPS
- Increased soluble CD25, CD30, FasL
- Decreased soluble Fas
- Expansion (elevated) α/β-DNT cells (see below)
- Expansion of other lymphocyte subsets: γ/δ-DNT cells, CD8+ T cells, HLA-DR+ T cells, CD57+ T cells, CD5+ B cells
- Central nervous system involvement—occurs occasionally: organic brain syndrome (mental status changes, headaches, seizures), Guillain-Barré syndrome
- Age—occurs in both children and adults; however, it manifests in the first few years of life.

Pathophysiology

ALPS has been attributed to defective apoptosis (programmed cell death) of lymphocytes, most often arising as a result of mutations in the gene encoding the lymphocyte apoptosis receptor FAS/APO-1/CD95. Because of the failure of the affected lymphocytes to die after their response to antigen has been completed, there is an accumulation and buildup of an excessive number of polyclonal lymphocytes, which leads to hepatosplenomegaly and lymphadenopathy. The mechanism underlying the induction of autoimmunity is unclear at the present time.

There are subtypes of ALPS on the basis of phenotypic and genotypic differences:

ALPS 0: It is caused by complete deficiency of Fas, resulting from homozygous null mutations of *fas* (TNFRSF-6, tumor necrosis factor receptor superfamily member 6) gene. Clinically, it manifests with lymphoproliferation with or without autoimmune complications. Its mouse mutant model counterpart is *lpr/lpr,* Fas ko (knock out).

ALPS Ia: This is the most common type of ALPS. It is caused by heterozygous mutations of *fas* (*TNFRSF-6*) gene. Mutant Fas exerts a transdominant effect on wild-type Fas. Clinically, it manifests with lymphoproliferation with or without autoimmune complications. Its mouse mutant model counterpart is *lpr^cg^/lpr^cg^.*

ALPS Ib: It is caused by a dominant mutation of Fas L (Fas ligand). Clinically, it manifests with features of systemic lupus erythematosus and chronic lymphoproliferation. However, it lacks the classical features of ALPS, that is, expansion of DNT cells and splenomegaly. Its mouse mutant counterpart is *gld/gld.*

ALPS II: It is caused by caspase 8 or caspase 10 deficiency. When it is due to caspase 10 deficiency, it is associated with T-, B-, and dendritic cell-proliferation. Clinically, it manifests with severe autoimmune complications. Caspase 8 deficiency is associated with lymphoproliferation and combined immune defects of T- and B-cell activation.

ALPS III: Molecular defect to account for this subtype of ALPS is unknown.

The following criteria have been recommended by the National Institutes of Health (NIH) ALPS Group to diagnose patients with ALPS:

Required criteria:

1. Chronic nonmalignant lymphoproliferation
2. Defective lymphocyte apoptosis *in vitro*
3. Greater than or equal to 1% TCR α/β+, CD4−, CD8−, T cells (α/β⁺-DNT cells) in peripheral blood, and/or presence of DNT cells in lymphoid tissue.

Supporting criteria:

1. Autoimmunity/autoantibodies
2. Mutations in TNFRSF6, FasL, or caspase 10 gene.

Mechanism of Autoimmunity

Although the mechanism of autoimmunity is not fully understood, it is known that DNT cells are not responsible for its manifestations. IL-10 is a likely cytokine playing a role in autoimmune manifestations in ALPS. IL-10 induces T-cell differentiation toward the Th₂-cell type and these cells in turn stimulate autoreactive B cells to make autoantibodies. IL-10 also causes increased expression of BCL-2 proteins, which contributes to inhibition of the mitochondrial pathway of apoptosis.

The Origin of α/β-DNT Cells

These cells in ALPS originate from cytotoxic CD8+ T cells that are chronically activated *in vivo* and anergic *in vitro*. Also, α/β-DNT cells of ALPS express uniform phenotype. In contrast, the minor population of α/β-DNT cells in healthy individuals contains multiple subpopulations.

Treatment

Hypersplenism: Splenectomy may be indicated.

Pre- and postsplenectomy: Normal precautions are warranted. Avoid splenectomy in children under 2 years of age.

Autoimmune disorder (e.g., ITP, AIHA): This should be treated in the standard way as follows.

Prednisone: If prednisone is required for a prolonged period of time, azathioprine or mycophenolate mofetil (MMF), or cyclosporine may be utilized for their prednisone-sparing effect. Occasionally, anti-CD20 antibody (rituximab) and vincristine have been used to treat resistant cases of ITP.

Autoimmune neutropenia: G-CSF can be used.

Fansidar (a combination of pyrimethamine 25 mg/sulfadoxine 500 mg per tablet): Has been found to be effective in a few patients. It induces apoptosis in activated lymphocytes through activation of the mitochondrial apoptotic pathway. Correction of hematologic abnormalities, shrinkage of lymphadenopathy, decrease in hepatomegaly and/or splenomegaly, and decrease in serum IL-10 levels occur in some patients.

Allogeneic stem cell transplantation is occasionally necessary.

Vaccines: It is important to decrease the frequency of infection, which can aggravate ALPS due to the recruitment of lymphocytes. B-cell responses to infections and vaccinations are mostly intact. All routine immunizations and influenza vaccines should be given. B-cell responses to pneumococcal polysaccharides and blood group antigens are abnormal.

Prognosis

Most patients require splenectomy. ALPS improves with age as children become older. The severity of ALPS varies from mild to severe within the same family. This may be because other pathways of apoptosis are compensating for the FAS pathway.
The following malignancies have been reported in ALPS families:

Burkitt lymphoma, T-cell-rich B-cell lymphoma, and atypical lymphoma
Nodular lymphocyte predominance Hodgkin disease
Breast cancer, lung cancer, basal cell carcinoma of the skin, squamous cell carcinoma of the tongue, and colon cancer.

Most of the cases of lymphoma occur in families with intracellular mutations of TNFRSF-6.

Dianzani Autoimmune Lymphoproliferative Disease

Dianzani autoimmune lymphoproliferative disease (DALD), an ALPS-like syndrome, is characterized by:

1. Defective function of the Fas receptor
2. Autoimmune conditions, predominantly involving blood cells; ITP, AIHA, and autoimmune neutropenia
3. Polyclonal accumulation of lymphocytes in the spleen and lymph nodes.

However, it differs from ALPS in that it lacks expansion of DNT cells. DALD patients have a high level of osteopontin (OPN) due to increases in the haplotype frequencies of B and C types of haplotypes of OPN. These haplotypes are responsible for the increased levels of OPN. *In vitro*, observations show that high levels of OPN decrease activation-induced T-cell apoptosis. For this reason, high levels of OPN have been implicated in the apoptotic defect of DALD.

Lymphomatoid Papulosis in Children

Lymphomatoid papulosis (LyP) is a clinically benign skin disorder characterized by chronic and recurrent self-healing papulonodular lesions. This disorder occurs rarely in children. The sites of lesions include the limbs and/or trunk. The eruption recurs episodically, often ulcerates, and heals spontaneously in 3–8 weeks, leaving an atrophic scar occasionally. LyP results from a clonal T-cell proliferation, which may explain its evolution or coexistence with Hodgkin disease, mycosis fungoides, or anaplastic large cell lymphoma (ALCL).

Histology

LyP is characterized by superficial and deep infiltrates consisting of atypical lymphocytes with a hyperchromatic, pleomorphic nucleus that can obscure the dermoepidermal junction. Similar cellular infiltrates can also be found in the epidermis along with spongiosis, parakeratosis, and neutrophils. Two types of activated T-cell infiltrates are found:

1. *LyP type A lesions:* LyP lesions of this cell type predominantly contain Ki-1+ (CD30+), Reed–Sternberg–type cells with a pale staining, convoluted nucleus, prominent nucleoli, and moderately basophilic cytoplasm.

2. *LyP type B lesions:* LyP lesions of this cell type contain the Sezary-type cell with a cerebriform, hyperchromatic nucleus and scant cytoplasm. Only some of these cells are CD30+.

The atypical cells of LyP have been shown to be of T-cell origin, in most cases expressing CD2, CD3, and CD4. However, these cells lack the expression of some of the usual pan-T-cell antigens, such as CD5, CD7, or both. Clonal rearrangement of the T-cell antigen receptor has been demonstrated in most of the cases studied. Thus, LyP serves as an example of a benign lymphoproliferative disorder in spite of the evidence of clonal T-cell receptor gene rearrangement.

A lymphoma evolving from lymphomatoid papulosis can be recognized by enlarging or persistent skin lesions, peripheral lymphadenopathy, or circulating atypical lymphocytes. A biopsy of suspicious skin lesions or enlarged lymph nodes for histologic, immunologic, cytogenetic, or gene rearrangement studies is indicated. It has also been suggested that a thorough physical examination every 6 months in children with lymphomatoid papulosis with attention to growth and development (as a tool in assessing occult malignancies in children), skin lesions, and lymph nodes should be carried out. Additional studies such as bone marrow examination and radioimaging studies should be performed as needed.

Table 13-8 shows the clinical and histologic differences among cutaneous CD30+ non-Hodgkin lymphoma (NHL) (including ALCL), borderline cases, and LyP.

Treatment

Treatment involves oral antibiotics, systemic corticosteroids, low-dose methotrexate, psoralen with ultraviolet radiation (PUVA), topical steroids, or ultraviolet beam.

Prognosis

The duration of LyP ranges from 1 to 40 years. Approximately 23 children have been described with Lyp and evolution to lymphomas has occurred in 2 of the 23 cases.

MYELODYSPLASTIC SYNDROME

Myelodysplastic syndrome (MDS) results from acquired clonal disorders of the pluripotent (i.e., a stem cell involved in myelopoiesis, erythropoiesis, megakaryopoiesis, and lymphopoiesis) or multipotent (i.e., a stem cell restricted to myelopoiesis, erythropoiesis, and megakaryopoiesis) hematopoietic progenitor cell. It is characterized by absolute and/or functional cytopenias with usually a hypercellular or normocellular bone marrow containing greater than 1 and less than 20% blasts. It has the propensity to evolve into acute myeloid leukemia.

Table 13-9 provides minimal diagnostic criteria for MDS, and Table 13-10 provides a list of investigations for the diagnosis and pertinent differential diagnosis of myelodysplasia. Table 13-11 shows the French–American–British (FAB) classification of MDS, and Table 13-12 the WHO classification and criteria of MDS. However, these two classifications are unsuitable for children with MDS. A classification of MDS in children that conforms to the WHO suggestions and also allows for the special problems of MDS in children has not yet been developed. Table 13-13 shows diagnostic categories of MDS and myeloproliferative diseases in children.

Recently, a consensus was reached among international MDS experts in pediatric hematology and oncology on some of the issues:

Table 13-8. Clinical and Histologic Differences among Cutaneous CD30+ NHL (Including ALCL), Borderline Cases, and LyP

Variable	Cutaneous CD30+ NHL (including ALCLs)	Borderline cases	LyP
Clinical criteria			
Extent of skin lesion	Solitary > regional > generalized	Regional	Regional or generalized
Type of skin lesion	Nodule, tumor	Nodule	Papules or papulonodular
Spontaneous regression	Rare	Frequent	Always
Extracutaneous disease	Possible	Rare	Rare
Histology			
Wedge shape of infiltrates	Never	Sometimes	Regular
Infiltration of subcutis	Regular	Rare	Rare
Inflammatory infiltrate (with neutrophils)	Infrequent	Regular, admixed	Regular, admixed
Epidermotropism	Infrequent	Epidermis infiltrated by small cells and large atypical CD30+ cells	Epidermis infiltrated by small cells, occasionally by large CD30+ cells
CD30 expression	>80% of tumor cells	Small clusters of CD30+ cells	Scattered CD30+ cells

Abbreviation: NHL, non-Hodgkin lymphoma.
Modified from Paulli M, Berti E, Rosso R, Boveri E, et al. CD30/Ki-1 positive lymphoproliferative disorders of the skin—clinicopathological correlation and statistical analysis of 86 cases: a multicentric study of the European Organization of Research and treatment of cancer cutaneous lymphoma project groups. J Clin Oncol 1995;13:1343–54, with permission.

Table 13-9. Minimal Diagnostic Criteria for MDS

At least two of the following:
- Sustained unexplained cytopenia (neutropenia, thrombocytopenia, or anemia)
- At least bilineage morphologic myelodysplasia
- Acquired clonal cytogenetic abnormality in hematopoietic cell
- Increased blasts (5%)

From Hasle H, et al. A pediatric approach to the WHO classification of myelodysplastic and myeloproliferative diseases. Leukemia 2003;17:277–82, with permission.

Table 13-10. Investigation for the Diagnosis and Pertinent Differential Diagnosis (D/D) of Myelodysplasia

Blood
  Hemoglobin level and red cell indices:
  Macrocytosis D/D—drugs, folate or B_{12} deficiency, congenital bone marrow failure syndromes, MDS, JMML
  Microcytic and ring sideroblasts: unlikely to be MDS, exclude mitochondrial diseases
  Normocytic:
  White cell count, differential count, platelet count
  Blood film
  Fetal hemoglobin concentration[a] D/D: MDS, JMML, congenital bone marrow failure syndromes
  Immunodeficiencies: occasionally, immunodeficiency may be associated with MDS or vice versa
  Pertinent tests to be performed on peripheral blood in the context of above D/D:
  Fetal hemoglobin (HbF)
  Cytogenetics (mitomycin C or di-epoxybutane [DEB] study for excessive chromosomal breakage)[b]
  Erythrocyte adenosine deaminase (ADA) level
  Leukocyte alkaline phosphatase
  Vitamin B_{12} and folate levels
  Quantitative immunoglobulin levels and T- and B-lymphocyte quantitation
Bone marrow
  Aspirate and trephine biopsy[c]
  Cytochemistry and iron stain
  Cytogenetics: conventional and fluorescent *in situ* hybridization for chromosome 7, 8, and BCR/ABL (Ph chromosome)
  Molecular analysis: RT-PCR for BCR/ABL
Additional tests
  Neutrophil function
  Platelet function
  Colony-forming unit assay for various lineages on bone marrow cells
  Sugar water test
  Assays for expression of CD 55 and CD 59 antigens on erythrocytes

Note: If bone marrow is hypocellular, aplastic anemia and/or paroxysmal nocturnal hemoglobinuria should be considered. Hepatomegaly or splenomegaly, or hepatosplenomegaly favors diagnosis of JMML or AML.

[a]Draw blood for hemoglobin electrophoresis, sugar water test, CD55 and CD59 antigen tests, and adenosine deaminase (if macrocytosis) before transfusing patient with red blood cells.

[b]Patients with Fanconi anemia may present with myelodysplasia. The significance of this observation is that all patients with myelodysplasia should have chromosomal breakage analysis performed to exclude Fanconi anemia because Fanconi anemia is a recessive disorder and warrants genetic counseling. Additionally, the preparative regimen for HSCT is different for patients with Fanconi anemia

[c]Bone marrow trephine biopsy. Two additional types of MDS have been recognized recently: (1) hypoplastic MDS and (2) MDS with myelofibrosis. Also, in some reports emphasis is placed on recognizing abnormal location of immature precursor cells (ALIP), i.e., presence of blasts in intertrabecular areas in bone marrow biopsy specimens, since it may have prognostic significance. However, no significance has been found thus far, in the major reports of pediatric MDS series.

Table 13-11. French–American–British Classification of Myelodysplastic Syndromes

Myelodysplastic syndrome	Peripheral		Marrow	
	Blasts	Other	Blasts	Other
Refractory anemia (RA)	<1%	Reticulocytopenia Oval macrocytes Rarely, platelets and polymorphonuclear cells (PMN) decreased or dysplastic	<5%	Erythroid hyperplasia Dyserythropoiesis
RA with ringed sideroblasts	<1%	As in RA, plus Basophilic stippling Dimorphic erythrocytes (hypo- and normochromic)	<5%	Erythroid hyperplasia Dyserythropoiesis 15% ringed sideroblasts
Chronic myelomonocytic leukemia	<5%	As in RA, plus Monocytes ↑Mature granulocytes Thrombocytopenia Pelger–Huët PMNs Hypogranular PMNs	≤20%	Monocytic hyperplasia Erythroid hyperplasia
RA with excess blasts (RAEB)	<5%	As in RA, plus Dysplasia and cytopenia of at least two cell lines Pelger–Huët PMNs Hypogranular PMNs Hypogranular and abnormal-sized platelets	5–20%	Granulocytic hyperplasia Erythroid hyperplasia Dyserythropoiesis Dysgranulocytopoiesis Dysmegakaryopoiesis
RAEB in transformation	>5%, <10%		20–30%	Auer rods

From Schwartz EL, Cohen HJ. Myeloproliferative and myelodysplastic syndromes. In: Pizzo P, Poplack DG, editors. Principles and Practice of Pediatric Oncology. 3rd ed. Philadelphia: Lippincott-Raven, 1997.

Table 13-12. WHO Classification and Criteria for the Myelodysplastic Syndromes

Disease	Blood findings	Bone marrow findings
Refractory anemia (RA)	Anemia No or rare blasts	Erythroid dysplasia *only* <5% blasts <15% ringed sideroblasts
Refractory anemia with ringed sideroblasts (RARS)	Anemia No blasts	Erythroid dysplasia *only* ≥15% ringed sideroblasts <5% blasts
Refractory cytopenia with multilineage dysplasia (RCMD)	Cytopenias (bicytopenia or pancytopenia) No or rare blasts No Auer rods <1 × 10⁹/L monocytes	Dysplasia in ≥10% of cells in two or more myeloid cell lines <5% blasts in marrow No Auer rods <15% ringed sideroblasts
Refractory cytopenia with multilineage dysplasia and ringed sideroblasts (RCMD-RS)	Cytopenias (bicytopenia or pancytopenia) No or rare blasts No Auer rods <1 × 10⁹/L monocytes	Dysplasia in ≥10% of cells in two or more myeloid cell lines ≥15% ringed sideroblasts <5% blasts No Auer rods
Refractory anemia with excess blasts 1 (RAEB-1)	Cytopenias <5% blasts No Auer rods <1 × 10⁹/L monocytes	Unilineage or multilineage dysplasia 5% to 9% blasts No Auer rods
Refractory anemia with excess blasts 2 (RAEB-2)	Cytopenias 5–19% blasts Auer rods ± <1 × 10⁹/L monocytes	Unilineage or multilineage dysplasia 10% to 19% blasts Auer rods ±
Myelodysplastic syndrome, Unclassified (MDS-U)	Cytopenias No or rare blasts No Auer rods	Unilineage dysplasia in granulocytes or megakaryocytes <5% blasts No Auer rods
MDS associated with isolated del (5q)	Anemia <5% blasts Platelets normal or increased	Normal to increased megakaryocytes with hypolobated nuclei <5% blasts No Auer rods Isolated del (5q)

Note: ± denotes that Auer rods may or may not be present.

From Vardiman JW, Harris NL, Brunning RD. The World Health Organization (WHO) classification of the myeloid neoplasms. Blood 2002;100:2292–302, with permission.

1. The concept of monosomy 7 as a distinct syndrome has been abandoned.
2. Myeloid leukemia in children with Down syndrome (DS) is distinct from the disease in non-DS children. MDS often precedes acute myeloid leukemia (AML) in DS. In some children with DS, AML is preceded by a transient myeloproliferative disorder. MDS and AML in DS are highly chemosensitive and have an excellent prognosis when treated on a modified AML protocol.
3. Nonclonal disorders with dysplastic morphology should not be considered to be MDS.

Epidemiology

Incidence: 1.8 per million children per year in age group 0–14 years.
Constitutes 4% of all hematologic malignancies.

Table 13-13. Diagnostic Categories of Myelodysplastic and Myeloproliferative Diseases in Children

I. Myelodysplastic/myeloproliferative disease
  • Juvenile myelomonocytic leukemia (JMML)
  • Chronic myelomonocytic leukemia (CMML) (secondary only)
  • BCR/ABL negative chronic myeloid leukemia (Ph⁻ CML)
II. Down syndrome (DS) disease
  • Transient abnormal myelopoiesis (TAM)
  • Myeloid leukemia of DS
III. Myelodysplastic syndrome (MDS)
  • Refractory cytopenia (RC) (peripheral blood blasts less than 2% and bone marrow blasts less than 5%)
  • Refractory anemia with excess blasts (RAEB) (peripheral blood blasts 2–19% and bone marrow blasts 5–19%)
  • RAEB in transformation (RAEB-T) (peripheral blood or bone marrow blasts 20–29%)

Abbreviation: RAEB, refractory anemia with excess blasts.
From Hasle H, et al. A pediatric approach to the WHO classification of myelodysplastic and myeloproliferative diseases. Leukemia 2003;17:277–82, with permission.

Constitutional abnormalities are present in 30% of children with MDS. The most common is Down syndrome.

Table 13-14 lists constitutional abnormalities associated with juvenile myelomonocytic leukemia (JMML) and MDS in children. Familial MDS is observed in 10% of children with MDS, associated with 7- or 7q-chromosome abnormalities.

Therapy-related MDS:

Alkylating agent-induced MDS is characterized by deletions or the loss of a whole chromosome. Latency period: 3–5 years.

Epipodophyllotoxin-induced MDS is characterized by translocations involving chromosome band 11q23. Latency period: 1–3 years.

Incidence of therapy-related MDS; represents 5% of all childhood MDS and occurs in 13% of children treated for malignancies.

Table 13-14. Constitutional Abnormalities Associated with JMML and MDS in Children

A. Associated with JMML
   Constitutional conditions
     Neurofibromatosis type 1 (NF-1)
     Noonan syndrome
     Trisomy 8 mosaicism
B. Associated with MDS
   Constitutional conditions
     Congenital bone marrow failure
       Fanconi anemia
       Kostmann syndrome
       Shwachman–Diamond syndrome
       Diamond–Blackfan syndrome
     Trisomy 8 mosaicism
     Familial MDS (at least one first-degree relative with MDS/AML)
   Acquired conditions
     Prior chemotherapy/radiation
     Aplastic anemia

From Hasle H, et al. A pediatric approach to the WHO classification of myelodysplastic and myeloproliferative diseases. Leukemia 2003;17:277–82, with permission.

Children with therapy-induced MDS or therapy-induced AML (t-MDS/t-AML) compared to children with *de novo* AML or MDS, have the following characteristics:

1. Older at presentation, have lower white blood cell (WBC) counts, and are less likely to have hepatomegaly or splenomegaly or hepatosplenomegaly
2. More likely to have trisomy 8 and less likely to have classic AML translocations
3. Less likely to attain remission after induction therapy (50% versus 72%) and less likely to have a longer overall survival (26% versus 47%) and event-free survival (21% vs 39%).

However, their disease-free survival after attaining remission is similar to that of children with *de novo* AML or MDS (45% versus 53%).

Pathophysiology

MDS is a clonal disease arising either in a pluripotent or multipotent hematopoietic stem cell. It is a heterogeneous disease with different pathophysiologic mechanisms playing roles in its initiation and progression. It has been postulated that initially apoptosis dominates the process and with time, as more genetic abnormalities accumulate in the MDS cells, arrest of maturation and proliferation occurs, resulting in transformation to AML. There is not much information regarding the pathophysiologic mechanisms of MDS in childhood.

Clinical Features

Clinical features are related to cytopenias (e.g., pallor, bruises, petechiae, infections). Usually, there is no lymphadenopathy or hepatosplenomegaly. Children with refractory anemia may not present with low hemoglobin levels, but they have macrocytosis and elevated fetal hemoglobin levels. The presence of hepatosplenomegaly and a WBC greater than $20,000/mm^3$ is strongly suggestive of AML.

Cytogenetics

Monosomy 7 is the most common cytogenetic abnormality in childhood MDS. Trisomy 8 and 21 are the second most common abnormalities. Monosomy 7 has no prognostic significance in childhood MDS.

If AML-specific chromosomal abnormalities are present, then these patients are considered to have AML and are treated for AML.

Differential Diagnosis

1. Clinical course and the response to therapy for M6 (erythroleukemia), M7 (acute megakaryoblastic leukemia), and AML with monosomy 7 are more similar to MDS than the other types of AML. For this reason, it is important for these conditions to be diagnosed accurately. AML with monosomy 7 has a poor prognosis, whereas it is not an unfavorable prognostic factor in MDS.
2. In a borderline case with 30% blasts, bone marrow examination should be performed after 2 weeks and 400 cells should be counted. If greater than 30% blasts are present in the second bone marrow sample, then a diagnosis of AML is made.
3. It is difficult to distinguish hypoplastic MDS (refractory anemia [RA]) from aplastic anemia in the absence of laboratory abnormalities. The majority of children, who develop MDS following a diagnosis of aplastic anemia, present with MDS within the first 3 years from the diagnosis of aplastic anemia. Patients with mild to moderate aplastic anemia may be more likely to develop a clonal disease than a patient with severe aplastic anemia. Repeated evaluation for both

conditions including bone marrow examinations may become necessary to reach a diagnosis.

4. In a case of RA with ringed sideroblasts (RARS) a search for mitochondrial disease is warranted because this subtype of MDS is rare in children.

Prognosis

The International Prognostic Scoring System (IPSS) for MDS is given in Table 13-15 but its applicability to MDS in children remains to be determined. The FPC (hemoglobin F, platelet counts, cytogenetics)-based scoring system for prognostic classification of childhood MDS is listed in Table 13-16.

Table 13-17 shows the IPSS for childhood MDS and JMML. Also, in an analysis reported by the European Working Group on MDS in childhood, preliminary data on childhood MDS revealed poor prognosis in patients with two to three lineage cytopenia and a blast count greater than 5% in bone marrow (see Table 13-17).

Table 13-15. International Prognostic Scoring System for MDS: Survival and AML Evolution

Prognostic variable	Score value				
	0	0.5	1.0	1.5	2.0
BM blasts (%)	<5	5–10	—	11–20	21–30
Karyotype[a]	Good	Intermediate	Poor		
Cytopenias	0/1	2/3			

Scores for risk groups are as follows: low, 0; intermediate 1, 0.5–1.0; intermediate 2, 1.5–2.0; and high, ≥2.5.

[a]Good, normal, -Y, del (5q), del (20q); poor, complex (≥3 abnormalities) or chromosome 7 anomalies; intermediate, other abnormalities.

From Greenberg P, Cox C, LeBeau MM, et al. International scoring system for evaluating prognosis in myelodysplastic syndromes. Blood 1997;89:2074–88, with permission.

Table 13-16. FPC Scoring System for Prognostic Classification of Childhood MDS[a]

Criteria (before treatment)	Points
Hemoglobin F (HbF) >10%	1
Platelet count ≤40,000/mm³	1
Cytogenetic studies	
No detectable clonal abnormalities	0
Simple abnormalities arising from one event, i.e., single translocation, other structural abnormalities, or gain or loss of one chromosome	1
Complex abnormalities arising from two or more structural or numerical events	2

Conclusion

Score	5-Year survival
0	61%
1	20%
2 or 3	0%

[a]Patients included: MDS as per FAB classification, juvenile chronic myeloid leukemia, infantile monosomy 7 syndrome, MDS with eosinophilia.

Data tabulated from information available from Passmore SJ, et al. article Blood 1995;85:1742–50.

Table 13-17. International Prognostic Scoring System (IPSS)[a] for Childhood MDS and JMML (European Working Group on MDS in Childhood)

IPSS risk group	5-Year survival (%)
Low	100
Intermediate 1	72
Intermediate 2	40
High	40

[a]Refer to Table 13-15 for definitions of IPSS risk groups for MDS, which was generated on the basis of a series of adult patients. Cytopenia and bone marrow blasts >5% correlated with poor survival; however, cytogenetic studies were not informative.

Data tabulated from information available from Hasle H, et al. article Leukemia 2000;14:968.

Treatment

- *Refractory anemia or refractory cytopenia:* Children with RA have a long and stable clinical course without treatment, the median time to RA with excess blasts (RAEB) being 47 months. For this reason, it is generally recommended that until children with RA become susceptible to infections, usually due to neutropenia, or become transfusion dependent they be observed with supportive therapy. Once these events set in, then, as soon as possible, they should be treated with a matched related stem cell donor transplantation. If a matched related donor is not available, then alternate donor transplant should be considered. Chemotherapy prior to stem cell transplant is not necessary.
- *Refractory anemia with excess blasts (RAEB):* Although controversial, AML-like therapy (see DCTER therapy in Chapter 14 on acute leukemias) is generally recommended before HSCT in children with RAEB, because without cytoreduction, prior to HSCT, there is a high relapse rate. If chemotherapy fails to induce remission or if minimal residual disease (MRD) exists, it is not known whether more chemotherapy should be given or HSCT performed without the use of prior cytoreductive chemotherapy. A suitable matched related donor is preferred for HSCT. If a suitable matched related donor is not available, then an alternate donor should be considered.
- *Refractory anemia with excess blasts in transformation (RAEB-T):* These patients are treated like patients with AML, that is, with AML-like chemotherapy (see DCTER in Chapter 14 on acute leukemias) followed by HSCT from a suitable matched related donor. In the absence of availability of a suitable matched related donor, HSCT from an alternate donor should be considered.

Allogeneic HSCT is the only curative treatment for MDS. Other therapies are ineffective.

Results of HSCT—disease-free survival
de novo pediatric MDS patients:

HLA-matched family donor	50%
Matched unrelated donor	35%
Children with secondary MDS	20–30%.

MDS in Children with Down Syndrome

Incidence

It has been suggested that approximately 1 in 150 children with DS develop MDS/AML by the age of 3. DS children are at 10–20 times the risk of developing

MDS/AML compared with non-DS children. The most common form of AML in DS children is acute megakaryoblastic leukemia (M7).

Ten percent of DS infants develop transient myeloproliferative disorder (TMD) at birth. TMD is characterized by accumulation of immature megakaryoblasts in blood and bone marrow. The majority of patients attain spontaneous remission in 3 months. However, 30% of TMD patients develop M7 AML by age 3 years.

Biology

Recently, it has been discovered that acquired mutations in GATA1 (a hematopoietic transcription factor gene) are uniquely associated with M7 AML and TMD of DS.

Treatment

Treatment of MDS/AML in DS

The DCTER regimen (see Chapter 14 on acute leukemias) is highly effective. However, conventional standard timing of chemotherapy is used; that is, after each cycle of chemotherapy the bone marrow should be allowed to recover before starting the subsequent course of chemotherapy. DFS at 4 years is 88%.

Treatment of Transient Myeloproliferative Disorder

Generally, supportive treatment is given. In the case of severe organ dysfunction, exchange transfusion, leukapheresis, and chemotherapy are used. Chemotherapies of various intensities with cytosine arabinoside (Ara-C) have been used.

Uncommon complications of TMD include hydrops fetalis, renal failure, organ infiltration, pleural effusion, respiratory failure, hepatic fibrosis and disseminated intravascular coagulopathy.

If bone marrow is hypocellular aplastic anemia and/or paroxysmal nocturnal hemoglobinuria should be considered. Hepatomegaly, splenomegaly, or hepatosplenomegaly favors a diagnosis of JMML or AML.

JUVENILE MYELOMONOCYTIC LEUKEMIA

Epidemiology

Incidence: 1.2 per million children per year
Median age at diagnosis: 1.8 years; 35% below 1 year of age, and only 4% above 5 years of age
Male:female ratio of 2:1
Association with neurofibromatosis type 1 (NF-1): Children with NF-1 have more than a 200-fold increased risk of JMML. Fifteen percent of children with JMML have NF-1.

Children with Noonan syndrome or trisomy 8 mosaicism are at increased risk of developing JMML. Most cases of neonates with Noonan syndrome with JMML-like presentation resolve spontaneously.

Clinical Features

JMML usually occurs before 2 years of age. Physical findings include:

Skin: eczema, xanthoma, café-au-lait spots, macular-papular rash
Lymphadenopathy
Hepatosplenomegaly

Bleeding
Respiratory symptoms: chronic tachypnea, cough, wheezing
Fever, infection.

Laboratory Features

Blood:
    WBC count: The majority of patients have >25,000/mm³ WBC counts.
    Monocytosis may be present for months before overt symptoms of JMML appear.
    Thrombocytopenia
    Immature myeloid cells with orderly maturation in peripheral blood
    Nucleated red blood cells
Bone marrow: increased cellularity, increased myeloid series, increased monocytes,
    less than 20% blasts
Cytogenetics:
    Monosomy 7: 25–30%, patients with monosomy 7 show lower WBC counts, higher
        percent monocytes in the blood, decreased myeloid:erythroid ratio in the bone
        marrow, high mean corpuscular volume, and normal to moderately high fetal
        hemoglobin levels. Monosomy 7 occurs with the same frequency in JMML,
        whether it is associated with NF-1 or not
    7q–: 5%
    Normal karyotype: 60%
    Other cytogenetic abnormalities: 5%.

    Table 13-18 lists diagnostic guidelines for JMML.

Differential Diagnosis

It is important to distinguish JMML from chronic active viral infections such as EBV,
cytomegalovirus, and human herpes virus 6 (HHV-6) infections. All of these infections

Table 13-18. Diagnostic Guidelines for Juvenile Myelomonocytic Leukemia (JMML)[a]

Suggestive clinical features	Hepatosplenomegaly
	Lymphadenopathy
	Pallor
	Skin rash
	Fever
Laboratory criteria:	
Minimum criteria for tentative diagnosis (all three must be fulfilled)	No Philadelphia chromosome and no BCR/ABL rearrangement
	Peripheral blood monocyte count greater than 1×10^9/L
	Blasts less than 20% of bone marrow cells
Criteria for definite diagnosis (at least two must be fulfilled)	Hemoglobin F increased for age
	Myeloid precursors in peripheral blood smear
	White blood cell count greater than 10×10^9/L
	Clonal abnormality
	Granulocyte monocyte colony-stimulating factor hypersensitivity of myeloid progenitors *in vitro*

[a]JMML includes patients with monosomy 7. There are no major clinical differences in children with JMML, with or without monosomy 7. The main difference is that JMML without monosomy 7 is associated with high fetal hemoglobin as compared to JMML with monosomy 7.

From Niermeyer CM, et al. Differentiating juvenile myelomonocytic leukemia from infectious disease. Blood 1998;91:365–7, with permission.

can present with hepatosplenomegaly, lymphadenopathy, leukocytosis, thrombocytopenia, and elevated hemoglobin F levels. The following tests are useful:

1. Bone marrow examination to see if hemophagocytosis is present. If present, then it favors viral illness.
2. Viral antibody titers.
3. Polymerase chain reaction (PCR) for viruses.
4. Bone marrow colony-forming units granulocyte macrophage (CFU-GM) studies for granulocyte macrophage colony-stimulating factor (GM-CSF) sensitivity.

Biology

JMML is a clonal disorder that arises from a pluripotent hematopoietic stem cell. The leukemic progenitor cell of JMML is capable of producing erythroid, myeloid, monocytic, megakaryocytic, and possibly lymphoid lineages. It is probably a heterogeneous disease in the context of clonal involvement of different lineages.

The distinct characteristic of JMML mononuclear cells, of both blood and bone marrow, is that they yield excessive numbers of granulocyte-macrophage colonies when cultured in a semisolid system, even without the addition of exogenous growth factors. The endogenous production of interleukin 1 (IL-1), GM-CSF, and tumor necrosis factor α (TNF-α) by monocytes accounts for the exuberant spontaneous growth of CFU-GM growth.

TNF-α exerts bidirectional actions:

1. It inhibits normal hematopoiesis.
2. It induces proliferation of the JMML clone-derived monocyte-macrophage elements.

The inhibitory effect of TNF-α on normal hematopoiesis causes bone marrow suppression and results in anemia and thrombocytopenia. Splenomegaly also contributes to the development of anemia and thrombocytopenia. IL-1 stimulates accessory cells to produce more GM-CSF.

Molecular Events

The constitutive activation of the RAS signaling pathway plays a central role in the proliferative responses to growth factors in JMML. RAS signaling proteins regulate cellular proliferation by switching between an active guanosine triphosphate state (RAS-GTP) and an inactive guanosine diphosphate state (RAS-GDP). In JMML, there may be mutations of *RAS* gene or there may be defective regulation of *RAS* gene, which results in the aberrant transmission of proliferative signals from GM-CSF to the nucleus. The conversion of RAS-GTP to the RAS-GDP is induced by GTP-ase-activating proteins (GAPS); thus, GAPS acts as a negative regulator of Ras. There are two GAPS; RAS-GAP and neurofibromin, the protein made by *nf-1* gene. An understanding of the crucial role of RAS in the pathogenesis of JMML has led to the trials with molecularly targeted therapies.

Figure 13-2 shows the biology of JMML and its correlation with hematologic findings.

Natural History

Spontaneous remission occurs in a few cases. The majority of patients progress, if untreated.

Blastic transformation occurs in 15% of patients and is associated with additional cytogenetic abnormalities in some patients.

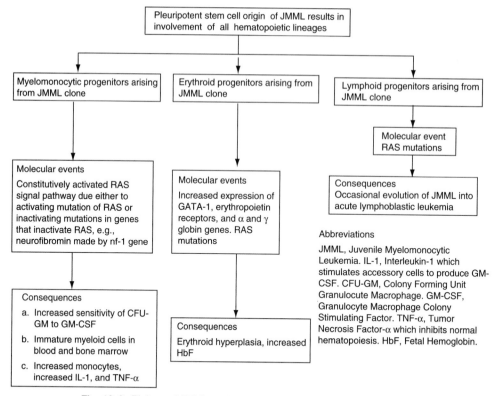

Fig. 13-2. Biology of JMML and its correlation with hematologic findings.

Most often patients die of respiratory failure, due to leukemic infiltrates and/or infections.

Erythroleukemia-like phase with anemia, erythroid hyperplasia, and megaloblastoid cells may develop in some patients.

Occasionally, pre-B ALL develops.

Prognosis

Adverse factors include:

Age at diagnosis: 2 years or more
High fetal hemoglobin level at diagnosis
Platelet count below 33,000/mm^3 at diagnosis (considered to be the strongest indicator of prognosis).

Treatment

JMML responds poorly to chemotherapy.

13-Cis Retinoic Acid

13-Cis retinoic acid (CRA; Isotretinoin, Accutane) is used to induce durable responses. CRA reduces spontaneous growth of JMML cells *in vitro*. Additionally, it induces maturation of normal and JMML hematopoietic cells.

Dose: 100 mg/m^2/day or 3 mg/kg/day for children less than 1 year of age.
Note: Each dose of CRA must be drawn from the caplet into a tuberculin syringe and given immediately to the patient.

Hematopoietic Stem Cell Transplantation

HSCT is the only curative treatment available for children with JMML. If a suitable family member donor is available, the patient is treated with HSCT. Splenectomy is usually recommended before HSCT. Allogeneic HSCT cures 30% of the patients with JMML. If a suitable family member donor is not available, an unrelated donor should be employed, if available. Treatment with CRA should be given in the interim.

Chemotherapy

If there is progression of the disease treatment with intensive chemotherapy may be required. However, the responses are usually short lived. The following chemotherapy is suggested:

Ara-C 100 mg/m^2/day by continuous infusion (days 0–4)
Etoposide 100 mg/m^2/day intravenously (days 0–4)
Low-dose Ara-C 15 mg/m^2/day subcutaneously (days 6–15)

Note that there are no standard chemotherapy regimens available for treatment of JMML. Ara-C–based regimens appear to be used most often.

Farnesyl Protein Transferase Inhibitor

RAS protein is synthesized as a cytosolic precursor that undergoes post-translational enzymatic processing in what is known as the *prenylation process.* Prenylation of RAS protein allows it ultimately to localize to the inner leaflet of plasma membrane. The first obligatory step in prenylation of RAS protein is the addition of farnesyl moiety catalyzed by farnesyl transferase. Farnesylation of RAS protein is essential for the function of RAS. For this reason, a clinical trial of farnesyl protein transferase (FPTase) inhibitor is being conducted in a phase II setting by the Children's Oncology Group (COG) in the United States for treatment of JMML, in sequential combination with fludarabine and Ara-C chemotherapy, splenectomy, and ultimately HSCT.

Other Investigational Therapies

Other investigational therapies include the use of analogues of GM-CSF and the use of GM-CSF/diphtheria fusion molecule.

CHRONIC MYELOPROLIFERATIVE DISEASES

Table 13-19 shows WHO classification of chronic myeloproliferative diseases.

CHRONIC MYELOGENOUS LEUKEMIA

Chronic myelogenous leukemia (CML) is a clonal myeloproliferative disorder of the primitive hematopoietic stem cell and is characterized by the presence of the Philadelphia (Ph^1) chromosome. This abnormal chromosome results from reciprocal translocation involving the long arms of chromosome 9 and 22, t(9;22)(q34;q11).

Incidence

One per 100,000 for persons younger than 20 years and 1–3% of all childhood leukemia. One hundred cases of CML are diagnosed in the United States per year.

Table 13-19. WHO Classification of Chronic Myeloproliferative Diseases

Chronic myelogenous leukemia (Ph chromosome, t[9;22] [q34;q11], BCR/ABL positive)
Chronic neutrophilic leukemia
Chronic eosinophilic leukemia (and the hypereosinophilic syndrome)
Polycythemia vera
Chronic idiopathic myelofibrosis (with extramedullary hematopoiesis)
Essential thrombocythemia
Chronic myeloproliferative disease, unclassifiable

From Vardiman JW, Harris NL, Brunning RD. The World Health Organization (WHO) classification of the myeloid neoplasms. Blood 2002;100:2292–302, with permission.

Clinical Phases

Chronic Phase

Blood or bone marrow contains less than 5% leukemic blasts.
Clinically stable for several years.

Signs and symptoms

Nonspecific complaints: fever, night sweats, abdominal pain, bone pain
Symptoms resulting from hyperviscosity:
    Neurologic dysfunction: headache, strokes
    Visual disturbances: retinal hemorrhages, papilledema
    Priapism
Hepatomegaly, splenomegaly
Pallor.

Laboratory Findings

Hematologic findings
Mild normocytic, normochromic anemia
Leukocytosis with shift to left characterized by sequential orderly maturation of myeloid series in all stages starting from myeloblasts to segmented neutrophils
Increased absolute eosinophil and basophil counts
Thrombocytosis
Decreased leukocyte alkaline phosphatase score
Deterioration of neutrophil function progressively
Bone marrow examination: hypercellularity, myelogenous bulge with sequential order maturation, increased eosinophilic and basophilic series, increased megakaryocytes. There may be myelofibrosis. Gaucher-like cells or sea-blue histiocytes may be present.
Cytogenetics: presence of Ph[1] chromosome.

Blood chemistry
Elevation of lactic dehydrogenase, uric acid, vitamin B_{12}, and transcobalamin 1 levels.

Accelerated Phase

Poorly defined intermediate phase characterized by increasing blood and bone marrow leukemic blasts (10–19%) and cytopenias

Dyspoiesis, rising basophil count, progressive myelofibrosis, or refractoriness to therapy Clonal karyotypic evolution.

Signs and symptoms

Fever, night sweats, weight loss.

Table 13-20 lists the WHO criteria for diagnosis of the accelerated phase of CML.

Blast Phase

Table 13-20 lists WHO criteria for diagnosis of the blast phase of CML.

Blasts greater than 20% in blood or bone marrow; or extramedullary or intramedullary clusters of blasts.

Myeloid blast crisis: most common type of blast crisis (80%); may be myeloblastic or myelomonocytic. Associated karyotypic evolution: duplication of Ph[1] chromosome, trisomies of 8, 19, or 21 chromosomes, i(17q), t(7;11), acute myelogenous leukemia specific rearrangements, for example, t(15;17).

Lymphoid blast crisis: less common type of blast crisis (15–20%), more often B lineage than T. Associated karyotypic evolution: duplication of Ph[1] chromosome, trisomy 21, inv(7), t(14;14).

Multilineage blast crisis: mixed myelocytic, erythrocytic, megakaryoblastic, and lymphocytic. Blasts may coexpress antigens of different lineage or two distinct populations of blasts may be present (uniclonal with bilineages).

Erythrocytic blast crisis: rare in pure form.

Megakaryoblastic blast crisis: rare in pure form, associated with inv(3)(q21;q26) or t(3)(q21;q26).

Mast cell crisis: extremely rare.

Signs and symptoms:

Pallor, easy bruisability, pruritis, urticaria, bone pain.

Table 13-20. WHO Criteria for Diagnosis of Accelerated and Blast Phases of CML

Accelerated phase
  Diagnose if one or more of the following is present:
    Blasts 10–19% of peripheral blood white cells or bone marrow cells
    Peripheral blood basophils at least 20%
    Persistent thrombocytopenia ($<100 \times 10^9$/L) unrelated to therapy, or persistent thrombocytosis ($>1000 \times 10^9$/L) unresponsive to therapy
    Increasing spleen size and increasing WBC count unresponsive to therapy
    Cytogenetic evidence of clonal evolution (i.e., the appearance of an additional genetic abnormality that was not present in the initial specimen at the time of diagnosis of chronic phase CML)
    Megakaryocytic proliferation in sizable sheets and clusters, associated with marked reticulin or collagen fibrosis, and/or severe granulocytic dysplasia, should be considered suggestive of accelerated phase. They often occur simultaneously with one or more of the other features listed.

Blast phase
  Diagnose if one or more of the following is present:
    Blasts 20% or more of peripheral blood white cells or bone marrow cells
    Extramedullary blast proliferation
    Large foci or clusters of blasts in bone marrow biopsy

From Vardiman JW, Harris NL, Brunning RD. The World Health Organization (WHO) classification of the myeloid neoplasms. Blood 2002;100:2292–302, with permission.

Biology of CML

Molecularly targeted therapies have revolutionized cancer therapeutics and are much more selective in their actions than traditional chemotherapy agents. CML is a disease that exemplifies how the discoveries in molecular biology have helped design molecularly targeted therapies.

Figure 13-3 depicts the Ph^1 chromosome, the molecular genetic studies of which have revealed that the ABL (Abelson) segment from chromosome 9 is translocated to chromosome 22 at its major breakpoint cluster region (BCR) and thus forms a novel fusion gene termed the *BCR-ABL*. The *BCR-ABL* fusion gene usually makes an oncoprotein having a 210-kDa molecular weight. The following are some of the functional domains of BCR-ABL oncoprotein:

Domain	Location	Function
Oligomerization domain	BCR	Activation of ABL kinase.
Y^{177}	BCR	Y^{177} regulates the Ras and P13K pathways through recruitment of GRB2-SOS and GAB2-P13K. These pathways are important for transformation and proliferation.
Serine-threonine kinase	BCR	Activation of signal transduction proteins.
Y kinase (SH1)	ABL	Constitutive tyrosine kinase activity that is responsible for phosphorylation of signal and adaptor proteins and plays a central role in leukemogenesis.
Actin binding domain	ABL	Interference with adhesion.

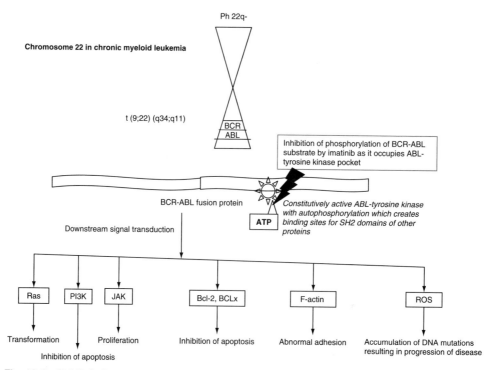

Fig. 13-3. t(9;22), fusion gene BCR-ABL, fusion protein BCR-ABL, cellular effects of BCR-ABL, and inhibition of BCR/ABL by imatinib in chronic myeloid leukemia.

The BCR/ABL oncoprotein activates—directly or indirectly—many downstream signal transduction pathways, for example, RAS, P13K, JAK-STAT, Bcl-2, BCLx, and ROS, which induce transformation, proliferation, inhibition of apoptosis, and oxidative damage to DNA. Additionally, cytoskeletal proteins are tyrosine phosphorylated and this results in alteration of cytoskeletal function. CML cells are less adherent and egress from the marrow into circulating blood prematurely. Figure 13-3 also depicts various cellular effects of BCR/ABL oncoprotein through downstream transduction pathways.

Several mechanisms play roles in disease progression, which lead eventually to blast crisis of CML. They include:

- Drug resistance: The mechanisms of drug resistance include (1) *BCR/ABL* gene amplification, (2) overexpression of BCR/ABL transcripts, (3) mutations in the ABL tyrosine kinase domain at the ATP binding site, (4) clonal evolution, and (5) drug efflux.
- Genomic instability.
- Impaired DNA repair.
- Tumor suppressor gene inactivation.
- Differentiation block.
- BCR/ABL-independent activation of more oncogenes and, thus, participation of more oncoproteins resulting in redundant pathways for proliferation, decreased apoptosis, and differentiation block.

Treatment

Treatment of Chronic Phase of CML

Supportive measures at diagnosis
Metabolic problems:

Tumor lysis syndrome: Hydration, alkalinization, and allopurinol are employed (see Chapter 26).

Hyperleukocytosis: Marked hyperleukocytosis (leukocyte count >200,000/mm^3 or blast count >50,000/mm^3) or, if patient is symptomatic, leukapheresis is performed and hydroxyurea (50–75 mg/kg/day) is started. Imatinib is started after the diagnosis of Ph-positive CML is established. If there is an unsatisfactory response to imatinib then IFN-α or IFN-α and Ara-C may be employed. Hydroxyurea may then be gradually tapered and discontinued.

Thrombocytosis: Anagrelide is used.

Priapism: Leukapheresis, analgesics, hydration, and cytoreductive therapy; hydroxyurea or imatinib should be used.

Cytoreduction in chronic phase: Cytoreduction is achieved with the use of imatinib.

Imatinib

Imatinib mesylate (Gleevec, Glivec, ST1571) treatment has ushered in a new era in the treatment of CML. However, imatinib is not curative and allogeneic HSCT is still the treatment of choice, aimed at cure in children and young adult patients.

Mechanism of action
Imatinib inhibits ABL-tyrosine kinase by occupying the adenosine triphosphate (ATP)-binding site in the kinase domain of the ABL component of the BCR/ABL oncoprotein (see Figure 13-3). As a result of this, phosphorylation of ABL-tyrosine kinase-substrates fails to occur, and activation of downstream leukemogenic signal transduction is prevented.

Dose
- In adults: Chronic phase of CML 400 mg/day orally
  Accelerated phase of CML 600 mg/day orally
  Blastic transformation of CML 600 mg/day orally
- In children: Chronic phase of CML 340 mg/m^2/day orally.

Management of side effects

Myelosuppression. Monitor complete blood counts (CBC) weekly during the first month of therapy. If absolute neutrophil count (ANC) remains greater than 1500/mm^3 and platelet count greater than 100,000/mm^3, then CBC can be obtained every 2 weeks until 12 weeks of therapy. Thereafter, it may be obtained once a month.

If ANC <1000/mm^3 and platelet count <50,000/mm^3, imatinib should be withheld until the ANC >1500/mm^3 and platelet count >100,000/mm^3. If recovery occurs in <4 weeks, imatinib is resumed at 400 mg/day. If recovery takes more than 4 weeks, imatinib is resumed at 300 mg/day and then increased to 400 mg/day if myelosuppression does not occur for more than 4 weeks.

Gastrointestinal toxicity. Nausea and vomiting can be avoided if imatinib is taken with food. If it persists, antiemetics such as ondansetron or prochlorperazine can be given. Use of antidiarrheal drug may be indicated.

Edema and fluid retention. Use of diuretics may be necessary. If water retention is severe, imatinib should be discontinued until edema is controlled.

Muscle cramps, bone pain, and arthralgia. Calcium and magnesium supplements are effective in controlling muscle cramps, in spite of normal serum levels of ionized calcium and magnesium. Use of nonsteroidal anti-inflammatory drugs is effective in controlling bone pain and arthralgia. They should be given only if the platelet count is greater than 100,000/mm^3. For patients with platelet counts of less than 100,000/mm^3, acetaminophen may be tried cautiously or a mild narcotic could be used. *A patient taking imatinib and high doses of acetaminophen has been reported to die of hepatic failure.*

Skin rashes. Use of antihistamines and/or topical steroids may control rashes. Occasionally, Stevens–Johnson syndrome may develop. In that case, imatinib should be discontinued and systemic steroids started.

Hepatotoxicity. If transaminases are greater than five times the upper limit of normal (grade 3 toxicity), discontinue imatinib. It could be restarted at a reduced dose when transaminases are less than 2.5 times the upper limit of normal or bilirubin less than 1.5 times the upper limit of normal.

With recurrent grade 3 hepatotoxicity, imatinib should be permanently discontinued. If there is persistent grade 2 hepatotoxicity, screening for viral hepatitis, ferritin levels, α_1-antitrypsin levels, and sonogram of liver should be performed. A liver biopsy may be indicated in some patients.

Drug interactions

Imatinib is metabolized in the liver by the CYP3A4/5 cytochrome P450 enzyme system. Main inducers of CYP3A4/5 activity, which causes a decrease in the level of imatinib, include carbamazepine, dexamethasone, phenytoin, phenobarbital, progesterone, rifampin, and St. John's wort. Drugs that inhibit CYP3A4/5 activity, which causes an increased level of imatinib, include cimetidine, erythromycin, fluoxetine, ketoconazole, ritonavir, itraconazole, verapamil, cyclosporine, clotrimazole, clarithromycin, azithromycin, isoniazid, and metronidazole. Grapefruit juice should also be avoided.

Imatinib is an inhibitor of CY2D6 and CYP2C9 isoenzymes. Warfarin is a substrate for these two enzymes. Therefore, when anticoagulation is needed, low-molecular-weight heparin (LMWH) should be used instead of warfarin. A physician should consult a pharmacist for drug interactions with other drugs as needed.

Hydroxyurea, busulfan, IFN-α, and IFN-α with Ara-C have been previously used for the treatment of CML, but at present imatinib is preferred for the treatment of a newly diagnosed patient in the chronic phase of CML.

Figure 13-4 shows an algorithm for the management of CML in the chronic phase in children, based on the guidelines for young adults with CML in the chronic phase, since no evidence-based guidelines are yet available for children with CML.

If IFN-α or IFN-α with Ara-C therapy is used in place of imatinib, because of unsatisfactory response to imatinib or as a matter of choice, the following guidelines are suggested.

Treatment with IFN-α

Timing of initiation of therapy: at the start of treatment.
Hydroxyurea is used to reduce the WBC count to 10,000–20,000/mm³.
Then IFN-α is started, following which hydroxyurea is tapered and discontinued.
Dose of IFN-α: 5×10^6 (5 million) units/m² per day subcutaneously or intramuscularly. Given daily as long as it is effective.
Note: Early flulike side effects (fever, chills, postnasal drip, anorexia) are minimized by starting IFN-α at 50% of dose for the first week of treatment.

The IFN-α dose is reduced to 50% if any of the following indications of toxicity are observed:

- Development of neurologic symptoms of parkinsonism, memory change, reduced attention span
- Increase in liver enzymes more than five times the upper limit of normal
- Increase in serum creatinine to 2.5 mg/dL or more
- Decline in performance status to 80% or less on the Karnofsky scale.

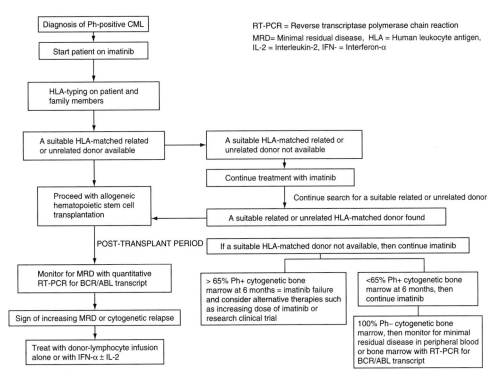

Fig. 13-4. Algorithm for management of chronic-phase CML in pediatric patients.

IFN-α is discontinued when the ANC is less than $750/mm^3$ or the platelet count is less than $50,000/mm^3$ or the WBC count is less than $2000/mm^3$, or serious systemic toxicity develops.

Treatment with IFN-α and Ara-C

Dose of interferon-α: 5×10^6 units/m^2 per day. Dose of IFN-α is modified, as per above-mentioned guidelines.

Dose of Ara-C: 20 mg/m^2 per day for 10 days per month. Ara-C is discontinued when ANC is less than $1000/mm^3$ or platelet count is below $60,000/mm^3$.

Combination therapy with IFN-α and Ara-C is superior to IFN-α alone because it induces higher major cytogenetic responses (35% versus 21% at 12 months) and higher 8-year survival (56% versus 45%).

Monitoring Response to Therapy

Hematologic criteria:

Complete response:	WBC less than $9000/mm^3$
	Morphology normal
	Splenomegaly absent
Partial response	WBC less than $20,000/mm^3$
	Splenomegaly present
Failure	WBC greater than $20,000/mm^3$
	Splenomegaly present.

Cytogenetic criteria:

	Complete[a]	Partial[a]	Minor	None
% Ph-positive cells in bone marrow	0	1–34	35–95	100

Note: Usually 20–50 metaphases are counted; cytogenetic abnormality is not detected unless it is present in 2–5% of cells.

[a]Major cytogenetic response = 66–100% Ph-negative cells in bone marrow.

Minimal Residual Disease

Although the response to therapy is measured initially on the basis of hematologic and cytogenetic criteria, it is necessary to perform more sensitive studies when a complete cytogenetic response is attained. The following BCR/ABL studies are used to monitor the presence of minimal residual disease:

Study on bone marrow[a]	Sensitivity[b]	Comment
FISH on interphase cells	1 per 1000 cells	False-positive rate 10%
Southern blot	1 per 100 cells	Low sensitivity, so rarely used
Western blot	1–10 per 1000 cells	Low sensitivity, so rarely used
RT-PCR[c]	1 per 10^5–10^6 cells	Most commonly used method

Note: Even when reverse transcriptase polymerase chain reaction (RT-PCR) is negative for the detection of BCR/ABL transcripts, a patient may still have up to a million leukemic cells.

[a]When RT-PCR on bone marrow sample becomes negative, peripheral blood sample can be used in place of bone marrow for the test.

[b]Lowest level of detection, i.e., number of leukemic cells per number of normal bone marrow cells.

[c]Three types of RT-PCR: (1) qualitative, (2) quantitative, and (3) real-time (FISH): fluorescence *in situ* hybridization.

Treatment of Advanced Phases of CML

Most of the information regarding treatment of various phases of CML is mainly derived from experience in adult patients.

Objectives of treatment:

- To attain cytogenetic response
- To achieve a complete hematologic remission
- To achieve a second chronic phase, followed by HSCT, if a suitable donor is available.

Treatment of CML in accelerated phase:

- Imatinib: 600 mg/day in adult patients (dose for children not yet established) OR
- IFN-α as a single agent or in combination with Ara-C (see above for dosages) OR
- Decitabine 15 mg/m^2 intravenously daily for 10 days OR
- Investigational drugs; farnesyl transferase inhibitors, retinoids, nucleoside analogs, and imatinib in combination with other drugs.

Treatment of CML in nonlymphoid blastic phase:

- Decitabine: 15 mg/m^2 intravenously daily for 10 days OR
- Fludarabine 30 mg/m^2 intravenously daily for 5 days and Ara-C 1 g/m^2 intravenously daily for 5 days OR
- Idarubicin 12 mg/m^2 intravenously daily for 3 days and Ara-C 1.5 g/m^2 intravenously daily for 4 days OR
- Fludarabine 30 mg/m^2 intravenously daily for 3 days, Ara-C 1 g/m^2 intravenously daily for 3 days, and mitoxantrone 10 mg/m^2 intravenously daily for 4 days OR
- Vincristine 0.4 mg daily for 4 days by continuous infusion, doxorubicin 12 mg/m^2 daily for 4 days by continuous infusion, and dexamethasone 40 mg daily on days 1–4, days 9–12, and days 17–20 OR
- Investigational agents including imatinib in combination with other agents.

Treatment of CML in lymphoid blastic phase:
Treated with the use of pre-B ALL protocol as outlined in chapter on acute leukemias. The remission rates in the blast cell phase of CML are low and duration of remission is usually short.

Allogeneic Stem Cell Transplantation for Chronic Myeloid Leukemia

The graft versus leukemia effect (GVL) results from a genetic disparity between donor and recipient. Therefore, greatest GVL effect occurs when the donor is unrelated to the recipient because of a greater number of incompatible minor histocompatibility antigens and also because of disparities between more major histocompatibility antigens.

Strongest GVL occurs when the transplantation is performed during the chronic phase in the presence of minimal residual disease, detectable by molecular testing. Weakest GVL effect occurs when the transplant is performed in a blastic phase and/or T-cell depletion is used for prevention of GVHD.

Figure 13-5 depicts some of the cellular mechanisms involved in GVL reaction following allogeneic HSCT in CML.

1. CML cells display antigens to antigen presenting cells (APCs).
2. APCs recognize leukemia-related antigens and present them to CD4+ and CD8+ cytotoxic T cells in the context of major histocompatibility (MHC) class

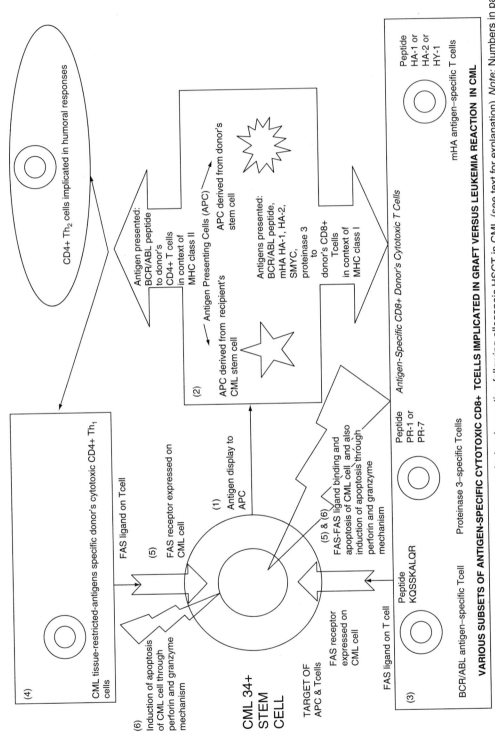

Fig. 13-5. Some of the cellular mechanisms involved in graft versus leukemia reaction following allogeneic HSCT in CML (see text for explanation). *Note:* Numbers in parentheses correspond to description in text.

II and MHC class I, respectively. APCs may be derived from recipient's CML stem cells or from donor's stem cells.

3. The immune response generates expanded population of antigen-specific CD8+ cytotoxic T cells. Specific antigens implicated in the GVL response in CML are as follows:

Antigen	Protein	Peptide
Minor histocompatibility antigens	—	HA-1
	—	HA-2
	SMYC	HY-1
Tissue-restricted	Proteinase 3	PR-1
		PR-7
Leukemia specific	BCR/ABL	KQSSKALQR

4. The immune response also generates CD4+ Th_1 and CD4+ Th_2 cells. Th_1 cells make IL-2, IFN-γ, and TNF, which induce proliferation of T cells (induced by IL-2) and apoptosis of CML cells (induced by IFN-γ and TNF). BCR/ABL-specific Th_1 cells exist in circulating blood, but they do not recognize the CML cells, indicating involvement of antigens other than BCR/ABL in a GVL effect induced by Th_1 cells. In this regard, Th_1 cells exhibit leukemia-specific cytotoxicity through tissue-restricted antigens. Th_2 cells make IL-4, IL-5, and IL-10 and are implicated in humoral responses.

5. FAS ligand, expressed on cytotoxic T cells (Th_1 and CD8+ T cells), binds to FAS receptor on CML 34+ stem cells and induces apoptosis of CML cells.

6. Additionally, cytotoxic T cells make perforin, which perforates the CML cells, and then they release granzyme into the CML cells, which induces cell death.

The results of allogeneic HSCT are listed below:

Cohort characteristics	Donor	DFS
CP <1 year	HLA-matched sibling	70%
CP >1 year	HLA-matched sibling	60%
CP <1 year	HLA-matched unrelated	60%
CP #1	HLA-haploidentical family member	25%

Abbreviations: CP, chronic phase; CP #1, first chronic phase; HLA, human leukocyte antigen; DFS, disease-free survival.

Treatment of post-transplant relapse:

- Donor leukocyte infusion (DLI)
- DLI plus IFN-α plus/minus IL-2
- If the patient relapses with accelerated or blast phase, intensive chemotherapy followed by a stem cell transplant may be performed.

Novel Therapies for CML

Currently, several novel targeted therapeutic strategies are being investigated. They include Troxacitabine (a nucleoside analogue), Decitabine (a hypomethylating agent), R15777 SCH66336 (farnesyl transferase inhibitor), Homoharringtone (a plant alkaloid), PS-341(a proteosome inhibitor), BCR/ABL junction peptide vaccine, proteinase 3 peptide PR1 vaccine, polyethylene glycol IFN-α preparations, and inhibitor of heat shock protein 90 (a molecular chaperone required for stability of signal proteins).

Essential Thrombocythemia

See Chapter 10.

Polycythemia Vera

See Chapter 8.

Agnogenic Myeloid Metaplasia with Myelofibrosis

Agnogenic myeloid metaplasia with myelofibrosis (AMM) is a clonal myeloprolif-erative disorder characterized by leukoerythroblastosis, myeloid metaplasia, and varying degrees of myelofibrosis. It is a rare disease in children and they have a better outlook than adults. Its etiology is unknown.

Clinical Features

Malaise, night sweats, weight loss, and discomfort from splenomegaly.

Hematologic Findings

Blood smear: teardrop cells, leukoerythroblastosis, Pelger–Hüet cells.
Bone marrow is difficult to aspirate. Bone marrow biopsies show fibrosis.
Cytogenetic abnormalities may be present in bone marrow cells.

Differential Diagnosis

Myelofibrosis secondary to metastatic disease to bone marrow. This diagnosis is more common in children than AMM.

Complications

Thrombocytosis, bleeding.
Splenomegaly; hypersplenism, refractory thrombocytopenia, hemolytic anemia; some children may not have hepatosplenomegaly.
Portal hypertension.
Transformation into leukemia.

Treatment

In children, wait and see if spontaneous remission occurs. In case of progression of disease consider the following options:
Hydroxyurea
IFN-α
Splenectomy for hypersplenism and/or severe discomfort and mechanical problems
Hematopoietic stem cell transplantation should be considered.

SUGGESTED READINGS
Lymphoproliferative Disorders

Bleesing JJH, Brown MR, et al. A composite picture of TcRα/β+, CD4−, CD8− T cells (α/β-DNTCs) in humans with autoimmune lymphoproliferative syndrome. Clin Immun 2002;104:21–30.

Bleesing JJH, Straus SE, et al. Autoimmune lymphoproliferative syndrome. A human disorder of abnormal lymphocyte survival. Pediatr Clin North Am 2000;47: 1291–1310.

Chiocchetti A, Indelicato M, et al. High levels of osteopontin associated with polymorphisms in its gene are a risk factor for development of autoimmunity/lymphoproliferation. Blood 2004;103:1376–82.

Cohen JI. Benign and malignant Epstein–Barr virus-associated B-cell lymphoproliferative diseases. Semin Hematol 2003;40:116–23.

Ganne V, Siddiqi N, et al. Humanized anti-CD20 monoclonal antibody (rituximab) treatment for post-transplant lymphoproliferative disorder. Clin Transplant 2003;17:417–22.

Garrett TJ, Chadburn A. Posttransplantation lymphoproliferative disorders treated with cyclophosphamide-doxorubicin-vincristine-prednisone chemotherapy. Cancer 1993;72:2782–85.

Hsueh C, Gonzalez-Crussi F, Murphy SB. Testicular angiocentric lymphoma of post thymic T-cell type in a child with T-cell acute lymphoblastic leukemia in remission. Cancer 1993;72:1801–5.

Medcinos LJ, Harris NL. Immunohistologic analysis of small lymphocytic infiltrates of the orbit and conjunctiva. Hum Pathol 1990;21:1126–31.

Paulli M, Berti E, Rosso R, Boveri E, et al. CD30/Ki-1 positive lymphoproliferative disorders of the skin—clinicopathological correlation and statistical analysis of 86 cases: a multicentric study of the European Organization of Research and treatment of cancer cutaneous lymphoma project groups. J Clin Oncol 1995;13:1343–54.

Peiper SC. Angiocentric lymphoproliferative disorders of the respiratory system: incrimination of Epstein–Barr virus in pathogenesis. Blood 1993;82:687–90.

Peterson BA, Frizzera G. Multicentric Castleman's disease. Semin Oncol 1993;636–47.

Seemayer TA, Gross TG, et al. X-linked lymphoproliferative diseases: twenty-five years after the discovery. Pediatr Res 1995;38:471–78.

Steinberg AD, Seldin MF, Jaffe ES, Smith MR, et al. Angioimmunoblastic lymphadenopathy with dysproteinemia. Ann Intern Med 1998;108:575–84.

Straathof KCM, Bollard CM, et al. Immunotherapy for Epstein–Barr virus-associated cancers in children. Oncologist 2003;8:83–98.

Sumegi J, Huang D, et al. Correction of mutations of the SH2D1A gene and Epstein–Barr virus infection with clinical phenotype and outcome in X-linked lymphoproliferative disease. Blood 2000;96:3118–25.

Tsatalas C, Margaritis D, et al. Successful treatment of angioimmunoblastic lymphadenopathy with dysproteinemia-type T-cell lymphoma with fludarabine. Acta Haematol 2001;105:106–8.

Uphouse WJ, Woods JC. Angioimmunoblastic lymphadenopathy with dysproteinemia. Cancer 1987;60:2161–4.

Van Der Werff Ten Bosch J, Schotte P, et al. Reversion of autoimmune lymphoproliferative syndrome with an antimalarial drug: preliminary results of a clinical cohort study and molecular observations. Br J Haematol 2002;117:176–88.

Zirbel GM, Gellis SE, Kadin ME, Esterly NB. Lymphomatoid papulosis in children. J Am Acad Dermatol 1995;33:741–8.

MDS and JMML

Arico M, Biondi A, et al. Juvenile myelomonocytic leukemia. Blood 1997;90:479–88.

Barnard DR, Lange B, et al. Acute myeloid leukemia and myelodysplastic syndrome in children treated for cancer: comparison with primary presentation. Blood 2002;100:427–34.

Flotho C, Valcmonica S, et al. RAS mutations and clonality analysis in children with juvenile myelomonocytic leukemia (JMML). Leukemia 1999;13:32–7.

Hasle H, Fenu S, et al. International prognostic scoring system for childhood MDS and JMML. Leukemia 2000;14:968.

Hasle H, Niemeyer C. Myelodysplastic syndrome and juvenile myelomonocytic leukemia in children. In: Bennett JM, editor. The Myelodysplastic Syndromes: Pathophysiology and Clinical Management. New York: Marcel Dekker, 2002;299–344.

Kang JH, Shin HY, et al. Novel regimen for treatment of juvenile myelomonocytic leukemia (JMML). Leukemia Res 2004;28:167–70.

Lange BJ, Kobrinsky N, et al. Distinctive demography, biology, and outcome of acute myeloid leukemia, and myelodysplastic syndrome in children with Down syndrome: Children's Cancer Group Studies 2861 and 2891. Blood 1998;91:608–15.

Luna-Fineman S, Shannon KM, et al. Myelodysplastic and myeloproliferative disorders of childhood: a study of 167 patients. Blood 1999;93:459–66.

Macmillan ML, Davies SM, et al. Haematopoietic cell transplantation in children with juvenile myelomonocytic leukemia. Br J Haematol 1998;103:552–8.

Passamore SJ, Hann CA, et al. Pediatric myelodysplasia: a study of 68 children and a new prognostic scoring system. Blood 1995;85:1742–50.

Woods WG, Barnard DR, et al. Prospective study of 90 children requiring treatment for juvenile myelomonocytic leukemia or myelodysplastic syndrome. J Clin Oncol 2002;20:434–40.

Myeloproliferative Disorders

Carella AM, Beltrami G, et al. Allografting in chronic myeloid leukemia. Semin Hematol 2003;72–8.

Deininger MWN, O'Brien SG, et al. Practical management of patients with chronic myeloid leukemia receiving imatinib. J Clin Oncol 2003;21:1637–47.

Sacchi S, Kantarjian HM, et al. Chronic myelogenous leukemia in nonlymphoid blastic phase. Analysis of the results of the first salvage therapy with three different treatment approaches for 162 patients. Cancer 1999;86:2632–41.

Sattler M, Griffin JD. Molecular mechanisms of translocation by the BCR-ABL oncogene. Semin Hematol 2003;40:4–10.

Schwartz J, Pinilla-Ibarz J, et al. Novel targeted and immunotherapeutic strategies in chronic myeloid leukemia. Semin Hematol 2003;40:87–96.

Sekhar M, Pretice HG, et al. Idiopathic myelofibrosis in children. Br J Hematol 1996;93:394–7.

Shet AS, Jahangir BN, et al. Chronic myelogenous leukemia: mechanisms underlying disease progression. Leukemia 2002;16:402–14.

14

LEUKEMIAS

Acute leukemias represent a clonal expansion and arrest at a specific stage of normal myeloid or lymphoid hematopoiesis. It constitutes 97% of all childhood leukemias and consists of the following types:

- Acute lymphoblastic leukemia (ALL)—75%
- Acute myeloblastic leukemia (AML), also known as acute nonlymphocytic leukemia (ANLL)*—20%
- Acute undifferentiated leukemia (AUL)—<0.5%
- Acute mixed-lineage leukemia (AMLL).

Chronic myeloid leukemias constitute 3% of all childhood leukemias (Chapter 13) and consist of:

1. Philadelphia chromosome–positive (Ph^1-positive) myeloid leukemia
2. Juvenile myelomonocytic leukemia (JMML).

Incidence

1. ALL: Three to four cases per 100,000 white children, 2500–3000 children diagnosed in the United States per year; AML—500 new cases in the United States per year.
2. Peak incidence between 2 and 5 years of age.
3. Accounts for 25–30% of all childhood cancers.

Etiology

The etiology of acute leukemia is unknown. The following factors are important in the pathogenesis of leukemia:

1. Ionizing radiation.
2. Chemicals (e.g., benzene in AML).
3. Drugs (e.g., use of alkylating agents either alone or in combination with radiation therapy increases the risk of AML).
4. Genetic considerations:
   a. Identical twins—If one twin develops leukemia during the first 5 years of life, the risk of the second twin developing leukemia is 20%.

---

*AML and ANLL are used interchangeably in this chapter and refer to the same disorder.

b. Incidence of leukemia in siblings of a leukemia patient is four times greater than that of the general population.

c. Chromosomal abnormalities:

Group	Risk	Time interval
Trisomy 21 (Down syndrome)	1 in 95	<10 years of age
Bloom syndrome	1 in 8	<30 years of age
Fanconi anemia	1 in 12	<16 years of age

d. Increased incidence with the following genetically determined conditions:
   (1) Congenital agammaglobulinemia
   (2) Poland syndrome
   (3) Shwachman–Diamond syndrome
   (4) Ataxia telangiectasia
   (5) Li–Fraumeni syndrome (germline p53 mutation)—the familial syndrome of multiple cancers in which acute leukemia is a component malignancy
   (6) Neurofibromatosis
   (7) Diamond–Blackfan anemia
   (8) Kostmann disease.

Most cases of leukemia do not stem from an inherited genetic predisposition but from somatic genetic alterations.

Clinical Features of Acute Lymphoblastic Leukemia

Table 14-1 shows the common clinical and laboratory presenting features of ALL.

General Systemic Effects

1. Fever (60%)
2. Lassitude (50%)
3. Pallor (40%).

Hematologic Effects Arising from Bone Marrow Invasion

1. Anemia—causing pallor, fatigability, tachycardia, dyspnea, and sometimes congestive heart failure
2. Neutropenia—causing fever, ulceration of buccal mucosa, and infection
3. Thrombocytopenia—causing petechiae, purpura, easy bruisability, bleeding from mucous membrane, and sometimes internal bleeding (e.g., intracranial hemorrhage)
4. One to 2% of patients present initially with pancytopenia and may be erroneously diagnosed as having aplastic anemia or bone marrow failure (represents 5% of acquired aplastic anemia) and ultimately develop acute leukemia. In these cases the illness is characterized by:
   Pancytopenia or single cytopenia
   Hypocellular bone marrow
   No hepatosplenomegaly
   Diagnosis of leukemia 1–9 months after onset of symptoms.

The treatment consists of supportive transfusions initially and specific antileukemic chemotherapy, when leukemia is diagnosed

**Table 14-1. Clinical and Laboratory Features at Diagnosis
in Children with Acute Lymphoblastic Leukemia**

Clinical and laboratory findings	Percentage of patients
Symptoms and physical findings	
Fever	61
Bleeding (e.g., petechiae or purpura)	48
Bone pain	23
Lymphadenopathy	50
Splenomegaly	63
Hepatosplenomegaly	68
Laboratory features	
Leukocyte count (mm^3)	
<10,000	53
10,000–49,000	30
>50,000	17
Hemoglobin (g/dL)	
<7.0	43
7.0–11.0	45
>11.0	12
Platelet count (mm^3)	
<20,000	28
20,000–99,000	47
>100,000	25
Lymphoblast morphology	
L1	84
L2	15
L3	1

From Pizzo PA, Poplack DG. Principles and Practice of Pediatric Oncology. 3rd ed.
Philadelphia: Lippincott-Raven, 1997, with permission.

Clinical Manifestations Arising from Lymphoid System Invasion

1. Lymphadenopathy—sometimes mediastinal lymphadenopathy causing superior vena cava syndrome
2. Splenomegaly
3. Hepatomegaly.

Clinical Manifestations of Extramedullary Invasion

Central nervous system (CNS) involvement occurs in less than 5% of children with ALL at initial diagnosis. It may present with the following:

1. Signs and symptoms of raised intracranial pressure (e.g., morning headache, vomiting, papilledema, bilateral sixth-nerve palsy).
2. Signs and symptoms of parenchymal involvement (e.g., focal neurologic signs such as hemiparesis, cranial nerve palsies, convulsions, cerebellar involvement—ataxia, dysmetria, hypotonia, hyperflexia).
3. Hypothalamic syndrome (polyphagia with excessive weight gain, hirsutism, and behavioral disturbances).
4. Diabetes insipidus (posterior pituitary involvement).
5. Chloromas of the spinal cord—(very infrequent in ALL) may present with back pain, leg pain, numbness, weakness, Brown–Séquard syndrome, and bladder and bowel sphincter problems.

6. CNS hemorrhage—complication that occurs more frequently in patients with AML than in those with ALL. It is caused by:
   a. Leukostasis in cerebral blood vessels, leading to leukothrombi, infarcts, and hemorrhage
   b. Thrombocytopenia and coagulopathy, contributing to CNS hemorrhage.

Genitourinary Tract Involvement

Testicular Involvement

1. Usually presents with painless enlargement of the testis.
2. Occurs in 10–23% of boys during the course of the disease at a median time of 13 months from diagnosis.
3. Occult testicular involvement recognized in 10–33% of boys undergoing bilateral wedge biopsies.
4. Risk factors for the development of testicular involvement:
   a. T-cell ALL
   b. Leukocytosis at diagnosis (>20,000/mm^3)
   c. Presence of a mediastinal mass
   d. Moderate to severe hepatosplenomegaly and lymphadenopathy
   e. Thrombocytopenia (<30,000/mm^3).

Ovarian Involvement

Occurs very rarely.

Priapism

Occurs rarely. It is due to involvement of sacral nerve roots or mechanical obstruction of the corpora cavernosa and dorsal veins by leukemic infiltrates or by the coagulation of the platelet-rich leukemic blood in the corpora cavernosa.

Renal Involvement

1. Occasionally may present with hematuria, hypertension, and renal failure.
2. Evaluated in many patients by ultrasonography; more common in T-cell ALL or mature B-cell ALL.

Gastrointestinal Involvement

1. The gastrointestinal (GI) tract is frequently involved in ALL. The most common manifestation is bleeding.
2. Leukemic infiltrates in the GI tract are usually clinically silent until terminal stages when necrotizing enteropathy might occur. The most common site for this is the cecum, giving rise to a syndrome known as typhlitis (Chapter 26).

Bone and Joint Involvement

Bone pain is one of the initial symptoms in 25% of patients. It may result from direct leukemic infiltration of the periosteum, bone infarction, or expansion of marrow cavity by leukemic cells. Radiologic changes seen most frequently include:

1. Osteolytic lesions involving medullary cavity and cortex
2. Transverse metaphyseal radiolucent bands
3. Transverse metaphyseal lines of increased density (growth arrest lines)
4. Subperiosteal new bone formation.

Skin Involvement

Skin involvement occurs most commonly in neonatal leukemia or AML.

Cardiac Involvement

One half to two thirds of patients have demonstrated cardiac involvement at autopsy, although symptomatic heart disease occurs in less than 5% of cases. Pathologic findings include leukemic infiltrates and hemorrhage of the myocardium or the pericardium.

Lung Involvement

This may be due to leukemic infiltrates or hemorrhage.

Diagnosis

Laboratory Studies

1. *Blood count:*
   a. *Hemoglobin:* Moderate to marked reduction. Normocytic; normochromic red cell morphology. Low hemoglobin indicates longer duration of leukemia; higher hemoglobin indicates a more rapidly proliferating leukemia.
   b. *White blood cell (WBC) count:* Low, normal, or increased.
   c. *Blood smear:* Blasts. Very few to none (in patients with leukopenia). When the WBC count is greater than $10,000/mm^3$, blasts are usually abundant. Eosinophilia is occasionally seen in children with ALL; 20% of patients with AML have an increased number of basophils.
   d. *Thrombocytopenia:* 92% of patients have platelet counts below normal. Serious hemorrhage (GI or intracranial) occurs at platelet counts less than $25,000/mm^3$.
2. *Bone marrow:* Bone marrow is usually replaced by 80–100% blasts. Megakaryocytes are usually absent. Leukemia must be suspected when the bone marrow contains more than 5% blasts. The hallmark of the diagnosis of acute leukemia is the blast cell, a relatively undifferentiated cell with diffusely distributed nuclear chromatin, one or more nucleoli, and basophilic cytoplasm. Special bone marrow studies, which help in detailed cell classification, include the following:
   a. Histochemistry
   b. Immunophenotyping
   c. Cytogenetics.
3. *Chest radiograph:* Mediastinal mass in T-cell leukemia.
4. *Blood chemistry:* Electrolytes, blood urea, uric acid, liver function tests, immunoglobulin levels.
5. *Cerebrospinal fluid:* Chemistry and cells. Cerebrospinal fluid findings for the diagnosis of CNS leukemia require:
   a. Presence of more than 5 $WBCs/mm^3$
   b. Identification of blast cells on cytocentrifuge examination. CNS involvement in leukemia is classified as follows:
      CNS 1 <5 $WBCs/mm^3$, no blasts on cytocentrifuge slide
      CNS 2 <5 $WBCs/mm^3$, blasts on cytocentrifuge slide
      CNS 3 >5 $WBCs/mm^3$, blasts on cytocentrifuge slide
   c. TdT stain for suspicious cells
   d. If a lumbar puncture is traumatic in a patient with peripheral blasts, the following formula can be helpful in defining the presence of CNS leukemia. CNS disease is present if:

<u>CSF WBC</u>	is greater	<u>Blood WBC</u>
CSF RBC	than	Blood RBC

6. *Coagulation profile:* Decreased coagulation factors that frequently occur with AML are hypofibrinogenemia, factors V, IX, and X.
7. *Cardiac function:* Electrocardiogram (ECG) and echocardiogram.
8. *Infectious disease profile:* Varicella antibody titer, cytomegalovirus (CMV) antibody titer, herpes simplex antibody, hepatitis antibody screening.
9. *Immunologic screening:* Serum for immunoglobulin levels, C3 and C4.

Classification

Acute leukemia can be classified based on morphologic characteristics (Tables 14-2 and 14-3), cytochemical features (Table 14-4), immunologic characteristics (Figure 14-1), and cytogenetic and molecular characteristics (Table 14-5 and Figure 14-2).

Table 14-2. Morphologic Characteristic of Lymphoblasts and Myeloblasts

Characteristic	Lymphoblasts	Myeloblasts
Size	10–20 μm	14–20 μm
Nucleus		
Shape	Round or oval	Round or oval
Chromatin	Smooth, homogeneous	Spongy, loose, finely developed meshwork
Nucleoli	0–2 and indistinct	2–5 and distinct "punched-out"
Nuclear membrane	Smooth, round	Irregular
Nuclear–cytoplasmic ratio	High	Low
Cytoplasm		
Color	Blue	Blue-gray
Amount	Thin rim	More abundant
Granules	Absent	Present
Auer rods	Absent	Present

Table 14-3. Cytologic Features of the Morphologic Types of Acute Lymphoblastic Leukemias

Cytologic features[a]	L1	L2	L3[b]
Cell size	Small cells predominate	Large, heterogeneous in size	Large and heterogeneous
Nuclear chromatin	Homogeneous	Variable, heterogeneous	Finely stippled and homogeneous
Nuclear shape	Regular occasional clefting or indentation	Irregular, clefting, and indentation common	Regular oval to round
Nucleoli	Not visible or small and inconspicuous	One or more present, often large	Prominent, one or more vesicular
Amount of cytoplasm	Scanty	Variable, often moderately abundant	Moderately abundant
Basophilia of cytoplasm	Slight or moderate, rarely intense	Variable, deep in some	Very deep
Cytoplasmic vacuolation	Variable	Variable	Often prominent

[a]For each of the features considered, up to 10% of the cells may depart from the characteristic of the type.

[b]The only immunologically pure type of ALL that can be consistently recognized morphologically and invariably carries IgM surface receptor on its membrane.

From Bennett JM, Catovsky D, Daniel MT, et al. Proposals for the classification of the acute leukemias. Br J Haematol 1976;33:451, with permission.

Table 14-4. Cytochemical Features of the Acute Leukemias

Staining reaction	ALL	Acute nonlymphoblastic leukemia			
		AML	Acute myelomonocytic leukemia	Erythroleukemia	Megakaryoblastic leukemia
Nonenzymatic					
PAS	Present as coarse granules or blocks in a variable number of cells	Negative or diffusely positive	Negative or fine granulation	Strongly positive granular	Positive or negative
Sudan black	Negative	Positive	Positive	Positive	Negative
Enzymatic					
Peroxidase	Negative	Positive[a]	Usually negative	Positive	Negative
Alkaline phosphatase	Normal	Low	High	Normal or high	—
Esterases					
Naphthol AS-D chloroacetate	Negative	Positive	Negative	Negative	—
Naphthol AS-D acetate	Negative or weakly positive	Positive (not inhibited by fluoride)	Strongly positive (inhibited by fluoride)	Weakly positive	Positive or negative
α-Naphthyl acetate	Negative	Negative	Strongly positive	Strongly positive	Positive or negative
Acid phosphatase	Positive in T-ALL	Negative	Negative	Negative	Positive (localized pattern)

[a]The peroxidase reaction, when positive, is considered to indicate the presence of myeloblastic rather than lymphoblastic elements. Unfortunately, myeloblasts that contain no specific granules will be peroxidase negative. It is these cells that cause the greatest difficulty in morphologic classification. Generally, when morphologic classification is difficult, these histochemical tests are of little help. However, demonstration of MPO (myeloperoxidase) by immunologic techniques or expression of MPO by molecular methods can be performed in specialized research laboratories.

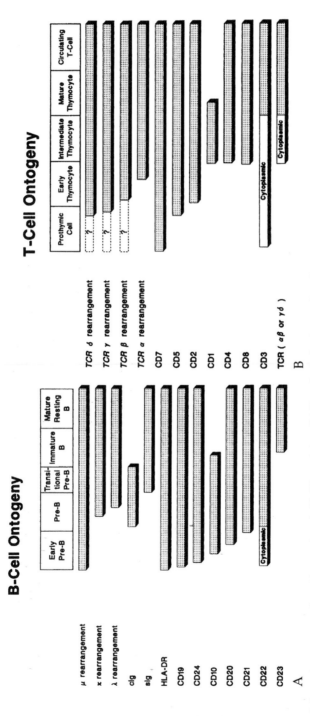

Fig. 14-1. Schematic representation of human lymphoid differentiation. (A) Hypothetical schema of marker expression and gene rearrangement during normal B-cell ontogeny. (B) Hypothetical schema of marker expression and gene rearrangement during normal T-cell ontogeny. (From Pui CH, Behm FG, et al. Clinical and biologic relevance of immunologic marker studies in childhood acute lymphoblastic leukemia. Blood 1993;82:343, with permission.)

Table 14-5. Common Nonrandom Chromosomal Translocations in Childhood ALL

Chromosomal translocation	Frequency (%)	Genetic alteration	Associated features
Acute lymphoblastic leukemia			
t(1;19)(q23;p13.3)	5 or 6	E2A-PBX1 fusion	Pre-B-cell phenotype, increased leukocyte count, black race, central nervous system leukemia, unfavorable prognosis with antimetabolic therapy
t(9;22)(q34;q11)	3–5	BCR-ABL fusion	Predominant B-lineage phenotype, older age, increased leukocyte count, dismal outcome with chemotherapy
t(4;11)(q21;q23)	2	MLL-AF4 fusion	CD10-B lineage phenotype, infancy, hyperleukocytosis, dismal outcome with chemotherapy
t(8;14)(q24;q32.3)	1 or 2	MYC-IGH fusion	B-cell phenotype, predominantly in boys, L3 morphology, bulky extramedullary disease, favorable prognosis with short-term intensive therapy
t(11;14)(p13;q11)	1	TTG2-TCRD fusion	T-cell phenotype, predominantly in boys, hyperleukocytosis, extramedullary disease
dic(9;12)(p11-p12;?p12)	1	?	B-lineage phenotype, predominantly in boys, excellent outcome with antimetabolic therapy

Modified from Pui CH. Childhood leukemias. N Engl J Med 1995;332:1618–30.

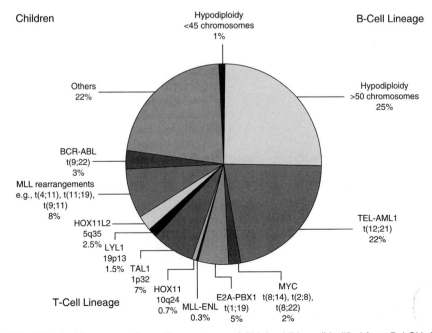

Fig. 14-2. Estimated frequency of specific genotypes of ALL in children. (Modified from Pui CH, Relling MV, Downing JR. Acute lymphoblastic leukemia. N Engl J Med 2004;350:1535–48.)

Light microscopy, cytochemistry, immunophenotyping, and cytogenetics are necessary studies to characterize leukemic subtypes.

Morphology

Light Microscopy

Certain morphologic criteria have been established to differentiate lymphoblasts from myeloblasts (Table 14-2). Acute lymphoblastic leukemia can be further subclassified according to the French–American–British (FAB) classification as L1, L2, and L3 morphologic types (Table 14-3).

Uncommon ALL subtypes:

1. *B-cell ALL with L1 morphology:* ALL patients have been described with lymphoblasts having L1 morphology but displaying B-cell ALL immunophenotype. The blast cells are TdT+ in some cases. L3 lymphoblasts generally express immunoglobulin on their cell surface, whereas L1 do not.
2. *Transitional pre-B ALL:* This is characterized by:
   a. Blasts cells that may express cytoplasmic and surface heavy chains but not Ig κ or λ light chains, indicating that these cells are in transition between pre-B and B stages of differentiation
   b. Blast cells that lack FAB L3 morphology or chromosomal translocations associated with B-cell ALL
   c. Very good clinical outcome.

Cytochemistry

The cytochemical characteristics of the various types of leukemia are listed in Table 14-4.

Immunology*

The putative immunologic classification and cellular characteristics of B-lineage ALL and T-cell ALL are shown in Figure 14-1.

A panel of antibodies is used to establish the diagnosis of leukemia and to distinguish among the immunologic subclones. The panel should include at least one marker that is highly lineage specific, for example, CD19 for B lineage, CD7 for T lineage, and CD13 or CD33 for myeloid cells. In addition, the use of cytoplasmic CD79a for early pre-B-cell lineage, cytoplasmic CD3 for T lineage, and cytoplasmic myeloperoxidase for myeloid cells can be helpful in differentiating unclear immunophenotypes.

Immunophenotype Distribution of Acute Lymphoblastic Leukemia

Pre-B-cell accounts for 80% of ALL cases and is subdivided on the basis of cytoplasmic immunoglobulin into transitional pre-B or common ALL antigen (CALLA positive).

Mature B-cell type accounts for 1–2% of ALL cases. These have surface immunoglobulin positivity and are treated as Burkitt lymphoma. The prognosis has improved and is now similar to other subtypes of high-risk ALL.

T-cell type accounts for 15–20% of ALL cases. This subtype is associated with:

- Older age at presentation
- High initial WBC count

---

*For CD antigen nomenclature, refer to Appendix 2.

- Presence of extramedullary disease
- Poor prognosis (treatment on high-risk intensive therapies has improved the prognosis).

Cytogenetics and Molecular Characteristics

The cytogenetic abnormalities observed in leukemia have biologic and prognostic significance. The realization of the biologic significance of leukemia cytogenetics has resulted in the application of molecular methods to understand various mechanisms of leukemogenesis. Specific cytogenetic abnormalities have been shown to have prognostic significance (Table 14-6).

Molecular Genetics of Leukemia of ALL

Table 14-5 lists and Figure 14-2 shows the distribution of molecular rearrangements and chromosomal translocations in childhood acute lymphoblastic leukemia. Seventy-five percent of childhood ALL cases have evidence of chromosomal translocations. The following translocations result in activation of protein kinases by oncogenes and activation of transcription factors:

1. Tel-AML1 fusion gene t(12;21)(p13q;q22). t(12;21) is detected by standard cytogenetics in less than 1 in 1000 cases, whereas, using molecular techniques, it is detected in 25% of pre-B cases. This translocation is associated with an excellent prognosis.
2. *BCR-ABL* fusion gene t(9;22)(q34;q11). t(9;22) occurs in only 3–5% of pediatric ALL cases. This is in contrast to adult ALL where this translocation is present in 25% of cases and 95% of adult chronic myelogenous leukemia (CML) cases. In pediatric *BCR-ABL*–positive ALL, the BCR breakpoint produces a 190-kb protein (p190) in contrast to CML where a different protein (p210) is usually produced. The t(9;22) in pediatric ALL is usually associated with older age, higher WBC count, and frequent CNS involvement at diagnosis.
3. *E2A-PBX1* fusion gene t(1;19)(q23;p13.3). t(1;19) is frequently associated with an elevated WBC at diagnosis and occurs in 25% of cases with a pre-B cytoplasmic immunoglobulin-positive phenotype. Intensive therapy is necessary in this subtype.
4. MLL gene rearrangement at chromosome band 11q23 affects 80% of ALL cases in infants, 3% of ALL cases in older children, and 85% of secondary AML

Table 14-6. **Prognostic Significance of Chromosomal Abnormalities in ALL**

Chromosomal abnormalities	5-year event-free survival (confidence level)
Hyperdiploidy	
>50 chromosomes	80% (65–90%)
47–50 chromosomes	90% (50–98%)
Near triploid, 66–73 chromosomes	Not known, but probably good
Near tetraploid, 82–94 chromosomes (clinical peculiarities: more often T-ALL; L2 morphology; expression of one or more myeloid antigens)	Not known, but probably less than 60%
Normal diploid, 46 chromosomes	80% (65–90%)
Hypodiploidy, <46 chromosomes	71% (55–85%)
Pseudodiploid	73% (55–85%)
t(1;19)	53%
t(4;11)	45%
t(9;22)	14%

involving the topoisomerase II inhibitor. This translocation carries a very poor prognosis with a survival of less than 20%, despite intensive therapy.

5. B-cell ALL translocations involve *MYC* genes on chromosome 8q24. Eighty percent of B-ALL cases contain t(8;14)(q24;q32); the remaining cases have t(2;8) (p12;q24) or t(8;22)(q24;q11). All of these translocations deregulate *MYC* expression and need to be treated intensively with the same agents used to treat Burkitt lymphoma.

Some examples of the prognostic significance of chromosomal abnormalities in ALL are listed in Table 14-6.

Prognostic Factors

Patients who are between ages 1 and 9 with an initial WBC <50,000/mm³ (standard risk), which includes two thirds of pre-B ALL patients, have a 4-year event-free survival of 80%. The remaining patients (high risk) have a 4-year event-free survival of 65%. Factors that should be included in risk classification are:

1. Age: Patients under 1 year of age and greater than 10 years of age have a worse prognosis than children >1 years and <10 years of age. Infants under 1 year of age have the worst prognosis.
2. White cell count: Children with the highest WBC tend to have a poor prognosis (Table 14-7).
3. Immunophenotype: Early pre-B-cell ALL has the best prognosis. Mature T-cell ALL has a worse survival due to its association with older age and higher WBC at diagnosis. Mature B-cell ALL previously had a poor prognosis with early relapses and CNS involvement but recent aggressive therapies have improved prognosis.
4. DNA index >1.16 hyperdiploid ALL with greater than 50 chromosomes has been associated with good outcome due to increased apoptosis and increased sensitivity to chemotherapeutic agents.
5. Cytogenetics: The combinations of trisomies of chromosomes 4, 10, and 17 have been associated with a very low risk of treatment failure and good outcome. Translocations involving the MLL rearrangement on 11q23 have been associated with a worse prognosis. The Philadelphia chromosome t(9;22)(q34;q11) ALL is the most difficult translocation to treat and has a bad prognosis. Hypodiploid ALL is also associated with a poor prognosis.
6. CNS disease: The presence of CNS disease at diagnosis is an adverse prognostic factor despite intensification of therapy with CNS irradiation and additional intrathecal therapy. The presence of blast on cytospin without an increased WBC (CNS2 status) is also associated with poor outcome.
7. Early response to induction therapy: Patients who are not in remission at the end of induction therapy have a very poor prognosis. Bone marrow results on day 7 and day 14 of induction therapy have also been used to estimate response to therapy. In future clinical trials the presence of minimal residual disease at day 28 of induction therapy will be used in addition to day 7 and day 14 bone marrow blasts percentages in determining rapid early response and subsequent therapy. Table 14-8 lists the classification of bone marrow remission status in ALL.

Table 14-7 lists a proposed risk classification system.

Future Directions in ALL Classifications

1. Gene expression profiling using DNA microassay technology can define biologically and prognostically distinctive ALL subsets, can identify genes that

Table 14-7. Proposed Risk Classification System of Pre-B-Cell ALL

Risk Group	Features
Low (treated same as standard risk)	Age >1 year to <10 years of age WBC count <50,000/mm^3 tel-AML or trisomy 4, 10, 17
Standard	Age >1 year to <10 years of age WBC count <50,000/mm^3 Not tel-AML or trisomy 4, 10, 17
High risk	Age >10 years WBC ≥50,000/mm^3 CNS 3 or testicular disease MLL translocation
Very high risk	Ph+ leukemia Hypodiploidy ≤ 45 chromosomes Induction failure

Table 14-8. Classification of Bone Marrow Remission Status in ALL

Classification	% Blasts in bone marrow
M$_1$ bone marrow	≤5%
M$_2$ bone marrow	≤25%
M$_3$ bone marrow	>25%

Based on 200 cell count, true remission requires M$_1$ marrow status with normal marrow cellularity and presence of all cell lines.

may be responsible for leukemogenesis, and may identify genes for which targeted therapy could be developed.

2. Host pharmacogenomics: Gene polymorphisms for genes that encode drug-metabolizing enzymes can influence the efficacy and toxicity of chemotherapy.
   a. Gene polymorphism for thiopurine methyltransferase (TPMT) is a gene that catalyzes the inactivation of mercaptopurine. Ten percent of the population carries at least one variant allele. This results in high levels of active metabolites of mercaptopurine. These patients, especially homozygous patients, have an increased risk of side effects and require marked reduction of 6-mercaptopurine doses.
   b. Gene polymorphism for thymidylate synthetase (target of methotrexate) has been associated with increased enzyme expression and poor outcome in ALL.

Treatment

General Care

In addition to the following information, more details on supportive medical care are given in Chapter 26.

At presentation, patients may be dehydrated, infected, bleeding, and anemic and may have impaired renal and hepatic functions due to leukemic infiltration. Blood urea, creatinine, electrolytes, calcium, phosphorus, serum glutamic pyruvic transaminase (SGPT), serum protein, and uric acid levels should be determined, as well as cultures of the blood, cerebrospinal fluid (CSF), and urine.

Supportive care including the use of packed red cells, platelet transfusions, and human recombinant granulocyte colony-stimulating factor (G-CSF), are required fairly frequently, especially when aggressive multiagent chemotherapy is employed, resulting in temporary bone marrow failure. When high fever and possible septicemia occur in the presence of neutropenia, antibiotic therapy should be started after taking appropriate blood cultures and chest radiographs. Platelet transfusions (1 unit of random donor platelets per 10 kilograms of body weight up to 6 units) should be administered to patients with overt bleeding or when the platelet count is below 10,000/mm^3.

A total of 10 mg/kg/day of allopurinol in divided doses is given in all cases before the commencement of antileukemic drugs. Because allopurinol interferes with the metabolism of 6-mercaptopurine, these two drugs must not be given together. When the blast cell count is more than 50,000/mm^3 or there are large tumor masses, allopurinol is obligatory, together with a fluid intake of 2–3 L/m^2/day and 3 g/m^2/day of oral bicarbonate in divided doses to keep the urine alkaline. These measures are aimed at preventing hyperuricemic acidosis and uric acid nephropathy, which could be fatal. Lactic acidosis, hyperkalemia, and hypocalcemia may also occur during induction.

Recombinant urate oxidase (rasburicase) is also used to prevent tumor lysis syndrome and uric acid nephropathy. The decrease in uric acid is very rapid with the use of 0.2 mg/kg daily as a single infusion for up to 5–7 days. The beneficial effect of urate oxidase is most dramatic in B-cell ALL and stage III, IV B-cell non-Hodgkin lymphoma (III/IV B-NHL) (see Chapter 16) and should be used at the time of initial therapy of B-cell ALL or stage III/IV B-NHL with a high uric acid or high white cell T-cell ALL. The drug should not be used in patients with glucose-6-phosphate dehydrogenase (G6PD) deficiency and allopurinol should be withheld during urate oxidase treatment.

In cases involving hyperleukocytosis (WBC >100,000/mm^3), it has been the practice in the author's clinic to do a partial exchange transfusion to remove a considerable amount of cell burden. This also corrects metabolic abnormalities (e.g., hyperphosphatemia, hypocalcemia, and hyperuricemia) that might occur following effective tumoricidal therapy, reduces the increased blood viscosity, and corrects the anemia. The level of circulating blast cells can also be rapidly reduced within 2–4 hours by leukapheresis. Leukapheresis, however, does not correct the metabolic problems or correct the anemia (see Chapter 26 and Table 26-1).

Live vaccines are contraindicated. There is evidence that the altered immune mechanism existing in the leukemic child may impair the child's ability to handle such antigenic stimuli; therefore, inactivated vaccine should be employed. Eighty percent of leukemic children who received intensive chemotherapy at our institution have at least one defect in cellular or humoral immunity. Fifty percent have two or more unprotective specific antibody responses to measles, mumps, rubella, polio, *Haemophilus influenzae* B, or pneumococcus. Therefore, children with ALL in long-term continuous remission may be at risk for developing serious life-threatening infections and should be evaluated for immune competence at the end of therapy. When protective specific antibody responses are absent, they should be revaccinated. This is a "Swiss cheese–like" humoral immune defect caused by the disease and/or chemotherapy.

Psychosocial support of child and family should be addressed but a detailed discussion of this subject is beyond the scope of this book.

Aims of Therapy

The aims of therapy in acute leukemia are cure and include the following:

1. To induce a clinical and hematologic remission
2. To maintain remission by systemic chemotherapy and prophylactic CNS therapy
3. To treat the complications of therapy and of the disease.

A complete remission is defined as:

1. No symptoms attributable to the disease (e.g., fever and bone pain)
2. No hepatosplenomegaly, lymphadenopathy, or other clinical evidence of residual leukemic tissue infiltration; normal CSF examination (including cytocentrifugation)
3. A normal blood picture, with minimal levels of 500/mm^3 granulocytes, 75,000/mm^3 platelets, and 12 g/dL hemoglobin with no blast cells seen on the blood smear
4. A moderately cellular bone marrow with a moderate number of normal granulocytic and erythroid precursors, together with adequate megakaryocytes and less than 5% blast cells, none possessing frankly leukemic features.

Relapse is defined by the appearance of any of the following:

1. More than 50% lymphoblasts in a single bone marrow aspirate
2. Progressive repopulation of lymphoblasts in excess of 5%, culminating in more than 25% in two or more bone marrow samples separated by 1 week or more
3. More than 25% lymphoblasts in the bone marrow and 2% or more circulating lymphoblasts
4. Leukemic cell infiltration in extramedullary organs, for example, CNS or gonads (biopsy proven) (for the diagnosis of isolated extramedullary relapse, the bone marrow should contain less than 5% blasts)
5. Lymphoblasts in the CSF with a cell count greater than 5 WBC/mm^3.

Minimal Residual Disease and Its Implication in the Management of Leukemia

Remission status in leukemia is usually determined on the basis of morphologic findings alone. However, methods with increased sensitivities are being utilized in some centers for the detection of minimal residual disease (MRD), and application of these techniques may have a profound influence on the management of leukemia for the following reasons:

1. A more precise definition of remission can be obtained based on morphologic, cytogenetic, immunologic, and molecular findings.
2. Treatments may be modified, depending on the level of MRD.
3. Recent studies have attempted to define the prognostic significance of positive MRD. Patients who have a molecular or immunologic remission (defined as leukemic cells less than 0.01% of nucleated bone marrow cells) are predicted to have a better outcome.

Table 14-9 shows the levels of detection of MRD by various methods. Future protocols will use MRD to determine remission status.

Treatment of Newly Diagnosed Acute Lymphoblastic Leukemia

Many successful treatment regimens are available for ALL management. All modern ALL regimens include certain treatment elements: remission induction, consolidation (intensification of remission), prevention of overt CNS leukemia, and maintenance therapy. Remission induction rates with three or four drugs (i.e., vincristine, prednisone, L-asparaginase, intrathecal chemotherapy with or with anthracyclines, depending on the risk classification) produce a 95% remission induction rate.

Acute Lymphoblastic Leukemia (ALL) trials of the Children's Oncology Group (COG) have determined the following therapeutic principles:

1. Initial response to therapy is an important predictor of outcome.
2. Postinduction intensification improves outcome for standard- and higher-risk patients.

Table 14-9. Levels of Detection of Minimal Residual Disease in Leukemia

Method	Lowest levels of detection[a]
Morphology	5 per 100
Conventional cytogenetics	2 per 100
Karyotyping of flow cytometry	1 per 100
Southern blot for receptor gene rearrangement	1 per 100
Karyotyping by fluorescent *in situ* hybridization (FISH)	1 per 1000
Double immunological marker analysis (leukemia-associated phenotype)	1 per 100,000
Polymerase chain reaction (PCR)	1 per 1,000,000
Combining the use of above methods (in theory)	Unknown (theoretically may increase sensitivity)

[a]Number of leukemic cells per number of normal bone marrow cells.

3. Standard-risk patients who receive delayed intensification (DI) do not receive additional benefit from intensive induction other than dexamethasone, vincristine, and L-asparaginase.
4. The augmented regimen (see Table 14-11 later in chapter) rescues higher-risk patients with >25% blasts on day 7.
5. Improved systemic therapy eliminates cranial irradiation for standard-risk patients.
6. Substitution of dexamethasone for prednisone improves outcome for standard-risk patients.

Table 14-10 lists the protocol used for standard-risk pre-B-cell ALL. Pre-B-cell ALL event-free survival (EFS) at 5 years is nearly 80%. Table 14-11 lists a protocol for the treatment of high-risk pre-B-cell ALL that includes an augmented therapy protocol for slow early responders (i.e., greater than 25% blasts at day 7 of therapy after drug induction). Table 14-12 lists a protocol for treatment of B-cell ALL (LMB 89 protocol), which has an EFS of 84% at 5 years using this protocol, and Table 14-13 lists the protocol for treatment of T-cell ALL, which has an EFS of approximately 75% at 5 years using this protocol.

Infant Leukemia

Infant ALL accounts for 2–5% of childhood leukemias. Infants under 12 months of age with ALL have an extremely poor prognosis, worse than that of any other age

Table 14-10. Therapy for Standard-Risk Pre-B-Cell ALL

Induction (1 month)	Oral dexamethasone for 28 days (6 mg/m²/day in 3 divided doses), IV vincristine (1.5 mg/m² on days 0, 7, 14, and 21), intramuscular L-asparaginase (6000 Units/m², 3 times weekly for 9 doses, starting on days 2–4), and age-adjusted intrathecal methotrexate (age 1 to less than 2 years, 8 mg; age 2 to less than 3 years, 10 mg; older than 3 years, 12 mg on days 0 and 14).
Consolidation (3 months)	Oral 6-mercaptopurine (75 mg/m²/day on days 0–70 of consolidation), IV vincristine (1.5 mg/m² on days 0, 28, and 56), oral methotrexate (20 mg/m² on days 28, 35, 42, 49, 56, 63, and 70), and age-adjusted (see above) intrathecal methotrexate on days 0, 7, 14, and 21 for patients without CNS disease at diagnosis. Dexamethasone 6 mg/m²/day on days 28–32 and 56–60.

(Continues)

Table 14-10. (Continued)

Delayed intensification (2 months)	Oral dexamethasone in all patients (10 mg/m^2/day for 21 days plus a 7-day taper), IV vincristine (1.5 mg/m^2 on days 0, 7, and 14), intramuscular L-asparaginase (6000 Units/m^2 for 6 doses given M/W/F on days 3–17), doxorubicin (25 mg/m^2, IV push, on days 0, 7, and 14), IV cyclophosphamide (1000 mg/m^2 over 30 minutes on day 28), oral 6-thioguanine (60 mg/m^2/day on days 28–41), cytarabine (75 mg/m^2/day, IV push, on days 29–32 and 36–39), and age-adjusted intrathecal methotrexate on day 28.
Maintenance (girls, 20 months; boys, 32 months)	Dexamethasone (6 mg/m^2/day on days 0–4, 28–32, and 56–60), oral mercaptopurine (75 mg/m^2/day on days 0–83), IV vincristine (1.5 mg/m^2 on days 0, 28, and 56), weekly oral methotrexate (20 mg/m^2 beginning on day 7 of each course), and age-adjusted intrathecal methotrexate (see above) on day 0 of each course.

Modified from Bostram BC, Sensel MR, Sather HN, Gaynon PS, Mei K, Johnston K, Erdman GR, Gold S, Heerema NA, Hutchinson RJ, Provisor AJ, Trigg ME. Blood 2003;101:3809–17.

group. Patients go into remission but have a high incidence of early bone marrow or extramedullary relapse. These patients have a high incidence of the following poor prognostic features:

- High initial WBC
- Massive organomegaly
- Thrombocytopenia
- CNS leukemia
- Failure to achieve complete remission by day 14.

Infant ALL is biologically unique. The leukemia arises from a very early stage of commitment to B-cell differentiation and has the following characteristics:

The leukemic cells are usually CALLA (CD10) negative.
A chromosomal abnormality on chromosome 11, particularly band 11q23 where the MLL/ALL1 gene is located, is commonly found in infant ALL and is associated with a poor prognosis.
The cells frequently express myeloid antigens.
Blasts have fetal characteristics and have a greater resistance to therapy.

Independent adverse prognostic features in this group are:

- Age <3 months
- WBC >75,000/mm^3
- CD10 negative
- Slow response to induction
- Presence of translocation 11q23.

Infant ALL requires very intensive therapy with advanced supportive care. Most centers advocate that after remission is attained, an allogeneic stem cell transplant be performed for infant ALL with an 11q23 cytogenetic abnormality or a molecular MLL abnormality. Intensive chemotherapy protocols have an event-free survival of 40%. The COG is studying an intensive therapy that may make stem cell transplantation unnecessary.

Bone Marrow Relapse in Children with ALL

Despite current intensive front-line treatments, 25–30% of children with ALL experience bone marrow relapse. Relapse may be an isolated event in the bone marrow or may be combined with relapse in other sites. Children who have a bone marrow

Table 14-11. High-Risk Pre-B-Cell ALL Protocol (for Rapid Early Responders [RER] and for Slow Early Responders [SER])

	RER (day 7 bone marrow <25% blasts)		SER-augmented regime (day 7 bone marrow >25% blasts)		
Phase	Treatment	Dose	Phase	Treatment	Dose
Induction	Prednisone	60 mg/m²/day PO for 28 days	Induction	Prednisone	60 mg/m²/day PO for 28 days
	Vincristine	1.5 mg/m² week IV, days 1, 8, 15, 22		Vincristine	1.5 mg/m² week IV, days 1, 8, 15, 22
	Daunomycin	25 mg/m² week IV, days 1, 8, 15, 22		Daunomycin	25 mg/m² week IV, days 1, 8, 15, 22
	Asparaginase	6000 units/m²/day IM, days 3, 5, 7, 10, 12, 14, 17, 19, 21		Asparaginase	6000 units/m²/day IM, days 3, 5, 7, 10, 12, 14, 17, 19, 21
	Cytarabine[a]	Age-adjusted IT, day 0		Cytarabine[a]	Age-adjusted IT, day 0
	Methotrexate[a]	Age-adjusted IT, day 14		Methotrexate[a]	Age-adjusted IT, day 14
Consolidation	Prednisone	7.5 mg/m²/day 0; 3.75 mg/m²/day, days 1, 2	Consolidation	Cyclophosphamide	1000 mg/m²/day IV, days 0, 28
	Cyclophosphamide	1000 mg/m²/day IV, days 0, 14		Cytarabine	75 mg/m²/day SC or IV, days 1–4, 8–11, 29–32, 36–39
	Mercaptopurine	60 mg/m²/day PO, days 0–27		Mercaptopurine	60 mg/m²/day PO, days 0–13, 28–41
	Vincristine	1.5 mg/m²/day IV, days 14, 21, 42, 49		Vincristine	1.5 mg/m²/day IV, days 14, 21, 42, 49
	Cytarabine	75 mg/m²/day IV, days 1–4, 8–11, 15–18, 22–25		Asparaginase	6000 units/m²/day IM, days 14, 16, 18, 21, 23, 25, 42, 44, 46, 49, 51, 53
	Methotrexate[a]	IT, days 1, 8, 15, 22		Methotrexate[a]	IT days 1, 8, 15, 22
	Radiotherapy[b]	Cranial, 1800 cGy Cranial, 2400 cGy, and spinal, 600 cGy		Radiotherapy[b]	Cranial, 1800 cGy Cranial, 2400 cGy, and spinal, 600 cGy Testicular, 2400 cGy
Interim maintenance (8 weeks)	Mercaptopurine	60 mg/m²/day PO, days 0–41	Interim maintenance I (8 weeks)	Vincristine	1.5 mg/m²/day IV, days 0, 10, 20, 30, 40
	Methotrexate	15 mg/m²/day PO, days 0, 7, 14, 21, 28, 35		Methotrexate	100 mg/m²/day IV, days 0, 10, 20, 30, 40 (escalate by 50 mg/m²/dose)
				Asparaginase	15,000 units/m²/day IM, days 1, 11, 21, 31, 41
Delayed intensification (7 weeks)			Delayed intensification I (8 weeks)		
Reduction (4 weeks)	Dexamethasone	10 mg/m²/day PO, days 0–20 then taper for 7 days	Reinduction (4 weeks)	Dexamethasone	10 mg/m²/day PO, days 0–20, then taper for 7 days
	Vincristine	1.5 mg/m²/day IV, days 0, 7, 14		Vincristine	1.5 mg/m²/day IV, days 0, 7, 14
	Doxorubicin	25 mg/m²/day IV, days 0, 7, 14		Doxorubicin	25 mg/m²/day IV, days 0, 7, 14
	Asparaginase	6000 units/m²/day IM, days 3, 5, 7, 10, 12, 14		Asparaginase	6000 units/m²/day IM, days 3, 5, 7, 10, 12, 14

Phase	Drug	Dose and schedule
Reconsolidation (3 weeks)	Vincristine	1.5 mg/m²/day IV, days 42, 49
	Cyclophosphamide	1000 mg/m²/day IV, day 28
	Thioguanine	60 mg/m²/day PO, days 28–41
	Cytarabine	75 mg/m²/day SC or IV, days 29–32, 36–39
	Methotrexate[a]	IT, days 29, 36
Maintenance (12 weeks)[c]	Vincristine	1.5 mg/m²/day IV, days 0, 28, 56
	Prednisone	40 mg/m²/day PO, days 0–4, 28–32, 56–60
	Mercaptopurine	75 mg/m²/day PO, days 0–83
	Methotrexate	20 mg/m²/day PO, days 7, 14, 21, 28, 35, 42, 49, 56, 63, 70, 77
	Methotrexate[a]	IT, day 0
Reconsolidation (4 weeks)	Vincristine	1.5 mg/m²/day IV, days 42, 49
	Cyclophosphamide	1000 mg/m²/day IV, day 28
	Thioguanine	60 mg/m²/day PO, days 28–41
	Cytarabine	75 mg/m²/day SC or IV, days 29–32, 36–39
	Methotrexate[a]	IT, days 29, 36
	Asparaginase	6000 units/m²/day IM, days 42, 44, 46, 49, 51, 53
Interim maintenance II (8 weeks)	Vincristine	1.5 mg/m²/day IV, days 0, 10, 20, 30, 40
	Methotrexate	100 mg/m²/day IV, days 0, 10, 20, 30, 40 (escalate by 50 mg/m²/dose)
	Asparaginase	15,000 units/m²/day IM, days 1, 11, 21, 31, 41
	Methotrexate[a]	IT, days 0, 20, 40
Delayed intensification II (8 weeks)	Same as for delayed intensification I	
Maintenance (12 weeks)[c]	Vincristine	1.5 mg/m²/day IV, days 0, 28, 56
	Prednisone	60 mg/m²/day PO, days 0–4, 28–32, 56–60
	Mercaptopurine	75 mg/m²/day PO, days 0–83
	Methotrexate	20 mg/m²/day PO, days 7, 14, 21, 28, 35, 42, 49, 56, 63, 70, 77
	Methotrexate[a]	IT, day 0

Abbreviations: IV, intravenously; PO, orally; IT, intrathecally; SC, subcutaneously; IM, intramuscularly.

[a]The doses are age adjusted as follows: Methotrexate: age 1 to 1.9 years, 8 mg; age 2 to 2.9 years, 10 mg; age ≥3 years, 12 mg. Patients with central nervous system disease at diagnosis do not receive intrathecal methotrexate on days 15 and 22 of consolidation therapy. Cytarabine: age 1 to 1.9 years, 30 mg; age 2 to 2.9 years, 50 mg; age ≥3 years, 70 mg.

[b]During the first 2 weeks of consolidation therapy, patients without central nervous system disease at diagnosis receive 1800 cGy of cranial radiotherapy in 10 fractions; patients with central nervous system disease at diagnosis receive 2400 cGy to the cranial midplane in 12 fractions and 600 cGy to the spinal cord in 3 fractions. In the augmented-therapy group, patients with testiculomegaly at diagnosis receive 2400 cGy bilateral testicular radiation in 8 fractions.

[c]The cycles of maintenance therapy are repeated until the total duration of therapy, beginning with the first interim maintenance period, reached is 2 years for girls and 3 years for boys.

Notes: Most other protocols delete cranial irradiation when CNS leukemia is not present at diagnosis with irradiation only for SER patients.

From Nachman JB, Sather HN, Sensel MG, Trigg ME, Cherlow JM, Lukens JN, Wolff L, Uckun FM, Gaynon PS. Augmented post-induction therapy for children with high-risk acute lymphoblastic leukemia and a slow response to initial therapy. N Engl J Med 1998;338:1663–71, with permission.

Table 14-12. Protocol for B-Cell ALL and B-Cell NHL with Marrow Involvement with or without CNS Involvement (LMB 89 Protocol)

Reduction phase
  COP

Cyclophosphamide	300 mg/m² IV, day 1
Vincristine	1 mg/m² (maximum dose, 2 mg) IV, day 1
Prednisone	60 mg/m²/day PO or IV, days 1–7
Methotrexate (MTX) and hydrocortisone (HC)	15 mg IT, days 1, 3, and 5 (dose adjusted for patients <3 years of age)[a]
Ara-C	30 mg IT, days 1, 3, and 5 (dose adjusted for patients <3 years of age)[a]
Folinic acid	15 mg/m² q6h PO, days 2 and 4

Induction: 2 courses, COPADM1 and COPADM2, started on day 8 after first day of reduction (COP) phase
  COPADM1:

Vincristine	2 mg/m² (maximum dose, 2 mg) IV, day 1
MTX high dose (HD)	8 g/m² (over 4 hours) IV, day 1
Folinic acid	15 mg/m² PO q6h × 12 doses, days 2–4 MTX level at 72 hours, <0.1 µmol/L
MTX and HC	15 mg IT days 2, 4, and 6 (dose adjusted for patients <3 years of age)[a]
Ara-C	30 mg IT, days 2, 4, and 6 (dose adjusted for patients <3 years of age)[a]
Cyclophosphamide	500 mg/m²/day IV, days 2–4 (in 2 injections per day q12h and hydration)
Adriamycin	60 mg/m² IV, day 2
Prednisone	60 mg/m² PO or IV, days 1–6

  COPADM2 (after hematologic recovery)
  Same as COPADM1 except

Cyclophosphamide	Doses doubled (1 g/m²/day, always in 2 injections per day at 12-h intervals)
Second vincristine	Day 6

Consolidation: 2 courses of CYVE (after hematologic recovery)
  CYVE

Cytarabine (Ara-C)	50 mg/m²/12-hour continuous infusions (hours 1–12), days 1–5
Cytarabine HD	3 g/m²/day (in 3 hours) IV (hours 12–15), days 1–4
VP16	200 mg/m²/day (in 2 hours) IV (hours 15–17), days 1–4

Maintenance: Four courses monthly in succession
  Course 1

Prednisone	60 mg/m² PO in 2 divided doses, days 1–5
MTX HD	8 g/m² (in 4 hours) IV, day 1
Folinic acid	15 mg/m² q6h IV, days 2–4
MTX IT and HC	15 mg IT, day 2 (doses adjusted for patients <3 years of age)[a]
Ara-C	30 mg IT, day 2 (doses adjusted for patients <3 years of age)[a]
Cyclophosphamide	500 mg/m²/day IV, days 1 and 2 (in 2 divided doses q12h per day)
Adriamycin	60 mg/m² IV, day 2
Vincristine	2 mg/m² (maximum dose, 2 mg) IV, day 1

(Continues)

Table 14-12. (*Continued*)

Cranial irradiation	2400 cGy to commence on day 8 in case of initial meningeal involvement (except in case of isolated compression of spinal cord)
Course 2 (after hematologic recovery)	
Cytarabine	100 mg/m^2/day SC, days 1–5 (in 2 injections q12h)
VP16	150 mg/m^2/day IV, days 1–3 (over 2 hours)
Course 3 (after hematologic recovery)	
Same as course 1 except without MTX HD and without IT	
Course 4 (after hematologic recovery)	
Same as course 2	

^{a}Age-adjusted doses for intrathecal use (triple intrathecal):

Age	MTX	HC	Ara-C
<1 year	8 mg	8 mg	15 mg
1 year	10 mg	10 mg	20 mg
2 years	12 mg	12 mg	25 mg
>3 years	15 mg	15 mg	30 mg

Notes: MTX and HC, methotrexate and hydrocortisone; Ara-C, cytarabine, cytosine arabinoside; IT, intrathecal; HD, high dose; SC, subcutaneous.

Modified from Patte C, Auperin A, Michon J, Behrendt H, et al. The Societe Francaise d' Oncologie Pediatrique LMB89 protocol: highly effective multiagent chemotherapy tailored to the tumor burden and initial response in 561 unselected children with B-cell lymphomas and L3 leukemia. Blood 2001;97:3370–9.

Table 14-13. Protocol for T-Cell ALL

Induction	
4 weeks	Vincristine 1.5 mg/m^2 weekly
	Prednisone 40 mg/m^2/day × 28 days
	Doxorubicin 30 mg/m^2 on days 5 and 6
	IT Ara-C (dosed by age) on days 5 and 19
	MTX 4 gm/m^2 on day 5 eight hours after 2nd dose of doxorubicin with leukovorin rescue beginning at hour 36
CNS treatment	Cranial XRT 1800 cGy with IT medications 4 doses during
3 weeks	cranial radiation
Intensification	Prednisone 120 mg/m^2/day × 5 days every 3 weeks
6–9 months	Doxorubicin 30 mg/m^2 every 3 weeks until cumulative dose of doxorubicin reaches 360 mg/m^2 and then substitute methotrexate as in continuation
	6-Mercaptopurine 50 mg/m^2/day PO × 14 days
	L-Asparaginase 25,000 IU/m^2 every week × 20 weeks
	Vincristine 2.0 mg/m^2 IV every 3 weeks
	IT Ara-C and methotrexate every 18 weeks
Continuation until	Prednisone 120 mg/m^2/day × 5 days
2 years continual	6-Mercaptopurine 50 mg/m^2/day po × 14 day
complete remission	Vincristine 2.0 mg/m^2 IV every 3 weeks ⎱ Every 3 weeks
	Methotrexate 30 mg/m^2 IV weekly
	IT Ara-C and methotrexate every 18 weeks

IT doses: IT Ara-C 15 mg <1 year, 1–2 years 20 mg, 2–3 years 30 mg, ≥3 years 40 mg. Methotrexate 8 mg ages 1–2, 10 mg ages 2–3, 12 mg ages >3 years.

Modified from Goldberg JM, Silverman LB, Levy DE, Dalton VK, Gelber RD, Lehmann C, Cohen HS, Sallan SE, Asselin BC. Childhood T cell acute lymphoblastic leukemia. The Dana-Farber Cancer Institute. Acute Lymphoblastic Leukemia Consortium experience. J Clin Oncol 2003;21:3616–22.

relapse before completing therapy or within 6 months after completing therapy have a very poor long-term survival (early relapse). Allogeneic stem cell transplantation should be considered for these patients.

Children whose bone marrow relapse occurs after 6 months after completion of therapy have a significantly longer second remission. Figure 14-3 lists suggested algorithms for treatment of ALL relapse.

The authors have used the Memorial Sloan-Kettering New York 2 protocol (Table 14-14) to treat ALL bone marrow relapses with satisfactory results, and Table 14-15 lists an alternative induction regimen for recurrent ALL if doxorubicin cannot be employed because of cardiotoxicity. When the alternative induction regimen is utilized, then the maintenance treatment is continued as indicated in Table 14-14.

Central Nervous System Relapse

Rationale of Therapy

1. Intrathecal chemotherapy alone fails to cure CNS leukemia. However, temporary remission can be achieved with intrathecal chemotherapy alone.
2. Bone marrow relapse occurs in more than 50% of patients achieving CNS remission, regardless of the use of intensified chemotherapy at the time of CNS relapse.

One of the recommended regimens in children relapsing only in the CNS who have not previously received cranial irradiation is listed in Table 14-16. This protocol should be employed alone in CNS relapses occurring after 18 months of first remission. However, early CNS relapses (<18 months first remission) should be treated with chemotherapy followed by allogeneic stem cell transplantation.

Toxicity of CNS Treatment

1. Significant decline in mean values on global IQ scale
2. Possibility of increased risk of leukoencephalopathy.

For these reasons recent protocols have further delayed radiation therapy to permit more extensive chemotherapy to be delivered prior to radiation therapy and have decreased cranial radiation therapy to 1800 cGy.

The 4-year event-free survival after CNS relapse for patients with a first complete remission ≥18 months is 83%, whereas for those with a first complete remission less than 18 months it is 46%.

Testicular Relapse

The principles of therapy for isolated testicular relapse include:

1. Local radiotherapy to both testes
2. Reinduction and continuation of systemic chemotherapy and CNS chemoprophylaxis.

Future trials will investigate the use of high-dose methotrexate to intensify therapy in an attempt to eliminate testicular radiation therapy.

Future Drugs in ALL Therapy

1. Imatinib mesylate (see Chapter 13) inhibits the BCR/ABL tyrosine kinase and is currently being tested in conjunction with chemotherapy in newly diagnosed Ph+ ALL.
2. Arabinosylguanine (506 U) is effective in T-cell ALL and is being studied in conjunction with other chemotherapy in T-cell ALL.

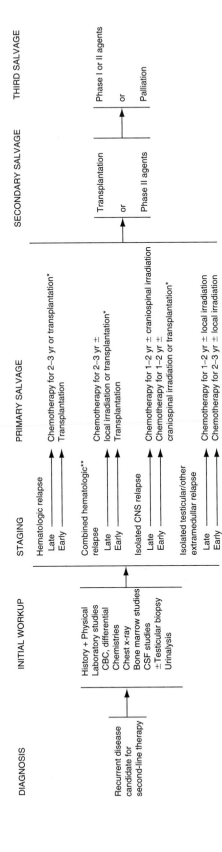

Fig. 14-3. Comprehensive Cancer Network recommendations for treatment of ALL relapse. (Modified from Pui CH. NCCN pediatric acute lymphoblastic leukemia practice guide-lines. Oncology 1996;10:1787–94, with permission.)

Table 14-14. Memorial Sloan-Kettering New York 2 Protocol for Acute Lymphoblastic Leukemia Relapse

Induction

Day 0: cytosine arabinoside 20, 30, 50, or 70 mg IT for ages <1, 1–2, 2–3, >3 years, respectively

Daunorubicin

Days 0, 1: daunorubicin 60 mg/m^2/day × 2 or daunorubicin 120 mg/m^2 over 48 hours continuous infusion

Day 2: cyclophosphamide 1200 mg/m^2 IV

Days 2, 9, 16, 23: vincristine 1.5 mg/m^2 IV days 2–23: prednisone 60 mg/m^2/day PO and 9-day tapering dose

Day 4 and every Monday, Wednesday, and Friday thereafter: L-asparaginase 6000 units/m^2/day IM

Days 15, 22: methotrexate 6, 8, 10, or 12 mg IT for ages <1, 1–2, 2–3, and >3 years, respectively

Days 0–3: 6-mercaptopurine 300 mg/m^2/day PO

Day 4: cyclophosphamide 600 mg/m^2 IV

Days 4, 11, 18, 25, 32, 39, 46, 53, 60: L-asparaginase 25,000 units IM

Days 11, 18, 25: vincristine 1.5 mg/m^2 IV

Days 18 to 25: prednisone 180 mg/m^2/day PO

Day 25: methotrexate 150 mg/m^2 IV over 4 hours

Days 40, 41: daunorubicin 20 mg/m^2/day IV or daunorubicin 40 mg/m^2 over 48 hours infusion intravenous

Days 42–44: cytosine arabinoside 100 mg/m^2/day, 72-hour continuous infusion

Days 42–44: thioguanine 40 mg/m^2/day PO every 12 hours × 6

Consolidation (begins on the nearest Monday to day 28 or when ANC >500/mm^3 and platelet count >100,000/mm^3)

Days 28, 29: cytosine arabinoside 3000 mg/m^2 over 3 hours IV

Days 28, 30, 32, 37, 39, 42, 44, 46, etc. until the beginning of maintenance: L-asparaginase 6000 units/m^2/day IM

Day 31: methotrexate 150 mg/m^2 IV over 4 hours

Days 32 and 39: vincristine 1.5 mg/m^2 IV

Days 32–39: prednisone 180 mg/m^2/day PO

First maintenance (day 56 of consolidation is day 0, begins with ANC >1000/mm^3 and platelet count >100,000/mm^3)

Days 0, 7, 15, 22: methotrexate IT

Subsequent maintenance cycles

Day 60/0: methotrexate IT

Days 0–3: 6-mercaptopurine 300 mg/m^2/day PO

Day 4: cyclophosphamide 1200 mg/m^2 IV

Days 11, 18, 25: vincristine 1.5 mg/m^2 IV

Days 18–25: prednisone 180 mg/m^2/day PO

Day 25: methotrexate 200 mg/m^2 IV over 4 hours, escalate dose by 50 mg/m^2 each subsequent cycle until mucositis or ANC <500/mm^3 occurs

Days 40, 41: daunorubicin 20 mg/m^2/day IV or daunorubicin 40 mg/m^2 over 48 hours Infusion intravenously or dactinomycin 750 μg/m^2 IV day 41 (1 day only instead of 2-day daunorubicin) once the limit of anthracycline has been reached

Days 42–44: cytosine arabinoside 100 mg/m^2/day 72-hour continuous infusion

Days 42–44: thioguanine 40 mg/m^2/dose PO every 12 × 6 hours

Duration of maintenance therapy: 2 years

Abbreviations: IT, intrathecal; IV, intravenous; PO, oral; IM, intramuscular; CNS, central nervous system; ANC, absolute neutrophil count.

From Steinherz PG, Redner A, Steinherz L, Meyers P, Tan C, Heller G. Development of a new intensive therapy for acute lymphoblastic leukemia in children at increased risk of early relapse. Cancer 1993;72:3120–30, with permission.

Table 14-15. Alternate Induction Regimen for Recurrent Acute Lymphoblastic Leukemia in Bone Marrow (MSKCC Protocol)

Cytosine arabinoside	3 g/m^2 IV over 3 hours, days 0 and 3
Methotrexate	200 mg/m^2 IV over 4 hours, day 1
Asparaginase	6000 units/m^2 IM, days 0, 2, 4, 7, 9, 11, 14, 16, 18, 21, 23, and 25
Vincristine	1.5 mg/m^2 IV, days 4 and 11
Prednisone	180 mg/m^2/day PO, days 4–11

Note: MSKCC, Memorial Sloan-Kettering Cancer Center, New York.

Table 14-16. Treatment Schema for ALL Patients with CNS Relapse

Induction (weeks 1–4)
    DEX: 10 mg/m^2 orally daily × 28
    VCR: 1.5 mg/m^2 IV weekly × 4
    DNR: 25 mg/m^2 weekly × 3
    TIT: MTX/HC/Ara-C (age-adjusted dose)[a] IT weekly × 4
Consolidation (weeks 5–10)
    Ara-C: 3 g/m^2 IV q12h × 4, followed by L-asp 10,000 IU/m^2 IM weeks 5 and 8
    L-ASP: 10,000 IU/m^2 IM on days 1 and 4 of weeks 6 and 9
    TIT: MTX/HC/Ara-C (age-adjusted dose) IT week 10
Intensification (weeks 11–22)
    MTX: 1000 mg/m^2 IV over 24 hours, followed by
    MP: 1000 mg/m^2 IV over 8 hours weeks 11, 14, 17, and 20
    VP-16: 300 mg/m^2 IV, followed by
    CYC: 500 mg/m^2 IV weeks 12, 15, 18, and 21
    TIT: MTX/HC/Ara-C (age-adjusted dose)[a] IT weeks 13, 16, 19, and 22
Irradiation (weeks 23–26)
    Cranial radiation: 2.4 Gy
    Spinal radiation: 1.5 Gy
    DEX: 10 mg/m^2 orally daily × 21
    VCR: 1.5 mg/m^2 IV weekly × 3
    L-ASP: 10,000 IU/m^2 IM thrice weekly × 9
Maintenance (weeks 27–102)
    MP: 75 mg/m^2 orally daily × 42
    MTX: 20 mg/m^2 IM weekly × 6
    Alternate with
    VCR: 1.5 mg/m^2 IV weekly × 4
    CYC: 300 mg/m^2 IV weekly × 4

[a]See Table 14-13 for age-adjusted doses for intrathecal therapy.

Abbreviations: DEX, dexamethasone; VCR, vincristine; DNR, daunomycin; TIT, triple intrathecal therapy; HC, hydrocortisone; Ara-C, cytarabine; L-asp, L-asparaginase; MP, 6-mercaptopurine; VP-16, etoposide; CYC, cyclophosphamide; IV, intravenously; IT, intrathecally; IM, intramuscularly.

    The authors have substituted 6-mercaptopurine 50 mg/m^2 day orally for 7 days instead of IV 6-mercaptopurine.

    Adapted from Ritchey AK, Pollock BH, Lauer SJ, Andejeski Y, Buchanan GR. Improved survival of children with isolated CNS relapse of ALL. A POG study. J Clin Oncol 1999;17:3745–52, with permission.

ACUTE MYELOID LEUKEMIA

The age incidence of AML in childhood is constant except for a peak of incidence in the neonatal period and a slight increase in incidence during adolescence. The following inherited disorders predispose a patient to AML:

Down syndrome
Fanconi anemia
Kostmann syndrome
Bloom syndrome
Diamond–Blackfan anemia.

Secondary AML can evolve from:

Myelodysplastic syndromes and myeloproliferative syndromes (Chapter 13)
Exposure to ionizing radiation treatment with chemotherapy agents. The following are chemotherapy agents associated with secondary AML:
Nitrogen mustard
Cyclophosphamide
Ifosfamide
Chlorambucil
Melphalan
Etoposide.

Clinical Features of AML

Many of the clinical features of AML are similar to those described in ALL in this chapter. The morphologic features of myeloblasts and the cytochemical features of AML are tabulated in Tables 14-2 and 14-4, respectively.

Classification of AML

WHO classification of AML defines that 20% blasts are required for the diagnosis of AML. In addition, patients with clonal cytogenetic abnormalities t(8;21)(q22;q22), inv(16)(p13q22) or t(16;16)(p13;q22) and t(15;17)(q22;q12) are considered to have AML regardless of the blast percentage.

FAB classification of AML:

- *Type M0*—acute undifferentiated leukemia
- *Type M1*—myeloblastic leukemia without maturation; morphologically indistinguishable from L2 morphology (Table 14-3)
- *Type M2*—myeloblastic leukemia with differentiation
- *Type M3*—acute promyelocytic leukemia (APML); most cells abnormal hypergranular promyelocytes; cytoplasm contains multiple Auer rods
- *Type M3V*—microgranular variant of APML; cells with deeply notched nucleus; typical hypergranular promyelocytes less frequent (see page 441)
- *Type M4*—both myelocytic and monocytic differentiation present in varying proportions
- *Type M4EOS*—associated with prominent proliferation of eosinophils
- *Type M5*—monocytic leukemia containing poorly differentiated and/or well-differentiated monocytoid cells (The M4 and M5 subtypes are particularly common in children under 2 years of age.)
- *Type M6*—erythroleukemia (Diguglielmo disease)
- *Type M7*—megakaryoblastic leukemia; associated with myelofibrosis; frequently observed in children with trisomy 21.

M7 Leukemia

1. Blast morphology: In M7 the blast morphology is heterogeneous in appearance, resembling L1 or L2 cells with or without granules and having one to three nucleoli; the cytoplasm has blebs.

2. Immunophenotype: CD41, CD42, CD61 positivity, in addition to CD13 and CD33 positivity.
3. Electron microscopy:
   a. Demonstration of platelet peroxidase (PPO)
   b. Positive PPO reaction localized exclusively on the nuclear membrane and the endoplasmic reticulum.

FAB M5 and M7 are more common in early childhood, whereas older children are more likely to have M0, M1, M2, and M3.

The quantitative bone marrow criteria for the diagnosis of acute myeloblastic leukemia are summarized in Table 14-17.

Uncommon subtypes of AML leukemia:

1. *AML with erythrophagocytosis*—M4 or M5 morphology with prominent erythrophagocytosis; fibrinolysis and consistent karyotype t(8;16)(p11;p13); associated with a poor prognosis.
2. *M0*—Lymphoblastic (L2) morphology; negative myeloperoxidase (MPO) and Sudan black by conventional histochemical methods, despite the positivity for myeloid antigens (CD13 and/or CD33). MPO detected by the monoclonal antibody method (which detects the α-chain as well as the inactive proenzyme form) or by electron microscopy may be positive. Lymphoid markers other than TdT and CD7 are negative.
3. *M3V-microgranular variant of acute promyelocytic leukemia (APML)*—M3V is characterized by bilobed cells, multilobular cells, or cells with reniform nucleus and cytoplasm with minimal or no granulation; generally associated with a few typical M3 cells. It presents with hyperleukocytosis and severe coagulopathy. Prognosis is poor as a result of fatal hemorrhages in vital organs during induction therapy. It displays the same cytochemical (MPO+), cytogenetic t(15;17), phenotypic (HLA-DR, CD13+, CD15+, CD33+), and molecular (RAR and PML rearrangements) features as the hypergranular (M3) APML. Morphologic diagnosis can be difficult.

Table 14-17. Quantitative Bone Marrow Criteria for the Diagnosis of Acute Myeloblastic Leukemia Subtypes[a]

Bone marrow cells	M1 (%)	M2 (%)	M4 (%)	M5 (%)	M6 (%)
Blasts					
All nucleated cells	—	>30	>30	—	<30 or >30
Nonerythroid cells	90	>30	>30	>80[c]	>30
Erythroblasts, all nucleated cells	—	<50	<50	—	>50
Granulocytic component,[b] nonerythroid cells	<10	>10	>20[d]	<20	Variable
Monocytic component,[c] nonerythroid cells	<10	<20	>20	>80[e]	Variable

[a]Lysozyme estimations and cytochemical tests are required if the peripheral blood monocyte count is 5×10^9/L or more, but the marrow suggests M2, and marrow suggests M4, but the peripheral blood monocyte count is less than 5×10^9/L.

[b]Promyelocytes, myelocytes, metamyelocytes, and neutrophils.

[c]Promyelocytes and monocytes.

[d]May include myeloblasts.

[e]Monoblasts in M5a; in M5b; the predominant cells are promonocytes and monocytes.

From Bennett JM, Catovsky D, Daniel MT, et al. Proposed revised criteria for the classification of acute myeloid leukemia. Ann Intern Med 1985;103:626, with permission.

Table 14-18. Relationship among Immunologic Surface Markers with FAB Subtypes of Acute Myeloblastic Leukemia

FAB subtype of AML	Immunologic surface marker										
	HLA-DR	CD11b	CD13	CD14	CD15	CD33	CD34	Glyco-phorin	CD41	CD42	CD61
M1/M2	+				+	+	+				
M3/M3V		+	+		+	+	+				
M4/M5	+	+	+	+	+	+	+				
M6	+		+			+	+	+			
M7	+		+			+	+		+	+	+
M0			+			+	+				

Immunophenotype of AML

Antibodies to cell surface proteins are useful in the diagnosis of AML and can be correlated with the FAB subtypes. Table 14-18 lists the relationship among immunologic surface markers with FAB subtypes of AML.

Molecular Genetics of AML

1. Fifteen percent of AML have a t(8;21)(q22q22), which is associated with FAB M2. The translocation creates an AML1-ETO fusion gene. The translocation seems to interfere with the expression of a myeloid-specific gene.
2. A related myeloid transcription factor is also altered by the cytogenetic inv(16) and t(16;16), which occurs in 15% of AML cases. These cases are associated with myelomonocytic differentiation with abnormal bone marrow eosinophils and a favorable progression. They result in a chimeric protein (CBFB-MYH11).
3. Acute promyelocytic leukemia is associated with a balanced translocation of the retinoic acid receptor α (RARα gene at 17q21) and the PML gene at 15q21. RARα is a transcription factor that binds retinoids and interacts directly with DNA.

These molecular abnormalities have clinical importance. APML can be treated with *trans*-retinoic acid due to its binding to the RARα receptor. Detection of AML-ETO or CBFB-MYH11 is associated with a high rate of long-term remission after treatment with high-dose cytosine arabinoside.

Table 14-19 lists the common translocations in pediatric AML, the FAB subtype associations, the affected genes, and the frequency of clinical presentations of these subtypes. Figure 14-4 identifies the distribution of translocations in pediatric AML.

Gene expression profiling by microassay technology has been able to define distinct expression profiles of leukemias based on their genetic mutations. These profiles may in the future be able to uncover links between molecular subclass and clinical outcome that cannot be identified by standard cytogenetic analysis and clinical variables at present.

Receptor tyrosine kinase mutations (FLT 3 mutations) have been described in pediatric AML. FLT 3 is a receptor tyrosine kinase that is highly expressed on myeloid blasts. FLT 3 internal tandem duplications (FLT 3-ITD) have been identified in up to 16.5% of pediatric AML patients. Patients with FLT 3-ITD mutations have a poorer prognosis.

Future chemotherapy trials will attempt to study this mutation to identify poorer risk subgroups. FLT 3 tyrosine kinase inhibitors are in development and will be tested in AML.

Treatment of Newly Diagnosed AML

The general supportive treatment described under ALL should be employed in the management of AML. The intensification of the induction therapy in AML has led to

Table 14-19. Cytogenetic Abnormalities in Childhood Acute Myelogenous Leukemia (AML)[a]

Chromosome abnormality	AML French–American–British type	Affected genes	Functions	Frequency	Comments
t(8;21)(q22;q22)	M1, M2	ETO-AML1	Transcription factors	5–15%	Auer rods common; chloromas
t(15;17)(q22;q12)	M3, M3v	PML-RARA	Transcription factor; hormone receptor	6–15%	Coagulopathy; ATRA responsiveness
t(11;17)(q23;q21)	M3	PLZF-RARA	Transcription factor; hormone receptor	Rare	Coagulopathy; ATRA unresponsiveness
inv(16)(p13q22); t(16;16)(p13;q22)	M4Eo	MYH11-CBFB	Muscle protein; transcription factor	2–11%	CNS leukemia; eosinophilia with basophilic granules
t(8;16)(p11;p13)	M5b	MOZ-CBP	Transcription factors	1%	Infants or young adults; high WBC; chloromas; erythrophagocytosis; secondary leukemia after epipodophyllotoxins
t(9;11)(p22;q23)	M4, M5a	AF9-MLL	Homeodomain proteins	5–13%	Infants or young adults; high WBC; chloromas; erythrophagocytosis; secondary leukemia after epipodophyllotoxins
t(10;11)(p12;q23)	M5	AF10-MLL	Homeodomain proteins	Rare	Infants or young adults; high WBC; chloromas; erythrophagocytosis; secondary leukemia after epipodophyllotoxins

(Continues)

Table 14-19. (*Continued*)

Chromosome abnormality	AML French–American–British type	Affected genes	Functions	Frequency	Comments
t(11;17)(q23;q25)	M5	MLL-AF17	Homeodomain proteins	Rare	Infants or young adults; high WBC; chloromas; erythrophagocytosis; secondary leukemia after epipodophyllotoxins
t/del(11)(q23)[b]	M4, M5	MLL, other partners	Homeodomain proteins	2–10%	Infants; high WBC, CNS, and skin involvement; poor prognosis often associated with these, especially t(4;11)
t(1;22)(p13;q13)	M7	?	?	2–3%	M7 AML in infants with Down syndrome; myelofibrosis
t(6;9)(p23;q34)	M2, M4, MDS	DEK-CAN	Transcription factor; nuclear protein	<1%	Basophilia
inv(3)(q21q26)t(3;3)(q21;q26)	M2, M4, MDS	EV11	Transcription factor	<1%	Prior MDS; thrombocytosis and abnormal platelets
−7/del(7)(q22-q36)	All subtypes, MDS	?	?	2–7%	Toxic exposure; prior MDS; more common in other adults, bacterial infections common
−5/del(5)(q11-q35)	All subtypes, MDS	?	?	Rare	Toxic exposure; prior MDS; more common in older adults
+8	All subtypes	?	?	5–13%	Prior MDS; older patients

Abbreviations: ATRA, all-*trans*-retinoic acid; CNS, central nervous system; MDS, myelodysplastic syndrome; MLL, malignant lymphoma, lymphoblastic; WBC, white blood cell count.
[a]This table is not a complete list of all chromosomal abnormalities associated with childhood AML, but represents some of the more common abnormalities or those with important phenotypic characteristics.
[b]11q23 translocations involving the MLL gene have been shown to have many different fusion partners.
Adapted from Pizzo P, Poplack D. Principles and Practice of Pediatric Oncology. Vol 4. Philadelphia: Lippincott Williams and Wilkins, 2002.

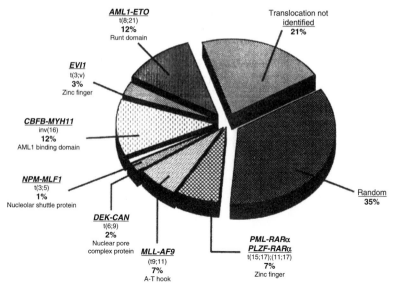

Fig. 14-4. Distributions of translocations in pediatric AML. (From Rubnitz JE, Look AT. Molecular genetics of childhood leukemia. J Pediatr Hematol Oncol 1998;20:1–11, with permission.)

an increased risk of sepsis and fungal infection. Rapid initiation of broad-spectrum intravenous antibiotics and possibly antifungal therapy is necessary for any febrile episodes while neutropenic. It has been suggested that newly diagnosed AML patients should remain hospitalized during induction therapy.

AML should be treated with intensive shortened therapy such as the DCTER regimen (Table 14-20) or MRC 10 (Table 14-21). The DCTER protocol results in a 75% remission rate and a 57% long-term survival. Patients receiving HLA-matched sibling donor allogeneic stem cell transplant have a 70% long-term survival.

The authors recommend that if a suitable family HLA-matched donor is available, all patients with AML, with the exception of the M3 subtype (acute promyelocytic leukemia) and Down syndrome patients, receive an allogeneic stem cell transplant in the first remission. In the absence of a suitable matched donor, patients should be treated with intensive chemotherapy.

Prognosis

Factors associated with poor prognosis in AML:

- WBC >100,000/mm^3
- Monosomy 7
- Secondary AML (see Chapter 13)
- FLT 3 ITD
- Minimal residual disease present after induction.

The MRC 10 protocol has produced a 48% event-free survival at 7 years. Factors associated with prognosis associated with the MRC 10 can be subdivided into:

1. Favorable karyotypes: t(8;21), t(15;17), inv 16—survival 72%
2. Intermediate karyotype: normal karyotype or karyotype that is abnormal but not in favorable or unfavorable group—survival 43%
3. Unfavorable karyotype: monosomy 5, monosomy 7, del (5q), and (3q) or other complex karyotypes—survival 17%.

Table 14-20. Intensive Shortened Therapy for Newly Diagnosed AML-DCTER Regimen

DCTER chemotherapy is administered on days 0–4 and on days 10–14 (cycle 1) regardless of bone marrow suppression following first course of DCTER.

↓

Days 0–4 and 10–14 DCTER induction [cycle 1]

Dexamethasone 6 mg/m^2/day (0.2 mg/kg/day) thrice daily for 4 days

Cytarabine 200 mg/m^2/day (6.7 mg/kg/day) continuous infusion for 4 days

Thioguanine 100 mg/m^2/day (3.3 mg/kg/day) twice daily for 4 days

Etoposide 100 mg/m^2/day (3.3 mg/kg/day) continuous infusion for 4 days

Rubidomycin (daunorubicin) 20 mg/m^2/day (0.67 mg/kg/day) continuous infusion for 4 days

Cytarabine intrathecal (age-based doses) on day 0 and 10 (0–1 year, 20 mg; 1–2 years, 30 mg; 2–3 years, 50 mg; >3 years, 70 mg)

After the two cycles of DCTER chemotherapy postremission therapy is administered as follows:

1. Conventional chemotherapy
   a. Course 1. Days 0–2 cytarabine, 3 g/m^2/dose (100 mg/kg) IV over 3 hours every 12 hours × 4 doses; L-asparaginase 6000 units/m^2 (200 units/kg) IM, hour 42. Days 7–9 cytarabine and L-asparaginase repeated exactly as administered days 0–2.
   b. Courses 2 and 3. Two 28-day cycles 6-thioguanine 75 mg/m^2 (2.5 mg/kg) PO daily, days 0–27; vincristine 1.5 mg/m^2 (0.05 mg/kg) IV, day 0; cytarabine 75 mg/m^2 (2.5 mg/kg) IV every day × 4, days 0–3; cyclophosphamide 75 mg/m^2 (2.5 mg/kg) IV every day × 4, days 0–3; 5-azacytidine 100 mg/m^2 (3.3 mg/kg) IV every day × 4, days 0–3.
   c. Course 4. Cytarabine 25 mg/m^2/dose (0.83 mg/kg) SC or IV every 6 hours × 5 days, days 0–4; daunomycin 30 mg/m^2 (1 mg/kg) IV, day 0; etoposide 150 mg/m^2 (5 mg/kg) IV/dose × 2, days 0 and 3; 6-thioguanine 50 mg/m^2/dose (1.67 mg/kg) PO every 12 hours × 5 days, days 0–4; dexamethasone 2 mg/m^2/dose (0.067 mg/kg) PO every 8 hours × 4 days, days 0–3.
2. Allogeneic HLA-matched donor stem cell transplant.

Notes: Doses in parentheses are used for children less than 3 years of age.

From Woods WG, Kobrinsky N, Buckley JD, et al. Timed-sequential induction therapy improves postremission outcome in acute myeloid leukemia: a report from the Children's Cancer Group. Blood 1996;87:4979–89, with permission.

Table 14-21. Therapy for Newly Diagnosed AML-Protocol (MRC 10)

Course 1	ADE	Daunorubicin 50 mg/m^2 IV days 1, 3, 5
		Cytosine arabinoside 100 mg/m^2 IV bolus every 12 hours days 1–10
		Etoposide 100 mg/m^2 IV (1-hour infusion) days 1–5
Course 2	ADE	Daunorubicin 50 mg/m^2 IV days 1, 3, 5
		Cytosine arabinoside 100 mg/m^2 IV bolus every 12 hours days 1–8 (16 doses)
		Etoposide 100 mg/m^2 IV (1-hour infusion) days 1–5
Course 3	MACE	Amsacrine 100 mg/m^2 IV (1-hour infusion) days 1–5
		Cytosine arabinoside 200 mg/m^2/d IV (continuous infusion) days 1–5
		Etoposide 100 mg/m^2 IV (1-hour infusion) days 1–5
Course 4	MidAC	Mitoxantrone 10 mg/m^2 IV (short infusion) days 1–5
		Cytosine arabinoside 1.0 gram/m^2 12-hourly IV (2 hour infusion) days 1–3

All doses are reduced by 25% for children less than 1 year of age.

Adapted from Stevens RF, Hann IM, Wheatley K, Gray RG. Marked improvement in outcome with chemotherapy alone in paediatric acute myeloid leukemia: results of the United Kingdom Medical Research Council's 10th AML trial. Br J Haematol 1998;101:130–40.

Treatment of Acute Promyelocytic Leukemia (APML) (Type M3) with *trans*-Retinoic Acid

The induction of remission of APML by *trans*-retinoic acid (ATRA) is associated with the differentiation of immature promyelocytes into mature granulocytes, followed by the restoration of normal hematopoiesis as the patient enters remission. Data in support of this mechanism include:

- The absence of bone marrow hypoplasia during induction with ATRA
- The persistence of Auer rods in morphologically mature granulocytes
- The persistence of t(15;17) in morphologically mature granulocytes
- The appearance of immunophenotypically unique intermediate cells that express both mature and immature cell surface antigens (CD33+, CD16+ cells), indicating their origin from leukemic promyelocytes.

Dose of *trans*-Retinoic Acid

Dose range: 10–100 mg/m^2/day.
Most commonly employed dose: 45 mg/m^2/day in a single or two equally divided doses
Time required to induce remission: 1–3 months (median time to remission, 44 days); resolution of APML-associated coagulopathy is frequently the first sign of response to ATRA
Range of duration of remission: 1–23 months (median duration of remission, 3–5 months).

The unique pharmacologic feature of ATRA leads to the resistance of APML cells to ATRA and, for this reason, ATRA is not useful as a maintenance agent in the therapy of APML. ATRA does not cross the blood–brain barrier. Therefore, ATRA is ineffective in the treatment of CNS involvement with APML.

Side Effects

The side effects of ATRA include skin dryness, itching, peeling, angular stomatitis, headache, pseudotumor cerebri, hypertriglyceridemia, and hypercholesterolemia. The following side effects occur only in patients with APML:

1. Fever
2. Hematologic
   a. Marked leukocytosis
   b. Thrombosis
3. Gastrointestinal: Hepatic liver enzymes and bilirubin level elevations
4. Cardiovascular
   a. Congestive heart failure
   b. Fluid overload
   c. Pericardial effusion
5. Pulmonary: Retinoic acid syndrome, which is characterized by respiratory distress, fever, pulmonary infiltrates radiographically, pleural effusion, weight gain, death due to progressive hypoxemia, and multiple-organ failure. Prompt treatment with dexamethasone (12 mg every 12 hours for 3 days) stops the progression of this syndrome.

Leukocytosis Following the Use of ATRA

ATRA treatment is associated with leukocytosis involving a count of 20,000/mm^3 or more leukocytes in 50% of patients with APML. The peripheral WBCs comprise myeloblasts, promyelocytes, intermediate cells (CD33+, CD16+ cells), and neutrophils. Nuclear shrinkage, nuclear elongation, and marked nuclear and cytoplasmic vacuolation characterize the granulocytic cells.

Management of Acute Promyelocytic Leukemia with ATRA

1. Treat with ATRA as described previously (45 mg/m^2/day in a single or equally divided doses).
2. Perform surveillance coagulation studies periodically and treat as follows:
   a. *Disseminated intravascular coagulation (DIC):* Treat with platelet and fresh frozen plasma transfusion to maintain a platelet count of $50,000/\text{mm}^2$ or more and a fibrinogen level of at least 100 mg/dL. Heparin is indicated for patients with marked or persistent elevation of fibrin degradation products.
   b. *Fibrinolysis:* The use of epsilon-aminocaproic acid is reserved for patients with life-threatening hemorrhages.
3. After the induction of remission with ATRA, the patient should be treated with three cycles of the cytosine arabinoside and anthracycline regimen commonly employed in the treatment of AML. Daunorubicin 60 mg/m^2/day IV bolus for 3 days and cytarabine 200 mg/m^2/day by continuous infusion IV for 7 days. This chemotherapy is repeated after hematologic recovery. After recovery then the second course is followed by daunorubicin 45 mg/m^2/day IV bolus for 3 days with cytarabine 1 g/m^2 every 12 hours for 4 days. Maintenance therapy consists of ATRA 45 mg/m^2/day for 15 days every 3 months and 6-mercaptopurine 90 mg/m^2/day and methotrexate 15 mg/m^2/week orally for 2 years.

Assessment of MRD

The use of reverse transcriptase polymerase chain reaction (RT-PCR) for detecting PML–RARα fusion transcripts may be helpful for the identification of patients with MRD, and it is possible that they may benefit from further antileukemic therapy.

Studies are now under way to investigate the use of arsenic as a differentiation inducer in APML.

Treatment of Refractory or Recurrent Acute Myeloblastic Leukemia

Treatment of these patients is difficult. However, induction of remission may be attempted with a high-dose Ara-C and L-asparaginase regimen (Table 14-22) or an intermediate-dose Ara-C, mitoxantrone, and etoposide regimen (Table 14-23). The reinduction protocol of Table 14-23 achieves a remission rate of 76% in relapsed or refractory AML.

Allogeneic stem cell transplantation should be carried out once a remission is attained. In the absence of a suitable matched donor, a search for a matched unre-

Table 14-22. High-Dose Ara-C Regimen (Capizzi Regimen)

Course 1
　Ara-C 3 g/m^2 IV over 3 hours every 12 hours × 4 doses followed by L-asparaginase
　　6000 units/m^2 IM 3 hours after the completion of the fourth dose of Ara-C. Decadron
　　eyedrops[a] every 4 hours beginning before, during, and 1 day after the Ara-C treatment.
Course 2
　Same as course 1, beginning on day 8. Decadron eyedrops every 4 hours as above.

　[a]To prevent severe conjunctivitis, which can cause pain and photophobia.

Table 14-23. Reinduction Protocol for Relapsed AML

Cytarabine (Ara-C) 1000 mg/m² as a 2-hour infusion every 12 hours for 4 days (8 doses) starting hour 0 day 0

Mitoxantrone 12 mg/m² as 1-hour infusion every 24 hours for 4 days beginning day 2 hour 11

Cytarabine (Ara-C) intrathecally on day 0 with age-adjusted doses

Decadron eyedrops every 4 hours during and for 48 hours after completion of cytosine arabinoside

Granulocyte colony-stimulating factor 5 µg/kg subcutaneously starting 24 hours after last dose of mitoxantrone

Adapted from Wells RJ, Adams MT, Alonzo TA, Arceci RJ, Buckley J, Whitlock JA. Mitoxantrone and cytarabine induction, high dose cytarabine and etoposide intensification for pediatric patients with relapsed or refractory acute myeloid leukemia: Children's Cancer Group study 2951. J Clin Oncol 2003;21:2940–7, with permission.

lated donor should be made. Use of a mismatched stem cell transplant may also need to be considered.

The prognosis of children with AML who fail to enter remission or relapse is very poor. Chemotherapy alone results in a less than 10% 1-year disease-free survival, whereas autologous or allogeneic stem cell transplant in second remission leads to a 30–50% long-term survival.

Monoclonal Antibody Targeted Therapy for AML

CD33 antigen is expressed on myelomonocytic precursor cells, monocytes, and most myeloid blasts and is absent from hematopoietic stem cells and nonhematopoietic tissues. Gemtuzumab ozogamicin (Mylotarg) is a new drug being used to treat AML. The drug is a humanized monoclonal antibody conjugated to an antitumor antibiotic calicheamicin. We have used gemtuzumab ozogamicin 6–9 mg/m² to induce remission in relapsed AML prior to allogeneic stem cell transplantation. Side effects are fever, chills, prolonged pancytopenia, abnormalities in liver function tests, and raised bilirubin. Veno-occlusive disease (VOD) of the liver has been seen in some patients treated with gemtuzumab ozogamicin. Care should be taken in allogeneic stem cell transplant of these patients because they have an increased risk of VOD. Ongoing trials are investigating the use of this agent in conjunction with chemotherapy for relapsed and newly diagnosed AML patients.

Acute Undifferentiated Leukemia Subtypes (M0)

In some patients with acute leukemia, assignment to a specific lineage is not possible because of the lack of lineage-associated antigens on the cell surface. These leukemias arise from clonal expansion of poorly differentiated hematopoietic cells and are referred to as acute undifferentiated leukemia (AUL). The prognosis for AUL is generally poor.

Acute Mixed-Lineage Leukemia (AMLL)

Acute mixed-lineage leukemia consists of:

1. Acute lymphoblastic leukemia expressing two or more myeloid-associated antigens (My⁺ALL)—6% of ALL cases
2. Acute myeloid leukemia expressing two or more lymphoid-associated antigens (Ly⁺AML)—17% of AML cases.

True AMLL displays the unequivocal features of more than one lineage on the same blast (as in acute biphenotypic leukemia) or separately on two populations of blasts (as in acute bilineal and acute biclonal leukemia). Bilineal leukemia may exist synchronously or develop metachronously. To distinguish bilineal metachronous leukemia as a result of spontaneous lineage switch, from therapy-induced second primary leukemia, the reappearance of the original clone must be demonstrated by the presence of identical cytogenetic abnormalities or identical gene rearrangements. Lineage switch from ALL to AML is observed more commonly than vice versa.

Therapy of AMLL should be initially based on the predominant cell population, either myeloid or lymphoid (see AML or ALL therapy earlier in this chapter) and then followed by therapy for the second lineage.

Leukemias that express a single marker of another lineage do not qualify for the mixed-lineage category.

Acute biphenotypic lymphoblastic leukemia exhibiting features of both T and B lineages has also been described (e.g., CD2+, CD19+ ALL, putatively originating from its normal [CD2+, CD19+] counterpart).

Congenital Leukemias

Leukemia diagnosed from birth to 6 weeks of age is defined as congenital leukemia. This is a rare disease. Its etiology is unknown. Congenital leukemia has been associated with:

- Trisomy 21
- Turner syndrome
- Mosaic trisomy 9
- Mosaic monosomy 7.

A few examples of congenital JMML have been reported.

Clinical Features

- Nodular skin infiltrates (bluish, fibroma-like tumors, leukemia cutis)
- Hepatosplenomegaly
- Lethargy, poor feeding, pallor
- Purpura/petechiae
- Respiratory distress.

Laboratory Studies

1. Usually monocytic subtype of ANLL
2. Occasionally ALL (pre-B immunophenotype).

Management

1. Congenital leukemia in Down syndrome or congenital leukemia with normal blast cell karyotype:
   a. Therapy should be withheld as long as possible, because spontaneous remission may occasionally occur.
   b. If disease progresses or hematologic or clinical condition deteriorates, appropriate chemotherapy should be administered.
2. Congenital leukemia with chromosomal anomalies in blast cells: This leukemia progresses clinically and hematologically and requires institution of therapy.

SUGGESTED READINGS

Areci RJ. Progress and controversies in the treatment of pediatric acute myelogenous leukemia. Curr Opin Hematol 2002;9:353–60.

Bostrom BC, Sensel MR, Sather HN, Gaynon PS, La MC, Johnston K, Erdmann GR, Gold S, Heerema NA, Hutchinson RJ, Provisor A, Trigg ME. Dexamethasone versus prednisone and daily oral versus weekly intravenous mercaptopurine for patients with standard risk acute lymphoblastic leukemia: a report from the Children's Cancer Group. Blood 2003;101:3809–3817.

Cavé H, Bosch JWDW, Suciu S, Guidal C, Waterkeyn C, Otten J, Bakkus M, Thelemans K, Grandchamp B, Vilmer E. Clinical significance of minimal residual disease in childhood ALL. N Engl J Med 1998;339:591–8.

Chessells JM. Relapsed lymphoblastic leukemia in children: a continuing challenge. Br J Haematol 1998;102:423–38.

Clark JJ, Smith FO, Arceci RJ. Update in childhood acute myeloid leukemia: recent developments in the molecular basis of disease and novel therapies. Curr Opin Hematol 2003;10:31–9.

de Boton S, Coiteux V, Chevret S, Rayon C, Vilmer E, et al. Outcome of childhood acute promyelocytic leukemia with all-*trans*-retinoic acid and chemotherapy. J Clin Oncol 2004;15;22(8):1404–12.

Gaynon PS, Qu RP, Chappell RJ, Willoughby RLN, Tubergen DG, Steinherz PG, Trigg ME. Survival after relapse in childhood acute lymphoblastic leukemia: impact of site and time to first relapse—the Children's Cancer Group experience. Cancer 1998;82:1387–95.

Gaynon PS, Trigg ME, Heerema NA, Sensel MG, Sathei HN, Hammond GD, Bleyer WA. Children's Cancer Group trials in childhood acute lymphoblastic leukemia: 1983–1995. Leukemia 2000;14:2223–33.

Goldberg JM, Silverman LB, Levy DE, Dalton VK, Gelber RD, Lehmann L, Cohen HJ, Salan SE, Asselin BL. Childhood T-cell acute lymphoblastic leukemia: the Dana Farber Cancer Institute. Acute lymphoblastic leukemia consortium experience. J Clin Oncol 2003;21:3616–22.

Golub TR, Areci RJ. Acute myelogenous leukemia. In: Pizzo PA, Poplack DG, editors. Principles and Practice of Pediatric Oncology. Philadelphia: Lippincott–Williams and Wilkin, 2002;545–90.

Harris RE, Sather HN, Feig SA. High dose cytosine arabinoside and L-asparaginase in refractory acute lymphoblastic leukemia: the Children's Cancer Group experience. Med Pediatr Oncol 1998;30:233–9.

Margolin JF, Poplack DG. Acute lymphoblastic leukemia. In: Pizzo PA, Poplack DG, editors. Principles and Practice of Pediatric Oncology. Philadelphia: Lippincott–Williams and Wilkin, 2002;489–544.

Nachman JB, Sather HN, Sensel MG, Trigg ME, Cherlow JM, Lukens JN, Wolff L, Uckun FM, Gaynon PS. Augmented post-induction therapy for children with high-risk acute lymphoblastic leukemia and a slow response to initial therapy. N Engl J Med 1998;338:1663–71.

Patte C, Auperin A, Michon J, Behrendt, H et al. The Societe Francaise d'Oncologie Pediatrique LMB89 protocol: highly effective multiagent chemotherapy tailored to the tumor burden and initial response in 561 unselected children with B cell lymphomas and L3 leukemia. Blood 2001;97:3370–9.

Pui CH. NCCN pediatric acute lymphoblastic leukemia practice guidelines. Oncology 1996;10:1787–94.

Pui CH, Gaynon PS, Boyett JM, Chesells JM, Baruchel A, Kamps W, Silverman LB, Biondi A, Harms DO, Vilmer E, Schrappe M, Camitta B. Outcome of treatment in childhood acute lymphoblastic leukemia with rearrangements of the 11q23 chromosomal region. Lancet 2002;359:1909–15.

Pui CH, Relling MV, Downing JR. Mechanisms of disease: acute lymphoblastic leukemia. N Engl J Med 2004;350:1535–48.

Ritchey AK, Pollock BH, Lauer SJ, Andejeski Y, Buchanan GR. Improved survival of children with isolated CNS relapse of acute lymphoblastic leukemia: a Pediatric Oncology Group Study. J Clin Oncol 1999;17:3745–52.

Rubnitz JE, Look AT. Molecular genetics of childhood leukemia. J Pediatr Hematol Oncol 1998;20:1–11.

Rubnitz JE, Pui CH. Recent advances in the treatment and understanding of childhood acute lymphoblastic leukemia. Cancer Treatment Rev 2003;29:31–44.

Sievers EL. Antibody-targeted chemotherapy of acute myeloid leukemia using gemtuzumab ozogamicin (Mylotarg). Blood Cells Mol Dis 2003;31:7–10.

Silvermann LB, Sallen SE. Newly diagnosed childhood acute lymphoblastic leukemia: update on prognostic factors and treatment. Curr Opin Hematol 2003;10:290–6.

Smith M, Arthur D, Camitta B, Carroll AJ, Crist W, Gaynon P, Gelber R, Heerema N, Korn EL, Link M, Murphy S, Pui CH, Pullen J, Reaman G, Sallan SE, Sather H, Shuster J, Simon R, Trigg M, Tubergen D, Uckun F, Ungerleider R. Uniform approach to risk classification and treatment assignment for children with acute lymphoblastic leukemia. J Clin Oncol 1996;14:18–24.

Steinherz PG, Redner A, Steinherz L, Meyers P, Tan C, Heller G. Development of a new intensive therapy for acute lymphoblastic leukemia in children at increased risk of early relapse. Cancer 1993;72:3120–30.

Stevens RF, Hahn IM, Wheatley K, Grayon RG. Marked improvements in outcome with chemotherapy alone in paediatric acute leukemia: results of the United Kingdom Medical Research Councils 10th AML trial. Br J Haematol 1998;101:130–40.

Vardiman JW, Harris NL, Brunning RD. The World Health Organization (WHO) classification of the myeloid neoplasms. Blood 2002;100:2292–2300.

Webb KH, Harison G, Stevens RF, Gibson BG, Hann IM, Wheatley K. Relationships between age at diagnosis, clinical features, and outcome of therapy in children treated in the Medical Research Council AML 10 and 12 trials for acute myeloid leukemia. Blood 2001;98:1714–20.

Wells RJ, Adams MT, Alonzo TA, Arceci RJ, Buckley J, Buxton AB, Dusenbery K, Gamis A, Masterson M, Vik T, Warkentin P, Whitlock JA. Mitoxanthrone cytarabine induction, high-dose cytarabine and etoposide intensification for pediatric patients with relapsed or refractory acute myeloid leukemia. Children's Oncology Study Group 2951. J Clin Oncol 2003;21:2940–7.

Wofford MM, Smith SD, Shuster JJ, Johnson W, Buchanan GR, Wharam MD, Richey AK, Rosen D, Haggard ME, Golembe BL, Rivera GK. Treatment of occult or late overt testicular relapse in children with acute lymphoblastic leukemia: a Pediatric Oncology Group study. J Clin Oncol 1992;10:624–30.

Woods WG, Kobrinsky N, Buckley JD, Lee JW, Sanders J, Neudorf S, Gold S, Barnard DR, DeSwarte J, Dusenbery K, Kalousek D, Arthur DC, Lange BJ. Timed-sequential induction therapy improves postremission outcome in acute myeloid leukemia: a report from the Children's Cancer Group. Blood 1996;87:4979–89.

Woods WG, Neudorf S, Gold S, Sanders J, Buckley JD, Barnard DR, Dusenbery K, DeSwarte J, Arthur DC, Lange BJ, Kobrinsby NL. A comparison of allogeneic bone marrow transplantation and aggressive chemotherapy in children with acute myeloid leukemia in remission: a report from the Children's Cancer Group. Blood 2001;97:56–61.

15

HODGKIN DISEASE

Hodgkin disease (HD) is characterized by progressive enlargement of the lymph nodes. It is considered unicentric in origin and has a predictable pattern of spread by extension to contiguous nodes.

ETIOLOGY AND EPIDEMIOLOGY

1. Cause unknown
2. Variation in incidence: 1–10 per 100,000 population
3. Bimodal age: incidence curve with one peak at 15–35 years of age and the other above 50 years of age
4. Sex ratio in children: 3:1 (males to females)
5. Incidence increased among consanguineous family members and among siblings of patients with HD
6. Immunologic disorders: HD is associated with systemic lupus erythematosus (SLE), rheumatoid arthritis, ataxia telangiectasia, and Swiss-type agammaglobulinemia
7. Association with Epstein–Barr virus (EBV).

ASSOCIATION OF EPSTEIN–BARR VIRUS WITH HODGKIN DISEASE

EBV has been associated with HD by epidemiologic and serologic studies. EBV has been detected in HD by Southern blotting. When the terminal repeats of EBV were analyzed, the infection was found to be monoclonal. Study of these tissues by *in situ* hybridization has shown that the EBV-positive cells are Reed–Sternberg cells and Hodgkin cells. Studies utilizing the polymerase chain reaction (PCR), with amplification of the internal repetitive fragment, also show that EBV genome fragments can be found in Reed–Sternberg cells in up to 58% of HD specimens, most commonly in the mixed cellularity and lymphocyte depletion and frequently with nodular sclerosis subtype of Hodgkin disease. Nodular lymphocyte predominance cases virtually never contain EBV in the lymphocytic and histiocytic cells. The EBV genome is temporarily stable because it can be found at diagnosis and in relapse. The identification of EBV in Reed–Sternberg cells might suggest a B-cell origin for HD. However, Reed–Sternberg cells can also have characteristics of T lymphocytes and interdigitating reticulum cells. Such evidence for the multilineage origin of the Reed–Sternberg cell may be explicable by postulating that the Reed–Sternberg cell is a hybridoma resulting from fusion of different cell lines, caused by a virus or other agents.

Age is also associated with EBV positivity in HD. Several studies have found an increased incidence in children less than 15 years with HD in both developed and developing countries. There is also an increased incidence of EBV positivity in cases in adults more than 50 years of age opposed to cases in patients between the ages of 15 and 50 years. EBV positivity appears to correlate with geographic, cultural, genetic, and/or socioeconomic influences, all of which are difficult to separate. Among persons from the United States, most parts of Europe, and Israel, approximately 40–50% of cases of HD have been shown to contain EBV-positive Reed–Sternberg cells. In contrast, among populations from less developed regions, particularly those with large numbers of cases of HD in children (e.g., populations from Central and South America, specifically in the Indian population from underdeveloped areas of Peru), a very high prevalence (about 94%) of EBV has been found in the Reed–Sternberg cells. The incidence of EBV positivity in the Reed–Sternberg cell in Kenyan HD patients is 92%. These results suggest that at least in Kenya, EBV may play a role similar to its role in endemic Burkitt lymphoma. Other countries with a very high prevalence of EBV positivity in HD include Iran and Greece (90% of children).

FAMILIAL HODGKIN DISEASE

Clustering of cases of HD within families or races may suggest a genetic predisposition to the disease or a common exposure to an etiologic agent. Analysis of familial HD kindred fails to reveal a germline mutation. However, studies of affected families have suggested an increased association of HD with specific HLA antigens. The concordance of HD in first-degree relatives (including siblings), particularly of the same gender, and in parent–child pairs has been noted in numerous reports. In families in which twins are concordant, the elevated risk of HD ranges from three-fold among first-degree relatives to sevenfold in siblings.

PATHOLOGY
Macroscopic Features

The spread of HD occurs mostly by contiguity from one chain of lymph nodes to another. Involvement of the left supraclavicular nodes often follows abdominal para-aortic node involvement, whereas involvement of the right supraclavicular nodes tends to be associated with mediastinal adenopathy. Para-aortic node involvement commonly occurs in association with involvement of the spleen, which in turn is commonly followed by liver or bone marrow involvement, or both. Nodular sclerosis of all histologic types shows the greatest propensity to spread by contiguity, whereas noncontiguous dissemination, when it occurs, is more than twice as frequent in the mixed cellularity and lymphocyte depletion histologic types.

Histopathology

The diagnosis of HD is based on the recognition of tumor giant cells (Reed–Sternberg cells) surrounded by benign-appearing host inflammatory cells composed singly or in a combination of lymphocytes, histiocytes, and granulocytes, including eosinophils, plasma cells, and fibroblasts. For purposes of diagnosis, tumor cells must have two or more nuclei or nuclear lobes and two or more large, inclusion-like nucleoli. Important exceptions to this rule apply to the categories of nodular sclerosing type and nodular variant lymphocyte predominance type in which peculiar variant forms of the tumor giant cells can be used to establish the diagnosis (lacunar cell variants). The histologic variants in HD are described in Table 15-1.

A revised European–American Classification of Lymphoid Neoplasms (REAL classification) has been proposed. In the REAL classification, HD is subdivided into

---

Table 15-1. Histopathologic Variants of Hodgkin Disease

Nodular lymphocyte predominance, with or without diffuse areas (LP)

A mixture of lymphocytes and histiocytes, particularly epithelioid histiocytes, is characteristic of nodular lymphocyte-predominant HD. Epithelioid histiocytes are preferentially found in the outer rim of nodular infiltrates. They are arranged in small groups or clusters, and well-formed granulomas may be present in rare cases. Eosinophils and neutrophils are rare. Plasma cells are not common and are seen only between follicles. The neoplastic cells of nodular lymphocyte predominance are the lymphocytic and histiocytic (L&H) cells (popcorn cells) usually found in and around the nodules. In diffuse areas, the L&H cells are still often arranged in a vaguely nodular pattern. Characteristically, L&H cells resemble centroblasts but are larger and have lobulated nuclei and small to moderate-sized basophilic nucleoli, often present and adjacent to the nuclear membrane. The cytoplasm is broad and only slightly basophilic. Ultrastructural studies demonstrate that L&H cells have the appearance of centroblasts of germinal centers. In addition, follicular dendritic cells characteristic of the B-cell follicle can be found in the vicinity of the L&H cells. Classic Hodgkin and Reed–Sternberg cells are few in number or completely lacking. In some cases, L&H cells may resemble lacunar cells because both cell types show irregularly shaped or lobulated nuclei, small nucleoli, and broad pale to slightly basophilic cytoplasm.

Nodular sclerosis (NS)

The nodular sclerosis subtype is characterized by collagenous bands and lacunar cells. The presence of one or more sclerotic bands is the defining feature. These bands usually radiate from a thickened lymph node capsule often following the course of a penetrating artery. These bands are composed of mature, laminated, relatively acellular collagen. They are birefringent in polarized light. In most cases, several broad collagenous bands can be identified, or fibrosis can be so extensive that isolated nodules of lymphoid tissue remain.

The collagenous bands of nodular sclerosis enclose nodules of lymphoid tissue containing variable numbers of Hodgkin cells and reactive infiltrates. Lacunar cells are the most common type of Hodgkin cells present and may be found in large numbers or in sheets. They tend to aggregate at the center of nodules, sometimes forming a rim around central areas of necrosis. Diagnostic Reed–Sternberg cells are usually not easily identified and may not be found in small biopsy specimens. Eosinophils and neutrophils are often numerous but histiocytes and plasma cells are usually less conspicuous.

Mixed cellularity (MC)

This intermediate subtype falls between lymphocyte-rich classical HD and lymphocyte depletion. The capsule is usually intact and of normal thickness. A vague nodularity may be present at low magnification, but the presence of any definite fibrous bands would warrant classification as nodular sclerosis rather than mixed cellularity. At high magnification, a heterogeneous mixture of Hodgkin cells, small lymphocytes, eosinophils, neutrophils, epithelioid and nonepithelioid cells, histiocytes, plasma cells, and fibroblasts is present. Diagnostic Reed–Sternberg cells and mononuclear variants are usually easy to find. Small foci of necrosis may be present, but the extent is much less than that seen in nodular sclerosis.

(Continues)

Table 15-1. (*Continued*)

Lymphocyte depletion (LD)

Lymphocyte-depletion HD encompasses two variants: diffuse fibrosis and reticular. The most characteristic features are a marked degree of reticulin fibrosis surrounding single cells along with lymphocyte depletion. In contrast to nodular sclerosis, this subtype is not characterized by the presence of thick fibrous bands, and the fibrosis envelops individual cells, not nodules of cells. Hodgkin cells are usually easily identified, but increased numbers of Hodgkin cells are not essential to the diagnosis. In the reticular variant, sheets of Hodgkin cells, often showing pleomorphic features, are found.

Lymphocyte-rich classical HD, nodular or diffuse

Many cases of lymphocyte-rich classical HD have a close resemblance to mixed cellularity HD, with a diffuse or vaguely nodular low-magnification appearance. Hodgkin and Reed–Sternberg cells are relatively rare, and the background is dominated by small mature lymphocytes. Eosinophils and neutrophils are usually restricted to blood vessels. Reed–Sternberg cells and variants are not easy to find but when encountered have identical features to the Hodgkin cells of mixed cellularity. Some cases of lymphocyte-rich HD may show a distinctly nodular appearance that may closely mimic nodular lymphocyte predominance HD and often contain relatively small germinal centers, with Hodgkin and Reed–Sternberg cells present in and near the mantle zone, a pattern that has been called *follicular* HD.

Unclassified Cases (UC)

UC is defined as histopathology that does not fit into a definite or provisional category (they may be T cell, B cell, or undefined; they may be borderline between HD and NHL).

---

lymphocyte-predominant, nodular (with or without diffuse areas), and the other forms of classical HD: nodular sclerosis, mixed cellularity, lymphocyte-depletion types, and lymphocyte-rich classic disease. Table 15-2 compares the REAL and Rye classifications. Lymphocyte-rich classic HD is a new subtype of HD (World Health Organization) in which the HD blast immunophenotypically resembles classic HD. A histopathologic classification depicting frequency by age is shown on Table 15-3. With modern treatment, the prognostic significance of these subtypes has diminished although the presenting characteristics and natural history remain significant, particularly for the nodular subtype of lymphocyte-predominant HD (see REAL classification in Table 15-2).

Immunophenotypic Features

Carl Sternberg in 1898 and Dorothy Reed in 1902, independently of each other, reported the cytologic features of the multinucleated giant cells, which have since

Table 15-2. Comparison of Revised European–American Classification (REAL) and Rye Classification of Hodgkin Disease

REAL classification	Rye classification	
Lymphocyte predominant, nodular (with or without diffuse)	Lymphocyte predominance, nodular Lymphocyte predominance, diffuse	} (5–15%)[a]
Classic Hodgkin disease	Nodular sclerosis (40–60%)	
Lymphocyte-rich classic disease	Mixed cellularity (15–30%)	
Nodular sclerosis	Lymphocyte depletion (<5%)	
Mixed cellularity		
Lymphocyte depletion		

[a]Parentheses indicate relative frequency of disease.

From DeVita VT Jr, Mauch PM, Harris NL. Hodgkin's disease. In: DeVita VT Jr, Hellman S, Rosenberg SA, editors. Cancer Principles and Practice of Oncology. Philadelphia: Lippincott–Raven, 1997:2242–83, with permission.

Table 15-3. Histopathologic Classification of Hodgkin Disease by Age Group

Age group	LP (%)	NS (%)	MC (%)	LD (%)	UC/IF (%)
<10 years	14	45	32	0	9
11–16 years	7	78	11	1	3
≥17 years	5	72	17	1	5

Abbreviations: LP, lymphocyte predominant; NS, nodular sclerosis; MC, mixed cellularity; LD, lymphocyte depletion; UC, unclassifiable Hodgkin disease; IF, interfollicular Hodgkin disease. From Donaldson SS, Link MP. Pediatr Clin North Am 1991;38:457–73, with permission.

been known as Reed–Sternberg cells. The mononucleated blasts have been designated as Hodgkin cells. In 1955, Lukes and Butler described a multilobated variant of the Hodgkin and Reed–Sternberg cells that occurs mainly in the nodular lymphocyte-predominant type of Hodgkin disease. These multilobated blasts were called lymphocytic and/or histiocytic (L&H) cells because in lymphocyte-predominant Hodgkin disease the cellular background consists of lymphocytes and histiocytes. The multilobated nuclear morphology of these cells causes them to be referred to as "popcorn cells."

Immunohistologic studies have shown that two distinct immunophenotypes of atypical blasts exist in HD (Table 15-4):

1. Immunophenotype I is characterized by the consistent expression of CD20 and J chain, and the constant absence of CD30 and CD15 with the presence of L&H cell (LPHD).
2. Immunophenotype II is characterized by the constant expression of CD30, frequent expression of CD15, and constant absence of J chain with presence of Reed–Sternberg and Hodgkin cells (classic Hodgkin disease).

Table 15-5 lists the immunophenotypic markers in HD compared with other lymphomas.

Table 15-4. The Two Immunophenotypes of Neoplastic Cells Encountered in Hodgkin Disease and Their Correlation with the Morphologically Distinct L&H Cell and Classic Hodgkin and Reed–Sternberg Cell Types

	Immunophenotype I lymphocyte-predominant Hodgkin disease	Immunophenotype II classic Hodgkin disease
Antigen		
J chain	+	−
CD20	+	−/+
CD79a	+	−/+
CD30	−	+
CD15	−	+/−
Cell type		
L&H	+	−
HRS	−	+

Abbreviations: CD, cluster of differentiation; L&H, lymphocytic and histiocytic; HRS, Hodgkin and Reed–Sternberg. Adapted from Stein H, Diehl V, Marafioti T, et al. The nature of Reed–Sternberg cells, lymphocytic and histiocytic cells and their molecular biology in Hodgkin disease. In: Mauch PM, Armitage JO, Diehl V, Hoppe RT, Weiss LM, eds. Hodgkin Disease. Philadelphia: Lippincott Williams & Wilkins, 1999:121, with permission.

Table 15-5. Immunophenotypic Markers in Various Lymphomas

	CD15	CD30	CD45	T cell	B cell	EMA
Hodgkin disease	±	+	−	∓	∓	−
Nodular, LPHD	−	±	+	−	+	±
Lymphomatoid papulosis[a]	±	+	+	+	−	−
Anaplastic (Ki-1) lymphomas	−	+	+	±	±	+
Immunoblastic lymphomas	−	∓	+	+	+	−

Abbreviations: CD-15, Leu-M1; CD-30, Ki-1 (Ber H2); CD-45, leukocyte common antigen; EMA, epithelial membrane antigen.

[a]Skin manifestation of systemic involvement in malignant lymphoma.

Cytogenetics of Hodgkin Disease

The results of single-cell PCR analysis of Reed–Sternberg cells suggest that most Reed–Sternberg cells are derived from germinal-center B cells with rearranged immunoglobulin genes. The absence of t(12:5) in Hodgkin disease is consistent with its derivation from B cells and supports the notion that it is different from anaplastic large-cell lymphoma, which is likely derived from cytotoxic T cells. The paucity of cases of Hodgkin disease with t(14:18) suggests a lack of relationship between HD and follicular center-cell lymphomas. This is consistent with the molecular evidence that reveals the presence of clonal crippling mutations in the immunoglobulin receptor in Reed–Sternberg cells, compared with somatic hypermutation in follicular center-cell lymphomas.

CLINICAL FEATURES
Lymphadenopathy (90% of All Cases)

- Painless swelling of one or more groups of superficial lymph nodes; rarely painful.
- Cervical nodes involved in 60–80% of cases; associated with mediastinal involvement in 60% of cases.
- Axillary, inguinal, and retroperitoneal nodes also frequently involved.
- Involved nodes are discrete, elastic, and usually "rubbery"; tenderness rare.
- The bulk of palpable lymph nodes is defined by the single largest dimension (in centimeters) of the single largest lymph node or conglomerate node mass in each region of involvement. A node or nodal mass ≥10 cm is defined as *bulky*. Abdominal nodal bulk is defined by the largest dimension of a single node or conglomerate nodal mass using computed tomography (CT), magnetic resonance imaging (MRI), or ultrasonography.

Figure 15-1 depicts the lymph node regions, and Table 15-6 lists the frequency of the initial involved sites in children with HD.

Mediastinal Adenopathy (60% of All Cases)

The term *mediastinal adenopathy* includes the following nodal subgroups:

- Prevascular, aortopulmonary
- Paratracheal, subcarinal
- Posterior mediastinal.

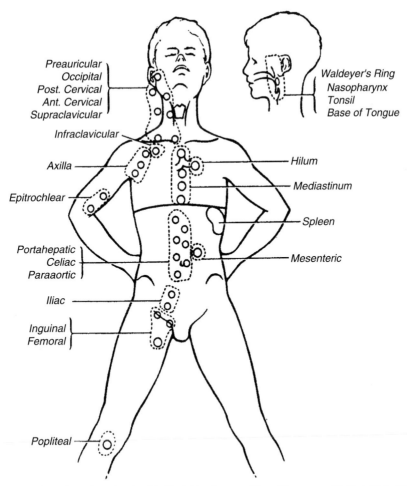

Fig. 15-1. Lymph node regions involved in Hodgkin disease. (From Thompson El. Hodgkin's disease. In: Fernbach DJ, Vietti TJ, editors. Clinical Pediatric Oncology. 4th ed. St. Louis: Mosby, 1991;355–75, with permission.)

A mediastinal mass is defined as bulky (*bulky mediastinal disease*) on a posteroanterior chest radiograph when the maximum width is equal to or greater than one third of the internal transverse diameter of the thorax at the level of the T5–6 interspace (mass/thoracic ratio ≥0.33). The chest radiograph should be taken with maximal inspiration in the upright position at a source–skin distance of 2 m. Relapse occurs more frequently in bulky mediastinal disease than in those with small masses. The principal sites of relapse are the margins of the radiation ports and adjacent organs.

The following nodes should be recorded separately:

- Hilar (bronchopulmonary) nodes are outside the mediastinum.
- Disease within the chest is usually in the anterior mediastinum (often at the site of thymus). The thymus may occasionally be the sole site of HD. This occurs as a variant of nodular sclerosing HD in younger patients.
- Internal mammary nodes are part of the lymphatic system of the chest wall and they drain the diaphragm.
- Paravertebral nodes, although in the posterior mediastinum, drain the chest wall and diaphragm.
- Anterior extension of a mediastinal mass into the sternum or chest wall or extension to lung or pericardium should be recorded as extranodal extension.

Table 15-6. Frequency of the Initial Sites of Involvement in Children with Hodgkin Disease

Site	Percentage
Neck (cervical, supraclavicular, occipital, preauricular)	76
Mediastinum	60
Spleen	26
Axilla–pectoral	24
Hilar	24
Para-aortic, celiac, splenic hilar	22
Lung	15
Iliac	7
Bone marrow	5
Inguinal–femoral	5
Infraclavicular	5
Pericardium	4
Pleura	2
Liver	2
Mesenteric	2
Bone	2
Popliteal	<1
Epitrochlear–brachial	<1
Thyroid	<1
Waldeyer's ring	<1
Pancreas	<1

From A survey of pediatric Hodgkin's disease at Stanford University: results of therapy and quality of survival. In: Malignant Lymphomas: Etiology, Immunology, Pathology, and Treatment. New York: Academic, 1982.

Clinical Presentation

- Persistent nonproductive cough; however, this site is often asymptomatic.
- Superior vena cava syndrome (enlargement of the vessels of the neck, hoarseness, dyspnea, and dysphagia).

Splenomegaly

- The spleen is commonly enlarged on physical examination or by ^{99m}Tc-sulfur colloid scan. However, its size is not indicative of splenic involvement with HD.
- In 13% of cases, the spleen is the only site of subdiaphragmatic disease. Spleen is involved in 26% of spleens resected in staging laparotomy. It is very important to determine splenic disease. On CT the accuracy of the "splenic index"* is only 59%. Fluorodeoxyglucose–positron emission tomography (FDG-PET) scan appears to be more sensitive (about 92% accuracy) in the identification of splenic HD.
- The frequency of splenic involvement correlates with the histopathologic type:
  Lymphocyte predominance—16%
  Nodular sclerosis—35%
  Mixed cellularity—59%
  Lymphocyte depletion—83%
- Both the para-aortic and splenic hilar nodes are involved in approximately 50% of patients with involved spleens.

---

*The splenic index is defined as the measurement of the spleen on CT scan. It is the product of the length × width × thickness of the spleen. If the splenic index (in cm³) exceeds 500 + 20 × age (in years) it is considered positive for splenic enlargement.

Systemic Symptoms (30% of All Cases)

- Intermittent fever (Pel–Ebstein), anorexia, fatigue, weakness, nausea, night sweats, and weight loss.
- Mild itching may be seen in 15–25% of patients with HD, although severe itching is less common. Pruritus is generally more common in patients with advanced-stage disease and frequently accompanies other systemic symptoms. Itching may be severe enough that excoriations are produced from scratching. Itching may be the first manifestation of HD. Patients with significant pruritus do have inferior overall survival and the importance of pruritus is similar to that of other B symptoms. Nonspecific therapy for itching is generally ineffective, although pruritus resolves when HD is successfully treated. Return of itching in treated patients may be the initial symptom of relapse.
- Alcohol-induced pain has been reported to occur in fewer than 5% of cases. The pain may begin within minutes of alcohol ingestion and usually occurs in areas of nodal enlargement. Pain may occur in the chest with radiation to the arms, back, and legs. The onset of alcohol-induced pain may precede the diagnosis of HD. The pain diminishes with treatment of HD and may recur before other signs or symptoms of relapse. The mechanism of alcohol-induced pain is unknown, but edema of lesions, vasodilation, and release of histamine have been proposed as causes.

Pulmonary Disease (17% of All Cases)

The mediastinal and hilar nodes are the pathway to the lungs for the spread of HD. Pulmonary HD does not occur without mediastinal or hilar disease. About two thirds of patients with HD have intrathoracic involvement. For this reason, lung CT scans should be carried out in patients with hilar or mediastinal adenopathy. There is a striking predilection of the nodular sclerosis type for mediastinal involvement. There are four forms of pulmonary involvement:

- Contiguous lesions
- Peribronchovascular disease
- Subpleural spread with plaque-like pleural thickening or effusion
- Intraparenchymal involvement, either nodular or alveolar in nature.

Uncommonly, these lesions may present radiographically as single or multiple cavitating lesions. The radiologic differential diagnosis in these cases is tuberculosis and fungal disease.

Pleural effusion occurs because of lymphatic obstruction in the mediastinum or hilum. Pleural invasion occurs but is relatively rare in comparison with its incidence in non-Hodgkin lymphoma.

Neurologic Manifestations

Neurologic dysfunction is usually a late manifestation. The disease can reach the nervous system in the following ways:

- Spread from paravertebral lymph nodes along nerve roots, blood vessels, or perineural lymphatics into the spinal canal by way of the intervertebral foramina and similarly into the intracranial region
- Hematogenous dissemination.

Involvement of the central neuroaxis is epidural and produces compression symptoms, which vary according to the area of the nervous system involved.

Intracranial disease may present with signs and symptoms of increased intracranial pressure or with hemiparesis, hemisensory defects, focal seizures, or occasionally papilledema. When the base of the brain is involved, there may be palsies of the cranial nerves.

Nonmetastatic neurologic complications may occur as a result of the following mechanisms:

- *Metabolic disorders:* These include hypercalcemia, hypoglycemia, hyponatremia, hepatic and renal failure, and pulmonary insufficiency.
- *Infections:*
  a. Herpes zoster is the most commonly encountered infection.
  b. Meningitis of bacterial, viral, fungal, or protozoal origin must be considered in every patient with headache, stiff neck, or unexplained fever. The most common causative organisms are *Cryptococcus, Listeria monocytogenes, Diplococcus pneumoniae, Toxoplasma gondii,* and varicella-zoster virus.
  c. Brain abscess is uncommon.
- *Chemotherapy-related neurotoxicity:* The most common of these occurs with vincristine, but steroids, procarbazine, and vinblastine may produce neurologic dysfunction as well.
- *Radiotherapy:* In about 5% of patients receiving treatment to the cervical, supraclavicular, and mediastinal region, a transient myelopathy (Lhermitte syndrome) develops. The incidence of this finding is reduced with the use of posterior cervical spine blocks. This is characterized by brief tingling and electric shock–like sensations down the back into the extremities on flexion or extension of the neck. This condition is not associated with motor dysfunction, and permanent myelopathy does not develop. A more serious complication of spinal radiation, radiation necrosis of the cord, occurs following dosages in excess of 4000 cGy over 4 weeks.

Paraneoplastic Manifestations Specific to Hodgkin Disease

These symptoms are usually associated with autoimmunity, and it is postulated that tumor cells express antigens that are similar to molecules on neurons. The following paraneoplastic neurologic manifestations of HD occur:

- Subacute cerebellar degeneration
- Limbic encephalitis
- Subacute necrotic myelopathy
- Subacute motor neuropathy
- Guillain–Barré syndrome and central pontine myelinolysis.

Bone Disease (2% of All Cases)

Osseous HD typically presents with bone pain, and the majority of patients have concurrent nonosseous lesions detected at staging. The radiographic features of osseous HD vary but indicate an aggressive malignant process. The histologic diagnosis may be problematic and immunohistochemical stains aid in establishing the diagnosis of HD in bone. Skeletal HD carries an ominous prognosis but survival of patients with osseous HD has improved in the last 10 years.

The major complication of vertebral involvement is spinal compression resulting from collapse of a vertebral body or from extension of the tumor into the epidural area.

Bone Marrow Involvement (5% of All Cases)

Symptomatic patients, particularly those with anemia, leukopenia, or thrombocytopenia, may have bone marrow involvement. Multiple biopsies are indicated, because HD tends to involve the marrow in a focal fashion. Choosing a site for bone marrow biopsy in such patients may be facilitated by MRI or bone marrow scintigraphy using [111]In. HD may mimic or be complicated by myelofibrosis, immune thrombocytopenic purpura, Coombs'-positive hemolytic anemia, or polycythemia.

Liver Disease (2% of All Cases)

Because the spleen appears to be the portal of entry into the liver, HD rarely affects the liver without concomitant splenic disease. Mild hepatomegaly, nonspecific abnormalities on liver scan, and abnormal liver function tests do not correlate with actual histologic involvement of the liver.

Liver biopsy is the only method for accurate diagnosis of liver involvement. To establish liver involvement, the following findings should be present:

- Evidence of discrete lesions that feature one of the histologic subtypes of HD
- Conclusive evidence of a Reed–Sternberg cell or one of its variants.

Nonspecific histologic findings are common and do not constitute evidence of invasion of the liver.

The presence of jaundice in patients is an ominous prognostic sign and may be terminal or preterminal. However, other possible causes of jaundice should be excluded (e.g., hemolytic anemia, viral hepatitis, toxic hepatitis, toxoplasmosis, and cholestasis of unknown etiology).

When jaundice is due to hepatic involvement, it is important to differentiate between parenchymal HD and obstruction of the porta hepatis by lymph nodes. In most instances, however, the jaundice is secondary to intrahepatic obstruction by portal peribiliary infiltration.

Cutaneous Manifestation

Cutaneous manifestations of HD may appear in several forms:

- Specific skin lesions: primary cutaneous HD
- Paraneoplastic lesions.

Cutaneous involvement of HD associated with nodal sites of disease occurs in 0.5–7.5% of cases. Skin involvement in these patients is felt to be caused by obstruction of regional lymphatics, direct extension from underlying nodes, or hematogenous dissemination. Lesions usually consist of erythematous nodules or papules. Dermal involvement of HD is often accompanied by extensive involvement at other sites and has been associated with a poor prognosis.

A large number of nonspecific erythematous, urticarial, vesicular, and bullous cutaneous manifestations of HD are true paraneoplastic phenomena, because they may be present at the time of diagnosis and remit with therapy. Reappearance of the lesions after treatment heralds relapse. The simultaneous appearance of skin lesions in association with HD may be secondary to cytokine secretion by tumor cells and is responsible for the development of cutaneous paraneoplastic syndromes.

Erythema nodosum consists of inflammatory nodules that appear most commonly on the anterior surface of the legs. These lesions are usually associated with infections, drugs, or inflammatory bowel disease, but they have also been described in association with HD and appear to respond to treatment for HD. The lesions may be seen several months before relapse and respond to chemotherapy.

Other skin lesions in HD include:

- Ichthyosiform atrophy of the skin
- Acrokeratosis paraneoplastica, a paraneoplastic dermatosis that responds to chemotherapy
- Granulomatous slack skin, which occurs in HD as well as in non-Hodgkin lymphoma.

All of these skin lesions are very uncommon in HD and especially in children with HD.

Renal Manifestations

HD may directly involve the kidney in 13% of cases. Renal involvement may be unilateral or bilateral and may be present as diffuse involvement, discrete nodules, or microscopic disease. Renal involvement with HD may result from ureteral obstruction, and patients with HD may also have renal dysfunction related to renal vein thrombosis, hypercalcemia, and hyperuricemia.

HD may be associated with glomerulonephritis. HD most commonly has minimal change disease. Membranous glomerulonephritis, focal glomerulosclerosis, membranoproliferative glomerulonephritis, proliferative glomerulonephritis, and crescentic glomerulonephritis have all been described in patients with HD.

Nephrotic syndrome generally occurs early in the course of disease, may predate the diagnosis of HD, uniformly remits with successful treatment of HD, and will often return in association with relapse of HD. Hodgkin disease and nephritic syndrome frequently have mixed-cellularity histology.

Hematologic Manifestations

- Myelosuppression in HD may be caused by hypersplenism or bone marrow infiltration. Bone marrow aplasia in patients with HD has been reported and may respond to therapy.
- A positive Coombs' test may or may not be associated with overt hemolysis. Patients with a positive Coombs' test frequently have advanced-stage disease and systemic symptoms. Cyclic hemolysis with exacerbations coinciding with Pel–Ebstein fever has been described.
- Immune thrombocytopenia may accompany HD in 1–2% of cases. Thrombocytopenia may develop before, concurrently with, or after the diagnosis of HD.
- Thrombotic thrombocytopenic purpura (TTP) has also been described in HD, and microangiopathic hemolytic anemia must be considered in any patient with thrombocytopenia.
- Autoimmune neutropenia has also been described in patients with HD. Neutropenia may occur before the diagnosis.
- Eosinophilia is frequently associated with HD. This occurs in 15% of patients. The presence of eosinophilia is not related to stage or histology. Interleukin-5 (IL-5) production by Reed–Sternberg cells may explain the etiology of eosinophilia accompanying HD.

Endocrine and Metabolic Manifestations

- The most common endocrine abnormality associated with HD is hypercalcemia. The incidence of hypercalcemia in HD ranges between 1% and 5%. Hypercalcemia is frequently associated with advanced stage and poor prognostic features. The etiology of hypercalcemia in HD appears related to altered 1,25-(OH)$_2$-D$_3$ (calcitriol) levels. Elevated calcitriol levels and hypercalcemia may be associated with relapse, and levels return to normal following chemotherapy. Infiltrating nonmalignant macrophages are the source of excess calcitriol. In some cases, hypercalcemia may be related to excess calcitriol. Hypercalcemia may be related to excess production of parathyroid hormone-related peptide, and normalization of calcium levels with indomethacin suggests that prostaglandin synthesis may play a role in hypercalcemia.

- The development of lactic acidosis at the time of HD relapse has been described. Chemotherapy resolves the metabolic abnormality. Other metabolic abnormalities associated with HD include the syndrome of inappropriate secretion of antidiuretic hormone.

Miscellaneous Abnormalities

- Patients with HD frequently have noncaseating granulomas in uninvolved tissues as well as in those containing lymphoma. This finding may be associated with improved survival. Granulomatous angiitis of the brain is a rare manifestation of HD.
- Polymyositis and scleroderma have been associated with HD. HD has been associated with aortitis and hypertension. Blood pressure normalizes when chemotherapy is initiated and then rises when HD recurs.

LABORATORY FEATURES
Hematologic Findings

1. *Anemia:* normocytic and normochromic in character
2. *Neutrophilia:* 50% of patients
3. *Eosinophilia:* 15% of patients
4. *Lymphocytopenia:* sign of advanced disease
5. *Bone marrow findings:* generally normal; focal or diffuse involvement of marrow may occur.

Biochemical Findings

Indices of active disease or extent of disease or prognosis of disease:

1. Elevated serum copper level. This is indicative of active HD, but serum copper levels are also elevated in infections, inflammatory disorders, pregnancy, and individuals on birth control pills.
2. Elevated serum ferritin and decreased serum transferrin levels. This is significantly associated with the advanced stages of HD.
3. Elevated sedimentation rate (ESR). This is also indicative of active HD and a persistently raised ESR is evidence of poor prognosis. ESR could also be elevated as a result of concomitant infectious or inflammatory disorders.
4. Elevated fibrinogen level.
5. Elevated haptoglobin level.
6. Elevated serum alkaline phosphatase level. This may indicate bone or liver involvement of HD. However, alkaline phosphatase is less useful in children because it is characteristically elevated as a function of active bone growth.

7. Elevated serum soluble interleukin-2 receptor (sIL-2R) level. A high level at diagnosis correlates with a higher risk of treatment failure.

8. Elevated β_2-macroglobulin (β_2 M): This correlates with tumor stage in patients with HD, and elevated levels predict a less favorable prognosis.

Immunologic Features

Cellular Immunity

Table 15-7 lists the immune profiles of patients with HD. Patients with HD, at presentation or in remission, exhibit a persistent defect in T-cell function. Natural killer cell–mediated cytotoxicity is depressed in untreated patients. The cellular immune defect appears to be the result of enhanced sensitivity to suppressor monocytes and T-suppressor cells, in addition to abnormal IL-2 production. Patients with advanced disease have an inherent T-lymphocyte defect. Reed–Sternberg cells function as antigen-presenting cells for mitogen-induced and mixed-lymphocyte T-cell proliferation. Immunologic parameters usually return toward normal with successful therapy of the disease, although abnormalities of T-cell function may persist for years. This deficiency of T cells has been postulated to be secondary to the production of cytokines by Hodgkin cells, which could render T cells unresponsive despite normal numbers. Table 15-8 lists the cytokines produced by Hodgkin cells and related clinical and pathologic features.

Humoral Immune Function

B-lymphocyte function is transiently reduced following treatment. It is important to immunize patients with pneumococcal vaccine and *Haemophilus influenzae* B (HIB) vaccine before splenectomy if splenectomy is going to be carried out, because, following splenectomy, normal immune response to these antigens is impaired.

Lymphocytopenia

Lymphocytopenia observed in patients with advanced HD results from depletion of both T and B lymphocytes.

Table 15-7. Immune Profiles in Hodgkin Disease

Activity	Untreated active disease	Disease-free survivors
Antigen-induced antibody production	Normal	Transiently depressed
Polymorphonuclear function		
Chemotaxis	Decreased	Decreased
Metabolic	Decreased	Decreased
Delayed-hypersensitivity skin tests		
Recall antigens	Anergic	Reactive
Neoantigens	Anergic	Anergic
E-rosette formation	Decreased	Decreased
Mitogen-induced T-cell proliferation	Decreased	Decreased
Mixed lymphocyte-induced proliferation		
Autologous	Decreased	Decreased
Allogeneic	Slightly decreased	Slightly decreased
Sensitivity to suppressor monocytes	Enhanced	Enhanced
Sensitivity to suppressor T cells	Enhanced	Enhanced
CD4/CD8 ratio	Slightly decreased	Decreased

From Slivnick DJ, Ellis TM, Nawrochi JF, Fisher RI. The impact of Hodgkin disease on the immune system. Semin Oncol 1990;17:673, with permission.

Table 15-8. Correlation of Clinical and Pathologic Presentation of Hodgkin Disease with Detection of Cytokines in Hodgkin Disease Tumors: Characteristic of a Tumor of Cytokine-Producing Cells

Clinical and pathologic features of HD	Cytokines
1. Constitutional "B" symptoms	TNF, LT- α, IL, IL-6
2. Polykaryon formation	IFN-γ, IL-4
3. Sclerosis	TGF-β, LIF, PDGF, IL-1, TNF
4. Acute-phase reactions	IL-1, IL-6, IL-11, LIF
5. Eosinophilia	IL-5, GM-CSF, IL-2, IL-3
6. Plasmacytosis	IL-6, IL-11
7. Mild thrombocytosis	IL-6, IL-11, LIF
8. T/H-RS cell interaction	IL-1, IL-2, IL-6, IL-7, IL-9, TNF, LT-α, CD30L, CD40L, B7 ligands (CD80 and CD86)
9. Immune deficiency	TGF-β, IL-10
10. Autocrine growth factors (?)	IL-6, IL-9, TNF, LT-α, CD30L, M-CSF
11. Increased alkaline phosphatase	M-CSF
12. Neutrophil accumulation/activation	IL-8, TNF, TGF-β

TNF, tumor necrosis factor; LT, lymphotoxin; IL, interleukin; IFN, interferon; PDGF, platelet-derived growth factor; TGF, transforming growth factor; LIF, leukemia inhibitory factor; GM-CSF, granulocyte macrophage colony-stimulating factor; T, T cells; H-RS, Hodgkin and Reed–Sternberg cells; M-CSF, macrophage colony-stimulating factor.

From Gross HJ, Kadin ME. Pharmacology of Hodgkin's Disease. Paris: Bailliere, 1996, with permission.

MANAGEMENT OF CRITICAL AIRWAY OBSTRUCTION IN A CHILD WITH A LARGE MEDIASTINAL MASS

Large mediastinal masses can result in the following:

1. Airway compression, causing dyspnea, which is aggravated in the supine position.
2. Encasement of the heart by a tumor, causing a hemodynamic effect similar to pericardial tamponade. The fixed, low cardiac output is aggravated by the following:
   a. Supine position (further compression by tumor)
   b. Straining at stool (Valsalva maneuver)
   c. Myocardial depressant effects of general anesthesia
   d. Induction of anesthesia, which may result in collapse of the trachea by the tumor and complete airway occlusion if the action of the voluntary respiratory muscles is paralyzed (decrease in intrathoracic negative pressure).

The preoperative assessment of patients with mediastinal masses, particularly those who are symptomatic (dyspnea, intolerance of supine position), should include studies to assess airway patency and cardiac status. These studies should include:

1. Chest radiograph, including posteroanterior and lateral views for evidence of airway compression. High-kilovolt-magnified radiographs of the airway and/or CT scans of the chest should be performed to assess the status of the patency of the trachea.
2. Chest CT.
3. Electrocardiogram (ECG).
4. Echocardiography.

5. Pulmonary function studies in upright and supine positions. If there is any evidence of cardiac or airway impairment, local anesthesia in the sitting position for cervical node biopsy should be carried out.

In children with large mediastinal masses in which general anesthesia is obligatory, endotracheal intubation or tracheostomy may not suffice to relieve the obstruction. In these cases, a system that will independently ventilate each lung beyond the sites of obstruction is needed.

STAGING

Table 15-9 outlines the modified Ann Arbor classification of HD, and Table 15-10 lists the investigations in HD.

Abdominal and pelvic CT are useful modalities to evaluate spread of the disease in the abdomen and pelvis including the retroperitoneum. The limitations of CT include:

- Difficulty in detecting splenic hilar, mesenteric, celiac, or porta hepatis lymph node disease, and because children, compared to adults, have little or no retroperitoneal fat there may be difficulty recognizing retroperitoneal lymph nodes.

Table 15-9. Modified Ann Arbor Classification of Hodgkin Disease

Stage	Description
I	Involvement of a single lymph node region (I) or of a single extralymphatic organ or site (IE) by direct extension
II	Involvement of two or more lymph node regions on the same side of the diaphragm (II) or localized involvement of an extralymphatic organ or site and of one or more lymph node regions on the same side of the diaphragm (II_E); optionally, the number of node regions involved is indicated by a subscript
III_1	Involvement of lymph node regions on both sides of the diaphragm (III); may or may not be accompanied by localized involvement of an extralymphatic organ or site (III_{SE}); abdominal disease is limited to the upper abdomen: spleen, splenic hilar node, celiac node, porta hepatis node
III_2	Involvement of lymph node regions on both sides of the diaphragm; abdominal disease includes para-aortic, mesenteric, iliac, or inguinal lymph node involvement with or without disease in the upper abdomen
III_3	Pelvic node involvement with or without any other abdominal disease
IV	Diffuse or disseminated involvement of one or more extralymphatic organs or tissues with or without associated lymph node enlargement; extralymphatic organs are defined as those other than lymph nodes, spleen, thymus, Waldeyer ring, appendix, and Peyer patches; liver or bone marrow involvement always indicates stage IV disease; biopsy—document involvement of stage IV sites is also denoted by letter suffixes: marrow, M+; lung, L+; liver, H+; pleura, P+; bone, O+; skin and subcutaneous tissue, D+

Subclassification
A: Denotes no specific symptoms
B: Denotes specific symptoms as follows:
    1. Unexplained body weight loss of more than 10% over a 6-month period
    2. Unexplained recurrent fever with temperature above 38°C
    3. Night sweats

From Carbone PP, Kaplan HS, Musshoff K, et al. Report of the Committee on Hodgkin's Disease Staging Classification. Cancer Res 1971;31:1860, with permission.

Table 15-10. Investigations in Hodgkin Disease

History: fever, night sweats, weight loss, pruritus

Physical examination: peripheral nodes, liver, spleen, bone tenderness, Waldeyer ring

Hematologic studies:

  Complete blood count

  Erythrocyte sedimentation rate

Biochemical studies:

  Liver function tests (serum glutamic-oxaloacetic transaminase, serum glutamic pyruvic transaminase, alkaline phosphatase, total protein/albumin, lactic dehydrogenase, bilirubin)

  Renal function studies (blood urea nitrogen, creatinine, serum electrolytes, urinalysis)

  Serum copper

  Fibrinogen

  Haptoglobin

  Immunoglobulins

  Serum ferritin and transferrin

  Serum β_2-macroglobulin

  Serum-soluble interleukin-2 receptor (sIL-2R)

  T_4/TSH

  LH/FSH

Immunologic evaluation:

  Absolute lymphocyte count

  T- and B-cell counts

  T-cell function studies

Anthropomorphic measurements and Tanner staging

Radiologic studies:

  Chest radiograph (posterior, anterior, and lateral)[a]

  CT scan—neck for soft tissue (in presence of high cervical node to evaluate Waldeyer ring involvement)

  CT scan—chest (with intravenous contrast) (special attention to thoracic inlet, axillae, and crura of diaphragm)

  CT of abdomen and pelvis (with oral and intravenous contrast)

  MRI of bones (if bone marrow or bony involvement suspected)

  CT or MRI of spine (if bony tenderness or symptoms of cord compression suspected)

  Bone scan (optional)

  Gallium scan (for all patients and specifically the cases with mediastinal mass)

  FDG-PET scan

  Ultrasound examination of abdomen (special attention to liver and spleen)

Exploratory laparotomy for surgical staging.[b] Rarely, if ever, required.

  Multiple lymph node biopsies—para-aortic, mesenteric, celiac, porta hepatis, pancreatic, splenic hilar, iliac

  Splenectomy

  Liver biopsy—needle and wedge (from both lobes)

Bone marrow biopsy (minimum two biopsies from each side of iliac bones)

Midline transposition of ovaries and oophoropexy (out of radiation port) in girls and young women if there is a possibility of future pelvic irradiation

---

[a]Radiograph should be taken with maximal inspiration in the upright position at a source–skin distance of 2 m.

[b]Bone marrow needle biopsy (from multiple sites, i.e., anterior and posterior both iliac bones) and percutaneous liver biopsy should be performed prior to surgical staging in patients suspected of having stage IV disease.

- CT reveals splenic disease, with only a 19% sensitivity. However, when the splenic index (SI) is utilized, accurate determination of splenic HD is about 59%. FDG-PET scans can identify splenic HD with 92% accuracy.
- MRI has limited value and is only useful in identifying nodes from loops of bowel when doubt exists on CT.

Radionuclide scanning with ^{67}Ga citrate provides true-positive data in only 40% of patients, with false-negative rates of 60% in patients, thus limiting its usefulness for assessing the subdiaphragmatic area in children.

Staging laparotomy is a major surgical procedure. Potential complications include wound infection, retroperitoneal hematoma, subphrenic abscess, pancreatitis, and acute pulmonary complications (e.g., atelectasis and pneumonia). Late complications such as adhesions, leading to intestinal obstruction, may occur even in those patients who do not receive abdominal radiation. The incidence is 3–12% in children.

When radiation alone is used, surgical staging is helpful to define subdiaphragmatic disease in anticipation of abdominopelvic radiation. When chemotherapy is used, either alone or in combination with radiation (which is the preferred mode of treatment of HD in most cases), the current trend is to rely on clinical staging because it has been shown that effective chemotherapy is sufficient to eradicate occult microfoci of subdiaphragmatic disease.

Surgical staging is no longer necessary because of the following:

- Increased use of systemic therapy in children.
- Advances in diagnostic imaging technology, which permit more accurate evaluation of retroperitoneal lymph nodes.
- Recognition of life-threatening sequelae, including overwhelming bacterial infections in asplenic children. Overwhelming sepsis with encapsulated bacteria occurs in 1–2% of patients with HD who have undergone splenectomy. The management of the splenectomized patient is described in Chapter 26.

For these reasons, surgical staging is rarely utilized today and in an ongoing Children's Oncology Group (COG) study, surgical staging is not recommended.

TREATMENT

Treatment of HD in children usually consists of combined modality treatment (CMT), consisting of chemotherapy and low-dose (20–25 Gy) involved field radiotherapy (IFRT) (Table 15-11). Standard chemotherapy in HD is six cycles of alternating MOPP (or MOPP derivatives) and ABVD (or ABVD derivatives) (see Tables 15-12 and 15-13). In selected patients, chemotherapy alone may be curative treatment. Non–cross-resistant chemotherapy alone without radiation therapy prevents:

- Radiation-induced growth complications
- Thyroid and cardiopulmonary dysfunction
- Solid tumor carcinogenesis (radiotherapy-induced secondary malignancies).

MOPP is the prototype alkylator combination that provided the first effective systemic therapy for HD. The alkylating agents in the regimen may cause secondary acute myeloid leukemia (s-AML) and infertility. Efforts to reduce the leukemogenic and gonadotoxic effects of MOPP have led to the development of MOPP derivatives that exclude mechlorethamine derivatives (Table 15-12). Mechlorethamine is a more potent leukemogen than cyclophosphamide as evidenced by the incidence of s-AML. Following MOPP-based therapy there is a 15-year cumulative incidence rate of 4–8% of s-AML compared with less than 1% after cyclophosphamide, vincristine, procarbazine, and prednisone-based therapy. Germ-cell function may also be preserved if treatment is limited to no more than three cycles of alkylating therapy.

The development of the ABVD combination provides a systemic therapy that produces superior disease-free survival compared with MOPP and is not associated with an excess risk of secondary leukemia or infertility. Treatment with bleomycin, however, is associated with an increased risk of pulmonary fibrosis and chronic

Table 15-11. Involved Field Regions

Mantle	Supradiaphragmatic disease involving mediastinum, as well as one or both cervical, supraclavicular, infraclavicular, or axillary lymph nodes
Minimantle	Bilateral supramediastinal disease involving cervical, supraclavicular, infraclavicular, or axillary lymph node chains
Hemiminimantle	Unilateral supramediastinal disease involving cervical, supraclavicular, infraclavicular, or axillary lymph node chains
Mediastinum	Disease in mediastinum, one or both hilar
Para-aortic-splenic hilar-spleen	Subdiaphragmatic disease in spleen, splenic hilar, or para-aortic areas
Spade[a]	Subdiaphragmatic disease in spleen, splenic hilar, para-aortic, and iliac areas
Pelvis	Disease in bilateral iliac and inguinal- femoral areas
Hemipelvis	Disease in unilateral iliac and inguinal-femoral areas
Inverted-Y	Subdiaphragmatic disease in spleen, splenic hilar, para-aortic, and pelvic areas

[a]Spade field: The para-aortic-splenic hilar-splenic field extends inferiorly beyond the bifurcation to include the common iliac nodes. The lateral borders should follow an oblique line from the lateral tip of each transverse process of L-5 to a point 1–2 cm lateral to the widest point of the pelvis.

From Hudson MM, Donaldson SS. Hodgkin's disease. In: Pizzo PA, Poplack DG, editors. Principles and Practice of Pediatric Oncology. 3rd ed. Philadelphia: Lippincott-Raven, 1997;523–43, with permission.

Table 15-12. Chemotherapy Regimens for Hodgkin Disease in Children

MOPP and derivatives

MOPP	Mechlorethamine, vincristine, procarbazine, prednisone
COPP	Cyclophosphamide, vincristine, procarbazine, prednisone
ChlVPP	Chlorambucil, vincristine, procarbazine, prednisone
CVPP	Cyclophosphamide, vinblastine, procarbazine, prednisone

ABVD and derivatives

ABVD	Doxorubicin, bleomycin, vincristine, dacarbazine
OPPA	Vincristine, procarbazine, prednisone, doxorubicin
VAMP	Vinblastine, doxorubicin, methotrexate, prednisone
DBVE	Doxorubicin, bleomycin, vincristine, etoposide
DBVE-PC	Doxorubicin, bleomycin, vincristine, etoposide, prednisone, cyclophosphamide

pneumonitis that may be enhanced by thoracic radiation. Cumulative bleomycin doses exceeding 400 U/m^2 produce the highest risk for developing pulmonary toxicity. In HD in children bleomycin in doses ranging from 60 to 100 U/m^2 commonly produces asymptomatic pulmonary restriction and diffusion deficits. Monitoring pulmonary function studies during therapy and withholding bleomycin in patients with significant declines in pulmonary function does not compromise disease control and may reduce the risk of further pulmonary injury. Several ABVD derivatives have been generated to reduce the risk of cardiopulmonary toxicities (Table 15-12).

Regimens containing etoposide with alkylating agents and anthracycline enhance treatment response. Treatment with etoposide and doxorubicin, however, is associated with s-AML but it differs from the features of alkylator-related s-AML. It is characterized by a shorter duration from the onset of the primary diagnosis, absence of a preceding myelodysplastic phase, monoblastic and myelomonoblastic histology, and

Table 15-13. Chemotherapy Regimens Used for Children with Hodgkin Disease

Drugs	Dosage	Route	Day(s)
MOPP			
Nitrogen mustard (mechlorethamine)	6 mg/m^2	IV	1, 8
Vincristine (Oncovin)	1.4 mg/m^2	IV	1, 8
Procarbazine	100 mg/m^2	PO	1–14
Prednisone	40 mg/m^2	PO	1–14
Repeat every 28 days			
ABVD			
Adriamycin (doxorubicin)	25 mg/m^2	IV	1, 15
Bleomycin	10 units/m^2	IV	1, 15
Vinblastine (Velban)	6 mg/m^2	IV	1, 15
Dacarbazine (DTIC)	375 mg/m^2	IV	1, 15
Repeat every 28 days			
MOPP/ABVD			
Alternating MOPP cycle with ABVD cycle			
MOPP/ABV hybrid			
Nitrogen mustard	6 mg/m^2	IV	1
Vincristine (Oncovin)	1.4 mg/m^2	IV	1
Procarbazine	100 mg/m^2	PO	1–7
Prednisone	40 mg/m^2	PO	1–14
Adriamycin	35 mg/m^2	IV	8
Bleomycin	10 units/m^2	IV	8
Vinblastine	6 mg/m^2	IV	8
Repeat every 28 days			
MVPP			
Nitrogen mustard	6 mg/m^2	IV	1, 8
Vinblastine	6 mg/m^2	IV	1, 8
Procarbazine	100 mg/m^2	PO	1–14
Prednisone	40 mg/m^2	PO	1–14
Repeat every 28 days			
MVOPP			
Nitrogen mustard	0.4 mg/kg	IV	1
Vinblastine	6 mg/m^2	IV	22, 29, 36
Vincristine (Oncovin)	1.4 mg/m^2	IV	1, 8, 15
Procarbazine	100 mg/m^2	PO	22–43
Prednisone	40 mg/m^2	PO	2–22, tapered 23–36, cycle One only
Repeat every 56 days ×3 courses			
COPP			
Cyclophosphamide	500–600 mg/m^2	IV	1, 8
Vincristine (Oncovin)	1.5 mg/m^2	IV	1, 8
Procarbazine	100 mg/m^2	PO	1–14
Prednisone	40 mg/m^2	PO	1–14
Repeat every 28 days			
COMP			
Methotrexate substituted for procarbazine in COPP	40 mg/m^2	IV	1, 8
ACOPP			
Adriamycin	20 mg/m^2	IV	1–3
Cyclophosphamide	1200 mg/m^2	IV	42
Vincristine (Oncovin)	1.5 mg/m^2	IV	14, 21, 28, 35
Procarbazine	50–100 mg/m^2	PO	13–42
Prednisone	30 mg/m^2	PO	14–42
Repeat every 8–9 weeks			

(Continues)

Table 15-13. (*Continued*)

OPPA

Vincristine (Oncovin)	1.5 mg/m²	IV	1, 8, 15
Procarbazine	100 mg/m²	PO	1–15
Prednisone	60 mg/m²	PO	1–15
Adriamycin	40 mg/m²	IV	1, 15
Repeat every 28 days			

OEPA

Vincristine	1.5 mg/m²	IV	1, 8, 15
Etoposide	125 mg/m²	IV	3–6
Prednisone	60 mg/m²	PO	1–15
Doxorubicin	40 mg/m²	IV	1, 15
Repeat every 28 days			

OPA

OPPA without procarbazine

COP/ABVD

C-Cyclophosphamide	200 mg/m²	IV	Weekly
O-Vincristine (Oncovin)	1.0 mg/m²	IV	Weekly
P-Procarbazine	100 mg/m²	PO	1–4
A-Adriamycin	25 mg/m²	IV	1, 15
B-Bleomycin	10 units/m²	IV	1, 15
V-Vinblastine	6 mg/m²	IV	1, 15
D-Dacarbazine	250 mg/m²	IV	1, 15
COP is given months 1, 3, 7, 9, and 11			
ABVD is given months 2, 6, 8, and 10			
CO is given months 4 and 5 with radiotherapy			

ChlVPP

Chlorambucil (Leukeran)	6 mg/m²	PO	1–14
Vinblastine	6 mg/m²	IV	1, 8
Procarbazine	100 mg/m²	PO	1–14
Prednisone	40 mg/m²	PO	1–14
Repeat every 28 days			

CVPP

Cyclophosphamide	600 mg/m²/day		1
Vinblastine	6 mg/m²/day		1
Procarbazine	100 mg/m²/day		1–14
Prednisone	40 mg/m²/day		1–14
Repeat every 28 days			

VAMP

Vinblastine	6 mg/m²/day		1 and 15
Adriamycin (doxorubicin)	25 mg/m²/day		1 and 15
Methotrexate	20 mg/m²/day		1 and 15
Prednisone	40 mg/m²/day		1–14
Repeat every 28 days			

translocations involving the *MLL* gene at chromosome band 11q23. Studies of childhood leukemia patients suggest a relationship between intermittent weekly or twice weekly dosing schedules of etoposide resulting in transforming mutations of myeloid progenitor cells. The risk of leukemogenesis after cumulative etoposide doses of 5 g/m² or less is not in excess of the risk associated with other agents used.

Modern therapy of HD can either be based on stage and response (stage and response–adapted therapy) or based on risk (risk-adapted therapy).

Stage and Response–Adapted Therapy

The Pediatric Oncology Group (POG) has recently completed two studies: one for *early-stage disease* (POG 9426) consisting of stages I, IIA and IIIA$_1$ and one for *advanced-stage disease* (POG 9425) consisting of stages IIB, IIIA$_2$, IIIB, IV, and bulk disease. These treatments employed fewer cycles of chemotherapy in a shorter period of time.

Early-Stage Disease (Table 15-14)

Doxorubin, bleomycin, vincristine, and etoposide (DBVE) are employed in 4-week cycles with granulocyte colony-stimulating factor (G-CSF) rescue. Following the initial two cycles of DBVE, the patients who have complete response (CR) and negative FDG-PET/gallium scans, receive only IFRT (25 Gy). After two cycles of DBVE, the patients who have only a partial response (PR) receive two more cycles of DBVE followed by IFRT (25 Gy).

Advanced-Stage Disease (Table 15-14)

Doxorubicin, bleomycin, vincristine, etoposide, prednisone, and cyclophosphamide (DBVE-PC) are employed with G-CSF rescue. After three cycles of DBVE-PC,

Table 15-14. Stage and Response Adapted Therapy

Drugs	Dosage	Route	Day(s)
		Early-Stage DBVE	
D: Doxorubicin	25 mg/m^2	IV	1, 15
B: Bleomycin	10 units/m^2	IV	1, 15
V: Vincristine	1.5 mg/m^2	IV	1, 15
E: Etoposide	100 mg/m^2	IV	1–5
G-CSF	5 µg/kg/day, SC from day 6 (24–36 hours after fifth dose of etoposide) until day 13; G-CSF is not administered on days 14 and 15 and restarted on day 16 until myeloid recovery occurs.		

DBVE is repeated after a 4-week interval.
After two courses of DBVE, patients in CR receive IFRT (25 Gy), whereas those in PR receive two additional courses of DBVE followed by IFRT (25 Gy).

		Advanced-Stage DBVE-PC	
D: Doxorubicin	30 mg/m^2	IV	1, 2
B: Bleomycin	10 units/m^2	IV	1, 8
V: Vincristine	1.4 mg/m^{2a}	IV	1, 8
E: Etoposide	75 mg/m^2	IV	1–5
P: Prednisone	40 mg/m^2	PO	1–10
C: Cyclophosphamide	800 mg/m^2	IV	1
G-CSF	5 µg/kg/day SC from day 6 until myeloid recovery; G-CSF is not administered on day 8 and restarted on day 9 until myeloid recovery.		

After three courses of DBVE-PC, patients in CR receive IFRT (21 Gy) and those in PR receive two additional courses of DBVE followed by IFRT (21 Gy).

Abbreviations: CR, complete response (disappearance of all clinical and imaging evidence of active disease; patients must be free of any symptoms related to disease); PR, partial response; IFRT, involved field radiation therapy.
[a]Maximum dose, 2.8 mg.

patients who have CR and negative FDG-PET/gallium scans receive only IFRT (21 Gy). After three cycles of DBVE-PC, patients who have only PR receive two more cycles of DBVE-PC followed by IFRT (21 Gy).

In the early-stage disease, the overall 3-year event-free survival (EFS) and survival rates are 88.8% and 97.6%, respectively. In the advanced stage, the overall 3-year EFS and survival rates are 86.5% and 92.5%, respectively. Zinecard (dexrazoxane), a possible cardiopulmonary protective agent, is associated with severe mucositis and an increased rate of secondary malignancies. For these reasons it is not recommended.

Risk-Adapted Therapy

Treatment for children and adolescents with HD may also be based on a risk-adapted approach that considers presenting features at diagnosis. The parameters considered in the risk assessment include:

- Presence of B symptoms
- Mediastinal and peripheral lymph node bulk (see pages 458–459).
- Extranodal extension of disease to contiguous structures
- Number of involved nodal regions
- Ann Arbor stage.

Low Risk

Low risk is defined as localized (stage I and II) nodal involvement without B symptoms and nodal bulk.

Intermediate Risk

Intermediate risk is defined as localized (stage IA and IIA) disease that has one or more unfavorable features and patients with stage IIIA disease. The criteria for unfavorable clinical presentation include:

- Presence of B symptoms
- Bulky lymphadenopathy
- Hilar lymphadenopathy
- Involvement of three to four or more nodal regions
- Extranodal extension to contiguous structures.

High Risk

High risk is defined as advanced-stage disease (stages IIIB and IV).

Treatment for Low-Risk Patients

Patients with low-risk disease are treated the same as those with early-stage disease (DBVE) (Table 15-14).

Chemotherapy alone appears to be an effective treatment for a low-risk and early-stage (IA and IIA) pediatric HD. The Multicenter German-Austria Pediatric Non-Randomized (GPOH) HD95 trial showed good results in low-risk patients who are in CR after two cycles (8 weeks) of OPPA (vincristine, prednisone, procarbazine, and Adriamycin) for females and OEPA (vincristine, etoposide, prednisone, and Adriamycin) for males (Table 15-13). Once a patient achieves CR, he or she receives two further courses (for a total of four courses) and no radiation therapy.

The COG is presently investigating the treatment of children and adolescents with newly diagnosed low-risk HD with three cycles of AVPC (Adriamycin, vincristine, prednisone, and cyclophosphamide) chemotherapy without radiation therapy. This therapeutic regime is aimed at reducing long-term toxicity.

Treatment for Intermediate-Risk Patients

The most effective chemotherapy strategies for children and adolescents with inter-mediate- or high-risk presentations include combinations derived from both ABVD and MOPP (Table 15-12). Low-dose radiation in most regimens has proven success-ful with long-term follow-up.

An ongoing COG study (AHOD0031) is evaluating a regimen of ABVE-PC (Adriamycin, bleomycin, vincristine, etoposide, prednisone, and cyclophosphamide) in the treatment of intermediate-risk HD (Table 15-15). This protocol combines dose

Table 15-15. Dose-Intensive Response-Based Treatment for Intermediate-Risk Children and Adolescents with Hodgkin Disease

ABVE-PC (2 courses)
   Evaluation with CT scan and FDG-PET/gallium scans and depending on response patient
    is assigned to rapid early response (RER) or slow early response (SER).

Rapid early response (RER) ABVE-PC (2 courses)
   CR: IFRT (21 Gy) or no RT[a]
   PR: IFRT

Slow early response (SER)
   Standard arm: ABVE-PC (2 courses) + IFRT (21 Gy)[b]
               or
   Augmented arm: DECA (2 courses) + ABVE-PC (2 courses) + IFRT (21 Gy)[b]

		ABVE-PC	
A: Doxorubicin	25 mg/m^2/day	IV	Days 1 and 2
B: Bleomycin	5 units/m^2/day	IV	Day 1
Bleomycin	10 units/m^2/day	IV	Day 8
V: Vincristine	1.4 mg/m^2/day	IV	Days 1 and 8
E: Etoposide	125 mg/m^2/day	IV	Days 1, 2, and 3
P: Prednisone	40 mg/m^2/day		Days 1–7
C: Cyclophosphamide	800 mg/m^2/day		Day 1
G-CSF		5 μg/kg/day subcutaneously 24 hours after etoposide and continuing until ANC >1500/mm^3 post nadir (do not administer on day 8)	
		DECA	
D: Dexamethasone	10 mg/m^2/day	IV	Days 1 and 2
E: Etoposide	100 mg/m^2/day	IV	Days 1 and 2
C: Cytarabine	3000 mg/m^2/day	IV	Days 1 and 2
A: Cis-platin	90 mg/m^2/day	IV	Day 1
G-CSF		5 μg/kg/day subcutaneously to start day 3 and to continue until ANC >1500/mm^3 post nadir.	

   Abbreviations: RER, rapid early response: at least 60% reduction in the sum of the products of the perpen-dicular diameters (SPPD) of measurable disease with negative FDG-PET/gallium scan, after 2 cycles of ABVE-PC. CR, complete response: at least 80% regression in their SPPD after 4 cycles of ABVE-PC. PR, <80% regression in their SPPD after 4 cycles of ABVE-PC. SER, slow early response: <60% reduction in SPPD after 2 cycles of ABVE-PC.
   [a]The benefit of IFRT in RER in CR has not yet been determined.
   [b]Optimum regime for SER has not yet been determined.

intensity with response-based augmentation and reduction in therapy to improve the outcome for all intermediate-risk pediatric patients with HD and decrease the risk of delayed effects of treatment.

The standard arm for this protocol is two cycles of ABVE-PC, followed by an evaluation with CT and FDG-PET/gallium scans to determine if the patient is a rapid early responder (RER) or slow early responder (SER). Rapid early responders then continue to complete two further cycles of chemotherapy (for a total of four cycles) and receive IFRT (ongoing study randomizes IFRT or no RT). SERs are randomized to the standard arm, or the augmented therapy arm (Table 15-15).

Treatment for High-Risk Patients

Treatment for high-risk patients is the same as that for intermediate-risk patients, but all patients receive IFRT (21 Gy).

Lymphocyte-Predominant Hodgkin Disease

Lymphocyte-predominant Hodgkin disease (LPHD) is a relatively uncommon histologic subtype of HD. LPHD appears to be distinct from classical HD with regard to clinical and biological features. Most patients present with localized disease (stage I or II) without B symptoms. Patients with LPHD generally have an excellent prognosis when treated on protocols for HD that include chemotherapy and/or radiation therapy. However, conventional treatment for HD exposes patients with LPHD to the risk of late effects including second malignant neoplasms as well as cardiac, pulmonary, and endocrine toxicity. There are reports in the literature of patients with LPHD who have been treated with surgery alone; some relapsed and received chemotherapy with or without radiotherapy, while others had no evidence of recurrence with long-term follow-up. The following approach for treatment of LPHD is suggested:

Stage I LPHD may be treated with complete surgical resection alone with long-term observation. At the time of recurrence patients should be treated with four cycles of chemotherapy that contains no alkylating agents as in VAMP (vinblastine, doxorubicin, methotrexate, prednisone) chemotherapy (Table 15-13) with or without low-dose IFRT (21 Gy).

Stage I that is not completely resected and stage II LPHD should be treated with four cycles of chemotherapy as in VAMP with or without low-dose IFRT (21 Gy).

Advanced-stage LPHD patients should be treated like other HD patients with advanced-stage disease.

PROGNOSIS

Combined modality therapy (CMT), that is, chemotherapy and radiotherapy, will result in cure of up to 90% of patients with HD. About 10–20% of patients with advanced-stage HD may relapse after treatment. Table 15-16 summarizes the treatment results in children with early-stage HD (stages I, IIA, IIIA, and no bulky mediastinal disease), and Table 15-17 lists the treatment results in children with advanced-stage HD (stages IIB, IIIB, IV, and bulky mediastinal disease) attained prior to the present-day approach to the treatment of HD, which has been designed to reduce long-term toxicity.

Table 15-16. Treatment Results in Children with Early-Stage Hodgkin Disease

Group/institution	Number of patients	Stage	Therapy RT	Therapy CT	Percentage survival Overall	Percentage survival RF	Follow-up interval (year)
Radiotherapy alone (full-dose IF or EF)							
Children's Hospital of Philadelphia	31	PS IA, IIA	EF		83	64	10
Joint Center/Harvard	50	PS I, IIA	EF		97	82	11
St. Bartholomew's/Great Ormond Street	28	CS[a] I, II	IF		96	79	10
Stanford University	48	PS[b] I, II	EF		86	82	10
Intergroup Hodgkin's Study	39	PS I, II	IF		95	41	5
	58	PS I, II	EF		96	67	5
University of Toronto	23	CS/PS I	IF[c]		95	87	10
	42	PS IIA, IIIA	EF		85	45	10
Full-dose RT and chemotherapy							
Hospital Saint-Louis	52	CS I, II	IF	MOPP×3–6	94	88	10
Intergroup Hodgkin's Study	97	PS I, II	IF	MOPP×6	90	95	5
St. Bartholomew's/Great Ormond Street	39	CS[a] I, II	IF	ChlVPP or MOPP or MVPP×3–8	86	84	10
German (DAL)							
HD78	73	PS I–IIA	EF	OPPA×2	97	90	10
HD82	100	CS/PS I, IIA	IF	OPPA×2	100	96	12
HD85	53	CS/PS I, IIA	IF	OPA×2	98	85	5
Low-dose RT and chemotherapy							
Stanford University	27	PS I, II		MOPP×6	100	96	10
University of Toronto	44	CS/PS I, II, III		MOPP×3/ABVD×3	100	100	10
	27	CS II, III		MOPP×6	93	89	10
Children's Hospital of Philadelphia	30	CS I, II		COPP×6 or ABVD×6 or MOPP×3/ABVD×3	90	68	10

	No. of patients	CS/PS	RT field	Chemotherapy			
German (DAL)							
HD87	104	CS/PS I–IIA	IF[a]	OPA×2	99	85	5
HD90	115 (female)	CS IA, IIA	IF[a]	OPPA×2		96	5
	159 (male)	CS IA, IIA	IF[a]	OEPA×2		93	5
Italian Multicenter Study	58	CS IA, IIA	IF	ABVD×3	·	95	7
French National Study	67	CS IA, IIA	IF	MOPP×2 ABVD×2		[a]	6
	65	CS IA, IIA	IF[a]	ABVD×4		[c]	6
	133	CS I, II	IF[a]	VBVP×4±OPPA×2	96	92	3
St. Jude Children's Research Hospital	28	CS I–IIB	IF	COP(P)×4–5 or ABVD×3–4	96	96	5
Chemotherapy alone							
Uganda	38	CS I–II		MOPP×6	100	100	5
Australia/New Zealand	38	CS IA–IIIA		MOPP×6 ChIVPP×608	94	92	4
Costa Rica	52	CS IA–IIIA		CVPP×6	100	90	5

Abbreviations: RT, radiotherapy; CT, chemotherapy; RF, relapse free; PS, pathologic stage; CS, clinical stage: full-dose radiotherapy, minimum dose to any nodal field ≥30 Gy; low dose to any nodal field ≤25.5 Gy; IF, involved field; EF, extended field; MOPP, nitrogen mustard, vincristine, procarbazine, prednisone; ChlVPP, chlorambucil, vincristine, prednisone, procarbazine; MVPP, nitrogen mustard, vinblastine, procarbazine, prednisone; OPPA, vincristine, procarbazine, prednisone, doxorubicin; OPA, vincristine, prednisone, doxorubicin; COPP, cyclophosphamide, vincristine, procarbazine, prednisone; ABVD, Adriamycin, bleomycin, vinblastine, dacarbazine; OEPA, vincristine, etoposide, prednisone, doxorubicin; VBVP, vinblastine, bleomycin, vincristine, prednisone; CVPP, cyclophosphamide, vinblastine, procarbazine, prednisone.

[a]Some patients pathologically staged.
[b]Some patients clinically staged.
[c]Some patients received chemotherapy.
[d]Boost to 35–40 Gy allowed.
[e]The relapse-free survival was 89% for both therapy regimens combined.

From Constine LZ, Quazi R, Rubin P. Rubin P. Malignant lymphomas. In: Rubin P, McDonald S, Quazi R, editors. Clinical Oncology: A Multidisciplinary Approach for Physicians and Students. Philadelphia: WB Saunders, 1993:217–50, with permission.

479

Table 15-17. Treatment Results in Advanced-Stage Hodgkin Disease

Stage	Chemotherapy	Radiotherapy	Number	Survival (%) Overall	DF (year)
CS IIB, IIA₂, IIIB, IV	4 MOPP/4 ABVD	None	80	94	78 (6)
CS IIB, IIA₂, IIIB, IV	4 MOPP/4 ABVD	21 Gy, IF	70	88	78 (6)
CS IIIB, IV	6 CVPP/6 EBO	None	24	81	60 (5)
CS I, II (M/T ≥0.33), III, IV	6 VEPA	15–25 Gy, IF	56	62	61 (N/A)
CS/PS IV	3 MOPP/3 ABVD	15–25 Gy, IF	13	85	69 (10)
CS IIA_E, IIB, IIIA	2 OPPA/2 COPP (F)	25 Gy, IF	N/A	100	91 (3)
	2 OEPA/2 COPP (M)	25 Gy, IF	N/A	98	84 (3)
CS IIB_E, IIA_E, IIIB, IV	2 OPPA/2 COPP (F)	20 Gy, IF	N/A	100	91 (3)
	2 OEPA/4 COPP (M)	20 Gy, IF	N/A	98	84 (3)
PS/CS IIB_E, IIIA_E, IIIB, IV	2 OPPA/4 COPP	20–36 Gy, IF	65	94	82 (5)
CS III/IV	4–5 COP(P)/3–4 ABVD	20 Gy, IF	57	93	93 (5)
CS IIIB, IV	5 MOPP/5 ABVD	20–25 Gy, EF	38	N/A	60 (N/A)
CS III	3 ABVD/3 MOPP	20–40 Gy, EF	40	N/A	82 (6)
CS IV	3 ABVD/3 MOPP	20–40 Gy, EF	21	N/A	62 (6)
PS/CS IIB_E, IIIA_E, IIIB, IV	2 OPPA/4 COPP	25 Gy, IF	50	N/A	88 (4.5)
	2 OPA/4 COMP	25 Gy, IF	N/A	100	54 (4.5)
PS/CS IIA_E, IIB, IIIA	2 OPPA/2 COPP	30 Gy, IF	53	N/A	94 (9)
	2 OPA/2 COMP	30 Gy, IF	N/A	N/A	55 (9)
PS III, IV	4 MOPP/4 ABVD	21 Gy, TN	62	95	77 (3)
CS IV	6 MOPP	25–35 Gy, EF	15	80	82 (5)
PS III, IV	12 ABVD	21 Gy, R	65	89	87 (3)
CS I–II, III, IV	6–8 MOPP or 6 CHlVPP	None	53	94	92 (4)
PS III, IV	6 MOPP	15–25 Gy, IF	28	78	84 (5)

Abbreviations: EF, extended field; IF, involved field; R, regional; TN, total nodal; CVPP, cyclophosphamide, vinblastine, procarbazine, prednisone; EBO, epirubicin, bleomycin, vincristine (Oncovin); OEPA, vincristine (Oncovin), etoposide, prednisone, doxorubicin (Adriamycin); VEPA, vinblastine, etoposide, prednisone, doxorubicin (Adriamycin); ChlVPP, chlorambucil, vinblastine, procarbazine, prednisone; treatment described in Table 15-13; other chemotherapy; F, female; M, male; N/A, not available; DF, disease free; CS, clinical staging; PS, pathological staging.

From Hudson MM, Donaldson SS. Hodgkin's disease. In: Pizzo PA, Poplack DG, editors. Principles and Practice of Pediatric Oncology. 3rd ed. Philadelphia: Lippincott–Raven, 1997:523–43, with permission.

RELAPSED DISEASE

Most relapses in patients with HD occur within the first 3 years, although some patients relapse as long as 10 years after their initial diagnosis. There is a significant salvage rate in patients who relapse after initial therapy. Progression of disease during induction therapy and/or within 12 months of completion of treatment results in a very poor prognosis. The 5-year EFS is less than 20%. Patients who relapse more than 12 months after initial treatment can be salvaged with conventional chemotherapy with an overall survival rate of 20–50%. Numerous conventional salvage chemotherapy regimens (Table 15-18) have been evaluated; however, most trials have reported a low 5-year disease-free survival rate. Response to high-dose chemotherapy prior to stem cell transplantation in patients with relapsed or refractory HD determines the EFS. Minimal disease status at the time of transplantation is a major predictor of improved EFS.

Table 15-18. Alternative Salvage Combination Chemotherapy Regimens for Relapsed and Resistant Hodgkin Disease

VABCD
 Vinblastine 6 mg/m^2, IV, every 3 weeks
 Doxorubicin 40 mg/m^2, IV, every 3 weeks
 Dacarbazine 800 mg/m^2, IV, every 3 weeks
 Lomustine (CCNU) 80 mg/m^2 PO, every 6 weeks
 Bleomycin 15 units IV, every 1 week
ABDIC
 Doxorubicin 45 mg/m^2 IV, day 1
 Bleomycin 5 units/m^2 IV, days 1 and 5
 Dacarbazine 200 mg/m^2, IV, days 1–5
 Lomustine 50 mg/m^2 PO, day 1
 Prednisone 40 mg/m^2 PO, days 1–5
 Cycle repeats every 28 days
CBVD
 Lomustine (CCNU) 120 mg/m^2 PO, day 1
 Bleomycin 15 units IV, days 1–22
 Vinblastine 6 mg/m^2 IV, days 1–22
 Dexamethasone 3 mg/m^2 PO, days 1–21
 Cycle repeats every 6 weeks
PCVP
 Vinblastine 3 mg/m^2, every 2 weeks
 Procarbazine 70 mg/m^2 PO, every 2 days
 Cyclophosphamide 70 mg/m^2 PO, every 2 days
 Prednisone 8 mg/m^2 PO, every 2 days
 Therapy lasts 1 year
CEP
 Lomustine (CCNU) 80 mg/m^2 PO, day 1
 Etoposide 100 mg/m^2 PO, days 1–5
 Prednimustine 60 mg/m^2 PO, days 1–5
EVA
 Etoposide 100 mg/m^2 IV, days 1–3
 Vinblastine 6 mg IV, day 1
 Doxorubicin 50 mg/m^2 IV, day 1

MIME
 Methyl GAG 500 mg/m^2 IV, days 1–14
 Ifosfamide 1 g/m^2 IV, days 1–5
 Methotrexate 30 mg/m^2 IV, day 3
 Etoposide 100 mg/m^2 IV, days 1–3, every 3 weeks
MOPLACE
 Cyclophosphamide 750 mg/m^2 IV, day 1
 Etoposide 80 mg/m^2 IV, days 1–3
 Prednisone 60 mg/m^2 PO, days 1–14
 Methotrexate 120 mg/m^2 IV, days 15, 22, with rescue
 Cytarabine 300 mg/m^2 IV, days 15, 22
 Vincristine 2 mg IV, days 15, 22, every 4 weeks
MINE
 Mitoguazone 500 mg/m^2, days 1 and 5
 Ifosfamide 1500 mg/m^2, days 1–5
 Vinorelbine (Navelbine) 15 mg, days 1 and 5
 Etoposide 150 mg/m^2, days 1–3
 Each cycle at 4-week intervals
MXT-CHOP
 Methotrexate 30 mg/m^2 IV, every 6 hours for 4 days, days 1 and 8 with rescue
 Cyclophosphamide 750 mg/m^2 IV, day 15
 Vincristine 1 mg/m^2 IV, days 15, 22
 Prednisone 100 mg/m^2 PO, days 22–26
 Doxorubicin 50 mg/m^2 IV, day 15, every 4 weeks
CEVD
 Lomustine (CCNU) 80 mg/m^2 PO, day 1
 Etoposide 120 mg/m^2 PO, days 1–5, 22–26
 Vindesine 3 mg/m^2 IV, days 1 and 22
 Dexamethasone 3 mg/m^2 PO, days 1–8, then 1.5 mg/m^2 PO, days 9–26, every 6 weeks

(Continues)

Table 15-18. (*Continued*)

CAVP
  Lomustine (CCNU) 90 mg/m² PO, day 1
  Melphalan 7.5 mg/m² PO, days 1–5
  Etoposide 100 mg/m² PO, days 6–10
  Prednisone 40 mg/m² PO, days 1–10,
    every 6 weeks
EVAP
  Etoposide 120 mg/m² IV, days 1, 8, 15
  Vinblastine 4 mg/m² IV, days 1, 8, 15
  Cytarabine 30 mg/m² IV, days 1, 8, 15
  Cisplatin 40 mg/m² IV, days 1, 8, 15,
    every 4 weeks
EPOCH
  Etoposide 200 mg/m² CIV, days 1–4
  Vincristine 1.6 mg/m² CIV, days 1–4
  Doxorubicin 40 mg/m² CIV, days 1–4
  Cyclophosphamide 750 mg/m² IV, day 6
  Prednisone 60 mg/m² PO, days 1–6
APE
  Cytarabine (Ara-C) 375 mg/m² IV bolus,
    followed by 375 mg/m² infusion over
    3 hours

Cisplatin 15 mg/m² IV infusion; starts
  1 hour after cytarabine and continues
  for 2 hours
Etoposide 20 mg/m² IV at end of
  cytarabine, cisplatin infusion
Repeat APE every 12 hours for 3–4 doses
Cycle repeats every 3–6 weeks
CEM
  Lomustine (CCNU) 100 mg/m² PO, day 1
  Etoposide 100 mg/m² PO, days 1–3, 21–23
  Methotrexate 30 mg/m² PO, days 1–8,
    21, 28, every 6 weeks
CVB
  Lomustine (CCNU) 100 mg/m² PO, day 1
  Vinblastine (Velban) 6 mg/m² IV, days 1, 8
  Bleomycin 10 mg/m² IV, days 1, 8
  Cycle repeats 4–6 weeks

Abbreviation: CIV, continuous intravenous infusion.

Ifosfamide, carboplatin, etoposide (ICE) (see page 556) chemotherapy can be utilized for attaining a remission in relapsed HD prior to the preparative ablative chemotherapy (Tables 16-13 and 16-14 in Chapter 16) for HSCT.

Because alkylating agents and etoposide (VP-16), which are highly active agents in the salvage treatment for HD, are associated with the development of myelodysplastic syndrome (MDS) and s-AML, alternative therapeutic approaches for reinduction with novel agents are presently being studied, such as ifosfamide (IF) with vinorelbine (VRB) and gemcitabine (GEM) with VRB.

Reinduction Therapy with Ifosfamide and Vinorelbine

Vinorelbine, a semisynthetic alkaloid, has shown marked clinical activity in HD. The mechanism of action of VRB is similar to that of other vinca alkaloids causing inhibition of microtubule formation. However, the degree of neurotoxicity with VRB is less than with vinca alkaloids. Maximum-tolerated dose range is from 30–35 mg/m²/wk. VRB has limited severe toxicities. However, granulocytopenia (grade 3 or 4) is common in 60% of patients. A pilot study is under way to evaluate IF/VRB as a novel reinduction regimen for patients with relapsed or refractory HD before stem cell transplantation. Acceptable hematologic toxicity and acceptable stem cell mobilization rates are realized. The overall response rate is 80% (40% CR and 40% PR). Table 15-19 shows a regimen of IF and VRB therapy in relapsed or refractory HD.

Reinduction Therapy with Gemcitabine and Vinorelbine

Gemcitabine (2¹,2¹-difluorodeoxycytosine; Gemzar) is a deoxycytidine analogue that inhibits DNA synthesis and repair. GEM as a single agent has been utilized in

Table 15-19. Regimen of Ifosfamide (IF) and Vinorelbine (VRB) in Relapsed or Refractory Hodgkin Disease

IF	$300 \text{ mg/m}^2/\text{day}$	Days 1–4 with MESNA 3000 mg/kg/day, day 1–5
VRB	$25 \text{ mg/m}^2/\text{day}$	Days 1, 5
G-CSF	$5 \mu\text{g/kg/day}$ starting on day 6 and until ANC >1500/mm^3 for 3 days or the ANC >10,000/mm^3	

- Next cycle is administered 21 days later (ANC >1000/mm^3 after discontinuation of G-CSF and platelet count >75,000/mm^3)
- Evaluation: If CR, peripheral stem cell harvest should be carried out after 2 cycles of IF/VRB. This should be followed by HSCT preparatory regimen (Chapter 25) and peripheral stem cell transplantation.
- Evaluation: If stable disease is attained and/or PR, peripheral stem cell harvest should be carried out followed by two more cycles of IF/VRB, HSCT preparatory regimen (cyclophosphamide, etoposide, and BCNU-CBV [Table 16-13] or BCNU, etoposide, Ara-C, melphalan-BEAM [Table 16-14]), and peripheral stem cell transplantation.

the treatment of patients who have relapsed or refractory HD. A response rate of 40% has been attained with GEM alone. There is an additive effect with GEM and VLB with little increase in toxicity. Combined GEM and VLB has produced disease stabilization or response in about 60% of cases. Table 15-20 shows a regimen of VRB and GEM therapy in relapsed or refractory HD.

Other Reinduction and Salvage Chemotherapy

See Table 15-18.

Autologous Stem Cell Transplantation

Preparative Regimes

A variety of high-dose chemotherapy regimens, including cyclophosphamide, etoposide, and BCNU (CBV) (Table 16-13 in Chapter 16) and BCNU, etoposide, Ara-C, and melphalan (BEAM) (Table 16-14 in Chapter 16), are being utilized as preparative regimens for stem cell transplantation.

Table 15-20. Regimen of Vinorelbine (VRB) and Gemcitabine (GEM) in Relapsed or Refractory Hodgkin Disease

VRB	$25 \text{ mg/m}^2/\text{day}$	Days 1 and 8
GEM	$1000 \text{ mg/m}^2/\text{day}$	Days 1 and 8
G-CSF	$5 \mu\text{g/kg/day}$ starting on day 9 for a minimum of 7 days and until the ANC >1500/mm^3 for 3 days or the ANC >10,000/mm^3.	

- Two cycles—second cycle is administered 21–28 days later.
- Evaluation: If CR, peripheral stem cell harvest should be carried out after 2 cycles of VRB/GEM. This should be followed by HSCT preparatory regimen (Chapter 25) and peripheral stem cell transplantation.
- Evaluation: If stable disease is attained and/or PR, peripheral stem cell harvest should be carried out followed by two more cycles of VRB/GEM, HSCT preparatory regimen (cyclophosphamide, etoposide, and BCNU-CBV [Table 16-13] or BCNU, etoposide, Ara-C, melphalan-BEAM [Table 16-14]), and peripheral stem cell transplantation.

Indications

- Relapse within 1 year of completion of conventional treatment (except stage I or IIA where only radiotherapy has been employed, in which case the patient can be treated with chemotherapy)
- Patients refractory to initial treatment who do not achieve complete remission.

For these patients, autologous bone marrow transplantation (AuBMT) or autologous peripheral stem cell rescue may be utilized after two or three cycles of conventional chemotherapy.

Post–Stem Cell Transplantation Management

There seems to be a beneficial role of immunotherapy following stem cell transplantation. Immune modulation with interferon γ (IFN-γ) and IL-2 after autologous stem cell rescue has been demonstrated to reduce the rate of relapse and to improve survival. Currently, COG is conducting a study that incorporates immunotherapy with cyclosporine, IFN-γ, and IL-2 during recovery after autologous stem cell rescue.

Prognosis

The early transplant-related mortality is 10% and the predominant reason for failure in patients who undergo salvage therapy is relapse.

Experience in children is limited. However, a report from the European Bone Marrow Transplant Group showed that 81 children with HD who underwent AuBMT had a long-term (>5 years) disease-free survival rate of 40%. A 1999 report from the Autologous Blood and Bone Marrow Registry (ABMTR) showed that 50% of patients who failed to achieve complete remission after one or more conventional therapy regimens achieved complete remission after autotransplantation.

Molecular Targeted Therapies

Studies of single-cell DNA amplification have documented the importance of signaling through NF-κB transcription factor both in the proliferation of Hodgkin and Reed–Sternberg (H/RS) cells and in suppression of apoptosis. Inhibition of proteosome and NF-κB in particular is an attractive biologic strategy in the therapy of HD. The focus of future targeted studies in HD will incorporate novel agents (chemotherapeutic and biologic agents) and therapeutic strategies that perturb the NF-κB pathway.

PS-341 is a highly selective inhibitor of NF-κB activation, as a result of induction of apoptosis. Strategies for incorporation of P-341 with effective therapeutic regimens for patients with relapsed/refractory pediatric HD are under way.

PROGNOSTIC FACTORS

- *Age:* Survival is significantly better in younger compared with older patients.
- *Sex:* The prognosis is better in females than in males.
- *Systemic symptoms:* Fever, weight loss, and night sweats are associated with a more unfavorable prognosis.
- *Complete remission:* The life expectancy is longer in patients with complete remission (CR) than in those with partial remission (PR) or no remission (NR).

- *Histopathology*
  a. The prognosis in lymphocyte-predominant (LP), nodular sclerosis (NS), mixed cellularity (MC), and lymphocyte-depleted (LD) HD is proportional to the ratio of lymphocytes to abnormal cells: LP > NS > MC > LD.
  b. Nodular, LPHD without diffuse type: This is an indolent, yet relapsing disease with patients rarely succumbing to their disease. Up to 10% of patients may develop non-Hodgkin lymphoma of B-cell origin.
  c. Nodular, LPHD with diffuse type: Relapses are uncommon, but once a relapse occurs the HD is often more aggressive histologically, resulting in decreased survival.
  d. Lymphocyte-depleted nodular sclerosing HD: This is associated with poor survival.
  e. Lymphocyte-depleted HD (LDHD): This is the most aggressive type of HD. It is frequently seen in older patients and is more common in men than women; it often presents as stage III or IV disease. This type must be distinguished from large-cell non-Hodgkin lymphoma. LDHD responds to modern therapy, although, in the past, prognosis was very poor.
- *Stage:* Survival correlates with the anatomic extent of the disease; bulky mediastinal disease in nodal and extranodal sites carries an unfavorable prognosis.

Factors of High Risk for Stages I and II

1. Presence of B symptomatology (fever, weight loss, and night sweats or fever and weight loss only)
2. Presence of bulky mediastinal disease
3. Presence of extralymphatic site involvement.

Factors of High Risk for Stage III

1. More than five nodal sites involved, including those above and below the diaphragm
2. Extensive splenic involvement (more than four nodules detected in the splenectomy specimen)
3. Stage III_1B
4. Stage III_2A or B
5. Stage III with bulky mediastinal disease
6. Pruritus.

Factors of High Risk for Stage IV

1. B symptomatology
2. Pruritus
3. More than one documented site of extranodal disease (all patients with more than one extranodal site of involvement usually have bone marrow disease).

Prognostic Score for Advanced Hodgkin Disease

Two-thirds of patients with advanced HD are cured with current approaches to treatment. Prediction of the outcome is important to avoid overtreating some patients and to identify others in whom standard treatment is likely to fail. For these reasons, prediction of the outcome of treatment may allow the identification of patients who are unlikely to have a sustained response to standard treatment.

The following prognostic factors have been found to be independently associated with a poor prognosis by the International Prognostic Factors (IPF) Project in which 5141 patients were evaluated:

1. Serum albumin level <4 g/dL
2. Hemoglobin level <10.5 g/dL
3. Male sex
4. Age greater than 45 years
5. Stage IV disease
6. Leukocytosis (leukocyte count >15,000/mm^3)
7. Lymphopenia (absolute lymphocyte count <600/mm^3) or lymphocytes <8% of white blood cells.

Each factor was found to add about 8% less tumor-free survival for the group. Use of the IPF data could potentially serve to select patients for more intensive therapy.

COMPLICATIONS

Complications from Disease

Complications arising from disease are described under the clinical and laboratory manifestations of Hodgkin disease.

Complications from Therapy

The modern treatment of HD, consisting of greater reliance on chemotherapy, reduced doses of radiation, and not doing staging laparotomy as standard care, has resulted in fewer complications from therapy compared to historic regimens of HD treatment.

1. *Pulmonary damage* (radiation induced and/or chemotherapy [bleomycin] induced): These complications consist of
   a. Pneumonitis
   b. Pulmonary fibrosis
   c. Decreased pulmonary function (as many as 40% of patients)
   d. Increased mediastinal width
   e. Infiltrates extending beyond radiation port
   f. Spontaneous pneumothorax
   g. Pleural effusion.
2. *Cardiac damage* (radiation induced and/or chemotherapy [doxorubicin] induced): These complications (about 13% of patients) consist of
   a. Cardiomyopathy, resulting in congestive heart failure
   b. Cardiac arrhythmias with conduction defects
   c. Pericarditis, resulting in pericardial effusion and cardiac tamponade
   d. Valvular damage to aorta and pulmonary artery
   e. Coronary artery disease and myocardial infarction.
3. *Spinal cord damage:* These complications consist of
   a. Lhermitte sign—a postradiation syndrome of numbness, tingling, and "electric shock" in extremities; self-limiting, subsiding within 10 months
   b. Radiation-induced transverse myelitis—more severe.
4. *Radiation nephritis*
5. *Azoospermia:* The quality of sperm may be poor in many patients with HD because of the disease itself before exposure to any therapy. Azoospermia induced by alkylating agents such as nitrogen mustard is almost always

permanent in postpubertal patients. However, the prognosis of this complication in prepubertal patients is unknown. Many adolescent boys with HD are azoospermic prior to initiation of therapy; thus, sperm banking itself is not always a suitable strategy to guarantee future reproduction among these patients. However, patients should be given the option for bank-cryopreserved sperm. Emerging data now suggest that recovery of spermatogenesis has been seen after three or fewer cycles of MOPP.

6. *Amenorrhea:* Radiation-induced ovarian damage can be avoided by performing oophoropexy during laparotomy. Among this group, a number of normal pregnancies and normal offspring have been observed. There has been no increase in fetal wastage or abortions. Chemotherapy (MOPP)-induced ovarian dysfunction and amenorrhea occur in 13% of patients under 25 years of age. The younger the patient is when treated, the higher the probability of maintaining regular menses following treatment. The younger the patient, the greater the complement of oocytes at the time of treatment and, hence, the greater the likelihood of maintaining fertility.

7. *Hypothyroidism:* This results from radiation therapy. Among children who receive neck radiation in doses of 2600 cGy or less, there is a 17% incidence of thyroid dysfunction as compared to a 78% incidence among patients who receive doses in excess of 2600 cGy. Surveillance studies, including tri-iodothyronine (T_3), thyroxine (T_4), and thyroid-stimulating hormone (TSH) levels and neck examination for thyroid swelling, are important in recognizing this complication. Euthyroid patients with high TSH (biochemical hypothyroidism) are treated with T_4 to prevent the development of thyroid adenoma.

8. *Damage to soft tissue and bone growth:* High doses (more than 3500 cGy) and large-volume irradiation administered to the axial skeleton result in a disproportionate alteration in sitting height as compared with standing height and a small thorax. The risk of this complication is particularly high in children under 6 years of age or in adolescence (11–13 years of age) when bone growth is very active at the time of treatment. Shortening of the interclavicular distance (small clavicles as well as atrophy of soft tissues of the neck) often occurs following high doses of radiation in children.

   Doses less than 2500 cGy have resulted in no standing height abnormalities greater than one standard deviation from the mean; thus, 2000–2500 cGy appears to be the threshold beyond which growth abnormalities are more likely to occur.

   With the use of radiotherapy, slipped femoral capital epiphysis may also occur. This can be minimized when routine humeral and femoral head blocks are used and when low radiation doses are administered.

9. *Postsplenectomy infection:* The incidence of significant infections and mortality in children splenectomized as part of a staging laparotomy for HD is 8.0% and 4.0%, respectively. The organisms reported to produce overwhelming sepsis in splenectomized children with HD are *Streptococcus pneumoniae, Neisseria meningitidis,* and *Haemophilus influenzae.* The risk of these infections can be decreased with the use of pneumococcal vaccine and HIB vaccine before splenectomy and with the use of penicillin prophylaxis after splenectomy for several years. Compliance with penicillin prophylaxis is of crucial importance.

10. *Secondary malignant neoplasms:* The risk of secondary malignancies is a problem of major concern in selecting therapy for children with HD. Overall, the risk of developing a secondary neoplasm is 2% at 5 years, 5% at 10 years, and 9% at 15 years; the probability of developing s-AML or a secondary non-Hodgkin lymphoma is reported as 1%, 3%, and 4% at 5, 10, and 15 years, respectively; and the probability of developing a solid tumor is reported as 0.4%, 2%, and

6% at 5, 10, and 15 years, respectively. The median time to development of s-AML after chemotherapy and solid tumors after radiotherapy is about 5 and 12 years, respectively. The risk increases among those who have had a relapse. A relationship between leukemia and prior splenectomy has been suggested in the past. Alkylating agent therapy is strongly associated with subsequent development of s-AML with a significant dose–response relationship. Among the agents most often linked to leukemia are nitrogen mustard (mechlorethamine), cyclophosphamide, chlorambucil, and procarbazine. s-AML is almost always refractory to treatment, whereas secondary lymphomas and sarcomas respond better to therapy, and about 50% may attain cures. The actuarial risk of breast cancer at 20 years is 9.2%. The other secondary neoplasms associated with treatment of HD are thyroid carcinoma, skin carcinomas, brain tumor, malignant fibrous histiocytoma, and breast cancer.

FOLLOW-UP EVALUATIONS
During Therapy

- *History and physical examination:* special reference to lymph nodes, liver, spleen, and indication of response
- *Complete blood count (CBC):* weekly with chemotherapy and radiotherapy
- *Erythrocyte sedimentation rate (ESR):* prior to each cycle of chemotherapy and radiotherapy
- *Serum copper:* prior to each cycle of chemotherapy and radiotherapy
- *Liver function tests:* prior to each cycle of chemotherapy and radiotherapy
- *Chest radiograph (posteroanterior and lateral):* for patients with mediastinal disease, prior to each chemotherapy and just prior to radiotherapy as well as 8 weeks after the completion of therapy; for patients with non–chest primary, at the end of therapy
- *Cardiac function studies (ECG, echocardiogram, or radioisotope ejection fraction):* prior to third cycle of the use of an anthracycline (e.g., ABVD [doxorubicin]) and prior to radiation therapy
- *CT scan of primary site:* prior to third cycle of chemotherapy and prior to radiation therapy
- *MRI of the chest (with mediastinal disease):* prior to third course of chemotherapy and prior to radiotherapy
- *FDG-PET and gallium scan:* prior to third cycle of chemotherapy and prior to radiation therapy
- *Pulmonary function tests:* prior to third cycle of the use of bleomycin (e.g., ABVD [bleomycin]) and prior to radiation therapy.

After Completion of Therapy

All patients should be followed for a minimum of 10 years.

- *History and physical examination, CBC, ESR, serum copper, chest radiograph (if chest primary):*
  Year 1—monthly
  Year 2—every 2 months
  Year 3—every 3 months
  Years 4 and 5—every 6 months
  Yearly thereafter
- *Anthropomorphic measurements and Tanner stage:* yearly until puberty is complete

- T_4, *TSH (if neck was irradiated):* every 6 months
- *Follicle-stimulating hormone (FSH) and luteinizing hormone (LH) (if pubertal):* yearly
- *Chest radiograph*
  Non–chest primary—every 3 months first year; yearly thereafter
  CT (with contrast), MRI, and FDG-PET and gallium scan of primary, if initially positive: years 1 and 2—every 3 months; year 3—every 6 months
- *Pulmonary function studies:* if abnormal, repeat yearly for 10 years
- *Cardiac function studies:* yearly for 10 years.

Dental Evaluation and Care

Supervision of oral health care is mandatory for patients who receive chemotherapy or radiotherapy to the neck and particularly if they receive both. All patients must undergo dental evaluation and prophylactic treatment and must receive instructions in home care of the teeth, including the use of fluoride prophylactically. Wisdom teeth, including those that are unerupted, and irreparable carious teeth must be removed. Patients must be followed closely during the second dentition to ensure prompt treatment of oral infections and other complications that can occur during the tooth-shedding process. Dental surveillance must continue after the patient is off therapy.

SUGGESTED READINGS

Ambinder R, Mann R. Epstein–Barr encoded RNA *in situ* hybridization. Hum Pathol 1994;25:602.

Aygun B, Karakas SP, Leonidas J, Valderrama E, and Karayalcin G. Reliability of splenic index to assess splenic involvement in pediatric Hodgkin's disease. J Pediatr Hematol Oncol 2004;26:74.

Bonadonna G, Valagussa P, Santoro A. Alternating non–cross-resistant combination chemotherapy or MOPP in stage IV Hodgkin's disease: a report of 8-year results. Ann Intern Med 1986;104:746.

Carbone PP, Kaplan HS, Husshoff K, et al. Report of the committee on Hodgkin's disease staging classification. Cancer Res 1971;31:1860.

De Vita VTJ, Canellos G, Moxley J. A decade of combination chemotherapy of advanced Hodgkin's disease. Cancer 1972;30:1495.

Donaldson SS, Hudson M, Lamborn R, et al. VAMP and low-dose, involved-field radiation for children and adolescents with favorable, early-stage Hodgkin disease: results of a prospective trial. J Clin Oncol 2002;20:3081.

Harris NL, Jaffe ES, Diebold J, et al. Wood Health Organization classification of neoplastic diseases of hemapoietic and lymphoid tissues: report of the clinical of neoplastic diseases of hemapoietic and lymphoid tissues. Report of the Clinical Advisory Committee Meeting, Virginia, Airlie House, November 1997. JCO 1999;17:3835.

Harris NL, Jaffe ES, Stein H, et al. A revised European–American classification of lymphoid neoplasms: a proposal from the International Lymphoma Study Group. Blood 1994;84:1361.

Kadin ME, Liebowitz. Cytokines and cytokine receptors in Hodgkin's disease. In: Mauch PM, Armitrage J, Diehl V, Hoppe RT, Weiss LM, editors. Hodgkin's Disease. Philadelphia: Lippincott Williams & Wilkins, 1999;139–57.

Karayalcin G, Behm FG, Geiser PW, et al. Lymphocyte predominant Hodgkin's disease; clinicopathologic features and results of treatment—the Pediatric Oncology Group experience. Med Pediatr Oncol 1997;29:516.

Lukes RJ, Butler JJ. The pathology and nomenclature of Hodgkin's disease. Cancer Res. 1966;26:1063.

Nachman JB, Sposo R, Herzog P, et al. Randomized comparison of low-dose involved-field radiotherapy and no radiotherapy for children with Hodgkin's disease who achieve a complete response to chemotherapy. J Clin Oncol 2002;20:3765.

Rini JN, Manalili EY, Hoffman M, Karayalcin G, Mechatra B, Thomas B, Palestro CJ. F-18 FDG versus Ga-67 for detecting splenic involvement in Hodgkin's disease. Clin Nucl Med 2002;27:572.

Ruhl U, Albrecht M, Dieckmann K, et al. Response-adapted radiotherapy in the treatment of pediatric Hodgkin's disease: an interim report at 5 years of the German GPOH-HD 95 trial. Int J Radiat Oncol Bio Phys 2001;51:1209.

Schellong G. Treatment of children and adolescents with Hodgkin's disease: the experience of the German-Austrian Paediatric Study Group. Baillieres Clin Haemotol 1996;9:619.

Schmitz N, Pfister B, Sextro M, et al. Aggressive conventional chemotherapy compared with high-dose chemotherapy with autologous stem-cell transplantation for relapsed chemo-sensitive Hodgkin's disease. A randomized trial. Lancet 2002;341:1051.

Stein H, Diehl V, Marafieti T, et al. The nature of Reed–Sternberg cells, lymphocytic and histiocytic cells and their molecular biology in Hodgkin's disease. In: Mauch PM, Armitage J, Diehl V, Hoppe RT, Weiss LM, editors. Hodgkin's Disease. Philadelphia: Lippincott Williams & Wilkins, 1999;121–37.

Weiner MA, Leventhal BG, Marcus R, et al. Intensive chemotherapy and low-dose radiotherapy for the treatment of advanced-stage Hodgkin's disease in pediatric patients: a Pediatric Oncology Group study. J Clin Oncol 1991;9:1591.

16

NON-HODGKIN LYMPHOMA

Non-Hodgkin lymphoma (NHL) results from malignant proliferation of cells of lymphocytic lineage. Although malignant lymphomas are generally restricted to lymphoid tissue such as lymph nodes, Peyer's patches, and spleen, it is not uncommon to find bone marrow involvement in children. Bone and primary central nervous system (CNS) lymphomas are rare presentations.

INCIDENCE AND EPIDEMIOLOGY
Incidence

1. NHL accounts for 6–7% of malignant diseases in childhood in Europe and the United States. It is the third most common childhood malignancy with an overall incidence of 10.5 per million.
2. The incidence of NHL is higher in the Middle East, Nigeria, and Uganda (150 per million children under 5–10 years of age) as a result of their increased incidence of endemic Burkitt lymphoma.
3. NHL accounts for 45% of all lymphomas in children and adolescents less than 20 years of age.
4. There has been a stable incidence for children less than 15 years of age during the last two decades, but in adolescents 15–19 years of age there has been an increase of 50% to 16.3 per million in 1990–1995.
5. Isolated cases of familial NHL occur.

Epidemiology

1. *Sex*: Male:female is 2.5:1 overall, and over 3:1 in ages 5–14.
2. *Age*: Relatively similar across all ages, but peaks at ages 15–19 years, largely because of a significant increase in the incidence of diffuse large-cell lymphoma.
3. *Risk factors*:
   a. Genetic: immunological defects (Bruton's type of sex-linked agammaglobulinemia, common variable agammaglobulinemia, ataxia telangiectasia, Wiskott–Aldrich syndrome, autoimmune lymphoproliferative disorder, and severe combined immune deficiency)

b. Post-transplant immunosuppression, for example, post–bone marrow transplantation (especially with use of T-cell depleted marrow); post–solid organ transplantation

c. *Drugs*: diphenylhydantoin

d. *Radiation*: children treated with chemotherapy and radiotherapy for Hodgkin disease

e. *Viral*: Epstein–Barr virus (EBV), human immune deficiency virus (HIV).

PATHOLOGIC CLASSIFICATION

Table 16-1 presents the World Health Organization (WHO) classification for NHL from the International Lymphoma Study Group. This classification for NHL is based on the currently recognized histologic (morphologic), immunophenotypic and genetic features, their clinical presentation and course. This updates the Revised European–American Lymphoma (REAL) classification and is the preferred classification for NHL.

Table 16-1. WHO Classification of Neoplastic Diseases of Hematopoietic and Lymphoid Tissues

Precursor B-cell neoplasms
  Precursor B-lymphoblastic leukemia/lymphoma

Mature (peripheral) B-cell neoplasms
  B-CLL/small lymphocytic lymphoma
  B-cell prolymphocytic leukemia
  Lymphoplasmacytic lymphoma
  Mantle-cell lymphoma
  Follicular lymphoma (grade 1, 2, or 3)
  Nodal marginal zone B-cell lymphoma (+/− monocytoid B cells)
  Extranodal marginal zone B-cell lymphoma of MALT type
  Splenic marginal zone B-cell lymphoma (+/− villous lymphocytes)
  Hairy cell leukemia
  Plasma cell myeloma/plasmacytoma
  Diffuse large-B-cell lymphoma
    Morphologic variants
    - Centroblastic
    - Immunoblastic
    - T-cell/histiocyte-rich
    - Anaplastic large B-cell
    - Plasmablastic
    Clinical variants
    - Mediastinal (thymic) large B-cell lymphoma
    - Primary effusion lymphoma
    - Intravascular large B-cell lymphoma
    - Lymphomatoid granulomatosis type
  Burkitt lymphoma/Burkitt cell leukemia
    Morphologic variants
    - Burkitt-like or typical Burkitt
    - With plasmacytoid differentiation (AIDS-associated)
    Clinical and genetic variants
    - Endemic
    - Sporadic
    - Immunodeficiency-associated

(Continues)

Table 16-1. (*Continued*)

Precursor T-cell neoplasms
  Precursor T-lymphoblastic leukemia/lymphoma

Mature (peripheral) T-cell neoplasms
  Predominantly leukemic/disseminated
    T-cell prolymphocytic leukemia
    T-cell granular lymphocytic leukemia
    Aggressive NK-cell leukemia
    Adult T-cell lymphoma/leukemia (HTLV1+)
  Predominantly nodal
    Angioimmunoblastic T-cell lymphoma
    Peripheral T-cell lymphoma, not otherwise characterized
    Anaplastic large-cell lymphoma, T/null cell, primary systemic disease
  Predominantly extranodal
    Mycosis fungoides/Sézary syndrome
    Anaplastic large-cell lymphoma, T/null cell, primary cutaneous type
    Subcutaneous panniculitis-like T-cell lymphoma
    Extranodal NK/T-cell lymphoma, nasal type
    Enteropathy-type T-cell lymphoma
    Hepatosplenic gamma-delta T-cell lymphoma

Table 16-2 lists the histologic classification, relative frequency of histologic types, correlation with immunophenotype, common sites of involvement, and genetic features in childhood NHL. Fifty percent of NHL in children are small, noncleaved, 30% lymphoblastic, and 20% large-cell types.

CLINICAL FEATURES

The presenting symptoms of NHL depend mainly on the location of the tumor. It may present in a variety of ways, occasionally providing a diagnostic dilemma because of the protean manifestations of its presentation.

Burkitt lymphoma (BL) may be of the endemic or sporadic variety. Table 16-3 lists the epidemiologic, immunologic, and molecular features of endemic and sporadic BL.

Abdomen

The primary site in 35% of cases is abdominal—the ileocecal region, appendix, ascending colon, or some combination of these sites. These patients usually present with:

- Abdominal pain
- Nausea and vomiting
- Constipation or diarrhea
- Abdominal distention
- Palpable mass
- Intussusception
- Peritonitis
- Ascites
- Acute gastrointestinal bleeding
- Obstructive jaundice
- Hepatosplenomegaly
- Right iliac fossa mass.

Table 16-2. Histologic Classification, Relative Frequency of Histologic Type, Correlation with Immunophenotype, Common Sites of Involvement and Genetic Features in Childhood Non-Hodgkin Lymphoma

Histology	Immunophenotype	Common Sites of Involvement	Frequency	Genetic Features
Lymphoblastic lymphoma (LBL): Convoluted Non-convoluted		Anterior mediastinum (50–70%), pleural effusion, sometimes cervical, axillary, inguinal lymphadenopathy. Occasional abdominal involvement.	30–35%	t(10;14), t(11;14), t(1;14), TCR/TAL1, t(1;19), t(8;14), (q24;q11), *c-myc*/TCRα TCR/RHOMB2, TCR/LCK
Precursor T (90% of LBL)	CD 2, 3, 4, 5, 7, 8 HLA-DR ,TdT positive			
Precursor-B (10% of LBL)	CD 10, 19, 20, 22, HLA-DR, TdT positive			
Small non-cleaved cell lymphomas (diffuse undifferentiated):	B-cell SIgM, (SIgG, SIgA occasionally)	Abdomen with or without ascites (90%). Most frequent pathology causing intussusception in children >6 years of age.	40-50%	BL: t(8;14), c-myc/ IgH t(8;22), c-myc/ Ig Lambda t(2;8), Ig Kappa/c-myc P53 mutation BLL: bcl-2 rearrangement 30%, bcl-6 rearrangement
Burkitt lymphoma (BL) Burkitt-like (BLL)	CD 10, 19, 20, 22, 38, 77, 79a TdT negative	Endemic BL: jaw		
Large cell Lymphomas Subtypes Diffuse large cell: B; T		Usually abdomen but may present with unusual sites of involvement e.g., mediastinum.	15-20%	

| Anaplastic large cell: usually T, NPM/ALK sometimes B-lineage. | CD 30 (Ki-1), 25, 71 Ia | Often skin, CNS, lymph nodes, lung, testes, muscle, GI tract, bone | t(2;5) (p23;q35), t(1;5) |

Synonyms in various classifications:

1. ML lymphoblastic synonyms: WHO/REAL: precursor T-lymphoblastic lymphoma/leukemia (T-LBL); Rappaport: poorly differentiated lymphocytic; Kiel: T-lymphoblastic; Lukes-Collins: convoluted T-lymphocytic; working formulation: lymphoblastic, convoluted, or nonconvoluted.

2. ML small noncleaved Burkitt synonyms: WHO: Burkitt lymphoma/Burkitt cell leukemia, typical Burkitt; subtype of mature B-cell neoplasms; REAL: Burkitt lymphoma subtype of peripheral B-cell lymphoma; Rappaport: undifferentiated lymphoma, Burkitt type; Kiel: Burkitt lymphoma; Lukes-Collins: small noncleaved follicular center cell; working formulation: small noncleaved cell, Burkitt type.

3. ML small noncleaved Burkitt-like synonyms: WHO: Burkitt lymphoma/Burkitt cell leukemia, Burkitt-like variant; REAL: a subtype of peripheral B-cell neoplasms assigned as a provisional entity of high-grade B-cell lymphoma Burkitt-type: Rappaport: undifferentiated non-Burkitt; Kiel: not listed; Lukes-Collins: small non-cleaved follicular center cell; working formulation: small noncleaved cell, non-Burkitt.

4. ML large-cell synonyms: WHO/REAL: diffuse large-B-cell lymphoma, a subtype of peripheral B-cell neoplasm (multiple variants); Rappaport: diffuse histiocytic; Kiel: centroblastic, B-immunoblastic, large-cell anaplastic B-cell; Lukes-Collins: large-cell cleaved, noncleaved, or immunoblastic; working formulation: large-cell lymphoma.

5. Anaplastic large-cell lymphoma: WHO: anaplastic large-cell lymphoma (T/null), a subtype of mature T-cell neoplasms, predominantly nodal and predominantly extranodal; REAL: anaplastic large-cell (CD30+) lymphoma (T/null), a subtype of peripheral T-cell and NK cell neoplasm; Rappaport: not listed; Lukes-Collins: T-immunoblastic sarcoma; working formulation; not listed.

Abbreviation: ML, malignant lymphoma.

495

Table 16-3. Epidemiologic, Immunologic, and Molecular Features of Endemic and Sporadic Burkitt Lymphoma

Feature	Endemic	Sporadic
Epidemiologic		
Population affected	African	Worldwide
Age affected	Children (peak age 7 years)	Young adults (peak age: 11 years)
Organ involvement	Jaw, orbit, paraspinal, abdomen, ovary	Abdomen, marrow, nasopharynx, ovary
Epstein–Barr virus	Present in >97% of cases	Present in 15–20% of cases
CNS involvement	More frequent than bone marrow involvement	Less frequent than bone marrow involvement
Immunologic		
IgM secretion	Little or none	Prominent
Fc and C3	+	−
CALLA	±	+
IgH gene rearrangement	DH or JH	IgH switch region
Molecular		
Breakpoints on chromosome 8	Upstream of c-*myc*	Within c-*myc*
Site of cell origin	Germinal center of lymph node	Bone marrow

Bleeding and perforation of the intestine occur infrequently in patients with Burkitt lymphoma.

Lymphoma is the most frequent anatomic lesion causing intussusception in children over 6 years of age. When this disease presents insidiously, it may clinically and radiologically resemble Crohn disease.

Head and Neck

In 13% of cases, the head and neck are involved, causing enlargement of the cervical node(s) and parotid gland, jaw swelling, and unilateral tonsillar hypertrophy. The disease may present with nasal obstruction, rhinorrhea, hypoacousia, and cranial nerve palsies.

Mediastinum

The frequency of involvement of the mediastinum is 26%. Patients may present with superior vena cava (SVC) syndrome (distended neck veins, edema of the neck and face, marked dyspnea, orthopnea, dizziness, headache, dysphagia, epistaxis, altered mental status, and syncope associated with bending). In this condition a large anterior mediastinal mass compresses the SVC because of the thinness of its wall and its close apposition to the vertebral column. The rapid growth of the mass does not permit enough time to develop effective collateral circulation to compensate and results in signs and symptoms of SVC compression.

Tumors of the mediastinum have a marked tendency to involve the bone marrow, transform to acute lymphoblastic leukemia, and develop meningeal and gonadal involvement. Many of these tumors are composed of cells of T-lymphocyte lineage. Pleural effusion may be produced by direct pleural involvement and/or may result from the compression of lymphatics by the mediastinal mass. The presence of pericardial effusion may cause cardiac tamponade.

Tumors may compress the trachea. Patients with significant tracheal compression may occlude their airway and die if forced to lie supine or are given general anesthesia due to a reduction in the negative intrapleural pressure (see pages 467–468, Chapter 15).

Other Primary Sites

Other sites involved (11%) include skin and subcutaneous tissue, orbit, thyroid, bone (with or without hypercalcemia), kidney, epidural space, breast, and gonads. The peripheral nodes are affected in 14% of cases.

Constitutional Symptoms

Fever and weight loss are relatively uncommon except in anaplastic large-cell lymphoma. Weight loss may also occur secondary to mechanical bowel obstruction.

DIAGNOSIS

Table 16-4 lists the diagnostic tests required to evaluate NHL. Excellent cytologic and histologic preparations are essential for precise diagnosis and accurate classification

Table 16-4. Evaluation of Patient with Non-Hodgkin Lymphoma

History and physical examination
Blood count
Serum electrolytes: calcium, phosphorus, magnesium
Evaluation of renal function (urinalysis, BUN, uric acid, creatinine)
Evaluation of hepatic function (bilirubin, alkaline phosphatase, alanine aminotransferase [ALT], aspartate aminotransferase [AST], serum protein electrophoresis)
Lactic dehydrogenase (LDH) levels
Soluble interleukin-2 receptor (IL-2R) levels (if possible)
Adequate surgical biopsy for cytochemical, immunologic, cytogenetic, and molecular studies
Viral studies: HIV antibody, hepatitis A, B, C serology, CMV antibody, varicella antibody, HSV antibody
Bone marrow aspiration and biopsy[a] (bilateral)
Spinal fluid, peritoneal,[a] pericardial or pleural[a] fluid examination: cytochemical, immunologic, cytogenetic, and molecular
Chest radiograph
CT scan of the chest (when indicated)
Ultrasonography of abdomen
CT scan of the abdomen with contrast (optional if abdominal ultrasound and gallium scans performed)
Plain radiograph and CT scan of affected site as deemed necessary on clinical grounds
Gallium scan
Diphosphonate bone scan prior to gallium scan, since gallium will obscure the diphosphonate (if bone scan positive, radiographs or CT scan of bone or MRI of involved area indicated)
Magnetic resonance imaging (MRI) when clinically indicated, especially for bone involvement (e.g., vertebrae)
Dental evaluation in patients with Burkitt lymphoma

Note: Avoid undue delay in carrying out investigations because of risk of rapid dissemination of the disease, especially to the bone marrow. In urgent medical situations (e.g., critical airway obstruction, cord compression, cranial nerve palsy, or renal failure), minimum investigations prompted by the patient's particular clinical problems should be carried out and patient should be treated on day of admission.
[a]May establish diagnosis without lymph node biopsy.

of lymphomas and special precautions must be taken in handling the specimen. Most diagnostic problems result from improperly and poorly prepared material and crushing artifacts. Selection of the appropriate node and histologic material is important. Histologic material that is obviously necrotic and that has been subject to vascular compromise creates major diagnostic problems.

STAGING

Staging of NHL requires an expeditious investigation to determine the clinical extent of the disease, the degree of organ impairment and biochemical disturbance present. Staging laparotomy to determine precise pathologic staging of the disease is not indicated.

Chemotherapy is the therapeutic mainstay because of the multicentric origin of NHL. Radiation therapy alone, with fields determined by an anatomic staging system, is not employed. Testicular involvement is present in less than 4% of males at diagnosis. Table 16-5 lists a staging system that enables a uniform interpretation of results of various treatment regimens. This classification recognizes the common occurrence of dissemination to either the bone marrow or the CNS, or both, and the fact that it is indicative of a poor prognosis.

Table 16-5. Staging System for Childhood Non-Hodgkin Lymphoma: Murphy Classification

Stage I
 A single tumor (extranodal) or single anatomic area (nodal) with the exclusion of mediastinum or abdomen

Stage II
 A single tumor (extranodal) with regional lymph node involvement
 Two or more nodal areas on the same side of the diaphragm
 Two single (extranodal) tumors with or without regional lymph node involvement on the same side of the diaphragm
 A resectable primary gastrointestinal tract tumor, usually in the ileocecal area, with or without involvement of associated mesenteric nodes only[a]

Stage III
 Two single tumors (extranodal) above and below the diaphragm
  Two or more nodal areas above and below the diaphragm
  All primary intrathoracic (mediastinal, pleural, thymic) tumors
  All extensive primary intra-abdominal disease[a]
  All paraspinal or epidural tumors, regardless of other tumor site (or sites)

Stage IV
 Any of the above with initial involvement of central nervous system or bone marrow[b] or both

[a]A distinction is made between apparently localized GI tract lymphoma versus more extensive intra-abdominal disease because of their quite different pattern of survival after appropriate therapy. Stage II disease typically is limited to a segment of the gut plus or minus the associated mesenteric nodes only, and the primary tumor can be completely removed grossly by segmental excision. Stage III disease typically exhibits spread to para-aortic and retroperitoneal areas by implants and plaques in mesentery or peritoneum, or by direct infiltrations of structures adjacent to the primary tumor. Ascites may be present, and complete resection of all gross tumor is not possible.

[b]Bone marrow involvement is defined as greater than 5% and less than 25% replacement of marrow elements by tumor without circulating blast cells.

From Murphy SB: Current concepts in cancer: Childhood non-Hodgkin's lymphoma. N Engl J Med 299:1446, 1978, with permission.

TREATMENT

Two potentially life-threatening complications are seen in children with NHL:

1. Superior vena cava syndrome or critical airway obstruction with a large mediastinal tumor. This is most often seen in lymphoblastic lymphoma.
2. Tumor lysis syndrome, due to metabolic complications of chemotherapy most often seen in Burkitt or Burkitt-like (BL/BLL) NHL.

General Management

Management of Intrathoracic Lesions

Always maintain patient in an inclined or sitting position and avoid use of general anesthesia. Diagnostic procedures should include:

- Chest radiograph to evaluate:
  Size of the mass
  Degree of airway compression
  Presence of significant amounts of pleural and/or pericardial effusions
- Echocardiogram for evaluation of pericardial effusion and cardiac function
- Biopsy of a clinically involved peripheral lymph node under local anesthesia or from the cytology of pleural effusion aspirate when present.

If the disease is present exclusively in the anterior mediastinum, a biopsy (under local anesthesia) through a small suprasternal incision should be performed or, if possible, obtain a core-needle biopsy.

It is possible that all of the preceding procedures may be prohibitive because of the patient's poor clinical condition. Under this circumstance, the patient should be treated with corticosteroids with or without a limited radiation field until the mass is sufficiently small to permit safe biopsy under general anesthesia. Corticosteroid and/or local radiotherapy can bring about rapid resolution of SVC obstruction.

Management of Pericardial Effusion

Pericardial effusion can cause life-threatening cardiac tamponade. A pericardial rub, S-T segment elevation on EKG, a globular-shaped heart on a chest radiograph, and cardiac ultrasonography establish the diagnosis. When signs of cardiac tamponade (pulsus paradoxus, elevated venous pressure or hypotension) are present, pericardiocentesis should be performed. The cytology of the fluid should be examined. Prompt treatment with chemotherapy is necessary to prevent reaccumulation of fluid.

Management of Gastrointestinal Complications

Abdominal disease is more commonly observed in patients with BL or BLL. The following complications are of immediate significance:

- *Small bowel obstruction:* NHL of the gastrointestinal (GI) tract commonly involves the terminal ileum and the cecum. The tumor can cause bowel obstruction, either by compression of the bowel lumen, or by intussusception. In about 25% of the patients, the tumor can be resected completely. Chemotherapy should begin within a few days of surgery.
- *Gastric bleeding or perforation:* Endoscopic examination should be performed to identify patients at high risk of massive bleeding and/or perforation by noting extent of involvement of the stomach wall and the degree of ulceration and necrosis. High-risk patients should be treated with resection of the tumor

(involving total or partial gastrectomy depending on the extent of the tumor) before starting chemotherapy.

Management of Tumor Lysis Syndrome

Management of tumor lysis syndrome and its metabolic complications is detailed in Chapter 26.

TREATMENT

Proliferation of lymphoblasts may be extremely rapid, with doubling times as short as 24 hours in some histologic types, such as Burkitt lymphoma. Successful therapy of NHL is realized with the recognition that short intervals between drugs (measured in hours) does not allow regrowth of the tumor to its original size. The use of divided-dose cyclophosphamide and other continuous infusions (doxorubicin, cytarabine) with corticosteroids is integral to successful NHL therapy.

Treatment groups can be divided into the following categories:

- Localized (stage I and II) lymphoblastic lymphoma (LL)
- Advanced (stage III and IV) LL
- Localized (completely resected stage I and abdominal stage II) B-lineage NHL BL, BLL, and diffuse B-cell, large-cell lymphoma (DLCL)
- Intermediate risk (see below)
- BL, BLL, and DLCL with CNS involvement or bone marrow with ≥25% lymphoblasts
- Large-cell anaplastic NHL.

Localized Lymphoblastic Lymphoma

Patient eligibility criteria:

- B or T lineage LL
- Stage I or II (Table 16-5).

Treatment

Table 16-6 and Figure 16-1 show treatment in stage I or II localized lymphoblastic lymphoma. Patients with localized LL receive induction protocol I, consolidation

Table 16-6. Therapy of Non-B-Cell Lymphoma (BFM-NHL Protocol) (to be read in conjunction with Figure 16-1)

Drug	Dose	Days when administered[a]
Induction protocol I[b]		
Prednisone (PO)	60 mg/m^2	1–28, then taper over 9 days
Vincristine (IV)	1.5 mg/m^2 (maximum dose, 2 mg)	8,15,22,29
Daunorubicin (IV over 1 h)	30 mg/m^2	8,15,22,29
Asparaginase (IV over 1 h)	10,000 units/m^2	12,15,18,21,24,27,30,33
Cyclophosphamide (IV over 1 h)[c]	1000 mg/m^2	36,64
Cytarabine (IV)	75 mg/m^2	38–41,45–48,52–55,59–62
Mercaptopurine (PO)	60 mg/m^2	36–63
MTX (IT)[d,e]	12 mg	1,15,29,45,59

(Continues)

Table 16-6. (*Continued*)

Consolidation protocol M[f]		
Mercaptopurine (PO)	25 mg/m^2	1–56
MTX (24-h infusion)[g]	5 gram/m^2	8,22,36,50
MTX (IT)[e]	12 mg	8,22,36,50
Reinduction protocol II		
Dexamethasone (PO)	10 mg/m^2	1–21, then taper over 9 days
Vincristine (IV)	1.5 mg/m^2 (maximum dose, 2 mg)	8,15,22,29
Doxorubicin (IV)	30 mg/m^2	8,15,22,29
Asparaginase (IV)	10,000 units/m^2	8,11,15,18
Cyclophosphamide (IV over 1 h)[c]	1000 mg/m^2	36
Cytarabine (IV)	75 mg/m^2	38–41, 45–48
Thioguanine (PO)	60 mg/m^2	36–49
MTX (IT)[e]	12 mg	38,45
Maintenance		
Mercaptopurine (PO)	50 mg/m^2/day	Daily[h]
Methotrexate (PO)	20 mg/m^2/day	Weekly[h]

[a]Adjustments of time schedule are made for clinical condition and marrow recovery.

[b]Patients with less than 70% response at day 33 $\left(\dfrac{\text{Initial tumor volume} - \text{tumor volume day 33}}{\text{Initial tumor volume}} \times 100\right)$ are treated as high-risk ALL.

[c]With Mesna.

[d]Additional doses at days 8 and 22 for CNS-positive patients.

[e]Doses adjusted for children less than 3 years of age as follows:

Methotrexate intrathecal

Age (years)	Dose (mg)
>3	12
2–3	10
1–2	8
Up to 1	6

[f]If residual tumor present after induction, it should be resected. If viable tumor present, treat with high-risk ALL therapy.

[g]Methotrexate with leucovorin (CF) rescue.

Methotrexate (MTX): 5 g/m^2 is administered IV over 24 hours as follows: 10% of the MTX dose of 5 g/m^2 (500 mg/m^2) is administered IV over 30 minutes and 90% of the dose (4500 mg/m^2) is administered over 23.5 hours as a continuous infusion.

CF rescue: 30 mg/m^2 IV at hour 42 followed by 6 doses of 15 mg/m^2 every 6 hours IV/PO until serum MTX level is <0.4μ molar.

[h]Total duration of therapy: 24 months.

Cranial radiation (CRT): Postpone CRT for patients <1 year of age with overt CNS involvement until second year of life and give a total dose of 18 Gy. Older children receive 24 Gy. Prophylactic CRT is given to all patients without CNS involvement using 12 Gy. Infants under 1 year are not irradiated prophylactically. Timing: CRT is delivered during the second phase of the reinduction protocol, i.e., 27–29 weeks from the time of initial diagnosis. Note that CRT is given only for patients with stage III and IV disease.

Testicular involvement: In males with biopsy-proven persistent testicular involvement after protocol M, deliver 20 Gy to the testes.

From Reiter A, Shrappe M, Ludwig W, et al. Intensive ALL-type therapy without local radiotherapy provides a 90% event-free survival for children with T-cell lymphoplasmacytic lymphoma: a BFM group report. Blood 2000;95:416–21, with permission.

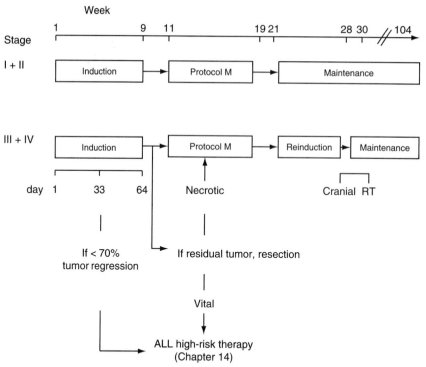

Fig. 16-1. General treatment strategy. RT indicates radiotherapy. The composition of treatment protocols is given in Table 16-6.

protocol M, and then proceed directly to maintenance therapy. They do not receive prophylactic cranial radiation.

Results

- Localized B-lymphoblastic lymphoma: 5-year event-free survival (EFS) approximates 85%. Even in localized B-lymphoblastic lymphoma, maintenance therapy is required in order to prevent two thirds of patients relapsing.
- Localized T-lymphoblastic lymphoma: 5-year EFS is 100%.

Stage III and IV Lymphoblastic NHL

Patient eligibility criterion: stage III or IV lymphoblastic lymphoma.

Treatment

Table 16-6 and Figure 16-1 show treatment in stage III or IV lymphoblastic lymphoma. Patients all receive induction protocol I, consolidation protocol M, reinduction protocol II, maintenance therapy, and either prophylactic or therapeutic cranial irradiation except patients under age 1 without CNS disease.

Results

Stage III and stage IV EFS at 6 years is 90% ± 3% and 95% ± 5%, respectively.

Localized BL, BLL, and DLCL

Patient eligibility criterion: completely resected stage I or abdominal stage II disease.

Treatment

Two cycles of COPAD, second cycle given when ANC >1000/cm^3 and platelet count >100,000/cm^3:

C	Cyclophosphamide	250 mg/m^2/dose every 12 hours as a 15-minute IV infusion for 6 doses on days 1–3. First dose prior to doxorubicin infusion on day 1. Hydration at 125 mL/m^2/hour until 12 hours after last cyclophosphamide.
O	Vincristine	2 mg/m^2 (maximum 2 mg) IV on days 1 and 6
P	Prednisone	60 mg/m^2 divided twice daily PO/IV days 1–5 inclusive, then taper over 3 days
AD	Doxorubicin	60 mg/m^2 as a 6-hour infusion on day 1
G-CSF		5 µg/kg/day subcutaneously 7 until ANC >3000/mm^3

Results

The 3-year EFS and overall survival rates are 98.5% (95% CI 96.4–100%) and 99.2% (95% CI 97.8–100%), respectively.

Intermediate-Risk BL, BLL, and DLCL

Patient eligibility criteria:

- Incompletely resected stage I
- All other stage II (except completely resected abdominal stage II)
- Stage III
- Stage IV (CNS negative, bone marrow with less than 25% blasts).

Treatment

See Table 16-7.

Results

A 90% 3-year EFS rate for all stages.

- Stage I and II nonresected: 98% 3-year EFS
- Stage III, LDH less than twice normal: 92% 3-year EFS
- Stage III, LDH greater than twice normal: 86% 3-year EFS
- Stage IV: 89% 3-year EFS.

Advanced-Stage BL, BLL, and DLCL Including B-Cell Acute Lymphoblastic Leukemia and B-Cell NHL

This category includes advanced-stage BL, BLL, and DLCL including B-cell acute lymphoblastic leukemia (ALL) and B-cell NHL with marrow involvement with or without CNS involvement.

Patient eligibility criteria:

- Greater than 25% lymphoblasts present in bone marrow.
- CNS involvement demonstrated by any of the following:
    Presence of any L3 lymphoblasts in the CSF
    Cranial nerve palsy without other explanation
    Spinal cord compression
    Parameningeal disease
    Intracerebral mass

Table 16-7. Protocol for Intermediate-Risk BL, BLL, and DLCL (LMB-96 Protocol)

Reduction phases

COP:

Cyclophosphamide	300 mg/m² IV	Day 1
Vincristine	1 mg/m² (maximum 2 mg) IV	Day 1
Prednisolone	60 mg/m² day PO or IV	Days 1–7
Methotrexate (MTX) and hydrocortisone (HC)	15 mg IT[a] (dose adjusted for patients <3 years of age)	Day 1

Induction: 2 courses of COPADM started on day 8 after first day of reduction (COP) phase

COPADM 1 & 2

Vincristine	2 mg/m² (maximum 2 mg) IV	Day 1
MTX high dose (HD)	3 g/m² (over 3 hours) IV	Day 1
Folinic acid (FA)	15 mg/m² PO q6h × 12 doses[b]	Days 2–4
MTX and HC	15 mg IT[a]	Days 2 and 6
Cyclophosphamide	250 mg/m²/dose IV q12h	Days 2–4 (6 doses total)
Doxorubicin	60 mg/m² IV 6-h infusion	Day 2 (after cyclophosphamide)
Prednisolone	60 mg/m² day PO or IV	Days 1–5
G-CSF	5 µg/kg/day SQ	Day 7 until ANC >3000/mm³

CYM 1 & 2

MTX high dose (HD)	3 g/m² (over 3 hours) IV	Day 1
Folinic acid (FA)	15 mg/m² PO q6h × 12 doses[b]	Days 2–4
Cytarabine	100 mg/m²/day 24 continuous IV infusion	Days 2–6, inclusive
MTX	15 mg IT[a]	Day 2
HC	15 mg IT[a]	Days 2 and 7
Cytarabine	30 mg IT[a]	Day 7
G-CSF	5 µg/kg/day SQ	Day 7 until ANC >3000/mm³

[a]Age-adjusted doses for intrathecal use:

Age	MTX	HC	Cytarabine
<1 year	8 mg	8 mg	15 mg
1 year	10 mg	10 mg	20 mg
2 years	12 mg	12 mg	25 mg
>3 years	15 mg	15 mg	30 mg

[b]If serum methotrexate level at 72 hours is >0.1 µM/L, continue FA until serum methotrexate level is <0.1 µM/L.

Treatment

See Table 16-8.

Results

A 90% 3-year EFS.

- B-ALL did significantly better than CNS-positive patients.
- CNS patients who received high-dose methotrexate (without cranial RT) had similar overall survival to those on LMB-89 who received cranial RT.
- Dose reduction by reducing the number of maintenance courses resulted in significantly worse outcome for those on the LMB-96 regimen. The full therapy outlined in Table 16-8 remains the standard.

Table 16-8. Protocol for Advanced-Stage BL, BLL, and DLCL (LMB-96 Protocol)

Reduction phase
   COP:

Cyclophosphamide	300 mg/m^2 IV (over 15 minutes)	Day 1
Vincristine	1 mg/m^2 (maximum 2 mg) IV	Day 1
Prednisolone	60 mg/m^2/day PO or IV	Days 1–7 (then 3-day taper)
Methotrexate (MTX)	15 mg IT^a (age adjusted)	Days 1, 3, 5
Hydrocortisone (HC)	15 mg IT^a (age adjusted)	Days 1, 3, 5
Cytarabine	30 mg IT^a (age adjusted)	Days 1, 3, 5
Folinic acid	15 mg/m^2 PO q12h	Days 2 and 4

Induction: 2 courses of COPADM started on day 8 after first day of reduction (COP) phase
   COPADM 1

Vincristine	2 mg/m^2 (maximum 2 mg) IV	Day 1
MTX high dose (HD)	8 g/m^2 (over 4 hours) IV	Day 1
Folinic acid (FA)	15 mg/m^2 PO q6h 12 doses^b	Days 2–4
MTX and HC	15 mg IT^a (age adjusted)	Days 2, 4, 6
Cytarabine	30 mg IT^a (age adjusted)	Days 2, 4, 6
Cyclophosphamide	250 mg/m^2/dose IV q12h	Days 2–4
Doxorubicin	60 mg/m^2 IV 6-h infusion	Day 2 (after cyclophosphamide)
Prednisolone	60 mg/m^2/day PO or IV	Days 1–5 (then 3-day taper)
G-CSF	5 µg/kg/day SQ	Day 7 until ANC >3000/mm^3

COPADM 2 Begin when ANC >1000/mm^3 and platelet count >100,000/mm^{3c,d}
CYVE 1 & 2 Begin when ANC >1000/mm^3 and platelet count >100,000 mm^{3c}

Cytarabine	50 mg/m^2/day as 12-h infusion (hours 1–12)	Days 1–5, inclusive
Cytarabine (HD)	3000 mg/m^2/day over 3 hours (hours 13–15)	Days 2–5, inclusive
Etoposide	200 mg/m^2/day IV over 2 hours (hours 17–19)	Days 2–5, inclusive
G-CSF	5 µg/kg/day SQ	Day 7 until ANC >3000/mm^3

Maintenance 1: Begin when ANC >1000/mm^3 and platelets >100,000/mm^{3b}

Vincristine	2 mg/m^2 (maximum 2 mg) IV	Day 1
MTX high dose (HD)	8 g/m^2 (over 4 hours) IV	Day 1
Folinic acid (FA)	15 mg/m^2 PO q6h × 12 doses^b	Days 2–4
MTX and HC	15 mg IT^a (age adjusted)	Day 2
Cytarabine	30 mg IT^a (age adjusted)	Day 2
Cyclophosphamide	500 mg/m^2 IV over 30 minutes	Days 2 and 3
Doxorubicin	60 mg/m^2 IV 6-h infusion	Day 2 (after cyclophosphamide)
Prednisolone	60 mg/m^2/day PO or IV	Days 1–5 (then 3-day taper)

Maintenance 2: Begin when ANC >1000/mm^3 and platelet count >100,000/mm^3

Cytarabine	50 mg/m^2/dose SQ injection every 12 hours	Days 1–5, inclusive
Etoposide	150 mg/m^2 IV over 90 minutes	Days 1–3, inclusive

Maintenance 3: Begin when ANC >1000/mm^3 and platelet count >100,000/mm^3

Vincristine	2 mg/m^2 (maximum 2 mg) IV	Day 1
Cyclophosphamide	500 mg/m^2 IV over 30 minutes	Days 1 and 2
Doxorubicin	60 mg/m^2 IV 6-h infusion	Day 1 (after cyclophosphamide)
Prednisolone	60 mg/m^2/day PO or IV	Days 1–5 (then 3-day taper)

(Continues)

Table 16-8. (*Continued*)

Maintenance 4: Begin when ANC >1000/mm^3 and platelet count >100,000/mm^3

Cytarabine	50 mg/m^2/dose SQ injection every 12 hours	Days 1–5, inclusive
Etoposide	150 mg/m^2 IV over 90 minutes	Days 1–3, inclusive

[a]Age-adjusted doses for intrathecal use:

Age	MTX	HC	Cytarabine
<1 year	8 mg	8 mg	15 mg
1 year	10 mg	10 mg	20 mg
2 years	12 mg	12 mg	25 mg
>3 years	15 mg	15 mg	30 mg

[b]If serum methotrexate level at 72 hours is >0.1 µM/L then continue FA until serum methotrexate level is <0.1 µM/L.

[c]G-CSF should not be administered for 48 hours prior to beginning of next course.

[d]If no hematologic recovery by day 25, perform bone marrow aspirate. If blasts present, begin COPADM2.

Ki-1+ Anaplastic Large-Cell Lymphoma

Diagnosis

Must carefully distinguish Hodgkin disease from the Hodgkin-like variant of anaplastic large-cell lymphoma (ALCL) and differentiate from malignant histiocytosis.

Treatment

Table 16-9 and Figure 16-2 show the treatment protocol for Ki-1+ ALCL.

- Stages I and II resected treatment use strategy 1, which consists of a cytoreductive chemotherapy phase followed by three courses of alternating chemotherapy courses A, B, A.

Table 16-9. Treatment of Ki-1+ Anaplastic Large-Cell Lymphoma (BFM-NHL 90 Protocol) (to be read in conjunction with Figure 16-2)

Drug	Dose	Days administered
Cytoreductive phase[a] (course)		
Prednisone (orally/IV)	30 mg/m^2	1–5
Cyclophosphamide (IV)	200 mg/m^2	1–5
Course A		
Dexamethasone (orally)	10 mg/m^2	1–5
Ifosfamide (1-hour infusion)	800 mg/m^2	1–5
Methotrexate (24-hour infusion)[b]	500 mg/m^2	1
Methotrexate (IT)[a]	12 mg[a]	1
Cytarabine (IT)[a]	30 mg[a]	1
Prednisolone (IT)[a]	10 mg[a]	1
Cytarabine (1-hour infusion)	150 mg/m^2 q12h	4, 5
Etoposide (1-hour infusion)	100 mg/m^2	4, 5
Course B		
Dexamethasone (orally)	10 mg/m^2	1–5
Cyclophosphamide (1-hour infusion)	200 mg/m^2	1–5
Methotrexate (24-hour infusion)	500 mg/m^2	1
Methotrexate (IT)[a]	12 mg[a]	1

(Continues)

Table 16-9. (*Continued*)

Drug	Dose	Days administered
Cytarabine (IT)[a]	30 mg[a]	1
Prednisolone (IT)[a]	10 mg[a]	1
Doxorubicin (1-hour infusion)	25 mg/m^2	4, 5
Course AA		
Dexamethasone (orally)	10 mg/m^2	1–5
Ifosfamide (1-hour infusion)	800 mg/m^2	1–5
Vincristine (IVP)	1.5 mg/m^2 (maximum, 2 mg)	1
Methotrexate (24-hour infusion)[b]	5 g/m^2	1
Methotrexate (IT)[a]	6 mg[a]	1, 5
Cytarabine (IT)[a]	15 mg[a]	1, 5
Prednisolone (IT)[a]	5 mg[a]	1, 5
Etoposide (1-hour infusion)	100 mg/m^2	4, 5
Course BB		
Dexamethasone (orally)	10 mg/m^2	1–5
Cyclophosphamide (1-hour infusion)	200 mg/m^2	1–5
Vincristine (IV)	1.5 mg/m^2 (maximum, 2 mg)	1
Methotrexate (24-hour infusion)[b]	5 g/m^2	1
Methotrexate (IT)[a]	6 mg[a]	1, 5
Cytarabine (IT)[a]	15 mg[a]	1, 5
Prednisolone (IT)[a]	5 mg[a]	1, 5
Doxorubicin (1-hour infusion)	25 mg/m^2	4, 5
Course CC		
Dexamethasone (orally)	20 mg/m^2	1–5
Vindesine (IV)[c]	3 mg/m^2 (maximum, 5 mg)	1
Cytarabine (3-hour infusion)	2 gram/m^2 q12h	1, 2
Methotrexate (IT)[a]	12 mg[a]	5
Cytarabine (IT)[a]	30 mg[a]	5
Prednisolone (IT)[a]	10 mg[a]	5
Etoposide (1-hour infusion)	150 mg/m^2	3–5

[a]Doses adjusted for children <3 years of age; given 2 hours after beginning of methotrexate infusion.
Age-adjusted doses of IT methotrexate (MTX), Ara-C, and prednisolone in courses AA, BB:

Age	MTX	Ara-C	Prednisolone
<1 year	3	8	2 mg
1–2 years	4	10	3 mg
2–3 years	5	13	4 mg
≥3 years	5	15	5 mg

Age-adjusted dose of IT methotrexate (MTX), Ara-C, and prednisolone in courses A, B, CC:

Age	MTX	Ara-C	Prednisolone
<1 year	6	16	4 mg
1–2 years	8	20	6 mg
2–3 years	10	26	8 mg
≥ 3 years	12	30	10 mg

[b]Infusion of MTX and leucovorin (CF) rescue:

In courses A and B, 10% of the MTX dose of 500 mg/m^2 (= 50 mg/m^2) is administered IV over 30 minutes and 90% (= 450 mg/m^2) as a 23.5-hour continuous IV infusion. Leucovorin 15 mg/m^2 is administered as a bolus at 48, 51, and 54 hours.

In courses AA and BB, the MTX dose is increased to 5 g/m^2. The infusion schedule and leucovorin rescue are the same as in protocol for non-B-cell lymphoma (see Table 16-6 footnote).

[c]May be replaced with vinblastine 6 mg/m^2 if vindesine is not commercially available.

From Seidemann K, Tiemann M, Schrappe M, et al. Short-pulse B-non Hodgkin lymphoma–type chemotherapy is efficacious treatment for pediatric anaplastic large cell lymphoma: a report of the Berlin-Frankfurt-Munster Group Trial NHL-BFM 90. Blood 2001;97:3699-3706, with permission.

Strategy	Stage	Therapy Course

Fig. 16-2. Therapy strategy and stratification criteria for the ALCL therapy group (NHL-BFM 90 protocol). (Read in conjunction with Table 16-9.)
Note: v = cytoreductive phase

- Stage II unresected and stage III treatment use strategy 2, which consists of a cytoreductive chemotherapy phase followed by six alternating chemotherapy courses A and B.
- Stage IV (or multiple bone involvement) Ki-1+ ALCL uses the strategy 3 treatment of a cytoreductive chemotherapy phase followed by six alternating chemotherapy courses AA, BB, and CC.

Hematologic parameters for starting a course are as follows: platelet count >50,000/mm^3; ANC >200/mm^3 for courses 2, 3, and 4; and ANC >500/mm^3 for courses 4, 5, and 6 (minimum interval between first day of two courses is 2 weeks).

Results

By intent to treat analysis:

- Patients stratified to strategy 1 have 100% 5-year EFS.
- Patients stratified to strategy 2 have a 73% ± 6% 5-year EFS.
- Patients stratified to strategy 3 have a 79% ± 11% 5-year EFS.

Radiation Therapy

Generally, radiotherapy is not indicated on an elective basis. It is only indicated for acute life-threatening complications refractory to initial chemotherapy, such as superior vena cava syndrome. Doses and fields should be limited. In B-cell-NHL with CNS disease, cranial irradiation should not be used. The use of cranial irradiation for CNS prophylaxis is controversial. However, it is used in many of the protocols to treat advanced-stage lymphoblastic lymphoma.

Surgical Therapy

The role of surgery in NHL treatment is limited. It should be performed on patients in whom there is good reason to believe that total resection can be achieved (e.g., localized bowel disease) without a mutilating procedure (e.g., amputation, extensive maxillofacial surgery, exenterations) or an excessively risky procedure. Patients with widespread lymphoma are not eligible for surgical resection, but the presence of a single nonresectable mass in addition to a totally resectable mass will not exclude patients from surgical treatment.

Prognosis

Prognosis depends on the appropriateness of protocols. Expected EFS has been mentioned with each category of treatment in the preceding discussion. Table 16-10

Table 16-10. Factors Associated with Favorable and Unfavorable Prognosis[a]

Favorable prognosis
  Primary site
  Stages I and II: Head and neck (nonparameningeal)
  Peripheral nodes
  Abdominal site: 80% or greater 2-year survival (recurrence after 2 years rare)
Unfavorable prognosis
  Stage of disease:
    Stage III or IV
    Stage IV with CNS involvement: worst prognosis
  Site of disease:
    Parameningeal stage II
    All stages of extranodal, extralymphatic NHL in head and neck area (sinus, jaw, orbit,
      scalp)
    Presence of pleural effusion in stage III small noncleaved cell lymphoma
  Incomplete initial remission within 2 months
  Soluble IL-2 R level
    >1000 U/mL
  LDH level
    >1000 U/L
  Uric acid level
    >7.1 mg/dL

[a]All of the above variables essentially reflect tumor burden—the higher the burden the worse the prognosis. IL-2R is a more specific marker of lymphoid malignancy than LDH and can be used as a marker to differentiate small round cell tumors of lymphoid origin from nonlymphoid origin.

lists clinical and biological factors associated with favorable and unfavorable prognosis.

Management of Relapse

A relapse indicates a poor prognosis, regardless of the site of relapse, tumor histology, other original prognostic factors, prior therapy, or time from diagnosis to relapse. For this reason, the selection of the most effective front-line treatment is critical. Relapsed patients are first treated to induce remission. For lymphoblastic lymphoma and B-cell lymphomas, see Table 16-11. Chemotherapy with ifosfamide, carboplatin, and etoposide (VP-16) is a useful salvage regimen following which autologous stem cell harvest is generally easily achieved. After induction of complete or very good partial remission, consolidation with stem cell transplantation is indicated. Patients who are chemotherapy resistant are unlikely to be cured using autologous stem cell transplantation. Patients with B-lineage lymphomas that are CD20+ may benefit from the addition of rituximab to help induce remission. ALCL may require less aggressive salvage (see Table 16-12). Autologous transplant does not provide added benefit. Patients who have a second relapse may benefit from therapy with vinblastine 6 mg/m²/week for 12–18 months. *Cis*-retinoic acid, with or without interferon-α, has maintained prolonged remissions in some patients.

Adoptive immunotherapy using allogeneic stem cell transplantation is theoretically preferable because numerous studies demonstrate a substantially lower relapse rate as a result of graft versus lymphoma effects. There is a tendency toward improved survival with allogeneic compared to autologous transplantation; however, the increased risk of allogeneic transplant–related mortality reduces this advantage somewhat. As transplantation techniques improve, it is likely that these differences will become statistically significant. Disease-free survival for allogeneic

Table 16-11. Treatment for Relapsed NHL

- Ifosfamide 1800 mg/m^2/day IV over 1 hour with Mesna 1800 mg/m^2/day IV (in 5 divided doses of 360 mg/m^2 given as a bolus: immediately before, as a 3-hour infusion immediately after ifosfamide, and as a bolus at hours 3, 6, and 9 post-ifosfamide) on days 1–5.
- Carboplatin 300 mg/m^2/day IV over 1 hour on days 1–3.
- Etoposide, 100 mg/m^2/day IV over 1 hour on days 1–5.
- Repeat second cycle 3 weeks from the first cycle, then reevaluate radiographically. If in complete remission or very good partial remission, proceed to consolidation with transplantation. If responsive, may give 3rd cycle prior to consolidation with transplantation.
  If resistant, alternate therapies such as rituximab or phase I/II therapy are indicated.

Table 16-12. Treatment of Relapsed Anaplastic Large Cell Lymphoma

Six-week cycles repeated for 12 months:
- CCNU 100 mg/m^2 PO day 1
- Vinblastine 6 mg/m^2 IV days 1, 8, 15, 22
- Cytarabine 100 mg/m^2 IV days 1–5

transplants range from 24% to 68%, and in autologous transplants from 22% to 46%. Although these numbers are encouraging, they represent patients transplanted, excluding those who could not be transplanted because of prior toxicity or lack of response.

Myeloablative chemotherapy regimens, including CBV (Table 16-13) or BEAM (Table 16-14), have been utilized followed by stem cell transplantation. Other mye-

Table 16-13. CBV Regimen for Stem Cell Transplantation in Non-Hodgkin Lymphoma

Days	Chemotherapy
–8, –7, –6	BCNU: 100 mg/m^2/day IV over 3 hours (total dose = 300 mg/m^2) Etoposide 800 mg/m^2/day IV as a 72-hour continuous infusion (total dose = 2400 mg/m^2)
–5, –4, –3, –2	Cyclophosphamide: 1500 mg/m^2/day IV over 1 hour. Use MESNA (total dose = 2200 mg/m^2 IV every 24 hours)
–1	No treatment
0	Stem cell infusion

Methylprednisolone 1 mg/kg/day in divided doses given every 6 hours for pulmonary protection from BCNU toxicity on days –9 to –2. Wean by 20% every 2 days for an 8-day taper.

Table 16-14. BEAM Regimen for Stem Cell Transplantation in Non-Hodgkin Lymphoma

Day	Chemotherapy
–6	BCNU: 300 mg/m^2 IV over 3 hours
–5, –4, –3, –2	Etoposide 200 mg/m^2/day IV over 1 hour (total dose = 800 mg/m^2)
–5, –4, –3, –2	Cytosine arabinoside: 400 mg/m^2/day IV over 1 hour (total dose = 1600 mg/m^2)
–1	Melphalan 140 mg/m^2 IV over 30 minutes
0	Stem cell infusion

Methylprednisolone 1 mg/kg/day in divided doses given every 6 hours for pulmonary protection from BCNU toxicity on days –7 to –2. Wean by 20% every 2 days for an 8-day taper.

loablative regimens that have been utilized consist of total body irradiation, etoposide, and cyclophosphamide. Post-transplantation interleukin-2 may be used to reduce recurrence rate.

SUGGESTED READINGS

Brugieres L, Quartier P, Le Deley MC, et al. Relapses of childhood anaplastic large-cell lymphoma: treatment results in a series of 41 children—a report from the French Society of Pediatric Oncology. Ann Oncol 2000;11:53–8.

Cairo MS, Gerrard M, Sposto R, et al. Results of a randomized FAB LMB 96 international study in children and adolescents with advanced B-NHL: patients with L3 leukemia/CNS have an excellent prognosis. Proc Am Soc Clin Oncol 2003;22:796.

Cairo MS, Sposto R, Perkins S, et al. Burkitt's and Burkitt-like lymphoma in children and adolescents: a review of the Children's Cancer Group Experience. Br J Haematol 2003;120:660–70.

Diebold J. World Health Organization classification of malignant lymphomas. Exp Oncol 2001;23:101–3.

Gerrard M, Cairo M, Weston C, et al. Results of the FAB international study in children and adolescents with localized, resected B cell lymphoma. Proc Am Soc Clin Oncol 2003;22:795.

Goldman SC, Holcenberg JS, Finklestein JZ, et al. A randomized comparison between rasburicase and allopurinol in children with lymphoma or leukemia at high risk for tumor lysis. Blood 2001;97(10):2998–3003.

Link MP, Shuster JJ, Donaldson SS, Berard CW, Murphy SB. Treatment of children and young adults with early stage non-Hodgkin's lymphoma. New Engl J Med 1997;337:1259–66.

Magrath IT. Malignant non-Hodgkin's lymphomas in children. In: Pizzo PA, Poplack DG, editors. Principles and Practice of Pediatric Oncology. 4th ed. Philadelphia: Lippincott Williams & Wilkins, 2002.

Neth O, Seidemann K, Jansen P, et al. Precursor B-cell lymphoblastic lymphoma in childhood and adolescence: clinical features, treatment, and results in trials NHL-BFM 86 and 90. Med Pediatr Oncol 2000;35:20–7.

Patte C, Gerrard M, Auperin A, et al. Results of the randomized international trial FAB LMB 96 for the "intermediate risk" childhood and adolescent B cell lymphoma: reduced therapy is efficacious. Proc Am Soc Clin Oncol 2003;22:796.

Reiter A, Schrappe M, Ludwig WD, et al. Intensive ALL-type therapy without local radiotherapy provides a 90% event-free survival for children with T-cell lymphoblastic lymphoma: a BFM Group report. Blood 2000;95(2):416–21.

Seidemann K, Tiemann M, Schrappe M, et al. Short-pulse B-non-Hodgkin lymphoma-type chemotherapy is efficacious treatment for pediatric anaplastic large-cell lymphoma: a report of the Berlin-Frankfurt-Munster Group Trial NHL-BFM 90. Blood 2001;97(12):3699–3706.

17

CENTRAL NERVOUS SYSTEM MALIGNANCIES

Tumors of the central nervous system (CNS) are frequently encountered in children: approximately 35 cases per 1 million in children under 15 years of age. Brain tumors are the second most common group of malignant tumors in childhood, accounting for 20% of all childhood malignancies.

Most childhood brain tumors (60–70%) arise from glial cells and tend not to metastasize outside the CNS unless there is operative intervention. The relative frequency with regard to specific tumor types can be seen in Table 17-1. Most are infratentorial in location.

There is an association between primary CNS tumors and the following conditions:

- Neurofibromatosis type 1 (NF-1)
- Tuberous sclerosis
- von Hippel–Lindau syndrome
- Children of families with Li–Fraumeni syndrome (families with an excess occurrence of breast, brain, and lung cancer, soft tissue sarcomas and adrenocortical carcinoma, osteosarcoma, and leukemia associated with a germline mutation of p53, a suppressor oncogene)
- Turcot syndrome (polyposis of colon and CNS malignancy)
- Gorlin syndrome (nevus basal cell carcinoma syndrome [NBCCS]), which is characterized by multiple basal cell carcinomas, odontogenic jaw cysts, palmar and plantar pits, and skeletal abnormalities.

PATHOLOGY

Supratentorial lesions:

1. *Cerebral hemisphere:* low- and high-grade glioma, ependymoma, meningioma, primitive neuroectodermal tumor (PNET)
2. *Sella or chiasm:* craniopharyngioma, pituitary adenoma, optic nerve glioma
3. *Pineal region:* pineoblastoma, pineocytoma, germ cell tumors, glioma.

Infratentorial lesions:

1. Posterior fossa: medulloblastoma, glioma (low grade more frequent than high grade), ependymoma, meningioma
2. Brain stem tumors: low- and high-grade glioma, PNET

Table 17-1. Relative Frequency of Common
Childhood Brain Tumors

Location and histology	Frequency (%)
Supratentorial	
Low-grade glioma	16
Ependymoma	3
High-grade glioma	5
PNET[a]	3
Other	2
Sella/chiasm	
Craniopharyngioma	6
Optic nerve glioma	5
Total	40
Infratentorial	
Cerebellum	
Medulloblastoma	20
Astrocytoma	18
Ependymoma	6
Brain stem	
Glioma	14
Other	2
Total	60

[a]Primitive neuroectodermal tumor.

The most useful pathologic classification for brain tumors is based on embryonic derivation and histologic cell of origin. Tumors are further classified by grading the degree of malignancy within a particular tumor type. This grading is useful in astrocytoma and ependymoma. Criteria that are useful microscopically in grading the degree of malignancy include:

1. Cellular pleomorphism
2. Mitotic index
3. Anaplasia and necrosis
4. MIB-1 index.

Molecular Pathology of CNS Neoplasms

The majority of CNS neoplasms are sporadic. Only a small percentage is associated with the inherited genetic disorders listed above.

Chromosomal abnormalities have been identified in many brain tumors in children. These chromosomal abnormalities are helpful in the pathologic classification, especially in the differentiation of PNET from atypical teratoid rhabdoid tumors. Identification of the genes involved and how they contribute to tumor genesis is ongoing.

Table 17-2 describes common cytogenetic abnormalities identified in brain tumors.

CLINICAL MANIFESTATIONS

Intracranial Tumors

Symptoms and signs are related to the location, size, and growth rate of the tumor:

1. Slow-growing tumors produce massive shifts of normal structures and may become quite large by the time they first become symptomatic.

Table 17-2. Cytogenetic loci implicated in malignant brain tumors in children

Tumor	Chromosome	Disorder
PNET/MB	5q21	Turcot syndrome
	9q22.3	NBCCS
	17p13.3	
	17q	
Astrocytoma, grades III–IV	7p12	
	17p13.1	Li–Fraumeni syndrome
	17q11.2	Neurofibromatosis-1
Subependymal giant cell tumor	9q34, 16p13	Tuberous sclerosis
Meningioma	22q	
	22q12	Neurofibromatosis-2
ATT/Rhabdoid tumor	22q11.2	

Abbreviations: PNET/MB, prototype primitive neuroectodermal tumor, medulloblastoma; ATT/RT, atypical teratoid rhabdoid; NBCCS, nevoid basal cell carcinoma syndrome.

Adapted from Biegel JA. Genetics of pediatric central nervous system tumors. J Pediatr Hematol Oncol 1997; 19:492–501, with permission.

   2. Rapidly growing tumors produce symptoms early and present when they are relatively small.

The most common presenting signs and symptoms of an intracranial neoplasm are increased intracranial pressure (ICP) and focal neurologic deficits. If symptoms and signs of increased ICP precede the onset of localized neurologic dysfunction, a tumor of the ventricles or deep midline structures is most likely. If localizing signs (seizures, ataxia, visual field defects, cranial neuropathies, or corticospinal tract dysfunction) are predominant in the absence of increased ICP, it is more probable that the tumor originates in parenchymal structures (cerebral hemispheres, brain stem, or cerebellum).

General signs and symptoms of intracranial tumors:

   1. Headache. In young children headache can present as irritability. Often worse in the morning, improving throughout the day.
   2. Vomiting (often early morning).
   3. Disturbances of gait and balance.
   4. Cranial nerve abnormalities.
   5. Impaired vision:
      a. Diplopia (6th nerve palsy). In young children diplopia may present as frequent blinking or intermittent strabismus.
      b. Papilledema from increased ICP may present as intermittent blurred vision.
      c. Parinaud syndrome (failure of upward gaze and setting-sun sign, large pupils and decreased constriction to light).
   6. Mental disturbances: somnolence, irritability, personality or behavioral change, or change in school performance.
   7. Seizures, usually focal.
   8. Endocrine abnormalities: Midline supratentorial tumors may cause endocrine abnormalities due to effects on the hypothalamus or pituitary and visual field disturbances due to optic pathway involvement.
   9. Cranial enlargement (characteristic of increased ICP in infants).
 10. Diencephalic syndrome can be seen in patients aged 6 months to 3 years with brain tumors who present with sudden failure to thrive and emaciation. The syndrome is caused by a hypothalamic tumor in the anterior portion of the hypothalamus or the anterior floor of the third ventricle.

Spinal Tumors

Spinal tumors of children may be found anywhere along the vertebral column. They cause symptoms by compression of the contents of the spinal canal. Localized back pain in a child or adolescent should raise suspicion of a spinal cord tumor, especially if the back pain is worse in the recumbent position and relieved when sitting up. The major signs and symptoms of spinal cord tumors are listed in Table 17-3. Most spinal cord tumors have associated muscle weakness, and the muscle group affected corresponds to the spinal level of the lesions.

Spinal tumors can be divided into three distinct groups:

1. *Intramedullary:* These tumors tend to be glial in origin and are usually gliomas or ependymomas.
2. *Extramedullary, intradural:* These tumors are likely to be neurofibromas often associated with neurofibromatosis. If they arise in adolescent females, meningiomas are more likely.
3. *Extramedullary, extradural:* These tumors are most often of mesenchymal origin and may be due to direct extension of a neuroblastoma through the intervertebral foramina or due to a lymphoma. Tumors of the vertebra may also encroach on the spinal cord, leading to epidural compression of the cord and paraplegia (e.g., PNET or Langerhans cell histiocytosis occurring in a thoracic or cervical vertebral body).

Table 17-3. Major Signs and Symptoms of Spinal Tumors

Back pain (50% of cases); increased in supine position or with Valsalva maneuver
Resistance to trunk flexion
Paraspinal muscle spasm
Spinal deformity (especially progressive scoliosis)
Gait disturbance
Weakness, flaccid or spastic
Reflex changes (especially decreased in arms and increased in legs)
Sensory impairment below level of tumor (30% of cases)
Decreased perspiration below level of tumor
Extensor plantar responses (Babinski sign)
Sphincter impairment (urinary or anal)
Midline closure defects of skin or vertebral arches
Nystagmus (with lesions of upper cervical cord)

DIAGNOSTIC EVALUATION

Computed Tomography

Computed tomography (CT) scan is an important procedure in the detection of CNS malignancies. Scans performed both with and without iodinated contrast agents detect 95% of brain tumors. However, tumors of the posterior fossa, which are common in children, are better evaluated with magnetic resonance imaging (MRI). CT scans should be performed using thin sections (usually 5 mm). Sedation is often necessary to avoid motion artifact. CT is more useful than MRI in:

- Evaluating bony lesions
- Detection of calcification in tumor
- Investigating unstable patients because of the shorter imaging time.

Magnetic Resonance Imaging

MRI provides the following advantages:

- No ionizing radiation exposure (especially important in multiple follow-up examinations)
- Greater sensitivity in detection of brain tumors especially in the temporal lobe and posterior fossa (these lesions are obscured by bony artifact on CT)
- Ability to directly image in multiple planes (multiplanar), which is of value to neurosurgical planning (CT is usually only in axial planes)
- Ability to apply different pulse sequences, which is useful in depicting anatomy (T_1-weighted images) and pathology (T_2-weighted images)
- Ability to map motor areas with functional MRI.

MRI specificity is enhanced with the contrast agent gadolinium diethylenetri-aminepentaacetic acid dimeglumine (Gd-DTPA), which should be used in the evaluation of childhood CNS tumors and has the following advantages:

- Highlights areas of blood–brain barrier breakdown that occur in tumors
- Useful in identifying areas of tumor within an area of surrounding edema
- Improves the delineation of cystic from solid tumor elements
- Helps to differentiate residual tumor from gliosis (scarring).

The major difficulty with MRI in infants and children is the long time required to complete imaging and for this reason adequate sedation is required.

Magnetic Resonance Angiography

Magnetic resonance angiography (MRA) may aid in the preoperative evaluation of the normal anatomic vasculature (e.g., dural sinus occlusion) and in the assessment of tumor vascularity.

Magnetic Resonance Spectroscopy

Magnetic resonance spectroscopy is a new technique that may be helpful in both diagnosing brain tumors in children and during follow-up investigations. This technique is able to distinguish between malignant tumors and areas of necrosis by comparing creatine/choline ratios with *N*-acetyl aspartate/choline ratios. This technique in combination with tumor characteristics as identified by MRI, tumor site, and other patient characteristics may be able to more accurately predict the tumor type preoperatively. In addition, it may be helpful in identifying postoperatively residual tumor from postoperative changes.

Positron Emission Tomography

Positron emission tomography (PET) is a potentially useful technique for evaluating CNS tumors. The F-18-labeled analogue of 2-deoxyglucose (FDG) can be used to image the metabolic differences between normal and malignant cells. Astrocytomas and oligodendrogliomas are generally hypometabolic, whereas anaplastic astrocytomas and glioblastoma multiforme are hypermetabolic.

PET is useful to determine:

- Degree of malignancy of a tumor
- Prognosis of brain tumor patients
- Appropriate biopsy site in patients with multiple lesions and large homogeneous and heterogeneous lesions

- Recurrent tumor from necrosis, scar, and edema in patients who have undergone radiation therapy and chemotherapy
- Recurrent tumor from postsurgical change.

Evaluation of the Spinal Cord

MRI and Gd-DTPA have replaced myelography in the evaluation of meningeal spread of brain tumors in the spinal column and delineating spinal cord tumors.

Cerebrospinal Fluid Examination

The cerebrospinal fluid (CSF) should have the following studies performed:

1. Cell count with cytocentrifuge slide examination for cytology of tumor cells
2. Glucose and protein content
3. CSF α-fetoprotein (AFP)
4. CSF human chorionic gonadotropin (hCG).

Polyamine assays in the CSF are of value in the evaluation of tumors that are in proximity to the circulating CSF (medulloblastoma, ependymoma, brain stem glioma). The assay is not useful in glioblastoma multiforme and not predictive in astrocytomas. AFP and hCG of the CSF may be elevated in CNS germ cell tumors.

Bone Marrow Aspiration and Bone Scan

These studies are indicated in medulloblastoma and high-grade ependymomas because a small percentage of these patients have systemic metastases at the time of diagnosis.

GENERAL CONSIDERATIONS

Surgery

The purpose of neurosurgical intervention is threefold:

1. To provide a tissue biopsy for purposes of histopathology and cytogenetics
2. To attain maximum tumor removal with the fewest neurologic sequelae
3. To relieve associated increased ICP due to CSF obstruction.

Use of preoperative dexamethasone can significantly decrease peritumoral edema, thus decreasing focal symptoms and often eliminating the need for emergency surgery. For patients with hydrocephalus that is moderate to severe, endoscopic or standard ventriculostomy can decrease ICP. Tumor resection is safer when performed 1–2 days following reduction in edema and ICP by these means.

Technical advances in neurosurgery that have improved the success of surgery include ultrasonic aspirators; image guidance, which allows 3-D mapping of tumors; functional mapping and electrocorticography, which allow pre- and intraoperative differentiation of normal and tumor tissue; and neuroendoscopy. Stereotactic biopsies allow biopsy of deep-seated midline tumors. The ideal goal is gross total resection of the tumor (probably leaving microscopic residual) because removal of a margin of normal tissue would cause devastating neurologic sequelae.

Radiotherapy

Most patients with high-grade brain tumors require radiotherapy to achieve local control of microscopic or macroscopic residual tumor. Radiation therapy for intracranial tumors consists of external beam irradiation using conventional fields or, now more commonly, 3-D conformal radiotherapy, which conforms to the margins of the tumor. The latter decreases radiation to normal brain tissue by up to 30%. Intensity modulation radiation therapy (IMRT) uses more complex computerized planning and intensity modulation of the radiation to further decrease radiation to normal tissue under certain circumstances.

The wider use of ionizing radiation in brain tumors in children has resulted in improved long-term survival. However, the significant long-term effects on cognition and growth, especially in patients requiring craniospinal irradiation (e.g., PNET), can be devastating. The total dose of radiotherapy depends on:

- Tumor type (which also influences volume of treatment)
- Age of the child
- Volume of the brain or spinal cord to be treated.

Current efforts seek to decrease radiation by conforming better to the tumor (conformal radiotherapy) and by using chemotherapy in addition. Children under 3 years of age are most drastically affected. In this group, newer strategies that avoid or delay radiation therapy by initial treatment with chemotherapy have promising preliminary results, but require further evaluation. In medulloblastoma therapy, this approach allows one-third diminution in the dose of craniospinal irradiation.

Brachytherapy, stereotactic radiosurgery, and fractionated stereotactic radiosurgery are alternatives to conventional radiation therapy presently under study and may prove useful in relapsed patients.

Chemotherapy

Chemotherapy plays an expanding role in the management of recurrent disease and in many newly diagnosed patients. Two anatomic features of the CNS make it unique with respect to the delivery of chemotherapeutic agents:

1. The tight junction of the endothelial cells of the cerebral capillaries, that is, the blood–brain barrier
2. The ventricular and subarachnoid CSF.

The blood–brain barrier inhibits the equilibration of large polar lipid-insoluble compounds between the blood and brain tissue, whereas small nonpolar lipid-soluble drugs rapidly equilibrate across the blood–brain barrier. The blood–brain barrier is probably not crucial in determining the efficacy of a particular chemotherapeutic agent, because in many brain tumors the normal blood–brain barrier is impaired. Factors such as tumor heterogeneity, cell kinetics and drug administration, distribution, and excretion play a more significant role in determining the chemotherapeutic sensitivity of a particular tumor than does the blood–brain barrier. Tumors with a low mitotic index and small growth fraction are less sensitive to chemotherapy; tumors with a high mitotic index and larger growth fraction are more sensitive to chemotherapy.

The CSF circulates over a large surface area of the brain and provides an alternate route for drug delivery; it can function as a reservoir for intrathecal administration or as a sink after systemic administration of chemotherapeutic agents. The rationale of instillation of chemotherapy into the CSF compartment is that significantly higher drug concentrations can be attained in the CSF and surrounding brain tissue. This mode of administration is most applicable in cases of meningeal spread or in those tumors in which the risk of spread through the CSF is high.

Adjuvant chemotherapy is used in select primary brain tumors and for recurrent disease (Table 17-4). In certain cases it allows for decreased radiation doses with equal or improved cure rates. In others, adjuvant chemotherapy improves outcome with standard radiation therapy. Trials of new agents, combinations of agents, and standard drugs as radiosensitizing agents are ongoing.

MANAGEMENT OF SPECIFIC TUMORS
Astrocytomas

Astrocytomas account for approximately 50% of the CNS tumors with peaks between ages 5–6 and 12–13 years. The World Health Organization (WHO) grades these tumors I–IV in increasing malignancy. Low-grade tumors (WHO I and II) are distinguished histologically from high-grade astrocytomas (WHO III and IV) by the absence of cellular pleomorphism, high cell density, mitotic activity, and necrosis. The following are the histologic subtypes:

- *Pilocytic astrocytoma* has a fibrillary background, rare mitoses, and, classically, Rosenthal fibers. It usually behaves in a benign fashion. These tumors are well circumscribed and grow slowly (WHO grade I).
- *Diffuse or fibrillary astrocytoma* is more cellular and infiltrative and more likely to undergo anaplastic change (WHO grade II).
- *Anaplastic astrocytoma* is highly cellular with significant cellular atypia. It is locally invasive and aggressive (WHO grade III).

Table 17-4. Chemotherapy Regimens for Brain Tumors

Regimen	Dosage/route	Frequency
CCNU	100 mg/m² PO, day 1	Every 6 weeks for 8 cycles
Vincristine[a]	1.5 mg/m² IV, days 1, 8	
Prednisone	40 mg/m² PO, days 1–14	
	OR	
CCNU	100 mg/m² PO, day 1	Every 6 weeks for 8 cycles
Vincristine[a]	1.5 mg/m² IV, days 1, 8	
Procarbazine	100 mg/m² PO, days 1–14	
	OR	
CCNU	75 mg/m² PO, day 1	Every 6 weeks for 8 cycles
Vincristine[a]	1.5 mg/m² IV, days 1, 8, 14	
Cisplatin	75 mg/m² IV, day 1 over 6 hours	
	OR	
Temozolomide	90 mg/m²/day PO × 42 days	During radiation therapy
Temozolomide	150–200 mg/m²/day PO × 5 days	Every 28 days for 6–12 cycles
	OR	
Vincristine[b]	0.065 mg/kg IV, days 1, 8, 29, 36	Every 12 weeks for 4 cycles for children ages 24–36 months
Cyclophosphamide	65 mg/kg IV, days 1, 29	
Cisplatin	4 mg/kg IV over 6 hours, day 57	For children less than 24 months of age at diagnosis for 8 cycles
Etoposide	6.5 mg/kg IV over 1 hour, days 59, 60	

[a]Maximum dose 2 mg.
[b]Maximum dose 1.5 mg.

- *Glioblastoma multiforme* demonstrates increased nuclear anaplasia, pseudopalisading, and multinucleate giant cells (WHO grade IV).

The majority of cerebellar astrocytomas remain confined to the cerebellum. Very rarely do they have neuraxis dissemination.

Low-Grade Astrocytomas

Low-grade astrocytomas present with hydrocephalus, focal signs, or seizures.

Surgery

Surgical excision is the initial treatment. Gross total resection is desirable. Pilocytic astrocytomas are slow growing and well circumscribed with a distinct margin. These features permit complete resection in 90% of patients with posterior fossa tumors, and a majority of hemispheric tumors. By contrast, diffuse low-grade astrocytomas are infiltrative and are less often completely resected. Diencephalic tumors are amenable to gross total resection in less than 40% of cases. If removal is complete, no further treatment is recommended. Patients with significant residual tumor postoperatively may require further therapy if the risk of subsequent surgery to remove progressive tumor is too great.

Radiotherapy

The role of radiation is undecided. The ability to re-resect hemispheric lesions usually allows postponement of adjuvant therapy. Current trends use radiotherapy when chemotherapy has failed in unresectable symptomatic tumors. Dosing is 5000 to 5500 cGy, depending on age, to the original tumor bed with a 2-cm margin.

In deep midline locations, chemotherapy tends to be used to avoid the long-term effects of radiation to vital areas, including the pituitary.

Chemotherapy

The carboplatin-vincristine regimen is the best studied regimen in patients with newly diagnosed, progressive low-grade astrocytoma (Table 17-5). Responses occur in 56% of patients. Patients less than 5 years of age have a 3-year progression-free survival (PFS) of 74% compared with 39% in older children. A previous study demonstrated a response rate of 52% in patients with recurrent disease. The Children's Oncology Group is currently comparing the carboplatin-vincristine regimen with 6-thioguanine, procarbazine, CCNU, and vincristine. Use of single-agent

Table 17-5. Chemotherapy for Low-Grade Astrocytomas and Optic Gliomas

Induction (one 12-week cycle):

Week	1	2	3	4	5	6	7	8	9	10	11-12
	V	V	V	V	V	V	V	V	V	V	REST
	C	C	C	C			C	C	C	C	

Maintenance (eight 6-week cycles)

Week	1	2	3	4	5-6
	V	V	V		REST
	C	C	C	C	

C: Carboplatin, 175 mg/m^2 IV
V: Vincristine, 1.5 mg/m^2 IV (maximum dose 2 mg)

vinblastine is also now being studied for recurrent disease with promising prelimi-nary results.

Prognosis

The 5- and 10-year survival rate for completely resected low-grade supratentorial astrocytomas treated with surgery alone is 76–100% and 69–100%, respectively. In the posterior fossa, these rates approach 100%. In patients with partially resected low-grade astrocytomas who are observed without treatment or who are treated with postoperative radiotherapy, the 5- and 10-year survival rate is 67–87% and 67–94%, respectively.

Recurrence

Recurrent low-grade astrocytomas should be approached surgically when possible. If not completely resectable, chemotherapy and/or radiation should be given, depending on prior therapy received.

High-Grade Astrocytomas

Surgery

Complete surgical removal of these tumors is rarely accomplished because of their infiltrative nature. In about 20–25% of cases, the contralateral hemisphere may be involved, due to spread through the corpus callosum. The main purpose of surgery in these cases is to reduce the tumor burden. Patients who have total or near-total resection have longer survival than do patients who have partial resection or simple biopsy. Maximal surgical debulking is recommended unless the neurologic sequelae are too devastating.

Radiotherapy

Postoperative irradiation increases survival in high-grade astrocytomas. The port should include the tumor bed and a 2-cm margin of normal surrounding tissue. The dose is 5000–6000 cGy in children over 5 years of age. The use of stereotactic radio-therapy is being investigated as a technique to increase local tumor doses.

Chemotherapy

In children, multiagent adjuvant chemotherapy added to postoperative radiation results in a significant (but modest) improvement in disease-free survival compared with postoperative radiation alone. CCNU, vincristine, and procarbazine (or pred-nisone) (Table 17-4) is the current standard, but without reasonable resection, chemotherapy is ineffective. PFS is approximately 33% at 5 years. Temozolomide sig-nificantly improves survival in adults when given for six cycles after radiotherapy (Table 17-4) and its efficacy is currently being investigated in children.

Medulloblastoma

Medulloblastoma (posterior fossa PNET) is the most common CNS tumor in chil-dren, representing approximately 20% of all childhood brain tumors, with 80% of cases presenting before the age of 15 years. The tumor presents in the posterior fossa, and widespread seeding of the subarachnoid space may occur. The frequency of CNS spread outside the primary tumor can be as high as 40% at the time of diagnosis.

Extraneural spread to bone, bone marrow, lungs, liver, or lymph nodes occurs in approximately 4% of patients.

Staging studies should include MRI of the spine (preferably preoperatively), lumbar CSF cytology, bone scan, liver function tests, and bone marrow examination. Histology and cytogenetics of the original tumor are essential to evaluate for large-cell anaplastic subtype and for monosomy 22, which is characteristic of *atypical teratoid/rhabdoid tumor*. These more aggressive tumors fare poorly when treated as typical medulloblastoma. The Chang staging system (Table 17-6), which evaluates tumor size, local extension, and metastases is used to assess prognosis. Patients are divided into average and high-risk categories based on extent of disease (i.e., CSF cytology or spinal cord involvement), volume of residual tumor, histology, and age of diagnosis (Table 17-7).

Surgery

Surgical excision is employed as the initial therapy with an objective of gross total resection or near-total resection with less than 1.5 cm^2 of residual tumor. Disease-free

Table 17-6. Chang Staging System for Posterior Fossa Medulloblastoma (PNET)

Classification	Description
T1	Tumor less than 3 cm in diameter and limited to the classic midline position in the vermis, the roof of the fourth ventricle, and less frequently to the cerebellar hemispheres
T2	Tumor 3 cm or greater in diameter, further invading one adjacent structure or partially filling the fourth ventricle
T3	Divided into T3a, and T3b:
T3a	Tumor further invading two adjacent structures or completely filling the fourth ventricle with extension into the aqueduct of Sylvius, foramen of Magendie, or foramen of Luschka, producing marked internal hydrocephalus
T3b	Tumor arising from the floor of the fourth ventricle or brain stem and filling the fourth ventricle
T4	Tumor further spreading through the aqueduct of Sylvius to involve the third ventricle or midbrain or tumor extending to the upper cervical cord
M0	No evidence of gross subarachnoid or hematogenous metastasis
M1	Microscopic tumor cells formed in cerebrospinal fluid
M2	Gross nodular seeding demonstrated in cerebellar, cerebral subarachnoid space, or in the third or lateral ventricles
M3	Gross nodular seeding in spinal subarachnoid space
M4	Metastasis outside the cerebrospinal axis

From Laurent J. Classification system for primitive neuroectodermal tumors (medulloblastoma) of the posterior fossa. Cancer 1985;56:1807, with permission.

Table 17-7. Medulloblastoma Risk Categories

Risk Category	Average	High
Extent of disease	Negative CSF cytology Normal MRI of spine	Positive CSF cytology Positive MRI of spine with Gd-DTPA
Volume of residual tumor*	≤1.5 cm^2	>1.5 cm^2
Histology	Undifferentiated	Large-cell anaplastic
Age at diagnosis	>3 years	<3 years

* On a 2-dimensional measurement.

survival improves for patients who have had a radical resection of their tumor. Occasionally a child presents with life-threatening raised intracranial pressure due to obstruction of the fourth ventricle. In these cases, preoperative endoscopic third ventriculostomy or shunting should be performed to reduce the intraoperative mortality of definitive tumor resection in the presence of increased ICP.

Radiation Therapy

Radiation therapy plays a critical role in treatment. Medulloblastomas are one of the most radiosensitive primary CNS tumors of childhood. The standard dose of radiotherapy is 5400–5580 cGy to the area of the primary tumor, with 2340 cGy given to the neuroaxis for localized disease, 3600 cGy for disseminated disease. Use of IMRT to spare the cochlea is important in decreasing therapy-induced hearing loss.

Radiation therapy to children under 3 years of age with medulloblastoma is controversial. Chemotherapy should be utilized so that radiation can either be omitted or postponed in this young age group (see pages 528–529).

Chemotherapy

The relatively rapid rate of growth and high mitotic index of medulloblastoma result in this tumor's responsiveness to a number of chemotherapeutic agents:

1. Adjuvant chemotherapy improves the disease-free survival for medulloblastoma patients who have high-risk disease (Table 17-7). Accordingly, adjuvant chemotherapy is clearly recommended in combination with craniospinal radiation. The current Children's Oncology Group (COG) trial tests the utility of carboplatin with vincristine as a radiosensitizer, followed by vincristine and cyclophosphamide with or without cisplatin. Preliminary results using aggressive multiagent chemotherapy for 4 months, followed by autologous stem cell rescue with carboplatin, thiotepa, and etoposide (Table 17-8), are encouraging. The use of second-look surgery when appropriate is being investigated.
2. Patients with average-risk disease (Table 17-7) have a greater than 60% 5-year disease-free survival with surgery and radiotherapy. A recent study utilizing craniospinal irradiation following surgery and adjuvant CCNU, vincristine, and cisplatin (Table 17-4) chemotherapy has demonstrated an 89% PFS rate in nondisseminated posterior fossa medulloblastoma with a decreased craniospinal irradiation dose. Trials are now under way to compare various chemotherapy regimens in an attempt to decrease local recurrences and to attempt to further decrease radiation therapy dosages.

Prognosis

Survival for patients with average-risk medulloblastoma treated with adjuvant radiation and chemotherapy is 89% at 5 years. In high-risk patients using craniospinal radiation with chemotherapy, 45–50% of patients are disease free at 5 years. When

Table 17-8. Conditioning Regimen for Autologous Stem Cell Transplantation

Carboplatin	500 mg/m^2/day IV[a]	Days −8 to −6
Thiotepa	300 mg/m^2/day IV	Days −5 to −3
Etoposide	250 mg/m^2/day IV	Days −5 to −3
Rest		Days −2 to −1
Stem cell infusion		Day 0
G-CSF	5 µg/kg/day	Day 1 to neutrophil engraftment

[a]Modified to AUC of 7 mg/mL/min by pediatric Calvert formula.

chemotherapy dose intensity is increased with more aggressive regimens and high-dose chemotherapy with autologous stem cell rescue (Table 17-8), 2-year disease-free survival is 73–78%.

Relapsed Medulloblastoma

Surveillance scanning is very important after therapy because it can detect most recurrences prior to the onset of symptoms. Recent studies show some improvement of survival in relapsed patients using high-dose carboplatin, thiotepa, and etoposide followed by autologous stem cell rescue (Table 17-8), with salvage rates up to 30%.

Brain Stem Tumors

Brain stem gliomas compose 15–20% of all childhood CNS tumors. The median age at presentation is 6–7 years of age. Fifty percent of the patients present with cranial nerve and long tract signs.

The majority of patients have diffuse, infiltrating pontine tumors, sometimes with an exophytic component. These are typically WHO grade II–IV gliomas with a median survival of less than 1 year, and 2-year survival rates of <10–20%. A subset of patients have focal lesions that are usually grade I tumors who have 2-year survival rates of about 60% or greater. Localized brain stem tumors may also be PNETs. Although sensitivity to chemotherapy as well as radiation is common, prognosis remains poor, at around 10%.

Surgery

Surgical resection is not usually possible because of the proximity to vital structures, limited room for expansion and swelling, and possible damage to medullary structures. There is no apparent benefit from a surgical biopsy when the imaging and clinical picture are indicative of a diffuse infiltrating pontine glioma. For focal tumors (nontectal), complete resection may be safe and may not require any further therapy. Partial resection of exophytic tumors will establish the diagnosis and reduce the obstructing mass within the fourth ventricle. If hydrocephalus is present, a CSF diversion should be performed.

Radiotherapy

Limited field irradiation is standard palliative care in patients with infiltrative pontine gliomas. A tumor dose of approximately 5400 cGy is standard. The treatment field should include the extent of the defined tumor and a 2-cm margin around the tumor. In irradiating these tumors, precaution should be taken to minimize brain stem edema, especially in patients who have not been shunted. The use of high-dose steroids is valuable during treatment and may be required throughout the treatment period. Children with diffusely infiltrating pontine gliomas often initially respond to radiation therapy but progressive disease is usually seen within 8–12 months. Timing of radiation for partially resected focal lesions is unclear. It is not known whether immediate adjuvant therapy is superior to observation and chemotherapy when progression occurs.

Chemotherapy

The use of combination chemotherapy after radiotherapy has not improved the disease-free survival in brain stem tumors. Until some chemotherapeutic regimen confirms a survival advantage in newly diagnosed patients, chemotherapy plays a palliative role.

Prognosis

The overall prognosis for brain stem tumors is poor. Most centers report a 5–20% 5-year survival rate when high doses of irradiation are employed. Children with diffusely infiltrating pontine gliomas often respond initially to radiation therapy but progressive disease is usually seen within 8–12 months. Improved survival is seen in focal low-grade brain stem astrocytomas especially those seen in patients with NF-1 and those in the tectal area.

Ependymomas

Fifty percent of all ependymomas occur during childhood and adolescence and constitute approximately 9% of all primary childhood CNS tumors. The tumors occur either infratentorially or supratentorially. The fourth ventricle is the most common location. Ependymomas can also occur in the spinal cord and account for 25% of spinal cord tumors. Obstructive hydrocephalus is the most common presenting condition.

Surgery

Total removal of these tumors is difficult to accomplish, especially in tumors originating from the fourth ventricle. However, because gross total or near total (residual <1.5 cm^2) tumor resection predicts a greatly improved outcome, this should be attempted. In the posterior fossa, the use of evoked potentials helps to make this process safer, but patients may still have multiple cranial nerve palsies and may require tracheostomy and gastrostomy for months until normal swallowing recovers. In the current COG study, patients with a subtotal resection receive two courses of neoadjuvant chemotherapy to improve resectability before potential second-look surgery.

Radiotherapy

The recurrence rate with surgery alone is extremely high, and postoperative radiotherapy results in a significant increase in survival. Local disease without evidence of subarachnoid spread should receive local irradiation with a margin (which should include extension to lateral ventricles or superior cervical spine when appropriate). Use of 3-D conformal radiation or IMRT may be appropriate and is currently under investigation. Dose is 5000–6000 cGy.

Chemotherapy

No advantage has been demonstrated from the use of adjuvant chemotherapy. However, even though platinum agents are the most active, they are not currently part of standard therapy. In infants <3 years of age, chemotherapy (Table 17-4) may be used to induce and maintain remission for months to years and to postpone radiotherapy.

Should the patient progress, radiotherapy would then be used when the child is older and the late effects less severe.

Prognosis

The overall prognosis for ependymomas is dependent on the initial extent of resection. Patients with total resection who receive radiation have a 5-year survival of 67–80% compared to a 5-year survival rate of 22–47% for patients who receive radiation after subtotal resection.

Optic Glioma

Optic gliomas constitute 5% of the primary CNS tumors in childhood and the majority are diagnosed by 5 years of age. Involvement of the optic chiasm is usually seen in older children. Neurofibromatosis is present in up to 70% of patients with tumors of the optic nerve or chiasmatic tumors, although chiasmatic tumors are more commonly seen in patients without NF-1. Patients may present with decreased vision, proptosis, optic atrophy, and papilledema. In young children asymmetric nystagmus may be the presenting sign of a chiasmatic tumor. Tumors that extend beyond the optic pathway may be associated with hypothalamic dysfunction. Histologically, approximately 90% are low-grade astrocytomas.

Surgery

MRI and CT should be used to make a clinical diagnosis because biopsy may compromise vision. Biopsy should be used for unusual circumstances. Surgery should be reserved for tumor extension into the optic canal or increasing visual compromise.

Radiotherapy

The role of radiotherapy in optic gliomas has not been completely established but it may have a beneficial role in preserving vision. Radiation may be indicated in patients with progressive disease instead of surgery, especially for chiasmatic-hypothalamic lesions. Patients with NF-1 may have exacerbation of moya moya, which must be considered before recommending radiation. A local field to the tumor of 4500–5000 cGy over 5–6 weeks is usually recommended.

Chemotherapy

Chemotherapy has been used to treat progressive disease. Regimens used include:

1. Actinomycin D and vincristine. Actinomycin D 0.015 mg/kg/day for 5 days (0.5 mg maximum per dose) IV every 12 weeks for six cycles. Vincristine 1.5 mg/m² (2 mg maximum dose) IV weekly for 8 weeks with a 4-week rest between cycles. Four-year PFS is 62.5%, but 7-year PFS is only about 33% OR
2. Carboplatin 560 mg/m² IV every 4 weeks for up to 18 months with an approximately 30% response rate OR
3. Carboplatin 175 mg/m² IV weekly for 4 weeks followed by a 2-week rest and then four more weekly doses of carboplatin. Vincristine 1.5 mg/m² (maximum dose 2 mg/weekly) for 10 weeks is given concurrently with the carboplatin course. If a response or stabilization is obtained, maintenance therapy is given consisting of courses of carboplatin 175 mg/m² weekly for 4 weeks with vincristine 1.5 mg/m² (maximum dose 2 mg) weekly for the first 3 weeks of each 4-week cycle. A 3-week rest period is provided between each maintenance cycle. In children with stable or improved disease, the regimen is continued for 8–12 cycles (Table 17-5).

Recommendations

Because optic glioma can run an indolent course, the decision for therapeutic intervention should be based on radiographic findings and assessment of visual acuity, visual fields, and visual-evoked response. The following treatment plan is recommended:

- *Evidence of optic nerve tumor and normal visual assessment:* No therapeutic intervention is recommended. CT scan and visual assessments are performed every 6 months to monitor progression of disease.

- *Evidence of progression on visual assessment, with tumor extending posteriorly into the optic canal:* A trial of chemotherapy is recommended.
- *Evidence of progression on visual assessment, without tumor extension into the optic canal:* A trial of chemotherapy is recommended in an attempt to preserve useful vision.

Prognosis

Progression-free survival rates with carboplatin and vincristine are 68% at 3 years.

Craniopharyngiomas

Craniopharyngiomas may involve the pituitary gland. They account for 6–9% of all CNS tumors in children. The peak incidence is 5–10 years of age. Patients present with symptoms of increased ICP, visual loss, and endocrine deficiencies. They typically require replacement therapy with cortisone, thyroxine, growth hormone, and sex hormones. These tumors are slow-growing benign lesions amidst vital anatomic structures.

Surgery

Craniopharyngiomas should be completely removed if possible without producing untoward neurologic sequelae. Complete excision is possible in 60–90% of cases. If radical excision can be accomplished without significant postoperative morbidity, a primary surgical approach is warranted. However, controversy exists over whether subtotal resection followed by radiation will produce less morbidity and be an equally effective strategy. Complete tumor removal is most easily accomplished in cystic tumors and is most difficult in solid or mixed tumors larger than 3 cm in size.

Radiotherapy

In tumors in which conservative surgery consisting only of drainage or subtotal removal is performed, the addition of radiotherapy reduces the local recurrence rate and improves long-term survival. For children older than 5 years, 5000–5500 cGy are given. The dose is reduced to 4000–4500 cGy in children less than 5 years of age.

Chemotherapy

At present there is no established role for chemotherapy in craniopharyngioma. A recent study demonstrated that 25% of patients (primarily those with cystic lesions) treated with interferon-alpha 2a responded.

Prognosis

The long-term survival of patients treated with radical and total removal is 80–90% at 5 years and 81% at 10 years. The 5-year recurrence-free survival after subtotal removal is approximately 50%. Survival after partial removal and radiation therapy is 62–84%.

Intracranial Germ Cell Tumors

Primary intracranial germ cell tumors (GCT) comprise 1–3% of primary pediatric brain tumors. The peak age is between 10 and 21 years of age. Multiple tumor types can be seen: the majority are germinomas (~55%), teratomas, and mixed germ cell tumors (~33%), and the remaining 10% are malignant endodermal sinus tumors, embryonal cell carcinomas, choriocarcinomas, and teratocarcinomas. In these tumors serum and cerebrospinal fluid AFP and human chorionic gonadotropin (β-hCG) may be raised. MRI of the spine with Gd-DTPA should be performed, because leptomeningeal spread is relatively common.

The outcome of patients with pure germinoma is considerably better than with mixed germ cell tumors.

Surgery

Surgical biopsy is indicated in all germ cell tumors to make an appropriate diagnosis unless elevated serum or CSF tumor markers establish the diagnosis. For patients with benign tumors such as teratomas or dermoids, surgery can be curative.

Radiation Therapy

Conventional radiotherapy for a CNS germinoma includes doses to the primary tumor of 5000 cGy with 3000 cGy craniospinal therapy. However, several studies have demonstrated the ability to use chemotherapy to reduce the dose of radiation to between 3060 and 5040 cGy to gross tumor only (in nondisseminated disease) depending on response while maintaining outcomes of >90% event-free survival. Nongerminoma germ cell tumors (NGGCTs) respond poorly to radiation therapy but the use of chemotherapy with radiation appears to improve survival substantially.

Chemotherapy

In both germinomas and NGGCTs, cycles of cisplatin 20 mg/m^2/day IV days 1–5 with etoposide 100 mg/m^2/day IV days 1–5 alone or alternating with cyclophosphamide 1 g/m^2/day × 2 days with vincristine 1.5 mg/m^2/day weekly × 3 have been used. For high-risk disease (nongerminomatous disease, β-hCG >50 mIU/mL or elevated AFP) doses of cisplatin and cyclophosphamide have been doubled. These approaches are generally combined with graded doses of radiation depending on initial risk and response.

Prognosis

The germinomas have the best overall survival rate followed by teratomas and pineal parenchymal tumors. NGGCTs such as embryonal carcinoma, endodermal carcinoma, and choriocarcinoma have a worse survival rate. However, preliminary data from recent combined chemotherapy and radiation approaches are encouraging and indicate that survival may now approach 60–80%.

Malignant Brain Tumors in Infants and Children Less Than 3 Years of Age

Infants and very young children with brain tumors have a worse prognosis than older children. They are also at higher risk for neurotoxicity including mental retardation, growth failure, and leukoencephalopathy. Due to these factors there is reluctance to treat infants and young children with radiation therapy. Recent studies have been designed to use chemotherapy and to either withhold radiation therapy or postpone its use to a time when the patient is older. Postoperative chemotherapy with cyclophosphamide, vincristine, cisplatin, and etoposide in children under 36 months of age at diagnosis (Table 17-4) is utilized followed by delayed radiation. Chemotherapy is administered for 48–96 weeks, depending on age at diagnosis, to delay radiation until as close to age 3 as possible or beyond. Ongoing studies are evaluating adding high-dose methotrexate to higher-risk cases. Newer approaches using high-dose chemotherapy with autologous stem cell rescue (Table 17-8) to intensify the chemotherapeutic regimen have been employed in an attempt to avoid radiation altogether.

Average-risk medulloblastoma and other PNETs have a 5-year PFS of about 40% in those who received chemotherapy and delayed reduced craniospinal irradiation. This increases to 60% for patients with a gross total resection. Gliomas may not do as well with this therapy. The 5-year PFS is between 0 and 43% in completely resected disease. The 5-year PFS of ependymoma is 66%, decreasing to 25% for those with subtotal resection.

Trials of intensive chemotherapy followed by stem cell rescue have also been attempted in young children with malignant brain tumors with promising results with the avoidance of radiation therapy. The current COG study uses three tandem autologous stem cell rescues after three cycles of chemotherapy. These approaches require further research. Additionally, with 3-D conformal radiation and IMRT, the timing and use of radiation therapy in subsets of disease that do worse with poor prognoses (i.e., subtotal resections) should be studied. The use of second-look surgery is also being evaluated in current trials.

SUGGESTED READINGS

Balmaceda C, Heller G, Rosenblum M, Diez B, Villablance JG, Kellie S, Maher P, Vlamis V, Walker RW, Leibel S, Finlay JL. Chemotherapy without irradiation—a novel approach for newly diagnosed CNS germ cell tumors: results of an international cooperative trial. J Clin Oncol 1996;14:2908–15.

Biegel JA. Genetics of pediatric central nervous system tumors. J Pediatr Hematol Oncol 1997;19:492–501.

Duffner PC, Horowitz ME, Krischer JP, Friedman HS, Burger PC, Cohen ME, Sanford RA, Mulhern RK, James HE, Freeman CR, Seidel FG, Kun LE. Postoperative chemotherapy and delayed radiation in children less than 3 years of age with malignant brain tumors. N Engl J Med 1993;328:1725–31.

Fahlbusch R, Honegger J, Paulus W, Huk W, Buchfelder M. Surgical treatment of craniopharyngiomas: experience with 168 patients. J Neurosurg 1999;90:237–50.

Halperin EC, Constine LS, Tarbell NJ, Kun LE. Pediatric Radiation Oncology. 3rd ed. Philadelphia: Lippincott Williams and Wilkins, 1999.

Mason WP, Growas A, Halpern S, Dunkel IJ, Garvin J, Heller G, Rosenblum M, Gardner S, Lyden D, Sands S, Puccetti D, Lindsley K, Merchant TE, O'Malley B, Bayer L, Petriccione M, Allen J, Finlay JL. Intensive chemotherapy and bone marrow rescue for young children with newly diagnosed malignant brain tumors. J Clin Oncol 1998;16:210–21.

MacDonald TJ, Rood BR, Santi, MR, Vezina G, et al. Advances in the diagnosis, molecular genetics and treatment of pediatric embryonal CNS tumors. Oncologist 2003;8:174–86.

Packer RJ, Ater J, Allen D, Phillips P, Geyer R, Nicholson HS, Jakacki R, Kurczynski E, Needle M, Finlay J, Reaman G, Boyett JM. Carboplatin and vincristine chemotherapy for children with newly diagnosed progressive low-grade glioma. J Neurosurg 1997;86:747–54.

Reddy AT, Packer RJ. Pediatric central nervous system tumors. Curr Opin Oncol 1998;10:186–93.

Srother D, Pollack I, Fisher P, Hunter J, et al. Tumors of the central nervous system. In: Pizzo PA, Poplack DG, editors. Principles and Practice of Pediatric Oncology. 4th ed. Philadelphia: Lippincott Williams and Wilkins, 2002.

Stupp R, Dietrich P, Kraljevic SO, Pica A, et al. Promising survival for patients with newly diagnosed glioblastoma multiforme treated with concomitant radiation plus temozolomide, followed by adjuvant temozolomide. J Clin Oncol 2002;20:1375.

18

NEUROBLASTOMA

Neuroblastoma originates from primordial neural crest cells that normally give rise to adrenal medulla and the sympathetic ganglia. Compared to any other tumor, this tumor has a more varied clinical presentation of primary, or metastatic disease and paraneoplastic syndromes.

INCIDENCE

1. Neuroblastoma is the most common extracranial solid tumor in infancy, accounting for 8–10% of all childhood malignancies.
2. Annual incidence is 1 per 7000 live births.
3. At diagnosis, 36% of patients are under age 1, 75% under age 4, and 90% under age 10.
4. Conditions associated with neuroblastoma are listed in Table 18-1.
5. The incidence of *in situ* neuroblastomas is 1 in 259 autopsies among infants less than 3 months of age. This 400-fold increase in the autopsy incidence of neuroblastoma compared with the clinical incidence of the tumor indicates that involution or maturation of the tumor occurs spontaneously in most infants.
6. On rare occasions it has been diagnosed immediately after birth with metastases to the placenta.

The tumor is more common in boys than in girls; the male:female ratio 1.2:1.

PATHOLOGY

Comparison of prognostic groups according to the histologic classification of Shimada and Joshi is shown in Table 18-2.

CLINICAL FEATURES

Neuroblastomas are tumors of sympathetic nerve tissue, and a tumor mass can occur anywhere along the sympathetic neural pathway. Most primary tumors occur within the abdomen (65%) and the most common presenting feature is an asymptomatic abdominal mass. Metastases at the time of diagnosis may be as high as 75% of cases.

Table 18-1. Conditions Associated with Neuroblastoma

Neurofibromatosis
Hirschsprung disease with aganglionic colon
Pheochromocytoma in family
Fetal hydantoin syndrome
Fetal alcohol syndrome
Nesidioblastosis

Table 18-2. Comparison of Prognostic Groups According to the Histopathologic Classifications of Shimada and Joshi

Prognosis	Histopathologic features/age
Favorable	
Shimada	Stroma rich, all ages, no nodular pattern
	Stroma poor, age 1.5–5 yr, differentiated, MKI[a] <100
	Stroma poor, age <1.5 yr, MKI <200
Joshi	Grade 1,[b] all ages; grade 2,[c] ≤1 yr
Unfavorable	
Shimada	Stroma rich, all ages, nodular pattern
	Stroma poor, age >5 yr
	Stroma poor, age 1.5–5 yr, undifferentiated
	Stroma poor, age 1.5–5 yr, differentiated, MKI >100
	Stroma poor, age <1.5 yr, MKI >200
Joshi	Grade 2, age >1 yr, grade 3,[d] all ages

[a]MKI, mitosis-karyorrhexis index (number of mitoses and karyorrhexis per 5000 cells).
[b]Grade 1 = low mitotic rate (≤10/10 high-power fields) and calcification present.
[c]Grade 2 = either low mitotic rate or calcification present.
[d]Grade 3 = neither low mitotic rate nor calcification present.
From Brodeur GM, Castleberry RP. Neuroblastoma In: Pizzo PA, Poplack DG, editors. Principle and Practice of Pediatric Oncology. 2nd ed. Philadelphia: Lippincott, 1993;746, with permission.

ANATOMIC SITE

Clinical manifestations depend on the anatomic site of the primary tumor:

1. *Head and neck:*
   Unilateral palpable mass
   Horner syndrome (meiosis, ptosis, enophthalmos, anhydrosis)
2. *Orbit and eye:*
   Orbital secondaries with periorbital hemorrhage ("raccoon eyes")
   Exophthalmos, palpable supraorbital masses, ecchymosis, edema of eyelids and conjunctiva, ptosis
   Cerebral involvement: papilledema, retinal hemorrhage, optic atrophy, paresis of the external rectus muscle, and strabismus
   Cervical sympathetic involvement: heterochromia iridis, anisocoria, Horner syndrome
   Opsoclonus ("dancing eyes syndrome")
3. *Chest:*
   Upper thoracic tumors: dyspnea, pulmonary infections, dysphagia, lymphatic compression, Horner syndrome
   Lower thoracic tumors: usually no symptoms

4. *Abdomen:*
   Anorexia, vomiting
   Abdominal pain
   Palpable mass
   Massive involvement of the liver with metastatic disease with or without respiratory distress especially in the newborn
5. *Pelvis:*
   Constipation
   Urinary retention
   Presacral mass palpable on rectal examination
6. *Paraspinal area* (dumbbell- or hourglass-shaped neuroblastoma):
   Localized back pain and tenderness
   Limp
   Weakness of lower extremities
   Hypotonia, muscle atrophy, areflexia, or hyperreflexia of lower extremities
   Paraplegia
   Scoliosis
   Bladder and anal sphincter dysfunction
7. *Lymph nodes:* enlarged
8. *Bone:* pain, limping, and irritability in the young child associated with bone and bone marrow metastases.
9. *Lung:* lungs and pleura are rarely involved; incidence of 0.7% in all patients with neuroblastoma; because of its rarity, lung involvement should be proven by biopsy
10. *Brain:* rarely, metastatic involvement of the brain can occur.

NONSPECIFIC CONSTITUTIONAL SYMPTOMS

Nonspecific constitutional symptoms include lethargy, anorexia, pallor, weight loss, abdominal pain, weakness, and irritability.

PARANEOPLASTIC SYNDROMES

Unique paraneoplastic syndromes have been associated with both localized and disseminated neuroblastoma.

Manifestations

1. *Signs and symptoms of excessive catecholamine (VMA/HVA) secretion:* Intermittent attacks of sweating, flushing, pallor, headaches, palpitation, and hypertension. Hypertension is usually renin induced due to renovascular compromise and is seen in 1–5% of patients. Normal levels of VMA and HVA are listed in Table A1-29.
2. *Signs and symptoms of vasoactive intestinal peptide (VIP) secretion:* Intractable watery diarrhea resulting in failure to thrive, associated with abdominal distention and hypokalemia due to the secretion of an enterohormone, VIP, by the neuroblastoma cells (Kerner–Morrison syndrome). Most of the VIP-secreting tumors are mature histologically (ganglioneuroblastoma or ganglioneuroma) and have favorable outcome.
3. *Acute myoclonic encephalopathy:* The syndrome of opsoclonus and myoclonus (OM) consists of:
   a. Bursts of rapid involuntary random eye movements in all directions of gaze (opsoclonus)

b. Motor incoordination due to frequent, irregular jerking of muscles of the limbs and trunk (myoclonic jerking)

c. Symptoms may or may not resolve after the tumor is removed or symptoms may resolve only after several months. In some cases these symptoms are permanent.

d. Prognosis for survival is favorable because tumor usually displays favorable biological features. If tumor displays biologically unfavorable features the prognosis is unfavorable.

All children presenting with OM should be evaluated for the presence of neuroblastoma (because more than 30% of them have an occult tumor of neural crest origin). Meta-iodobenzylguanidine (MIBG) scan, octreoid (somatostatin receptor) scan, CAT scan of the neck, chest, abdomen, and pelvis, and urinary Vanillyl mandelic Acid (VMA), and Homovanillic Acid (HVA) measurement may help detect the presence of neuroblastoma.

Pathophysiology of OM

This syndrome is not due to direct involvement of the central nervous system (CNS) by tumor or due to the production of catecholamines. It is associated with well-defined IgG and IgM autoantibodies that bind to the cytoplasm of cerebellar Purkinje cells and to some axons in the white matter. They also bind to the large and small axons of the peripheral nerves. Western blot analysis shows a distinctive pattern of binding to several neural proteins of the neurofilaments. The role of these autoantibodies in the pathogenesis of OM is unclear at the present time. Diffuse and extensive lymphocytic infiltration with lymphoid follicles is a characteristic histologic feature of OM. This observation suggests an immune-mediated mechanism for this rare syndrome.

Treatment of OM

- Dexamethasone 0.9 mg/kg/day PO.
- If dexamethasone fails, high-dose Intravenous Immunoglobulin (IVIG) 150–500 mg/kg/day for 4–5 days. It may also provide a steroid-sparing effect.
- Chemotherapy: Children who receive chemotherapy, due to their advanced stages, have a better neurologic outcome of OM than patients who do not receive chemotherapy.

NEONATAL NEUROBLASTOMA

Neuroblastoma in the newborn can present in the following ways:

1. Subcutaneous nodules. If these nodules are massaged, a zone of pallor surrounding the nodules develops due to the discharge of catecholamines.
2. Extensive metastases to the liver, with or without respiratory distress.
3. Bone marrow involvement.
4. Massive adrenal hemorrhage into tumor.
5. Hydrops fetalis and/or signs of erythroblastosis fetalis.
6. Stage 4S neuroblastoma (see Table 18-5 later in this chapter).

Prenatal ultrasound may identify a neuroblastoma. Neuroblastomas identified prenatally usually follow a clinically favorable course and are cured by surgical resection, especially when they have many of the favorable factors of prognosis. In many of these patients, an abdominal mass is not palpable and only 50% of them have elevated urinary catecholamines.

DIAGNOSIS

Table 18-3 shows the recommended criteria from the International Neuroblastoma Staging System (INSS) conference for a diagnosis of neuroblastoma.

Table 18-3. Recommended Criteria at INSS Conference for a Diagnosis of Neuroblastoma

Established if:
(1) Unequivocal pathologic diagnosis[a] is made from tumor tissue by light microscopy (with or without immunohistology, electron microscopy), and/or increased urine or serum catecholamines or metabolites.[b]

OR

(2) Bone marrow aspirate or trephine biopsy contains unequivocal tumor cells[a] (e.g., syncytia or immunocytologically positive clumps of cells) and increased urine or serum catecholamines or metabolites.[b]

[a]If histology is equivocal, karyotypic abnormalities in tumor cells characteristic of other tumors [e.g., t(11;22)], excludes a diagnosis of neuroblastoma, whereas genetic features characteristic of neuroblastoma (1p deletion, MYCN amplification) would support this diagnosis.

[b]Includes dopamine, HVA, and/or VMA (levels must be >3.0 SD above the mean per-milligram creatinine for age to be considered increased, and at least two of these must be measured).

From Brodeur GM, Pritchard J, Bethold F, et al. Revisions of the International Criteria for Neuroblastoma Diagnosis, Staging, and Response to Treatment. J Clin Oncol 1993;11:1466, with permission.

Early Diagnosis of Neuroblastoma by a Screening Program

Results of screening tests using urinary catecholamine determinations suggest that the majority of infants identified by a mass screening program have low-risk neuroblastoma by stage (stages I, II, IV in 70–90% of cases) and biological tumor marker studies, favorable histology (93%), hyperdiploid (75–100%) with a normal MYCN copy number, chromosome 1p abnormality (13%), and Ha-ras p21 expression (60–80%). Only a few patients with unfavorable biologic features have been identified and they have had an unfavorable outcome. It remains to be determined if a mass screening program at 1, 1.5, and 2 years of age would identify patients with and without high-risk biologic features at the earliest possible time and if early treatment of these patients would improve their prognosis. This is illustrated in patients by false negativity for screening at 6 months of age who then develop aggressive neuroblastoma after 1 year of age. Widespread screening for neuroblastoma at or before the age of 6 months and perhaps even at later ages remains controversial.

If a screening test at or before 6 months of age is positive, then a search for a primary tumor is recommended. If a primary tumor is found, then studies for metastatic evaluation (CT scan, bone marrow aspiration and biopsy, and MIBG scan) should be performed. Patients with stage I and II disease should be followed periodically with urinary catecholamine determinations, CT scan, and MIBG scan. Assessment with urinary catecholamines and abdominal sonogram is needed once a month for 1 year and every 3 months thereafter.

For mediastinal tumors, urinary catecholamines and CT should be obtained at least once every 3 months. Patients with progressive disease or advanced-stage neuroblastoma diagnosed by screening at ≤6 months should always be resected and tumor samples tested for biologic features of prognosis. Intensity of treatment is then determined accordingly.

Table 18-4 shows the recommended studies for the assessment of extent of disease.

Table 18-4. Recommended Studies for Assessment of Extent of Disease

Tumor site	Recommended tests
Primary site	CT and/or MRI scan[a] with 3-D measurements; MIBG scan.[b]
Metastatic sites[b]	
Bone marrow	Bilateral posterior iliac crest marrow aspirates and trephine (core) bone marrow biopsies required to exclude marrow involvement. A single positive site documents marrow involvement. Core biopsies must contain at least 1 cm of marrow (excluding cartilage) to be considered adequate.
Bone	MIBG scan; ^{99}Tc scan required if MIBG scan negative or unavailable. Plain radiographs of positive lesions.
Lymph nodes	Clinical examination (palpable nodes), confirmed histologically. CT scan for nonpalpable nodes (3-D measurements).
Abdomen/liver	CT and/or MRI scan[a] with 3-D measurements.
Chest	AP and lateral chest radiographs. CT/MRI necessary if chest radiograph positive, or if abdominal mass/nodes extend into chest.

Abbreviation: AP, anteroposterior.

[a]Ultrasound considered suboptimal for accurate 3-D measurements.

[b]The MIBG scan is applicable to all sites of disease.

From Brodeur GM, Pritchard J, Bethold F, et al. Revisions of the International Criteria for Neuroblastoma Diagnosis, Staging, and Response to Treatment. J Clin Oncol 1993;11:1466, with permission.

STAGING

Table 18-5 shows a comparison of two staging systems—INSS and Children's Oncology Group (COG)–for neuroblastoma that are currently in use. Table 18-6 shows the modified International Neuroblastoma Response Criteria (INRC) definitions of response to treatment.

Table 18-5. Comparison of Staging Systems (INSS and COG) for Neuroblastoma

INSS system (International Staging System)	COG system (Children's Oncology Group)
Stage 1. Localized tumor with complete gross excision, with or without microscopic residual disease; representative ipsilateral lymph nodes negative for tumor microscopically (nodes attached to and removed with the primary tumor may be positive).	*Stage 1.* Tumor confined to organ or structure of origin.
Stage 2A. Localized tumor with incomplete gross excision; representative ipsilateral nonadherent lymph nodes negative for tumor microscopically.	*Stage 2.* Tumor extending in continuity beyond the organ or structure of origin, but not crossing the midline. Regional lymph nodes on the ipsilateral side may be involved.
Stage 2B. Localized tumor with or without complete gross excision, with ipsilateral nonadherent lymph nodes positive for tumor. Enlarged contralateral lymph nodes must be negative microscopically.	
Stage 3. Unresectable unilateral tumor infiltrating across the midline,[a] with or without regional lymph node	*Stage 3.* Tumor extending in continuity beyond the midline. Regional lymph nodes may be involved bilaterally.

(Continues)

Table 18-5. (*Continued*)

INSS system (International Staging System)	COG system (Children's Oncology Group)
involvement; or localized unilateral tumor with contralateral regional lymph node involvement; or midline tumor with bilateral extension by infiltration (unresectable) or by lymph node involvement.	
Stage 4. Any primary tumor with dissemination to distant lymph nodes, bone, bone marrow, liver, skin, and/or other organs (except as defined for stage 4S).	*Stage 4.* Remote disease involving the skeleton, bone marrow, soft tissue, and distant lymph node groups (see stage 4S).
Stage 4S. Localized primary tumor (as defined for stage 1, 2A, or 2B), with dissemination limited to skin, liver, and/or bone marrow[b] (limited to infants <1 yr of age).	*Stage 4S.* As defined in stage I or II, except for the presence of remote disease confined to the liver, skin, or bone marrow (without bone metastases).

Multifocal primary tumors (e.g., bilateral adrenal primary tumors) should be staged according to the greatest extent of disease, as defined above, and followed by a subscript letter M (e.g., 3_M).

[a]The midline is defined as the vertebral column. Tumors originating on one side and crossing the midline must infiltrate to or beyond the opposite side of the vertebral column.

A grossly resectable tumor arising in the midline from pelvic ganglia or the organ of Zuckerkandl is stage 1. A midline tumor extending beyond one side of the vertebral column that is unresectable is stage 2A. Ipsilateral lymph node involvement is stage 2B, whereas bilateral lymph node involvement is stage 3. A midline primary tumor with bilateral infiltration that was not resectable is stage 3. A tumor of any size with malignant ascites or peritoneal implants is stage 3 (but a thoracic tumor with malignant pleural effusion unilaterally is stage 2B).

[b]Marrow involvement in stage 4S should be minimal, i.e., <10% of total nucleated cells identified as malignant on bone marrow biopsy or on marrow aspirate. More extensive marrow involvement is stage 4. The MIBG scan should be negative in the marrow.

Table 18-6. Modified International Neuroblastoma Response Criteria (INRC) Definitions of Response to Treatment

Response	Primary tumor[a]	Metastatic sites[a,b]
CR	No tumor	No tumor; catecholamines normal.
VGPR	Decreased by 90–99%	No tumor; catecholamines normal; residual ^{99}Tc bone changes allowed.
PR	Decreased by >50%	All measurable sites decreased by >50%. Bones and bone marrow: number of positive bone sites decreased by >50%; no more than 1 positive bone marrow site allowed.[b]
MR	No new lesions; >50% reduction of any measurable lesion (primary or metastases) with <50% reduction in any other; <25% increase in any existing lesion.	
SD	No new lesions; <25% increase in any existing lesion; exclude bone marrow evaluation.	
PD	Any new lesion; increase of any measurable lesion by >25% previous negative marrow has become positive for tumor.	

Abbreviations: CR, complete response; VGPR, Very good partial response; PR, partial response; MR, mixed response; SD, stable disease; PD, progressive disease.

[a]Evaluation of primary and metastatic disease as outlined in Table 18-4.

[b]One positive marrow aspirate or biopsy allowed for PR if this represents a decrease from the number of positive sites at diagnosis.

From Brodeur GM, Pritchard J, Berthold F, et al. Revisions of the International Criteria for Neuroblastoma Diagnosis, Staging, and Response to Treatment J Clin Oncol 1993;11:1466, with permission.

PROGNOSIS

Table 18-7 describes factors of prognostic significance in children with neuroblastoma. Major advances have been made in the refinement of prognostic criteria, which may eventually help in planning treatment protocols. Table 18-8 lists risk groups for neuroblastoma therapy based on clinical and biologic tumor features.

GENERAL TREATMENT MODALITIES

The treatment modalities used in neuroblastoma are surgery, chemotherapy, and radiotherapy. The role of each is determined by the patient's age and the stage and biologic features (MYCN status, histopathology, and DNA ploidy) of the tumor.

Table 18-7. Factors of Prognostic Significance in Neuroblastoma[a]

Histology: favorable > unfavorable histology
Age: under 2 years > older than 2 years at diagnosis[b]
Neuron-specific enolase: normal level (1–100 ng/mL) > abnormal (>100 ng/mL)
Ferritin level: normal level (0–150 ng/mL) > abnormal (>150 ng/mL)
VMA/HVA ratio: high (>1) > low (<1)
Stage: I or II or IVs > III > IV[c]
Stage IVn (i.e., patients with only lymph node metastasis) > IV
Site of primary tumor: neck or posterior mediastinum or pelvis > abdominal primaries
Gallium uptake by tumor: absent > present
MYCN gene amplification: 1 MYCN gene copy > greater than 1 MYCN gene copies
Flow cytometric DNA analysis of neuroblastoma: favorable outcome associated with an aneuploid stem cell line and low percentage of tumor cells in S, G_2, and M phases of the cell cycle
Immunocytologic detection of bone marrow metastasis: immunocytologic analysis of bone marrow aspirates is more sensitive than conventional analysis in detection of tumor cells and is of prognostic significance.[d]
P-glycoprotein levels in tumor cells at diagnosis: expression of P-glycoprotein before treatment may be of prognostic significance.[e]
Expression of neural growth factor receptor (TRK) gene: high levels of messenger RNA of TRK gene in tumor cells is strongly predictive of a favorable outcome.
Lower LDH levels: (<1500 μ/mL) > high LDH levels (>1500 μ/mL)
Neuropeptide-Y: plasma levels of NPY can be useful in diagnosis and early detection of relapse of neuroblastoma.
Ha-ras p21 expression: aggressive tumors have a low expression of Ha-ras p21. High Ha-ras p21 correlates with higher disease-free survival.
BCL-2 oncogene[f]: associated with a poor prognosis
Telomerase: increased telomerase activity is associated with aggressive disease.
Chromosome 1p deletion: associated with poor survival

[a]>Represents better prognosis.
[b]Survival rate for patients under 1 year of age: 82%; for 1–2 years: 32%; for more than 2 years: 10%.
[c]Survival rate for stage I: 80–90%; for stage II: 60–80%; for stage III: 30–50%; for stage IV: 7%; for stage IVs: 75%. Stage IVs patients 6 weeks of age or younger without skin metastases have less favorable prognosis (38%) compared with skin metastases (85%) or age greater than 6 weeks irrespective of skin metastases (86%). Stage IV patients with bone metastasis fare worse than patients without bone metastasis.
[d]Survival according to immunocytologically detectable neuroblasts/100,000 marrow cells: For all patients with stage I, II, or III: no detectable tumor cells: 90%; <6 tumor cells: 70%; ≥6 tumor cells: 20%. For children >12 months age with stage I, II, or III: no detectable tumor cells: 80%; <6 tumor cells 50%; ≥6 tumor cells: 15%. For all patients with stage IV: no detectable tumor cells: 50%; 1–20 tumor cells: 35%; >20 tumor cells: 15%. For infants <12 months age with stage IV: no detectable tumor cells: 75%; >20 tumor cells: 0%.
[e]Survival according to P-glycoprotein level. For all patients with stages III, IV, and IVs: P-glycoprotein negative: 80%; P-glycoprotein positive: 0–15%.
[f]This is a novel class of oncogene that inhibits (apoptosis) expression of neuroblastoma because it renders neuroblastoma cells resistant to chemotherapy.

Table 18-8. COG Risk Group Assignment for Neuroblastoma According to Clinical and Biologic Factors

INSS stage	Age (yr)	MYCN status	Shimada histology	DNA ploidy	Risk/Group study
1	0–21	Any	Any	Any	Low
2A and 2B	<1	Any	Any	Any	Low
	≥1–21	Nonamplified[a]	Any	NA	Low
	≥1–21	Amplified[b]	Favorable	NA	Low
	≥1–21	Amplified	Unfavorable	NA	High
3	<1	Nonamplified	Any	Any	Intermediate
	<1	Amplified	Any	Any	High
	≥1–21	Nonamplified	Favorable	NA	Intermediate
	≥1–21	Nonamplified	Unfavorable	NA	High
	>1–21	Amplified	Any	NA	High
4	<1	Nonamplified	Any	Any	Intermediate
	<1	Amplified	Any	Any	High
	>1–21	Any	Any	NA	High
4S	<1	Nonamplified	Favorable	>1	Low
	<1	Nonamplified	Any	1	Intermediate
	<1	Nonamplified	Unfavorable	Any	Intermediate
	<1	Amplified	Any	Any	High

[a]MYCN copy number ≤10.
[b]MYCN copy number >10.
Abbreviations: INSS, International Neuroblastoma Staging System; NA, not applicable.
From Castleberry RP. Biology and treatment of neuroblastoma. Pediatri Clin North Am. 1997;44:919–39, with permission.

Surgery

The role of initial surgery before any other therapy is administered is to:

- establish the diagnosis and provide tissue for biologic studies
- stage the disease
- excise the tumor if possible without compromising vital structures.

Tumors are removed (except in infants with INSS stage 4S) if it is safe to remove at least 90% of the tumor; otherwise, only a biopsy should be obtained. If any residual tumor is left, it is monitored by appropriate imaging studies performed periodically while receiving chemotherapy.

Second-look surgery is performed to:

- assess response to chemotherapy
- remove any residual disease if possible.

Radiation Therapy

Radiation therapy is given to the following patients:

1. Those who have tumor progression despite chemotherapy and/or surgery.
2. Persistence of viable disease in patients with unfavorable biology after chemotherapy.
3. Persistence of disease after second-look surgery or partial response following surgery for local recurrence ≥3 months after completing initial therapy.

Chemotherapy

Chemotherapy protocols depend on the age of patient, stage of disease, biologic features of the tumor, and the risk group assignment, as described next.

RISK GROUP ASSIGNMENT

The COG has developed a system for neuroblastoma risk stratification. This system utilizes the following clinical factors:

- INSS stage
- Patient age at diagnosis (<1 year versus 1–21 years)
- MYCN status
- Shimada histopathology
- DNA index (DI).

These criteria assign patients to one of three risk groups: low, intermediate, and high risk (Table 18-8).

Low-Risk Group

The low-risk group consists of:

1. All patients with INSS stage 1
2. <1 year of age, INSS stage 2A and 2B
3. All ages INSS stage 2A, 2B, nonamplified MYCN, and favorable or unfavorable Shimada histology
4. All ages INSS stage 2A, 2B, or amplified MYCN and favorable Shimada histology
5. Infants with INSS stage 4S disease, favorable Shimada histology, nonamplified MYCN (single copy), and hyperdiploidy.

Treatment

1. All patients INSS stage 1:
   a. Surgical removal of the primary tumor
   b. Disease-free survival (DSF): 90% for all age groups
   c. Indication for chemotherapy: recurrence
   d. Chemotherapy: cyclophosphamide (CPM)/Adriamycin (ADR) as follows:
   Cyclophosphamide: 150 mg/m^2 PO, days 1–7
   Adriamycin: 35 mg/m^2 IV, day 8
   e. Repeat every 21 days for a total of five cycles
2. All patients who are <12 months with INSS stage 2A or 2B:
   In these cases incomplete surgical resection does not compromise the relapse-free survival in the setting of localized disease and favorable histologic features. This is a unique feature of neuroblastoma.
   Treatment: Surgery and chemotherapy. Chemotherapy consists of five cycles of low-dose sequential CPM/ADR (see above schema).
   Two-year disease-free survival: 85%. If a complete remission is not attained cisplatin/VM-26 chemotherapy should be used as follows:
   Cisplatin: 90 mg/m^2 IV over 6 hours, day 1.
   VM-26 (teniposide): 100 mg/m^2 IV over 1 hour, day 3.
   Repeat every 4 weeks for two cycles. Repeat imaging studies. If response occurs, then four more cycles should be administered.

3. All patients who are ≥12 months with stage 2A or 2B:
   If the initial tumor is unresectable or if gross residual tumor is present, chemotherapy should be used as follows (alternating courses of OPEC and OJEC every 21 days):
   a. *OPEC therapy courses 1, 3, and 5:*
      Vincristine 1.5 mg/m^2 IV bolus (max 2 mg) on day 1
      Cisplatin 80 mg/m^2 IV continuous infusion over 24 hours, day 1
      Etoposide 200 mg/m^2 IV over 4 hours, day 2.
   b. *OJEC therapy courses 2 and 4:*
      Vincristine 1.5 mg/m^2 (max 2 mg) IV bolus, day 1
      Cyclophosphamide 600 mg/m^2 over 20 minutes, day 1
      Etoposide 200 mg/m^2 IV over 4 hours, day 1
      Carboplatin 500 mg/m^2 IV over 1 hour, day 1.
      Second-look surgery should be done after course 5. Patients who are in complete remission following second-look surgery should receive one additional course each of OJEC and OPEC. Other patients should be treated with radiation therapy.
4. Infants with INSS stage 4S disease: Majority of patients with INSS stage 4S disease fall into the low-risk category with overall survival of 85%.
   a. A diagnostic biopsy is indicated for evaluation of the biologic features of the tumor to plan treatment according to its correlation with risk category.
   b. Tumors with favorable nonamplified MYCN usually regress spontaneously, especially in infants under 6 months of age, and should be observed closely without any treatment.
   c. However, it has been suggested that sometime during the course of the disease, the primary tumor be resected because of a small chance of a late recurrence at the site of the primary tumor.

Infants under 2 months of age with 4S disease are at higher risk for developing hepatomegaly and multiorgan compromise resulting in a fatal outcome. Neonates who die from 4S neuroblastoma are those who have extensive hepatic involvement, which causes respiratory compromise, disseminated intravascular coagulopathy, and renal, inferior vena cava or gastrointestinal compromise.

If a massively enlarged liver compromises respiratory function, a short course of low-dose oral cyclophosphamide (5 mg/kg/day for 5 days every 2–3 weeks as needed) can induce remission. In addition, low-dose radiation (150 cGy two or three times to the anterior two thirds of the liver through lateral oblique ports avoiding radiation to the kidneys, ovary, and spine) may be delivered to the tumor. This dose is generally sufficient to halt the progression of the tumor and induce regression. The disadvantage of delivering neonatal radiation to the liver is the possibility of subsequent hepatic fibrosis or cirrhosis.

The rare stage 4S patients with unfavorable biologic features (diploidy, unfavorable histology, MYCN amplification) should be considered for either intermediate-risk (diploidy or unfavorable Shimada histology) or high-risk (MYCN amplification) treatment protocols.

Intermediate-Risk Group:

The intermediate-risk group (Table 18-8) consists of patients with:

1. INSS stage 3, younger than 1 year, with nonamplified MYCN, favorable or unfavorable histology
2. INSS stage 3, older than 1 year, nonamplified MYCN and favorable Shimada histology

3. INSS stage 4 infants, younger than 1 year, with nonamplified MYCN and favorable or unfavorable Shimada histology
4. INSS stage 4S infants, younger than 1 year, with nonamplified MYCN, favorable or unfavorable histology and DNA index of 1
5. INSS stage 4S infants, younger than 1 year, with nonamplified MYCN, unfavorable Shimada pathology.

Patients with intermediate-risk neuroblastoma have a reported estimated 3-year survival of 75–98%.

Treatment

Surgery is indicated as described under general treatment modalities earlier in this chapter. Table 18-9 describes various induction chemotherapy and response rates from the Pediatric Oncology Group (POG), the Children's Cancer Group (COG), and the European Neuroblastoma Study Group (ENSG).

The recent cooperative COG, based on clinical INSS stage, age, and selected biologic features such as MYCN, Shimada histopathology, and ploidy, has developed a chemotherapy regimen designed to maintain or improve event-free survival of previous studies and to minimize acute and long-term morbidity for this group of patients. This regimen uses four of the most active agents in neuroblastoma treatment (carboplatin, etoposide, cyclophosphamide, and doxorubicin). Patients with intermediate-risk neuroblastoma and favorable biology get one course of four cycles of chemotherapy, and patients with unfavorable biology get two courses (eight

Table 18-9. Induction Chemotherapy Regimens and Response Rates from Pediatric Oncology Group, Children's Cancer Group, and European Neuroblastoma Study Group.

Study	Regimen[a]	CR + PR (%)[b]

POG-8742 (regimen 1)	Days 1–5, CDDP 40 mg/m²/day
	Days 2–4, VP-16 100 mg/m²/day
	Alternating every 21 days with
	  Days 1–7, CPM 150 mg/m²/day (PO)
	  Day 8, DOX 35 mg/m²
	Total of 5 cycles
	OR
		77

CCG-3891	Day 1, CDDP 60 mg/m² Day 3, DOX 30 mg/m² Days 3 and 6, VP-16 100 mg/m² Days 4 and 5, CPM 900 mg/m² Repeat every 28 days × 5 cycles **OR**	78
ENSG-3C	Days 1–5, CDDP 40 mg/m²/day Days 1–5, VP-16 100 mg/m²/day Days 21–23, Ifos 3 g/m²/day Day 21, VCR 1.5 mg/m² Day 23, DOX 60 mg/m² Repeat 3–4 weeks × 4 cycles	55

Abbreviations: CDDP, cisplatin; CPM, cyclophosphamide; CR, complete response; DOX, doxorubicin; PR, partial response; VCR, vincristine; VP-16, etoposide; Ifos, ifosfamide.
[a]All drugs are given intravenously unless noted otherwise.
[b]Responses all include surgery and 5–6 months of chemotherapy.
Adapted from Matthay KK, Castleberry RP. Treatment of advanced neuroblastoma: the U.S. experience. In: Brodeur GM, Sawada T, Tsuchida Y, et al., editors. Neuroblastoma. Amsterdam: Elsevier Science, 2000;437–52, with permission.

cycles). Each cycle is given every 3 weeks. For the details of this chemotherapy, see doses and schema as described next.

Treatment for Patients with Intermediate-Risk Favorable Biology

For children <1 year of age or who are ≤12 kg in weight, the doses of chemotherapy are adjusted and given as milligrams per kilogram. Each of four cycles is given at 3-week intervals.

1. Carboplatin 560 mg/m^2 or 18 mg/kg IV over 1 hour for 1 day
2. Etoposide 120 mg/m^2 or 4 mg/kg IV over 2 hours daily for 3 days
3. Cyclophosphamide 1000 mg/m^2 or 33 mg/kg over 1 hour daily for 1 day
4. Doxorubicin 30 mg/m^2 or 1 mg/kg IV over 60 minutes daily for 1 day.

The various drugs are given on the following days of the course.

Course number	Cycle number	Day	Agents
I	1	0	Carboplatin and etoposide
		1	Etoposide
		2	Etoposide
	2	21	Carboplatin, cyclophosphamide, and doxorubicin
	3	42	Cyclophosphamide and etoposide
		43	Etoposide
		44	Etoposide
	4	63	Carboplatin, etoposide, and doxorubicin
		64	Etoposide
		65	Etoposide

Treatment for Patients with Intermediate-Risk, Unfavorable Biology

These patients should receive an additional four cycles of chemotherapy in course II as follows:

Course number	Cycle number	Day	Agents (in doses listed earlier)
II	5	84–86	Repeat chemotherapy drugs in cycle 3
	6	105	Repeat cycle 2
	7	126–128	Repeat cycle 1
	8	147	Cyclophosphamide and doxorubicin

Growth factors (G-CSF or GM-CSF) should be given for infants less than 60 days of age. Older infants and children may also receive growth factors. G-CSF 5 µg/kg/day Subcutaneously (SC) or GM-CSF 250 µg/m^2/day SC starting 24 hours after chemotherapy administration until the absolute neutrophil count is ≥1,000/µL for 2 consecutive days.

Estimated 3-year relapse-free survival is 75–98%.

High-Risk Group

The high-risk group (Table 18-8) consists of patients with:

1. INSS stage 2A, 2B, older than 1 year, amplified MYCN, and unfavorable Shimada pathology

2. INSS stage 3, younger than 1 year, amplified MYCN, and favorable or unfavorable Shimada histology
3. INSS stage 3, older than 1 year, nonamplified MYCN, and unfavorable Shimada histology
4. INSS stage 3, older than 1 year, amplified MYCN, with favorable or unfavorable Shimada histology
5. INSS stage 4, younger than 1 year, amplified MYCN, and favorable or unfavorable histology
6. INSS stage 4, older than 1 year, amplified or nonamplified MYCN, and favorable or unfavorable histology
7. INSS Stage 4S with amplified MYCN and favorable or unfavorable histology.

Treatment

Surgery is indicated as described under general treatment modalities earlier in this chapter. The probability of long-term survival in this group of patients is less than 15%. Overall survival rates have been improved to 43–50% by employing comprehensive treatment approaches that include:

1. Induction chemotherapy
2. High-dose consolidation therapy with autologous stem cell rescue
3. Therapy for minimal residual disease:
   a. Radiation to tumor sites
   b. Noncytotoxic agents.

Induction Therapy

Because neuroblastoma is sensitive to chemotherapy (even with MYCN amplification) the goal of induction therapy is to induce maximum reduction in the primary tumor bulk and the metastatic sites. The efficacy of induction chemotherapy is assessed by the response rate, as generally determined by second-look surgery. Many treatment protocols are available for induction chemotherapy. The regimens with the best response rates to date are described in Table 18-9.

The duration of induction therapy in each protocol is about 4–5 months. There is substantial evidence that the quality of remission at the end of induction therapy correlates highly with long-term survival. The patients who achieve complete remission or very good partial response have a good chance of converting to complete remission with consolidation high-dose myeloablative chemotherapy.

Persistent bony lesions and bone marrow involvement are the only independent adverse prognostic factors.

Consolidation Therapy

The next phase of therapy is consolidation. The goal of this treatment is to eliminate any remaining tumor with myeloablative cytotoxic agents and stem cell rescue. The 3-year event-free survival for patients given a myeloablative regimen followed by stem cell rescue is far superior (38–50%) to that of chemotherapy alone (15%) (Table 18-10). This is especially true for patients at very high risk such as those older than 1 year of age and MYCN-amplified metastatic disease.

There are a few consolidation regimes (Table 18-10) currently in use. The COG is utilizing peripheral blood stem cell (PBSC) rescue because PBSC provides superior engraftment and less transplant-related morbidity compared to bone marrow grafts. In addition, PBSCs are less likely to contain tumor cells. Stem cell harvest occurs after two to three cycles of chemotherapy, thus allowing *"in vivo* purging" of the tumor cells.

Table 18-10. Consolidation Regimens and 3-Year Event-Free Survival from Recent Pediatric Oncology Group, Children's Cancer Group, and European Neuroblastoma Study Group

Study	Regimen[a]	3-year event-free survival[b]
CCG-3891	Day −8 to day −5 carboplatin 250 mg/m^2/day (8.33 mg/kg/day if child ≤12 kg) Day −8 to day −5 etoposide 160 mg/m^2/day (5.33 mg/kg/day if child ≤12 kg) Day −7 melphalan 140 mg/m^2 (4.7 mg/kg if child ≤12 kg) Day −6 melphalan 70 mg/m^2 (2.4 mg/kg if child ≤12 kg) Day −4 no therapy Day −3 to day −1 TBI 330 cGy each day Day 0 ABMT[c] OR	43
POG-8844	Day −6 to day −4 melphalan 60 mg/m^2/day Day −3 to day −1 TBI 200 cGy each day Day 0 ABMT[c] OR	38
CCG-321P3	Day −8 to day −5 carboplatin 300 mg/m^2/day Day −8 to day −5 etoposide 200 mg/m^2/day Day −7 melphalan 140 mg/m^2 × 1 day Day −6 melphalan 70 mg/m^2 × 1 day Day −4 no therapy Day −3 to day −1 TBI 333 cGy daily Day 0 ABMT[c]	50

Abbreviations: TBI, total body irradiation; ABMT, autologous bone marrow transplant.
[a]All studies used purged autologous bone marrow unless otherwise noted.
[b]Three-year event-free survival rate from time of autologous marrow infusion.
[c]The original studies were done with ABMT but currently patients receive peripheral stem cell transplant.

Minimal Residual Disease Therapy

Despite the effective induction and myeloablative consolidation therapy, the majority of high-risk neuroblastoma patients experience relapse. The aim of this phase of therapy is to eradicate any residual tumor cells using radiation to tumor sites and noncytotoxic agents, which are theoretically active against chemoresistant tumor cells that survive intensive induction and consolidation regimens. It is preferable to give radiation post-transplantation if the tumor volume was large at the time of diagnosis or liver metastases were present.

Several novel agents such as *cis*-retinoic acid, anti-GD2 monoclonal antibody, or interleukin-2 are targeted to the biology of neuroblastoma and are found to be effective in eradicating minimal residual disease. Measurable responses have been observed in refractory neuroblastoma patients. Such protocols are not yet available for routine clinical practice. These protocols are available only in multicenter clinical trials on an experimental basis.

Risk Factors for Specific Relapse at a Specific Site

1. For local relapse in primary site:
   a. Incomplete resection of the primary tumor. Aggressive complete surgical removal of the primary tumor is critically important in determining long-term prognosis.

2. For bone marrow relapse:
   a. Bone marrow tumor content at the time of bone marrow harvest >0.1%.
   b. Involvement of bone marrow at the time of initial diagnosis.
3. For bone relapse:
   a. Involvement of bone at the time of initial diagnosis.

Follow-Up Studies

Physical examination should be performed monthly in the first year, every second month in the second year, and every third month in the third year following diagnosis.

Table 18-11 lists follow-up laboratory studies to determine disease status.

TREATMENT OF PATIENTS WITH DUMBBELL NEUROBLASTOMA AND SPINAL CORD COMPRESSIONS

In children with dumbbell extension of neuroblastoma associated with spinal symptoms, spinal cord decompression is a neurologic emergency and can be accomplished by three methods: radiation, surgery, and chemotherapy.

If there is no loss of neurologic function or indication of progression of neurologic symptoms, the dose of dexamethasone 0.25–0.5 mg/kg orally every 6 hours should be given.

Table 18-11. Follow-Up Laboratory Studies to Determine Disease Status of Neuroblastoma

Study	Frequency during		
	1st year	2nd year	After 2nd year
For evaluation of anatomic disease status[a]			
a. Primary site:			
CT and/or MRI study	3 months or as indicated clinically	3 months or as indicated clinically	If indicated clinically
MIBG scintiography (when available)	6 months or as indicated clinically	6 months or as indicated clinically	If indicated clinically
b. Metastatic sites: Bone			
^{99m}Tc-diphosphonate scintiography	6 months	6 months	If indicated clinically
Bone marrow[b]			
2 biopsies and 2 aspirates from two separate sites (e.g., right and left posterior iliac spine)	3 months or as indicated clinically	6 months or as indicated clinically	If indicated clinically
For evaluation of tumor marker response 24-hour urinary VMA/ HVA and creatinine	3 months or as indicated clinically	6 months or as indicated clinically	If indicated clinically

[a]If surgery is performed repeat the studies for primary site before and after surgery. If stem cell transplantation (SCT) is performed repeat all of the above studies before and after SCT.

[b]Neuroblastoma-specific immunocytology is a more sensitive method when available.

Radiation

If there is rapidly progressive spinal cord dysfunction, the treatment of choice is immediate dexamethasone in a bolus dose of 1.0–2 mg/kg. Dexamethasone can be followed by radiation alone or in combination with laminectomy (see below) in order to rapidly reduce cord compression. The daily radiotherapy dose (180 and 400 cGy) is given with concomitant dexamethasone. The total dose of radiation depends on the response to initial therapy.

Surgery

Close follow-up of patients is necessary to determine appropriate indication (failure to get an immediate response to radiation and high-dose decadron or progression of neurologic symptoms or signs) for decompression by laminectomy. Neurologic improvement is observed in 65–70% of patients and complete neurologic recovery is observed in 30–40% of patients. Risks of laminectomy include failure of response and development of kyphoscoliosis and spinal column instability.

Chemotherapy

Intensity of chemotherapy is determined according to stage and age risk criteria as previously described. It is important to use dexamethasone in moderately high doses (1.0–2.0 mg/kg). Risks of the use of primary chemotherapy in case of neurologic deficit include the possibility of chemoresistance, a delay in effectiveness, and hematologic toxicity, making the condition suboptimal for surgical resection if chemotherapy fails. However, in general, the response in most patients (approximately 80–85%) is very good. It has the advantage of making surgery safer by reducing the size of the tumor.

Prognosis

The prognosis depends on the neurologic findings when treatment is begun. Patients who are ambulatory when treatment is started usually remain ambulatory. Fifty percent of the children who are nonambulatory at the beginning of treatment can regain the ability to walk after emergency treatment.

NEUROBLASTOMA IN THE YOUNG ADULT AND ADULTS

- The distribution of primary neuroblastoma sites in this group of patients is similar to that seen in pediatric age group patients.
- The tumor growth rates of neuroblastoma in young adults and adults are slower than in pediatric age group patients.
- Neuroblastomas in this group of patients are relatively more resistant to chemotherapy than in pediatric age group patients.
- At present, the best treatment approach remains to be determined, but intensive chemotherapy with peripheral blood stem cell rescue, surgery, and radiation may be considered to improve prognosis.

SUGGESTED READINGS

Bessho F. Colloquy on neuroblastoma screening: is there a future for neuroblastoma mass screening? Med Pediat Oncol 1998;31:106–110.

Bowman LC, Castleberry RP, Cantor A, et al. Genetic staging of unresectable or metastatic neuroblastoma in infants: a Pediatric Oncology Group study. J Natl Cancer Inst 1997;89(5):373–80.

Cheung NK. Monoclonal antibody-based therapy for neuroblastoma. Curr Oncol Rep 2000;2(6):547–53.

Cojean N, Entz-Werle N, Eyer D, et al. Dumbbell nephroblastoma: an uncommon cause of spinal cord compression. Arch Pediatr 2003;10(12):1075–8.

Cooper R, Khakoo Y, Matthay KK, et al. Opsoclonus-myoclonus—ataxia syndrome in neuroblastoma: histopathologic features—a report from the Children's Cancer Group. Med Pediatr Oncol 2001;36(6):623–9.

Hsu LL, Evans AE, D'Angio GJ. Hepatomegaly in neuroblastoma stage 4S: criteria for treatment of the vulnerable neonate. Med Pediatr Oncol 1996;27(6):521–28.

Katzenstein HM, Bowman LC, Brodeur GM, Thorner PS, Joshi VV, et al. Prognostic significance of age, MYCN oncogene amplification, tumor cell ploidy and histology in 110 infants with stage D(S) neuroblastoma: the Pediatric Oncology Group experience—a Pediatric Oncology Group study. J Oncol 1998;16:2007–17.

Kerbl R, Urban CE, Ambros IM, et al. Neuroblastoma mass screening in late infancy: insights into the biology of neuroblastic tumors. J Clin Oncol 2003;21(22):4228–34.

Kushner BH, Cheung NK, LaQuaglia MP, et al. International neuroblastoma staging system stage I neuroblastoma: a prospective study and literature review. J Clin Oncol 1996;14(7):2174–80.

Matthay KK. Stage 4S neuroblastoma: what makes it special? J Clin Oncol 1998;16:2003–6.

Matthay KK, Brisse H, Couanet D, et al. Central nervous system metastases in neuroblastoma: radiologic, clinical, and biologic features in 23 patients. Cancer 2003;98(1):155–65.

Matthay KK, Edeline V, Lumbroso J, et al. Correlation of early metastatic response by ^{123}I-metaiodobenzylguanidine scintigraphy with overall response and event-free survival in stage IV neuroblastoma. J Clin Oncol 2003;21(13):2486–91.

Matthay KK, Perez C, Seeger RC, et al. Successful treatment of stage III neuroblastoma based on prospective biologic staging: a Children's Cancer Group study. J Clin Oncol 1998;16(4):1256–64.

Pollono D, Tomarchia S, Drut R, et al. Spinal cord compression: a review of 70 pediatric patients. Pediatr Hematol Oncol 2003;20(6):457–66.

Reynolds CP, Villablanca JG, Stram DO, et al. 13-*cis*-retinoic acid after intensive consolidation therapy for neuroblastoma improves event-free survival: a randomized Children's Cancer Group (CCG) study. Proc Am Soc Clin Oncol 1998;17:A5, 2a.

Rubie H, Coze C, Plantaz D, et al. Localised and unresectable neuroblastoma in infants: excellent outcome with low-dose primary chemotherapy. Br J Cancer 2003;89(9):1605–9.

Seeger RC, Reynolds CP, Gallego R, et al. Quantitative tumor cell content of bone marrow and blood as a predictor of outcome in stage IV neuroblastoma: a Children's Cancer Group Study. J Clin Oncol 2000;18(24):4067–76.

Tchirkov A, Paillard C, Halle P, et al. Significance of molecular quantification of minimal residual disease in metastatic neuroblastoma. J Hematother Stem Cell Res 2003;12(4):435–42.

Woods WG, Tuchman M, Bernstein M, Lemieux B. Screening infants for neuroblastoma does not reduce the incidence of poor-prognosis disease. Med Pediatr Oncol 1998;31:450–4.

19

WILMS' TUMOR

Wilms' tumor (nephroblastoma) is the second most common malignant retroperitoneal tumor. It is the most common primary renal tumor of childhood.

CLINICAL FEATURES

Incidence

1. Six percent of all childhood cancers.
2. Fourth most common childhood malignancy in the United States. Occurs in 1 out of 10,000 children less than 15 years of age.
3. Nine new cases per million children diagnosed annually in the United States.
4. Male:female ratio 0.92:1.00 in unilateral disease and 0.6:1.00 in bilateral disease.
5. Seventy-eight percent of children are diagnosed at 1–5 years of age, with a peak incidence occurring between 3 and 4 years of age. Median age of presentation is 44 months in unilateral disease, 32 months in bilateral disease.
6. Usually sporadic, but 1% of cases are familial.

Associated Congenital Anomalies

Congenital anomalies occur in 12–15% of cases. The most frequently diagnosed congenital anomalies are aniridia, hemihypertrophy, Beckwith–Wiedemann syndrome, and genitourinary tract anomalies, including WAGR syndrome (Wilms' tumor, aniridia, genitourinary malformations, and mental retardation) and Denys–Drash syndrome (DDS; Wilms' tumor, renal disease, and pseudohermaphroditism). Table 19-1 lists the incidence of congenital anomalies in patients with Wilms' tumor.

Congenital Aniridia and Wilms' Tumor

1. Aniridia is present in 1 out of 70 children with Wilms' tumor.
2. A child with nonfamilial aniridia has a 1 in 3 chance of subsequently developing Wilms' tumor.
3. Associated anomalies of the nonfamilial bilateral aniridia–Wilms' tumor syndrome are listed in Table 19-2.
4. A chromosomal deletion has been consistently found in the short arm of chromosome 11 (11p13 deletion).

Table 19-1. Incidence of Congenital Anomalies in Patients with Wilms' Tumor

Anomaly	Incidence (%)
Genitourinary anomalies: horseshoe kidney, dysplasia of kidney, cystic disease of kidney, hypospadias, cryptorchidism, duplication of collecting system	4.4
Congenital aniridia	1.1
Congenital hemihypertrophy	2.9
Musculoskeletal anomalies: clubfoot, rib fusion, distal phocomelia, hip dislocation	2.9
Hamartomas: hemangiomas, "birthmarks," multiple nevi, café-au-lait spots	7.9

Table 19-2. Associated Anomalies in Patients with Nonfamilial Bilateral Aniridia–Wilms' Tumor Syndrome

Associated anomalies	Incidence (%)
Ocular anomalies	78
Cataract	
Glaucoma	
Central nervous system involvement	71
Mental retardation	
Microcephaly	
Craniofacial dysmorphism	
External ear anomalies	35
Deformed pinna	
Growth retardation	28
Reproductive system anomalies	28
Cryptorchidism	
Urinary tract anomalies	21
Hypospadias	
Horsehoe kidney	

Note. Mean age: 1 year, 10 months.

Hemihypertrophy and Wilms' Tumor

There is a definite relationship between hemihypertrophy, Beckwith–Wiedemann syndrome, and Wilms' tumor. Congenital hemihypertrophy has also been reported in association with other conditions:

- Adrenocortical tumors
- Hepatic tumors
- Hamartomas
- Neurofibromatosis
- Silver syndrome.

Beckwith–Wiedemann Syndrome

This syndrome consists of:

1. Hyperplastic fetal visceromegaly involving the kidney, adrenal cortex, pancreas, gonads, and liver
2. Macroglossia, abdominal wall defect (omphalocele, umbilical hernia, diastasis recti), hemihypertrophy, ear pits or creases, microcephaly, mental retardation, hypoglycemia, and postnatal somatic gigantism.

This syndrome is associated with an increased incidence of embryonal tumors of childhood, including:

- Wilms' tumor
- Neuroblastoma
- Rhabdomyosarcoma
- Adrenal carcinoma
- Hepatoblastoma.

Follow-Up of Patients with Sporadic Aniridia, Hemihypertrophy, and Beckwith–Wiedemann Syndrome

This group of children should have an abdominal ultrasound and a determination of α-fetoprotein (because of the rare association with hepatoblastoma) every 3 months until their fifth birthday and then yearly until full growth has occurred to evaluate for Wilms' tumor.

Signs and Symptoms of Wilms' Tumor

1. Initial signs and symptoms, in order of frequency, are listed in Table 19-3.
2. Abdominal mass is the most common presenting symptom and sign. Occasionally, there is abdominal pain, especially when hemorrhage occurs in the tumor following trauma.
3. Hematuria is not common but is more often seen microscopically than on gross examination.
4. Hypertension is seen in approximately 25% of patients due to elaboration of renin by tumor cells or, less commonly, due to compression of renal vasculature.
5. Polycythemia is occasionally present. Erythropoietin levels are usually increased but can also be normal. Polycythemia is usually associated with males, older age, and low clinical stage. All children with unexplained polycythemia should be investigated for Wilms' tumor.
6. Bleeding diathesis is due to the presence of acquired von Willebrand disease (reduced von Willebrand factor antigen level, prolonged bleeding time, decreased factor VIII, and factor VIII ristocetin cofactor activity).

Table 19-3. Initial Signs and Symptoms of Wilms' Tumor in Order of Frequency

Sign/symptom	Frequency (%)
Palpable mass in abdomen	60
Hypertension	25
Hematuria	15
Obstipation	4
Weight loss	4
Urinary tract infection	3
Diarrhea	3
Previous trauma	3
Other signs/symptoms: nausea, vomiting, abdominal pain, inguinal hernia, cardiac insufficiency,[a] acute surgical abdomen, pleural effusion, polycythemia, hydrocephalus[b]	8

[a]Due to propagation of tumor clot from inferior vena cava into right atrium.
[b]Intracerebral secondary-associated congenital anomaly or associated central nervous system tumor.

LABORATORY STUDIES

Table 19-4 lists investigations required in Wilms' tumor. The basic information required prior to surgery includes:

- Presence of a functioning kidney on the other side
- Presence of lung metastases
- Presence of bone or brain metastases if indicated by history or physical examination
- Presence of thrombi in inferior vena cava.

STAGING SYSTEM

Table 19-5 describes the clinicopathologic staging system as recommended by the National Wilms' Tumor Study (NWTS).

PATHOLOGY

Wilms' tumor is derived from primitive metanephric blastema and is characterized by histopathologic diversity. The classic Wilms' tumor is composed of persistent blastema, dysplastic tubules (epithelial), and supporting mesenchyme or stroma.

Table 19-4. Investigations in Wilms' Tumor

History: family history of cancer, congenital defects, and benign tumors

Physical examination: congenital anomalies (aniridia, hemihypertrophy, genitourinary anomalies), blood pressure, liver enlargement

Complete blood count: presence or absence of polycythemia

Urinalysis

Blood chemistries: blood urea nitrogen, creatinine, uric acid, serum glutamic-oxaloacetic transaminase, serum glutamic pyruvic transaminase, lactic dehydrogenase, alkaline phosphatase

Assessment of coagulation factors: prothrombin time, partial thromboplastin time, fibrinogen level, bleeding time (if abnormal, factor VIII level, von Willebrand factor antigen level, factor VIII ristocetin cofactor activity)[a]

Assessment of cardiac status: electrocardiogram and echocardiogram in all patients who receive Adriamycin; echocardiogram may be useful in detecting the presence of tumor in the right atrium

Abdominal ultrasound

Abdominal CT scan with special attention to:
  Presence and function of the opposite kidney
  Evidence of bilateral involvement
  Evidence of involvement of blood vessels with tumor
  Lymph node involvement
  Liver infiltration

Chest radiograph (posteroanterior and lateral)

Chest CT scan: helps recognize small metastases that may be hidden behind ribs, diaphragm, and heart and may be missed on chest radiograph

Skeletal scintigram: only in cases of clear-cell sarcoma—bone-metastasizing renal tumor of childhood

Magnetic resonance imaging and/or CT scan of brain: only in cases of rhabdoid tumors, which are frequently associated with CNS tumors, and clear-cell sarcoma of the kidney, which may metastasize to the brain

Peripheral blood for chromosomal analysis: in cases of congenital anomalies, such as aniridia, Beckwith–Wiedemann syndrome, hemihypertrophy

[a]To exclude associated acquired von Willebrand disease.

Table 19-5. Clinicopathologic Staging System[a]

Stage	Description
I	Tumor limited to the kidney and completely excised: The surface of the renal capsule is intact. The tumor is not ruptured before or during removal or has been biopsied. No residual tumor apparent beyond the margins of excision.
II	Tumor extends beyond the kidney but is completely excised: There is regional extension of the tumor (i.e., penetration through the renal capsule into the perirenal soft tissues). The vessels of the renal sinus are not involved nor is there extensive invasion of the renal sinus. Vessels outside the kidney are infiltrated or they contain tumor thrombus. The tumor may have been biopsied or there has been local spillage of the tumor confined to the flank. No residual tumor is apparent at or beyond the margins of excision.
III	Residual nonhematogenous tumor confined to the abdomen: Any of the following may occur: A. Involved lymph nodes (on biopsy) in the hilus, the periaortic chains, or beyond[b] B. Diffuse peritoneal contamination by the tumor due to spillage of tumor beyond the ipsilateral flank before or during surgery, or tumor growth that has penetrated the peritoneal surface C. Tumor implants found on the peritoneal surfaces D. Gross or microscopic tumor remains postoperatively (e.g., tumor cells are found at the margin of surgical resection on microscopic examination) E. Tumor not completely resectable because of local infiltration into vital structures.
IV	Hematogenous metastases: Metastases extend beyond those seen in stage III (e.g., lung, liver, bone, and brain).
V	Bilateral renal involvement at diagnosis: An attempt should be made to stage each side according to the preceding criteria on the basis of extent of disease prior to biopsy.

[a]Each case should be characterized according to favorable and unfavorable histology.
[b]Lymph node involvement in the thorax or other extra-abdominal sites would be criteria for stage IV.

The coexistence of epithelial, blastemal, and stromal cells has led to the term *triphasic* to characterize the classic Wilms' tumor. Each of the cell types may exhibit a spectrum of differentiation, generally replicating various stages of renal embryogenesis. The proportion of each cell type may also vary significantly from tumor to tumor. Some Wilms' tumors may be biphasic or even monomorphous in appearance.

Clear cell sarcoma of the kidney and rhabdoid tumor of the kidney are not Wilms' tumor variants.

ANAPLASTIC WILMS' TUMOR

The presence of anaplasia is the only criterion for "unfavorable" histology in a Wilms' tumor.

Criteria for Anaplasia

Anaplasia denotes the presence of gigantic polypoid nuclei within the tumor sample. Recognition of this change requires both of the following:

1. Nuclei with major diameters at least three times those of adjacent cells, with increased chromatin content
2. Multipolar or otherwise recognizably polypoid mitotic figures.

Both of these features must be identified in the sample.

Focal versus Diffuse Anaplasia

The criteria for distinguishing focal from diffuse anaplasia are dependent on the distribution of anaplasia. Focal anaplasia requires that anaplastic nuclear changes be confined to sharply restricted foci within the primary tumor. This definition restricts focal anaplasia to one or a few discrete loci within the primary tumor and with no anaplasia or marked nuclear atypia elsewhere.

A diagnosis of diffuse anaplasia requires the following characteristics:

- Anaplasia in any extrarenal site, including vessels of the renal sinus, extracapsular infiltrates, or nodal or distant metastases
- Anaplasia in a random biopsy specimen
- Anaplasia unequivocally expressed in one region of the tumor, but with extreme nuclear pleomorphism approaching the criteria of anaplasia (extreme nuclear unrest) elsewhere in the lesion
- Anaplasia in more than one tumor slide, unless (1) it is known that every slide showing anaplasia came from the same region of the tumor or (2) anaplastic foci on the various slides are minute and surrounded on all sides by nonanaplastic tumor.

CYTOGENETIC AND MOLECULAR FEATURES OF WILMS' TUMOR

Recessive cancer genes (suppressor genes) play an important role in the pathogenesis of Wilms' tumor. With the use of cytogenetic techniques and molecular analysis for restriction length polymorphism, homozygosity or hemizygosity for a small deletion on chromosome 11 (11p13) has been detected in the tumor cells of Wilms' tumor. This Wilms' tumor 1 (*WT1*) gene encodes a transcription factor that is important in normal kidney and gonadal development. Germ line mutations within the *WT1* gene have been identified in WAGR and DDS and some bilateral Wilms' tumors. Specific mutations of *WT1* have been found in only 10% or less of sporadic Wilms' tumors.

A second Wilms' tumor locus (*WT2*) maps to chromosome 11p15.5, based on tumor-specific loss of heterozygosity. The Beckwith–Wiedemann syndrome also maps to this location. The copy of 11p15 that is lost is derived from the mother, suggesting that the 11p15 locus is subject to genomic imprinting. Twenty percent of Wilms' tumor syndromes have allelic loss of the long arm of chromosome 16. It is felt that there are other yet unidentified loci where mutation may predispose to Wilms' tumor formation.

TREATMENT OF WILMS' TUMOR

Treatment of Wilms' tumor is based on the conclusions of the NWTS programs as shown in Table 19-6 and Figures 19-1 and 19-2.

Surgery

1. Complete exploration of the abdomen, including the liver and the contralateral kidney, should be done.
2. All lymph nodes removed should be identified and the site marked. If no abnormal lymph nodes are identified, one or more apparently normal lymph nodes should be removed.

Table 19-6. Treatment Recommendations for Wilms' Tumor

Stage	Histology	Surgery	Radiation therapy	Chemotherapy		
				Agents	Dose and schedules	Duration (weeks)
I and II	FH	Yes	No	AMD + VCR	Figure 19-1	18
I	FA-UH DA-UH	Yes	No	AMD + VCR	Figure 19-1	18
III and IV	FH	Yes	Yes 1080 cGy to tumor bed	AMD + VCR + ADR	Figure 19-2	24
II, III, IV	FA-UH	Yes	Yes 1080 cGy to tumor bed	AMD + VCR + ADR	Figure 19-2	24
II, III, IV	DA-UH	Yes	Yes 1080 cGy to tumor bed	ICE[a]	Page 556	

Abbreviations: FH, favorable histology; UH, unfavorable histology; DA, diffuse anaplasia; FA, focal anaplasia; AMD, dactinomycin (actinomycin D); VCR, vincristine sulfate; ADR, doxorubicin (Adriamycin).

Note: Babies <12 months of age should receive one-half the recommended dose of all drugs. Full doses lead to prohibitive hematologic toxicity in this age group. Full doses of chemotherapeutic agents should be administered to children >12 months of age.

[a]See page 556 for precise protocol for ICE treatment. Although this protocol is not universally recommended, it has been used successfully by the author followed by stem cell transplantation in diffuse anaplasia.

3. Radical excision is advised so that all tumor tissue can be completely removed. The junction of suspicious abnormal areas with normal kidney should be removed to facilitate the accurate diagnosis of small lesions.

Radiation Therapy

1. Radiation therapy (RT) is usually begun shortly after surgery (within 10 days), with the aim of eradicating tumor cells that may have spilled during surgery. The size of the field depends on the findings at surgery, but in all cases, the liver, spleen, and opposite kidney should be carefully shielded.
2. Stages III and IV favorable histology (FH) and stages II, III, and IV unfavorable histology (UH) disease require irradiation to the tumor bed at a dose of 1080 cGy as determined by the preoperative radiologic findings. The tumor bed is

```
WEEK 0  1  2  3  4  5  6  7  8  9  10 11 12 13 14 15 16 17 18
        A     A     A     A        A        A        A
        V  V  V  V  V  V  V  V  V  V     V*       V*       V*
```

A – Dactinomycin (45 µg/kg, IV)
V – Vincristine (0.05 mg/kg, IV)
V* – Vincristine (0.067 mg/kg, IV)

Fig. 19-1. Stage I favorable or anaplastic histology or stage II favorable histology.

```
WEEK 0    1  2  3   4  5  6  7  8  9   10 11 12 13 14 15 16 17 18 19 20 21 22 23 24
          A     D+     A     D+        A        D*       A        D*       A
          V  V  V  V  V  V  V  V  V  V  V     V*       V*       V*       V*       V*
        XRT
```

A – Dactinomycin (45 µg/kg, IV)   V – Vincristine (0.05 mg/kg, IV)
D* – Doxorubicin (1.0 mg/kg, IV)   V* – Vincristine (0.067 mg/kg, IV)
D+ – Doxorubicin (1.5 mg/kg, IV)   XRT – Radiation therapy

Fig. 19-2. Stages III and IV favorable histology or stage II–IV unfavorable histology.

defined as the outline of the kidney and any associated tumor. The portals should be extended to include areas of more diffuse involvement (e.g., the para-aortic chains) when those nodes are found to be involved. When there is peritoneal seeding or gross tumor spillage, total abdominal irradiation should be given through anterior and posterior portals from the diaphragmatic domes to the inferior margin of the obturator foramen, sparing the femoral heads. The contralateral kidney should be shielded.

3. Whole abdominal radiotherapy is unnecessary for patients with tumor spills confined to the flank or for those who had prior biopsy of the neoplasm.
4. Metastatic disease to lungs visible on chest x-ray require whole-lung RT 1200 cGy. Immediately after RT chemotherapy doses should be decreased 50%. *Pneumocystis carinii* prophylaxis with trimethoprim-sulfamethoxazole (Bactrim) or pentamidine should be instituted in patients receiving lung RT.

Treatment of Tumors Considered Inoperable Because of Size

Preoperative therapy should be used only in carefully selected cases after pathologic diagnosis is obtained. The following management plan is recommended:

- The chemotherapy regimen shown in Figure 19-2 should be administered.
- An abdominal computed tomography (CT) scan should be performed after approximately 5 weeks of therapy.
- Radiation therapy should be given if there is no reduction in the size of the tumor from chemotherapy.
- The suggested radiation dose is 1200–1260 cGy (150 cGy/day for 8 days or 180 cGy/day for 7 days). During radiation therapy, vincristine should be continued at weekly intervals.

Shrinkage usually occurs in 6 weeks. Surgery is planned according to tumor shrinkage and when a radiologic assessment suggests that the tumor can be totally excised.

The primary tumor should be considered stage III, regardless of the findings at surgery. Postoperative radiation therapy is required. If pathology at definitive surgery is consistent with diffuse anaplasia, chemotherapy should be changed.

TREATMENT OF ACQUIRED VON WILLEBRAND DISEASE

Occasionally, acquired von Willebrand disease occurs in Wilms' tumor. If this is identified either clinically or in the laboratory, treatment should be carried out as follows:

- Initially, administer 1-deamino-8-D-arginine vasopressin (DDAVP). If no response, administer Humate-P (see Chapter 11, Table 11-20).

Acquired von Willebrand disease disappears after treatment of Wilms' tumor is initiated.

POST-THERAPY FOLLOW-UP

1. Chest radiographs should be performed every 3 months during the first and second years and every 6 months for 5 years thereafter. In patients with pulmonary disease at diagnosis, chest CT scans should be performed at the same intervals.

2. Abdominal ultrasonography should be performed every 3 months during the first and second years post-therapy and then every 6 months until 5 years post-therapy.

Treatment of Relapse

Treatment of relapse is determined by the following factors:

Group I

Favorable factors are as follows:

1. Histology favorable at diagnosis
2. Stage I at time of diagnosis
3. Treatment initially with only dactinomycin and vincristine
4. Recurrence only in the lungs OR
5. Recurrence in the abdomen when radiotherapy was not initially given OR
6. Recurrence 12 months or more after diagnosis.

This group is treated with the regimen depicted in Figure 19-2.
Other types of relapse include:

Pulmonary relapse: radiation to both lungs, in addition to aforementioned chemotherapy

Liver relapse: surgery with partial hepatectomy if the tumor is localized to one lobe with or without radiotherapy, in addition to aforementioned chemotherapy

Local relapse in tumor bed: surgical excision and local radiotherapy, in addition to aforementioned chemotherapy.

Group II

Unfavorable factors are as follows:

1. Unfavorable histology at diagnosis (anaplastic clear cell and rhabdoid subtypes), regardless of other factors
2. Favorable histology at diagnosis, previously treated with dactinomycin, vincristine, and doxorubicin or tumor recurs in the abdomen after radiotherapy or in other nonpulmonary sites.

This group is treated as follows:

1. To induce complete response or good partial response, 2 courses at 3 weekly intervals of the following ICE therapy should be employed:
   Ifosfamide 1800 mg/m^2/IV mixed with mesna 360 mg/m^2/IV daily for 5 days. This is given over 60 minutes. A continuous infusion of mesna (total dose 360 mg/m^2/IV) is given during the second, third, and fourth hours. Mesna 360 mg/m^2/IV is then infused over 15 minutes at hours 8, 11, and 14.
   Carboplatin 400 mg/m^2/day IV over 1 hour × 2 days
   Etoposide 100 mg/m^2/day IV over 1 hour × 5 days
   G-CSF 5–10 µg/kg SC on day 6 (24 hours after completion of chemotherapy) daily until ANC >5000/mm^3.
2. Surgery and radiotherapy should be employed (or radiotherapy can be administered following autologous stem cell transplantation).
3. In chemotherapy-responsive disease ablative chemotherapy and autologous stem cell transplantation should be carried out. The ablative chemotherapy consists of the following:
   Etoposide 200 mg/m^2/day IV over 2 hours on days –7, –6, –5, –4, and –3

Carboplatin over 1 hour intravenously at a total dose required to attain an area under the curve (AUC) of 4 mg/min/mL over 1 hour for 5 days on days –7, –6, –5, –4, and –3 (the dose of carboplatin is calculated using the Calvert formula*)
Melphalan 180 mg/m^2/day IV on day –2
Autologous stem cell transplantation on day 0.

A trial of chemotherapy is recommended prior to surgery or radiotherapy for both groups to determine tumor responsiveness.

PROGNOSIS

Table 19-7 lists the percentage of event-free survival and overall survival at diagnosis in relationship to the stage of disease and histology. Positive prognostic factors include the following:

- Stages I and II
- Negative para-aortic nodes
- Absence of anaplastic or sarcomatous histology
- Absence of tumor rupture
- Site of metastases at relapse: lung better than liver
- Time of relapse: late better than early (>15 months from diagnosis).

BILATERAL WILMS' TUMOR

Presentation: abdominal mass synchronously (simultaneously) or metachronously (sequentially)
Associated findings: hypertension, aniridia, and genitourinary anomalies; may arise from renal dysplasia or nodular or diffuse nephroblastomatosis
Histology: usually favorable.

Prognostic Factors

1. Diagnosis at an early age (<2 years of age) carries a better prognosis (survival 70–75%) than diagnosis at more than 2 years of age (survival 20–45%).
2. Survival is better for patients with stage I or II disease (85%) compared to stage III or IV disease (0%).
3. Synchronous tumors have a better outlook than metachronous tumors.

Table 19-7. Percentage of Event-Free Survival (EFS) and Overall Survival (OS) for Favorable Histology

	EFS (%)	OS (%)
2 years		
Stage I–III	86	96
Stage IV	72	86
4 years		
Stage I–III	86	95
Stage IV	69	81

Modified from D'Angio GJ. Med Pediatr Oncol 2003;41:545–9.

---

*Calvert formula: For dose of carboplatin 4× (glomerular filtration rate +25) in mg.

Treatment

Objectives:

- Maximum preservation of renal tissue
- Tumor removal by partial nephrectomy.

Management:

1. A laparotomy and biopsy of both kidneys should be performed for purposes of staging and histology. Suspicious lymph nodes should be biopsied; each side is staged separately. Excision of the tumor(s) is performed at the initial operation only if all of the tumor can be removed with preservation of sufficient renal parenchyma for normal renal function on at least one side.
2. The chemotherapy regimen should be administered according to Figure 19-2.
3. Evaluation and abdominal CT scan should be carried out at week 5:
   a. At about week 6, if the radiologic evaluation demonstrates persistent but resectable tumor or the tumor has responded completely to chemotherapy, second-look surgery and biopsy are indicated.
   b. At the time of second-look surgery, complete excision of the tumor from the least involved kidney should be carried out. If the procedure leaves a viable and functioning kidney on one side, then the other kidney, if extensively involved with tumor, should be removed.
4. Postoperative chemotherapy should be adapted to renal function abnormalities:
   a. If second-look surgery demonstrates no gross or pathologic evidence of persistent tumor, the chemotherapy regimen should be administered as shown in Figure 19-2.
   b. If second-look surgery demonstrates gross or pathologic evidence of persistent disease that could not be resected, the patient should receive radiation therapy and consideration should be given to change the chemotherapy to ICE therapy (page 556).
5. Further surgery may be required, depending on the radiologic evidence of persistent disease.

NEPHROBLASTOMATOSIS

Nephroblastomatosis represents the persistence of embryonal renal tissue. It is a premalignant lesion with a potential to develop into Wilms' tumor. Management of nephroblastomatosis involves:

1. Conservative renal tissue–preserving surgery
2. Chemotherapy
3. Abdominal ultrasonography (follow-up should be done yearly until 10 years after diagnosis in patients with unilateral Wilms' tumor who have evidence of nephroblastomatosis in one or both kidneys).

CONGENITAL MESOBLASTIC NEPHROMA

Congenital mesoblastic nephroma is usually benign but may have perirenal extension. A nephrectomy with wide surgical margin alone is sufficient. However, incomplete resection and/or cellular congenital mesoblastic nephroma in children beyond 3 months of age at diagnosis indicates a higher rate of local recurrence and/or metastasis. Patients who experience a local recurrence or metastases require treatment with chemotherapy (vincristine, actinomycin, and doxorubicin) and radiation.

CLEAR CELL SARCOMA OF THE KIDNEY

1. Clear cell sarcoma of the kidney is the second most common pediatric renal neoplasm.
2. Bone metastases occurs in 40–60% of patients with clear cell sarcoma compared to 2% for Wilms' tumor.
3. Peak incidence between age 3 and 5 years.
4. Treatment consists of nephrectomy, radiation therapy, and chemotherapy with cyclophosphamide, etoposide, vincristine, and doxorubicin for 24 weeks (Figure 19-3).
5. 75% survival.

RHABDOID TUMOR OF THE KIDNEY

1. Occurs in 2% of renal tumors.
2. Chromosomal deletion of 22q11-12 is present in these patients.
3. More than 50% of patients are less than 1 year of age at diagnosis.
4. Metastases found in lung, liver, and brain.
5. Poor prognosis; mortality is over 80%. Responds poorly to current chemotherapy and radiotherapy. No satisfactory treatment available but intensive chemotherapy (ICE therapy; see page 556) followed by sublethal chemotherapy and peripheral stem cell rescue has been utilized with some success in our clinic.

RENAL CELL CARCINOMA

1. Two to 5% of primary renal tumors under 21 years of age
2. Most common renal neoplasm in adults
3. Survival for stage 1 disease after complete resection: 90%
4. Survival stage II and III: 50%

Week

0 1 2 3 4 5 6 7 8 9 10 11 12 13 14 15 16 17 18 19 20 21 22 23 24
C   D   C   D   C   D   C   D
D V V E V V V V V E V V V* V*   E   V*   E   V*
C*   C*   C*   C*

XRT

V – Vincristine 1.5 mg/m^2 (max 2 mg) or 0.05 mg/kg
V*– Vincristine 2.0 mg/m^2 (max 2 mg) or 0.067 mg/kg
D – Doxorubicin 45 mg/m^2 or 1.5 mg/kg
C – Cyclophosphamide 440 mg/m^2/day × 5 days or 14.7 mg/kg/day × 5 days
C*– Cyclophosphamide 440 mg/m^2 day × 3 days or 14.7 mg/kg/day × 3 days
E – Etoposide 100 mg/m^2 day × 5 days or 33 mg/kg/day × 5 days

Fig. 19-3. Clear-cell carcinoma stages I–IV. (Modified from Pizzo PA, Poplack DG, editors. Principles and Practice of Pediatric Oncology. 4th ed. Philadelphia: Lippincott Wilkins & Williams, 2002.)

5. Stage IV: 0% survival
6. Treatment: surgery. Not responsive to radiation therapy, poor chemotherapy response.

SUGGESTED READINGS

Abu-Gosh AM, Krailo MD, Goldman SC, Slack RS, Davenport V, Morris E, Laver JH, Reaman GH, Cairo W. Ifosfamide, carboplatin and etoposide in children with poor risk relapsed Wilms tumor: a Children's Cancer Group report. Ann Oncol 2002;13:460–9.

Beckwith JB, Zuppan CE, Browning NG, Moksness J, Breslow NE. Histological analysis of aggressiveness and responsiveness in Wilms' tumor. Med Pediatr Oncol 1996;27:422–8.

Calvert AH, Newell DR, Gumbrell LA, et al. Carboplatin dosage: prospective evaluation of a simple formula based on renal function. J Clin Oncol 1989;7:1748–56.

D'Angio GJ. Pre or post operative treatment for Wilms tumor? Who, what, when, where, how, why and which. Med Pediatr Oncol 2003;41:545–9.

Dome JS, Coppes MJ. Recent advances in Wilms' tumor genetics. Curr Opin Pediatr 2002;14:5–11.

Green DM. Wilms' tumor. Eur J Cancer 1997;33:409–18.

Green DM, Beckwith JB, Breslow NE, Faria P, Moksness J, Finkelstein JZ, Grundy P, Thomas PRM, Kim T, Shochat S, Haase G, Ritchey M, Kelalis P, D'Angio GJ. Treatment of children with stage II to IV anaplastic Wilms' tumor: a report from the National Wilms' Tumor Study Group. J Clin Oncol 1994;12:2126–31.

Green DM, Breslow NE, Beckwith JB, Finkelstein JZ, Grundy P, Thomas PRM, Kim T, Shochat S, Haase G, Ritchey M, Kelalis P, D'Angio G. Effect of duration of treatment on treatment outcome and cost of treatment for Wilms' tumor: a report from the National Wilms' Tumor Study Group. J Clin Oncol 1998;16:3744–51.

Green DM, Breslow NE, Beckwith JB, Finkelstein JZ, Grundy PE, Thomas PRM, Kim T, Shochat SJ, Haase GM, Ritchey MC, Kelalis PP, D'Angio GJ. Comparison between single dose and divided dose administration of dactinomycin and doxorubicin for patients with Wilms' tumor: a report from the National Wilms' Tumor Study Group. J Clin Oncol 1998;16:237–48.

Green DM, D'Angio GJ, Beckwith JB, Breslow NE, Grundy PE, Ritchey MI, Thomas PRM. Wilms' tumor CA Cancer J Clin 1996;46:46–63.

Kremens B, Gruhn B, Klingebiel T, Hasan C, Laws HJ, Koscielniak E, Hero B, Selle B, Niemeyer G, Finckenstein FG, Schulz A, Wawer A, Zinti F, Graf N. High dose chemotherapy with autologous stem cell rescue in children with nephroblastoma. Bone Marrow Transpl 2002;30:893–8.

Merguerian PA. Pediatric genitourinary tumors. Curr Opin Oncol 2003;15:222–6.

Pein F, Michon J, Valteau-Couanet D, Quintana E, Frappaz D, Vannier JP, Philip T, Bergeron C, Baranzelli MC, Thyss A, Stephan JL, Boutard P, Gentet JC, Zucker JM, Tournadi MF, Hartman O. High dose melphalan, etoposide, and carboplatin followed by autologous stem cell rescue in pediatric high risk recurrent Wilms' tumor: a French Society of Pediatric Oncology study. J Clin Oncol 1998;16:3295–301.

Pein F, Tournade MF, Zucker JM, Brunat-Mentigny M, Deville A, Boutard P, Dusol F, Gentet JC, Legall E, Mechinaud F, Plouvier E, Plantaz D, Pautard B, Rubie H, Lemerle J. Etoposide and carboplatin: a highly effective combination in relapsed or refractory Wilms' tumor, a phase II study by the French Society of Pediatric Oncology. J Clin Oncol 1994;12:931–6.

Petruzzi MJ, Green DM. Wilms' tumor. Pediatr Clin North Am 1997;44:939–51.

20

RHABDOMYOSARCOMA AND OTHER SOFT-TISSUE SARCOMAS

The soft-tissue sarcomas constitute a heterogeneous group of malignant tumors with a common origin in primitive mesenchyme. These tumors arise from muscle, connective tissue, supportive tissue, and vascular tissue. Rhabdomyosarcoma, the most common soft-tissue sarcoma of childhood, represents 48% of soft-tissue sarcomas in children under age 15. Nonrhabdomyosarcoma soft-tissue sarcomas increase in incidence throughout childhood. As a group, they are highly invasive locally and have a high propensity for local recurrence. When they metastasize, it is usually via the bloodstream and, less commonly, via the lymphatics. Collaborative studies of rhabdomyosarcoma (RMS) have dramatically improved cure rates. Nonrhabdomyosarcoma soft-tissue sarcomas (NRSTS) in children frequently have a better prognosis than in their adult counterparts. In infants and young children, these tumors often behave in a benign manner and have an excellent prognosis with surgery alone. Table 20-1 summarizes the clinical and biological features of the NRSTS.

EPIDEMIOLOGY

Rhabdomyosarcoma, a tumor of striated muscle, has the following epidemiologic characteristics:

- It is the most common pediatric soft-tissue sarcoma, with an incidence of 4.6 per million in children 0–14 years old, and it constitutes 5.8% of all malignant solid tumors in children.
- Among extracranial solid tumors, rhabdomyosarcoma is the third most common solid tumor, following neuroblastoma and Wilms' tumor.
- It accounts for 3.4% of all malignant neoplasms in children of the United States. Approximately 350 new cases are diagnosed in the United States each year. The male:female ratio is 1.1–1.5:1.
- There are two age peaks: 2–6 years and 15–19 years. Incidence in African-American females is half that of Caucasian females. Incidence is lower in Asian populations residing in Asia or the West.

Fibrosarcoma, the most common group of NRSTS tumors, is most common in infants, whereas others predominate in mid- to late adolescence.

Table 20-1. Clinical and Biological Features of the Nonrhabdomyosarcoma Soft Tissue Sarcomas (NRSTS)

Tumor[a]	Cell origin/cytogenetics	Common sites	Common ages	Good prognostic factors[b]	Outcome	Therapy
Synovial sarcoma	Mesenchymal cells/t(X;18)	Extremities (lower>upper)	Adolescence/young adulthood	Age <14 years, Size <5 cm, calcification	Stages I & II, 70%, Stages III & IV, poor	WLE[c] with/without RT[d], Chemo: ifosfamide/Adriamycin
Malignant fibrous histiocytoma	Fibroblast/19p+	Lower extremity, trunk, head, and neck	40–60 years, In children, 10–20 years	Extremity site	5 year survival, 27–53%	WLE, Chemo: no established role; responsive to VAC[e] +/– doxorubicin
Angiomatoid form		Extremity	Young children		Excellent with surgery alone	WLE
Malignant peripheral nerve sheath tumor	Schwann cell or fibroblast/17q, 22q loss or rearrangement	Extremity, retroperitoneum, trunk	Younger in patients with neurofibromatosis (NF)	Size <5 cm, no NF	53% survival without NF, 16% with NF	WLE with/without RT, Chemo: neoadjuvant role, ifosfamide and etoposide active
Fibrosarcoma	Fibroblast				Excellent with surgery alone	WLE, avoid amputation RT/chemo if WLE not possible
Congenital	t(12;15)	Extremity, trunk	Most <2 years	<5 years	5-year survival 84%	Neo-adjuvant VA[f] useful
Adult form	t(X;18), t(2;5), t(7;22)	Extremity (thigh, knee)	Adolescence		5-year survival 34–60%	WLE with/without RT, Chemo: no established role

Leiomyosarcoma	Smooth muscle t(12;14) Common in HIV+ children	Retroperitoneum GI tract, vascular tissue	40–70 years, when in children, any age	<5 cm	33% disease-free survival at 1–5 years	WLE Chemo: doxorubicin, ifosfamide, and dacarbazine
Epithelioid form[g]		Stomach			Excellent with surgery alone	WLE
Alveolar soft tissue sarcoma	Paraganglionic mesoderm (?), neuroepithelial (?), muscle (?) t(X;17)	Lower extremity, head and neck	15–35 years	Young age, orbital site, <5 cm	27–59% (indolent; death from disease after 10–20 years) 5-year survival	WLE Chemo or RT only after recurrence Chemo: doxorubicin based
Hemangiopericytoma[b]	Pericytes t(12;19), t(13;22)	Extremity, retroperitoneum, head and neck	20–70 years, when in children, 10–20 years	Low stage, <5 cm	Stage I & II, 30–70% 5-year survival with adjuvant therapy Stages III & IV, poor	WLE, with/without RT Chemo: no established role
Infantile form		Extremity, trunk	Rare, but typically <1 year		Excellent with surgery alone	WLE
Liposarcoma	Primitive mesenchyme t(12;16)	Extremity, retroperitoneum	0–2 years and second decade; sixth decade most common	Child, myxoid type	Very good with WLE, rarely metastasizes	WLE, with/without RT RT important in retroperitoneal lesions Chemo: no established role

[a]Listed in order of decreasing incidence.
[b]Low histologic grade and low stage are good prognostic factors.
[c]Wide local excision.
[d]Radiation therapy.
[e]Vincristine, actinomycin D, cyclophosphamide.
[f]Vincristine, actinomycin D.
[g]Carney triad: a condition consisting of gastric epithelioid leiomyosarcoma, pulmonary chondroma, functioning extra-adrenal paraganglioma.

PATHOLOGIC CLASSIFICATION

Table 20-2 lists the histologic subtypes with reference to their frequency, morphology, site of origin, and age distribution.

Specific assays may be necessary to aid in the differential diagnosis of rhabdomyosarcoma from the other small round cell tumors of childhood (i.e., lymphoma, Ewing's sarcoma, primitive neuroectodermal tumor, neuroblastoma). These assays include:

- Electron microscopy
- Immunocytochemistry
- Cytogenetics.

Table 20-2. Histologic Subtypes of Rhabdomyosarcoma and Undifferentiated Sarcoma

Pathologic subtype[a]	Morphology	Usual primary sites	Usual ages (years)
Rhabdomyosarcoma Embryonal (57%)	Resembles skeletal muscle in 7- to 10-week fetus. Moderately cellular with loose myxoid stroma. Actin and desmin positive.	Head and neck, orbit, genitourinary tract	3–12
Botryoid variant (6%)[b]	Cambial layer of tumor present, several cells thick. Loose myxoid stroma. Typically grapelike configuration is present grossly.	Bladder, vagina, nasopharynx, bile duct	0–8
Spindle cell variant (3%)	Spindle-shaped cells with elongated nuclei and prominent nucleoli. Low cellularity. Collagen rich and poor variants.	Paratesticular	2–12
Alveolar (24%)	Resembles skeletal muscle in 10- to 21-week fetus. Basic cell is round with scanty eosinophilic cytoplasm; alveolar pattern may be lost if densely packed; cross striations more common than embryonal variety.	Extremities, trunk, perineum (adolescents)	6–21
Undifferentiated (3.5%)	Cell of origin appears mesenchymal with no evidence of myogenesis or differentiation. Cells are round, larger than mature lymphocytes and have scanty or moderate cytoplasm; may be a heterogeneous group.	Extremities, trunk	Under 1 year
Other (6.5%)[c]	Heterogeneous.	Extremities, trunk	6–21

[a]Numbers in parentheses indicate frequency of histologic subtype.

[b]Forms within structures covered with mucosa and apposite to a body cavity.

[c]Reserved for tumors in which there is an inadequate amount of tissue for determination or in which no classification beyond that of a sarcoma is possible.

GENETICS OF RHABDOMYOSARCOMA
Molecular Genetics

1. Alveolar rhabdomyosarcoma (ARMS) has a characteristic translocation of the *FKHR* gene at 13q14 with *PAX3* at 2q35 or less commonly *PAX7* at 1p36.
2. Embryonal rhabdomyosarcoma (ERMS) has a loss of heterozygosity (LOH) at the 11p15 locus. This LOH involves loss of maternal genetic information with duplication of paternal genetic material.
3. RMS overproduces insulin-related growth factor 2 (IGF-2), potentially from loss of imprinting. IGF-2 stimulates growth of RMS, and blockade of the IGF-2 receptor inhibits RMS growth *in vivo*.
4. Other chromosomal abnormalities in rhabdomyosarcoma include 5q+; 9q+; 16p+; 12p+; del (1); and hyperdiploidy with multiple copies of 2, 6, 8, 12, 13, 18, 20, 21.
5. The DNA content or ploidy has been implicated in prognosis, particularly in tumors of embryonal histology. Diploid tumors may have a worse prognosis than hyperdiploid tumors. Hyperdiploid cells have 51 or more chromosomes.

Clinical Genetic Factors

1. Associated with germline mutations of the p53 tumor suppressor gene, as in familial multiple malignancy syndrome (Li–Fraumeni syndrome), which consists of an association between early-onset breast cancer in close relatives and sarcomas, brain tumors, and adrenocortical tumors in family members.
2. Associated with neurofibromatosis (as in the malignant triton tumor—a neurogenic sarcoma with evidence of rhabdomyosarcomatous differentiation within the mass), basal cell nevomatosis, lung adenomatosis, and nevus sebaceous of Jadassohn.
3. Associated with anomalies of the central nervous system (CNS), genitourinary system, gastrointestinal system, and cardiovascular system.
4. Associated with both maternal and paternal use of marijuana and cocaine, possibly as an environmental interaction with genetic predisposition.

CLINICAL FEATURES
Primary Sites

1. Rhabdomyosarcoma may occur in any anatomic location of the body where there is skeletal muscle, as well as in sites where no skeletal muscle is found (e.g., urinary bladder, common bile duct).
2. Table 20-3 lists the most commonly involved sites.

Signs and Symptoms

The most frequent presenting sign is a mass. Specific clinical manifestations vary with the site of origin of the primary lesion (Table 20-4).

An important clinical feature of parameningeal head and neck primary tumors (nasopharynx, sinuses, middle ear) is an approximate 25–35% incidence of CNS involvement that may present at diagnosis with cranial nerve palsies, meningeal symptoms, or respiratory difficulty due to brain stem infiltration. Up to 7% of non-parameningeal head and neck primary tumors may also have CNS involvement at diagnosis.

Table 20-3. Primary Sites of Rhabdomyosarcoma and Undifferentiated Sarcoma

Primary site	Relative frequency (%)	Regional spread and distant metastatic sites
Head and neck	40	
Orbit	8	Nodes rarely involved; rare lung metastasis
Parameningeal[a]	25	Regional spread to bone, meninges, brain; lung and bone metastases
Other[b]	7	Nodes rarely involved; lung metastases
Genitourinary tract	29	
Bladder, prostate	10	Nodes rarely involved; metastases to lung, bone, and bone marrow (primarily prostate primaries)
Vagina, uterus	5	Nodes rarely involved; metastases to retroperitoneal nodes (mainly from uterus)
Paratesticular	14	Retroperitoneal nodes in 50% of boys 10 or older; metastases to lung and bone
Extremities	14	Nodes involved in up to 50% of cases; metastases to lung, bone marrow, bone, CNS
Trunk	12	Nodes rarely involved; metastases to lung and bone
Other	5	Nodal involvement site dependent (increased in perineal/perianal primaries); metastases to lung, bone, and liver

[a]Parameningeal sites are adjacent to the meninges at the base of the skull; they consist of nasopharynx, middle ear, paranasal sinuses, and infratemporal and pterygopalatine fossae.

[b]Nonorbital, non-parameningeal sites consist of larynx, oropharynx, oral cavity, parotid, cheek, and scalp.

Table 20-4. Signs and Symptoms of Rhabdomyosarcoma in Various Anatomic Locations

Location	Signs and symptoms
Head and neck[a]	
Neck	Soft-tissue mass
	Hoarseness
	Dysphagia
Nasopharynx	Sinusitis
	Local pain
	Epistaxis
	Dysphagia
Paranasal sinus	Sinus obstruction/sinusitis
	Unilateral nasal discharge
	Local pain and swelling
	Epistaxis
Middle ear/mastoid	Chronic otitis media–purulent blood-stained discharge
	Polypoid mass in external canal
	Peripheral facial nerve palsy

(Continues)

Table 20-4. (*Continued*)

Orbit	Proptosis
	Ocular palsies
	Conjunctival mass
Genitourinary	
Vagina and uterus	Vaginal bleeding
	Grapelike clustered mass protruding through vaginal or cervical opening (i.e., sarcoma botryoides)
Urethra	Dysuria
Prostate	Hematuria
	Constipation
	Urinary obstruction
Bladder	Urinary obstruction
	Hematuria
	Tumor extrusion
	Recurrent urinary tract infections
Paratesticular	Painless scrotal or inguinal mass
Retroperitoneum	Abdominal pain
	Abdominal mass
	Intestinal obstruction
Pelvic	Constipation
	Genitourinary obstruction
Extremity/trunk	Asymptomatic or painful mass

*All can extend through multiple foramina and fissures into the epidural space and infiltrate the central nervous system with cranial nerve palsies, meningeal symptoms, and brain stem signs.

Rare primary sites for rhabdomyosarcoma include the gastrointestinal–hepatobiliary tract (3%), where it presents with obstructive jaundice and a large abdominal mass. These tumors arise in the common bile duct and may extend into both lobes of the liver. Other rare primary sites are the intrathoracic region (2%) and the perineal–perianal area (2%).

Rhabdomyosarcoma in children under 10 years of age generally involves the head and neck or genitourinary areas. Adolescents more commonly develop extremity, truncal, or paratesticular lesions.

DIAGNOSTIC EVALUATION

The diagnostic evaluation should delineate the extent of the primary tumor and the extent of metastatic disease and should consist of the following:

1. Complete history
2. Physical examination
3. Complete blood count
4. Urinalysis
5. Serum electrolytes, blood urea nitrogen (BUN), creatinine, alanine aminotransferase (ALT) and aspartate aminotransferase (AST), LDH, and alkaline phosphatase
6. Magnetic resonance imaging (MRI)* and/or computed tomography (CT) of primary lesion

---

*MRI may have value in predicting the extent and probability of surgical resection for extremity, abdominopelvic, and retroperitoneal tumors because of its enhanced ability to differentiate tumor from normal surrounding tissue compared to CT. It is useful for evaluating spinal cord involvement with retroperitoneal or paraspinal tumors.

7. Chest CT scan
8. Bone scan
9. Bilateral bone marrow aspiration and biopsy
10. Biopsy of suspicious lymph nodes and sentinel nodes for extremity primaries.

ADDITIONAL EXAMINATIONS FOR RHABDOMYOSARCOMA IN SPECIAL SITES

1. *Parameningeal head and neck:*
   a. Ear, nose, and throat examination under anesthesia
   b. Ophthalmologic examination
   c. Cerebrospinal fluid cytology
   d. Brain MRI
   e. Head CT scan (to evaluate bone involvement)
   f. Surgical intervention: incisional biopsy; except for orbital lesions, gross removal usually not feasible.
2. *Genitourinary, abdominal, pelvic:*
   a. Cystoscopy, vaginoscopy
   b. Ultrasonography
   c. CT scan of retroperitoneal nodes
   d. Surgical intervention: incisional or cystoscopic biopsy.
3. *Thorax:*
   a. Chest radiograph and CT
   b. MRI
   c. Surgical intervention: complete excision, if possible.
4. *Extremities:*
   a. Bone radiographs
   b. MRI
   c. Surgical intervention: biopsy of regional lymph nodes, wide local excision, if possible.
5. *Trunk:*
   a. MRI (or myelogram) if lesion is paraspinal
   b. Surgical intervention: complete excision, if possible.
6. *Gastrointestinal:*
   a. Liver scan
   b. Surgical intervention: complete excision, if possible.

STAGING

It is essential to fully stage the tumor because therapy and prognosis depend on the degree of regional spread, nodal involvement, and distant metastatic disease. The original staging system of the Intergroup Rhabdomyosarcoma Study (IRS) consists of four clinical groups, based on the extent of surgical resection (Table 20-5). The recently completed IRS trial, IRS-IV, incorporates the most significant prognostic variables (size, invasiveness, lymph node involvement, primary site) into a new TNM (tumor–node–metastasis) staging system (Table 20-6). This TNM staging system is defined as follows:

- *Stage I:* Favorable localized disease involving the orbit or head and neck (excluding parameningeal sites) or genitourinary system (excluding bladder and prostate)
- *Stage II:* Localized disease of any unfavorable primary site (primary tumor less than 5 cm in diameter; no regional node involvement)

Table 20-5. Intergroup Rhabdomyosarcoma Study Clinical Grouping System

Group	Definition
I	A. Localized, completely resected, confined to site of origin
	B. Localized, completely resected, infiltrated beyond site of origin
II	A. Localized, grossly resected, microscopic residual
	B. Regional disease, involved lymph nodes, completely resected
	C. Regional disease, involved lymph nodes, grossly resected with microscopic residual
III	A. Local or regional grossly visible disease after biopsy only
	B. Grossly visible disease after ≥50% resection of primary tumor
IV	A. Distant metastasis present at diagnosis

Table 20-6. TNM Staging of Rhabdomyosarcoma

T = Tumor	N = Regional nodes	M = Metastasis[a]
T1 = Confined to anatomic site of origin	N0 = Not clinically involved	M0 = No distant metastasis
T2 = Extension	N1 = Clinically involved	M1 = Distant metastasis present
a = ≤5 cm in diameter	NX = Clinical status unknown	
b = >5 cm in diameter		

TNM pretreatment staging classification for intergroup rhabdomyosarcoma study IV

Stage	Sites	T invasiveness	T Size	N	M
I	Orbit, head and neck (excluding parameningeal), Genitourinary (nonbladder/nonprostate)	T1 or T2	a or b	N0 or N1 or NX	M0
II	Bladder/prostate Extremity Cranial parameningeal Other (includes trunk, retroperitoneum, etc.)	T1 or T2	a	N0 or NX	M0
III	Bladder/prostate Extremity Cranial parameningeal Other (includes trunk retroperitoneum, etc.)	T1 or T2	a b	N1 N0 or N1 or NX	M0
IV	All	T1 or T2	a or b	N0 or N1	M1

[a]Distant metastatic disease consists of lung, liver, bones, bone marrow, brain, and distant muscle and nodes. The presence of positive cytology in CSF, pleural, or abdominal fluids, as well as implants on pleural or peritoneal surfaces, also constitutes stage IV disease.

From Mandell LR. Ongoing progress in the treatment of childhood rhabdomyosarcoma. Oncology 1993;7:71–84, with permission.

- *Stage III:* Localized disease of any unfavorable primary site (primary tumor greater than 5 cm in diameter and/or regional node involvement)
- *Stage IV:* Metastatic disease at diagnosis. The original grouping system, however, is retained to define the extent of radiation therapy.

TREATMENT

General Principles

Successful treatment of rhabdomyosarcoma requires achievement of both local and systemic control of disease. Local control is accomplished using surgery and/or radiotherapy. Systemic control is accomplished with chemotherapy. Patients with localized disease require systemic therapy to eradicate micrometastatic disease typically present at diagnosis.

Surgery

Surgery is most effective if the tumor can be completely excised with an adequate margin of uninvolved tissue. If the tumor cannot be resected because of proximity to blood vessels and nerves or because this would produce major functional or cosmetic sequelae, an incisional or debulking biopsy is performed. This is followed by induction chemotherapy and radiation to cytoreduce the tumor. Second-look surgery should then be performed to resect residual tumor, if possible.

For primary tumors arising in the orbit, head and neck, and certain extremity locations, aggressive surgical debulking, such as enucleation, head and neck dissection, and amputation, are not indicated. Instead, chemotherapy and radiotherapy should be relied on to control the tumor at the primary site. Radical surgical debulking is reserved for cases with residual disease after chemotherapy and radiation therapy.

The role of lymph node biopsy or dissection as part of the primary approach depends on the tumor site. Clinically suspicious nodes should be excised at any site. In addition, routine sampling of regional nodes is appropriate for most sites; search of a sentinel node in extremity lesions is advisable. Sites with a high incidence of regional node involvement include:

- Extremity (15%)
- Genitourinary (20%)
- Perirectal (33%)
- Paratesticular (40%).

Prophylactic regional radical node dissection is not necessary.

Radiotherapy

Rhabdomyosarcoma is only moderately radiation sensitive and, for this reason, high doses of radiation are required. The dose of radiation to most sites is not modified for patient age or tumor size, although modifications are recommended for young patients in the following instances:

- Limit of 1440 cGy to both lungs
- Limit of 2400 cGy to whole brain for children <3 years old with parameningeal tumors and positive CSF cytology (older children receive 3060 cGY)
- Lower daily doses (150 cGy) and total doses (1800 cGy) for large fields such as the whole abdomen.

The following are the radiation therapy guidelines (Table 20-7):

- Clinical group I tumors (TNM stages I and II) do not receive radiation therapy.
- Clinical group I (TNM stage III) and clinical group II tumors (all TMN stages) receive conventional external beam radiation at a total dose of 4140 cGy.
- Clinical group III tumors receive conventional radiation of 5040 cGy.
- Clinical group IV tumors receive conventional radiation of the primary tumor according to the extent of resection of the primary site (clinical group as noted

Table 20-7. Guidelines for Radiotherapy for Rhabdomyosarcoma

TNM stage	Clinical group I	Clinical group II (cGy)	Clinical group III (cGy)
Stage I	No RT	4140	5040
Stage II	No RT	4140	5040
Stage III	4140 cGy	4140	5040
Stage IV (primary)	No RT[a] 3600 cGy[b]	4140	5040
Stage IV (metastases)			5040

[a]Embryonal histology.
[b]Alveolar histology.

above). Patients also receive 5040 cGy to metastatic sites. One exception is that patients with alveolar histology and complete resection of the primary tumor (clinical group I, stages II and II) should receive 3600 cGy to the primary.

- Clinical group IV metastic tumor sites (TNM stage IV, metastases) receive a total dose of 5040 cGy.

The timing of radiation therapy is as follows:

1. Patients receive radiotherapy to the primary tumor and metastatic sites at week 9 (day 62).
2. Patients with parameningeal tumors with evidence of meningeal extension begin radiation to the primary tumor on day 0. Patients with parameningeal tumors without evidence of meningeal extension will receive radiation at week 9.
3. Patients who require emergency radiotherapy (e.g., spinal cord compression) receive radiation on day 0. The entire course of radiation therapy should be administered at this time.

Chemotherapy

All patients regardless of their initial stage or group receive combination chemotherapy. The effective agents in rhabdomyosarcoma are cyclophosphamide, ifosfamide, melphalan, actinomycin D, Adriamycin, cisplatin, carboplatin, vincristine, etoposide, topotecan, and irinotecan.

Treatment Regimens

Table 20-8 shows recommendations for therapy of rhabdomyosarcoma and undifferentiated sarcoma of childhood. Figure 20-1 shows the chemotherapy protocol for stage I, clinical group I paratesticular rhabdomyosarcoma and clinical groups I and II orbit and eyelid rhabdomyosarcoma. Figure 20-2 shows the chemotherapy regimens for other stage I, II, III, and IV disease.

Granulocyte colony-stimulating factor (G-CSF) is incorporated into these protocols to shorten the periods of neutropenia, which follow these myelosuppressive combinations.

Guidelines for Specific Anatomic Sites

Head and Neck (Extraorbital)

These tumors can be classified into two major clinical groups:

- *Superficial sites:* scalp, temporal region, facial structures, and neck
- *Parameningeal sites:* paranasal sinuses, nasopharynx, middle ear, and pterygopalatine fossa.

Table 20-8. IRS IV Recommendations for Therapy of Rhabdomyosarcoma and Undifferentiated Sarcoma in Childhood[a,b]

Site	TNM stage	Clinical group	Radiation therapy[c] (cGy)	Chemotherapy	Operative consideration/comments
Orbit and eyelid	I	I	None	VA × 32 weeks	Nonexcisional biopsy standard for orbital tumors
		II	4140 (begins at week 9)	VA	
		III	5040	VAC × 52 weeks	
Other head and neck (nonparameningeal)	I	I	None	VAC	Wide excision if feasible; routine sampling of clinically; uninvolved nodes not indicated
		II	4140	VAC	
		III	5040	VAC	
Paratesticular	I	I	None	VA	Inguinal incision, orchiectomy, resection of entire spermatic cord. Formal dissection of ipsilateral retroperitoneal lymph nodes not indicated in ages <10 years. Systematic sampling of bilateral high and low infrarenal and bilateral iliac nodes is recommended (although role in subsequent management is unclear). Positive inguinal nodes are considered distant spread (stage IV).
		II	4140	VAC	
		III	5040	VAC	
Vulva and vagina		I	None	VAC	Complete surgical excision rarely possible initially. Second-look operation at week 9, with radiation therapy based on results.
		II	4140	VAC	
		III	5040	VAC	
Uterus		I	None	VAC	
		II	4140	VAC	
		III	5040	VAC	
Cranial parameningeal	II/III	I	None for stage II 4140 for stage III	VAC	Wide resection rarely feasible. Cervical lymph node biopsy only if clinically suspicious nodes. Begin radiation therapy at day 0 for limited intracranial extension, base of skull invasion, bone erosion, or cranial neuropathy. Begin at week 9 if no intracranial extension. No whole-brain radiation therapy (tumor plus 2-cm margin).
		II	4140	VAC	
		III	5040	VAC	

Site	Stage	Group	Radiation dose (cGy)[c]	Chemotherapy[a,b]	Surgical considerations
Extremity	II/III	I	None for stage II 4140 for stage III	VAC	Limb-sparing wide or radical resection to remove all gross (and, ideally, microscopic) tumor. Pretreatment reexcision of residual tumor may improve outcome. Regional lymph node sampling should be performed. Involvement of ipsilateral supraclavicular (scalene) nodes (upper extremity) or iliac/para-aortic nodes (lower extremity) is considered distant spread (stage IV).
		II	4140	VAC	
		III	5040	VAC	
Genitourinary (bladder and prostate)	II/III	I	None for stage II 4140 for stage III	VAC	Dome of bladder tumors may be amenable to total resection (partial cystectomy). Most other tumors can only be biopsied with goal of preservation of bladder and urethral function. Regional lymph node sampling (iliac and para-aortic nodes) only if laparotomy performed. Extirpative procedures reserved for early treatment failure, progression or biopsy-proven residual viable tumor 6 months after completion of radiation therapy.
		II	4140	VAC	
		III	5040	VAC	
Chest wall, trunk, retroperitoneum, and other	II/III	I	None for stage II 4140 for stage III	VAC	Wide local excision if feasible. Pretreatment reexcision should be considered for residual tumor. Chest wall lesions involving rib cage should remove one rib above and below lesion plus attached envelope of soft tissue and/or lung.
		II	4140	VAC	
		III	5040	VAC	
Any site	IV	I	4140	VAC	Most patients have gross residual disease. Radiation therapy begins at week 18.5 (except for cranial parameningeal tumors). Role of pulmonary metastectomy unclear.
		II	4140	VAC	
		III	5040	VAC	

Abbreviations: A, actinomycin D; C, cyclophosphamide; V, vincristine.

Modified from Wexler L, Hellman L. Rhabdomyosarcoma and the undifferentiated sarcomas. In: Pizzo PA, Poplack DG, editors. Principles and Practice of Pediatric Oncology. 3rd ed. Philadelphia: Lippincott-Raven, 1997, with permission.

[a]The specific chemotherapeutic dosing and scheduling are shown in Figures 20-1, 20-2, and 20-3.

[b]The standard regimen is VA and VAC.

[c]All radiation is given as conventional fractionation.

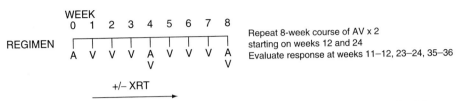

Fig. 20-1. Therapy for clinical group I paratesticular tumors and clinical groups I and II orbit or eyelid tumors. A = actinomycin D, 0.015 mg/kg/day IV × 5 (maximum single dose, 0.5 mg); V = vincristine 1.5 mg/m^2 (maximum single dose, 2 mg); ±XRT = no radiotherapy is given to group I patients; give conventional radiotherapy to group II patients. Prescribe G-CSF for dose-limiting hematopoietic toxicity.

Surgery

Wide excision with a normal margin of tissue is desirable, yielding superior survival rates, provided it does not cause significant cosmetic and functional deficits. This approach is not appropriate for orbital lesions, and is not usually possible in most head and neck sites. Incisional biopsy or debulking is warranted, with reliance on chemotherapy, second-look surgery, and radiation for local control and prevention of spread. Elective lymph node dissection is not recommended unless nodes are clinically palpable.

Radiotherapy

The primary tumor should be treated according to the guidelines in Figure 20-2 and Table 20-8.

Chemotherapy

Patients with parameningeal lesions or with superficial lesions receive chemotherapy as outlined in Figure 20-3 and in Table 20-8. Patients with parameningeal disease may require additional CNS therapy, depending on the extent of CNS involvement. This therapy may consist of irradiation to the meninges adjacent to a lesion, whole-brain irradiation, or spine and triple intrathecal chemotherapy.

Orbit and Eyelid

Tumors of the orbit tend to remain localized for a long period of time and are usually detected when small because of visual disturbances or proptosis.

Surgery

Surgical biopsy, followed by radiation and chemotherapy, is recommended as outlined in Figure 20-1. Orbital exenteration is recommended only for recurrent disease.

Radiotherapy

The volume to be irradiated should include the gross tumor volume plus a 1.5-cm margin. This need not include the entire orbit, and shielding of the cornea, lens, lacrimal gland, and optic chiasm should be attempted.

Paratesticular

Paratesticular lesions are commonly found in the scrotum, adjacent to the testes (80%). The remainder are found along the spermatic cord in the inguinal canal. All

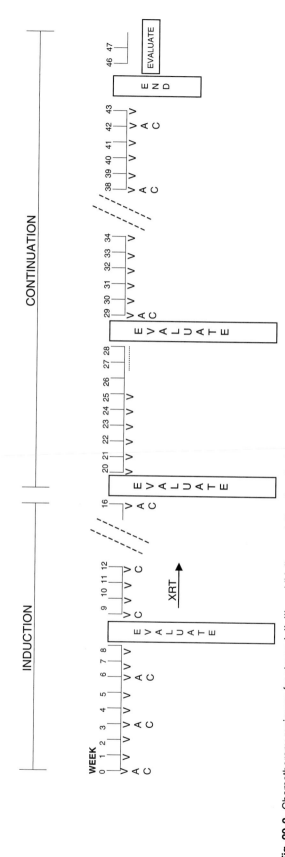

Fig. 20-2. Chemotherapy regimens for stages I, II, III, and IV disease (other than for those shown in Figures 20-1 and 20-3). V = vincristine, 1.5 mg/m² IV (maximum dose, 2 mg); A = actinomycin D, 0.015 mg/kg/day IV × 5 (maximum dose, 0.5 mg); C = cyclophosphamide: 2.2 g/m² IV with mesna.

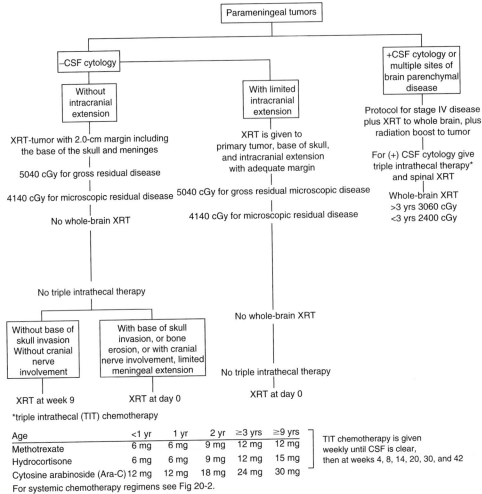

Fig. 20-3. CNS therapy in patients with parameningeal disease based on IRS-IV recommendations.

patients should have abdominal and pelvic CT with 5-mm cuts to evaluate nodal involvement.

Surgery

The following surgical approach is recommended:

1. The tumor is excised by orchiectomy, and the entire spermatic cord resected.
2. For stage I, group I, patients less than 10 years old with no evidence of lymph node involvement, retroperitoneal node biopsy or node sampling is not to be done. The risk of nodal involvement or relapse in this group is very small. Systematic retroperitoneal lymph node sampling is indicated for all other patients (stages II–IV and groups II–IV less than age 10; all patients age 10 or older) with tumors in this site. This entails evaluation of the ipsilateral nodes from the renal veins to the end of the ipsilateral common iliac artery (where it is crossed by the ureter). Inguinal nodes are rarely involved and should be biopsied only if enlarged or if the scrotum is invaded. Inguinal nodes are not considered regional and, if positive, the patient is placed in stage IV.

Radiotherapy

If complete microscopic excision is accomplished, no radiation is required. In patients with microscopic or gross residual tumor (about 25% of cases), radiotherapy is administered. If the retroperitoneal lymph nodes are involved, the radiation portal should encompass the positive nodes and immediate adjacent unaffected lymph node group.

Chemotherapy

Chemotherapy is given as outlined in Figure 20-1. If retroperitoneal irradiation is required for lymph node involvement, the myelosuppressive effects of chemotherapy may be exaggerated, because a significant portion of bone marrow may be in the irradiated field.

Extremities

Tumors in the extremities have a high rate of early dissemination and the worst outcome of any major site.

Surgery

Because high recurrence and mortality occur in patients with clinical group III extremity lesions, the surgeon should attempt to place these patients into clinical group I (preferably) or II by carrying out a gross resection. Some sacrifice in limb function should be accepted to attain this end, but amputation does not appear necessary for local disease control, nor does it improve overall disease-free survival. Delayed second surgical resection after diminution by chemotherapy and/or radiotherapy generally has unsatisfactory results and should be avoided.

Inguinal and axillary lymph nodes should be biopsied in lower and upper extremity lesions, respectively. If the immediate regional nodes are positive, the more proximal lymph node groups should be explored (i.e., supraclavicular for upper extremity lesions and iliac and/or periaortic for lower extremity lesions).

Radiotherapy

In patients in whom complete removal has been accomplished at diagnosis (clinical group I), radiotherapy is omitted. All others receive radiotherapy with a 2-cm margin as outlined in Table 20-7. If the regional nodes are involved with tumor, they should be irradiated with the portal encompassing the positive nodes and the immediate adjacent unaffected lymph node group.

Chemotherapy

Chemotherapy is given as outlined in Table 20-8.

Retroperitoneal Area

Surgery

These tumors often grow to a huge size before becoming clinically detectable. Complicating factors such as intestinal or genitourinary obstruction may be present. Surgery should aim to debulk as much tumor as can be safely removed and should rely on chemotherapy and radiotherapy for further cytoreduction. Most tumors will fall into group III.

Radiotherapy

The primary tumor should be treated as outlined in Table 20-7. In instances in which near total or total abdominal irradiation is required, adjustments in chemotherapy may be needed temporarily until the irradiated bone marrow recovers.

Chemotherapy

Chemotherapy is initiated at the start of therapy, as shown in Table 20-8. Most of these patients will be clinical group III. With the large volume of radiotherapy required, these patients will need careful monitoring of blood counts during chemotherapy.

Genitourinary tract

Tumors of the genitourinary tract include lesions of the vagina, uterus, bladder, and prostate. These tumors are generally of the embryonal variety. Nonbladder and non-prostate tumors have a better prognosis. The therapeutic approach depends on the site of the tumor.

Vagina, uterus, and bladder dome

Tumors in this area can be managed by a primary chemotherapy approach, as shown in Table 20-8. In patients in whom initial chemotherapy and surgery result in complete tumor removal, radiation therapy should be omitted. An exception to this primary chemotherapy approach is sarcoma of the uterus in adolescent females, which is histologically heterogeneous and clearly less sensitive to chemotherapy. These rare tumors should be managed by an initial hysterectomy, followed by chemotherapy. If the tumor is completely resected microscopically, radiotherapy can be omitted.

Bladder neck/trigone and prostate

Tumors in this area respond less well to chemotherapy. Radiation therapy is given routinely if the tumor is not completely resected initially, irrespective of the degree of chemotherapy response. Delayed conservative surgery may often be performed with good results.

Follow-Up after the Completion of Therapy

First Year after Completion of Therapy

- Physical examination every 2 months
- Chest radiograph every 2 months
- Appropriate imaging studies (i.e., CT or MRI of the involved region) every 4 months
- Echocardiogram 1 year after completion of therapy to follow possible anthracycline cardiotoxicity (if indicated)
- Appropriate studies outlined below.

Second and Third Years after Completion of Therapy

- Physical examination every 4 months
- Chest radiograph every 4 months
- Appropriate studies outlined below.

Fourth to Tenth Years after Completion of Therapy

- Annual visit for physical examination and studies outlined below.

Ten Years after Completion of Therapy

- Maintain yearly visit or phone contact.
- Record attainment of puberty, offspring, and development of second malignancies.

General Studies

- Height and weight at 6-month intervals
- Annual BP measurements
- Tanner staging annually until stage V
- Testicular size annually
- Onset of menses in girls
- Patients who receive cyclophosphamide: evaluation of gonadal function (FSH, LH, and testosterone/estradiol).

Studies for Specific Sites

Head and Neck

- Annual growth measurements
- Annual ophthalmologic examination
- Annual dental examination.

Trunk

- Radiographs of irradiated bones every 1–2 years
- Kidney function, urinalysis, creatinine annually
- Sitting height/standing height ratio
- If patient received radiotherapy to chest or lungs, history of exercise intolerance or shortness of breath.

Genitourinary Sites

- Kidney function evaluation every 1–2 years
- Girls—follow-up of sexual maturation and ovarian function
- Boys—history regarding ejaculatory function, semen analysis.

Extremities

- Annual bilateral limb length measurements
- Radiographs of primary sites for bone growth abnormalities.

PROGNOSIS

Rhabdomyosarcoma is curable in the majority of children receiving optimal therapy (>70% survival 5 years after diagnosis). The prognosis depends on the factors discussed below.

Extent of Disease

This is one of the most important prognostic factors. The 3-year failure-free survival (FFS) rates based on the IRS-IV experience are summarized in Table 20-9. Children with localized, completely resected disease do better than those with widespread or disseminated disease. Patients with gross residual disease after surgery (group III) have a statistically significantly lower 3-year FFS of 73% compared with 83% and 86% FFS for groups I and II, respectively. Five-year survival for patients with no residual tumor following surgery (clinical group I) is 83%.

**Table 20-9. Failure-Free Survival (%) of Children at 3 Years
by Stage and Group on IRS-IV**

	Clinical stage	Clinical group
I	86	83
II	80	86
III	68	73
IV	25	25

Tumor Burden at Diagnosis

Patients with smaller tumors (<5 cm) have improved survival compared to children
with tumors greater than 5 cm. Those with metastatic disease at diagnosis have the
worst prognosis. Among those with metastatic disease, two or fewer metastases is
significantly better than three or more.

Histologic and Cytologic Type

Patients with an alveolar histology have a worse prognosis (Table 20-10). The alveolar subtype is frequently associated with an extremity site, which is indicative of a
poor prognostic factor.

**Table 20-10. Failure-Free Survival (%) of Children at 3 Years
According to Histologic Subtype**

Histologic type	Nonmetastatic	Metastatic, ≤2 sites
Embryonal	83	40
Alveolar/unspecified	66	21

Primary Tumor Site

The outcome varies with the location of the primary tumor.

Favorable:

1. Head and neck, orbit (nonparameningeal)
2. Genitourinary (excluding prostate and bladder).

Unfavorable:

1. Extremity
2. Bladder and prostate
3. Cranial parameningeal
4. Other (trunk, pelvis-perineum, retroperitoneum, and paravertebral).

Based on site, extent of resection, and histology, patients are now stratified as low,
intermediate, or high risk and treated accordingly. Table 20-11 shows the 3-year FFS
and overall survival (OS) by risk stratification from IRS-III and IRS-IV data.

Age

Children between 1 and 9 years of age have a better prognosis than those older
than 9 years of age (83% versus 68% 3-year FFS on IRS-IV). This is due to the higher
incidence of advanced disease and (possibly) to alveolar type in older children.

Table 20-11. Risk Stratification and Survival Data from IRS-III and IRS-IV

Characteristics	Risk group	Number of patients	3 Year FFS	3 Year OS
Embryonal histology, favorable site	Low	279	88	94
Embryonal histology, unfavorable site, group I/II	Low	63	88	93
Embryonal histology, unfavorable site, group III	Intermediate	275	76	83
Embryonal histology, any site, group IV, <10 years old	Intermediate	98	55 (5-year)	59
Alveolar histology, any site, group I–III	Intermediate	165	55 (5-year)	—

Abbreviations: FFS, failure-free survival; OS, overall survival.

Response to Therapy

The most significant prognostic variable is the response to therapy. Those who do not attain a complete pathologic response do not survive.

Cellular DNA Content (Ploidy)

Tumors whose DNA content is 1.5 times normal (hyperdiploid) have a better prognosis.

Sites of Metastases

Most patients with rhabdomyosarcoma who fail to respond to a multiple-modality approach develop metastatic disease within 18 months of diagnosis. Table 20-12 shows the frequency of metastatic disease at autopsy according to primary site.

Table 20-12. Site of Metastases in Children Dying of Rhabdomyosarcoma

Primary tumor site	Lung	CNS	Lymph node	Bone	Liver	Bone marrow	Soft tissue
Head and neck (extraorbital)	25	70	16	—	—	—	—
Extremity	46	32	60	35	10	—	17
Trunk	40	40	—	—	—	—	—
Genitourinary	35	7	65	28	35	21	14
All sites combined	37	37	33	25	16	7	9

Frequency of metastatic disease at autopsy (%)

Recurrent Disease

Although some children do attain durable remissions with secondary therapy, the long-term prognosis for children with progressive or recurrent disease is poor. The 3-year survival following relapse for patients who were originally diagnosed as clinical groups II–IV is 15%.

When recurrent disease is suspected, biopsy should always be performed. After pathologic verification of recurrence, an extent of disease workup should be undertaken. In formulating a treatment plan, several factors should be considered:

1. The timing of recurrence (progression while on therapy, recurrence within 6–12 months after completion of therapy, or recurrence after more than 12 months after completion of therapy)
2. The extent of disease at recurrence (localized or disseminated)
3. The extent of disease at diagnosis
4. The nature of prior therapy:
    a. Duration and intensity of chemotherapy
    b. Fields and doses of radiation.

Durable remission is most difficult to attain in patients who have unresectable or widespread disease at diagnosis and in those who progressed on therapy or relapsed early.

Localized Recurrence

- Complete surgical resection, if feasible, improves outcome.
- Surgery should be followed by adjuvant chemotherapy and radiation (if further radiation is feasible).
- Durable remission in paratesticular and vaginal recurrences can be attained with the preceding approach.
- The drug combinations that are effective in patients who have not received these agents are:
    1. Ifosfamide/etoposide
    2. Carboplatin/etoposide
    3. Ifosfamide/carboplatin and etoposide.

Table 20-13 depicts a regimen that utilizes these agents. In patients who have previously received these agents, phase I and II agents should be considered.

Table 20-13. Chemotherapy for Recurrent Soft-Tissue Sarcomas[a,b,c]

Course A		
Carboplatin	150 mg/m²/day	Days 1, 2, 3, 4
Etoposide	150 mg/m²/day	Days 1, 2, 3, 4
Two courses of A are given		
Course B		
Etoposide	150 mg/m²/day	Days 1, 2, 3, 4
Ifosfamide	2000 mg/m²/day	Days 1, 2, 3, 4
Mesna	2000 mg/m²/day	Days 1, 2, 3, 4, 5, 6
After course B, give course A and another course B		
Course C		
Carboplatin	150 mg/m²/day	Days 1, 2, 3, 4
Ifosfamide	2000 mg/m²/day	Days 1, 2, 3, 4
Mesna	2000 mg/m²/day	Days 1, 2, 3, 4, 5, 6
Two courses of C are given		

[a]This therapy can be given without requiring stem cell rescue. G-CSF is utilized at the completion of each course.

[b]Subsequent courses are given when the absolute neutrophil count reaches 1000/mm³ and the platelet count reaches 75,000/mm³. The entire seven courses are given within 24 weeks.

[c]If the intent is to utilize stem cell transplant, then the myeloablative regimen in Table 20-14 can be utilized.

From Klingebiel T, Pertl U, Hess C, et al. Treatment of children with relapsed soft tissue sarcoma: report of the German CESS/CWS REZ 91 Trial. Med Pediatr Oncol 1998;30:269–75, with permission.

Disseminated Recurrence

- Disseminated recurrence is essentially incurable.
- Surgical resection of metastatic lesions is not curative, but may be palliative.
- Trials are under way using the preceding agents in very intensive regimens, followed by autologous stem cell rescue, but no large studies to date demonstrate any significant salvage rate.
- Use of etoposide 100 mg/m²/day IV three days weekly for 3 weeks with a 1-week interval between courses for up to 1 year was successful in a case report.
- Phase I and II agents should be considered.

Autologous Stem Cell Transplantation

To date, the use of high-dose chemotherapy with autologous stem cell rescue has been disappointing. Although this approach may provide equal results with a shorter, more intensive regimen, it has yet to demonstrate a statistically significant improvement in outcome of high-risk or relapsed patients in a large trial. It should therefore only be performed as part of a clinical study.

Future Perspectives

1. Survival has dramatically increased during the past 20 years; however, improvements in disease control are still needed, especially for the majority of patients (approximately 65%) with gross residual disease after resection or metastatic disease at the time of diagnosis.
2. Current areas of investigation include:
   a. Risk stratification into low-, intermediate-, and high-risk strata to reduce the short- and long-term toxicities of therapy in lower-risk patients and the use of novel approaches with the high-risk patients.
   b. High-dose therapy with autologous stem cell rescue for high-risk tumors.
   c. Brachytherapy with radioactive implants or radiosurgery to more precisely target the tumor.
   d. Studies of cytologic and molecular genetics, immunohistochemistry, and cultured tumor cell lines to advance understanding of rhabdomyosarcoma cell biology and to refine treatment according to specific prognostic factors.
   e. Studies of antitumor immunotherapies such as antitumor monoclonal antibodies or graft versus sarcoma effect.
   f. Studies of antiangiogenesis factors.

SUGGESTED READINGS

Blakely M, Spurbeck W, Pappo A, et al. The impact of margin of resection on outcome in pediatric nonrhabdomyosarcoma soft tissue sarcoma. J Pediatr Surg 1999;34:672.

Breneman J, Lyden E, Pappo A, et al. Prognostic factors and clinical outcomes in children and adolescents with metastatic rhabdomyosarcoma: a report from the Intergroup Rhabdomyosarcoma Study IV. J Clin Oncol 2003;21:78.

Cecchetto G, Modesto C, Alaggio R, et al. Fibrosarcoma in pediatric patients: results of the Italian Cooperative Group Studies (1979–1995). J Surg Oncol 2001;78:225.

Crist W, Anderson J, Meza J, et al. Intergroup Rhabdomyosarcoma Study IV: results for patients with nonmetastatic disease. J Clin Oncol 2001;19:3091.

Lawrence W, Gehan E, Hays D, et al. Prognostic significance of staging factors of the UICC staging system in childhood rhabdomyosarcoma: a report from the Intergroup Rhabdomyosarcoma Study (IRS-II). J Clin Oncol 1987;5:46.

Miser J, Pappo A, Triche T, et al. Other soft tissue sarcomas of childhood. In: Pizzo PA, Poplack DG, editors. Principles and Practice of Pediatric Oncology. 4th ed. Philadelphia: Lippincott Williams & Wilkins, 2002.

Wexler L, Crist W, Helman L. Rhabdomyosarcoma and the undifferentiated sarcomas. In: Pizzo PA, Poplack DG, editors. Principles and Practice of Pediatric Oncology. 4th ed. Philadelphia: Lippincott Williams & Wilkins, 2002

21

MALIGNANT BONE TUMORS

Malignant bone tumors constitute approximately 6% of all childhood malignancies. In the United States, the annual incidence in children under 20 years of age is 8.7 per million. Osteosarcoma (56%) and Ewing sarcoma (34%) comprise the most frequently encountered malignant bone tumors in children and adolescents. In the United States 650–700 children are diagnosed with malignant bone tumors each year. There are approximately 400 cases of osteosarcoma and 200 cases of Ewing sarcoma per year.

The peak incidence of bone cancer is age 15, coincident with the adolescent growth spurt, after which rates show a decline (Figure 21-1). Osteosarcoma incidence has a bimodal age distribution with peaks in early adolescence and in adults over 65 years of age. Ewing sarcoma is a disease of children and young adults; it is very rare in older adults.

OSTEOSARCOMA

Osteosarcoma (OS) is a tumor in which the malignant spindle cell stroma produces osteoid.

Epidemiology

The incidence is slightly higher in males. The incidence in African-American children is higher than in whites. Although the etiology of osteosarcoma is unknown, certain factors appear to correlate with its occurrence:

1. *Bone growth:* The development of osteosarcoma is correlated with linear bone growth as evidenced by the following:
   a. The peak incidence occurs during the pubescent growth spurt at 15–19 years of age.
   b. The patients are taller than average.
   c. The most common sites are metaphyses of the most rapidly growing bones (distal femur, proximal humerus, proximal tibia).
2. *Genetic factors:* The development of osteosarcoma is associated with genetic factors as evidenced by the following:
   a. The relationship between bilateral retinoblastoma and the development of a secondary osteosarcoma is independent of the therapeutic modalities or radiation field.

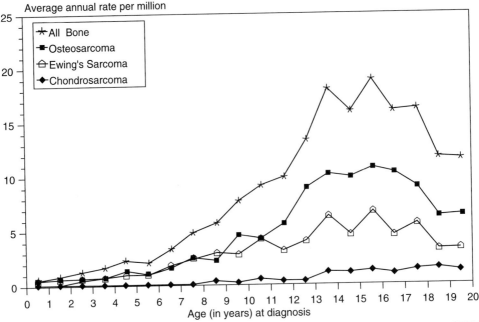

Fig. 21-1. Bone cancer age-specific incidence rate by histology for all races and both sexes, SEER, 1976–94 and 1986–94 combined. (From Gurney JG, Swensen AR, Bukterys M. Malignant bone tumors. Cancer incidence and survival among children and adolescents: United States SEER Program 1975–1995. NIH Pub No 99-4649. Bethesda, MD: National Cancer Institute, SEER Program, 1999:99–110, with permission.)

    b. A retinoblastoma recessive oncogene (Rb) on chromosome 13, band q14, is implicated in osteosarcoma, irrespective of a prior history of retinoblastoma. Deletions and rearrangements of the Rb gene, altered expression of the Rb transcripts, or altered Rb protein have been described in osteosarcoma tumors.

    c. A second recessive oncogene p53 on chromosome 17p13.1 has also been felt to play a role in the development and progression of osteosarcoma. Inactivation of the p53 gene product with the loss of a growth regulator that inhibits cellular proliferation is important in the growth of osteosarcoma. Twenty-five percent of patients have a germline mutation in the p53 gene.

    d. Osteosarcoma has been seen in families with Li–Fraumeni syndrome, in which members of the affected families have breast cancer, brain tumors, soft-tissue sarcomas, leukemia, and adrenal cortical carcinoma and osteosarcoma associated with a germline mutation of p53, a suppressor oncogene.

    e. There are nongermline mutations of both p53 and Rb in osteosarcoma tumors. Twenty-five percent have point mutation of p53, 10–20% have p53 rearrangements, 75% have loss of one 17q allele, and 60% of OS tumors have a loss of heterozygosity at 13q of the site of the Rb gene.

  3. *Environmental factors:* The environmental factor most commonly associated with the development of osteosarcoma is radiation therapy as evidenced by the following:

    a. Approximately 3% of osteosarcomas arise in previously irradiated bone.

    b. The interval between irradiation and the appearance of osteosarcoma has ranged from 4 to 40 years.

    c. Treatment with alkylating agents may lead to secondary bone cancer independent of radiation therapy.

    d. Bone diseases: Paget disease, osteochondroma, enchondroma, exostoses, fibrous dysplasia, metallic implants, bone infarcts, or chronic osteomyelitis have a higher incidence of osteosarcoma compared to the general population.

Pathology

The histologic diagnosis of osteosarcoma is dependent on the demonstration of osteoid material associated with anaplastic stromal cells. Table 21-1 lists the classification of osteosarcoma. Although the small cell type may be confused with Ewing sarcoma in osteosarcoma the anaplastic stromal cells produce osteoid.

Clinical Manifestations

The average duration of symptoms is 3 months. Patients commonly present with the following symptoms:

1. Local pain (90%)
2. Local swelling (50%)
3. Decreased range of motion (45%)
4. Pathologic fracture (8%)
5. Rapidly growing long bones most commonly affected (>50% involving the femur)
6. Joint effusion, suggesting extension of the tumor into the joint space
7. Multifocal presentation, with lesions in symmetric metaphyseal locations (1–2%).

The primary sites of origin in osteosarcoma are (Figure 21-2):

1. Femur (49%)
2. Tibia (26%)
3. Humerus (10%)
4. Fibula (5.5%)
5. Pelvis (4.5%)
6. Other (3%).

Diagnostic Evaluation

The diagnostic evaluation should delineate the extent of the primary tumor and the presence or absence of metastatic disease. All patients should have the following evaluation:

1. History
2. Physical examination

Table 21-1. Classification of Osteosarcoma

  I. Classic
    A. Osteoblastic
    B. Chondroblastic
    C. Fibroblastic
 II. Telangiectatic
III. Small cell
IV. Periosteal
 V. Parosteal

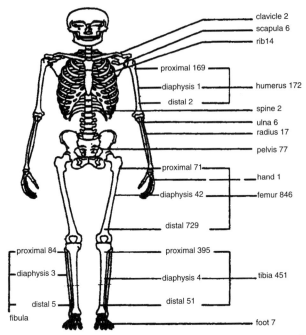

Fig. 21-2. Skeletal distribution of 1702 patients with osteosarcoma. (From Bielack SS, Kampf-Bielack B, Delling G, Exner GU, Flege S, Helmke K, Kotz R, Salzer-Kuntschik M, Werner M, Winkleman W, Zoubek A, Jurgens H, Winkler K. Prognostic factors in high grade osteosarcoma of the extremities or trunk: an analysis of 1,702 patients treated on neoadjuvant cooperative osteosarcoma study group protocols. J Clin Oncol 2002;20[3]:776–90, with permission.)

3. Blood count
4. Urinalysis
5. Blood urea nitrogen (BUN), creatinine, liver enzymes, alkaline phosphatase (approximately 50% of patients have elevated alkaline phosphatase), total bilirubin
6. Radiographs of the affected bone
7. Computed tomography (CT) or magnetic resonance imaging (MRI) of affected bone
8. Bone scan
9. Chest CT
10. Creatinine clearance to assess renal function prior to chemotherapy
11. Echocardiogram to assess cardiac function prior to chemotherapy
12. Baseline hearing test prior to chemotherapy.

Radiographically, osteosarcoma produces dense sclerosis in the metaphysis of the affected long bone along with the following findings:

1. Soft-tissue extension (75%)
2. Radiating calcification, or sunburst (60%)
3. Osteosclerotic lesion (45%)
4. Lytic lesion (30%)
5. Mixed lesion (25%).

MRI gives valuable information in planning limb salvage surgery, such as interosseous extent of tumor and involvement of muscle groups, subcutaneous fat, joints, and neurovascular structures around the tumor. Approximately 5% of patients will have evidence of bone metastases on bone scan. The use of chest CT is essential for staging patients, because it detects metastases not seen on chest radiographs. If a lesion detected on chest CT cannot be defined as metastatic, histologic confirmation is indicated.

Treatment

The two therapeutic modalities currently used in the primary treatment are surgery and chemotherapy. The use of surgery alone results in a 90% rate of recurrence of osteosarcoma. The tumor is radioresistant and radiation therapy does not play a primary role in management.

Surgery

The surgical approach to osteosarcoma includes surgical biopsy, followed by either amputation or limb salvage surgery.

A biopsy is required to confirm the diagnosis. An open biopsy is the preferred method. The biopsy should be performed with surgery in mind, by an orthopedic surgeon experienced in the management of malignant bone tumors. A poorly placed biopsy may jeopardize future limb salvage surgery. Because the biopsy tract and skin are contaminated with tumor cells, the biopsy site needs to be excised en bloc with the tumor during definitive surgery.

Surgery should remove all gross and microscopic tumor with a margin of normal tissue to prevent local recurrence. Appropriate surgical procedures are limb salvage surgery or amputation.

Definitive surgery may be done immediately after diagnosis (by biopsy) or following preoperative chemotherapy. Delaying definitive surgery until after preoperative chemotherapy is preferred, because an assessment of the chemotherapeutic responsiveness of the tumor can be determined.

The type of surgery is determined by tumor location, size, extramedullary extent, presence of metastatic disease, age, skeletal development, and patient's lifestyle choices. If complete excision cannot be accomplished with limb-sparing surgery, amputation is indicated.

Limb salvage surgery should be performed by orthopedic surgeons experienced with these techniques. Guidelines for the use of limb-sparing surgery include:

- No major neurovascular involvement by tumor
- Ability to have a wide resection of affected bone with a normal muscle cuff in all directions
- Ability to perform en bloc removal of all previous biopsy sites and all potentially contaminated tissue
- Adequate motor reconstruction
- Adequate soft-tissue coverage.

Contraindications to limb-sparing surgery include:

- Major neurovascular involvement
- Nonhealing pathologic fracture of bone affected by tumor
- Prior inappropriate biopsy with contamination of normal tissue planes and compartments
- Infection of biopsy site
- Young age with immature skeletal development
- Extensive muscle involvement.

Limb salvage has generally been applied to most upper extremity lesions and selected lower extremity lesions where en bloc resection permits adequate tumor margins with an intact joint.

Chemotherapy

The use of chemotherapy in a neoadjuvant (preoperative) or adjuvant (postoperative) fashion results in significant improvement in disease-free survival in patients with osteosarcoma. More than 90% of patients treated with surgery alone will develop metastatic disease. With the addition of multiagent chemotherapy, 60–70% of nonmetastatic extremity osteosarcoma patients will survive without evidence of recurrence. The agents most commonly used in the treatment of osteosarcoma are high-dose methotrexate, cisplatin, and doxorubicin. Addition of ifosfamide, alone or with etoposide, may enhance tumor response; however, its effect on overall and event-free survival (EFS) is less clear.

Although timing of chemotherapy (neoadjuvant versus adjuvant) does not affect EFS, neoadjuvant chemotherapy offers the following advantages:

1. Shrinkage of the tumor at the primary site so as to facilitate less radical surgery such as limb salvage
2. Initial attack on micrometastases present in 80% of patients
3. Assessment of sensitivity of primary tumor to chemotherapy so that poor responders can receive alternative treatment postsurgically.

The degree of tumor necrosis (Table 21-2) following neoadjuvant chemotherapy is an independent predictor of EFS and overall survival, presumably reflecting tumor resistance to chemotherapy. Patients whose tumors exhibit a good response (≥90% necrosis) have superior local tumor control as well as EFS and overall survival compared with poor responders (Figure 21-3). In patients whose response is suboptimal, attempts to improve outcome by modifying chemotherapy are continuing.

Figure 21-4 shows the Pediatric Oncology Group POG-8651 protocol for osteosarcoma. This protocol compares immediate surgery to chemotherapy followed by surgery. The presurgical chemotherapy group patients received high-dose methotrexate (12 g/m^2) and leucovorin rescue (15 mg every 6 hours for 10 doses) in weeks 0, 1, 5, 6, 13, 14, 18, 19, 23, 24, 37, and 38. For patients treated with immediate surgery this regimen was administered in weeks 3, 4, 8, 9, 13, 14, 18, 19, 23, 24, 37, and 38. Doxorubicin 37.5 mg/m^2/day for 2 days and cisplatin 60 mg/m^2/day for 2 days were administered in weeks 2, 7, 25, and 28 for the presurgical chemotherapy group and in weeks 5, 10, 25, and 28 for the immediate surgery group. The combination of cyclophosphamide 600 mg/m^2/day, bleomycin 15 mg/m^2/day, and dactinomycin 0.6 mg/m^2/day was administered for 3 days in weeks 15, 31, 34, 39, and 42 for both groups. A single course of doxorubicin 30 mg/m^2/day for 3 days was administered in week 20 for both groups. Both of the regimens have the same outcome with 65% EFS at 5 years and a similar incidence of limb salvage.

Table 21-2. Histologic Response of Osteosarcoma to Preoperative Chemotherapy

Grade	Description
I	Little or no effect of chemotherapy
II	Partial response to chemotherapy with more than 50% tumor necrosis but with areas of viable tumor still demonstrable
III	Near-complete response to chemotherapy with more than 90% tumor necrosis but with areas of viable tumor still demonstrable
IV	Complete response to chemotherapy with no viable tumor cells demonstrable

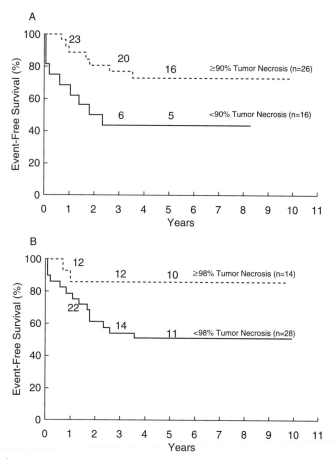

Fig. 21-3. Event-free survival comparing pathologic response at (A) less than 10% residual viable tumor versus ≥ residual viable tumor and (B) less than 2% residual viable tumor versus ≥2% residual viable tumor. Numbers on the curves represent patients still at risk. (From Goorin AM, Schwartzentruber DJ, Devidas M, Gebhardt MC, Ayala AG, Harris MB, Helman LJ,Grier HE, Link MP. Presurgical chemotherapy compared with immediate surgery and adjuvant chemotherapy for non-metastatic osteosarcoma: Pediatric Oncology Group Study POG-8651. J Clin Oncol 2003;21[8]:1574–80, with permission.)

An alternative treatment plan is outlined in Figure 21-5 as per Rizzoli's 4th protocol. This regimen consists of high-dose methotrexate, cisplatin, doxorubicin, and ifosfamide. The 5-year EFS and overall survival rates are 56% and 71%, respectively, for patients with localized disease. Patients with metastatic disease have an EFS of 17% and overall survival of 24%.

The use of high-dose methotrexate with citrovorum rescue requires the following precautions to avoid serious toxicity:

1. Normal creatinine clearance, CBC, and liver profile
2. Measurement of serum methotrexate levels at 24, 48, and 72 hours after administration
3. Vigorous hydration with alkalinization for 72 hours to keep the urine pH above 7.0.

Administration of High-Dose Methotrexate

The dose of methotrexate (MTX) is calculated at 12 g/m^2 with a maximum dose of 20 grams. All doses are rounded up to the next highest full gram of methotrexate.

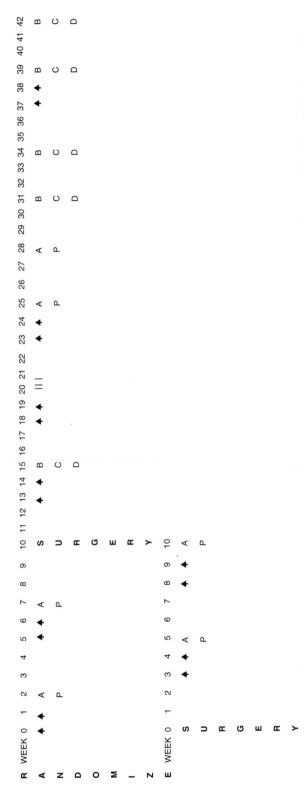

Fig. 21-4. Chemotherapy regimen. The timing of surgery was determined by randomization to be performed at either week 0 or week 10; ◢, administration of high-dose methotrexate and leucovorin rescue; AP, doxorubicin and cisplatin administration; BCD, cyclophosphamide, bleomycin, and dactinomycin; and |||, doxorubicin administration. (From Goorin AM, Schwartzentruber DJ, Devidas M, Gebhardt MC, Ayala AG, Harris MB, Helman LJ, Grier HE, Link MP. Presurgical chemotherapy compared with immediate surgery and adjuvant chemotherapy for non-metastatic osteosarcoma: Pediatric Oncology Group Study POG-8651. J Clin Oncol 2003;21[8]:1574–80, with permission.) An alternative regimen is outlined in Fig. 21-5.

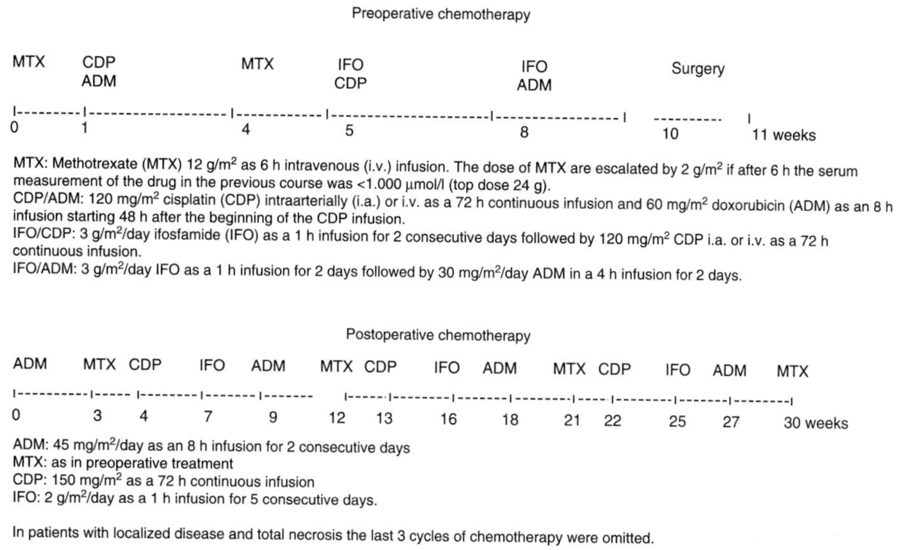

Preoperative chemotherapy

MTX	CDP ADM		MTX	IFO CDP		IFO ADM		Surgery	

```
|---------|-------------------|-------------|-----------------------|-----------------|  ---------  |
0         1                  4             5                       8                 10          11 weeks
```

MTX: Methotrexate (MTX) 12 g/m² as 6 h intravenous (i.v.) infusion. The dose of MTX are escalated by 2 g/m² if after 6 h the serum measurement of the drug in the previous course was <1.000 µmol/l (top dose 24 g).
CDP/ADM: 120 mg/m² cisplatin (CDP) intraarterially (i.a.) or i.v. as a 72 h continuous infusion and 60 mg/m² doxorubicin (ADM) as an 8 h infusion starting 48 h after the beginning of the CDP infusion.
IFO/CDP: 3 g/m²/day ifosfamide (IFO) as a 1 h infusion for 2 consecutive days followed by 120 mg/m² CDP i.a. or i.v. as a 72 h continuous infusion.
IFO/ADM: 3 g/m²/day IFO as a 1 h infusion for 2 days followed by 30 mg/m²/day ADM in a 4 h infusion for 2 days.

Postoperative chemotherapy

ADM	MTX CDP	IFO	ADM	MTX CDP	IFO	ADM	MTX CDP	IFO	ADM	MTX

```
|----------|-----|--------|-------|-------|     |-----|--------|-------|--------|----|-------|-------|--------|
0          3     4        7       9           12    13       16      18       21   22      25      27       30 weeks
```

ADM: 45 mg/m²/day as an 8 h infusion for 2 consecutive days
MTX: as in preoperative treatment
CDP: 150 mg/m² as a 72 h continuous infusion
IFO: 2 g/m²/day as a 1 h infusion for 5 consecutive days.

In patients with localized disease and total necrosis the last 3 cycles of chemotherapy were omitted.

Fig. 21-5. Chemotherapy regimen as per Rizzoli's 4th protocol. (From Bacci G, Briccoli A, Ferrari S, Longhi A, Mercuri M, Capanna R, Donati D, Lari S, Forni C, DePaolis M. Neoadjuvant chemotherapy for osteosarcoma of the extremity: long-term results of the Rizzoli's 4th protocol. Eur J Cancer 2001;37:2030–9, with permission.)

Methotrexate is administered in 1 L of D5W 1/4 NS with 50 mEq of sodium bicarbonate per liter over 4 hours after urine pH is over 7.0. Hydration is administered to achieve a urine output of 1400–1600 mL/m² for the first 24 hours after methotrexate and a minimum urine output of 2000 mL/m² for each 24-hour period after that. Sodium bicarbonate is administered to achieve a urine pH greater than 7.0. Oral leucovorin is begun 20 hours after the completion of the methotrexate infusion at a dose of 10 mg every 6 hours continuing until the 72-hour methotrexate level (and longer if necessary) is less than 1.0×10^{-7} mol/L. Patients whose methotrexate excretion is delayed require increased dose or duration of leucovorin (Figure 21-6).

Approximately 15–20% of patients with osteosarcoma present with metastatic disease. Etoposide and high-dose ifosfamide are effective neoadjuvant chemotherapy for metastatic osteosarcoma. The following is the management approach to patients who present with metastatic disease:

1. Preoperative induction chemotherapy is used to assess the chemoresponsiveness of the primary and metastatic lesions (Figure 21-7).
2. Surgical amputation or limb salvage surgery of the primary lesion is performed. Surgical removal of metastatic sites is recommended, if feasible.
3. Figure 21-8 depicts details of an appropriate continuation adjuvant regimen utilizing high-dose ifosfamide, etoposide, high-dose methotrexate, doxorubicin, and cisplatin (CDDP).
4. With the above-mentioned chemotherapy protocol, 2-year PFS for the patients with pulmonary metastases is 39% ± 11%. The projected 2-year PFS for the patients with bone metastases is 58% ± 17%.
5. When a tumor arises in a site that is not resectable, radiation may be used for local control, even though osteogenic sarcoma is usually not radiosensitive.

Treatment of Patients with Recurrent Disease

More than 85% of the recurrences are in the lung. In a significant proportion of the patients, lungs are the only site of metastases. Predictors of outcome at relapse:

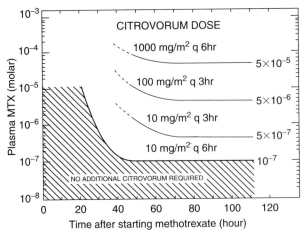

Fig. 21-6. Plasma MTX concentration. (From Pediatric Oncology Group Protocol 9351, with permission.)

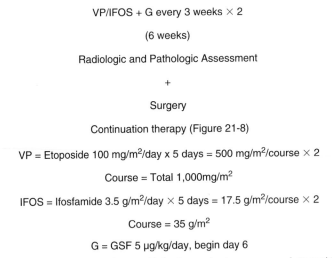

VP/IFOS + G every 3 weeks × 2

(6 weeks)

Radiologic and Pathologic Assessment

+

Surgery

Continuation therapy (Figure 21-8)

VP = Etoposide 100 mg/m²/day x 5 days = 500 mg/m²/course × 2

Course = Total 1,000mg/m²

IFOS = Ifosfamide 3.5 g/m²/day × 5 days = 17.5 g/m²/course × 2

Course = 35 g/m²

G = GSF 5 µg/kg/day, begin day 6

Fig. 21-7. Treatment plan for induction therapy. Patients receive two courses of etoposide and ifosfamide, then radiologic assessment and surgery of primary tumor. The pathologic assessment of tumor necrosis is performed after surgery. (From Goorin AM, Harris MB, Berstein M, Ferguson W, Devidas M, Siegal GP, Gebhardt C, Schwartz CL, Link MP, Grier HE. Phase II/III trial of etoposide and high dose ifosfamide in newly diagnosed metastatic osteosarcoma: a Pediatric Oncology Group trial. J Clin Oncol 2002;20[2]:426–33, with permission.)

1. Completeness of surgical resection
2. Late (more than 1-year post-treatment) versus early relapse
3. Unresectable pulmonary hilar involvement, malignant plural effusion, more than 16 nodules on CT or extrathoracic disease
4. Prior treatment (patients who relapse after multiagent chemotherapy have worse survival).

Although there are no controlled studies, adjuvant chemotherapy is recommended, preferably with the agents that patients have not received before such as ifosfamide, etoposide, cyclophosphamide, topotecan, and irinotecan.

Week	1	2	3	4	5	6	7	8	9	10	11	12	13	14	15	16	17	18
		M	M	A			M	M	I			M	M	A			M	M	I
		T	T	P			T	T	VP			T	T	P			T	T	VP
		X	X				X	X	G*			X	X				X	X	G*

Week	19	20	21	22	23	24	25	26	27	28	29	30	31	32	33	34
			A			I			A			M	M	A		
			P			VP			P			T	T			
						G*						X	X			

VP = Etoposide, 100 mg/m^{2}day × 5 days: 5 courses = Total 2,500 mg/m^2
MTX = Methotrexate, 12 g/m^2 over 4 hours, plus leucovorin, 15 mg q6h × 10 doses: 10 courses = 120 g/m^2
I = Ifosfamide, 2.4 g/m^2 + mesna/day × 5 days: 3 courses = Total 36 g/m^2. Total ifosfamide = 71 g/m^2
A = Doxorubicin, 37.5 mg/m^2/day × 2 days: 5 courses = Total 375 mg/m^2
P = CDDP, 60 mg/m^2/day × 2 days: 4 courses = Total 480 mg/m^2
*G = G – CSF 5 µg/kg/day

Fig. 21-8. Continuation chemotherapy regimen started 1–2 weeks after surgery. (From Goorin AM, Harris MB, Berstein M, Ferguson W, Devidas M, Siegal GP, Gebhardt C, Schwartz CL, Link MP, Grier HE. Phase II/III trial of etoposide and high dose ifosfamide in newly diagnosed metastatic osteosarcoma: a Pediatric Oncology Group trial. J Clin Oncol 2002;20[2]:426-433, with permission.)

Newer Agents under Investigation

Several cooperative groups and institutions have intensified the postoperative treatment to improve the outcome of patients who have a standard response (<90% necrosis) to neoadjuvant chemotherapy. Most of these studies show that the intensified treatment does not change the outcome for these patients. In addition, several institutions have intensified their neoadjuvant treatments to influence this outcome. Although the percentage of good responders increases, the event-free and overall survival rates have not changed. The degree of necrosis to chemotherapy appears to be an innate sensitivity of an osteosarcoma to chemotherapy, which is not altered by intensification of the chemotherapy. For this reason, targeted or biologically based therapies such as liposomal muramyl tripeptide-phosphatidylethanolamine (MTP-PE), interferon, trastuzumab, and granulocyte macrophage colony-stimulating factor are being investigated.

Follow-Up Studies

1. Chest radiograph monthly for 2 years after diagnosis; then less frequently
2. CT of the chest every 4–6 months for 2 years after diagnosis; then less frequently
3. Bone scan every 4–6 months for 2 years after diagnosis; then less frequently
4. Evaluation of the primary site every 4–6 months for 2 years after diagnosis; then less frequently.

Prognosis

The following factors have been associated with a poor prognosis:

1. Children less than 10 years of age
2. Axial skeletal primaries
3. Size of the tumor more than one third the size of the limb
4. Proximal location within the limb
5. Detectable metastatic disease at diagnosis

6. Incomplete resection
7. Poor response to chemotherapy.

Key prognostic factors are surgical resection and response to chemotherapy (Figure 21-3).

The actuarial disease-free survival for patients with nonmetastatic osteosarcoma treated with adjuvant chemotherapy is 60–80%. Patients who present with metastatic disease have a significantly worse prognosis of 10–40%.

EWING SARCOMA

Ewing sarcoma is a malignant tumor of bone in which the predominant feature is densely packed small cells with round nuclei without prominent nucleoli. It is the second most common malignant primary bone tumor of childhood.

Epidemiology

The etiology of Ewing sarcoma is unknown. Certain associations with Ewing sarcoma in children have been reported. Eighty percent of patients with Ewing sarcoma are younger than 20 years at diagnosis. Ewing sarcoma has a striking difference in racial incidence with an extremely low incidence in black and Asian children. It is not usually associated with familial cancer syndromes.

Pathology

Ewing sarcoma, atypical Ewing sarcoma, and peripheral primitive neuroectodermal tumor (PPNET) all derive from primitive, pluripotent, postganglionic parasympathetic primordial cells. Expression of neural markers increases with neural differentiation from Ewing sarcoma to atypical Ewing sarcoma to PPNET. Table 21-3 lists the distinction between Ewing sarcoma, atypical Ewing sarcoma, and PPNET.

The pathologic features of Ewing sarcoma are:

1. Highly cellular aggregates of small round cells compartmentalized by strands of fibrous tissue
2. Tumor cells have round or oval nuclei, occasionally with indistinct nucleoli
3. Nuclei containing finely dispersed chromatin (ground-glass appearance)
4. Fewer than two mitotic figures per high-power field.

Ewing sarcoma is one of the small round blue-cell tumors of childhood. To differentiate it from other small round blue-cell tumors, immunohistochemical studies are necessary (Table 21-4).

The presence of cytoplasmic glycogen supports the diagnosis of Ewing sarcoma, which is demonstrable in 75% of cases. Glycoprotein p30/32 mic2 (CD99) has proven useful in confirming the diagnosis of Ewing sarcoma and PPNET. CD99 reacts with the cytoplasmic membrane of Ewing sarcoma cells, giving a honeycomb staining pattern. It is also expressed by other tumors and normal tissues including the non-blastematous portion of Wilms' tumor, clear-cell sarcoma of the kidney, lymphoma and leukemia, pancreatic islet cell tumors, immature teratomas, testicular embryonal carcinoma, ependymomas, and choroid plexus papillomas. In contrast to Ewing sarcoma, the staining in other tissues is diffuse staining of the cytoplasm. A new immunocytochemical marker, β_1-integrin-linked protein kinase (ILK), has

Table 21-3. Ewing Sarcoma Family of Tumors: Histopathologic and Ultrastructural Features

Feature	Ewing sarcoma		PPNET
	Typical	Atypical	
Light microscopy			
Pattern	Sheets of cell	Usually nesting	Alveolar, rosettes, organoid, or lobular pattern
Extracellular matrix	Absent	Usually present	Present
Cell size	Small	Small to large	Small to large
Cell shape	Exclusively round	Predominantly round	Predominantly round
Cytoplasm	Scant	Scant to easily identifiable	Easily identifiable
Nucleus	Round smooth	Round, occasionally oval	Round, occasional oval
Mitoses	<2 per high-power field	≥2 high-power field	≥2 per high-power field
Electron microscopy			
Cell shape	Round smooth	Round to oval, irregular	Round to oval, irregular, cell processes
Nuclear shape	Round	Round to oval	Round to oval
Neurosecretory granules	Absent	Absent	Present
Organelles	Sparse	Moderate	Moderate to many
Filaments	Absent	Absent to few	May be present
Glycogen	Present	Present	Present
Attachments	Primitive	Primitive to moderately developed	Moderate to well developed
Basal lamina	Absent	Absent	Absent
Extracellular matrix	Absent	Variable	Variable

Abbreviation: PPNET, peripheral primitive neuroectodermal tumor.

From Ginsberg JP, Woo SY, Johnson ME, Hicks MJ, Horowitz ME. Ewing sarcoma family of tumors: Ewing sarcoma of bone and soft tissue and the peripheral primitive neuroectodermal tumors. In: Pizzo PA, Poplack DG, editors. Principles and Practice of Pediatric Oncology. 4th ed. Philadelphia: Lippincott–Raven, 2003, with permission.

shown intense cytoplasmic staining in Ewing sarcoma. It is thought to be a marker of neural differentiation and is present in 30% of neuroblastomas and all of medulloblastomas.

DNA Ploidy and Proliferative Indices

Patients with diploid tumors have prolonged survival compared to patients with aneuploid tumors. Individuals with higher proliferative indices such as Ki67 and proliferating cell nuclear antigen (PCNA) are more likely to die of their disease or to be alive with disease versus those with low proliferative markers who were more likely to have no evidence of disease.

Molecular Genetics

Table 21-5 lists the frequency of chromosomal translocations in Ewing sarcoma. The t(11;22) translocation that is characteristic of Ewing sarcoma and PPNET has been found to involve the juxtaposition of two normally distinct genes, *FL11* on

Table 21-4. Immunocytochemistry of Ewing Sarcoma Family of Tumors and Other Small Blue-Cell Tumors

| Marker | Ewing sarcoma | | PPNET | Neuroblas-toma | Rhabdo-myosarcoma | Lymphoma[a] |
	Typical	Atypical				
NSE	−	+/−	+	+	+/−	−
S-100	−	+/−	+	+	+/−	−
NFTP	−	−	−/+	+	+/−	−
Desmin	−	−	−/+	−	+	−
Actin	−	−	+/−	−	+	−
Vimentin	+	+	+/−	−	+	+
Cytokeratin	+/−	+/−	+/−	−	+/−	−
LCA	−	−	−/+	−	−	+
HNK-1	+/−	+/−	+	+	+	−
β$_2$-Microglobulin	+	+	+/−	−[b]	+/−	+
HBA71	+	+	+/−	−	+[c]	−

Abbreviations: PPNET, peripheral primitive neuroectodermal tumor; −, negative; +/−, positive in greater than 10% of cases; −/+, positive in less than 10% of cases; +, positive.

[a]Nonhistiocytic.

[b]Only in ganglion cells, Schwann cells, and stage IVS neuroblastoma.

[c]Only well-differentiated rhabdomyoblasts.

From Ginsberg JP, Woo SY, Johnson ME, Hicks MJ, Horowitz ME. Ewing sarcoma family of tumors: Ewing sarcoma of bone and soft tissue and the peripheral primitive neuroectodermal tumors. In: Pizzo PA, Poplack DG, editors. Principles and Practice of Pediatric Oncology. 4th ed. Philadelphia: Lippincott–Raven, 2003, with permission.

Table 21-5. Frequency of Chromosomal Translocations in Ewing Sarcoma

Chromosomal abnormality	Frequency
t(11;22)(q24;q12)	90–95%
t(21;22)(q2;q12)	5–10%
t(7;22)(p22;q12)	<1%
t(17;22)(q12;q12)	<1%
t(2;22)(q33;q12)	<1%

chromosome 11 and *EWS* on chromosome 22. The fused gene results in an EWS/FL11 chimeric protein. Ewing sarcoma and PPNET that do not have a t(11;22) and a detectable EWS/FL11 fusion frequently have variant translocations fusing *EWS* to other ETS family transcription factors such as t(21;22) and EWS/ERG fusion. It is felt that EWS/FL11 may play an important role in growth deregulation.

These translocations can be easily detected by reverse transcriptase–polymerase chain reaction (RT-PCR) and fluorescent *in situ* hybridization (FISH). Recent studies have utilized the RT-PCR method to detect metastatic disease in the blood and bone marrow.

Clinical Features

Patients commonly present with the following symptoms:

1. Local pain (96%)
2. Local swelling (61%)
3. Fever (21%)
4. Pathologic fracture (16%).

It is important to realize that, because fever is a frequent symptom of Ewing sarcoma, it may be initially mistaken for osteomyelitis. The previous symptoms may be present for long periods of time, and more than 5% of patients have had symptoms for over 6 months before the tumor is identified. The pain may be intermittent.

Ewing sarcoma most commonly involves the lower extremity, with the pelvis being the next most common site. Table 21-6 lists the primary sites of origin in Ewing sarcoma. In long bones, Ewing sarcoma usually begins in the diaphysis.

Askin tumor is a PPNET of the thoracopulmonary region that involves the chest wall. It is seen more commonly in adolescent women. It is thought to arise from pluripotent cells along the intercostal nerves.

Diagnostic Evaluation

The diagnostic evaluation should consist of the following:

1. History
2. Physical examination
3. Blood count
4. Erythrocyte sedimentation rate
5. Urinalysis
6. BUN, creatinine, liver enzymes, alkaline phosphatase, serum LDH
7. Bone marrow aspirate and biopsy
8. Radiographs of affected bone
9. Bone scan
10. CT scan with or without MRI of primary site
11. Chest CT.

Radiographically, Ewing sarcoma produces changes in the diaphysis of long bones with extension toward the metaphysis. Table 21-7 lists the radiographic findings in

Table 21-6. Distribution of Primary Site for 303 Patients with Ewing Sarcoma of Bone

Primary site	Percentage
Pelvic	20
Ilium	12.5
Sacrum	3.3
Ischium	3.3
Pubis	1.7
Lower extremity	45.6
Femur	20.8
Fibula	12.2
Tibia	10.6
Feet	2.0
Upper extremity	12.9
Humerus	10.6
Forearm	2.0
Hand	0.3
Axial skeleton/ribs	12.9
Face	2.3

From Grier HE. The Ewing family of tumors: Ewing sarcoma and primitive neuroectodermal tumors. Pediatr Clin North Am 1997;44:991–1004, with permission.

Table 21-7. Radiographic Findings in Ewing Sarcoma

Finding	Percentage
Bone destruction	75
Soft-tissue extension	64
Reactive bone formation	25
Lamellated periosteal reaction (onion skin)	23
Radiating spicules (sunburst)	20
Periosteal thickening	19
Sclerosis	16
Fracture	13

From Green DM. Diagnosis and Management of Solid Tumors in Infants and Children. Boston: Nijhoff, 1985, with permission.

Ewing sarcoma. About 5–8% of patients have a normal plain radiograph of the affected bone.

Approximately 20–30% of patients have evidence of metastases at diagnosis in the following sites:

1. Lung (38%)
2. Bone (31%)
3. Bone marrow (11%).

The site of the primary tumor bears a relationship to the incidence of metastases at diagnosis:

1. Central primary—40% incidence of metastases
2. Proximal primary—30% incidence of metastases
3. Distal primary—15% incidence of metastases.

Treatment

The treatment of Ewing sarcoma involves a multimodal approach, using surgery and radiation therapy for control of the primary lesion and chemotherapy for eradication of subclinical micrometastases. The preservation of function and the reduction of long-term sequelae should be taken into consideration in determining the treatment.

Because neuroectodermal differentiation does not affect outcome, patients with typical Ewing sarcoma and PPNET are treated with the same protocols as patients with Ewing sarcoma.

Surgery

Biopsy should be performed at the center at which ultimate surgical treatment will be rendered. The biopsy site should be chosen carefully and placed in line with the potential resection site or radiation portals. The biopsy should be preferably taken from the extraosseous component to prevent pathologic fracture. Frozen section analysis of all biopsy specimens is essential to ensure adequate material has been obtained for light microscopy, electron microscopy, immunohistochemistry, and cytogenetics. The biopsy site must be included en bloc with the resection or irradiation.

Surgical excision can be used for those tumors in which the removal of the affected bone is not associated with significant functional deficit and in which grossly complete excision can be technically accomplished. Amputation may be more appropriate for tumors involving neurovascular bundle, in young children when reconstruction is not technically feasible, or for tumors of the distal leg or foot.

The following is an approach to the management of the primary lesion in Ewing sarcoma:

1. Preoperative chemotherapy for approximately 9 weeks, if initially not resectable
2. Complete surgical removal after preoperative chemotherapy, if surgery does not cause significant functional impairment
3. Surgical debulking followed by radiation therapy, if complete removal would result in significant functional impairment.

Radiation

Ewing sarcoma is a radioresponsive tumor. Local control can be achieved in most patients, provided that:

1. A sufficient dose of radiation is administered
2. An adequate volume of normal tissue is in the radiation field.

Current recommendations for radiation of the primary site are doses ranging from 55 to 60 Gy. In the postoperative setting, gross disease requires 55.8 Gy; microscopic disease requires 45 Gy. The appropriate radiation volume is an involved field of the pretreatment tumor plus a 2- to 2.5-cm margin, followed by a boost to the postinduction tumor volume with margin.

Because the incidence of second bone tumors in the irradiated fields ranges from 10–30% at 20 years after therapy, if surgery can be completely performed with adequate function, it is the preferable modality for local control.

Chemotherapy

The major impact on improved long-term survival in Ewing sarcoma has been systemic chemotherapy. Addition of ifosfamide and etoposide has significantly increased the 5-year event-free (from 54±4% to 69±3%) and overall survivals (from 61±3.6% to 72±3.4%).

Treatment consists of vincristine 2 mg/m^2 (maximal dose 2 mg), doxorubicin 75 mg/m^2 and cyclophosphamide 1200 mg/m^2 followed by mesna alternating with ifosfamide 1800 mg /m^2/day for 5 days and etoposide 100 mg/m^2/day for 5 days. The courses are administered every 3 weeks for a total of 17 courses with a planned treatment duration of 49 weeks. Doxorubicin is substituted by actinomycin D 1.25 mg/m^2/dose when total doxorubicin dose of 375 mg/m^2 is reached (after 5 cycles of doxorubicin). Reevaluation and local control occurs at week 12 of chemotherapy.

Treatment of High-Risk and Metastatic Ewing Sarcoma at Presentation

Patients with Ewing sarcoma of the central axis or proximal location and those with metastatic disease at diagnosis have a worse prognosis. In these patients, intensive chemotherapy and radiation therapy are indicated.

In metastatic patients, studies have shown that, despite the addition of ifosfamide and etoposide and increased doses of chemotherapy, the survival has not been improved. Myeloablative regimens followed by autologous stem cell rescue have failed to improve the outcome for these patients.

Treatment of Relapsed Ewing Sarcoma

The prognosis for patients with recurrent disease is poor. The choice of chemotherapeutic agents depends on the patient's previous treatment. Patients initially treated with vincristine, doxorubicin, actinomycin D, and cyclophosphamide should receive high-dose chemotherapy containing ifosfamide and etoposide, followed by autologous stem cell transplantation.

Prognosis

The overall 5-year disease-free survival for localized Ewing sarcoma treated with surgery, radiation, and multiagent chemotherapy is approximately 55–70%. Patients with localized distal tumors have a 5-year survival of 75%. Patients who present with metastases at diagnosis have a 5-year survival rate of 20–30%.

Factors reported to have an adverse effect on survival in Ewing sarcoma include the following:

- Male sex
- Age older than 12 years
- Fever
- Anemia
- High serum LDH level
- Axial location
- Type of chemotherapy regimen.

In surgically treated patients, the most important prognostic factor is chemotherapy-induced necrosis.

SUGGESTED READINGS
Osteogenic Sarcoma

Bacci G, Briccoli A, Ferrari S, Longhi A, Mercuri M, Capanna R, Donati D, Lari S, Forni C, DePaolis M. Neoadjuvant chemotherapy for osteosarcoma of the extremity: long-term results of the Rizzoli's 4th protocol. Eur J Cancer 2001;37:2030–9.

Bielack SS, Kampf-Bielack B, Delling G, Exner GU, Flege S, Helmke K, Kotz R, Salzer-Kuntschik M, Werner M, Winkleman W, Zoubek A, Jurgens H, Winkler K. Prognostic factors in high grade osteosarcoma of the extremities or trunk: an analysis of 1,702 patients treated on neoadjuvant cooperative osteosarcoma study group protocols. J Clin Oncol 2002;20(3):776–90.

Ferguson WS, Goorin AM. Current treatment of osteosarcoma. Cancer Invest 2001;19(3):292–315.

Gaetano B, Forni C, Ferrari S, Longhi A, Bertoni F, Mercuri M, Donati D, Capanna R, Bernini G, Briccoli A, Setola E, Versari M. Neoadjuvant chemotherapy for osteosarcoma of the extremity: intensification of preoperative treatment does not increase the rate of good histologic response to the primary tumor or improve the final outcome. J Pediatr Hematol Oncol 2003;25(11):845–53.

Goorin AM, Harris MB, Berstein M, Ferguson W, Devidas M, Siegal GP, Gebhardt C, Schwartz CL, Link MP, Grier HE. Phase II/III trial of etoposide and high dose ifosfamide in newly diagnosed metastatic osteosarcoma: a Pediatric Oncology Group trial. J Clin Oncol 2002;20(2):426–33.

Goorin AM, Schwartzentruber DJ, Devidas M, Gebhardt MC, Ayala AG, Harris MB, Helman LJ, Grier HE, Link MP. Presurgical chemotherapy compared with immediate surgery and adjuvant chemotherapy for non-metastatic osteosarcoma: Pediatric Oncology Group Study POG-8651. J Clin Oncol 2003;21(8):1574–80.

Gorlick R, Meyers PA. Osteosarcoma necrosis following chemotherapy: innate biology versus treatment-specific. J Pediatr Hematol Oncol 2003;25(11):840-1.

Gurney JG, Swensen AR, Bukterys M. Malignant bone tumors. Cancer incidence and survival among children and adolescents: United States SEER Program 1975–1995. NIH Pub No 99-4649. Bethesda, MD: National Cancer Institute, SEER Program, 1999:99–110.

Link MP, Genhardt MC, Meyers PA. Osteosarcoma. In: Pizzo PA, Poplack DG, editors. Principles and Practice of Pediatric Oncology. 4th ed. Philadelphia: Lippincott–Raven, 2003.

Ewing Sarcoma

Donaldson SS. Ewing sarcoma: radiation dose and target volume. Pediatr Blood Cancer 2004;42:471–6.

Gaetano B, Ferrari S, Bertoni F, Rimondidni S, Longhi A, Bacchini P, Forni C, Manfrini M, Donati D, Picci P. Prognostic factors in nonmetastatic Ewing sarcoma of bone treated with adjuvant chemotherapy: analysis of 359 patients at the Istituto Ostopedico Rizzoli. J Clin Oncol 2000;18(1):4–11.

Ginsberg JP, Woo SY, Johnson ME, Hicks MJ, Horowitz ME. Ewing sarcoma family of tumors: Ewing sarcoma of bone and soft tissue and the peripheral primitive neuroectodermal tumors. In: Pizzo PA, Poplack DG, editors. Principles and Practice of Pediatric Oncology. 4th ed. Philadelphia: Lippincott–Raven, 2003.

Grier HE, Krailo MD, Tarbell NJ, Link MP, Fryer CJH, Pritchard DJ, Gebhardt MC, Dickman PS, Perlman EJ, Meyers PA, Donalson SS, Moore S, Rausen AR, Vietti TJ, Miser JS. Addition of ifosfamide and etoposide to standard chemotherapy for Ewing sarcoma and primitive neuroectodermal tumor of bone. N Engl J Med 2003;348:694–701.

Gurney JG, Swensen AR, Bukterys M. Malignant bone tumors. Cancer incidence and survival among children and adolescents: United States SEER Program 1975–1995. NIH Pub No 99-4649. Bethesda, MD: National Cancer Institute, SEER Program, 1999:99–110.

Kushner BH, Meyers PA. How effective is dose intensive/myeloablative therapy against Ewing sarcoma/primitive neuroectodermal tumor metastatic to bone or bone marrow? The Memorial Sloan-Kettering experience and a literature review. J Clin Oncol 2001;19(3):870–80.

Meyers PA, Krailo MD, Ladanyi M, Chan K, Sailer SL, Dickman PS, Baker DL, Davis JH, Gerbing RB, Grovas A, Herzog CE, Lindsley KL, Liu-Mares W, Nachman JB, Sieger L, Wadman J, Gorlick RG. High-dose melphalan, etoposide, total-body irradiation and autologous stem-cell reconstitution as consolidation therapy does not improve prognosis. J Clin Oncol 2001;19(11):2812–20.

22

HISTIOCYTOSIS SYNDROMES

The term *histiocytosis syndrome* identifies a group of disorders that have in common the proliferation of cells of the mononuclear phagocyte system and the dendritic cell system. In the context of histiocytosis syndromes, histiocytes are defined as a group of immune cells, including macrophages and dendritic cells.

Macrophages function predominantly as antigen-processing cells and dendritic cells function as accessory cells or antigen-presenting cells. Although the principal pathologic cells of these syndromes are histiocytes, the term *histiocytosis syndrome* is a very selective term in the sense that it does not include storage diseases, hyperlipidemic xanthomatosis, or granulomatous reaction in chronic infections such as tuberculosis or foreign body granuloma. Figure 22-1 shows the ontogeny of histiocytes. Table 22-1 lists the identifying features of various cells of the histiocyte system. Table 22-2 shows a contemporary classification of histiocytic disorders based on newer information regarding cell lineage and biological behavior, and Table 22-3 shows an older but clinically useful classification of histiocytosis syndromes.

LANGERHANS CELL HISTIOCYTOSIS

INCIDENCE

The ratio of male to female incidence is 2:1. Most cases occur in children between 1 and 15 years of age. The prevalence is 1 in 50,000 and the incidence is 1.08 in 200,000 per year.

PATHOLOGY

The Histiocyte Society established the criteria required for the histologic, histochemical, and electron microscopic diagnosis of Langerhans cell histiocytosis (LCH); see Table 22-4. The characteristic histopathology required for a "presumptive diagnosis" is well described. A "definitive diagnosis" of LCH requires the immunohistochemical identification of the presence of Langerhans cells by cell surface CD1a or by the presence of cells with Birbeck granules by electron microscopy. The CD1a surface antigen can now be identified routinely from paraffin-embedded specimens; thus, electron microscopy is only rarely needed.

The abnormal Langerhans cell is the characteristic cell of LCH. The Langerhans granules (Birbeck granules) are derived from the cytoplasmic membrane and appear as racquet-shaped structures in the cytoplasm on electron microscopy. They are

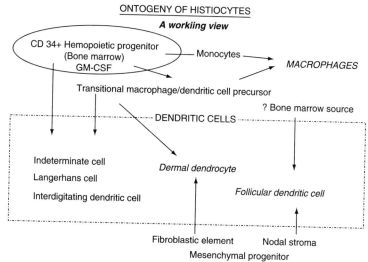

ONTOGENY OF HISTIOCYTES

A workiing view

Fig. 22-1. Much of the basis for this scheme of ontogeny derives from *in vitro* work in developing systems for the production of dendritic cells for immunotherapy. Cytokines (granulocyte macrophage colony-stimulating factor [GM-CSF], TNF-α, IL-4, etc.) play important roles in these pathways, and GM-CSF is fundamental to the differentiation of the Langerhans cells. Langerhans cells, indeterminate cells of the dermis, and interdigitating dendritic cells are considered to be in a cytologic continuum. Indeterminate cells are precursors to Langerhans cells. (From Favara BE, Feller AC, with members of the WHO Committee on Histiocyte/Reticulum Cell Proliferations, Pauli M, et al. Contemporary classification of histiocytic disorders. Med Pediatr Oncol 1997;29:157–66.)

Table 22-1. Immunologic, Cytochemical, and Histologic Identifying Features of Cells of the Histiocyte System

Macrophage	Lysozyme, CD45, CD14, and CD68 positive S100, CD1a, and factor XIIIa negative Langerhans cell (Birbeck) granules absent
Indeterminate cell	CD45, S100, and CD1a positive Factor XIIIa negative Langerhans cell granules absent
Langerhans cell	CD45, S100, and CD1a positive CD14 and factor XIIIa negative Langerhans cell granules present
Interdigitating dendritic cell	CD45 and S100 positive CD14, CD1a, and factor XIIIa negative Langerhans cell granules absent
Dermal dendrocyte	Factor XIIIa, CD45, and CD68 positive S100 and CD1a negative Langerhans cell granules absent
Follicular dendritic cell	KiM4, CD21, and CD35 positive S100 variable CD45 negative Langerhans cell granules absent

From Favara BE, Feller AC, with members of the WHO Committee on Histiocyte/Reticulum Cell Proliferations: Pauli M, et al. Contemporary classification of histiocyte disorders. Med Pediatr Oncol 1997;29:157–66, with permission.

Table 22-2. A Contemporary Classification of Histiocytic Disorders

Disorders of varied biologic behavior
  Dendritic cell related
    Langerhans cell histiocytosis
    Secondary dendritic cell processes
    Juvenile xanthogranuloma and related disorders
    Solitary histiocytomas of various dendritic cell phenotypes
  Macrophage related
    Hemophagocytic syndromes
      Primary hemophagocytic lymphohistiocytosis (familial and sporadic; commonly elicited by viral infections)
      Secondary hemophagocytic syndromes
        Infection associated
        Malignancy associated
        Other
    Rosai–Dorfman disease (sinus histiocytosis with massive lymphadenopathy)
    Solitary histiocytoma with macrophage phenotype
Malignant disorders
  Monocyte related
    Leukemias (FAB and revised FAB classifications)
      Monocytic leukemia M5A and B
      Acute myelomonocytic leukemia M4
      Chronic myelomonocytic leukemia
    Extramedullary monocytic tumor or sarcoma (monocytic counterpart of granulocytic sarcoma)
  Dendritic cell-related histiocytic sarcoma (localized or disseminated)
    Specify phenotype: follicular dendritic cell, interdigitating dendritic cell, etc.
  Macrophage-related histiocytic sarcoma (localized or disseminated)

From Favara BE, Feller AC, with members of the WHO Committee on Histiocyte/Reticulum Cell Proliferations: Pauli M, et al. Contemporary classification of histiocyte disorders. Med Pediatr Oncol 1997;29:157–66, with permission.

involved in receptor CD1a-mediated endocytosis, as well as in nonreceptor-mediated endocytosis.

Recent data strongly support the idea that LCH is a clonal, myeloproliferative disorder of the Langerhans cell similar in many ways to the transient myeloproliferative disease described in Down syndrome.

Table 22-3. Classification of Histiocytosis Syndromes in Children

Class	Syndrome
I	Langerhans cell histiocytosis
II	Histiocytosis of mononuclear phagocytes other than Langerhans cells
	Hemophagocytic lymphohistiocytosis (familial and reactive)
	Sinus histiocytosis with massive lymphadenopathy (Rosai–Dorfman disease)
	Juvenile xanthogranuloma
	Reticulohistiocytoma
III	Malignant histiocytic disorders
	Acute monocytic leukemia (FAB M5)
	Malignant histiocytosis
	True histiocytic lymphoma

From Writing Group of the Histiocyte Society (Chu T, D'Angio GJ, Favara B, Ladisch S, Nebit M, Pritchard J). Lancet 1987;1:208–9, with permission.

**Table 22-4. Histologic, Histochemical, and Electron Microscopic Diagnosis
of Langerhans Cell Histiocytosis**

1. Presumptive diagnosis: light morphologic characteristics
2. Designated diagnosis
   a. Light morphologic features plus
   b. Two or more supplemental positive stains for
      (1) Adenosine triphosphatase
      (2) S-100 protein
      (3) α-D-Mannosidase
      (4) Peanut lectin
3. Definitive diagnosis
   a. Light morphologic characteristics plus
   b. Birbeck granules in the lesional cell with electron microscopy and/or
   c. Staining positive for CD1a antigen on the lesional cell

From Writing Group of the Histiocyte Society (Chu T, D'Angio GJ, Favara B, Ladisch S, Nebit M, Pritchard J). Lancet 1987;1:208–9, with permission.

The following organs are commonly involved in LCH: bone (pelvis, femur, ribs, skull, and orbit), skin, lymph nodes, bone marrow, lungs, hypothalamic pituitary axis, spleen, and liver. The basic lesion is a granuloma formed by histiocytes, granulocytes, and lymphocytes. Early in the course of the disease, the lesions are usually proliferative and locally destructive. Later, the lesions undergo necrosis. The damaged tissue is cleared by macrophages, which eventually undergo xanthomatous change, and fibrosis ensues. These lesions may no longer contain demonstrable Langerhans cells.

CLINICAL FEATURES

Clinical manifestations depend on the site of lesions, number of involved sites, and extent to which the function of the involved organs is compromised.

Although replaced by more prognostically reliable systems (see Tables 22-10 and 22-12 later in this chapter) the classic designations—eosinophilic granuloma, Hand–Schuller–Christian disease, and Abt–Letterer–Siwe disease—are useful descriptions of the various clinical manifestations of LCH.

Eosinophilic granuloma, solitary (SEG) or multifocal (MEG), are found predominantly in older children, as well as in young adults, usually within the first three decades of life with the incidence peaking between 5 and 10 years of age. SEG and MEG represent approximately 60–80% of all instances of LCH. Patients with systemic involvement frequently have similar bone lesions in addition to other manifestations of disease.

Hand–Schuller–Christian disease (multisystem disease) consists of the clinical triad of lytic lesions of bone, exophthalmos, and diabetes insipidus. It is most commonly described in younger children aged 2–5 years and represents 15–40% of such patients, although this type of involvement is observed in all ages. Signs and symptoms include bony defects with exophthalmos due to tumor mass in the orbital cavity. This usually occurs from involvement of the roof and lateral wall of the orbital bones (although bony involvement is not necessary). Orbital involvement may result in vision loss or strabismus due to optic nerve or orbital muscle involvement, respectively. The most frequent sites of skeletal involvement include the flat bones of the skull, ribs, pelvis, and scapula. There may be extensive involvement of the skull, with irregularly shaped, lucent lesions, giving rise to the so-called geographic skull. Somewhat less frequently, long bones and lumbosacral vertebrae, usually the anterior portion of the vertebral body, are involved.

Oral involvement commonly affects the gums and/or palate. Erosion of the lamina dura gives rise to the characteristic "floating tooth" seen on dental radiographs. The entire mandible may be involved, with loss of bone leading to diminished height of the mandibular rami. Erosion of gingival tissue causes premature eruption, decay, and tooth loss. Parents of affected children, particularly infants, frequently report precocious eruption of teeth when, in fact, the gums are receding to expose immature dentition. Chronic otitis media, due to involvement of the mastoid and petrous portion of the temporal bone, and otitis externa are not uncommon.

Abt–Letterer–Siwe disease is the rarest (10% of cases) and most severe manifestation of LCH. Typically, patients are less than 2 years of age and present with a scaly seborrheic, eczematoid, sometimes purpuric rash involving the scalp, ear canals, abdomen, and intertriginous areas of the neck and face. The rash may be maculopapular or nodulopapular. Ulceration may result, especially in intertriginous areas. Ulcerated and denuded skin may serve as a portal of entry for microorganisms, leading to sepsis. Draining ears, lymphadenopathy, hepatosplenomegaly, and, in severe cases, hepatic dysfunction with hypoproteinemia and diminished synthesis of clotting factors can occur. Anorexia, irritability, failure to thrive, and significant pulmonary symptoms such as cough, tachypnea, and pneumothorax may occur as well. One of the most significant areas of involvement is that of the hematopoietic system, which may cause pancytopenia.

Other presentations of LCH are commonly seen. LCH can have a strictly *nodal presentation*, not to be confused with sinus histiocytosis with massive lymphadenopathy or Rosai–Dorfman disease. This presentation is characterized by significant enlargement of multiple lymph node groups, with little or no other signs of disease. In the *pulmonary syndrome* there is almost exclusive involvement of the lungs. This condition is usually seen in young adults in their third or fourth decade (and occasionally in adolescents) and may follow a severe and often chronic, debilitating course; patients may present with pneumothorax. In contrast, the pulmonary involvement in younger patients with system disease is frequently mild, although fulminant pulmonary disease may occur in this age group as well. *Cutaneous disease* with no evidence of dissemination has been described in children and adults. Rarely, patients present with deep subcutaneous skin nodules only (formerly described as Hashimoto–Pritzker syndrome).

Involvement by Site of Disease

Bone

Painful bone lesions affecting hematopoietically active bones are common. Radiographically, the lesions are lytic. They occur commonly in the skull as punched-out lytic lesions, without evidence of marginal sclerosis or periosteal reaction. Bone involvement of the mandible and maxilla and soft-tissue involvement of the gingivae may result in loss of teeth. Involvement of vertebrae can result in vertebral collapse (vertebra plana) and lesions of long bones could result in fractures. There is often an inability to bear weight and tender, sometimes warm swelling due to soft-tissue infiltrations overlying the bone lesions occur. Radionuclide bone scan (^{99m}Tc-polyphosphate) may show localized increased uptake at the site of involvement. Magnetic resonance imaging (MRI) shows bone lesions not identifiable by either radiographic or radionuclide scans. The differential diagnoses include osteomyelitis, malignant bone tumors, and bony cysts. Only rarely are the wrists, hands, bones of the feet, or cervical vertebrae involved. Table 22-5 lists the distribution of the sites of bone lesions.

Table 22-5. Distribution of Bone Lesions in
Langerhans Cell Histiocytosis

Site	Incidence (%)
Skull	49
Innominate bone	23
Femur	17
Orbit	11
Ribs	8
Humerus	7
Mandible	7
Tibia	7
Vertebra	7
Clavicle	5
Scapula	3
Fibula	2
Sternum	1
Radius	1
Metacarpal	1

Skin

Cutaneous eruptions consist of:

1. Diffuse papular scaling lesions, resembling seborrheic eczema (most common)
2. Petechiae and purpura
3. Granulomatous ulcerative lesions
4. Xanthomatous lesions
5. Bronzing of the skin.

Lungs

Lung involvement may result in pulmonary dysfunction with tachypnea and/or dyspnea, cyanosis, cough, pneumothorax, or pleural effusion. Radiographic densities or infiltrates consisting of diffuse cystic changes, nodular infiltrations, or extensive fibrosis can occur. The radiographic appearance may resemble miliary tuberculosis.

Liver

The liver may be enlarged. Liver dysfunction may consist of the following: hypoproteinemia (total protein less than 5.5 g/dL and/or albumin less than 2.5 g/dL), edema, ascites, and/or hyperbilirubinemia (bilirubin level greater than 1.5 mg/dL, not attributable to hemolysis).

Pretreatment liver biopsy more often reveals portal triaditis and less often fibrohistiocytic infiltrates or bile duct proliferation. Patients with triaditis alone are at less risk of having liver dysfunction and progressive liver disease than those who show fibrohistiocytic or cirrhotic changes.

Hematopoietic System

The pathophysiology of hematopoietic dysfunction can be due to hypersplenism as well as direct involvement by Langerhans cells and/or reactive macrophages. Hematopoietic system dysfunction may consist of the following:

1. Anemia (hemoglobin level less than 10 g/dL, not due to iron deficiency or superimposed infection), leukopenia (neutrophils less than $1500/mm^3$), or thrombocytopenia (platelets less than $100,000/mm^3$).
2. An excessive number of histiocytes in the marrow aspirate not considered evidence of dysfunction.

Lymph Nodes

Occasionally, massive lymph node enlargement of cervical or other nodes occurs without other evidence of histiocytosis.

Endocrine System

Short stature has been found in up to 40% of children with systemic LCH. Chronic illness and steroid therapy play an important role in its causation. However, short stature may also be a consequence of anterior pituitary involvement and growth hormone deficiency, which may occur in at least half of the patients with initial anterior pituitary dysfunction. Posterior pituitary involvement with diabetes insipidus is characteristic of systemic LCH. Other endocrine manifestations include hyperprolactinemia and hypogonadism due to hypothalamic infiltration. Pancreatic and thyroid involvement have also been reported.

Gastrointestinal System

Gastrointestinal tract disease has been identified. Two to 13% of patients have biopsy-proven gastrointestinal involvement and/or digestive tract symptoms.

Central Nervous System

Clinically, four groups of patients can be distinguished:

- Patients who present with a disorder of the hypothalamic pituitary system
- Patients who present with site-dependent symptoms of space-occupying lesions such as headache and seizures
- Patients who exhibit a neurologic dysfunction mostly following a cerebellar-primitive pathway, including reflex abnormalities, ataxia, intellectual impairment, tremor, or dysarthria with variable progression to severe central nervous system (CNS) deterioration
- Patients who present with an overlap of the aforementioned symptoms.

Patients who develop CNS disease are more likely to have multisystem disease and skull lesions.

Table 22-6 shows the clinical characteristics of patients with LCH who developed CNS disease compared to those who did not develop CNS disease. It reveals that patients who developed CNS disease are more likely to have multisystem disease with skull and temporal bone lesions, orbital involvement, diabetes insipidus, and endocrinopathies. Table 22-7 shows the classification of CNS lesions according to MRI morphology.

Histopathology

The four stages of LCH involvement of the CNS are as follows:

1. Hyperplastic proliferative
2. Granulomatous

Table 22-6. Extent of Langerhans Cell Histiocytosis and Organs Involved at Diagnosis in Patients Who Develop CNS Disease Compared to Those Who Do Not Develop CNS Disease

	Percentage in 38 CNS patients	Percentage in 275 LCH patients
Multisystem disease	72	40
Single-system bone disease	18	53
Single-system skin, lymph node	0	7
Primary CNS disease	10	0
Bone	84	79
Skull	74	40
Temporal bone	34	8
Skin	58	25
Diabetes insipidus	31	6
Orbits	24	2
Endocrinopathies	18	3
Lungs	16	6
Gastrointestinal tract	10	5
Liver	10	11
Spleen	10	9

From Grois NG, Favara BE, Mostbeck GH, Prayer D. Central nervous system disease in Langerhans cell histiocytosis. Hematol Oncol Clin North Am 1998;12:287–305, with permission.

Table 22-7. Classification of Central Nervous System Lesions According to MRI Morphology[a]

Type		Number	Percentage
Ia	White-matter lesions without enhancement	21	55
Ib	White-matter lesions with enhancement	9	24
IIa	Gray-matter lesions without enhancement	19	50
IIb	Gray-matter lesions with enhancement	3	8
IIIa	Extraparenchymal, dural based	12	32
IIIb	Extraparenchymal, arachnoidal based	2	5
IIIc	Extraparenchymal, choroid plexus based	3	8
IVa	Infundibular thickening	8	21
IVb	(Partial) empty sella	14	37
IVc	Hypothalamic mass lesions	4	10
Va	Atrophy, diffuse	10	26
Vb	Atrophy, localized	6	16
VI	Therapy-related with enhancement	6	15

[a]LCH-CNS Study, $n = 38$.

From Grois NG, Favara BE, Mostbeck GH, Prayer D. Central nervous system disease in Langerhans cell histiocytosis. Hematol Oncol Clin North Am 1998;12:287–305, with permission.

3. Xanthomatous
4. Fibrosis.

Lesions in the hyperplastic proliferative stage are most likely to contain the diagnostic LCH cells. In the cerebellum and cerebrum, white matter may show demyelination and there may also be destruction of Purkinje cells in the absence of histiocytes. Exuberant gliosis with plasma cell infiltrates may also be found.

Hypothalamic Pituitary Involvement

The signs and symptoms of hypothalamic pituitary involvement include:

- *Hypothalamic involvement:* disturbances in social behavior, appetite, temperature regulation, sleep pattern
- *Posterior pituitary involvement:* diabetes insipidus (DI), polyuria, polydipsia
- *Anterior pituitary involvement:* growth failure, precocious or delayed puberty, amenorrhea, hypothyroidism.

Of all these, DI is the most common manifestation. The incidence of this complication ranges from 5 to 50% depending on the extent and location of disease. Fewer than one third of children who ultimately develop DI have polydipsia and polyuria as a presenting symptom of LCH. Most children present within 4 years of diagnosis. DI is due to infiltration by Langerhans cells into the hypothalamus with or without involvement of the posterior pituitary gland. Local tissue damage may be a consequence of interleukin 1 (IL-1) and prostaglandin E2 production. Polydipsia and polyuria may develop at presentation, during active disease (even when there is improvement in other areas), or after therapy is discontinued and there is no other apparent active disease.

Laboratory studies for the diagnosis of DI include:

1. Water deprivation test
2. Measurement of urinary arginine vasopressin (ADH).

These tests discriminate partial from complete DI. Partial DI fluctuates spontaneously. However, partial DI is very rare in LCH.

Gadolinium-enhanced MRI studies show thickening of the hypothalamic pituitary stalk (>2.5 mm) and absence of a posterior pituitary "bright" signal in T_1-weighted images. These lesions are caused by the infiltration of LCH cells. There is no convincing evidence that established DI can be reversed by any treatment modality.

Replacement therapy with desmopressin (DDAVP) is recommended for patients with DI. The rapid institution of effective systemic chemotherapy for disseminated disease may prevent the occurrence of DI and might be responsible for the low frequency of DI.

A small pituitary, or "empty sella," indicates combined anterior and posterior pituitary insufficiency. This may be a result of disease or may be observed following cranial radiotherapy for DI.

Patients presenting with isolated idiopathic DI and morphologic changes in the suprasellar area should be observed very closely. Stereotactic biopsy performed because of an enlarged pituitary stalk can distinguish a variety of conditions such as sarcoidosis, granulomatosis, tuberculosis, nonspecific lymphocytic hypophysitis, and LCH. However, the biopsy is risky and should be avoided if possible. Treatment is determined by the histologic diagnosis.

Space-Occupying CNS Lesions

These lesions most often arise from adjacent bone lesions, brain meninges, or choroid plexus. They usually give rise to signs and symptoms of increased intracranial pressure. They are also site specific and size dependent. Such symptoms include headaches, vomiting, papilledema, optic atrophy, seizures, and other focal symptoms. Even diffuse meningitis-like manifestations can occur. These lesions may occur without any other evidence of LCH.

In some cases, the onset of CNS symptoms occurs many years after the initial diagnosis of LCH.

Mass lesions respond well to treatment, leaving minimal or even no residual defects.

Cerebellar Syndrome/Neurologic Degeneration

The cerebellum is the second most common site of LCH CNS involvement, the first being the hypothalamic–hypophyseal axis. Neurologic symptoms occasionally predate the diagnosis of LCH. The symptoms mainly follow the pontine–cerebellar pattern, beginning as a discrete reflex abnormality or gait disturbance, and/or nystagmus. They can progress to disabling ataxia. Pontine symptoms include dysarthria, dysphagia, and other cranial nerve deficits, ultimately leading to fatal CNS degeneration. On MRI, lesions in the pons, basal ganglion, and cerebellar peduncles show white matter lesions without enhancement. MRI of the cerebrum may show white-matter lesions in the periventricular area.

There is no effective treatment available and prognosis is poor. Aggressive early treatment may reduce the incidence of this syndrome. Biopsy shows a primarily inflammatory, lymphocytic response associated with gliosis, demyelination, and neuronal death. The etiology of this neurodegenerative process is unknown, but is believed to be an immune-mediated paraneoplastic response.

In addition to the above lesions, therapy-related CNS changes should also be taken into consideration in the differential diagnosis of LCH CNS lesions.

CLINICAL AND LABORATORY EVALUATION

Tables 22-8 and 22-9 list the tests necessary for clinical and laboratory evaluation and follow-up of LCH and evaluation required upon specific indication respectively. Every patient should have a thorough physical examination including temperature, height, weight and head circumference, pubertal status, skin and scalp for rash, pallor, or jaundice, external and middle ear, face and orbits, oropharynx, dentition, chest and lungs, abdomen for organomegaly, extremity, and spine.

Indications for diagnostic imaging studies are discussed next.

At Diagnosis

A chest radiograph and skeletal survey should be performed.

Follow-Up Radiograph

A chest radiograph should be performed monthly if the lungs are involved and every 6 months if the lungs are not involved. A follow-up chest film is not required when a monostotic lesion is found at presentation; however, a one-time skeletal survey should be obtained at 6 months in this situation. When multiple bones are affected, skeletal surveys are obtained every 6 months. No follow-up skeletal survey is required if bones are not involved at presentation.

Special Situations

- Presence of malabsorption, unexplained chronic diarrhea, or failure to thrive—endoscopic biopsy, upper gastrointestinal study with small-bowel follow-up; 72-hour stool fat
- Patients with hormonal, visual, or neurologic abnormalities—MRI scan or contrast-enhanced computed tomography (CT) scan of the brain and hypothalamic pituitary axis

Table 22-8. Required Laboratory and Radiographic Evaluation of New Patients with Langerhans Cell Histiocytosis

Test	Follow-up test interval when organ system is:		
	Involved	Not involved	Single-bone lesion
Hemoglobin and/or hematocrit	Monthly	6 months	None
White blood cell count and differential count	Monthly	6 months	None
Platelet count	Monthly	6 months	None
Ferritin, iron, transferritin ESR	Monthly	6 months	None
Liver function tests (SGOT, SGPT, alkaline phosphatase, bilirubin, total proteins, albumin)	Monthly	6 months	None
Coagulation studies (PT, PTT, fibrinogen)	Monthly	6 months	None
Chest radiograph (PA and lateral)	Monthly	6 months	None
Skeletal radiograph survey[a]	6 months	None	Once, at 6 months
Urine osmolality measurement after overnight water deprivation	6 months	6 months	None
Bone marrow aspirate and biopsy[b]			
HLA-typing[c]			

Abbreviation: SGOT, serum glutamic-oxaloacetic transaminase; SGPT, serum glutamic pyruvic transaminase; PT, prothrombin time; PTT, partial thromboplastin time; PA, posteroanterior.

[a]Radionuclide bone scan is not as sensitive as the skeletal radiograph survey in most patients. It may be performed optionally but should not replace the skeletal survey. If suspicion of lesion exists (e.g., pain) and both radiographic and radionuclide tests are negative, an MRI should be performed.

[b]From multisystem patients.

[c]From high-"risk" patients.

Modified from Broadbent V, Gadner H, Komp D, Ladish S. Histiocytosis in children II: approach to the clinical and laboratory evaluation of children with Langerhans cell histiocytosis. Med Pediatr Oncol 1989;17:492.

- Patients with oral involvement—panoramic dental radiographs of the mandible and maxilla every 6 months
- Patients with suspected spinal cord compression—MRI of the spine
- Patients with pulmonary symptoms or significant mediastinal widening of chest film—high-resolution CT of the lungs, pulmonary function tests
- Superior vena cava syndrome—CT with contrast
- Significant cervical lymphadenopathy—CT or MRI of the neck
- Ear involvement—CT of temporal bones
- Hepatosplenomegaly—ultrasound of the abdomen
- Soft-tissue tumors—MRI of involved tissue.

^{99m}Technetium labeled with methylene diphosphonate (MDP) scintography for bone lesions and routine radiographic skeletal examinations are complementary to each other, because radiography is more likely to detect older and quiescent lesions and scintography may detect early aggressive lesions. The ability of scintography to determine the activity of a lesion can be useful in the evaluation of a persistent radiographic abnormality.

TREATMENT OF LANGERHANS CELL HISTIOCYTOSIS

Solitary Bone Lesion

A generally accepted standard for the initial treatment of patients with LCH is to use an appropriate amount of the least toxic therapy to treat the disease. In patients

Table 22-9. Evaluation Required upon Specific Indication

Indications	Tests	Follow-up tests
Anemia, leukopenia, or thrombocytopenia	Bone marrow aspirate and trephine biopsy	6 months
Abnormal chest radiograph, tachypnea, intercostal retractions	Pulmonary function test Chest CT	Every 6 months
Patients with abnormal chest radiographs in whom chemotherapy is being considered, to exclude opportunistic infection	Bronchoalveolar lavage; if not helpful, lung biopsy necessary	None
Unexplained chronic diarrhea or failure to thrive, evidence of malabsorption	Small-bowel series and biopsy; 72-hour stool fat	None
Liver dysfunction, including hypoproteinemia not due to protein-losing enteropathy, to differentiate active LCH of the liver from cirrhosis	Liver biopsy	To be performed when all disease resolved but liver dysfunction persists to distinguish cirrhosis from continuing LCH
Hormonal, visual, or neurologic abnormalities	MRI of brain/hypothalamic pituitary axis	Every 6 months
Oral involvement	Panoramic dental radiograph of mandible and maxilla; oral surgery consultation	Every 6 months
Short stature, growth failure, diabetes insipidus, hypothalamic syndromes, galactorrhea, precocious or delayed puberty; CT or MRI abnormality of hypothalamus/pituitary	Endocrine evaluation	None
Aural discharge, deafness	Otolaryngology consultation and audiogram	Every 6 months

Abbreviations: CT, computed tomography; MRI, magnetic resonance imaging.

From Broadbent V, Gadner H, Komp D, Ladish S. Histiocytosis in children II: approach to the clinical and laboratory evaluation of children with Langerhans' cell histiocytosis. Med Pediatr Oncol 1989;17:492.

with potentially life-threatening disease at presentation, or in those developing life-threatening disease during the course of treatment, alternative and sometimes more aggressive treatment should be implemented. Whether more intensive therapy in lower risk patients with systemic disease reduces disease sequelae such as diabetes insipidus, CNS degeneration, or sclerosing cholangitis, or whether disease recurrence outweighs the risk of more intense therapy is under evaluation.

Specific Site

- *Solitary bone lesions:*
  Curettage (radical treatment is not indicated)
  Intralesional steroids (e.g., methylprednisolone acetate 40 mg/mL, 1–4 mL, depending on size of lesion)
  Radiotherapy (total 450 cGy for small lesions, 600–900 cGy for most lesions, and ≤1500 cGy for large lesions in 150–200-cGy fractions) is reserved for isolated lesions inaccessible to intralesional steroid treatment or lesions that have the potential to compromise vital structures (e.g., optic nerve, spinal cord)
  Systemic therapy for disease involving multiple bones.
- *Localized skin involvement:*
  Topical steroid application
  Systemic steroids for patients with skin and multisystem disease.
- *Severe or refractory skin disease:*
  Local application of 20% nitrogen mustard only to involved skin, avoiding the surrounding normal skin
  Psoralen and ultraviolet A irradiation
  Topical tacrolimus
  Electron beam radiotherapy
  Systemic therapy.
- *Solitary lymph node:* Excisional biopsy should be performed and observation of the patient.
- *Regional lymph node involvement:* Systemic therapy should be administered.
- *Meningeal disease and brain parenchyma disease:* Systemic therapy should be administered.
- *Multisystem disease:* For appropriate risk-adapted therapy, patients with multisystem disease are grouped as shown in Table 22-10.

Certain principles of treatment were derived from the Histiocyte Society–sponsored randomized studies, LCH-I and LCH-II:

- LCH-I showed that the rapidity of the initial response correlates with prognosis.
- Results from the LCH-II study suggest that there is no significant advantage from adding etoposide in terms of survival or the frequency of disease recurrence.
- In an attempt to improve the response rate and possibly reduce the frequency of recurring disease, the LCH-III trial is currently addressing whether the initial response rate is improved by the addition of intermediate-dose methotrexate to prednisone and vinblastine and whether overall outcome is improved using 6 or 12 months of continuation therapy.

Table 22-11 lists systemic therapy for patients with LCH and summarizes the LCH-III study.

RECURRENT OR REFRACTORY DISEASE

For patients with recurrent and/or refractory disease, alternative treatment has not been standardized. Patients with recurrent disease, that is, disease that reappears

Table 22-10. Risk Groups According to the Histiocyte Society LCH-III Trial

Group 1—Multisystem "Risk" Patients

Multisystem patients with involvement of one or more "risk" organs (i.e., hematopoietic system, liver, spleen, or lungs).

Group 2—Multisystem "Low-Risk" Patients

Multisystem patients with multiple organs involved but without involvement of "risk" organs.

Group 3—Single System "Multifocal Bone Disease" or Localized "Special Site" Involvement

Patients with multifocal bone disease, i.e., lesions in two or more different bones or patients with localized special site involvement, such as lesions with intracranial soft-tissue extension or vertebral lesions with intraspinal soft-tissue extension.

Table 22-11. Systemic Therapy for LCH[a]

	Initial treatment	Continuation treatment	Duration
Group 1	Prednisone[b] Vinblastine[c] ±Methotrexate[d]	6-MP[e] Prednisone[f] Vinblastine[g] ±Methotrexate[h]	12 months
Group 2	Same as group 1	Prednisone[f] Vinblastine[g]	Not yet established whether results with 12 months of therapy are better than 6 months
Group 3	Same as group 1	Same as group 2	6 months only

[a]Patients on systemic chemotherapy should receive standard supportive care including sulfamethoxazole/trimethoprim (5 mg/kg/day of trimethoprim) in 2 divided doses per day for 3 days per week (sulfamethoxazole/trimethoprim should not be administered during methotrexate administration).

[b]Oral prednisone 40 mg/m² daily in 3 divided doses as a 4-week course, followed by a tapering dose over a period of 2 weeks. Poor responders should receive a further 6-week course of prednisone 40 mg/m² daily on days 1–3 of each week for an additional 6 weeks.

[c]Vinblastine 6 mg/m² IV bolus on day 1 of weeks 1, 2, 3, 4, 5, and 6. This 6-week course of vinblastine is repeated for poor responders.

[d]Methotrexate 500 mg/m² 24 hours—infusion with folinic acid (leucovorin) rescue day 1 of weeks 1, 3, and 5. Ten percent of the dose is given as IV bolus over 30 minutes, followed by 90% of the dose as a 23.5-hour infusion with 2000 mL/m² hydration.

Folinic acid 12 mg/m² is given 24 and 30 hours after methotrexate infusion is completed (at 48 and 54 hours after methotrexate therapy is started).

It has not been established whether the addition of methotrexate improves results.

[e]Oral 6-mercaptopurine (6-MP) 50 mg/m² daily until the end of the 12th month from commencement of therapy.

[f]Pulses of oral prednisone 40 mg/m² daily in 3 doses on days 1–5 every 3 weeks, starting on day 1 of week 7 in patients who have no active disease after course 1 or on day 1 of week 13 in patients who have no active disease or the active disease is better after course 2, continued until the end of month 12.

[g]Vinblastine 6 mg/m²/day IV bolus once weekly for 3 weeks, starting on day 1 of week 7 in patients with no active disease after course 1 or on day 1 of week 13 in patients with no active disease or the active disease is better after course 2, continued until the end of month 12.

[h]Methotrexate 20 mg/m² orally, once weekly, until the end of month 12. It has not been established whether the addition of methotrexate improves results.

after a period of remission, often respond well to the drugs with which they were initially treated. A number of chemotherapeutic approaches have had limited success. There is anecdotal experience using tumor necrosis factor (TNF) inhibitors in recurrent or refractory disease as well as pamidronate for bone lesions. Several studies, however, have demonstrated significant activity to 2-chlorodeoxyadenosine (2-CdA) in recurrent and refractory LCH. In addition, the combination of 2-CdA and high-dose cytosine arabinoside (Ara-C) has been used in refractory patients. Our current approach is to treat refractory patients with two courses of 2-CdA (6 mg/m^2/day in 50 mL normal saline over 2 hours for 5 consecutive days every 4 weeks). If there is a good response, then the patient receives 2–4 additional courses of 2-CdA. If there is a poor initial response after two courses of 2-CdA, Ara-C (100 mg/kg in 75 mL normal saline every 12 hours for 4 doses to begin on first day of 2-CdA administration) is added to two to four more courses of the 2-CdA. Stem cell transplantation for high-risk or refractory patients warrants further evaluation.

Prognosis

Historic prognostic factors used to stratify therapy include:

1. Response to initial therapy
2. Age at diagnosis (<24 months, 55–60% mortality)
3. Number of organs involved at diagnosis:

Number of organs	Mortality (%)
1–2	0
3–4	35
5–6	60
7–8	100

4. Organ dysfunction (e.g., lung, liver, bone marrow) at diagnosis:

Organ dysfunction	Mortality (%)
Present	66
Absent	4

5. Natural history on treatment:

Group	Description	Mortality (%)
A	No disease progression over 6–12 months	0
B	Progressive disease without organ dysfunction	20
C	Development of organ dysfunction during course of disease	100

6. Congenital self-healing histiocytosis: condition that manifests in neonates with skin lesions, pulmonary nodules with or without bone lesions (these lesions may regress spontaneously and require no treatment)

Table 22-12 shows a clinical staging system based on age, number of organs involved, and presence of organ dysfunction.

SEQUELAE AND COMPLICATIONS

The risk factors for developing residual disabilities are:

1. Generalized disease with bony involvement
2. Smoldering disease for 5 years or longer.

Table 22-12. Clinical Staging System for Langerhans Cell Histiocytosis

Variable	Points
Age at presentation	
>2 years	0
<2 years	1
Number of organs involved	
<4	0
≥4	1
Presence of organ dysfunction[a]	
No	0
Yes	1

Stage[b]	Total points
I	0
II	1
III	2
IV	3

[a]Hepatic, pulmonary, or hematopoietic.
[b]Stage is determined by the addition of points for the three variables.
From Levin PT, Osband ME. Evaluating the role of therapy in histiocytosis-X. Hematol Oncol Clin North Am 1987;1:35, with permission.

Long-term complications include:

- *Pulmonary:* Progressive fibrosis, pulmonary cyst formation, and chronic pneumothoraces. There is no effective therapy for these complications and progression to cor pulmonale and respiratory failure occurs. Opportunistic infections are common.
- *Hepatic:* Cirrhosis and portal hypertension are associated with healing in LCH. Another serious sequela of LCH, sclerosing cholangitis, has been reported and may lead to secondary biliary cirrhosis and liver failure. The etiology is not understood. The only successful treatment for either has been liver transplantation. Sclerosing cholangitis joins severe central nervous dysfunction as one of the most devastating sequelae of LCH.
- *Neuropsychiatric:* CNS manifestations can occur without any relationship to radiotherapy or other treatments. This may manifest with learning disability, ataxia, pyramidal signs, and behavioral changes. MRI studies are helpful in localizing structural changes in the brain.
- *Endocrinal:* Diabetes insipidus and growth retardation are the most frequent complications. They result from histiocytic infiltration of the pituitary and hypothalamus. They are sometimes associated with panhypopituitarism.
- *Orthopedic:* Deformities of the spine can result in long-term disabilities.
- *Malignant:* Second primary malignancies associated with radiation therapy include astrocytoma, medulloblastoma, meningioma, hepatoma, osteosarcoma of the skull, and thyroid carcinoma.

OTHER HISTIOCYTIC DISORDERS

Secondary Dendritic Cell Processes

The accumulation of dendritic cells and Langerhans cells occurs in the lymph nodes in Hodgkin disease, lymphoma, and tumor of the lung, thyroid, and other sites. The secondary dendritic cell processes involute with control of the primary disease. This is a histopathologic finding of no clinical significance.

Juvenile Xanthogranuloma

Clinically, juvenile xanthogranuloma (JXG) is characterized by multiple cutaneous nodules consisting of dermal dendrocytes. These lesions involute spontaneously and no treatment is required. Occasionally there is systemic involvement. When this occurs therapy similar to that for LCH is used. The disorder is often misdiagnosed as LCH.

Solitary Histiocytomas with Dendritic Cell Phenotypes

These tumors are composed of dendritic cells without malignant features. They have variable phenotypes identified by various immunological and cytochemical markers (Table 22-1), for example, indeterminate cell or interdigitating dendritic cell phenotype. They occur in the cutaneous tissue and less often in the central nervous system. The location of the lesions and associated signs of systemic disease determine the prognosis because tumors may be the forerunners of more widespread and serious histiocytic disorders.

Hemophagocytic Lymphohistiocytosis (Hemophagocytic Syndromes)

Hemophagocytic lymphohistiocytosis (HLH) falls into two categories:

1. *Familial hemophagocytic lymphohistiocytosis (FHLH)* (familial or sporadic): This is an autosomal recessive disease that affects immune regulation. Although it is commonly termed familial HLH, because the disease has an autosomal recessive inheritance, sporadic cases with no obvious family inheritance occur. FHLH may be triggered by infections.
2. *Nonfamilial HLH:* A lymphohistiocytic proliferation with hemophagocytosis may also develop from marked immunological activation during viral, bacterial, and parasitic infections (see Infection-Associated Hemophagocytic Lymphohistiocytosis section). This may also be associated with malignancies, prolonged administration of lipids, rheumatoid arthritis (macrophage activation syndrome), immune deficiencies associated with cytotoxic T- and/or NK-cell dysfunction such as DiGeorge syndrome (del 22q11.2), Chédiak–Higashi syndrome, Griscelli syndrome,* X-linked lymphoproliferative disease (XLP), and lysinuric protein intolerance (LPI).

Table 22-13 lists the diagnostic guidelines for HLH. Note that there is no specific diagnostic feature for primary HLH (FHLH). For this reason, when the index of suspicion is strong for primary HLH, treatment may be started before extensive disease activity causes irreversible organ damage and the likelihood of a response to therapy decreases.

Familial Hemophagocytic Lymphohistiocytosis

Pathophysiology, Immunology, and Genetics

In the absence of perforin activity, the resulting inability to kill infected target cells results in sustained NK- and cytolytic T-cell (CTL) activity. This, in turn, results in the

---

*Type 2; mutation in RAB27A[15q21], decreased T- and NK-cell function, hypogammaglobulinemia, and partial albinism.

Table 22-13. Diagnostic Guidelines for Hemophagocytic Lymphohistiocytosis[a]

Clinical criteria
 Fever[b]
 Splenomegaly[b]
Laboratory criteria
 Cytopenia affecting at least two of three lineages in the peripheral blood[b]:
  Hemoglobin (<90 g/L)
  Platelets ($<100 \times 10^9$/L)
  Neutrophils ($<1.0 \times 10^9$/L)
 Hypertriglyceridemia and/or hypofibrinogenemia[b] (fasting triglycerides, >2.0 mmol/L or
  3 SD of the normal value for age; fibrinogen, ≤1.5 g/L or ≤3 SD)
Histopathologic criteria
 Hemophagocytosis in bone marrow or spleen or lymph nodes[b]
 No evidence of malignancy

[a]If hemophagocytic activity is not proven at the time of presentation, further search for hemophagocytic activity is encouraged. If the bone marrow specimen is not conclusive, material should be obtained from other organs, especially lymph nodes or spleen (fine-needle aspiration biopsy). Serial marrow aspirates over time may also be helpful.

The following findings may provide strong supportive evidence for the diagnosis:
1. Spinal fluid pleocytosis (mononuclear cells)
2. Histologic picture in the liver resembling chronic persistent hepatitis
3. Low natural killer cell activity.

Other abnormal clinical and laboratory findings consistent with the diagnosis are cerebromeningeal symptoms, lymph node enlargement, jaundice, edema, skin rash, hepatic enzyme abnormalities, hyperferritinemia, hypoproteinemia, hyponatremia, spinal fluid protein ↑, very low density lipoprotein (VLDL) ↑, high-density lipoprotein (HDL) ↓, circulation soluble interleukin-2 receptor ↑.

[b]All criteria required for the diagnosis of HLH. In addition, the diagnosis of FHLH is justified by a positive family history, and parental consanguinity is suggestive.

From Henter JI, Arico M, Elinder G, Imashuku S, Janka G. Familial hemophagocytic lymphohistiocytosis. Hematol Oncol Clin North Am 1998;12:417–33, with permission.

overexpression of inflammatory cytokines (soluble IL-2 receptor, IL-6, TNF-α, IL-10, and IL-12) leading to excessive macrophage activation, dissemination, and organ infiltration and the signs, symptoms, and laboratory abnormalities that characterize HLH.

Impaired NK-cell activity is key to the diagnosis. FHLH is inherited as an autosomal recessive disorder. FHLH type 1, in linkage with the 9q21.3 locus, represents approximately 10% of the cases and can be recognized by impaired NK-cell function not associated with the absence of perforin expression. The absence of intracytoplasmic perforin may be used as a reliable marker in the 20–40% of patients with familial HLH type 2 associated with the 10q21-22 mutations in the gene at chromosome 10q22 resulting in perforin gene (PRF1) mutations. Perforin functions by perforating the cytolytic target cell membrane, allowing for the entry of granzymes that in turn initiate the apoptotic cell death pathway. The pathways leading to the synthesis of perforin, subcellular compartmentalization, and directional targeting and release of cytolytic granules all represent potential points that could be mutated and contribute to different genetic causes of inherited HLH syndromes. One such is the description of mutations in the *Munc 13-4* gene, which is essential for cytolytic granule fusion. Inactivating mutations in this gene, located at chromosome 17q25, have now been shown to cause familial HLH, termed FHLH type 3. Those patients with absent perforin expression should undergo *PRF1* and more recently described *Munc 13-4* (FHLH type 3) mutation analysis.

A substantial proportion of familial cases of HLH are genetically completely uncategorized. Patients with an infection-associated HLH may have transiently impaired

NK activity; thus, mutation analysis will distinguish these cases from familial HLH. In the absence of a positive mutation analysis, reevaluation of NK function after successful treatment should be undertaken.

In summary, a wide array of immune dysfunction may result in defective NK and CTL target cell killing, resulting in the failure to eliminate infected cells, which, in turn, permits a sustained inflammatory response complete with excessive cytokine production and sustained systemic macrophage activation that characterizes a final pathway of HLH.

Clinical Features

1. The age of onset is less than 1 year of age in 70% of cases. There is no known upper age limit for the onset of disease.
2. Signs and symptoms of FHLH:
   a. Fever (91%), splenomegaly (98%), and hepatomegaly (94%) are the most common early findings.
   b. Lymph node enlargement (17%), skin rash (6%), and neurologic abnormalities (20%) may also occur. Neurologic findings include irritability, bulging fontanel, neck stiffness, hypotonia, hypertonia, convulsions, cranial nerve palsies, ataxia, hemiplegia, blindness, and unconsciousness.
   c. Multisystem involvement includes lungs, bone marrow, and leptomeninges. Occasionally, ocular, heart, skeletal muscles, and kidney involvement have been noted.

Treatment

Patients should be treated as per modern protocols (HLH 2004) according to the Histiocyte Society.* Nonfamilial disease is treated in a similar manner. The following treatment protocol has been utilized:

1. Dexamethasone 10 mg/m^2/day for 2 weeks followed by a decrease every 2 weeks to 5 mg/m^2, 2.5 mg/m^2, and 1.25 mg/m^2 for a total of 6 weeks
2. Etoposide IV (150 mg/m^2 IV 2-hour infusions daily) twice weekly for 2 weeks, then weekly
3. Cyclosporine A 3–5 mg/kg/day by continuous IV infusion starting week 8 to reach a blood trough level of 150–200 ng/mL and switching to oral administration of 6–10 mg/kg/day in two divided doses
4. Intrathecal methotrexate (IT MTX), age-adjusted doses of IT MTX weekly for 3–6 weeks as follows if there are progressive neurologic symptoms or if abnormal cells persist in the CSF:

Age (years)	IT MTX dose (mg)
<1	6
1–2	8
2–3	10
>3	12

5. Allogeneic stem cell transplantation (BMT) after cytotoxic chemotherapy (this is the only potentially curative treatment available) for all patients with familial disease or those with persistent nonfamilial disease.

---

*For details, contact the local chapter of the Histiocyte Society in various countries or the Histiocyte Society, 302 North Broadway, Pitman, NJ 08071. Fax: 1–609–589–6614; Telephone: 1–609–589–6606.

Without treatment, FHLH is usually rapidly fatal, with a median survival of about 2 months. Chemotherapy and immunosuppressive therapy may prolong survival in FHLH but only stem cell transplantation may be curative. Patients with known familial disease or severe or persistent acquired disease should receive hematopoietic stem cell transplantation (HSCT). The 3-year actuarial survival in familial HLH with this approach has been reported as 51% ± 20%.

Nonfamilial Hemophagocytic Lymphohistiocytosis

A number of inherited disorders associated with impaired cytotoxic T- or NK-cell function result in HLH. HLH may also be associated with a number of infectious agents and malignancies.

Infection-Associated Hemophagocytic Lymphohistiocytosis

The findings in children with infection-associated HLH (IAHLH) are similar to those in FHLH. However, decreased or absent NK cells are found more often in FHLH. NK-cell activity in IAHLH patients is reconstituted as soon as the infection is cleared.

Table 22-14 lists the triggering organisms and clinical outcomes for IAHLH. Viruses include Epstein–Barr virus, human herpes virus 6 (HHV-6), cytomegalovirus (CMV) (most common of the viruses), adenovirus, parvovirus, varicella zoster, herpes simplex virus (HSV), Q-fever virus, and measles.

Treatment

- Epstein–Barr virus (EBV)–related IAHLH: etoposide and immunoglobulin treatment
- Other infections: antibiotics for bacterial infections, antiviral drugs for viruses, in addition to corticosteroids and/or etoposide. Patients with persistent HLH may require FHLH treatment and HSCT. Patients with resolved disease may discontinue therapy at 8 weeks. If the syndrome recurs therapy should be restarted and HSCT should be employed.

Table 22-15 shows IAHLH in children by age and clinical outcome prior to the use of effective protocols.

Malignancy-Associated Hemophagocytic Syndrome

Table 22-16 shows the malignancies associated with the development of hemophagocytic syndromes.

Table 22-14. Infection-Associated Hemophagocytic Syndrome in Children: Associated Organisms and Clinical Outcome

Organism	Number of patients	Clinical outcome		
		Dead	Alive	No data
Epstein–Barr virus	121	72	27	22
Other viruses	28	11	13	4
Bacteria	11	2	9	0
Fungi	2	1	1	0
Protozoa	1	0	1	0
No organism	56	13	34	11

From Janka G, Imashuku S, Elinder G, Schneider M, Henter JI. Infection and malignancy associated hemophagocytic syndromes. Hematol Oncol Clin North Am 1998;12:435–43, with permission.

Table 22-15. Infection-Associated Hemophagocytic Syndrome in Children by Age and Clinical Outcome

Age	Number of patients	Clinical outcome		
		Dead	Alive	No data
<3 years	77	40	26	11
>3 years	82	29	47	6
"Children"[a]	60	34	22	4
Totals	219	103/198	95/198	

[a]Age unknown from records reviewed.

From Janka G, Imashuku S, Elinder G, Schneider M, Henter JJ. Infection and malignancy associated hemophagocytic syndromes. Hematol Oncol Clin North Am 1998;12:435–43.

Table 22-16. Malignancies Associated with the Development of Hemophagocytic Syndromes

1. Development of a hemophagocytic syndrome before and/or during the treatment for malignancy, such as
   Acute lymphoblastic leukemia
   Multiple myeloma
   Germ cell tumor
   Thymoma
   Carcinoma
2. Development of a hemophagocytic syndrome with a masked hematolymphoid malignancy in the background, such as
   T/NK-cell leukemia
   Lymphomas
      Angiocentric immunoproliferative lesion-like
      Large cell anaplastic lymphoma
      Adult B-cell lymphoma

From Janka G, Imashuku S, Elinder G, Schneider M, Henter JJ. Infection and malignancy associated hemophagocytic syndromes. Hematol Oncol Clin North Am 1998;12:435–43.

Treatment

If the malignancy-associated hemophagocytic syndrome (MAHS) occurs in an immunocompromised host before treatment, therapy of malignancy and infection is suggested. If it develops in association with an infection during chemotherapy, cessation of chemotherapy may be considered if the malignancy is under control. In addition, treatment for infectious agents, corticosteroids, and etoposide should be administered. Rapidly progressive MAHS may also need to be treated according to the HLH-2004 protocol (see page 622).

Macrophage Activation Syndrome in Systemic Juvenile Rheumatoid Arthritis and Other Chronic Conditions (Reactive Hemophagocytic Lymphohistiocytosis)

Macrophage activation syndrome (MAS) is caused by an excessive activation and proliferation of mature macrophages. It is observed in a number of conditions, including infections, neoplasms, and rheumatologic diseases. Triggers for MAS in juvenile rheumatoid arthritis (JRA) include gold therapy, aspirin, other nonsteroidal anti-inflammatory drugs, and viral infections. Typically, patients with such chronic conditions present with the following features of acute illness:

- Persistent fever
- Hepatosplenomegaly
- Pancytopenia
- Low erythrocyte sedimentation rate (ESR)
- Elevated liver enzymes
- Prolonged prothrombin time, prolonged partial thromboplastin time, hypofibrinogemia, and low levels of vitamin K–dependent clotting factors
- Easy bruisability and mucosal bleeding
- Fibrin degradation products (may be present)
- Elevated serum liver enzyme values
- Numerous, well-differentiated hemophagocytic histiocytes are a pathognomonic feature of this condition and are found in various organs.

In patients with systemic JRA, the acute deterioration is preceded by either a viral infection or major changes in therapy (e.g., administration of gold therapy or nonsteroidal anti-inflammatory drugs).

Macrophage activation syndrome as a complication of JRA is associated with considerable morbidity and death. Table 22-17 shows the clinical differentiation of macrophage activation syndrome associated with JRA from a typical acute exacerbation of systemic JRA. The presence of hemophagocytic histiocytes in the bone marrow and lymph nodes confirms the diagnosis.

Treatment

Because of its seriousness, this syndrome should be recognized promptly on the basis of the previously mentioned findings. Early treatment, consisting of the use of corticosteroids (after performing a bone marrow examination), should be instituted. This treatment usually results in a rapid resolution of symptoms. The dose should be tapered slowly to prevent relapse. If corticosteroids fail to improve this condition, cyclosporine A has been shown to be successful.

Table 22-17. Features That Differentiate Acute Exacerbation of Juvenile Rheumatoid Arthritis from Macrophage Activation Syndrome Complicating Juvenile Rheumatoid Arthritis

	Acute exacerbation of JRA	Macrophage activation syndrome in JRA[a]
Fever	One spike or two spikes daily	Persistent, unremitting
Generalized lymphadenopathy	Present	Not present
Hepatosplenomegaly	Present	Present
Laboratory findings		
Blood count	Marked polymorphonuclear leukocytosis and thrombocytosis	Pancytopenia
Clotting studies	Hyperfibrinogenemia	Hypofibrinogenemia, prolonged PT, prolonged PTT, increased D-dimers
ESR	Increased ESR	Decreased ESR
Liver enzymes	Mildly elevated	Moderately elevated

[a]Must be clearly differentiated from malignant histiocytic conditions.

Sinus Histiocytosis with Massive Lymphadenopathy (Rosai–Dorfman Disease)

Manifestations of sinus histiocytosis with massive lymphadenopathy (SHML) include the following:

- Worldwide occurrence with higher incidence among blacks
- Onset in first two decades of life
- Massive painless bilateral cervical lymphadenopathy with involvement of other groups of lymph nodes; snoring, when there is involvement of retropharyngeal lymphoid tissue; possibility of sleep apnea
- Extranodal infiltration in 25% of patients (skin, orbit, eyelid, liver, spleen, testes, CNS, salivary glands, bone, respiratory tract)
- Immunologic abnormalities with manifestations of autoimmune disorders (e.g., hematologic antibodies, glomerulonephritis, amyloidosis, or joint disease) in 10% of patients
- Fever
- Leukocytosis with neutropenia, mild anemia, elevated ESR
- Polyclonal hypergammaglobulinemia.

Complications

- Retropharyngeal involvement causing respiratory embarrassment
- Epidural involvement causing spinal cord compression.

Diagnosis

Lymph node shows marked dilatation of sinuses by proliferation of benign histiocytes with prominent phagocytosis of lymphocytes, plasma cells, and erythrocytes by sinus histiocytes. Plasma cell infiltrates in the medullary cords and capsular fibrosis may also be evident.

Prognosis

Twenty percent of patients have spontaneous resolution or improvement within 3–9 months. The majority of patients have stable and persistent disease lasting up to several years. Seven percent of patients have a fatal outcome, especially if immunologic abnormalities and extranodal involvement are present.

Treatment

No treatment is generally warranted because this is a self-limited disease. Prednisone 2 mg/kg PO may be administered for life-threatening complications. If prednisone fails, 6-mercaptopurine 60 mg/m^2/day PO and methotrexate 12 mg/m^2/week PO may be tried. α-Interferon has also been reported to be effective in some cases.

Malignant Histiocytic Disorders in Children

Table 22-2 shows a contemporary classification of malignant histiocytic disorders, based on recently available phenotypic and genotypic data.

Nosology

Figure 22-2 shows the nosology for malignant histiocytic disorders in children.

Histiocytes

(general term for cells of the mononuclear phagocytic system)

Antigen-processing cells
  (macrophages and monocytes)
Monocyte-related malignant
  histiocytic disorders:
  Leukemias: monocytic leukemia
    (M5A and B), acute myelomonocytic
    leukemia (M4), chronic myelomonocytic
    monocytic leukemia
  Extramedullary monocytic tumor
    or sarcoma (monocytic counterpart
    part of granulocytic sarcoma)
  Macrophage-related histiocytic
    sarcoma (localized or disseminated)

Antigen-presenting cells
  (dendritic cells)
Dendritic cell–related histiocytic
  sarcoma (localized sarcoma or
  disseminated):
Follicular dendritic cell sarcoma
Dermal dendrocyte sarcoma
Monocytic interdigitating dendritic
  cell sarcoma
Indeterminate cell sarcoma
Langerhans cell sarcoma

Fig. 22-2. Classification of histiocytic malignancies.

The previously mentioned malignant histiocytic disorders are categorized as monocyte–macrophage histiocytic sarcomas (MMHS). The term *sarcoma*, although not an ideal name, is used instead of lymphoma because lymphomas are malignant tumors of different lymphoid cell types and, thus, they cannot be "histiocytic." Table 22-18 lists the criteria for true malignant monocyte–macrophage–related disorders.

In about 20% of all anaplastic large-cell lymphomas (ALCLs), the cell of origin remains unclear. Some of these tumors, which lack lymphoid markers, show clear markers for monocytes and/or macrophages. These are considered to be macrophage-related histiocytic sarcomas.

Treatment

The following treatments are recommended for MMHS:

1. Monocyte-related leukemias and extramedullary monocytic sarcoma—same as the treatment for acute nonlymphocytic leukemias (see Chapter 14)

Table 22-18. Criteria for True Malignant Monocyte–Macrophage–Related Disorders

Immunophenotyping
  Cells are negative for T- and B-cell-associated antigens and express antigens associated
    with monocyte–macrophage origin including:
    Myelomonocytic antigen: Cd11b, CD11c, CD13, CD15, CD33, lysozyme
    Monocyte–macrophage antigens: CD36, CD68, MAC-387, α-1-antitrypsin,
      α-1-antichymotrypsin
    Antibodies associated with other lineages that may show reactivity cells of
      monocyte–macrophage lineage: HLA-DR, CD41, CD43, CD45RO, CD45 (LCA), CD74
Gene rearrangement studies
  Negative B immunoglobulin and T-cell antigen receptor gene rearrangement studies[a]

[a]It is generally assumed that Ig and TCR gene rearrangements are functional only in B and T cells, respectively. We are aware of the fact that such rearrangements have been described to occur occasionally in cells from other lineages as well, known as cross-lineage rearrangements.

Data from Egeler RM, Schmitz L, Sonneveld P, et al. Malignant histiocytosis: a reassessment of cases formerly classified as histiocytic neoplasms and a review of the literature. Med Pediatr Oncol 1995;25:1. From Bucsky P, Egeler RM. Malignant histiocytic disorders in children. Hematol Oncol Clin North Am 1998;12:465–71.

2. Macrophage-related histiocytic sarcomas (localized and disseminated)—the BFM-NHL protocol for Ki-1+ anaplastic large-cell lymphoma (ALCL) (see Chapter 16)
3. Dendritic cell–related histiocytic sarcoma
   a. Localized disease—wide excision only and observe (these tumors are only locally aggressive)
   b. Disseminated disease—the BFM-NHL protocol for Ki-1+ ALCL.

These recommendations are based on the observation of a small number of patients because these disorders are rare. The treatment for MHS is the same as the BFM-NHL 90 protocol for ALCL. (See Figure 16-2 and Table 16-9 in Chapter 16; the figure and the table must be read in conjunction with each other.) Treatment is stratified into three categories, depending on the stage of the disease.

- *Category I:* Stages I and II (Murphy staging system of NHL) with completely resected disease—three courses of A–B–A
- *Category II:* Stage II not resected and stage III (Murphy staging system of NHL)—six courses of A–B–A–B–A–B
- *Category III:* Stage IV (Murphy staging system of NHL)—six intensified courses with higher doses of methotrexate and cytarabine AA–BB–CC–AA–BB–CC.

SUGGESTED READINGS

Ambruso DR, Hays T, Zwartjes WJ, Tubergen DG, Favara BE. Successful treatment of lymphohistiocytic reticulosis with phagocytosis with epipodophyllotoxin VP 16-213. Cancer 1980;45:2516–20.

Arico M, Allen M, Brusa S, Clementi R, Pende D, Maccario R, Moretta L, Danesino C. Haemophagocytic lymphohistiocytosis: proposal of a diagnostic algorithm based on perforin expression. Br J Haematol 2002;119:180–8.

Arico M, Egeler RM. Clinical aspects of Langerhans' cell histiocytosis. Hematol Oncol Clin North Am 1998;12:247–58.

Broadbent V, Gadner H. Current therapy for Langerhans' cell histiocytosis. Hematol Oncol Clin North Am 1998;12:327–37.

Dufoureq-Lagelouse R, Pastural E, Barrat FJ, Feldmann J, Le Deist F, Fischer A, De Saint Basile G. Genetic basis of hemophagocytic lymphohistiocytosis syndrome (Review). Int J Mol Med 1999;4:127–33.

Egeler RM, D'Angio G. Langerhans' cell histiocytosis. J Pediatr 1995;127:1–11.

Favara BE, Feller AC, with members of the WHO Committee on Histiocytic/Reticulum Cell Proliferations, Pauli M, et al. Contemporary classification of histiocyte disorders. Med Pediatr Oncol 1997;29:157–66.

Feldmann J, Callebaut I, Raposo G, Certain S, Bacq D, Dumont C, Lambert N, Ouachee-Chardin M, Chedeville G, Tamary H, Minard-Colin V, Vilmer E, Blanche S, Le Deist F, Fischer A, de Saint Basile G. Munc 13-4 is essential for cytolytic granules fusion and is mutated in a form of familial hemophagocytic lymphohistiocytosis (FHL3). Cell 2003;115:461–73.

Grois NG, Favara BE, Mostbeck GH, Prayer D. Central nervous system disease in Langerhans' cell histiocytosis. Hematol Oncol Clin North Am 1998; 12:287–305.

Grom AA, Passo M. Macrophage activation syndrome in systemic juvenile rheumatoid arthritis. J Pediatr 1996;129:630–2.

Henter JI, Arico M, Elinder G, Imashuku S, Janka G. Familial hemophagocytic lymphohistiocytosis. Hematol Oncol Clin North Am 1998;12:417–33.

Henter JI, Samuelsson-Horne A, Arico M, Egeler RM, Elinder G, Filipovich AH, Gadner H, Imashuku S, Komp D, Ladisch S, Webb D, Janka G. Treatment of hemophagocytic lymphohistiocytosis with HLH-94 immunochemotherapy and bone marrow transplantation. Blood 2002;100:2367–73.

Janka G, Imashuku S, Elinder G, Schneider M, Henter JI. Infection and malignancy associated hemophagocytic syndromes. Hematol Oncol Clin North Am 1998;12:435–43.

Ladisch S, Gadner H, Arico M, Broadbent V, Grois N, Jacobson A, Komp D, Nicholson HS. LCH-1: a randomized trial of etoposide versus vinblastine in disseminated Langerhans' cell histiocytosis. Med Pediatr Oncol 1994;23:107–10.

Ladisch S, Jaffe ES. The histiocytoses. In: Pizzo PA, Poplack DG, editors. Principles and Practice of Pediatric Oncology. 3rd ed. Philadelphia: Lippincott–Raven, 1997; 615–31.

Lipton JM, Arceci RJ. Histiocytic disorders. In: Hoffman R, Benz EJ, Shattil SJ, Furie B, Cohen HJ, Silberstein LE, McGlave P, editors. Hematology: Basic Principles and Practice. 4th ed. New York: Churchill Livingstone, 2004.

Malone M. The histiocytoses of childhood. Histopathology 1991;19:105–19.

Munn S, Chu AC. Langerhans' cell histiocytosis of the skin. Hematol Oncol Clin North Am 1998;12:269–85.

Murakami I, Gogusev J, Fournet JC, Glorion C, Jambert F. Detection of molecular cytogenetic aberrations in Langerhans' cell histiocytosis of bone. Hem Pathol 2002;33:555–60.

Newell KA, Alonso EM, Kelly SM, Rubin CM, Thistlehwaite JR, Whitington PF. Association between liver transplantation for Langerhans' cell histiocytosis and development of post-transplant lymphoproliferative disease in children. J Pediatr 1997;131:98–104.

Reiter A, Schrappe M, Tiemann M, Parwaresch R, Zimmerman M, Yakisan E, Dopfer R, Bucsky P, Mann G, Gadner H, Riehm H. Successful treatment strategy for Ki-1 anaplastic large cell lymphoma of childhood: a prospective analysis of 62 patients enrolled in three consecutive Berlin–Frankfurt–Munster Group studies. J Clin Oncol 1994;12:899–908.

Ware R, Friedman HS, Kinney TR, Kurtzberg J, Chaffee S, Falletta JM. Familial erythrophagocytic lymphohistiocytosis: late relapse despite continuous high-dose VP-16 chemotherapy. Med Pediatr Oncol 1990;18:27–9.

William CL, McClain KL. An update on clonality, cytokines, and viral etiology in Langerhans' cell histiocytosis. Hematol Oncol Clin North Am 1998;12:407–16.

23

RETINOBLASTOMA

Retinoblastoma is a malignant tumor of the embryonic neural retina. It affects young children under the age of 5 years. Tumors may be unilateral or bilateral, unifocal or multifocal. There are hereditary and nonhereditary forms of the disease and the disease can be sporadic or familial. Intraocular growth occurs first, prior to invasion of structures within the globe or spread to metastatic sites. In developed nations, presentation with metastatic disease is unusual. However, metastatic disease is not uncommon in developing nations, where it is a significant cause of morbidity and mortality. Retinoblastoma is the paradigm for a genetically inherited cancer and provides the basis for Knudson's two-hit hypothesis of carcinogenesis.

INCIDENCE

1. Retinoblastoma is the most common intraocular malignancy of childhood, occurring at a rate of 1 in 20,000 live births.
2. The average annual incidence is 11.0 new cases per million under 5 years of age.
3. Approximately 200 new cases of retinoblastoma occur each year in the United States.
4. Retinoblastoma accounts for 11% of cancers developing in the first year of life, but for only 3% of all cancers diagnosed in children younger than 15 years of age.
5. The average age at diagnosis is 18 months.
6. Approximately 40% of cases are hereditary. The majority of these patients present with bilateral disease with an average of three tumors per eye and presents in the first year of life. Of these, only 15% have an established family history of retinoblastoma.
7. The remaining 60% of cases are nonhereditary, most often presenting with unilateral and unifocal disease in the second and third years of life.

CLASSIFICATION

There are three overlapping methods for classifying retinoblastoma:

1. *Laterality:* Tumors may be unilateral or bilateral
2. *Focality:* Tumors may be unifocal or multifocal
3. *Genetics:* Tumors may be hereditary or nonhereditary

The disease may be familial or sporadic.

Laterality

Bilateral Tumors

Patients have one or more tumors in both eyes. Tumor development can be synchronous or metachronous. It is presumed that these patients have the hereditary form of the disease even in the absence of a positive family history. These patients almost always present prior to age 2 years and most present in the first year of life. The severity of tumors may be variable in the two eyes, and this becomes important in weighing potential treatment options.

Unilateral Tumors

Patients have one or more tumors in one eye. Median age of presentation is 23 months, with few presenting under 1 year of age. Tumor development within the affected eye can be synchronous or metachronous. For those with unifocal unilateral disease, it is presumed that these patients have the nonhereditary form of the disease. Patients with multifocal unilateral disease or those who present at a younger age are more likely to have the hereditary form of the disease.

Focality

Unifocal Tumors

A single tumor focus exists. These tumors are more likely to be nonhereditary.

Multifocal Tumors

Multiple tumor foci are noted in one or both eyes. These tumors are more likely to be hereditary.

Genetics

Two-Hit Hypothesis

Knudson's two-hit hypothesis proposes that as few as two stochastic events are required for tumor initiation. The first can be either germline or somatic and the second occurs somatically in the individual retinoblast cells.

The *RB1* Gene

Retinoblastoma occurs as a result of mutations of the *RB1* gene located on chromosome 13q14. This is a tumor suppressor gene that spans 183 kilobases of genomic DNA, consisting of 27 exons and coding for a 110-kDa protein p110, with 928 amino acids. Positive and negative regulation of transcription and, thus, cell proliferation are linked to the phosphorylation of the RB protein. Involved in this process are E2F1, a transcription factor that regulates the cell cycle during G_1, histone deacetylase 1, and downstream cell cycle-specific kinases. Loss of function is the initiating event for retinoblastoma. Mutations may be germline or somatic and there is a broad array of types and locations of mutations, ranging from single base changes to large deletions. Hot spots of common mutation have not been identified.

Hereditary Retinoblastoma

Patients with hereditary retinoblastoma inherit a germline mutation in the *RB1* gene that is present in every cell of the body. Eighty-five percent of these are new spontaneous mutations (sporadic), while the remaining 15% have a positive family history (familial). For the sporadic cases, the paternal allele is affected in approximately 94% of cases. Postconception, a second somatic mutation occurs in the remaining *RB1* gene in one or more retinoblasts, leading to tumor development.

Nonhereditary Retinoblastoma

These patients inherit two normal copies of the *RB1* gene. Postconception, two somatic mutations occur, one in each copy of the *RB1* gene in a retinoblast and tumor results.

Genetic Counseling

The *RB1* gene is inherited in an autosomal dominant fashion. Penetrance is high, approximately 90–95%. Genetic counseling should be an integral part of the therapy for a patient with retinoblastoma, whether unilateral or bilateral. Genetic counseling, however, is not always straightforward. Families with retinoblastoma may have a founder with embryonic mutagenesis causing genetic mosaicism of gametes. A significant proportion (10–18%) of children with retinoblastoma have somatic genetic mosaicism, making the genetic story more complex and contributing to the difficulty of genetic counseling.

As a guide, the following schema can be applied to retinoblastoma genetic counseling, although this is far from absolute and exceptions exist.

Unilateral or bilateral disease with a positive family history of retinoblastoma:

1. Risk for parents to have another child with retinoblastoma is 40%.
2. Risk for the affected patient to have offspring with retinoblastoma is 40%.
3. Risk for a normal sibling of the affected patient to have offspring with retinoblastoma is 7%.

Bilateral disease without a positive family history of retinoblastoma:

1. Risk for parents to have another child with retinoblastoma is 6%.
2. Risk for the affected patient to have offspring with retinoblastoma is 40%.
3. Risk for a normal sibling of the affected patient to have offspring with retinoblastoma is 1%.

Unilateral disease without a positive family history of retinoblastoma:

1. Risk for parents to have another child with retinoblastoma is 1%.
2. Risk for the affected patient to have offspring with retinoblastoma is 8%.
3. Risk for a normal sibling of the affected patient to have offspring with retinoblastoma is 1%.

Prenatal Diagnosis and Further Genetic Counseling

With sequencing of the *RB1* gene available, prenatal diagnosis can be undertaken, particularly if there is a family history and the mutation has been identified. However, a negative result cannot categorically rule out disease, because 100% of mutations are not picked up by current screening methods. The positive predictive value of screening, however, is rapidly improving and this is now offered in some centers as a clinical service. This will also assist in the process of genetic counseling and remove some uncertainty in our predictions of risk for other cases in families.

OTHER EPIDEMIOLOGIC DATA

1. There is an identified 13q deletion syndrome associated with an increased risk of retinoblastoma. This led to the identification of the *RB1* gene. This occurs

in <0.05% of patients with retinoblastoma and is notable for the following features:

   a. Microcephaly

   b. Broad nasofrontal bones

   c. Hypertelorism

   d. Micro-ophthalmia

   e. Epicanthic folds

   f. Ptosis

   g. Micrognathia

   h. Hypoplastic or absent thumbs.

2. No known associations exist for race or gender.
3. There is no eye predilection.
4. Environmental and demographic risk factors that have been identified in some studies but are inconsistent or limited include:

   a. Increased paternal age

   b. Paternal employment in the military, in metal manufacturing, or as a welder machinist

   c. Maternal use of steroid hormones

   d. High birthweight.

RISK FOR SECOND MALIGNANT NEOPLASMS

1. Because the *RB1* gene is a tumor suppressor gene, individuals with heritable retinoblastoma are at high risk for the development of second and subsequent malignancies.
2. The most common second malignant neoplasms (SMNs) reported have been osteosarcoma, followed by soft-tissue sarcomas and melanoma. Leukemia, lymphoma, and breast cancer are also reported in excess of that expected.
3. The risk is highest for those children with the heritable form of the disease who are treated with full-dose, external beam radiotherapy delivered without use of conformal fields under the age of 12 months.
4. The 50-year-risk is 50% for those treated with radiotherapy and 28% for those treated without radiotherapy. Those who received radiotherapy at less than 1 year of age are at highest risk.
5. The risk for those patients with unilateral disease is approximately 5%, which is likely representative of the small fraction of genetic cases with only a single eye affected.
6. For those who survive a SMN, the risk of developing yet another primary malignancy is about 2% per year.
7. Approximately 60% of SMNs occur within the radiotherapy field, but the remainder occur outside the field.
8. Patients with retinoblastoma should be counseled carefully regarding their increased risk of SMN and should be followed by routine clinical evaluation. Any signs or symptoms potentially referable to an SMN should be promptly evaluated.

PATHOLOGY

Retinoblastoma

The tumor is composed mainly of undifferentiated anaplastic cells that arise from the nuclear layers of the retina. Histology shows similarity to other embryonal tumors of childhood, such as neuroblastoma and medulloblastoma, including features such as aggregation around blood vessels, necrosis, calcification, and Flexner-Wintersteiner rosettes. Retinoblastomas are characterized by marked cell proliferation as evidenced by high mitosis counts and extremely high MIB-1 labeling indices.

Retinocytoma

This is a benign variant of retinoblastoma that may be referred to as either retinoma or retinocytoma. These tumors are composed of benign-appearing cells with a high degree of photoreceptor differentiation. Eyes with such tumors have normal vision. These tumors behave in a benign manner. The main issue is that these tumors will not regress in the same way as retinoblastoma, when treated with chemotherapy or local ophthalmic therapy. Thus differentiating these benign variants from the malignant form of the tumor is essential so that unnecessary treatment is not employed.

CLINICAL FEATURES

Presenting Signs and Symptoms

1. Leukocoria
2. Strabismus
3. Decreased visual acuity
4. Inflammatory changes
5. Hyphema
6. Vitreous hemorrhage, resulting in a black pupil.

Patterns of Spread

Intraocular:

1. With endophytic growth, there is a white hazy mass.
2. With exophytic growth, there is retinal detachment.
3. Most tumors have combined growth.
4. Retinal cells frequently break off from the main mass and seed the vitreous or new locations on the retina.
5. Glaucoma may result from occlusion of the trabecular network or from iris neovascularization.

Extraocular:

1. Retinoblastoma spreads first to surrounding structures and then by hematogenous or lymphatic extension.
2. Retinoblastoma invades the optic nerve. From there it can spread directly along the axons to the brain or may cross into the subarachnoid space and spread via the cerebrospinal fluid to the brain.
3. Hematogenous spread leads to metastatic disease, most commonly to brain, bone marrow, or bone.
4. Lymphatic spread is rare because there is minimal lymphatic drainage of the orbit. Occasionally, retinoblastoma spreads lymphatically to the preauricular and submandibular nodes.

Trilateral Retinoblastoma

Trilateral retinoblastoma is a well-recognized syndrome that occurs in children under the age of 5 years. It consists usually of bilateral hereditary retinoblastoma associated with an intracranial neuroblastic tumor of the pineal gland, and occurs in approximately 5–15% of children with familial, multifocal, or bilateral retinoblastoma. With the onset of systemic neoadjuvant chemotherapy, the incidence of this syndrome appears to be decreasing.

DIAGNOSTIC PROCEDURES

Screening

All children should have screening performed as part of well-child checkups, primarily by eliciting red reflexes in the eye. However, most cases of retinoblastoma are diagnosed after a parent or other relative notices an abnormality of the eye and this prompts further evaluation.

Siblings of children with retinoblastoma should be screened by ophthalmology at regular intervals at least through age 2–3 years.

Diagnosis of Intraocular Retinoblastoma

Diagnosis is made by ophthalmologists, retinal specialists, or ocular oncologists using a combination of an ophthalmologic examination generally performed under sedation or anesthesia, together with retinal camera (RetCam) imaging, ultrasound, CT, or MRI. Due to concern about rupturing the tumor and causing both intraocular and extraocular spread, surgical biopsies are not performed for confirmation.

Defining Extent of Disease

The ophthalmologic examination will determine the extent of intraocular tumor and presence or absence of orbital extension. It is crucial that intraocular examination with a binocular indirect ophthalmoscope be performed on both eyes with the pupils maximally dilated. The ophthalmologist should use diagrams of the retina to show the number, size, and location of all tumors. These diagrams are now being supplemented by the use of RetCam images, which are helpful in determining not only the extent of disease, but response to treatment. When the binocular indirect ophthalmoscope is used, the location of the tumor(s) should be related to specific landmarks such as the optic nerve head, fovea, and ora serrata. Size of the lesion is estimated by comparison with the optic nerve head diameter.

Extraocular Extent of the Disease

All children with retinoblastoma should be referred to a pediatric oncologist for evaluation of extraocular disease. Table 23-1 summarizes the investigations to be performed.

STAGING

The standard staging system for intraocular retinoblastoma is not truly a staging system, but rather a grouping system and is the Reese–Ellsworth classification, which is shown in Table 23-2. This system was designed to predict outcome when disease was treated with external beam radiotherapy, and the prognosis associated with each group refers to the probability of retaining useful vision rather than survival.

Table 23-1. Investigations for Diagnosis of Retinoblastoma

Examinations	Imaging studies	Laboratory evaluations	Diagnostic studies
Examination under anesthesia by pediatric ophthalmologist Examination and consultation with pediatric oncologist Audiology evaluation if systemic carboplatin is considered	CT scan of brain and orbits	Complete blood count with differential blood chemistries, electrolytes and urinalysis if systemic chemotherapy is considered Creatinine clearance if systemic carboplatin is considered	Lumbar puncture only with radiographic or clinical suspicion of CNS disease Bone scan only with bone pain or other extraocular disease Bone marrow biopsy only with abnormal blood counts (without alternative explanation) or other extraocular disease Pathologic evaluation if enucleation is performed

Table 23-2. Reese–Ellsworth Staging for Intraocular Retinoblastoma

Group I: very favorable.
A. Solitary tumor, less than 4 disc diameters in size at or behind the equator
B. Multiple tumors, none over 4 disc diameters in size at or behind the equator

Group II: favorable
A. Solitary tumor, 4–10 disc diameters in size at or behind the equator
B. Multiple tumors, 4–10 disc diameters in size behind the equator

Group III: doubtful
A. Any lesion anterior to the equator
B. Solitary tumors larger than 10 disc diameters behind the equator

Group IV: unfavorable
A. Multiple tumors, some larger than 10 disc diameters
B. Any lesion extending anterior to the ora serrata

Group V: very unfavorable
A. Massive tumors involving more than one-half the retina
B. Vitreous seeding

With the advent of the use of systemic chemotherapy together with local ophthalmic therapies in the 1990s, it became evident that this grouping system was not useful in stratifying patients with respect to outcome following these newer treatment modalities. Therefore, newer treatment protocols are using the International Classification System for Intraocular Retinoblastoma, which is based on the extent and location of intraocular retinoblastoma. A preliminary version of this classification system is shown in Table 23.3.

TREATMENT

To maximize the preservation of useful vision, treatment should be undertaken in specialized centers, where there is collaboration between pediatric oncology and pediatric ophthalmology. The initial therapy for retinoblastoma is dependent on both

Table 23-3. International Classification System for Intraocular Retinoblastoma

GROUP A: Small intraretinal tumors away from foveola and disc
GROUP B: All remaining discrete tumors confined to the retina
GROUP C: Discrete local disease with minimal subretinal or vitreous seeding
GROUP D: Diffuse disease with significant vitreous or subretinal seeding
GROUP E: Presence of any one or more of these poor prognostic features:
Tumor touching the lens
Tumor anterior to the anterior vitreous face involving ciliary body or anterior segment
Diffuse infiltrating retinoblastoma
Neovascular glaucoma
Opaque media from hemorrhage
Tumor necrosis with aseptic orbital cellulites
Phthisis bulbi

the intraocular and extraocular extent of the disease. Therapeutic modalities include the following and a combined modality approach is not uncommon:

1. Systemic chemotherapy
2. External beam radiotherapy
3. Local ophthalmic therapy, including local administration of chemotherapy
4. Enucleation.

Treatment of Intraocular Retinoblastoma

Systemic Chemotherapy

For intraocular retinoblastoma, chemotherapy is used in a neoadjuvant setting, often in combination with local ophthalmic therapies, where its purpose is to decrease tumor size and volume to allow the successful utilization of local ophthalmic therapies. In this setting, it is often referred to as *chemoreduction*. Systemic chemotherapy can also be used in combination with enucleation, where one eye is enucleated and chemotherapy is delivered to treat tumors in the remaining eye. Chemotherapy regimens generally include vincristine, etoposide, and carboplatin (Table 23-4).

External Beam Radiotherapy

Standard of care for intraocular retinoblastoma for many years has included external beam radiotherapy with doses of 40–45 Gy. This resulted in a number of late effects and increased risk of second malignancies both in and out of the field of radiotherapy. Newer methods of delivering radiotherapy with more conformal fields are being used at present, so that the normal structures receive less scatter and thus the risk for

Table 23-4. Adjuvant Chemotherapy Protocol for Intraocular Retinoblastoma[a]

Six cycles of the following are given every 28 days:
Vincristine 0.05 mg/kg (1.5 mg/m^2 if ≥age 3 years) on day 1
Carboplatin 18.6 mg/kg (360 mg/m^2 if ≥age 3 years) on day 1
Etoposide 5 mg/kg (150 mg/m^2 if ≥age 3 years) on days 1 and 2

[a]Ongoing protocols are evaluating the utility of higher doses of carboplatin and etoposide for patients with group C or D disease. Ongoing protocols for patients with group B disease are evaluating the elimination of etoposide from this regimen. There are other protocols that include cyclosporin A aimed at decreasing drug resistance.

adverse long-term outcomes will be less. Conformal radiotherapy, stereotactic radiotherapy, proton beam radiotherapy, and intensity-modulated radiation therapy all use technology that minimizes doses to nontarget structures. In addition, there are current protocols testing doses of 23–36 Gy with encouraging results. Increased risk of secondary malignancy is reduced when radiation is given after 1 year of age to children with retinoblastoma. The use of systemic neoadjuvant chemotherapy may allow delay of external beam radiotherapy to until after 1 year of age.

Local Ophthalmic Therapies

Local therapy is used to eradicate local disease after reduction of the tumor volume by chemotherapy and may include cryotherapy, green laser, infrared laser, and/or radioactive plaque. The goal of local therapy is to achieve a type I regression pattern with calcification or type IV with flat chorioretinal scars, or avascular, linear, white gliosis.

Cryoablation

Cryotherapy can be utilized after chemotherapy for ablating tumor remnants/recurrences up to 3 mm in height that are located at or anterior to the equator. It is recommended that no more than four different sites be frozen in one eye at a single session. There is less likelihood of creating vitreous seeds with cryotherapy if a tumor has been previously treated with chemotherapy. Extensive cryotherapy has been associated with significant persistent retinal detachment, particularly if the retina was originally detached prior to chemotherapy. Retinal breaks can be caused by cryotherapy.

Green Laser Photoablation

Green laser (argon or 532-nm frequency-doubled YAG) photoablation can be used to directly coagulate tumors up to 8 mm in thickness, especially posterior to the equator following chemotherapy. The tumor is outlined with burns half on and half off the retina. There should be a 30% spot overlap. After outlining the tumor, the entire tumor should be covered with 30% overlapping spots. Complete coverage is considered "one laser treatment." Each numbered lesion should receive a minimum of three complete "laser treatments" with only one "complete laser treatment" given at each session. Laser-induced hemorrhage has been associated with vitreous seeding. Inadequate dilation of the pupil can cause laser burns to the iris.

Infrared Laser Photoablation

Infrared laser photoablation can be selected to treat tumors up to 8 mm in thickness that have an intact retinal pigment epithelium following chemoreduction. The use of excessive power may result in hemorrhage or vitreous dissemination of tumor, but starting with low power and gradually increasing avoids these problems.

Episcleral Plaque Radiotherapy

Plaque radiotherapy may be used to treat local recurrences up to 8 mm in thickness and 15 mm in base. Iodine-125 or ruthenium-106 can be utilized for plaques. The tumor dose is prescribed at the apex of the tumor. The total dose to the tumor apex is 30–35 Gy. Proliferative retinopathy secondary to plaque can occur.

Subtenon Chemotherapy

For patients with more advanced intraocular disease (Resse-Ellsworth group V; international classification groups C and D), pilot studies have been conducted using subtenon carboplatin in addition to systemic chemotherapy and other local ophthalmic therapies. The ophthalmologist makes a 3-mm incision in the conjunctiva and anterior tenons. A 5-cc syringe containing the carboplatin is fitted with an olive-tip irrigating cannula. The olive-tip cannula is placed through the conjunctival incision and is gently and bluntly passed through the posterior tenon's capsule while maintaining constant contact with the globe. Once the irrigating cannula has been passed posteriorly to its full extent, the opening in the conjunctiva and tenons is pulled tightly over the shank of the needle with a forceps and the carboplatin is slowly delivered into the retrobulbar space by gentle pressure on the syringe plunger. The cannula is withdrawn once the retrobulbar injection is complete. No sutures are necessary on the conjunctival incision but that is the surgeon's choice. A combination antibiotic ointment should be instilled into the conjunctival sac on completion of the injection. While the early results of such studies are promising, larger trials are required to fully evaluate efficacy.

Enucleation

Enucleation of the eye is recommended when there is no chance for useful vision even if the entire tumor is destroyed. It is also indicated with high features where risk of development of extraocular or metastatic disease is high.

Careful examination of the enucleated specimen by an experienced pathologist is necessary to determine if high-risk features for metastatic disease are present. These include:

1. Anterior chamber seeding
2. Choroidal involvement
3. Tumor beyond the lamina cribrosa
4. Intraocular hemorrhage or
5. Scleral and extrascleral extension.

External beam radiotherapy or systemic adjuvant therapy is generally required in patients with certain high-risk features assessed by pathologic review after enucleation to prevent the development of metastatic disease. Adjuvant therapy with external beam radiotherapy and chemotherapy is required if there is tumor at the cut end of the optic nerve.

Treatment of Extraocular Retinoblastoma

In the United States, a minority of patients with retinoblastoma presents with extraocular disease. Extraocular disease may be localized to the soft tissues surrounding the eye or to the optic nerve beyond the margin of resection. However, further extension may occur into the brain and meninges with subsequent seeding of the spinal fluid, as well as distant metastatic disease involving the lungs, bones, and bone marrow. In patients with the genetic form of retinoblastoma, central nervous system (CNS) disease is less likely the result of metastatic or regional spread than another primary intracranial focus, such as a pineoblastoma, associated with the trilateral retinoblastoma syndrome.

There is no clearly proven effective therapy for the treatment of extraocular retinoblastoma. Clinical trials are now under way to improve the overall dismal outcome (survival of approximately 10%) for this group of patients. Those with CNS metastases appear to do worse than those with other forms of extraocular disease. In the past, chemotherapy has included conventional doses of vincristine, cyclophosphamide, and doxorubicin, and, although they produce an initial response, relapse is common. Carboplatin, ifosfamide, and etoposide have shown more promise for remission and a regimen similar to that used for relapsed Wilms' tumor (see Chapter 19, page 556) can be employed. Other induction regimens include the use of cisplatin or carboplatin together with etoposide, cyclophosphamide, and vincristine. There is no recommended standard regimen, and it is largely based on institutional preference. Generally, induction chemotherapy is given for four cycles and this is followed by high-dose chemotherapy followed by stem cell rescue. Following recovery from stem cell transplantation, radiotherapy is generally given to sites of initial bulky disease. As with induction regimens, there is no standard stem cell transplant regimen. A regimen using etoposide, carboplatin, and melphalan such as that used to treat relapsed Wilms' tumor (see Chapter 19, pages 556–557) is used by some centers. Others use regimens of carboplatin, thiotepa, and etoposide or carboplatin, etoposide, and cyclophosphamide or carboplatin, thiotepa, and topotecan (Table 23-5).

Treatment of Recurrent Retinoblastoma

The prognosis for a patient with recurrent or progressive retinoblastoma depends on the site and extent of the recurrence or progression. Responses as high as 85% have been reported following treatment with etoposide and carboplatin. If the recurrence or progression of retinoblastoma is confined to the eye and is small, the prognosis for sight and survival may be excellent with local ophthalmic therapy only. If the recurrence or progression is confined to the eye but is extensive, the prognosis for sight is poor; however, the survival remains excellent. If the recurrence or progression is extraocular, the prognosis is more guarded and the treatment depends on many factors and individual patient considerations.

POST-TREATMENT MANAGEMENT
Disease-Related Follow-Up

Patients should be monitored for follow-up of the primary tumor. The majority of recurrences appears within 3 years of diagnosis and recurrences are extremely rare after 5 years of age. The follow-up schedule is largely dependent on the therapy used and the extent of original disease. For example, children who are treated with neoadjuvant chemotherapy and local ophthalmic therapies, who retain their eye and are

Table 23-5. Potential Preparative Chemotherapy Regimens for Stem Cell Transplant for Metastatic Retinoblastoma[a]

Carboplatin–etoposide–cyclophosphamide
   Carboplatin 250–350 mg/m^2/day on days 1–5
   Etoposide 350 mg/m^2 on days 1–5
   Cyclophosphamide 1.6 g/m^2/day on days 2–5

Carboplatin–thiotepa–etoposide
   Carboplatin 500 mg/m^2/day or dosed to attain an area under the curve
      of 7 mg/min/mL using the Calvert formula on days 1–3
   Thiotepa 300 mg/m^2/day on days 1–3
   Etoposide 250 mg/m^2 on days 1–3

   All are followed by infusion of autologous stem cells.
   [a]Many alternative preparative regimens are available and no current data to support any one as a standard of care.

not treated with external beam radiotherapy, require closer follow-up than children who have undergone an enucleation and for whom pathology failed to show any high-risk features.

For patients treated with chemotherapy for intraocular or extraocular disease, an evaluation under anesthesia (EUA) is recommended to be performed every 3–4 weeks until there is no active tumor seen on a minimum of three EUAs, then every 6–8 weeks until age 3 years, then every 4–6 months to age 10 years. Patients should be transitioned to an office exam without anesthesia when old enough to cooperate.

For patients who have undergone an enucleation and/or received external beam radiotherapy, an evaluation should be performed 4–6 weeks post-treatment, then every 2–3 months for the first year post-therapy, every 3–4 months the following year, every 6 months until age 5 years, and then annually. For patients with extraocular disease, assessment for recurrent metastatic disease should also be performed, which should include CT or MRI of the brain and orbits, CSF evaluation, bone marrow evaluation, and bone scan.

To screen for trilateral retinoblastoma, patients diagnosed with bilateral retinoblastoma, especially those diagnosed at less than 1 year of age, or those with positive family history are recommended to have a head CT or MRI every 6 months from the end of therapy, continuing until 5 years of age.

Toxicity-Related Follow-Up

This is largely dependent on the therapy received. For those treated with chemotherapy or radiation therapy, a history and physical examination should be performed at least every 3 months until 2 years off therapy, then every 6 months until 5 years off therapy, then yearly. A visual acuity assessment should be conducted at least yearly. Attention should be made for late effects of chemotherapy and radiotherapy, growth and development, and surveillance for SMNs. Parents (and patients as they get older) should be counseled regarding their risk of SMN and should have a comprehensive risk-directed evaluation annually lifelong.

If systemic chemotherapy has been used, follow-up laboratory studies may be indicated, dependent on the agent given. After treatment with the most common chemotherapy agents used now for retinoblastoma—vincristine, etoposide, and carboplatin—a complete blood count with differential, electrolytes, calcium, phosphorus, magnesium, transaminases, and bilirubin is generally conducted at least every 6 months for the first year off therapy and then yearly. If renal functions are abnormal, assessment of glomerular filtration should be performed. If carboplatin has been used, audiology should be performed at the end of therapy and yearly for 2 years. It should only be repeated thereafter if abnormal or if testing was suboptimal.

There is no clear screening known to be effective for SMNs. Patients who have received chemotherapy associated with the occurrence of secondary leukemia (etoposide, alkylating agents, doxorubicin, nitrosoureas) should have an annual blood count with differential performed throughout 10–15 years after exposure. Patients should be made aware of signs and symptoms of the most common second malignancies following retinoblastoma, osteosarcoma, and soft-tissue sarcomas, as well as skin cancers and breast cancer. At this point in time, no routine imaging studies are recommended for surveillance for skin and solid organ tumors. However, careful physical examinations by the patient and physician are clearly indicated for early detection and successful treatment. Guidelines for follow-up for patients treated with systemic chemotherapy for intraocular retinoblastoma are found in Table 23-6.

Table 23-6. Recommended Follow-Up for Patients Treated with Systemic Chemotherapy for Intraocular Retinoblastoma

Months from discontinuing chemotherapy	CT or MRI orbits and brain	Oncology evaluation with attention to growth/development and late effects	Labs	Audiology (if platinum therapy used)	Ophthalmology (at least every 4–6 weeks initially until no tumor progression, then at least every 3 months through age 3 years, then at least every 4–6 months until age 10 years, then at least annually
0	×	×	×	×	×
3		×			×
6	×	×	×		×
9		×			×
12	×	×	×	×	×
15		×			×
18	×	×			×
21		×			×
24	×	×	×	×[a]	×
30	×	×			×
36	×	×	×		×
42	×	×			×
48	×	×	×		×
54	×	×			×
60	×	×	×		×
72		×	×		×
84		×	×		×
96		×	×		×
108		×	×		×
120		×	×		×

[a]Repeat audiology after this point every 6 months until stable for at least 2 years.

FUTURE PERSPECTIVES

Until recently, retinoblastoma was largely a disease managed by ocular oncologists, pediatric ophthalmologists, and radiation oncologists. With the advent of neoadjuvant chemotherapy for intraocular disease and dose-intensive myeloablative protocols for extraocular disease, the role of the pediatric oncologist in the management of this disease is growing. Pediatric oncologists are also well versed in the late effects of therapy and surveillance for second malignant neoplasms. Table 23-7 summarizes the plans for studies within this group. Having a cooperative trials group committee for retinoblastoma will allow for accrual of sufficient numbers of patients across multiple institutions to rigorously test clinical and scientific hypotheses. Standardized databases regarding diagnosis, group and stage determination, treatment, and late effects will be established for the studies. The International Classification System will be validated. Uniform response criteria to local and systemic chemotherapy will be established that will be relevant to clinical outcomes. Long-term outcomes can be studied in a more systematic fashion.

The goal of neoadjuvant systemic chemotherapy is to avoid high-dose external beam radiotherapy and enucleation and the acute and long-term effects associated

Table 23-7. Initiatives of the Children's Oncology Group Retinoblastoma Committee

Patient population	Trial and goals	Current expected outcome
Unilateral enucleation pathology	Biology studies of specimens Adjuvant chemotherapy for those with high-risk features for development of metastatic disease	Fewer than 5% of patients will develop metastatic disease
Group B	Reduction in systemic chemotherapy to decrease late effects (ARET0331)	EFS[a] 96%
Group C/D	Intensification of systemic chemotherapy; inclusion of subtenon carboplatin; inclusion of lower dose radiotherapy using stereotactic or IMRT for selected patients to improve eye salvage (ARET0231)	EFS[a] Group C 70% EFS[a] Group D 30%
Extraocular disease	Intensification of systemic chemotherapy, using myeloablative therapy with stem cell support to improve patient survival	EFS[b] 0–40%

[a]Survival without requiring enucleation or external beam radiotherapy;
[b]typical event-free survival including relapse, death from disease.

with both. It is only with these cooperative group studies that long-term data can be systematically collected to demonstrate that changes in approach toward eye salvage provide an acceptable acute toxicity profile, while decreasing risks for adverse late outcomes. Biologic samples will be obtained to better understand retinoblastoma genetics and to test new treatment strategies.

SUGGESTED READINGS

Abramson DH, Frank CM, Dunkel IJ. A phase I/II study of subconjunctival carboplatin for intraocular retinoblastoma. Ophthalmol 1999;106(10):1947–50.

Bunin GR, Meadows AT, Emanuel BS, Buckley JD, Woods WG, Hammond GD. Pre- and postconception factors associated with sporadic heritable and nonheritable retinoblastoma. Cancer Res 1989;49(20):5730–5.

Dunkel IJ, Aledo A, Kernan NA, Kushner B, Bayer L, Gollamudi SV, Finlay JL, Abramson DH. Successful treatment of metastatic retinoblastoma. Cancer 2000;89(10):2117–21.

Friedman DL, Himelstein B, Shields CL, Shields JA, Needle M, Miller D, Bunin GR, Meadows AT. Chemoreduction and local ophthalmic therapy for intraocular retinoblastoma. J Clin Oncol 2000;18(1):12–7.

Gallie BL, Budning A, DeBoer G, Thiessen JJ, Koren G, Verjee Z, Ling V, Chan HS. Chemotherapy with focal therapy can cure intraocular retinoblastoma without radiotherapy. Arch Ophthalmol 1996;114(11):1321–8.

Hurwitz RL, Shields CL, Shields JA, Chevez-Barrios P, Hurwitz MY, Chintagumpala, MM. Retinoblastoma. In: Pizzo PA, Poplack DG, editors. Principles and Practice of Pediatric Oncology. 4th ed. Philadelphia: Lippincott Williams and Wilkins, 2002; 825–46.

Knudson AG. Cancer genetics. Am J Med Genet 2002;111(1):96–102.

Moll AC, Imhof SM, Schouten-Van Meeteren AY, Kuik DJ, Hofman P, Boers M. Second primary tumors in hereditary retinoblastoma: a register-based study, 1945–1997: is there an age effect on radiation-related risk? Ophthalmol 2001;108(6):1109–14.

Murphree AL, Villablanca JG, Deegan III WF, Sato JK, Malogolowkin M, Fisher A, Parker R, Reed E, Gomer CJ. Chemotherapy plus local treatment in the management of intraocular retinoblastoma. Arch Ophthalmol 1996;114(11):1348–56.

Namouni F, Doz F, Tanguy ML, et al. High-dose chemotherapy with carboplatin, etoposide, and cyclophosphamide followed by a haematopoietic stem cell rescue in patients with high-risk retinoblastoma: a SFOP and SFGM study. Eur J Cancer 1997;33(14):2368–75.

Rodriguez-Galindo C, Wilson MW, Haik BG, Lipson MJ, Cain A, Merchant TE, Kaste S, Pratt CB. Treatment of metastatic retinoblastoma. Ophthalmol 2003;110(6):1237–40.

Wong FL, Boice Jr. JD, Abramson DH, Tarone RE, Kleinerman RA, Stovall M, Goldman MB, Seddon JM, Tarbell N, Fraumeni Jr. JF, Li FP. Cancer incidence after retinoblastoma. Radiation dose and sarcoma risk. JAMA 1997;278(15):1262–7.

24

MISCELLANEOUS TUMORS

GERM CELL TUMORS

Germ cell tumors are neoplasms that develop from primordial germ cells of the human embryo, which are normally destined to produce sperm or ova. Primordial germ cells appear to originate in the yolk sac endoderm and migrate around the hindgut to the genital ridge on the posterior abdominal wall where they become part of the developing gonad. Figure 24-1 depicts the histogenesis of tumors of germ cell origin. Viable germ cells arrested along this path of migration may form neoplasia in midline sites, such as the pineal region (6%), mediastinum (7%), retroperitoneum (4%), and sacrococcygeal region (42%) or in the ovary (24%), testis (9%), and other sites (8%).

Incidence

Tumors of germ cell origin account for approximately 2–3% of childhood malignancies. The incidence of germ cell tumors is 2.5 per million in white children and 3.0 per million in African-American children under 15 years of age with a male:female ratio of 1.0:1.1. Germ cell tumors are more common in the ovaries and testes than extragonadal sites.

Pathology

The germ cells are the precursors of sperm and ova and retain the potential to produce all the somatic (embryonic) and supporting (extraembryonic) structures of a developing embryo. *Endodermal sinus tumors* are derived from a totipotential germ cell that differentiate to extraembryonic structures. *Teratomas* are embryonal neoplasms that contain tissues from all three germ layers (ectoderm, endoderm, and mesoderm). Teratomas are mature or immature and may occur with or without malignant germ cell elements (endodermal sinus tumor, choriocarcinomas, embryonal carcinomas, or germinoma) or rarely malignant somatic elements (such as neuroblastoma in children).

The malignant histologic variants of germ cell tumors in order of increasing malignant behavior are:

1. Germinoma
   a. Dysgerminoma (ovary)
   b. Seminoma (testis)
2. Immature teratoma

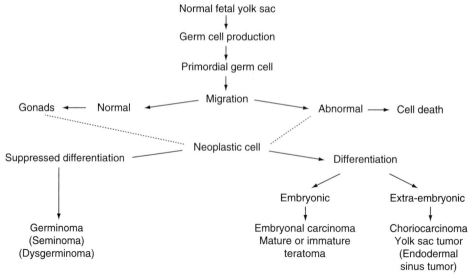

Fig. 24-1. Histogenesis of tumors of germ cell origin.

3. Embryonal carcinoma
4. Endodermal sinus tumor (yolk sac tumor)
5. Choriocarcinoma.

Table 24-1 describes the pathology of germ cell tumors and associated biochemical markers. Cytogenetic analysis has identified i(12p) as a specific abnormality in more than 80% of germ cell tumors.

Clinical Features

The signs and symptoms of germ cell tumors are dependent on the site of origin. Table 24-2 lists the clinical features of germ cell tumors at different sites. In addition, certain histologic variants may have associated clinical findings, as listed in Table 24-3.

Although germ cell tumors are a diverse group histologically, all originate from primordial germ cells and have a common pattern of spread, irrespective of the primary site as follows:

1. Lungs
2. Liver
3. Regional nodes
4. Central nervous system (CNS)
5. Bone and bone marrow (less commonly).

Most recurrences develop within 2 years.

Diagnostic Evaluation

The following evaluations should be carried out:

1. History
2. Physical examination
3. Complete blood count (CBC)
4. Liver function tests, electrolytes, blood urea nitrogen (BUN), creatinine
5. α-Fetoprotein (AFP)
6. Human chorionic gonadotropin (β-hCG)

Table 24-1. Pathology of Germ Cell Tumors and Associated Markers

Histologic variant	Morphology	Common sites of origin	Markers*		
			AFP	β-hCG	PLAP
Germinoma	Cells are round with discrete membranes, abundant clear cytoplasm. Round nucleus with one to several prominent nucleoli. Cells arranged in nest or lobules separated by fibrous stroma. Areas of necrosis with granulomatous reaction. Multinucleated giant cells may be present.	Ovary: dysgerminoma Testis: seminoma Anterior mediastinum	–	–	+
Mature teratoma	Mature tissue derived from Ectoderm: squamous epithelium, neuronal tissue Mesoderm: muscle, teeth, cartilage, bone Endoderm: mucous glands, gastrointestinal and respiratory tract lining No mitoses seen	Sacrococcygeal/presacral Gonads Mediastinum	–	–	–
Immature teratoma	Immature tissue derived from the three germinal layers. Lesions are graded histologically: Grade 1: Some immaturity with neuroepithelium absent or limited to a rare low magnification (×40) field and not more than one such field in any slide Grade 2: Immaturity and neuroepithelium present but does not exceed three low-power microscopic fields in any slide Grade 3: Immaturity and neuroepithelium prominent; occupying four or more low-magnification microscopic fields	Sacrococcygeal/presacral Gonads Mediastinum	–	–	–
Embryonal carcinoma	Tumor cells polygonal with abundant pink vacuolated cytoplasm with ill-defined cellular membranes. Nucleus irregular and pleomorphic with prominent nucleoli. Cells arranged in solid sheets with scanty stroma or in tubules, acini, or papillary structures. Typical and atypical mitoses present.	Testis (young adult)	–	±	±

(Continues)

647

Table 24-1. (*Continued*)

Histologic variant	Morphology	Common sites of origin	Markers*		
			AFP	β-hCG	PLAP
Endodermal sinus	Five characteristics are seen microscopically:	Testis (infant)	+	–	–
	1. Aggregates of small undifferentiated embryonal cells	Ovary			
	2. Areas of stellate mesodermal cells	Presacral			
	3. Areas of perivascular formation consisting of a mesodermal core with a capillary in the center lined by columnar cells (Schuller–Duvall body)				
	4. Cystic structures that form small cavities lined by flat cells continuous with the parietal lining of the endodermal sinuses				
	5. Intra- and extracellular hyaline globules that are PAS positive and that contain α-fetoprotein, α₁-antitrypsin, albumin, or transferrin as demonstrated by immunohistochemical staining				
Choriocarcinoma	Presence of	Ovary	–	+	–
	1. Syncytiotrophoblastic cells that have multiple hyperchromatic nuclei and abundant eosinophilic cytoplasm	Mediastinum			
	AND	Pineal region			
	2. Cytotrophoblasts that have a single nucleus with abundant clear cytoplasm and well-defined cell borders. The two cell populations are often arranged in biphasic plexiform pattern				

*AFP, α-Fetoprotein; β-hCG, human chorionic gonadotropin; PLAP, placental alkaline phosphatase.

Table 24-2. Clinical Features of Germ Cell Tumors

Tumor type	Median age (yr)	Relative frequency (%)	Features
Pediatric ovarian tumors			
Dysgerminoma	16	24	Rapidly developing; 14–25% with other germ cell elements; very radiosensitive
Endodermal sinus tumor	18	16	↑ AFP; 75% stage I; all patients require chemotherapy because of high risk of relapse even in low-stage disease
Teratoma			
Mature (solid, cystic)	10–15	31	Neuroglial implants may occur with cystic or solid teratomas, but do not affect prognosis; surgery is mainstay of treatment
Immature	11–14	10	Grading system based on amount of neuroepithelium present; prognosis inversely related to stage and grade; 30% with ↑ AFP
Embryonal carcinoma	14	6	47% prepubertal; ↑ β-hCG and precocious puberty common; chemotherapy indicated
Malignant mixed germ cell tumor	16	11	40% premenarchal; 30% sexually precocious; AFP/β-hCG may be increased
Gonadoblastoma	8–10	1	Associated with dysgenetic gonads and sexual maldevelopment; removal of both gonads is treatment of choice
Other (polyembryoma, choriocarcinoma)	NA	<1	Rare in children
Pediatric testicular tumors			
Endodermal sinus tumor	2	26	Most common of malignant germ cell tumors of the testes; ↑AFP; compared to adult cases, pediatric tumors are pure histologically; 85% stage I; chemotherapy reserved for higher stage or recurrent disease
Teratoma	3	24	Poorly differentiated histologic features do not impart a malignant course in children. Surgery alone is usually sufficient treatment
Embryonal carcinoma	Late teens	20	Uncommon in young children; ↑AFP ± β-hCG; managed as for adults, with retroperitoneal lymphadenectomy ± chemotherapy ± irradiation based on stage
Teratocarcinoma	Late teens	13	80% stage I with 75% survival after surgery alone; more advanced disease requires multimodality therapy
Gonadoblastoma	5–10	<1	Associated with sexual maldevelopment syndromes; bilateral involvement in 30%; bilateral removal of gonads is treatment of choice
Other (seminoma, mixed germ cell tumor, choriocarcinoma)	NA	16	Rare in children

Abbreviations: AFP, α-fetoprotein; β-hCG, human chorionic gonadotropin
From Pizzo PA, Poplack DG, editors. Principals and Practice of Pediatric Oncology. 4th ed. Philadelphia: Lippincott-Raven, 2002, with permission.

Table 24-3. Clinical Association of Different Histologic Variants of Germ Cell Tumors

Histology	Clinical association
Teratoma	Musculoskeletal anomalies
	Rectal stenosis
	Congenital heart disease
	Microcephaly
Ovarian dysgerminoma (postpubertal)	Amenorrhea
	Menorrhagia
	46XY (male pseudohermaphrodite)
Ovarian embryonal carcinoma	Precocious puberty
	Amenorrhea
	Hirsutism

7. Lactic dehydrogenase (LDH) isoenzyme 1
8. Radiographic evaluation of primary site and regional disease:
   a. Mediastinum—chest and upper abdominal computed tomography (CT)
   b. Ovary—pelvic and abdominal CT
   c. Sacrococcygeum—pelvic and abdominal CT
   d. Testis—ultrasound, pelvic and abdominal CT
9. Radiographic evaluation for distant metastases:
   a. Chest radiographs (posteroanterior and lateral)
   b. Chest CT
   c. Bone scan.

Tumor Markers

Certain histologic variants of germ cell tumors secrete the tumor markers AFP and β-hCG. The production of these markers can be assessed by immunohistologic staining of tissue sections or measurement of blood levels, and they have important diagnostic value.

AFP is a major serum protein of the human fetus. It is produced in the embryonic liver, in the yolk sac, and, in smaller amounts, in the gastrointestinal tract. In general, the highest AFP levels are seen in endodermal sinus tumor with embryonal carcinoma exhibiting intermediate levels.

The beta subunit of human chorionic gonadotropin (β-hCG) can serve as a tumor marker when positive. It may be positive when syncytiotrophoblasts are present in the tumor, and it is found to be elevated in embryonal carcinomas, endodermal sinus tumors, and choriocarcinomas. In choriocarcinoma, there is generally a marked elevation of β-hCG.

Tissue staining and/or measurements of the serum levels of AFP and β-hCG are extremely useful in evaluating teratomas. Pure teratomas are not associated with AFP or β-hCG production; elevation of either marker in association with teratoma indicates the presence of more malignant germ cell elements and requires review of the histologic material or study of more histologic sections. α-Fetoprotein is difficult to evaluate as an indicator of residual or recurrent germ cell tumors in infants less than 8 months of age. Some infants' malignant germ cell tumors do not produce it. The half-life of AFP also varies with age: 5.5 days at birth to 2 weeks of age, 11 days from 2 weeks to 2 months of age, and 33 days from 2 to 4 months of age. The half-life of AFP (beyond 8 months of age) and β-hCG is 5 days and 16 hours, respectively.

AFP and β-hCG levels are useful for clinical evaluation and for assessing disease activity. Table 24-4 lists the mean and standard deviation of normal serum AFP levels of infants at various ages. Increasing levels of serum AFP are not necessarily indicative of tumor progression because abrupt escalation in serum AFP can occur after chemotherapy-induced tumor lysis. Elevations of serum AFP could also be caused by alterations in hepatic function such as viral hepatitis, cirrhosis, hepatoblastoma, pancreatic and gastrointestinal (GI) malignancies, and lung cancers. β-hCG can also experience sudden increases secondary to cell lysis during chemotherapy or can be increased with malignancies of the liver, pancreas, GI tract, breast, lung, and bladder. The utility of CA-125 in monitoring ovarian germ cell tumors in children has not been thoroughly evaluated.

LDH may also correlate with disease activity such as:

- Tumor bulk
- Residual tumor after surgery
- Response to chemotherapy and radiotherapy
- Tumor recurrence.

Staging

The staging systems for germ cell tumors differ depending on the site of origin and are listed in Table 24-5.

Treatment

The treatment strategies for germ cell tumors depend on:

- Histologic subtype
- Site of origin
- Stage of disease.

Germinoma

Germinoma is the most common pure malignant germ cell tumor. It has been designated *seminoma* when it occurs in the testes, *dysgerminoma* when it involves the ovary,

Table 24-4. Mean and Standard Deviation of Normal Serum α-Fetoprotein of Infants at Various Ages

Age	Mean ± SD	(ng/mL)
Premature	134,734	± 41,444
Newborn	48,406	± 34,718
Newborn–2 weeks	33,113	± 32,503
2 weeks–1 month	9,452	± 12,610
2 months	323	± 278
3 months	88	± 87
4 months	74	± 56
5 months	46.5	± 19
6 months	12.5	± 9.8
7 months	9.7	± 7.1
8 months	8.5	± 5.5

Abbreviation: SD, standard deviation.

From Wu JT, Book L, Sudar K: Serum α-fetoprotein (AFP) levels in normal infants. Pediatr Res 1981;15:50–2, with permission.

Table 24-5. Staging Systems for Germ Cell Tumors

Stage	Extent of disease
Extragonadal	
I	Complete resection at any site, including coccygectomy for sacrococcygeal site; negative tumor margins; tumor markers positive but fall to normal or markers negative at diagnosis; lymphadenectomy negative for tumor
II	Microscopic residual disease; lymph nodes negative; tumor markers positive or negative
III	Gross residual or biopsy only; retroperitoneal nodes negative or positive; tumor markers positive or negative
IV	Distant metastases, including liver
Ovarian	
I	Limited to ovary or ovaries; peritoneal washings negative for malignant cells; no disease beyond ovaries; presence of gliomatosis peritonei[a] does not result in changing stage I disease to a higher stage; tumor markers normal after appropriate half-life decline (AFP, 5 days; β-hCG, 16 hours)
II	Microscopic residual or positive lymph nodes (≤2 cm); peritoneal washings negative for malignant cells; presence of gliomatosis peritonei does not result in changing stage II disease to a higher stage; tumor markers positive or negative
III	Lymph node involvement (metastatic nodule) >2 cm; gross residual or biopsy only; contiguous visceral involvement (omentum, intestine, bladder); peritoneal washings positive for malignant cells; tumor markers positive or negative
IV	Distant metastases, including liver
Testicular	
I	Limited to testes; complete resection by high inguinal orchiectomy or trans-scrotal orchiectomy with no spill at surgery; no clinical, radiographic, or histologic evidence of disease beyond the testes; tumor markers normal after appropriate half-life decline; patients with normal or unknown tumor markers at diagnosis must have a negative ipsilateral retroperitoneal node dissection to confirm stage I disease
II	Trans-scrotal orchiectomy with gross spill of tumor; microscopic disease in scrotum or high in spermatic cord (≤5 cm from proximal end); retroperitoneal lymph node involvement (≤2 cm); increased tumor markers after appropriate half-life decline
III	Retroperitoneal lymph node involvement (>2 cm) but no visceral or extra-abdominal involvement
IV	Distant metastases, including liver

[a]Peritoneal implants that contain only mature glial elements with no malignant elements.

and when it arises in extragonadal sites such the as pineal region, anterior mediastinum, and retroperitoneum, it is termed *germinoma*. Germinomas comprise 10% of ovarian tumors in children and 15% of all germ cell tumors. Germinomas are the most common malignancy found in undescended testes. Ovarian dysgerminomas are sometimes associated with precocious sexual development, but the majority of patients are developmentally normal.

Ovarian Dysgerminoma

Rapid development of signs and symptoms of an abdominal mass is the usual presentation. Abdominal pain is not common unless torsion is present. Seventy-five percent of patients have stage I disease at presentation. Patterns of spread include contiguous extension and metastasis to regional lymph nodes and rarely to liver and lungs.

Surgery

Dysgerminoma is the only germ cell tumor of the ovary in which there is a high incidence of bilateral ovarian involvement (5–10%). Bilateral involvement is particularly common in women with a Y chromosome and gonadal streaks. Conservative surgery consisting of unilateral salpingo-oophorectomy and wedge biopsy of the contralateral ovary and sampling of regional lymph nodes are recommended for patients with the following criteria:

1. Stage I unilateral encapsulated tumor less than 10 cm in diameter
2. Normal contralateral ovary
3. No evidence of retroperitoneal lymph node metastases
4. No ascites; negative cytology of peritoneal washing
5. Normal female 46XX karyotype.

Patients with stage I disease require no further postsurgical therapy. In the past the standard surgical management of patients with stage II and III disease had been total abdominal hysterectomy (TAH) and bilateral salpingo-oophorectomy (BSO) followed by postoperative radiotherapy. However, because the tumor most commonly affects children and young women, a program employing limited surgery, chemotherapy, and/or radiotherapy may be more appropriate. Such an approach preserves as much endocrine and reproductive function as possible without compromising survival, compared to TAH and BSO plus radiotherapy.

Chemotherapy

Dysgerminoma and seminoma (testicular tumor analogous to dysgerminoma) are responsive to combination chemotherapy. Tables 24-6 and 24-7 list the chemotherapy regimens used for the treatment of germ cell tumors.

The primary chemotherapy approach in patients with stage II and III disease, combined with limited surgery, has been effective in children. This approach has the advantage of preserving as much reproductive and endocrine function as possible without compromising long-term survival. It is recommended for pediatric and adolescent patients with 46XX karyotype.

Radiotherapy

Dysgerminoma is the most radiosensitive of the ovarian germ cell tumors. However, radiation therapy is reserved for patients with persistent disease after chemotherapy.

Table 24-6. Various Chemotherapy Regimens for Germ Cell Tumors

	<12 months of age (every 3 weeks)	≥12 months of age (every 3 weeks)
Regimen 1 (PEB)		
Cisplatin (P)	1.1 mg/kg/IV on days 1, 2, and 3	33.3 mg/m^2/IV on days 1, 2, and 3
Etoposide (E)	5.5 mg/kg/IV on days 1, 2, and 3	167 mg/m^2/IV over days 1, 2, and 3
Bleomycin (B)	0.5 units/kg/IV on day 1	15 units/m^2/IV on day 1
OR		
Regimen 2 (HDP/EB)		
Cisplatin	1.3 mg/kg/IV on days 1–5	40 mg/m^2/IV on days 1–5
Etoposide	3 mg/kg/IV on days 1–5	100 mg/m^2/IV on days 1–5
Bleomycin	0.5 units/kg on day 1	15 units/m^2 on day 1

Note: Disease is evaluated in week 12. If complete remission then discontinue chemotherapy; If partial remission then surgery (week 12) followed by two more cycles of chemotherapy as above (weeks 13 and 16).

Table 24-7. Chemotherapy Regimens for Malignant Germ Cell Tumors

Site	Histology	Therapy
Testicular	Stage I	Radical inguinal orchiectomy only
Testicular	Stage II	PEB or HDP/EB every 3 weeks, ×3 cycles
Testicular	Stages III and IV	PEB or HDP/EB every 3 weeks, ×3 cycles followed by surgery If no disease (CR), discontinue therapy; if PR, 3 more cycles and repeat surgery
Ovarian	Stages I and II	PEB or HDP/EB every 3 weeks ×3 cycles
Ovarian	Stages III and IV	PEB or HDP/EB every 3 weeks, ×3 cycles followed by surgery If CR, discontinue therapy; if PR, 3 more cycles and repeat surgery
Malignant Extragonadal germ cell tumor	Stages I–IV	PEB or HDP/EB every 3 weeks, ×3 cycles followed by surgery If CR, discontinue therapy; if PR, 3 more cycles and repeat surgery
Immature teratoma[a]		Surgery alone

Abbreviations: CR, complete remission; PR, partial remission.
[a]If AFP is increased, chemotherapy as per Table 24-6.

Occasionally, dysgerminomas occur in combination with other malignant germ cell elements such as malignant teratomas, yolk sac tumor, or embryonal carcinoma. Management should be based on the most malignant component present.

Prognosis

The prognosis for ovarian dysgerminoma correlates with extent of disease at diagnosis:

Extent of disease	Five-year survival (%)
Stage I	95
Stage II	75
Stage III	60
Stage IV	33

Extragonadal Germinoma

Incomplete migration of germ cells seems to be responsible for the origin of extragonadal germ cell tumors. Most extragonadal germinomas occur in the mediastinum. In contrast to other germ cell tumors in the mediastinum, hematogenous metastases are rare and the primary therapeutic strategy is aimed at local control.

Surgery

Although excellent cure rates of 70–80% have been reported with mediastinal germinomas treated by surgical excision, most tumors are not resectable because of their size and/or proximity to great vessels and vital structures. In most cases, biopsy or minimal debulking is the only feasible surgical approach.

Radiotherapy

These tumors are radiosensitive and radiation to the mediastinum in the range of 4500–5000 cGy cures approximately 50–60% of patients.

Chemotherapy

Combination chemotherapy has been employed in advanced extragonadal germinomas. Cisplatin is particularly effective with excellent results. The chemotherapy regimens employed are shown in Table 24-6. In patients with large bulky mediastinal masses, an approach using combination chemotherapy with or without radiotherapy (depending on the response to two to three courses of chemotherapy) may improve the results compared to patients treated with radiotherapy alone.

Teratoma

Pathologically, teratomas can be divided into three main groups for the purpose of therapeutic strategies:

1. *Mature teratomas:* These tumors contain mature tissue, and the treatment is surgical excision, irrespective of the site. It is critically important that multiple histologic sections be examined to exclude the presence of focal immature tissue and malignant germ cell elements.
2. *Immature teratomas:* These tumors contain elements of immature tissue and are graded histologically (see Table 24-1). If AFP is increased, chemotherapy, in addition to surgery, is employed.
3. *Teratomas with malignant germ cell elements:* These tumors contain foci of frankly malignant tissue—usually embryonal carcinoma, endodermal sinus tumor, or choriocarcinoma. These lesions are treated in an aggressive multimodal fashion. Chemotherapy improves local and metastatic control. Radiation therapy does not help. Table 24-7 lists the chemotherapy regimen utilized in malignant germ cell tumors.

Sacrococcygeal teratomas are the most common germ cell tumors of childhood and account for 44% of all germ cell tumors and 78% of extragonadal tumors. These tumors are relatively rare with an incidence of 1 in 40,000 live births. Females are more frequently affected. Seventeen percent are malignant at diagnosis and 5% have distant metastases. The average age at diagnosis in the 5% with metastatic disease is 22 months of age. Congenital anomalies and musculoskeletal and CNS defects are seen in up to 18–20% of patients. Sacrococcygeal tumors can be diagnosed antenatally on fetal ultrasound. Large tumors can be associated with congestive cardiac failure and hydrops fetalis due to arteriovenous shunting within the tumor. Because most of these neoplasms are exophytic and are visible externally, approximately 80% are diagnosed within the first month of life.

Tables 24-8 and 24-9 describe, respectively, the anatomic location and histologic grading of sacrococcygeal teratomas. The histology of the malignant component of sacrococcygeal teratomas is almost always embryonal, usually endodermal sinus tumor and embryonal carcinoma. Approximately 17% of sacrococcygeal teratomas are malignant in nature. The incidence of a malignant component of the tumor is related to the type of the tumor, 38% in type IV versus 8% in type I.

Surgery

Complete surgical excision should be performed, which necessitates removal of the entire coccyx. In almost all cases, the tumor is attached to the coccyx and failure to

Table 24-8. Anatomic Location of Sacrococcygeal Teratoma

Type	Location	Malignant histology (%)
I	Tumor predominantly external (sacrococcygeal) with only a minimal presacral component (the most common type)	8
II	Tumor presenting externally but with a significant intrapelvic extension (second in frequency to type I)	21
III	Tumor with minimal external component but with the predominant mass extending into the pelvis and abdomen	34
IV	Tumor internalized presacral tumor without external presentation	38

Table 24-9. Histologic Grading for Sacrococcygeal Teratoma

Grade	Description
0	All tissue mature; no embryonal tissue
1	Rare foci of embryonal tissue not exceeding 1 low-power field per slide
2	Moderate quantity of embryonal tissue and some atypia but not exceeding 3 lower-power fields per slide
3	Large quantity of immature tissue exceeding 3 lower-power fields per slide, with abundant mitoses and cellular atypia

remove the coccyx results in local tumor recurrence in 30–40% of cases. In patients with complete removal where tumors are histologic grade 0 or 1, no further therapy is required. However, continuous monitoring of these patients is required because malignant germ cell tumors can recur either from missed malignant tissue in the original tumor or malignant conversion of residual tumor. In patients with histologic grade 3 or with frankly malignant foci, postsurgical chemotherapy is required.

Radiotherapy

Radiotherapy can produce responses in immature teratoma, but the dose required is in the range of 4500–5000 cGy. Because most patients are under 1 year of age, such high-dose radiation therapy can have severe long-term sequelae. Radiotherapy is, therefore, only recommended for disease that persists after chemotherapy and attempted re-excision.

Chemotherapy

Sacrococcygeal teratoma grade 3 or with malignant foci of embryonal carcinoma or endodermal sinus tumor is responsive to combination chemotherapy. The regimens used are outlined in Table 24-6.

Prognosis

The prognosis of sacrococcygeal teratoma depends on the following factors:

- Age
- Surgical resectability
- Histologic grading.

Patients under 2 months of age have a favorable outlook, because only 7% of tumors in females and 10% in males are malignant. Patients over 2 months of age have a less favorable outlook; the incidence of malignancy is 48% in females and 67% in males. Patients whose tumors are initially resectable have a more favorable outcome. Patients whose disease precludes resectability do poorly, even though these lesions are initially responsive to chemotherapy.

The histologic grading is extremely important. Patients with grade 0, 1, and 2 lesions have a 90–95% cure rate with complete surgical excision (mortality of 5–10% from surgical complications or infection). Patients with grade 3 or malignant embryonal elements have an approximately 45–50% 2-year disease-free survival when treated with surgery and chemotherapy.

Ovarian Teratoma

These tumors comprise 40–50% of the ovarian tumors seen in childhood and adolescence. The clinical behavior of immature ovarian teratoma correlates well with the histologic grading but poorly with the stage.

Surgery

The surgical approach is similar to that for other ovarian tumors. The incidence of bilateral involvement is unusual, but the contralateral ovary should be inspected and biopsied if abnormalities are found on inspection and palpation.

Prognosis

Evidence of overt malignant elements (embryonal carcinoma, endodermal sinus tumor, choriocarcinoma) portends a poorer prognosis and intensive chemotherapy is required.

Mediastinal Teratoma

Mediastinal teratomas are located in the anterior mediastinum. The average age of the pediatric patient is 3 years. They are more common in males. Teratoma subtypes (mature, immature, or malignant) comprise the bulk of the tumor but yolk sac tumor and choriocarcinoma may occasionally be seen. Mediastinal teratomas occasionally have sarcomatous foci resembling rhabdomyosarcoma or undifferentiated sarcoma. These foci are extremely aggressive; therefore, appropriate metastatic survey including serum markers (AFP and β-hCG and LDH) is recommended. Most of these tumors are benign lesions (grade 0).

Surgery

Patients with benign lesions are treated successfully with surgical excision. Patients who have malignant lesions (grade 2 or 3) are not generally amenable to complete surgical excision because of infiltration of surrounding vital structures. In these cases, surgical debulking may be attempted after reduction with chemotherapy.

Chemotherapy

Aggressive chemotherapy is used for those with foci of malignant elements. The combinations appropriate for these patients are shown in Table 24-6.

Radiotherapy

Germ cell tumors of the mediastinum are not especially radiosensitive.

Prognosis

The two critical prognostic factors in mediastinal germ cell tumors are age and histology. In patients under 15 years of age, mediastinal teratomas tend not to metastasize and behave in a benign fashion. In older patients, these tumors behave in a malignant fashion with 50% of patients developing metastases within 1 year.

Immature mediastinal teratomas containing elements of endodermal sinus tumor or choriocarcinoma have a worse prognosis than do those for which only the immature elements are present.

Endodermal Sinus Tumor (Yolk Sac Tumor)

Also termed yolk sac tumor, the endodermal sinus tumor is characteristically pure in children. When present in an extragonadal site, endodermal sinus tumor behaves in a highly malignant fashion. It is important to recognize that foci of endodermal sinus tumor present in immature teratoma require aggressive therapy similar to that for pure endodermal sinus tumor. Endodermal sinus tumors are the most common malignant germ cell tumor in children. The sacrococcygeal area is the major site of involvement in the newborn and infant; the ovary is the most common location for endodermal sinus tumors in older children and adolescents. Testicular endodermal sinus tumors have two peaks of incidence in infancy and adolescence and are the most frequent malignant testicular tumors in children.

Testicular Endodermal Sinus Tumor

This tumor is localized (stage I) in 85% of cases. Overall survival rate is higher than 70%, which seems to correlate with age. The management of this tumor is considered separately in two age groups—under 2 years of age and over 2 years of age—because the clinical behavior of this tumor differs markedly between the two groups.

Patients under 2 years of age
   Surgery. The definitive surgical treatment is inguinal orchiectomy with high ligation of the spermatic cord. Retroperitoneal lymph node dissection is not indicated in young patients with disease limited to the testes because less than 5–6% will have positive retroperitoneal lymph nodes. Retroperitoneal lymph node inspection and dissection are only recommended in those infants who (1) have persistent elevation of AFP and/or β-hCG after radical orchiectomy or (2) have evidence of retroperitoneal disease on ultrasound or CT. In infants with a negative metastatic workup and normal AFP and β-hCG following orchiectomy, no further therapy is required. Close observation with serum AFP and radiologic evaluation of chest and abdomen are indicated because even with normalization of AFP in stage I disease 20–40% false-negative results have been seen and retroperitoneal disease has occurred before elevation of AFP.
   Prognosis. In infants with normal AFP and β-hCG following orchiectomy, the cure rate is 85–90% with surgery alone. In the small number of patients with recurrence, combination chemotherapy can produce subsequent cure.

Patients over 2 years of age
   Surgery. Radical orchiectomy combined with unilateral retroperitoneal lymphadenectomy is recommended for patients with disease clinically confined to the testes, but with an elevated AFP. If on exploration the ipsilateral nodes are clinically involved, the contralateral nodes should be examined. Contralateral nodal involvement is seen in 15–30% of cases when the ipsilateral nodes are involved. In patients with stage II or III disease, initial chemotherapy followed by surgical debulking and possibly retroperitoneal lymphadenectomy should be done.

Table 24-14. Clinical Features of the Various Pathologic Types of Hepatic Tumors

Feature	Hepatoblastoma	Hepatocellular carcinoma	Fibrolamellar variant
Usual age of presentation	0–3 yr	5–18 yr	10–20 yr
Associated congenital anomalies	Dysmorphic features Hemihypertrophy Beckwith–Wiedemann syndrome	Metabolic	None
Advanced disease at presentation	40%	70%	10%
Usual site of origin	Right lobe	Right lobe, multifocal	Right lobe
Abnormal liver function tests	15–30%	30–50%	Rare
Jaundice	5%	25%	Absent
Elevated AFP	60–70%	50%	10%
Positive hepatitis B serology	Absent	Present in some	Absent
Abnormal B$_{12}$-binding protein	Absent	Absent	Present
Chromosomal abnormalities	11p15.5, 18, 17p13, occasional loss of heterozygosity	17q11.2, 20p12, 11q22-23, rare presence of TP53 mutation	Not reported
Distinctive radiographic appearance	None	None	None
Pathology	Fetal and/or embryonal cells + mesenchymal component	Large pleomorphic tumor cells and tumor giant cells	Eosinophilic hepatocytes with dense fibrous stroma

From Pizzo PA, Poplack DG, editors. Principles and Practice of Pediatric Oncology. 4th ed. Philadelphia: JB Lippincott, 2002, with permission.

Table 24-15. Frequency of Signs and Symptoms in Children with Hepatoblastoma and Hepatocarcinoma

Sign/symptom	Hepatoblastoma (%)	Hepatocarcinoma (%)
Abdominal mass	80	60
Abdominal distention	27	34
Anorexia	20	20
Weight loss	19	19
Abdominal pain	15	21
Vomiting	10	10
Pallor	7	Rare
Jaundice	5	10
Fever	4	8
Diarrhea	2	Rare
Constipation	1	Rare
Pseudoprecocious puberty	Occasional	Not reported

All patients should have the following evaluations:

- History
- Physical examination
- Complete blood count (anemia with moderate leukocytosis is commonly seen; thrombocytosis with platelet counts greater than 500,000/mm^3 is the most frequent abnormality)
- Urinalysis
- Liver profile and electrolytes
- Fibrinogen, partial thromboplastin time (PTT), and prothrombin time (PT)
- Hepatitis B surface antigen (HB$_s$Ag), core antigen (HB$_c$Ag), and core antibody
- AFP
- β-hCG
- Carcinoembryonic antigen (CEA)
- Radiographic evaluation of intrahepatic disease: sonogram, abdominal CT, magnetic resonance imaging (MRI)
- Radiographic evaluation of extrahepatic disease: chest radiographs (PA and lateral), chest CT, bone scan
- Bone marrow aspirate/biopsy.

Approximately 90% of children with hepatoblastomas and 50% of children with hepatocarcinoma will have elevated AFP. AFP is a valuable marker for monitoring residual or metastatic disease following resection of the primary tumor or for monitoring the response of an unresectable primary tumor to therapy. AFP is normally elevated in the newborn period and then declines (Table 24-4). Concentrations greater than 500,000 ng/mL of AFP are not unusual in hepatoblastoma. Failure of AFP to return to normal after surgery is an indication of incomplete tumor removal or metastases. Serial determinations of AFP are the most precise measurement of the effectiveness of hepatoblastoma therapy.

β-hCG is measured for the occasional patient with hepatoma who has associated precocious puberty. Unlike AFP, β-hCG levels do not necessarily reflect the clinical course of the tumor.

MRI angiography and MRI cholangiogram are useful complements to CT for evaluation of intrahepatic disease because they aid in determining surgical resectability. In hepatoblastoma, the right lobe of the liver is more commonly involved than the left, but the tumor involves both lobes in 30% of patients.

Approximately 10% of patients with hepatoma will have demonstrable pulmonary metastases on plain radiographs. The widespread use of chest CT has increased the number of patients detected with lung metastases.

Staging

The staging of hepatoma relates to the degree of surgical resectability of the primary lesion and the presence or absence of metastatic disease. Table 24-16 describes the staging system for hepatoma on the basis of these criteria and the percentage of cases.

Treatment

The most effective therapeutic modality for hepatoma is complete resection, but this is possible in only 40–50% of patients. Chemotherapy plays an ancillary role in eradicating subclinical metastases in completely resected disease and chemotherapy plus radiation therapy may be effective in permitting initially unresectable disease to become resectable.

Surgery

The optimal management of hepatoma is complete resection. Patients who are suitable candidates for complete resection include those with:

1. Tumors confined to the right lobe
2. Tumors originating in the right lobe that do not extend beyond the medial segment of the left lobe
3. Tumors confined to the left lobe.

Patients who have tumor involvement of both lobes are not candidates for curative surgical resection. In these cases, biopsy should be performed.

Radical hepatic resection results in many potential postoperative complications, including the following:

- Hypovolemia
- Hypoglycemia
- Hypoalbuminemia
- Hypofibrinogenemia and deficiency of coagulation proteins.

Hyperbilirubinemia persists for 2–4 weeks after resection, and hepatic regeneration is complete by 1–3 months postsurgery.

Table 24-16. Staging of Hepatoma in Children and Percentage of Cases

Stage	Description	Percentage of cases by stage
I	Complete resection of tumor by wedge resection lobectomy or by extended lobectomy as initial treatment	25
II	Tumors rendered completely resectable by initial radiotherapy or chemotherapy	4
	A. Residual disease confined to one lobe	
III	A. Gross residual tumor involving both lobes of liver	48
	B. Regional lymph node involvement	
IV	Metastatic disease irrespective of extent of liver involvement	23

Chemotherapy

Combination chemotherapy plays several roles in the management of hepatoma:

1. Adjuvant therapy for patients who have undergone complete resection, because its use improves disease-free survival
2. Preoperative therapy for patients who have initial unresectable disease to shrink the primary tumor
3. Palliative therapy for patients with metastatic disease at diagnosis.

Table 24-17 lists three commonly used chemotherapy regimens for childhood hepatoma. Regimen 2 has recently been shown to be as effective as regimen 1 with an equivalent survival. Regimen 2 eliminates the use of anthracycline and has minimal toxicity.

Radiation

Radiotherapy is not curative for intrahepatic disease because the effective tumor dose exceeds hepatic tolerance. However, radiotherapy may have value in promoting shrinkage of unresectable disease or microscopic residual disease. Radiation dosages used to treat hepatic tumors have ranged from 1200 to 2000 cGy. Occasionally, higher doses to localized areas of tumor have been associated with tumor regression. Radiotherapy immediately after hepatic resection will limit hepatic regeneration.

Treatment Recommendations

The only patients who have a reasonable chance of cure are those in whom complete resection can be achieved. Every attempt should be made to resect the primary intra-hepatic tumor, even if this requires en bloc resection of contiguous structures.

In patients in whom a complete resection is initially performed, adjuvant chemotherapy should be administered. In patients in whom a complete resection is

---

Table 24-17. Various Combination Chemotherapy Regimens for Hepatomas

Regimen 1 (every 3–4 weeks)
  Adriamycin 25 mg/m^2/day ×3 continuous infusion by central line:
  Cisplatin 20 mg/m^2/day ×5 days continuous infusion, days 0–4 (6 cycles of chemotherapy)
  Patients less than 10 kg receive chemotherapy according to weight:
  Adriamycin 0.83 mg/kg ×3 days; cisplatin 0.66 mg/kg/day for 5 days (6 cycles of chemotherapy)
OR
Regimen 2 (every 3–4 weeks)
  Cisplatin 100 mg/m^2 IV infused over 6 hours, day 1;
  Vincristine 1.5 mg/m^2 IV (max 2 mg), days 3, 10, 17;
  Fluorouracil 600 mg/m^2 IV, day 3;
  Under 1 year of age, Cisplatin 3.3 mg/kg and Vincristine 0.05 mg/kg;
  After 4 cycles, attempt surgical resection, followed by 4 more cycles
OR
Regimen 3 (every 3–4 weeks)
  Cisplatin 90 mg/m^2 IV infused over 6 hours (hours 0–6), day 0;
  Adriamycin 20 mg/m^2/day continuous infusion × 4 days, days 0–3;
  Under 1 year of age, Cisplatin 3 mg/kg;
  Adriamycin 0.66 mg/kg;
  After 4 cycles, attempt surgical resection followed by 4 additional courses of chemotherapy

not possible (biopsy or incomplete removal), every attempt should be made to promote tumor shrinkage and resectability.

Liver Transplantation

Liver transplantation has been used in selected cases of hepatoblastoma that were unresectable.

Prognosis

The factors that determine prognosis include tumor resectability and histology. Using the staging system shown in Table 24-16, the 5-year survival rates are as follows:

Stage	Percentage
I	90
II	100
III	65
IV	40

Histology also influences prognosis, as shown below:

Pathology	Prognosis
Hepatoblastoma—fetal pattern Fibrolamellar carcinoma	Favorable histology
Hepatoblastoma—embryonal pattern Hepatocellular carcinoma	Unfavorable histology

The reduction in AFP level is a good predictor of outcome in patients with unresected tumors who undergo chemotherapy initially because of unresectability. A report from the Children's Cancer Group demonstrated that patients who showed a decline in AFP by 2 logs in the initial four courses of chemotherapy had a 75% survival.

Studies of DNA content have shown that diploid tumors with low proliferation index have a better prognosis than aneuploid tumors and high proliferative index.

SUGGESTED READINGS
Germ Cell Tumors

Ablin AR, Krailo MD, Ramsay NKC, Malogolowkin MH, Issacs H, Raney RB, Adkins J, Hays DM, Benjamin DR, Grosfeld JL, Leiken SL, Deutsch M, Hammond GD. Results of treatment of malignant germ cell tumors in 93 children: a report from the Children's Cancer Study Group. J Clin Oncol 1991;9:1782–92.

Balmaceda C, Heller G, Rosenblum M, et al. Chemotherapy without irradiation: a novel approach for newly diagnosed CNS germ cell tumors: results of an international cooperative trial. J Clin Oncol 1996;12:2908–15.

Beyer J, Kramar R, Mandanas W, et al. High-dose chemotherapy as salvage treatment in germ cell tumors: a multivariate analysis of prognostic variables. J Clin Oncol 1996;14:2638–45.

Cushing B, Giller R, Lauer S, et al. Comparison of high dose or standard dose cisplatin with etoposide and bleomycin (HDPEB versus PEB) in children with stage I–IV extragonadal malignant germ cell tumors (MGCT). Proc Am Soc Clin Oncol 1998;2017.

Cushing B, Giller R, Marina N, et al. Results of surgery alone or surgery plus cisplatin, etoposide and bleomycin (PEB) in children with localized gonadal malignant germ cell tumor (MGCT): a pediatric intergroup report (POG 9048/CCG 8891). Proc Am Soc Clin Oncol 1997;16:511a.

Cushing B, Perlman E, Marina N, Castleberry RP. Germ cell tumors. In: Pizzo PA, Poplack DG, editors. Principles and Practice of Pediatric Oncology. 4th ed. Philadelphia: Lippincott–Raven, 2002.

Hawkins EP. Pathology of germ cell tumors in children. Crit Rev Oncol Hematol 1990;10:165–79.

Malogolowkin MH, Ortega JA, Krailo M, Gonzalez O, Hossein Mahour G, Landing BH, Siegel SE. Immature teratomas: identification of patients at risk for malignant recurrence. J Natl Cancer Inst 1989;81:870–4.

Marina NM, Cushing B, Giller R, Cohen L, et al. Complete surgical excision is effective treatment for children with immature teratomas with or without malignant elements: a Pediatric Oncology Group/Children's Cancer Group intergroup study. J Clin Oncol 1999;17:2137–43.

Motzer RJ, Mazumdar M, Bosl GJ, et al. High-dose carboplatin, etoposide, and cyclophosphamide with autologous bone marrow transplantation in first-line therapy for patient with poor-risk germ cell tumors. J Clin Oncol 1997;15:2546–52.

Nichols CG, Fox EP. Extragonadal and pediatric germ cell tumors in children. North Am Hematol Oncol Clin 1990;5:1189–1209.

Nichols CR, Williams S, Loehrer PJ, et al. A randomized study of cisplatin dose intensity in advanced germ cell tumors: a southeastern and southwest oncology group protocol. J Clin Oncol 1991;9:1163–72.

Teinturier C, Gelez J, Flamant V, Habrand SL, Lemerle S. Pure dysgerminoma of the ovary in childhood: treatment results sequelae. Med Pediatr Oncol 1994;23:1–7.

Hepatoma

Bilk P, Superina R. Transplantation for unresectable liver tumors in children. Transplan Proc 1997;29:2834–6.

Buckley JD, Sather H, Ruccione K, Rogues PCJ, Haas JG, Henderson BE, Hammond GD. A case control study of risk factors for hepatoblastoma: a report from the Children's Cancer Study Group. Cancer 1989;64:1169–76.

Douglass EC, Reynolds M, Finegold M, Cantor AB, Glicksman A. Cisplatin, vincristine, and fluorouracil therapy for hepatoblastoma: a Pediatric Oncology Group study. J Clin Oncol 1993;11:96–9.

Ortega JA, Douglass E, Feusner J, et al. A randomized trial of cisplatin, vincristine, 5-fluorouracil versus cisplatin/doxorubicin IV continuous infusion for the treatment of hepatoblastoma: results from the Pediatric Intergroup Hepatoma study (CCG-8881/POG-8945). Proc Am Soc Clin Oncol 1994;13:A1421.

Ortega JA, Krailo MD, Haas JE, King DR, Ablin AR, Quinn JJ, Feusner J, Campbell JR, Lloyd DA, Cherlow J, Hammond GD. Effective treatment of unresectable or metastatic hepatoblastoma with cisplatin and continuous infusion doxorubicin chemotherapy: a report from the Children's Cancer Study Group. J Clin Oncol 1991;9:2167–76.

Raney B. Hepatoblastoma in children: a review. J Pediatr Hematol Oncol 1997; 19:418–22.

Tomilinson GE, Finegold MJ. Tumors of the liver. In: Pizzo PA, Poplack DG, editors. Principles and Practice of Pediatric Oncology. 4th ed. Philadelphia: Lippincott–Raven, 2002.

25

HEMATOPOIETIC STEM CELL TRANSPLANTATION

Hematopoietic stem cell transplantation (HSCT) has become an accepted therapeutic modality for a wide variety of diseases and is increasingly utilized for the treatment of malignant and nonmalignant disorders. Tables 25-1 and 25-2 list the indications for allogeneic and autologous stem cell transplantation, respectively. Preparation for HSCT involves delivery of high-dose chemotherapy with or without radiation to ablate normal (and abnormal) hematopoiesis and provide sufficient immunosuppression to allow donor cell engraftment.

The rationale for high-dose chemotherapy involves the theory of the steep dose–response curve for many chemotherapeutic agents. Most drugs exhibit a log-linear relationship between tumor cell kill and dose over a certain range, followed by flattening of the curve in the upper dose ranges. For this reason, small changes in dose can produce significant changes in response for chemotherapeutic agents whose major dose-limiting toxicity is myelosuppression. Hematopoietic growth factor support offers the potential to maximize the dose–response effort of high-dose therapy. A 3- to 10-fold increase in drug dose may result in a multiple log increase in tumor cell killing. Multidrug therapy, compared to a single agent, is necessary to overcome tumor heterogeneity and drug resistance.

The most common form of stem cell transplantation to treat leukemia is allogeneic, using a human leukocyte antigen (HLA)–matched histocompatible donor, usually a sibling. Solid tumors have been treated with high-dose chemotherapy followed by autologous bone marrow transplantation (purged or unpurged marrow, depending on whether the bone marrow is actually or potentially invaded with malignant cells) or peripheral blood stem cell transplantation (PBSCT) with concomitant use of hematopoietic growth factors, for example, granulocyte colony-stimulating factor (G-CSF), or granulocyte macrophage colony-stimulating factor (GM-CSF) (see Chapter 26), to reduce the effects of neutropenia caused by escalating doses of chemotherapy.* Exogenous erythropoietin is beneficial in correcting the anemia that may occur for up to 1 year post–allogeneic stem cell transplantation.

Table 25-3 lists the different sources of hematopoietic stem cells for transplantation. Tables 25-4 and 25-5 list the advantages and disadvantages of allogeneic and autologous HSCT, respectively.

---

*G-CSF and GM-CSF stimulate the production, maturation, and function of the myeloid and monocytic cell lineages.

Table 25-1. Indications for Allogeneic Hematopoietic Stem Cell Transplantation

Malignant disorders
Leukemias
1. Acute lymphoblastic leukemia (ALL) in first remission with high risk for relapse (e.g., failure to enter complete remission, Philadelphia chromosome-positive ALL) or in second remission
2. Acute nonlymphoblastic leukemia (AML, ANLL) (after first remission)[a]
3. Chronic myelogenous leukemia—Ph+
   a. Stable phase
   b. Accelerated phase
4. Juvenile chronic myeloid leukemia (JCML)
5. Juvenile myelomonocytic leukemia (JMML)
Lymphomas (second or subsequent complete remission or partial remission)
1. Hodgkin
2. Non-Hodgkin
Myelodysplasia
Myelofibrosis
Familial hemophagocytic lymphohistiocytosis

Nonmalignant disorders
Congenital
1. Immunodeficiency syndromes
   a. Severe combined immunodeficiency syndrome (SCID)
   b. Congenital agammaglobulinemia (Bruton disease)
   c. DiGeorge syndrome
   d. Wiskott–Aldrich syndrome
   e. Chronic mucocutaneous candidiasis
   f. Other immune-mediated disorders such as X-linked lymphoproliferative syndromes, ALPS (Chapter 13)
2. Hematologic disorders
   a. Hemoglobinopathies:
      Sickle cell anemia (selected cases)
      Thalassemia
   b. Fanconi anemia (progressive)
   c. Shwachman–Diamond syndrome
   d. Kostmann agranulocytosis[b]
   e. Diamond–Blackfan anemia
   f. Dyskeratosis congenita
   g. Thrombocytopenia absent radii syndrome (TAR)
   h. Chronic granulomatous disease
   i. Chédiak–Higashi syndrome
   j. CD11/19 deficiency (leukocyte adhesion deficiency)
   k. Neutrophil actin defects
3. Storage diseases (Gaucher disease)[c]
4. Lysosomal diseases
5. Mucolipidosis
6. Mucopolysaccharidoses
7. Infantile osteopetrosis
Acquired
1. Severe aplastic anemia
2. Paroxysmal nocturnal hemoglobinuria

[a]After initial remission in AML, investigators differ regarding the optimum treatment strategy. Comparison of HSCT for HLA-matched sibling donors with patients without such donors who receive chemotherapy demonstrates a significantly better disease-free survival for HSCT (50–57%) compared with those receiving chemotherapy (36–37%). Beyond first remission, HSCT from unrelated donor or mismatched family member is recommended.

[b]G-CSF may be successful in treatment and avoiding HSCT.

[c]Enzyme replacement may avoid HSCT.

Table 25-2. Indications for Autologous Hematopoietic Stem Cell Transplantation

Hematologic malignancies
1. Non-Hodgkin lymphoma
2. Hodgkin disease
3. AML[a] (investigational)
4. CML[a] (investigational)

Solid tumors
1. Neuroblastoma stage IV
2. Ewing sarcoma, primitive neuroectodermal tumor[b]
3. Rhabdomyosarcoma[b]
4. Germ cell tumor[b]
5. Brain tumor
6. Testicular cancer[b]
7. Wilms' tumor[b]

[a]When HLA-compatible donor is not available.

[b]Metastatic disease at presentation but achieved partial remission with conventional chemotherapy or relapsed but has chemosensitive disease.

Table 25-3. Sources of Hematopoietic Stem Cells for Transplantation

1. Allogeneic bone marrow or peripheral blood stem cell (PBSC) using HLA-matched sibling.
2. Allogeneic bone marrow or PBSC using HLA-DR–matched family members other than sibling donors.
3. Syngeneic bone marrow or PBSC (an identical twin).
4. Allogeneic bone marrow or PBSC using HLA-matched unrelated donors.
5. Autologous bone marrow: Patient's own marrow is cryopreserved and reinfused after patient has received aggressive chemotherapy and/or radiation therapy to treat the underlying malignancy *in vivo* purging or *ex vivo* purging.[a]
6. Peripheral blood stem cells. The number of circulating stem cells can be increased by the use of recombinant growth factors, which can increase stem cell numbers by 100-fold prior to apheresis. This induces a more rapid hematopoietic recovery after transplantation.[b]
7. Umbilical cord blood stem cells (always allogeneic). *Ex vivo* expansion of cells in culture to increase the number of CD34+ cells available for transplant has been employed experimentally.
8. Fetal liver stem cells administered to patients *in utero* (26- to 30-week gestation) with severe immunodeficiency and inborn errors of metabolism.

[a]*Ex vivo* purging for removing malignant cells from peripheral blood stem cells or marrow relies on physical (density or velocity sedimentation, filtration), pharmacologic (e.g., 4-hydroperoxycyclophosphamide [4HC]), or immunologic (monoclonal antibodies, magnetic immunobeads) principles.

[b]This is a useful method in patients who have received previous pelvic radiation therapy or because of tumor in the marrow. G-CSF 10 µg/kg/day or GM-CSF 500 mg/m² for 5–7 days can be used to mobilize progenitor cells. Blood progenitor cells can be collected for 2–5 days beginning on day 4 or 5 after initiation of growth factor.

INDICATIONS FOR HEMATOPOIETIC STEM CELL TRANSPLANTATION IN MALIGNANT DISORDERS

Leukemia

Leukemic patients eligible for allogeneic HSCT are divided into standard- and high-risk groups for transplantation.

Table 25-4. Advantages and Disadvantages of Allogeneic Hematopoietic Stem Cell Transplantation

Advantages
1. Lower relapse rate
2. Graft versus leukemia effect[a]

Disadvantages
1. Compatible donor availability limited (approximately 25–30% of siblings are compatible)
2. Graft versus host disease (GVHD), except in syngeneic (identical) twins
3. Increased risk with age
4. Increased risk of cytomegalovirus infection and interstitial pneumonia (this risk is 2.5 times greater in unrelated matched donors compared to matched siblings)
5. Risk of veno-occlusive disease greater in unrelated donors

[a]The relapse rate is 2.5 times lower in allogeneic recipients who have grade II–IV acute GVHD compared to recipients without GVHD. Leukemic cells have been reported to disappear during episodes of acute GVHD.

Table 25-5. Advantages and Disadvantages of Autologous Hematopoietic Stem Cell Transplantation

Advantages
1. No need for an allogeneic donor
2. No GVHD
3. Lower risk of opportunistic infection (e.g., CMV, *Pneumocystis carinii*)

Disadvantages
1. Increased risk of relapse (approximately 50%)
2. No graft versus leukemia effect
3. Graft failure due to:
    a. Effect of *in vitro* purging
    b. Effect of previous chemotherapy and radiotherapy

Standard-Risk Leukemia Group

This group includes patients under 21 years of age with any of the following:

1. Acute myeloblastic leukemia (AML) in first or second remission
2. Acute lymphoblastic leukemia (ALL) in second or subsequent remission
3. High-risk leukemia (Chapter 14) in first remission
4. Chronic myelogenous leukemia (CML) in:
    a. Chronic phase,
    b. Early accelerated stage, or
    c. Chronic phase after treatment for blast crisis
5. Juvenile chronic myelogenous leukemia (JCML) in first remission
6. Juvenile myelomonocytic leukemia (JMML)
7. Myelodysplasia.

High-Risk Leukemia Group

This group includes patients with any of the following:

1. Refractory acute leukemia (failed to achieve remission after two courses of conventional chemotherapy)
2. Acute leukemia in relapse
3. CML in accelerated or blastic phase.

Solid Tumors

Patients with solid tumors with less than a 30% chance of long-term survival with conventional chemotherapy, only if a chemotherapy dose–response relationship is established, should be considered for autologous or allogeneic (if bone marrow is invaded) stem cell transplantation in remission or for minimal residual disease.

ALLOGENEIC TRANSPLANTATION

Donor Selection

Table 25-6 lists the blood bank support necessary for bone marrow transplantation. Any HLA-identical sibling should be considered as a donor. ABO mismatch is not a contraindication, but if multiple donors are available, donors with the same ABO type should be used. Major ABO mismatch (A or B in O) requires removal of the red cells and plasma from the marrow prior to infusion. The HLA match can be

Table 25-6. Blood Bank Support in Bone Marrow Transplantation

Problem	Solution

Transfusion-associated graft versus host disease	Standard: gamma radiation (2500–3000 cGy)
	 Investigational:
	   a. Leukocyte depletion
	   b. Selective T-cell depletion
	   c. Ultraviolet radiation

CMV transmission (CMV-negative donor and recipient)	Standard: use of only CMV-negative blood products through an in-line filter to remove lymphocytes and leukocytes that may harbor latent viruses Alternative: leukocyte-depleted blood products

Alloimmunization
   1. Graft failure or rejection (especially aplastic anemia)
 	
   2. Refractory thrombocytopenia[a]
	Avoidance or minimizing of pretransplant transfusions; avoidance of transfusions from family members, especially potential donors
	 Most effective: leukocyte-depleted blood products
	   a. Single-donor platelets
	   b. Ultraviolet irradiation
	   c. HLA-matched donors
	   d. Cross-matched platelets

ABO incompatibility
   1. Major
     Patient O, donor A-IHT >1:16
     Patient O, donor B-IHT >1:16
   2. Minor
     Patient A, donor O-IHT >1:128
     Patient B, donor O-IHT >1:128
	Removal of red blood cells from donor marrow
	
	 Removal of plasma from donor marrow

Donor red cell transfusion requirements	Autologous red blood cell salvage Predeposition of autologous red blood cell units

Abbreviations: CMV, cytomegalovirus; IHT, isohemagglutinin titer.

From Rowe JM, et al. Recommended guidelines for the management of autologous and allogeneic bone marrow transplantation: a report from the Eastern Cooperative Oncology Group ECOG. Ann Int Med 1994;120:143–58, with permission.

[a]Nonalloimmunization causes of refractory thrombocytopenia include drugs, hepatic veno-occlusive disease, hypersplenism, or sepsis. Another more unusual cause of refractory thrombocytopenia is a syndrome resembling thrombotic thrombocytopenic purpura, often associated with the use of cyclosporine, total body irradiation, or the development of acute GVHD.

phenotypic or genotypic. Finding the right donor necessitates matching of HLA antigens or histocompatibility genes by serology or molecular methodology. The major histocompatibility complex (MHC) is divided into two groups. The class I molecules are HLA-A, HLA-B, and HLA-C and the class II molecules are HLA-DR, HLA-DQ, and HLA-DP. Currently, matching is generally confined to major class I and II loci. However, it is increasingly appreciated that minor histocompatibility antigens are also likely to play important roles in the outcome of allogeneic HSCT. One of the major obstacles in allogeneic HSCT is that 60–70% of patients have no acceptable donors within their families. In these cases, volunteer unrelated or related donors who are HLA, A, B, and DR compatible with the recipients may be available as bone marrow donors worldwide through the U.S. National Marrow Donor Program (NMDP). Partial HLA-matched donors are sometimes used. Immunosuppressive drugs are given after transplantation to inhibit or modify the graft versus host immune reaction.

Histocompatibility Testing

The MHC genes are mapped within a region called HLA (human leukocyte antigen system A) located on the short arm of chromosome 6. Disparity at major loci requires vigorous immunologic intervention to avoid rejection or, should engraftment occur, subsequent graft versus host disease (GVHD).

The class I molecules are composed of an α-chain and β_2-microglobulin, are highly polymorphic, and are expressed on most nucleated cells and on platelets. The HLA class II loci are also highly polymorphic and are involved in exogenous antigen processing. The HLA class II antigens are heterodimeric cell surface molecules formed by the α- and β-chains, each of which is polymorphic. HLA terminology is designated by the World Health Organization (WHO) nomenclature committee for factors of the HLA system and is updated at regular intervals. The broadest designation is on serologic typing, and the highest resolution is based on actual DNA sequence.

Typing of HLA class II alleles can be determined using nucleotide sequence polymorphism. The following different techniques have been used for identification of class I and II polymorphism for determination of bone marrow donor and recipient selection by:

- Sequence-specific oligonucleotide probe (SSOP)
- Sequence specific primer (SSP).

Medical evaluation of bone marrow donors includes:

- Physical examination
- Complete blood count
- Biochemistry profile
- Cytomegalovirus (CMV) antibody, Epstein–Barr virus (EBV) profile, herpes antibody titers, Human T-Lymphotropic Viruses antibody (HTLV)
- Human immunodeficiency virus (HIV) profile
- Hepatitis screen.

Further evaluation is required in 2–20% of donor candidates.

Bone Marrow Harvesting and Transplantation

Bone marrow harvesting is carried out under general or epidural anesthesia using sterile conditions. The posterior and/or anterior iliac crests of the donor are prepared and draped. Approximately 2 mL of bone marrow are aspirated from each site, avoiding dilution with blood by taking multiple aspirates from the anterior and posterior iliac crests. The marrow is collected in a heparinized saline container. The concentration of heparin (preservative free) is 3–5 units/mL of bone marrow. The quantity of nucleated bone marrow cells required to ensure engraftment is $2–5\times10^8$ cells per kilogram of recipient body weight. The usual volume of marrow required to achieve this cell yield is 10–20 mL/kg of recipient body weight. Marrow from children, especially infants, has a higher proportion of marrow-repopulating cells than marrow from older donors. The marrow is filtered through an apparatus that removes bone and tissue fragments and then placed in a blood transfer pack. In allogeneic transplants, the pack containing the bone marrow is then given to the recipient as an intravenous infusion over a period of a few hours.

For autologous bone marrow transplantation, some form of processing to remove the erythrocytes* is necessary prior to the collected marrow being cryopreserved at either –80°C or –139°C. At this temperature, the marrow can be preserved for periods of up to 10 years or possibly longer. The cryopreserved bone marrow is thawed at the bedside in a 37°C water bath and given intravenously to the recipient over a period of a few minutes to an hour, depending on the volume infused.

Peripheral blood stem cells (PBSC) have been collected from autologous donors after stimulation with G-CSF or GM-CSF and have been successfully used to reconstitute hematopoiesis in recipients of autologous, syngeneic, and allogeneic grafts who undergo a myeloablative preparative regimen. Patients who receive more than 5×10^6 CD34+ cells/kg engraft satisfactorily.

Umbilical cord blood (UCB) has been collected, cryopreserved, and used as the source of pluripotential hematopoietic stem cells when a related or unrelated stem cell donor is not available. UCB cells have increased proliferative capacity and decreased alloreactivity with a lower incidence of GVHD. This property, coupled with an absence of donor risk, is an advantage in the use of this source of hematopoietic cells but a disadvantage in the inability to evaluate the genetic history of these donors.

ABO incompatibility between donor and recipient is encountered in 25–30% of allogeneic transplants. A major incompatibility occurs when the recipient plasma contains isohemagglutinins directed against the donor red blood cell (RBC) antigens (e.g., group O recipient, group A donor), and minor incompatibility occurs when the donor plasma contains isohemagglutinins directed against recipient RBC antigens (e.g., group A recipient, group O donor). In both instances, appropriate anti-A or anti-B isohemagglutinin titers must be determined before infusion of the cells. After the transplant procedure, all patients should have immunohematologic testing for the appearance of donor-derived RBCs and changes in recipient isohemagglutinin titers.

Several techniques have been developed for special treatment of marrow before infusion or cryopreservation. This includes removal of T lymphocytes from allogeneic donor marrow in an attempt to decrease the risk of GVHD or to remove potentially or known malignant cells from autologous marrow (e.g., use of monoclonal antibodies combined with complement, monoclonal antibodies linked to toxins, and various chemotherapy drugs).

Table 25-7 lists the investigations to be carried out prior to HSCT.

---

*Generation of a "buffy coat" or sedimentation at unit gravity in hetastarch produces an erythrocyte-poor product that contains most of the nucleated cells, including mature granulocytes, whereas Ficoll–Hypaque density separation provides mononuclear cells depleted of erythrocytes and mature myeloid cells. Most investigators freeze cells in tissue culture medium containing 10% dimethyl sulfoxide (DMSO) and a colloid (autologous plasma or human serum albumin are common); use of bags for marrow cryopreservation simplifies thawing and allows direct infusion afterward. Because of the possibility of bag breakage, it is recommended that at least two bags (preferably more) be used for each patient.

**Table 25-7. Pretransplantation Investigation Required
for Evaluation of the Recipient**

Physical examination
Complete blood count
Biochemistry profile
24-Hour urine for creatinine clearance
Blood type including red cell antigen panel
HIV, HTLV profile
EBV, CMV, hepatitis, herpes titers
Echocardiogram and EKG
Pulmonary function test (PFT)
Chest and sinus radiographs
Dental evaluation
Bone marrow aspiration/biopsy if applicable
Psychosocial evaluation

Table 25-8. Stem Cell Transplantation Preparative Regimens

Drug	Total dose	Cyclophosphamide, total dose	Total body irradiation (cGv)
Cyclophosphamide	120 mg/kg	—	1200–1350
Cytosine arabinoside	36 g/m^2	—	1200
Etoposide	60 mg/kg	—	1200
Etoposide	30 mg/kg	120 mg/kg	1200
Busulfan	16 mg/kg	200 mg/kg	—
Melphalan	135 mg/m^2	—	1350

Pretransplantation Preparative Regimens

Pretransplantation conditioning is used both for the purpose of eradicating disease
and as a means of immunosuppressing the recipient sufficiently to allow the acceptance of a new immunologically disparate hematopoietic system. The current mainstay of the preparatory regimen for HSCT consists of ablative doses of total body
irradiation (TBI) and cyclophosphamide or busulfan (Bu) and cyclophosphamide.
Table 25-8 shows various preparative regimens. On completion of the preparative
regimen, the donor marrow, PBSC, or UCB is infused. During the subsequent pan-
cytopenic period, supportive care is critical.

Preconditioning Regimens

Leukemia

Two preconditioning regimes, which have antitumor as well as immunosuppressive
properties, are commonly used prior to stem cell transplantation. TBI (fractionated
doses) and cyclophosphamide are utilized in ALL. A combination of TBI and
cyclophosphamide or cyclophosphamide and busulfan is utilized in AML, CML,
myelodysplasia, JCML, and JMML as follows:

1. *Total body irradiation (TBI) and cyclophosphamide:*

Day	Schema I
−8	TBI 150 cGy twice daily
−7	TBI 150 cGy twice daily
−6	TBI 150 cGy twice daily

–5	TBI 150 cGy twice daily
–4	TBI 150 cGy once daily
–3	Cyclophosphamide 60 mg/kg/day IV over 1 hour
–2	Cyclophosphamide 60 mg/kg/day IV over 1 hour
–1	Rest day
0	Stem cells harvested and given intravenously over a period of 3–4 hours

2. *Busulfan* and cyclophosphamide:*

Day	Schema II
–9	Busulfan 0.8–1 mg/kg IV, 6 hourly
–8	Busulfan 0.8–1 mg/kg IV, 6 hourly
–7	Busulfan 0.8–1 mg/kg IV, 6 hourly
–6	Busulfan 0.8–1 mg/kg IV, 6 hourly
–5	Cyclophosphamide 50 mg/kg/day IV over 1 hour
–4	Cyclophosphamide 50 mg/kg/day IV over 1 hour
–3	Cyclophosphamide 50 mg/kg/day IV over 1 hour
–2	Cyclophosphamide 50 mg/kg/day IV over 1 hour
–1	Rest
0	Stem cell harvested and given intravenously over a period of 3–4 hours

Aplastic Anemia

Patients who have received fewer than five blood transfusions usually receive cyclophosphamide 50 mg/kg/day for 4 days, followed by 1 day of rest and stem cell transplantation on the following day.

In multiply transfused patients, rejection of the bone marrow is a major problem (can be as high as 20–25%). To improve long-term survival in these patients, pre-transplant conditioning requires more intensive immunosuppression, consisting of any of the following:

- Cyclophosphamide, antithymocyte globulin (ATG)
- Cyclophosphamide and total nodal irradiation
- Cyclophosphamide and TBI (according to above schedule)
- Busulfan and cyclophosphamide (according to above schedule).

Miscellaneous Conditions

In hemoglobinopathies and selected immunodeficiency and other inherited disorders, the conditioning regimen used is busulfan and cyclophosphamide (see above) with or without ATG. In Fanconi anemia, low-dose cyclophosphamide (5 mg/kg/day for 4 days) followed by 500–600 cGy of thoracoabdominal radiation are generally employed because these patients are extremely sensitive to cyclophosphamide in the pretransplantation regimen.

Non-myeloablative Regimens

These regimens are based on the ability of donor T cells to ablate the host hematopoiesis or malignancy or both. The object is to use the donor lymphoid cells to eradicate the disease in the host. This allows the use of decreased doses of myeloablative chemotherapy with less toxicity. However, aggressive immunosuppressive

---

*IV busulfan is preferred if available because of the difficulty taking oral busulfan and the unreliable absorption. It is recommended to measure the plasma levels of busulfan and adjust the dose as per area under the curve (AUC 900–1300 ng/mL) or as per concentration at steady state (CSS 600–900 ng/mL).

therapy is still required to eliminate the potential host rejection of the donor cells. This approach is referred to as a non-myeloablative or mini-transplant process.

The following regimens are being used:

- Low-dose TBI
- Antithymocyte globulin
- Low-dose busulfan
- Low-dose melphalan
- Fludarabine
- Low-dose cyclophosphamide.

At present this approach is still in the experimental stages and is being used in selected cases of:

- CML
- AML
- Lymphoma
- Hodgkin disease
- Second transplant following graft failure or relapse of disease.

Evidence of Engraftment

Evidence of engraftment is usually seen within 3 weeks following stem cell transplantation and is identified as follows.

Direct Evidence

1. Fluorescence *in situ* hybridization (FISH) in sex-mismatched transplantation
2. Variable number of tandem repeats (VNTR) in same-sex-matched transplantation
3. HLA typing: mismatched transplantation
4. Donor-type red cell antigens
5. Immunoglobulin allotypes of donor
6. In severe combined immunodeficiency disease (SCID): the presence of adenosine deaminase (ADA) in white blood cells.

Indirect Evidence

1. Aplastic anemia and leukemia:
   a. Adequate bone marrow cellularity
   b. Increase in white blood cells with normal morphology and increase in platelet counts
2. SCID: improved immunologic parameters.

Causes of Failure to Engraft

- Increased genetic disparity
- T-cell depletion or GVHD prophylaxis
- Inadequate stem cell dose
- History of multiple transfusions in aplastic anemia
- Disordered microenvironment in storage disorders and osteopetrosis.

Results

Table 25-9 lists the 5-year disease-free survival in different disorders following allogeneic stem cell transplantation using HLA-identical matched siblings. The disease-free survival varies among different published series.

Table 25-9. HLA-Identical Matched Sibling Allogeneic Stem Cell Transplantation 5-Year Disease-Free Survival

Disease	Disease-free survival (%)
ANLL, first remission	55–70
ALL, first or second remission	30–50
ANLL, transplant in relapse	10–30
CML, chronic phase[a]	60–80
CML, accelerated or blastic phase[a]	10–30
Lymphoma, Hodgkin disease, after failure of first-line therapy	15–40
Aplastic anemia, untransfused	85–90
Aplastic anemia, transfused	50–70
Thalassemia major	70–85

[a]Age dependent; DFS decreases with increasing age.

The probability of acute GVHD grade II–IV is approximately 70% in unrelated matched donors compared to 30% in patients with HLA-A, -B, and -DR matched sibling transplantation.

Graft versus Host Disease Prophylaxis

Methotrexate, cyclosporine, and methylprednisolone are the most common drugs used singularly or in combination for GVHD prophylaxis beginning immediately following stem cell infusion. The most commonly used combinations are cyclosporine plus methotrexate or cyclosporine plus methylprednisolone. The drugs are used in the dosages as follows.

Methotrexate (Short Course)

Methotrexate 15 mg/m^2 IV on day following transplantation and 10 mg/m^2 IV on days 3, 6, and 11 post-transplant.

Cyclosporine

Cyclosporine 1.5 mg/kg twice daily IV starting on the day before transplant and given until the patient can take oral medication. At that time, a dose of 12 mg/kg/day in two divided doses is given orally. Serum levels should be kept between 150 and 300 µg/mL. Cyclosporine is slowly tapered by 10% weekly to start from 60–180 days post-transplant.

The complications of cyclosporine include:

- Renal insufficiency (cyclosporine is adjusted if there is any abnormality in the blood urea nitrogen [BUN] and creatinine values)
- Gingival hyperplasia
- Hirsutism
- Hepatic dysfunction
- Hypertension with concurrent hypomagnesemia
- Seizures, tremors
- Syndromes resembling thrombotic thrombocytopenic purpura and hemolytic–uremic syndrome especially with concurrent hypomagnesemia.

Methylprednisolone

Methylprednisolone is administered in a dose of 0.5 mg/kg orally every 12 hours from day 5 until day 28 post-transplant and thereafter it is tapered slowly.

The other major technique to prevent GVHD is purging of the donor marrow of T lymphocytes.* Use of this technique has the following disadvantages:

- Increase in early and late engraftment failures
- Disease relapse
- Secondary tumors.

AUTOLOGOUS STEM CELL TRANSPLANTATION

Autologous stem cell transplantation offers a viable alternative when a matched sibling is not available for transplantation. Normal-appearing bone marrow is removed from the patient and may be treated *ex vivo* with cytotoxic drugs or monoclonal antibodies directed at the malignant cells. A concentrated selection of pluripotent hematopoietic cells can be obtained using CD34+ (stem cell antigen) as a marker for stem cells to reduce the volume of stem cells required for reinfusion. This is performed *in vitro* using CD34+-labeled columns. The stem cells are then cryopreserved. The patient then receives intensive chemotherapy with hematopoietic stem cell rescue (Table 25-3) and hematopoietic growth factor. Table 25-10 presents the results of autologous stem cell transplantation disease-free survival for various malignancies.

Indications for Autologous Stem Cell Transplantation

- Leukemia, where stem cell transplantation is indicated but a matched allogeneic bone marrow donor is not available
- Intermediate- and high-grade lymphomas in first relapse or partial remission
- Hodgkin disease in first relapse or partial remission
- High-risk tumors at the time of diagnosis where long-term survival is less than 30% and a chemotherapy dose–response is demonstrated (most consistent indicator of a poor prognosis is disseminated disease)
- Failure or partial response to initial therapy or recurrence of disease (i.e., progressive disease).

Table 25-10. Autologous Stem Cell Transplantation

Disease	Disease-free survival (%)
Lymphoma	30–60
Neuroblastoma	45–50
Ewing sarcoma	25–30
Rhabdomyosarcoma	30
Wilms' tumor	50
Brain tumor	50

---

*T-cell purging can be done by monoclonal antibodies accompanied by complement-mediated lysis, immunotoxins, or immunomagnetic beads. Physical methods of T-cell depletion include counter-elutriation and soybean lectin agglutination plus E-rosette depletion.

Drugs appropriate for high-dose chemotherapy should have the following properties:

- The drug should be active against the tumor type.
- The drug should be tolerable at 3–10 times nonmarrow-ablative dose.
- The drug should generate a steep and straight-line dose–response curve over many logs of tumor cell kills.
- The combination of drugs should have non-cross-resistance and nonoverlapping toxicities.
- The dose-limiting toxicity should be marrow ablation only with tolerable toxicity to other organs.

The following factors contribute to the outcome:

- Timing of intensive chemotherapy
- Chemotherapy schedule (dose and drugs) and expected toxicity
- Supportive care (appropriate use of antibiotics and other drugs for managing side effects)
- Appropriate use of peripheral stem cell transplant and growth factors, which can reduce the period of neutropenia and hospitalization.

Acute Lymphocytic Leukemia

Most of the HSCT in patients with ALL and acute nonlymphoblastic leukemia (ANLL) have been performed in second or subsequent remissions with or without purged bone marrow using the regimen of cyclophosphamide and total body irradiation or cyclophosphamide and busulfan. The long-term disease survival is 20–30% as reported in different series. Autologous SCT for ALL and ANLL is only recommended after second remission for patients with a long first remission.

Solid Tumors

See the relevant chapters for specific tumors. Table 25-11 lists high-risk solid tumors that may respond to intensive chemotherapy and autologous HSCT.

Table 25-11. High-Risk Solid Tumors That May Respond to Intensive Chemotherapy and Autologous Stem Cell Transplantation[a]

Tumor	Indication
Supratentorial astrocytoma	Recurrence
Medulloblastoma	Recurrence
Ependymoma	Recurrence
Ewing sarcoma/PNET	Primary metastatic
	Recurrence
Rhabdomyosarcoma	Primary stage IV
	Recurrence
Neuroblastoma	Stage IV n-myc positive
	Recurrence
Wilms' tumor	Recurrence
Retinoblastoma	Primary extraocular
	Recurrence

Abbreviation: PNET, primitive neuroectodermal tumor.

[a]All tumors must have demonstrated some response to initial chemotherapy prior to autologous SCT.

Blood Bank Support

The use of blood products is critical in the management of transplant patients. Table 25-6 lists the problems that arise in the use of blood products.

COMPLICATIONS OF HEMATOPOIETIC STEM CELL TRANSPLANTATION

Despite quantitative myeloid (neutrophil) recovery after bone marrow transplantation, the functional recovery of humoral and cellular immunity may take a year or longer. The type of graft used (autologous or allogeneic), the type and method of administration of immunosuppressive therapy after transplant (cyclosporine, corticosteroids, ATG), and whether GVHD has occurred (especially chronic GVHD) all influence the rate of lymphoimmunologic reconstitution.

After stem cell transplantation, a transient state of combined immunodeficiency develops in all patients. The natural history of immune reconstitution is similar for autologous and allogeneic transplants but often is altered in allogeneic transplants by GVHD as well as by immunosuppressive therapy. Although natural killer cells reconstitute to normal levels usually within the first month after transplantation, other immunologic defects may persist.

The importance of the recognition of the delayed overall immunologic reconstitution relates to the clinically observed incidence of recurrent bacterial (*Streptococcus pneumoniae*) and opportunistic infections (*Pneumocystis carinii*, fungal, herpes zoster, CMV) that can occur many months after transplantation. In addition to the use of prophylaxis against *P. carinii* infection, many centers add penicillin as a post-transplant prophylaxis against *S. pneumoniae* infection, particularly if the patient has chronic GVHD. The suppressed immunity also has major practical implications for consideration of the timing of vaccinations after HSCT. It is probably reasonable to consider the following approach:

1. At the end of 1 year, individuals who do not have chronic GVHD should receive influenza (yearly) and pneumococcal polysaccharide vaccines and should also have vaccinations with inactivated poliovirus and diphtheria–pertussis–tetanus (DPT). It is probably also safe to administer hepatitis B and *Haemophilus influenzae* conjugate vaccines.
2. Immunosuppressed patients with chronic GVHD are less likely to develop an adequate antibody response after vaccinations. If vaccines are administered, antibody titers should be checked after vaccination to determine the efficacy of the response.
3. For select patients who are 2 years post-HSCT, have no evidence of GVHD, and are not receiving immunosuppressive therapy, measles, mumps, and rubella (MMR) live vaccines can be given. Table 25-12 lists a reimmunization schedule after transplantation.

The risks of HSCT are related to the underlying disease, the pretransplantation conditioning with cytotoxic drugs or irradiation or both, post-transplantation

Table 25-12. Reimmunization Schedule after Stem Cell Transplantation

Vaccine	Time to begin reimmunization
Diphtheria–tetanus toxoid	6–12 months
Oral poliovirus	Not recommended
Inactivated poliovirus	6–12 months
Measles–mumps–rubella	24 months

immunosuppression (infections), and GVHD. The early mortality can be as high as 20%, depending on the conditioning regimens, the disease, and the patient's status. The potential complications post-transplant are discussed next.

Effects of Conditioning Regimens

The conditioning regimens can result in:

- Toxic vasculitis
- Severe mucositis
- Veno-occlusive disease of the liver
- Acute alveolitis
- Obliterative bronchiolitis
- Hemolytic–uremic syndrome
- Multiple organ failure.

Infections

Patients undergoing stem cell transplantation have increased risks of infection related to their disease and its status. Patients with more than two relapses who undergo stem cell transplantation develop more infectious complications than those who receive transplants during the first remission. The adequacy of treatment of any infection in the patient prior to marrow ablation influences the risk of subsequent complications. Prolonged duration of neutropenia, use of central venous catheters, and slow speed of marrow engraftment are important risk factors.

Table 25-13 lists prophylaxis and supportive care for stem cell transplantation. Table 25-14 lists the infections most frequently seen at different times post-transplantation.

Table 25-13. Prophylaxis and Supportive Care for Stem Cell Transplantation

1. Mouth care: Peridex or Biotin solution and Mycostatin every 3–4 hours daily
2. Recombinant hematopoietic growth factors: G-CSF or GM-CSF (Chapter 26)[a]
3. Prophylaxis against *Pneumocystis carinii*: trimethoprim/sulfamethoxazole 5 mg/kg in two divided doses (3 times per week) starting after engraftment; continue if chronic GVHD is present[b]
4. Prophylaxis against *Candida*: fluconazole 4–6 mg/kg once a day
5. Prophylaxis for herpes simplex and CMV: IV acyclovir 250 mg/m^2 every 8 hours for first 3–6 months or longer if patient continues to be on immunosuppressive drugs.
6. Additional prophylaxis for CMV:
   a. CMV-negative blood products should be used if patient and donor are CMV-negative patients; if CMV-negative blood is not available, leukocyte filters to remove leukocytes should be employed
   b. Ganciclovir 5 mg/kg/dose twice a day for 1 week followed by 5 mg/kg once a day until day 100 post-transplant. Ganciclovir should be started when absolute neutrophil count is above 1000/mm^3.[c]
7. IVIG (only in recipient of allogeneic stem cell transplant): 500 mg/kg every 2–3 weeks for first 3 months after transplant[d]; then check IgG levels periodically if less than within normal limits; then infuse accordingly
8. Nutrition: total parenteral nutrition given if enteral nutrition is not possible or inadequate

---

[a]Does not increase relapse and GVHD rates. Stimulates hematopoietic recovery.

[b]If patients are allergic to trimethoprim/sulfamethoxazole or if severe cytopenia is present, aerosolized pentamidine (300 mg) or intravenously 4 mg/kg once a month can be used.

[c]Drug-related neutropenia is a major side effect.

[d]For its immunomodulatory (decreased incidence of GVHD) effect and antimicrobial activity, especially CMV. It also decreases gram-negative sepsis.

Table 25-14. Infections Most Frequently Seen at Different Times Post-Transplantation

I. Infections in first 30 days post-transplantation
    A. Bacteremia
        Gram-positive organisms: *Staphylococcus epidermidis*
        Gram-negative aerobes and anaerobes
    B. Invasive fungal infections: *Aspergillus, Candida*
    C. Reactivation of herpes simplex I
II. Infections 30–120 days post-transplantation
    A. Protozoal infections
        Pneumocystis carinii
        Toxoplasma
    B. Viral infections
        Cytomegalovirus (CMV)
        Adenovirus
        Epstein–Barr virus (EBV)
        Human herpesvirus 6 (HHV-6)
    C. Fungal infections
        Candida (*C. albicans* and *C. tropicalis*)
        Aspergillus
        Trichosporon
        Fusarium
        Candida krusei
III. Infections after 120 days post-transplantation
    A. Sinopulmonary infections with encapsulated organisms
    B. Viral infections
        Cutaneous herpes zoster

During the first 30 days, the most frequently documented infection is coagulase-negative staphylococcal epidermidis infection associated with the use of indwelling central venous catheters. During the second and third months, infections with CMV and interstitial pneumonia occur. CMV infection occurs within approximately 20–100 days after transplantation, with the highest infection rate in patients who are CMV seropositive before transplantation or seronegative recipients receiving a seropositive graft. CMV infection arises from exogenous introduction of virus in blood products or from reactivation of endogenous virus.

The clinical manifestations of CMV infection are variable, ranging from asymptomatic viral excretion to fever, arthralgia, arthritis, hepatitis, secondary bone marrow hypoplasia with thrombocytopenia and leukopenia, retinitis, esophagitis, gastroenteritis, and pneumonia with up to 80% mortality.

Early treatment with the antiviral drug ganciclovir plus high-titer CMV intravenous gammaglobulin has reduced morbidity to less than 20%. Prophylactic or preemptive therapy in seropositive patients or patients receiving a seropositive graft is an effective way to prevent the development of CMV.

The following guidelines for the prophylaxis and treatment of CMV infections should be carried out (as recommended by the U.S. Centers for Disease Control and Prevention along with the American Society of Blood and Marrow Transplantation):

1. Allogeneic transplantation patients who are seronegative at the time of transplant and have a seronegative donor do not require additional CMV prophylaxis other than the strict use of CMV-negative blood products.

2. Allogeneic transplantation patients who are CMV positive at transplant or those who received a transplant from a CMV-positive donor should receive prophylactic or preemptive ganciclovir.

3. Allogeneic transplantation patients should have surveillance for CMV antigenemia assay or a polymerase chain reaction (PCR) assay and blood, urine, and throat cultures obtained weekly for the first 120 days post-transplant. Those patients with evidence of CMV cultured from blood, bronchial washings, the throat, or the gastrointestinal tract should be treated with ganciclovir and gammaglobulin at least until day 100 after transplant or for 2–3 weeks past the latest date of positive cultures.

4. Autologous transplantation patients who are seronegative at the time of transplant should preferably receive CMV-negative blood products but may, as an alternative, receive leukocyte-filtered blood products.

Interstitial Pneumonitis

Interstitial pneumonitis is an important complication and may be due to any of the following causes:

- CMV
- *Pneumocystis carinii*
- Undiagnosed infections (e.g., fungal)
- Drugs
- Radiation toxicity
- Immune reactions involving the lung
- Idiopathic (16%).

The mortality rate for interstitial pneumonitis is 60%. The use of prophylactic Bactrim has reduced *P. carinii* infection to less than 2%.

After 120 days post–HSCT, the most common infections are sinopulmonary infections with encapsulated organisms and cutaneous infections with herpes zoster. Other localized or disseminated viral infections that occur include adenovirus, herpes simplex virus, varicella virus, and respiratory syncytial virus.

Table 25-15 outlines the management of infection during stem cell transplantation and post-transplantation.

Pancytopenia

In addition to the corrections of anemia and thrombocytopenia by the use of irradiated leukocyte-depleted packed red cells and platelets, recombinant hematopoietic growth factors play the following roles:

1. It is safe and effective to administer growth factors to allogeneic transplantation patients. All allogeneic and autologous transplantation patients should receive G-CSF or GM-CSF therapy following stem cell infusion.

2. With the use of ganciclovir to prevent or treat CMV infections and other myelosuppressive therapies, growth factors may play an added role in the prevention or treatment of myelosuppression caused by these agents after stem cell transplantation.

Graft versus Host Disease

The incidence of acute GVHD varies among different transplant centers and depends on the primary diagnosis. In patients with primary immunodeficiency

Table 25-15. Management of Infections during First 30 Days Post–HSCT

Gram-negative infections
  Empiric combination therapy (Chapter 26)
Gram-positive infections
  Vancomycin
Fungal infections
  Amphotericin B
  Liposomal amphotericin
  Voriconazole
  Itraconazole
Removal of indwelling catheter
Management of interstitial pneumonia
  1. Bronchoalveolar lavage (BAL)
  2. Open lung biopsy
  3. Treatment depends on etiology
     a. *Pneumocystis:* Bactrim, pentamidine
     b. CMV: ganciclovir plus CMV high-titer gammaglobulin
     c. Idiopathic: supportive care, steroids
     d. Fungal: antifungals
Management of herpes zoster
  Acyclovir

and aplastic anemia, the incidence of GVHD may vary from 10% to 35%, whereas in patients with acute leukemia, it may be approximately 50%. In unrelated matched donor transplantation, it may vary from 50 to 70%. Approximately 10–30% of all patients with sustained allogeneic engraftment die of acute GVHD or its complications.

GVHD is caused by donor alloreactivity in an immunocompromised host and results from T lymphocytes contained in the stem cell graft that proliferate and differentiate in the host. These T cells recognize host alloantigens as foreign and through both direct effector mechanisms and by inflammatory mediators released by T cells, monocytes and production of cytokines especially interleukin 1 (IL-1) and tumor necrosis factor in the host may cause tissue damage.

Graft versus host disease is divided into two stages:

- Acute GVHD, which manifests in the first 100 days post-transplantation, usually observed within 30–40 days
- Chronic GVHD, which manifests 100 days after stem cell transplantation.

Acute GVHD

The clinical manifestations of acute GVHD range from a mild maculopapular eruption to generalized erythroderma, hepatic dysfunction, gastroenteritis, stomatitis, and lymphocytic bronchitis. Thrombocytopenia and anemia have been reported in GVHD. Ocular symptoms, including photophobia, hemorrhagic conjunctivitis, and pseudomembrane formation, have also been observed. It is occasionally difficult to separate the clinical manifestations of GVHD from other disorders in the post-transplant patient and, in these cases, a biopsy of the skin or liver may be required. Table 25-16 lists the clinical manifestations and stages of acute GVHD, and Table 25-17 describes the histologic grades of acute GVHD. Table 25-18 presents a comparison between acute and chronic GVHD.

Table 25-16. Clinical Manifestations and Stages of Acute Graft versus Host Disease

Clinical grade	Skin[a]	Liver (serum total bilirubin, mg/dL)[b]	Gut (diarrhea)[c]	
			Children (mL/kg/day)	Adults (mL/day)
I (mild)	Maculopapular rash, <25% body surface. May be pruritic or painful	1.5–3.0	10–15	500–1000 Nausea and vomiting
II (moderate)	Maculopapular rash, 25–50% body surface	3.0–6.0	16–20	1000–1500 Nausea and vomiting
III (severe)	Maculopapular rash, >50% body, or generalized erythroderma	6.0–15.0	21–25	>1500 Nausea and vomiting
IV (life-threatening)	Desquamation and bullae	>15	>25 Pain or ileus	>2500 Pain or ileus

[a]Differential diagnosis includes chemoradiotherapy-induced rash, drug allergy, and viral exanthem. Skin biopsies are informative for patients more than 21 days after HSCT.

[b]The degree of hyperbilirubinemia does not correlate well with clinical outcome. Differential diagnosis includes hepatotoxic drug reactions and viral infections. Liver biopsy is helpful in establishing the diagnosis.

[c]Diarrhea may be severe and associated with crampy abdominal pain. The diarrhea is green, mucoid, watery, and mixed with exfoliated cells that may form fecal casts. It may progress to bleeding and ileus. Intestinal radiographs show mucosal and submucosal edema with rapid barium transit time and loss of haustral folds. A variant of enteric GVHD in 13% of patients has presenting features of anorexia and dyspepsia. Patients with upper gastrointestinal disease may not manifest lower tract involvement. Gastrointestinal endoscopy and biopsy are mandatory for the diagnosis of upper gastrointestinal tract disease. Lower tract disease may be diagnosed with rectal biopsy, which shows necrosis of individual cells in crypts that may progress to dropout of entire crypts and loss of epithelium.

Table 25-17. Histologic Grades of Acute Graft versus Host Disease

Grade	Skin	Liver	Gut
I	Epidermal base cell vacuolar degeneration	Fewer than 25% small interlobular bile ducts abnormal (degeneration or necrosis)	Single-cell necrosis of epithelial cells
II	Grade I changes plus "eosinophilic bodies"	25–50% bile ducts abnormal	Necrosis
III	Grade II changes plus separation of the dermal–epidermal junction	50–75% bile ducts abnormal	Focal microscopic mucosal denudation
IV	Frank epidermal denudation	More than 75% bile ducts abnormal	Diffuse mucosal denudation

Table 25-18. Comparison of Acute and Chronic Graft versus Host Disease

Characteristic	Acute	Chronic
Incidence	40–60%	20–40%
Onset, days	7–60 (up to 100)	>100 (after >60)
Clinical manifestations		
Skin	Erythematous rash	Sclerodermatous changes
Gut	Secretory diarrhea	Dry mouth, esophagitis, malabsorption
Liver	Hepatitis	Cholestasis
Lung	Diffuse alveolar hemorrhage	Pulmonary dysfunction
Other	Fever	Contractures (due to sclerodermatous skin damage)
		Alopecia
		Thrombocytopenia
Target cells	Epidermal	Mesenchymal
Basis of clinical grading	Severity of disease	Extent of disease

Treatment

Prophylaxis

Complete matching of the donor and recipient at the level of HLA class I and II by DNA typing are the most important factors in preventing GVHD. Consideration of the sex and parity of the donor are advisable if there is a choice of donor. If the patient is CMV seronegative, use of a CMV-negative donor appears to reduce the risk of CMV infection as well as risk of GVHD. Table 25-19 lists additional measures that can be employed in the prophylaxis of GVHD, as mentioned earlier in this chapter. Prophylactic drugs have been used in an attempt to inhibit T-cell response by relying on *in vivo* immunosuppression. Currently, all agents are used in a combination that targets different molecular intermediates of T-cell signals.

Therapy

Grade II–IV GVHD requires therapeutic intervention with high-dose methylprednisolone 3–5 mg/kg/day ×7 days, after which the dose is decreased to 2 mg/kg/day. The progression of GVHD despite steroid therapy in these doses requires an increase in the dose of methylprednisolone to 20 mg/kg/day for 3 days, 10 mg/kg/day for

Table 25-19. Prophylaxis of Graft versus Host Disease

1. Major histocompatibility complex (MHC) matching
2. Irradiation of blood products
3. Prevention of infection
4. *In vivo* treatment of recipient[a]
   a. Cyclosporine
   b. Methotrexate
   c. Corticosteroids
   d. Tacrolimus
   e. Mycophenolate mofetil
   f. ATG
5. Depletion of donor T cells from marrow graft such as:
   a. Purging of marrow with monoclonal antibodies OK T3, T12
   b. Soybean lectin and E-rosette depletion
   c. Pretreatment of marrow with various antibody-ricin conjugates
   d. Magnetic beads

[a]Current prevention in many centers consists of methotrexate and cyclosporine.

3 days, 5 mg/kg/day for 3 days, 3 mg/kg/day with tapering doses of steroids, depending on the response or the use of ATG. ATG is usually given in doses of 10–15 mg/kg every other day for 7–14 days. Newer immunosuppressive agents like mycophenolate mofetil and methods targeting CD5, CD3, the interleukin-2 receptor, and tumor necrosis factor α and its receptor have been used with some success.

Chronic GVHD

Chronic GVHD occurs 100 days after transplantation. It either follows as a direct, progressive extension of acute GVHD, follows a quiescent period after acute GVHD has resolved, or occurs in a patient who did not have evidence of acute GVHD. In matched-sibling grafts, the incidence of chronic GVHD is 13% for children under 10 years of age and 28% for children 10–19 years of age. In unrelated-donor or mismatched-family-member donor, the incidence of chronic GVHD ranges from 42 to 56%.

The predictors for chronic GVHD are:

- Donor–recipient HLA disparity
- Increasing patient age
- Latent donor viral infection
- Female donor with a history of parity (sensitized)
- Source of allogeneic cells; number of T cells collected during pheresis is greater than that collected during bone marrow harvest.

One-third of patients who develop chronic GVHD are at risk for bacterial and opportunistic infections. The duration of chronic GVHD varies and the morbidity and mortality range from 10 to 15%. Chronic GVHD can be divided into limited and extensive tissue involvement (Table 25-20), as discussed next.

Limited tissue involvement (usually involving only one organ):

- Localized skin involvement: erythema, hyperkeratosis, patchy scleroderma-like lesions, reticular hyperpigmentation, desquamation, alopecia, nail loss; rash initially involving palms and soles, back of neck and ears, and later the trunk and extremities
- Hepatic dysfunction: predominantly cholestatic abnormalities.

Table 25-20. Classification of Chronic Graft versus Host Disease

Limited
   Either or both
      Localized skin involvement
      Hepatic dysfunction
Extensive
   Either
      Generalized skin involvement
      Hepatic dysfunction plus
      Ocular involvement (Schirmer's test, <5-mm wetting)
      Oral mucosal involvement (lip biopsy positive)
      Any other target organ

Extensive tissue involvement (associated with worse prognosis):

- Generalized skin involvement: resembling lichen planus or scleroderma; atrophy of skin with ulceration; fibrosis of skin with or without limitation of joint movement
- Hepatic dysfunction: liver histology showing chronic aggressive hepatitis, bridging necrosis, or cirrhosis
- Ocular symptoms: dry eyes, Schirmer's test with less than 5-mm wetting; keratoconjunctivitis sicca including burning, irritation, photophobia, and pain
- Buccal cavity: dry mouth, sensitivity to acidic or spicy foods and pain; oral atrophy with depapillation of tongue; erythema and lichenoid lesions of buccal and labial mucosa; involvement of minor salivary glands or oral mucosa demonstrated on labial biopsy specimen
- Gastrointestinal tract: malabsorption due to submucosal fibrosis of gastrointestinal tract; dysphagia, pain, and weight loss
- Genitourinary tract: vaginitis and vaginal strictures
- Polyarthritis, myositis, and fascitis leading to contractures
- Pulmonary complications: interstitial pneumonia and bronchiolitis obliterans.

Prognosis

Morbidity and mortality are highest in patients with progressive-onset chronic GVHD that directly follows acute GVHD, are intermediate in patients after resolution of acute GVHD, and are lowest in those with *de novo* onset. The median day of diagnosis of chronic GVHD in recipients of HLA-identical sibling BMT is 200 days, and the onset of the disease in recipients of bone marrow from an HLA-nonidentical or unrelated donor is approximately 145 days. Screening studies at day 100 with skin examination with biopsy, oral examination with lip biopsy, ocular examination with Schirmer's test, and liver function studies are useful in predicting patients at risk for the development of chronic GVHD. Even in the absence of signs or symptoms, a positive random skin biopsy or history of previous acute GVHD independently predicts a threefold increase in the relative risk of subsequent chronic GVHD.

Treatment

- Methylprednisolone 1–2 mg/kg alone or in combination with PO cyclosporine 10–12 mg/kg/day or tacrolimus 0.15–0.3 mg/kg/day in two divided doses or mycophenolate mofetil 600 mg/m^2/dose twice a day. Azathioprine 1.5 mg/kg once a day may also be utilized. The azathioprine dose is adjusted to keep the white blood cell count between 2500 and 3500/mm². This can have a steroid-sparing effect if unable to taper steroids.

- Thalidomide is also effective in chronic GVHD.

In addition, the following supportive care should be given:

- Intravenous gammaglobulin 500 mg/kg every 2–4 weeks (as per IgG levels)
- Bactrim prophylaxis for *P. carinii* infection
- Antibiotics for chronic sinopulmonary infection.

Therapy should be continued for a minimum of 9 months or until all clinical and pathologic evidence of chronic GVHD has cleared and when biopsies of the skin and lip have returned to normal.

Veno-Occlusive Disease

Veno-occlusive disease (VOD) occurs as a complication of chemotherapy and/or radiation in allogeneic stem cell transplant. It is a common life-threatening complication of preparative-regimen-related toxicity of stem cell transplantation. It occurs after approximately 20% of allogeneic stem cell transplantations and after about 10% of autologous stem cell transplantations. VOD is characterized by fibrous obliteration of small hepatic vessels. It usually occurs within the first 30 days.

Clinical Manifestations

- Jaundice
- Weight gain
- Ascites
- Hepatomegaly
- Right upper quadrant pain.

Because not all patients exhibit the full spectrum of the syndrome, a common clinical definition requires the presence of any two of the above-listed features with the onset occurring no later than 14 days from stem cell infusion. Because these clinical manifestations are not specific to VOD, all other causes of hepatic dysfunction must be excluded. Another condition that may mimic hepatic VOD is nodular regenerative hyperplasia of the liver, a diffuse nonfibrotic nodulation of the liver with areas of regenerative activity alternating with areas of atrophy. This syndrome effects the same transplantation population at risk for hepatic VOD, and both conditions are frequently associated with the development of ascites. Although no specific treatments are available for either entity, the mortality rate is considerably higher for patients who develop hepatic VOD than for those who develop nodular regenerative hyperplasia.

Predisposing Factors

The cause of VOD remains unknown; however, patients with the following have an increased risk:

- Preexisting hepatitis (one of the most strongly predictive risk factors)
- Elevated liver function tests
- Refractory leukemia
- Age over 15 years
- Underlying metastatic tumor in the liver
- Positive CMV serologic status

- Conditioning agents (such as TBI, busulfan, cytosine arabinoside)
- Mismatched or unrelated allogeneic transplants
- Certain antimicrobial agents (especially vancomycin and acyclovir when given before transplantation) have also been implicated.

Prophylaxis

Lower or fractionated doses of BCNU (carmustine), lower total doses of TBI or shielding of the liver during TBI, use of T-cell–depleted marrow, use of ursodeoxycholic acid, and continuous infusion of low-dose heparin have been used to reduce toxicity.

Treatment

- Supportive care
- Sodium restriction
- Spironolactone therapy
- Thrombolytic therapy (continuous infusion of heparin during pretransplant conditioning and through the first 2 weeks post-transplant in a dose of 100–150 units/kg/day or recombinant human tissue plasminogen activator [t-PA] and heparin or antithrombin [AT] infusion if AT levels are low)*
- Prostaglandin E (may be a promising agent in prophylaxis)
- Portacaval shunting
- Liver transplantation.

Late Sequelae of Stem Cell Transplantation

Table 25-21 lists the late sequelae of allogeneic stem cell transplantation in children.

Post–Stem Cell Transplantation Therapy

Post–stem cell transplantation patients do not require any chemotherapy with the exception of certain patients with lymphoma, who may require localized radiotherapy to the primary site. Because the relapse rate is about 50%, a number of investigators have considered the following post-transplant therapy:

1. Use of double autologous HSCT to eradicate the few remaining logs of tumor cells. Sufficient stem cells can be cryopreserved from a single harvest for two transplants. Non-cross-resistant regimens, each with activity, if not causing considerable toxicity, would be advantageous.
2. Use of cytokines to enhance hematopoietic (shortening the period of neutropenia) and immunologic recovery. Cytokines are also used for their antitumor effects, which include the following:
   a. Stimulation of host antitumor effector cells
   b. Direct cytotoxic effect
   c. Cytostatic effect on tumor cells
   d. Interference with nutrient and oxygen supply to tumor by acting on tumor vasculature.
3. Use of differentiation inducers (e.g., 13-*cis*-retinoic acid). These agents can arrest cell proliferation and induce terminal differentiation and may prove

---

*These approaches are limited by the risk of fatal intracerebral and pulmonary bleeding. Heparin has little effect on the overall incidence of VOD but may reduce the severity of the clinical illness. A dose of 100 units/kg/day of heparin has been shown to be safe.

Table 25-21. Late Sequelae of Allogeneic Stem Cell Transplantation in Children

1. Chronic GVHD
2. Multiple endocrine disorders (hypothyroidism, delayed pubescence, gonadal failure, growth hormone deficiency)[a]
3. Second malignancies (incidence of 0.6 per 100 person-years)[b]
4. Sterility due to gonadal failure
5. Cataracts (secondary to radiation therapy); 20–50% incidence at 5–6 years
6. Renal insufficiency (nephrotoxic antibiotics and cyclosporine)
7. Obstructive and restrictive pulmonary disease (occurs in 10–15% of patients with chronic GVHD)
8. Cardiomyopathy
9. Aseptic necrosis of bone
10. Leukoencephalopathy (especially with IT MTX)
11. Immunologic dysfunction
12. Post-transplant lymphoproliferative disorders (PTLD) (occasionally seen in T-cell-depleted stem cell graft recipients)
13. Disturbance in dental development (from TBI) particularly if HSCT takes place in patients less than 6 years of age

Note: The frequency and severity of these sequelae vary considerably with the conditioning required preceding SCT.

[a]Associated with the use of TBI.

[b]At 15 years after HSCT, 6% develop second malignancies if not prepared with TBI and 20% for those prepared with TBI regimens.

effective against minimal disease after autologous HSCT. They do not have hematopoietic toxicity and should be well tolerated in autologous HSCT.

4. Use of antimyeloid monoclonal antibody in myeloid leukemia such as gemtuzumab ozogamicin (Mylotarg).
5. Use of low-dose cyclosporine to induce GVHD, which also has a beneficial effect on graft versus leukemia reaction and thus might reduce the relapse rate.
6. For treatment of post-transplant lymphoproliferative disorder, see Chapter 13.

SUGGESTED READINGS

Anderson KC. The role of the blood bank in hematopoietic stem cell transplantation. Transfusion 1992;32(3):272–85.

Arico M, Valsecchi MG, Camitta B, et al. Outcome of treatment in children with Philadelphia chromosome-positive acute lymphoblastic leukemia. N Engl J Med 2000;342(14):998–1006.

Bearman SI, Lee JL, Baron AE, McDonald GB. Treatment of hepatic veno-occlusive disease with recombinant human tissue plasminogen activator and heparin in 42 marrow transplant patients. Blood 1997;89(5):737–44.

Bodmer JG, Marsh SG, Albert ED, et al. Nomenclature for factors of the HLA system, 1998. Hum Immunol 1999;60(4):361–95.

Brunet S, Urbano A, Ojeda E, et al. Favourable effect of the combination of acute and chronic graft versus host disease on the outcome of allogeneic peripheral blood stem cell transplantation for advanced hematological malignancies. Br J Haematol 2001;114(3):544–45.

Champlin R, Khouri I, Kornblau S, et al. Allogeneic hematopoietic transplantation as adoptive immunotherapy. Induction of graft-versus-malignancy as primary therapy. Hematol Oncol Clin North Am 1999;13(5):1041–57.

Champlin R, Khouri I, Kornblau S, et al. Reinventing bone marrow transplantation: reducing toxicity using nonmyeloablative, preparative regimens and induction of graft-versus-malignancy. Curr Opin Oncol 1999;11(2):87–95.

Essell JH, Schroeder MT, Harman GS, et al. Ursodiol prophylaxis against hepatic complications of allogeneic bone marrow transplantation. Ann Intern Med 1998;128:975–81.

Gluckman E, Devergie A, Bourdeau EH, et al. Transplantation of umbilical cord blood in Fanconi's anemia. Nouv Rev Fr Hematol 1990;32(6):423–5.

Gluckman E. Umbilical cord blood hematopoietic stem cells; biology and transplantation. Curr Opin Hematol 1995;2(6)413–16.

Guruangan S, Dunkel IJ, Goldman S, et al. Myeloablative chemotherapy with autologous bone marrow rescue in young children with recurrent malignant brain tumors. J Clin Oncol 1998;16(7):2486–93.

Hongeng S, Krance RA, Bowman LC, et al. Outcomes of transplantation with matched-sibling and unrelated-donor bone marrow in children with leukemia. Lancer 1997;350(9080):767–71.

Levine JE, Harris RE, Fausto R, et al. A comparison of allogeneic and autologous bone marrow transplantation for symptomatic lymphoma. Blood 2003;101(7):2476–82.

Majolino I, Pearce R, Taghipour G, Goldstone AH. Peripheral blood stem-cell transplantation versus autologous bone marrow transplantation in Hodgkin's and non-Hodgkin's lymphomas: a new matched-pair analysis of the European Group for Blood and Marrow Transplantation Registry Data. Lymphoma Working Party of the European Group for Blood and Marrow Transplantation. J Clin Oncol 1997;15(2):509–17.

Matthay KK, Villablanca JG, Seeger RC, et al. Treatment of high-risk neuroblastoma with intensive chemotherapy, radiotherapy, autologous bone marrow transplantation, and 13-*cis*-retinoic acid. Children's Cancer Group. N Engl J Med 1999;341(16):1165–73.

Mehta J, Powles R, Singhal S, et al. Transfusion requirements after bone marrow transplantation from HLA-identical siblings: effects of donor–recipient ABO incompatibility. Bone Marrow Transpl 1996;18(1):151–6.

Morrison VA, Peterson BA. High-dose therapy and transplantation in non-Hodgkin's lymphoma. Semin Oncol 1999;26(1):84–98.

Neudorf S, Sanders JE, Howells W, et al. The beneficial role of autologous bone marrow transplantation in the treatment of childhood acute myelogenous leukemia: a report from the Children's Cancer Group. Blood 1998;92[Suppl 1]:294a.

Porter DL, Antin JH. The graft-versus-leukemia effects of allogeneic cell therapy. Ann Rev Med 1999;50:369–86.

Rosenthal J, Sender L, Secola R, et al. Phase II trial of heparin prophylaxis for veno-occlusive disease of the liver in children undergoing bone marrow transplantation. Bone Marrow Transpl 1996;18:185–91.

Sable CA, Donowitz GR. Infections in bone marrow transplant recipients. Clin Infect Dis 1994;18:273–84.

Slavin S, Nagler A, Naparstek E, et al. Nonmyeloablative stem cell transplantation and cell therapy as an alternative to conventional bone marrow transplantation with lethal cytoreduction for the treatment of malignant and nonmalignant hematologic diseases. Blood 1998;91(3):756–63.

Walters MC, Storb R, Patience M, et al. Impact of bone marrow transplantation for symptomatic sickle cell disease. Blood 2000;95(6):1918–24.

Woolfrey AE, Gooley TA, Sievers EL, et al. Bone marrow transplantation for children less than 2 years of age with acute myelogenous leukemia or myelodysplastic syndrome. Blood 1998;92(10):3546–56.

Zecco M, Prete A, Rondelli R, et al. Chronic graft versus host disease in children: incidence, risk factors, and impact on outcome. Blood 2003:100(4):1192–200.

26

SUPPORTIVE CARE AND MANAGEMENT OF ONCOLOGIC EMERGENCIES

Survival in children with cancer has increased dramatically during the past four decades. This progress is due not only to advances in specific oncologic therapies, but also to advances in supportive care and an ability to manage oncologic emergencies.

Cancer therapy requires supportive care in the following areas:

- Management of infectious complications
- Blood component therapy
- Hematopoietic growth factors
- Pain management
- Management of nausea and vomiting
- Nutritional support
- Psychosocial support.

ONCOLOGIC AND METABOLIC EMERGENCIES

Oncologic emergencies arise from:

1. Metabolic and endocrine disturbances that result from malignancy or are secondary to therapy
2. Space-occupying lesions that can press on or obstruct vital organs and cause mechanical/surgical emergencies
3. Pancytopenia secondary to bone marrow replacement or chemotherapy that may result in hemorrhage, anemia, and susceptibility to overwhelming infection.

Metabolic and Endocrine Emergencies

Hyperleukocytosis

A total white cell count greater than $100,000/mm^3$ is considered hyperleukocytosis. It is seen in 9–13% of children with acute lymphocytic leukemia (ALL) and 5–22% of children with acute myeloid leukemia (AML) at presentation. It occurs in almost all children with chronic myeloid leukemia. Hyperleukocytosis leads to increased blood viscosity and emboli in the microcirculation. Hemorrhage and leukostasis leading to intracranial hemorrhage or thrombosis, pulmonary hemorrhage, and leukostasis are far more prevalent in AML than in ALL because myeloblasts are larger than lymphoblasts and are more easily trapped in the microcirculation. Tumor lysis syndrome and metabolic abnormalities occur almost exclusively in ALL because lymphoblasts are more sensitive than myeloblasts to chemotherapy. The mortality rate is 23% in AML and 5% in ALL.

Clinical Features

1. *Central nervous system (CNS):* blurred vision, confusion, delirium, and papilledema; computed tomography (CT) may reveal hemorrhage or leukemic plaques
2. *Pulmonary:* tachypnea, dyspnea, hypoxia; chest radiograph may reveal pneumonitis or leukemic emboli
3. *Genitourinary:* oliguria, anuria, priapism.

Therapy

Table 26-1 outlines the management of hyperleukocytosis and tumor lysis syndrome.

Table 26-1. Management of Hyperleukocytosis and Tumor Lysis Syndrome

Management/objective	Guidelines
Hydration and alkalinization	D_5 1/4 NS + 50–100 mEq/L NaHCO$_3$ at 2–4× maintenance to maintain: Urine specific gravity <1.010 Urine output >100 mL/m^2/h Urine pH 6.5–7.5
Diuresis	Furosemide 0.5–1 mg/kg Mannitol 0.5 g/kg can be used if patient has oliguria unresponsive to increased hydration and furosemide
Uric acid reduction	Allopurinol 300 mg/m^2/day or 10 mg/kg/day PO OR 200 mg/m^2/day IV OR Rasburicase (recombinant urate oxidase) 0.2 mg/kg/day IV
Leukocyte reduction	Leukopheresis or exchange transfusion can be used if the initial white cell count is greater than 100,000/mm^3 Because of the volume of blood required to prime the pump, leukopheresis is usually used for children >4 years of age
Transfusion	Transfuse platelets to keep platelet count over 20,000/mm^3 to decrease the risk of intracranial hemorrhage. Avoid packed RBC transfusions, because it will increase the viscosity. Maintain hemoglobin less than 10 g/dL.
Chemotherapy	Started when patient is stabilized and has adequate urine output
Dialysis	Indicated for progressive renal failure with potassium >6 mEq/L, phosphate >10 mg/dL, oliguria, anuria, and volume overload unresponsive to the above measures
Monitor	Electrolytes; calcium, phosphorus, uric acid, BUN, creatinine every 6 hours Complete blood counts every 6 hours Urine output, pH, specific gravity Respiratory, CNS, and cardiac monitoring if there is hyperkalemia or hypocalcemia

Tumor Lysis Syndrome

In patients with high tumor burden—especially with stage III and stage IV Burkitt or Burkitt-like, B-cell acute lymphoblastic leukemia and T-cell leukemia or lymphoma, uric acid nephropathy may commence prior to initiating therapy. Extremely rapid cell proliferation is accompanied by significant cell death and release of intracellular ions, and may result in the following metabolic complications before starting chemotherapy:

- Hyperuricemia
- Hyperkalemia
- Hyperphosphatemia
- Hypocalcemia
- Hypercalcemia
- Renal failure.

These complications are observed in the above-mentioned conditions because these tumors have high growth fractions and they are exquisitely sensitive to chemotherapy. As a consequence there is rapid release of intracellular metabolites (such as phosphorus, potassium, and uric acid) in quantities that exceed the excretory capacity of the kidneys. If not successfully treated, tumor lysis syndrome can result in cardiac arrhythmias, renal failure, seizures, coma, disseminated intravascular coagulation (DIC), and death. Management of tumor lysis syndrome is outlined in Table 26-1.

Hyperuricemia (>8 mg/dL)

1. *Allopurinol:* 300 mg/m^2/day orally divided tid or 200 mg/m^2/day IV.
2. *Urate oxidase:* Recombinant urate oxidase (rasburicase) reduces uric acid levels to well below normal levels. It is indicated for patients with pretreatment hyperuricemia and in Burkitt or Burkitt-like or T-cell lymphoblastic lymphoma prophylactically, or for any patient with evidence of urate nephropathy. The dose is 0.2 mg/kg/day as single daily infusion over 30 minutes for up to 5 days. Allopurinol may be stopped and resumed at cessation of rasburicase.
3. *Hydration:* Hydration should be given at the rate of 3000 mL/m^2 over 24 hours and increased as needed to maintain urine output at >100 mL/m^2/h or ≥5 mL/kg/h before initiating chemotherapy and at ≥3 mL/kg/h once chemotherapy is begun. Strict measurement of intake and output should be carried out and verified every 2–4 hours. A Foley catheter should be inserted for continuous monitoring of urinary output. If urine output falls (i.e., less than 75% of input), hydration fluid should be increased and/or diuretics (furosemide 0.5–1 mg/kg/dose or mannitol 5–15 g/m^2 or 0.5 g/kg as 25% solution over 5–10 minutes repeated every 6 hours as necessary) should be administered. If response to bolus furosemide is insufficient, continuous infusion furosemide, beginning at 0.05 mg/kg/h may be used and titrated upward to desired effect. If at 10 hours from the start of treatment, BP is less than 130/90 and urinary output is still inadequate, dopamine infusion of 5 µg/kg/min should be started.
4. *Alkalinization of urine:*
   a. To increase solubility of urates, urine should be alkalinized with sodium bicarbonate (NaHCO$_3$) aimed at maintaining urine pH between 6.5 and 7.5. Urine pH >7.5 should be avoided because it is associated with precipitation of hypoxanthine and calcium phosphate in renal tubules.
   b. Administer NaHCO$_3$ 120 mEq/m^2 over 24 hours in IV hydration fluid.
   c. If urine pH is less than 6.5 increase NaHCO$_3$ and/or start Diamox 300 mg/m^2 every 6 hours.

Hyperkalemia (>6.0 mEq/L)

High potassium results from tumor cell lysis and/or renal failure.

1. Potassium should not be administered until tumor lysis is controlled.
2. The following measures to drive potassium into the cells are utilized:
   a. $NaHCO_3$: 1–2 mEq/kg/IV. For every increase in 0.1 pH unit, potassium is decreased about 1 mEq/L. The onset of action is within 30 minutes and the duration of activity lasts several hours.
   b. Insulin and glucose: Use dextrose 0.5 g/kg/h with insulin 0.1 units/kg/h. Monitor serum glucose closely. In case of an emergency, 50% dextrose can be used at 1 mL/kg through a central line. The onset of action is within 20–30 minutes and the duration of activity lasts several hours.
3. For life-threatening arrhythmias, calcium as calcium chloride 10 mg/kg IV is administered. The onset of action is within minutes and the duration of action lasts about 30 minutes. (*Caution:* Do not administer calcium in the same line as $NaHCO_3$.)
4. Sodium polystyrene sulfonate (Kayexalate) is administered to remove 1 mEq of potassium per liter per gram of resin over 24 hours. One gram per kilogram is given orally every 6 hours with Sorbitol 50–150 mL. The duration of action depends on the rate of endogenous potassium release.
5. Dialysis can be employed if the aforementioned measures fail.

Hyperphosphatemia (>6.5 mg/dL)

1. A low-phosphate diet should be prescribed.
2. Aluminum hydroxide 150 mg/kg/day divided every 4–6 hours should be administered.
3. Urine output should be maintained ≥3 mL/kg/hour.

Hypocalcemia (Ionized Calcium <1.5 mEq/L)

As the product of serum calcium and phosphate increases over 60 due to hyperphosphatemia, a compensatory hypocalcemia occurs to maintain the calcium phosphate product at 60; otherwise metastatic calcification can occur and exacerbate renal damage.

For symptomatic hypocalcemia (e.g., tetany), 10 mg/kg of elemental calcium (i.e., 0.5–1.0 mL/kg of 10% calcium gluconate) should be given. Calcium administration should be discontinued when symptoms resolve. Dialysis should be carried out if hyperphosphatemia persists. (*Caution:* Do not administer calcium in the same line as $NaHCO_3$.)

Hypercalcemia

Hypercalcemia has three main causes:

1. Osteolytic bone lesions (particularly in T-cell leukemia and lymphoma)
2. Bone demineralization secondary to parathyroid-like factors (paraneoplastic syndrome)
3. Immobilization.

Patients become symptomatic when serum calcium exceeds 12 mg/dL. Symptoms include:

- Nausea, vomiting, constipation
- Weakness

- Coma
- Pruritus
- Polyuria, nephrogenic diabetes insipidus
- Bradycardia, arrhythmias
- Dehydration, impaired renal function
- DIC.

Treatment
1. Dehydration and electrolyte disturbances should be corrected.
2. Renal calcium excretion should be increased by inducing diuresis with normal saline at two- to threefold maintenance and furosemide 1–2 mg/kg/dose every 6 hours.
3. Calcium mobilization from bone should be decreased by:
   a. Bisphosphonates such as pamidronate 0.5–1 mg/kg IV over 4 hours
   b. Prednisone 1.5–2.0 mg/kg daily (in lymphoproliferative disorders)
   c. Calcitonin 0.5–1.0 units/kg daily
   d. Mithramycin 10–25 µg/kg daily.

Renal Failure

Mechanisms of renal failure
- Precipitation of urates in the acid environment of urine
- Precipitation of hypoxanthine when the urine pH exceeds 7.5
- Increase in the hypoxanthine levels after starting treatment with allopurinol
- Precipitation of calcium phosphate in renal microvasculature and renal tubules when the product of serum calcium and phosphate values exceeds 60. Lymphoblasts contain four times the amount of phosphate present in normal lymphocytes.

Treatment
Hemodialysis or hemofiltration should be used when renal failure occurs. Peritoneal dialysis should not be used. Chemotherapy such as cyclophosphamide is given immediately after dialysis and not before. Renal dialysis usually needs to be repeated every 12 hours because of continuous rapid tumor lysis. Indications for renal dialysis are:

- An estimated glomerular filtration rate (GFR) less than 50%.

$$\text{Estimated GFR} = \frac{\text{Height in cm} \times 0.5 \text{ (children/adolescent girls) or 0.7 (adolescent boys)}}{\text{Serum creatinine in mg/dL}}$$

- Congestive heart failure
- Anuria
- Symptomatic hypocalcemia with hyperphosphatemia
- Hyperkalemia with QRS internal widening and/or potassium level of >6.0 mEq/L
- High creatinine with poor urinary output
- BP >150/90 and inadequate urinary output at 10 hours from the start of treatment.

Syndrome of Inappropriate Antidiuretic Hormone Secretion

- Involves continuous pituitary release of antidiuretic hormone (ADH), irrespective of plasma osmolality
- Leads to hypo-osmolality and water intoxication

- Results from physiologic stress, pain, surgery, mechanical ventilation, infections, CNS and pulmonary lesions, lymphomas, and leukemias
- Occurs as a side effect of vincristine, cyclophosphamide, ifosfamide, cisplatin, and melphalan.

Clinical Features

- Oliguria, weight gain
- Fatigue, lethargy, confusion, seizures, coma.

Laboratory Features

- Hypo-osmolality (<280 mOsm/L)
- Hyponatremia (sodium, <135 mEq/L)
- Increased urine specific gravity.

Treatment

Fluid restriction; hydrate with normal saline limited to insensible losses (500 mL/m²/24 hours) plus ongoing losses.

In case of severe neurologic involvement (seizures or coma):

1. Hydrate with hypertonic saline 3%.
2. Furosemide 1 mg/kg should be administered to increase diuresis.
3. The rate of sodium correction should be limited to 2 mEq/L/h. Correction that takes place too rapidly causes a sodium diuresis and can lead to further neurologic deterioration and death.

Oncologic Emergencies by Anatomic Region

Thoracic Emergencies

- Superior vena cava syndrome (SVCS) consists of the signs and symptoms of superior vena cava (SVC) obstruction.
- Superior mediastinal syndrome (SMS) consists of tracheal compression.

In pediatrics, SVCS and SMS usually occur together.

Etiology

1. Intrinsic causes: vascular thrombosis following the introduction of a catheter
2. Extrinsic causes: malignant anterior mediastinal tumors
   a. Hodgkin lymphoma
   b. Non-Hodgkin lymphoma
   c. Teratoma or other germ cell tumor
   d. Thyroid cancer
   e. Thymoma.

Clinical Features

1. SVC obstruction:
   a. Swelling, plethora, and cyanosis of the face, neck, and upper extremities
   b. Suffusion of the conjunctiva
   c. Engorgement of collateral veins
2. SMS: cough, hoarseness, dyspnea, orthopnea, wheezing, stridor, and chest pain. Supine position worsens symptoms.

Management

1. Extreme care in handling the patient. The following may precipitate respiratory arrest: supine position; stress; sedation, conscious sedation, or anxiolytics; or general anesthesia. The patient may have to be intubated. Extubation may not be possible until the anterior mediastinal mass has significantly decreased in size.
2. Diagnosis should be made quickly in the least invasive manner.
   a. Radiograph and CT of the chest.
   b. CBC, bone marrow aspirate and biopsy.
   c. A tissue diagnosis is desirable. Because of the risk of anesthesia, the least invasive technique possible (such as fine-needle aspiration, pleurocentesis, pericardiocentesis) should be used.
   d. If vascular and infectious causes can be eliminated, the most likely cause is lymphoma.
   e. Serum markers such as α-fetoprotein and β-hCG can help to diagnose teratoma and rule out lymphoma.
3. Therapy:
   a. For thrombosis, a continuous infusion of tissue plasminogen activator (tPA) 0.1–0.6 mg/kg/hour for 6 hours followed by heparin 75 units/kg bolus followed by 20 units/kg/hour may be successful in lysing the clot.
   b. Establishing a tissue diagnosis may not be possible and patients may need empiric treatment as a life-saving measure. Treatment options are radiotherapy and steroids. Both treatments may confound the diagnosis. Patients should undergo biopsy as soon as the mass shrinks and patients are stable.
   c. Specific chemotherapy should be instituted after a biopsy has been obtained.

Abdominal Emergencies

- *Esophagitis:* the most common gastrointestinal (GI) problem in oncology patients
- *Gastric hemorrhage:* especially in patients on corticosteroid therapy
- *Typhlitis:* seen only in neutropenic patients
- *Perirectal abscess:* in prolonged neutropenia
- *Hemorrhagic pancreatitis:* especially in patients on L-asparaginase therapy
- *Massive hepatic enlargement from tumor:* especially in infants with stage IVS neuroblastoma.

Evaluation and Diagnosis

1. History regarding onset, timing, location, and radiation of pain
2. Observation and gentle examination including rectal examination (the classic signs of an acute abdomen may be muted in a neutropenic patient or a patient on steroids)
3. Serial blood counts to evaluate for hemorrhage, inflammation, infection
4. Blood cultures
5. Electrolyte monitoring
6. Vital signs monitoring
7. Abdominal sonography, radiography, CT, and magnetic resonance imaging (MRI).

Typhlitis

Typhlitis, a necrotizing colitis localized in the cecum, occurs in the setting of severe neutropenia, particularly in patients with leukemia and in stem cell transplant recipients.

It should be strongly suspected in patients with right lower quadrant pain and the development of a partially obstructive right lower quadrant mass. Healing can occur with fibrosis and stricture formation.

Bacterial invasion of the mucosa can progress from inflammation to full-thickness infarction to perforation, peritonitis, and septic shock. The responsible pathogens include *Pseudomonas* species, *Escherichia coli*, other gram-negative bacteria, *Staphylococcus aureus*, α-hemolytic *Streptococcus*, *Clostridium*, *Aspergillus*, and *Candida*.

Diagnosis
- Typhlitis is usually diagnosed clinically when a neutropenic patient presents with right lower quadrant pain or a right lower quadrant mass.
- Radiograph of the abdomen may reveal pneumatosis intestinalis or bowel wall thickening.
- Ultrasonography may reveal thickening of the bowel wall in the region of the cecum.
- CT scan may demonstrate diffuse thickening of the cecal wall.
- Barium enema may show severe mucosal irregularity, rigidity, loss of haustral markings, and occasional fistula formation.

Treatment
Medical management is the initial treatment, consisting of:

- Discontinuation of oral intake
- Nasogastric tube suctioning
- Broad-spectrum antibiotics
- Intravenous fluid and electrolytes
- Packed red cell and platelet transfusions, as indicated
- Vasopressors, as needed (hypotension is associated with a poor outcome).

Indications for surgical intervention:

- Persistent GI bleeding despite resolution of neutropenia and thrombocytopenia
- Evidence of free air in the abdomen on abdominal radiograph (indicating perforation)
- Clinical deterioration requiring fluid and pressor support, indicating uncontrolled sepsis from bowel infarction.

Surgery consists of removing necrotic portions of the bowel and diversion via colostomy.

Perirectal Abscess

Inflammation and infection of the rectum and perirectal tissue occur commonly in patients receiving chemotherapy or radiation therapy, especially in patients with prolonged neutropenia. Presentation includes anorectal pain, tenderness, and painful bowel movements. An abscess or draining fistula may be present; however, in the neutropenic patient, pus will be absent and the patient will present with a brawny edema and dense cellulitis.

Management
1. Initial therapy with intravenous antibiotics to cover gram-negative organisms and anaerobes
2. Granulocyte colony-stimulating factor (G-CSF) to shorten period of neutropenia
3. Sitz baths four times a day, and meticulous attention to perirectal hygiene
4. Surgical incision and drainage of obviously fluctuant areas or draining fistulas that do not resolve with medical management.

Neurologic Emergencies

Spinal Cord Compression

Incidence and etiology
- Three to five percent of children with cancer develop acute spinal cord or cauda equina compression. Sarcomas account for about half of the cases of spinal cord involvement in childhood; the remainders are caused by neuroblastoma, germ cell tumor, lymphoma, leukemia, and drop metastasis of CNS tumors.
- The spinal cord can be compressed by tumor in the epidural or subarachnoid space or by metastases within the cord parenchyma.

The mechanisms of tumor spread to the spinal cord include:

- Direct extension of the tumor
- Metastatic spread to the vertebrae with secondary cord compression
- Spread to the epidural space via infiltration of the vertebral foramina
- Subarachnoid spread down the spinal cord from primary CNS tumor (such as medulloblastoma).

Clinical presentation
- Back pain with localized tenderness occurs in 80% of patients.
- Incontinence, urinary retention, and other abnormalities of bowel or bladder function are frequent.
- Loss of strength and sensory deficits with a sensory level may also occur.
- Any child with cancer and back pain should be presumed to have spinal cord involvement until further workup indicates otherwise.

Evaluation
- A thorough history and neurologic examination should be included in the evaluation.
- MRI with and without gadolinium is necessary to detect the presence and extent of epidural involvement.
- Lumbar puncture myelography is usually not necessary if MRI is available.
- Spine radiographs may be helpful, but they miss epidural disease in 50% of cases.
- Cerebrospinal fluid (CSF) analysis is important in the evaluation of subarachnoid disease, but it is not helpful in localizing epidural disease.

Treatment
Because the potential for permanent neurologic damage is high, it is crucial to initiate treatment immediately.

1. Dexamethasone is initiated prior to diagnostic studies.
   a. For progressive dysfunction and significant deficits, administer 1–2 mg/kg/day loading dose. Follow with 1.5 mg/kg/day divided q6h.
   b. For mild stable deficits, administer 0.25–1 mg/kg/dose every 6 hours.
2. Emergency MRI with and without gadolinium enhancement is performed after the administration of dexamethasone.
3. If an epidural mass is identified, treatment is aimed at rapid decompression. Chemotherapy, radiation therapy, or surgical decompression may be used.
   a. If tumor is known to be radiosensitive, give local radiation including the full volume of the tumor plus one vertebra above and below the lesion. Three daily doses of 400 cGy are given. Additional daily doses of 200 cGy are given for a total of 2000–3000 cGy, depending on the responsiveness of the tumor.

  b. Surgical intervention may be indicated for rapid decompression.

  c. Specific chemotherapy can be instituted in addition to the use of radiation and dexamethasone in lymphoma, leukemia, and neuroblastoma.

SUPPORTIVE CARE

Management of Infectious Complications

Children being treated for cancer are rendered significantly immunocompromised through the use of chemotherapy. For this reason, it is extremely important to expeditiously evaluate and treat the febrile oncology patient. Any delay in antibiotic therapy while waiting culture results may lead to uncontrolled progression of infection in the neutropenic patient.

Several factors lead to the susceptibility of oncology patients to infections:

1. *Underlying cancer:* Patients with leukemia, advanced-stage lymphoma, and uncontrolled tumors are more prone to infections.
2. *Type of therapy:* Dose-intensive therapies, high-dose cytosine arabinoside, and stem cell transplant render patients more susceptible to infections.
3. *Degree and duration of neutropenia:* The most important determinant of susceptibility to bacterial and fungal infections is the number of circulating neutrophils. Patients who are neutropenic (absolute neutrophil count [ANC] <1000/mm^3) are more susceptible to infection. Neutropenia can be secondary to disease (leukemia, aplastic anemia) or chemotherapy. Neutrophil function may also be impaired by disease and by chemotherapy.
4. *Disruption of normal barriers:* The normal mechanical barriers to infection in the skin, respiratory, GI, and genitourinary systems are disrupted.
5. *Nutritional status:* Malnutrition affects lymphocyte function, neutrophils, mononuclear cells, and complement system.
6. *Humoral immunity:* Defects in humoral immunity produce susceptibility to encapsulated bacteria including *Streptococcus pneumoniae, Haemophilus influenzae,* and *Neisseria meningitidis.*
7. *Cell-mediated immunity:* Defects in cellular immunity produce susceptibility to viruses, fungi, and intracellularly replicating bacteria (e.g., *Listeria* and *Salmonella).* Patients with Hodgkin disease and non-Hodgkin lymphoma have impaired cell-mediated immunity. Chemotherapy, radiation, and steroids induce defects in lymphocyte function. Lymphopenia may persist after completion of chemotherapy.
8. *Colonizing microbial flora:* Many bacterial infections arise from endogenous microflora.
9. *Foreign bodies:* Indwelling central catheters, ventriculoperitoneal shunts.

Table 26-2 lists the predominant pathogens in cancer patients.

Management of Fever in the Oncology Patient

Fever is defined as a temperature greater than 38°C three times in 24 hours or greater than 38.5°C once. There are four categories of febrile patients:

1. Nonneutropenic patients
2. Patients with an indwelling catheter
3. Neutropenic patients
4. Splenectomized patients.

Table 26-2. Predominant Pathogens in Children with Cancer

Gram-positive bacteria
Staphylococci (coagulase-negative, *Staphylococcus aureus*)
Streptococci (α-hemolytic)
Enterococci
Corynebacteria
Listeria sp.
Clostridium difficile

Gram-negative bacteria
Enterobacteriaceae (*Escherichia coli, Klebsiella, Enterobacter, Serratia*)
Pseudomonas aeruginosa, Stenotrophomonas maltophilia
   (and similar oxidase-positive multiresistant gram-negative organism)
Anaerobes

Fungi
Candida sp.
Aspergillus sp.
Zygomycetes
Cryptococci

Other
Pneumocystis carinii
Toxoplasma gondii
Strongyloides stercoralis
Cryptosporidium

Viruses
Herpes simplex virus
Varicella-zoster virus
Cytomegalovirus
Epstein-Barr virus
Respiratory syncytial virus
Adenovirus
Influenza virus
Parainfluenza virus

From Alexander SW, Walsh TJ, Freifield AG, Pizzo PA. Infectious complications in pediatric cancer patients. In: Pizzo PA, Poplack DG, editors. Principles and Practice of Pediatric Oncology. 4th ed. Philadelphia: Lippincott Williams & Wilkins, 2002;1239–84, with permission.

Febrile Nonneutropenic Patients

The nonneutropenic patient remains susceptible to infections secondary to lymphocyte dysfunction. Evaluation should include a careful history and physical examination. Blood and urine cultures should be obtained. In addition, patients with localized findings should undergo the appropriate diagnostic procedures (e.g., throat culture, stool culture, chest radiograph). If they do not have an indwelling catheter, empiric antibiotic therapy is rarely indicated. They should be followed for clinical or microbiological evidence of infection. If infection is documented, they should be treated with appropriate antibiotics.

Patients with Indwelling Venous Catheters

If the patient with a subcutaneously tunneled catheter such as a Broviac, a Hickman, or a totally implantable venous access device or "port" (e.g., Mediport) is neutropenic, follow the guidelines for the neutropenic patient. If the patient is not neutropenic, manage as follows:

1. Examine the site for evidence of inflammation at the exit site or on the skin overlying the subcutaneously tunneled portion of the catheter. If there is pus at the exit site, collect and send for culture.
2. Obtain cultures from each lumen of the catheter and from a peripheral venous site.
3. A broad-spectrum, third-generation cephalosporin (ceftriaxone) is appropriate if there is no sign of tunnel infection. If there is tunnel infection, the catheter should be removed and patients should be treated with intravenous antibiotics.
4. Follow cultures for 48–72 hours; if they are negative, antibiotics should be discontinued.
5. If cultures are positive, a 10- to 14-day course of the appropriate antibiotic is indicated.

Febrile Neutropenic Patients

Patients with an ANC of less than $500/mm^3$ and those with an ANC of less than $1000/mm^3$ and decreasing are considered neutropenic. Because of the high risk of morbidity and mortality in the febrile neutropenic patient, the workup should be thorough and expeditious and empiric broad-spectrum antibiotics should be started as soon as possible.

1. Management includes careful history and physical examination with special attention to important sites of infection in the neutropenic patient:
   a. Oral mucosa and periodontium
   b. Pharynx
   c. Lower esophagus
   d. Lungs
   e. Skin including sites of vascular access, bone marrow aspiration sites, tissue around the nails
   f. Perineum and anus.
2. In the neutropenic patient, even subtle signs of inflammation must be considered as potential sources of infection and should be cultured appropriately.
3. Obtain a complete blood count, serum chemistries, urinalysis, and urine culture.
4. Obtain blood cultures from all lumens of indwelling catheters and from a peripheral vein.
5. Obtain a chest radiograph.
6. Start broad-spectrum antibiotic therapy. Broad-spectrum therapy is required in the neutropenic patient even if a single source or pathogen is isolated, because the occurrence of infection with a second pathogen during continuing neutropenia is not infrequent.

Empiric antibiotic therapy
The prompt initiation of antibiotic therapy in febrile neutropenic patients has decreased the mortality rate for gram-negative infections significantly. Table 26-3 shows the frequently used antimicrobial drugs, their dosages, route of administration, and dosage schedules. Figure 26-1 provides an algorithm for the management of the febrile neutropenic patient. The choice of antibiotics should depend on the predominant organisms and antibiotic sensitivity patterns. Any initial antibiotic regimen should include drugs with antipseudomonal activity. Initial therapy with oral antibiotics alone is not recommended for children.

Table 26-3. Frequently Used Antibiotics for Fever and Neutropenia

Drug	Dose	Route	Schedule
Aminoglycosides			
Amikacin	15 mg/kg/day	IV	Divided q8h
Gentamicin	6.0–7.5 mg/kg/day	IV	Divided q8h
Tobramycin	6.0–7.5 gm/kg/day	IV	Divided q8h
β-Lactam drugs			
Antipseudomonal, semisynthetic penicillins			
Azlocillin	300 mg/kg/day (maximum 24 g/day)	IV	Divided q4–6h
Mezlocillin	300 mg/kg/day (maximum 24 g/day)	IV	Divided q4–6h
Piperacillin	300 mg/kg/day (maximum 24 g/day)	IV	Divided q4–6h
Piperacillin/tazobactam	300 mg/kg/day of piperacillin component	IV	Divided q6h
Ticarcillin	300 mg/kg/day (maximum 24 g/day)	IV	Divided q4–6h
Carbenicillin	500 mg/kg/day	IV	Divided q4–6h
Cephalosporins			
Ceftazidime	100–150 mg/kg/day	IV	Divided q8h
Cefazolin	50–100 mg/kg/day (maximum 6 g/day)	IV	Divided q8h
Cefepime	50 mg/kg per dose (maximum 2 g)	IV	q8h
Carbapenem			
Imipenem/cilastatin	50 mg/kg/day (maximum 4 g/day)	IV	Divided q6–8h
Meropenem	60–120 mg/kg/day (maximum dose 6 g/day)	IV	Divided q8h
Penicillinase-resistant penicillin			
Nafcillin	100–200 mg/kg/day	IV	Divided q4–8h
Other			
Vancomycin	40 mg/kg/day (maximum 2 g/day)	IV	Divided q6–8h
Anaerobic coverage			
Clindamycin	40 mg/kg/day	IV	Divided q6–8h
Metronidazole	30 mg/kg/day (loading dose initially 15 mg/kg)	IV	Divided q6h

From Wolff LJ, Altman AJ, Berkow RL, Johnson FL. The management of fever and neutropenia. In: Altman AJ, editor. Supportive care of children with cancer. Current therapy and guidelines from the Children's Oncology Group. 3rd ed. Baltimore: The Johns Hopkins University Press, 2004;200–20, with permission.

Antibiotic regimens

Because gram-positive, gram-negative, and mixed infections occur, broad-spectrum coverage must be provided. Initial regimens include:

1. Monotherapy with cefepime, ceftazidime, or imipenem
2. Two-drug regimen: aminoglycoside and antipseudomonal penicillin, cefepime, or ceftazidime.

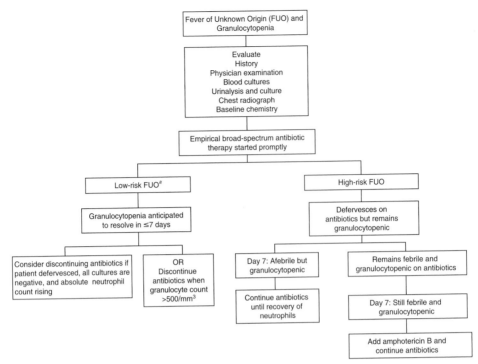

Fig. 26-1. Algorithm for the initial management of the child who has an unexplained fever or neutropenia. From Alexander SW, Walsh TJ, Freifeld AG, Pizzo PA. Infectious complications in pediatric cancer patients. In Pizzo PA, Poplock DG, editors. Principles and Practice of Pediatric Oncology. 4th ed. Philadelphia: Lippincott, Williams; Wilkins, 2002; 1239–84, with permission.
[a]Nutropenia resolves within one week.

Vancomycin is not recommended for empiric therapy because its use promotes the emergence of resistant strains such as vancomycin-resistant enterococci. Vancomycin should only be added to the initial regimen if the following is present:

1. Obvious central line infection
2. Intensive chemotherapy causing mucositis (such as high-dose cytosine arabinoside for AML)
3. Patients colonized with resistant organisms that are treatable only with vancomycin
4. Hypotension
5. Patients who have developed fever despite quinolone prophylaxis.

Management of Fever of Unknown Origin

Many febrile neutropenic patients have no identifiable cause for their fever. It is likely that a significant percentage of these patients have occult infections. These patients should be carefully reassessed including review of previous culture results, a meticulous physical examination, chest radiography, diagnostic imaging of any organ suspected of having infection, examination of the status of vascular catheters, and additional cultures. Patients with fever of unexplained origin can be divided into two groups:

1. *Low-risk patients.* Neutropenia resolves within 1 week of starting antibiotics. In these patients, antibiotics may be stopped when the absolute neutrophil count reaches 500/mm^3.
2. *High-risk patients.* Neutropenia persists for more than 1 week, and there is no evidence of bone marrow recovery. If the patient is continuously febrile, antifungal

treatment should be added. If the patient is afebrile but remains granulocy-topenic, antibiotics should be continued for a 14-day course and then discontin-ued. If the patient subsequently becomes febrile, antibiotics should be resumed.

Antibiotic therapy may need to be modified according to patient's clinical status (Table 26-4).

Empiric Institution of Antifungal Therapy

Up to one third of febrile neutropenic patients who do not respond to a 1-week course of antibiotics have systemic fungal infections. In most cases, these infections are caused by *Candida* and *Aspergillus* species. For this reason and because of the high morbidity and mortality of fungal infections, we recommend systemic antifungal therapy for the neutropenic patient who is persistently febrile after 4–7 days on broad-spectrum antibiotics. Amphotericin B 0.5–1 mg/kg/day IV is the standard drug for this purpose. Lipid formulations of amphotericin B can be used as alterna-tives. They do not appear to be more effective; however, there is less drug-related toxicity.

Table 26-4. Modifications of Initial Antimicrobial Regimen for Febrile Neutropenic Cancer Patients

Status of symptom	Modifications of primary regimen
Fever	
Persistent for >5 days	Add empiric antifungal therapy.
Recurrence after ≥5 days in patient with persistent neutropenia	Add empiric antifungal therapy.
Persistent or recurrent fever at time of recovery from neutropenia	Evaluate liver and spleen using computed tomography, ultrasonography, or magnetic resonance imaging for hepatosplenic candidiasis, and evaluate need for antifungal therapy.
Bloodstream	
Cultures before antibiotic therapy	
Gram-positive organism	Add vancomycin pending further identification.
Gram-negative organism	Maintain regimen if patient is stable and isolate is susceptible. If *Pseudomonas aeruginosa, Enterobacter, Serratia,* or *Citrobacter* is isolated, add an aminoglycoside or if resistant to cephalosporin, add a carbapenem.
Organism isolated during antibiotic therapy	
Gram-positive organism	Add vancomycin.
Gram-negative organism	Change to new combination regimen (e.g., imipenem plus gentamicin or vancomycin, or gentamicin plus piperacillin).
Head, eyes, ears, nose, throat	
Necrotizing or marginal gingivitis	Add specific antianaerobic agent (clindamycin or metronidazole) to empiric therapy.
Vesicular or ulcerative lesions	Suspect herpes simplex infection. Culture and begin acyclovir therapy.
Sinus tenderness or nasal ulcerative lesions	Suspect fungal infection with aspergillus or mucor.

(Continues)

Table 26-4. (*Continued*)

Status of symptom	Modifications of primary regimen
Gastrointestinal tract	
Retrosternal burning pain	Suspect *Candida*, herpes simplex, or both. Add antifungal therapy and, if no response, acyclovir. Bacterial esophagitis is also a possibility. For patients who do not respond within 48 hours, endoscopy should be considered.
Acute abdominal pain	Suspect typhlitis, as well as appendicitis, if pain in right lower quadrant. Add specific antianaerobic coverage to empirical regimen and monitor closely for need for surgical intervention.
Perianal tenderness	Add specific antianaerobic drug to empirical regimen and monitor need for surgical intervention, especially when patient is recovering from neutropenia.
Respiratory tract	
New focal lesion in patient recovering from neutropenia	Observe carefully, because this may be a consequence of inflammatory response in concert with neutrophil recovery.
New focal lesion in patient with continuing neutropenia	*Aspergillus* is the chief concern. Perform appropriate cultures and consider biopsy. If patient is not a candidate for procedure, administer high-dose amphotericin B (1.5 mg/kg/day) or liposomal formulation.
New interstitial pneumonitis	Attempt diagnosis by examination of induced sputum or bronchoalveolar lavage. If not feasible, begin empiric treatment with trimethoprim sulfamethoxazole or pentamidine. Consider noninfectious causes and the need for open lung biopsy if condition has not improved after 4 days of therapy.

From Alexander SW, Walsh TJ, Freifeld AG, Pizzo PA. Infectious complications in pediatric cancer patients. In: Pizzo PA, Poplack DG, editors. Principles and Practice of Pediatric Oncology. 4th ed. Philadelphia: Lippincott Williams & Wilkins, 2002; 1239–84, with permission.

Antiviral drugs are indicated only if there is clinical or laboratory evidence of viral infection.

Therapy with G-CSF at a dose of 5 µg/kg/day SC is recommended under certain conditions in which worsening of the clinical course is predicted and there is an expected long delay in the recovery of the marrow. It should also be considered for patients who remain severely neutropenic and have documented infections that do not respond to appropriate antibiotic treatment. There are no specific indications for standard use of granulocyte transfusions. Granulocyte transfusions may be useful in patients with profound neutropenia, in whom the infections progress despite optimal antibiotic treatment and G-CSF and in cases of severe uncontrollable fungal infections. Significant side effects include transmission of cytomegalovirus, alloimmunization, progressive platelet refractoriness, and respiratory insufficiency associated with concomitant administration of amphotericin B.

Febrile Splenectomized Patients

The spleen acts both as a mechanical filter and as an immune effector organ. Immune functions of the spleen are as follows:

1. Production of antibodies to polysaccharide antigens
2. Removal of damaged cells and opsonin-coated organisms from the circulation.

Splenectomized patients are immunocompromised in the following ways:

1. They are deficient in antibody production when challenged with particulate antigens.
2. They have decreased levels of immunoglobulin M (IgM) and properdin.
3. They are deficient in the phagocytosis-promoting protein tuftsin.

They are at risk for fulminant and rapidly fatal septicemia due to encapsulated bacteria, including *S. pneumoniae*, *H. influenzae* type b, and *N. meningitidis*.

Management
To decrease the risk of overwhelming postsplenectomy infection, the following measures are recommended:

1. Before splenectomy, administer the *H. influenzae* type B (HIB) vaccine, the 23-valent pneumococcal vaccine, and the quadrivalent meningococcal vaccine. If the splenectomy is elective, the vaccines should be given 2 weeks before surgery to increase the likelihood of eliciting an optimal antibody response.
2. Prophylaxis with oral penicillin (125 mg twice daily for children under 5 years; 250 mg twice daily for children 5 years and older) is commonly prescribed. It should be continued at least into adulthood.
3. If the splenectomized patient becomes febrile:
   a. Obtain two blood cultures.
   b. Start broad-spectrum IV antibiotic therapy (the currently recommended drug is ceftriaxone 2 g IV every 24 hours for adults or 75 mg/kg IV every 24 hours for children).
   c. Continue antibiotic therapy until the blood cultures are negative for 72 hours and the patient is afebrile for 24–48 hours.
   d. If the patient is febrile and neutropenic, manage as for the febrile neutropenic patient, but include an antibiotic with excellent activity against pneumococci.

Bacterial Infections

Table 26-3 lists the doses, routes, and schedules for frequently used antibiotics, Table 26-4 modifications of initial antimicrobial therapy, and Table 26-5 various infections, common pathogens encountered, and their appropriate treatment.

Fungal Infections

Table 26-6 shows the common fungal infections and their treatment. Table 26-7 shows the recommended doses and routes of administration of the antifungal drugs. Invasive fungal infections are a significant cause of morbidity and mortality. Neutropenia is the most important predisposing factor.

Viral Infections

Children on chemotherapy can tolerate many common viral infections, but defects in cellular immunity predispose them to unusually severe infections with certain viruses, particularly of the herpes virus group. Primary varicella infection, in particular, can produce serious morbidity, including encephalitis and pneumonitis, and mortality in 7% of patients.

Table 26-5. Common Pathogens and Treatment in Various Infections in Children with Cancer

Infection	Common pathogens	Treatment
Bacteremia	*S. aureus, S. epidermidis, Streptococcus* sp., *Enterococcus* sp., *E. coli, K. pneumoniae, Enterobacter*	Cefepime or ceftazidime and gentamicin followed by appropriate antibiotics for the isolate
Catheter-associated bacteremia	*S. epidermidis*, other gram-positive and gram-negative bacteria, fungi	Vancomycin or appropriate antibiotics for 7–10 days. Antibiotic infusion should be rotated through each lumen of the catheter. If infected with vancomycin resistant enterococci, *Candida*, or multiple organisms, if cultures are persistently positive despite antibiotics, if there is recurrent bacteremia with the same organism, remove the catheter.
Local catheter infections: exit site infection, tunnel infection	Gram-positive cocci, gram-negative bacilli	Vancomycin or appropriate antibiotic for 7–10 days. If there is tunnel infection, remove the catheter.
Otitis media	*S. pneumonia, H. influenzae*, other gram-positive and gram-negative bacteria	10–14 days of amoxicillin-clavulanic acid
Sinusitis	*S. pneumonia, H. influenzae, Moraxella catarrhalis, S. aureus*, gram-negative aerobes, anaerobes, fungi (*Aspergillus, Candida*, mucor)	If patient not neutropenic, amoxicillin, clavulanic, acid or TMP/SMX. If patient neutropenic, ticarcillin/clavulanate or clindamycin and gentamicin. If no improvement in 72 hours, perform biopsy to rule out fungal infection.
Localized pulmonary infiltrate	Gram-positive and gram-negative bacteria, *Aspergillus* sp., *P. boydii, Fusarium* sp., *Trichosporon beigelii, Zygomycetes, Candida* sp., *H. capsulatum*	Cefepime or ceftazidime and gentamicin AND azithromycin. If there is no improvement within 72 hours, a BAL or open lung biopsy should be performed.
Diffuse pulmonary infiltrate	PCP	TMP/SMX or pentamidine and short course of steroids
	CMV	Ganciclovir and IVIG
	HSV or VZV	Acyclovir
	RSV	Ribavirin
	Adenovirus, parainfluenza, influenza, HHV-6	
Infections in oral cavity:		
Thrush	*C. albicans*	Topical antifungal agents, fluconazole
Mucositis	HSV	Acyclovir
Periodontal disease	Anaerobic bacteria, mixed aerobic	Clindamycin, metronidazole, imipenem
Esophagitis	Candida	Fluconazole, amphotericin B
	HSV	Acyclovir
Typhlitis	Anaerobes, gram-negative bacilli	Ticarcillin/clavulanate or clindamycin and gentamicin
Peritonitis	*Clostridium*	Penicillin, cephalosporins, clindamycin, vancomycin

(Continues)

Table 26-5. (*Continued*)

Infection	Common pathogens	Treatment
Colitis	*C. difficile*	Oral vancomycin or metronidazole
Hepatitis	Hepatitis A, B, C	
	HSV	Acyclovir
	CMV	Ganciclovir, foscarnet
	EBV, coxsackie B, adenovirus	
	Toxoplasmosis	
	C. albicans, Aspergillus	Amphotericin B
	Bacterial sepsis	Appropriate antibiotics
Perianal cellulitis	Aerobic gram-negative bacilli (*P. aeruginosa, K. pneumoniae, E. coli*), enterococci, bowel anaerobes	Cefepime or ceftazidime AND gentamicin AND clindamycin/metronidazole
Intraventricular shunt and ommaya reservoir	Coagulase-negative and positive staphylococci, *Corynebacterium sp., Propionibacterium acnes,* gram-negative bacilli	Vancomycin followed by appropriate antimicrobials for the isolate
Meningitis	*S. epidermidis,* α-hemolytic streptococci, *Enterococcus, E. coli, K. pneumoniae, P. aeruginosa, C. albicans, Aspergillus*	Ceftriaxone and vancomycin followed by appropriate antimicrobials for the isolate
Urinary tract infections	*E. coli, Klebsiella sp., Proteus sp., P. aeruginosa,* enterococci, *C. albicans, Candida tropicalis, Candida glabrata,* adenovirus, polyomavirus (BK virus)	Cefepime or ceftazidime and gentamicin followed by appropriate antimicrobials for the isolate
Skin infections	*P. aeruginosa, Aeromonas hydrophilia, S. marcenses, Aspergillus, Candida,* HSV, VZV	Appropriate antimicrobials for the organism Acyclovir

Table 26-8 lists the indications, route of administration, and recommended dosages for the current antiviral therapies.

Protozoan Infections

Two protozoan infections occur relatively frequently:

- *Toxoplasma gondii*
- *Pneumocystis carinii.*

Pneumocystis carinii is a ubiquitous organism that causes severe or fatal pneumonitis in immunocompromised patients.

Clinical Features

1. Rapid onset of symptoms with fever and tachypnea
2. Progressive respiratory distress with nasal flaring and intercostal retractions

Table 26-6. Drugs for Invasive and Other Serious Fungal Infections[a]

Disease	Intravenous amphotericin B	Oral, absorbable			Intravenous or oral		
		Caspofungin[b]	Flucytosine	Ketoconazole[b]	Itraconazole	Fluconazole	Voriconazole
Aspergillosis	P	A	—	—	A, M	—	A
Blastomycosis	P	—	—	A, M	M, (P)	A, M	—
Candidiasis:							
Chronic, mucocutaneous	A	—	—	A	A	P	—
Oropharyngeal, esophageal	A (severe cases)	—	—	A	A	P	—
Systemic	P, S	—	S	—	—	(P), A, M	—
Coccidioidomycosis	P	—	—	A, M	A, M	(P), A, M	—
Cryptococcosis	P, S	—	P, S	—	A	A, M	—
Histoplasmosis	P	—	—	A, M	(P), A	A, M	—
Mucormycosis (zygomycosis)	P	—	—	—	—	—	—
Paracoccidioidomycosis	(P)[c]	—	—	M	P, M	—	—
Pseudallescheriasis	—	—	—	A	P	—	A
Sporotrichosis	(P)	—	—	—	P	A, M	—

[a] P indicates preferred treatment in most cases (parentheses indicate drug is considered preferred treatment by some experts); A, efficacy less well established or alternative drug; M, for mild and moderately severe cases; S, combination recommended if infection is severe or central nervous system is involved.

[b] Efficacy and safety have not been established for children.

[c] Usually in combination with itraconazole or a sulfonamide.

From Pickering LK, editor. Red Book: 2003 Report of the Committee on Infectious Diseases. 26th ed. Elk Grove Village, IL: American Academy of Pediatrics, 2003;725, with permission.

Table 26-7. Antifungal Agents and Doses

Drug	Route	Dose
Amphotericin B (Fungizone)	IV	Test dose 0.1 mg/kg to a maximum dose of 1 mg over 1 hour; if tolerated, may use 0.4 mg/kg and increase to 1 mg/kg/day
Amphotericin B lipid complex (Abelcet)	IV	5 mg/kg/day
Amphotericin B liposomal (AmBisome)	IV	3–5 mg/kg/day
Amphotericin B colloidal dispersion (Amphotec)	IV	3–5 mg/kg/day
Flucytosine	PO	50–150 mg/kg/day divided every 6 hours
Fluconazole	IV, PO	3–12 mg/kg/day (maximum dose 600 mg/day)
Itraconazole	IV, PO	3–10 mg/kg/day has been used, but dose yet to be established
Voriconazole	IV, PO	6 mg/kg every 12 hours, IV for first 24 hours and then 4 mg/kg every 12 hours. Oral dose: >40 kg, 200 mg bid, may increase to 300 mg bid, <40 kg 100 mg bid, may increase to 150 mg bid
Caspofungin	IV	35–70 mg/day IV. Not adequately studied in patients <18 years of age

From Wolff LJ, Altman AJ, Berkow RL, Johnson FL. The management of fever and neutropenia. In: Autumn AJ, editor. Supportive care of children with cancer. Current therapy and guidelines from the Children's Oncology Group. 3rd ed. Baltimore: The Johns Hopkins University Press, 2004;25–38, with permission.

3. Absence of rales on physical examination
4. Hypoxemia on arterial blood gas
5. Development of bilateral pneumonitis on chest radiograph
6. Rapid progression of respiratory distress/respiratory failure over a few days; usually fatal if untreated.

Diagnosis

1. Typical clinical syndrome
2. Demonstration of the organism in sputum or material from endobronchial washing or percutaneous needle biopsy or open lung biopsy
3. Identification of organism by Gomori methenamine silver stain.

Treatment

Start treatment as soon as the patient develops tachypnea and hypoxemia, even if there is no laboratory confirmation of the organism:

1. Trimethoprim/sulfamethoxazole (TMP/SMX) 20 mg/kg/day of TMP component IV divided into four doses is the treatment of choice. Treatment should continue for 21 days. TMP/SMX causes myelosuppression.
2. If TMP/SMX is not tolerated, treat with pentamidine 4 mg/kg/day IV or TMP 5 mg/kg PO every 6 hours and dapsone 100 mg/day PO for 21 days.

Monitor carefully for hypotension. Pentamidine is recommended if patients fail to respond to TMP/SMX in 72 hours or if they develop *Pneumocystis* in spite of TMP/SMX prophylaxis.

Table 26-8. Antiviral Drugs for Viral Infections in Children with Cancer

Generic (trade name)	Indication	Route	Usually recommended dosage
Acyclovir[a,b] (Zovirax)	Varicella in immuno-compromised host	IV	For children <1 year of age: 30 mg/kg/day in 3 divided doses for 7–10 days; some experts also recommend this dose for children ≥1 year of age.
		IV	For children ≥1 year of age: 1500 mg/m² of body surface area per day in 3 divided doses for 7–10 days.
Foscarnet[a] (Foscavir)	CMV retinitis in patients with acquired immuno-deficiency syndrome	IV	180 mg/kg/day in 3 divided doses for 14–21 days, then 90–120 mg/kg once a day as maintenance dose
	HSV infection resistant to acyclovir in immuno-compromised host	IV	80–120 mg/kg/day in 2–3 divided doses until infection resolves
Ganciclovir[a] (Cytovene)	Acquired CMV retinitis in immunocompromised host[c]	IV	10 mg/kg/day in 2 divided doses for 14–21 days; for long-term suppression, 5 mg/kg/day for 5–7 days/week.
	Prophylaxis of CMV in high-risk host	IV	10 mg/kg/day in 2 divided doses for 1 wk, then 5 mg/kg/day in 1 dose for 100 days.
Lamivudine (Epivir-HBV)	Treatment of chronic hepatitis B	Oral	For people ≥2 years of age, 3 mg/kg/day (maximum 100 mg/day).

Abbreviations: IV, intravenous.

[a]Dose should be decreased in patients with impaired renal function.

[b]Oral dosage of acyclovir in children should not exceed 80 mg/kg/day.

[c]Some experts use ganciclovir in immunocompromised host with CMV gastrointestinal tract disease and CMV pneumonitis (with or without CMV immune globulin intravenous).

For more information on individual drug see *Physician's Desk Reference* (Greenwood Village, CO: Thomson Micromedex) or http://pdrel.thomsonhc.com/pdrel/librarian/action/command.command)

Prophylactic Antibiotics

Pneumocystis carinii **Prophylaxis**

1. TMP/SMX 5–10 mg/kg/day divided into 2 daily doses for 3 days per week. TMP/SMX may cause rash, neutropenia, and GI symptoms.
2. Dapsone 2 mg/kg/day.
3. Pentamidine 4 mg/kg administered intravenously once a month
4. Atovaquone 30 mg/kg/day in children 1–3 months and those older than 2 years. The recommended dose is 45 mg/kg/day for children between 3 and 24 months of age.

Antiviral Prophylaxis

Acyclovir prophylaxis is used against reactivations of HSV in seropositive stem cell transplant patients.

Antifungal Prophylaxis

1. Nystatin oral swish and swallow; 2 mL twice daily in infants, 5 mL twice daily in children and adults
2. Clotrimazole troche one bid
3. Fluconazole 2 mg/kg/day; maximum 200 mg.

Varicella Exposure

Patients who had continuing household exposure to active varicella, or have been in the same room with an individual for at least 1 hour in the contagious state of varicella (1–2 days before and 5 days after eruption of vesicles), should receive varicella immune globulin (VZIG) 1 vial/10 kg IM (maximum of 5 vials) within 96 hours of exposure. Children who have been vaccinated and have positive titers do not need to receive VZIG with exposures.

Blood Component Therapy

The two main causes of pancytopenia in children with malignancies are:

1. Invasion or replacement of the bone marrow by malignant cells
2. Myelosuppression due to chemotherapeutic agents.

Blood component administration is an integral component of management. The risks associated with transfusions (Table 26-9) are:

1. Transfusion reactions (febrile and hemolytic reactions)
2. Development of alloimmunization and refractoriness
3. Transmission of infectious agents
4. Development of graft versus host disease (GVHD).

Transfusion reactions include:

1. Acute hemolytic transfusion reactions
2. Delayed hemolytic transfusion reactions
3. Febrile nonhemolytic transfusion reactions
4. Allergic reactions
5. Transfusion-related acute lung injury (TRALI).

Most hemolytic reactions are *acute hemolytic transfusion reactions* and result from blood group incompatibility (both major and minor red cell antigens) between the donor and the recipient. They can be prevented by thorough typing and cross-matching of all packed red cell transfusions. Acute hemolytic transfusion reactions present with fever, chills, back or abdominal pain, dark urine, pallor, bleeding, or shock during the

Table 26-9. Relative Risks of Transfusion Complications per Unit

Risk	Risk ratio
Hepatitis C	1:1,600,000
HIV	1:1,900,000
Wrong blood in tube	1:1,000
Wrong recipient of auto unit	1:16,000
TRALI	1:5,000
Hemolysis from ABO-incompatible plasma in an apheresis platelet	1:10,000–46,000

Abbreviation: TRALI, transfusion-related acute lung injury.

transfusion. Laboratory investigations show positive direct antiglobulin test, spherocytes, decreased haptoglobin, hyperbilirubinemia, and hemoglobinuria. The transfusion should be stopped immediately. The unit and a sample of the patient's blood should be sent to the blood bank for investigation. The patient should be vigorously hydrated. *Delayed hemolytic transfusion reactions* occur 2–14 days after the transfusion. Patients present with low-grade fever, decreased hemoglobin, and jaundice.

Febrile reactions are almost always caused by sensitization to leukocyte antigens. They can be largely prevented by two measures:

1. Leukocyte-depleted products (usually through the use of leukocyte filters). Prestorage leukocyte filtration offers the most effective approach. Inflammatory cytokines (interleukin [IL]-1, IL-6, and tumor necrosis factor α [TNF-α]) secreted from leukocytes cannot be filtered by post-storage filtration and may still lead to febrile reactions.
2. Premedication of the recipient with Tylenol 10–15 mg/kg and Benadryl 1 mg/kg.

Allergic reactions are due to plasma proteins. Mild cutaneous hypersensitivity reactions (itching, rash, redness) respond to antihistamines. Severe allergic reactions are often due to development of anti-IgA in IgA-deficient patients. Patients may require epinephrine and parenteral steroids.

Transfusion-related acute lung injury occurs within 4–6 hours of transfusions. Leukoagglutinins in the donor blood interact with recipient white cells and lead to sequestration of the white cell complexes in the pulmonary vasculature. This results in increased vascular permeability and exudation of fluid and protein into the alveoli. The clinical picture of TRALI resembles adult respiratory distress syndrome. Patients present with dyspnea, hypoxia, fever, and noncardiogenic pulmonary edema. Treatment is supportive. Table 26-10 lists the clinical benefits from using leukoreduced blood products.

Alloimmunization and Refractoriness

To some extent, all transfusion recipients become sensitized to foreign leukocyte antigens. However, the use of leukocyte filters helps to prevent this problem.

The problem of refractoriness applies particularly to platelet transfusions. Patients who are refractory show no rise or significantly less than the expected rise in platelet count following a platelet transfusion. In some patients, refractoriness occurs much sooner than in others. Specific factors affecting platelet survival will be discussed in the section on platelet transfusions.

Transmission of Infectious Agents

The agents that can be transmitted by transfusions are viruses, including cytomegalovirus (CMV), hepatitis, and human immunodeficiency virus (HIV),

Table 26-10. Clinical Benefits from Using Leukoreduced (LR) Blood Products

Prevention of recurrent febrile nonhemolytic transfusion reactions
Prevention of primary HLA-alloimmunization and resulting complications, including
    platelet refractoriness
Prevention of transfusion-transmitted cytomegalovirus infection in at-risk patients
Reduction of prion (vCJD) transmission
Reduction of transmission of other leukotropic viruses (HTLV I-II and EBV)
Reduction of viral reactivation
Reduction of parasitic or bacterial infections
Reduction of transfusion-related acute lung injury

Abbreviation: CJD, Creutzfeldt-Jakob disease

(Table 26-11) bacteria, and protozoa. Careful donor selection and improvements in screening and blood product testing have largely eliminated this problem. The other infectious risk is bacterial contamination of the donor units of blood. Infection is most commonly due to *Yersinia enterocolitica* and other gram-negative organisms. Platelet units are most commonly contaminated with *S. aureus, Klebsiella pneumoniae, Serratia marcenses,* and *Staphylococcus epidermidis.* Parasitic infections that can be transmitted through blood transfusion are malaria, Chagas disease, and *Babesia.*

Donated blood is screened for hepatitis B and C and HIV. Positive units are discarded. CMV may be transmitted via CMV antibody-positive blood. Eighty-five percent of the population is positive for CMV antibodies. It is, therefore, impossible to discard all CMV-positive units. Because of the high risk of CMV interstitial pneumonitis in severely immunocompromised patients, it is recommended that patients who will be undergoing allogeneic stem cell transplantation and who are CMV antibody negative receive CMV antibody-negative products. Patients who will not be undergoing transplant or transplant patients who are already CMV positive can receive CMV-positive, leuko-depleted products. Leuko-depletion reduces the risk of CMV and, in theory, Creutzfeldt-Jakob disease.

Graft versus Host Disease

GVHD has been observed to arise 4–30 days after the administration of nonirradiated blood products to immunocompromised patients. It results from viable donor precursor cells or stem cells engrafting in the immunocompromised host's marrow. The clinical manifestations are fever, erythematous maculopapular skin rash, anorexia, nausea, vomiting, diarrhea, elevated liver enzymes, and hyperbilirubinemia. A very high morbidity and mortality rate is associated with transfusion-acquired GVHD. Measures to prevent GVHD include irradiating all blood products with 2500 cGy and depleting the blood products of leukocytes.

General Guidelines

All oncology patients should receive leukocyte-filtered, irradiated blood products. CMV-negative products should be used according to the previously mentioned guidelines.

Red Cell Transfusions

Causes of anemia in cancer patients in children include:

1. Replacement of the bone marrow with malignant cells
2. Chemotherapy-induced myelosuppression
3. Anemia of inflammation

Table 26-11. Risk Estimates of Viral Transmission by Transfusion

Virus/infection	Estimated risk in 2002
Human immunodeficiency virus (HIV)	1:2,135,000
Hepatitis C (HCV)	1:1,935,000
Hepatitis B (HBV)	1:1,205,000
Human T-cell lymphotropic virus (HTLV-I/II)	1:641,000

From Jamali F, Ness PM. Infectious complications. In: Hillyer CD, Strauss RG, Luban NLC, editors. Handbook of Pediatric Transfusion Medicine. San Diego: Elsevier Academic Press, 2004;329–39.

4. Blood loss due to thrombocytopenia
5. Iatrogenic blood loss
6. Hemolysis.

Packed red cell transfusions are indicated for patients whose hemoglobin is less than 8 g/dL or those whose hemoglobin is greater than 8 g/dL but who are cardiovascularly unstable and have respiratory failure or bleeding.

Patients should receive 10–15 mL/kg of packed red cells over 3 hours. Each transfusion should be completed within 4 hours after the unit or aliquot has been started.

Patients who are profoundly anemic (Hgb, <5 g/dL) should be transfused at a slower rate (3–5 mL packed red cells/kg over 3–4 hours) with careful monitoring of vital signs. Repeat transfusions can be given.

The expected increment can be estimated as follows: 1 mL/kg of packed red cells increases the hematocrit by 1%.

Platelet Transfusions

The causes of thrombocytopenia in children who have cancer are:

1. Decreased production
2. Increased destruction
3. Hypersplenism
4. Consumption due to brisk bleeding or massive transfusion.

Serious bleeding episodes and spontaneous bleeding occur when the count is below 15,000–20,000/mm^3. For this reason, platelet transfusions are given when:

1. The platelet count is less than 15,000–20,000/mm^3.
2. The platelet count is greater than 20,000/mm^3, but the patient is bleeding (e.g., prolonged epistaxis, GI bleeding, or CNS bleeding).
3. The patient is scheduled for an invasive procedure and the platelet count is less than 50,000/mm^3.

Platelets are collected in two ways:

1. Platelets are collected from units of routinely donated whole blood and pooled (random-donor) platelets; 1 unit of random-donor platelets has $5–10 \times 10^{10}$ platelets.
2. Platelet concentrates can be collected from a single donor by platelet apheresis; 1 unit of single-donor platelets has $3–6 \times 10^{11}$ platelets (roughly equivalent to 6 units of random donor platelets).

The dose of platelets given per transfusion is 1 unit random-donor platelets/10 kg or 1 unit single-donor platelets/50 kg. Apheresis units may be divided for smaller patients. Use ABO-type-specific platelets. The expected platelet increment can be calculated by corrected platelet count index (CCI) as follows:

$$CCI = \frac{\text{Post-transfusion platelet count} - \text{pretransfusion platelet count} \times \text{body surface area}}{\text{Number of platelets transfused } (\times 10^{11})}$$

One unit of random-donor platelets per 10 kg of body weight should increase the platelet count by 40,000–50,000/mm^3 within 1 hour after the infusion. In the average-sized adolescent or adult, 6 units of platelet concentrates or 1 single-donor apheresis unit will increase the platelet count by 50,000/mm^3 or greater. If the post-transfusion platelet count is below the expected count, the patient is refractory. Table 26-12 lists the factors leading to decreased platelet transfusion response and approaches to platelet refractoriness.

Table 26-12. Factors Leading to Decreased Platelet Transfusion Response

Age of transfused platelets
Washing platelets
Fever, infection
Disseminated intravascular coagulation
Graft versus host disease
Hepatosplenomegaly, hypersplenism
Alloantibodies/autoantibodies
Massive blood loss
Hemolytic uremic syndrome/thrombotic thrombocytopenic purpura
    (platelet transfusions discouraged/contraindicated)
Necrotizing enterocolitis
Medications (amphotericin, vancomycin, ciprofloxacin)

Approaches to platelet refractoriness
Transfuse ABO identical platelets
Use fresh platelets
HLA-Matched platelets
Cross-matched platelets
Intravenous gammaglobulin 1 g/kg prior to transfusion
Plasmapheresis
Corticosteroids

Other measures to prevent bleeding in patients with severe thrombocytopenia include:

1. Avoid invasive procedures: nasogastric tube or urinary catheter insertion, rectal examination, intramuscular injections, deep venipunctures.
2. Apply local pressure for wounds and epistaxis.
3. Avoid aspirin and other drugs that interfere in platelet function (Chapter 10).
4. Epsilon-aminocaproic acid or prednisone can be used as adjunct treatment in bleeding patients.
5. Estrogen or high-dose birth control pills may be used for menometrorrhagia.

Granulocyte Transfusions

Neutropenia (ANC <1000/mm^3) and severe neutropenia (ANC <500/mm^3) commonly occur in patients on chemotherapy. Severe neutropenia greatly increases the risk for overwhelming sepsis and for invasive fungal infections. Most neutropenic patients are treated with G-CSF to shorten the period of neutropenia (see later section titled Hematopoietic Growth Factors). Occasionally, however, patients are treated with granulocyte transfusions.

Indications

1. Serious bacterial (particularly gram-negative) or fungal infection with persistent (48 hours or more) positive cultures despite appropriate antibiotic coverage in severely neutropenic patients (ANC <200/mm^3).
2. The ANC is not expected to increase to more than 500/mm^3 for several days.
3. Prolonged survival of the patient is reasonably expected if the infection is controlled.
4. In addition, patients with severe granulocyte dysfunction (e.g., chronic granulomatous disease) who have severe infection.

Risks

1. CMV infection
2. Graft versus host disease
3. Respiratory distress with pulmonary infiltrates (particularly in patients concurrently receiving amphotericin)
4. Alloimmunization
5. Hemolytic reactions.

Precautions to Be Observed

1. Use granulocytes from an ABO–Rh compatible donor.
2. If the patient is on amphotericin, leave 4–6 hours between amphotericin and granulocyte transfusion.
3. Do not administer with a leukocyte-depleting filter.
4. Administer granulocytes as soon as possible after collection to maximize effectiveness. If not used immediately, store at room temperature.
5. Premedicate with diphenhydramine and hydrocortisone.
6. Granulocytes are always irradiated to prevent transfusion-associated GVHD.

Dose and Duration

1. The dose is usually greater than $0.75–1.0 \times 10^{10}$ granulocytes
2. The transfusion is administered through a 170-μm filter at a rate of 150 mL/m^2/hour.
3. Granulocytes are usually administered for 5–7 days or until the ANC has risen to more than 500/mm^3. (Transfused granulocytes have a half-life of 6–10 hours and do not increase the ANC.)

Hematopoietic Growth Factors

Basic Biology of Growth Factors

Hematopoietic cells are derived from self-renewing, pluripotent stem cells. Pluripotent stem cells are able to differentiate into committed progenitor cells. The most primitive form of committed progenitor is termed a *colony-forming unit granulocyte, erythrocyte, macrophage, and megakaryocyte* (CFU-GEMM). This cell is capable of producing colonies containing neutrophils, macrophages, erythrocytes, megakaryocytes, eosinophils, and basophils. CFU-GEMMs appear to have a limited capacity for self-renewal, and therefore, are not true "stem cells." The committed hematopoietic progenitors (erythroid burst-forming unit [BFU-E], erythroid colony-forming unit [CFU-E], granulocyte macrophage colony-forming unit [CFU-GM], granulocyte colony-forming unit [CFU-G], macrophage colony-forming unit [CFU-M], eosinophil colony-forming unit [CFU-Eo], basophil colony-forming unit [CFU-Baso], and megakaryocyte colony-forming unit [CFU-Meg]) are capable of giving rise to colonies containing cells of only one or two types.

The hematopoietic growth factors and interleukins are cytokines that regulate the growth, differentiation, and functional activities of progenitor cells in peripheral blood, bone marrow, and placental-cord blood. A second important action of many of these factors is augmentation of the function of mature cells. Some growth factors are specific for one type of progenitor, whereas others affect many types of progenitors. Figure 26-2 illustrates the hierarchy of hematopoietic progenitor cells and the sites of responsiveness of growth factors and interleukins. Table 26-13 lists the uses of hematopoietic growth factors.

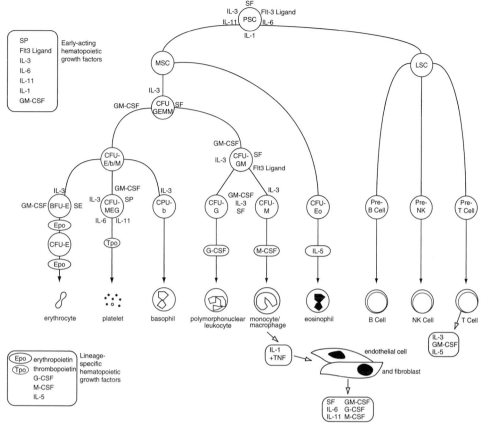

Fig. 26-2. Major cytokine sources and actions. Cells of the bone marrow microenvironment such as macrophages (ma), endothelial cells (ec), and reticular fibroblastoid cells (fb) produce macrophage colony-stimulating factor (M-CSF), granulocyte-macrophage colony-stimulating factor (GM-CSF), granulocyte colony-stimulating factor (G-CSF), interleukin (IL)-6, and probably Steel factor (SF; cellular sources not yet precisely determined) after induction with endotoxin (ma) or IL-1/tumor necrosis factor (TNF) (ec, fb). T cells produce IL-3, GM-CSF, and IL-5 in response to antigenic and IL-1 stimulation. These cytokines have overlapping actions during hematopoietic differentiation, as indicated, and for all lineages optimal development requires a combination of early- and late-acting factors. PSC, pluripotent stem cells; MSC, myeloid stem cells; CFU-E/b/M, erythrocyte, basophil, and megakaryocyte colony-forming unit; CFU-E, erythroid colony-forming unit; CFU-G, granulocyte colony-forming unit; CFU-M, macrophage colony-forming unit; CFU-Eo, eosinophil colony-forming unit; NK = natural killer. (From Clark SC, Nathan DG, Sieff CA. The anatomy and physiology of hematopoiesis. In: Nathan DG, Gingburg ND, Orkin SH, Look AS, editors. Hematology of Infancy and Childhood. 6th ed. Philadelphia: Saunders, 2003;180, with permission.)

Table 26-13. Uses of Hematopoietic Growth Factors

Enhances hematopoietic recovery, lowers hospital cost, permits increased cytotoxic drug dose

Early hematopoietic recovery reduces nonhematologic toxicity (e.g., infection, mucositis, pneumonia)

Mobilizes peripheral-blood progenitor cells

Augments transplant using smaller number of hematopoietic cells

Expands hematopoietic cells

Clinical Use of G-CSF, GM-CSF, Erythropoietin, and IL-11

Recombinant Human G-CSF

Indications for use
1. Prophylactic use in patients in whom the expected incidence of neutropenia following chemotherapy is greater than or equal to 40%. It accelerates myeloid recovery when the expected duration of severe neutropenia is 7 or more days.
2. After a prior episode of febrile neutropenia.
3. After high-dose chemotherapy with autologous progenitor stem cell support to accelerate myeloid recovery.
4. Mobilization of peripheral blood progenitor cells for harvesting prior to autologous stem cell transplant.
5. To increase granulocyte count in patients with aplastic anemia, myelodysplastic syndromes, congenital neutropenia, and other congenital neutropenic disorders.

Contraindication
1. Hypersensitivity to G-CSF or to *E. coli*–derived proteins.

Dose and duration
1. Start with a dose of 5 μg/kg/day SC or IV. When given intravenously, it is diluted with albumin and given over 15–30 minutes. The dose is 10 μg/kg/day SC or IV for peripheral blood stem cell mobilization in preparation for autologous transplant. A PEGylated form of G-CSF (pegfilgrastim) is used at a dose of 6 mg SC once per chemotherapy cycle in patients over 45 kg. There is no experience with pegfilgrastim in pediatrics.
2. Continue until the ANC is greater than $10,000/mm^3$.
3. Start G-CSF 24 hours after the last dose of chemotherapy.
4. Do not resume chemotherapy until 24–48 hours after discontinuing G-CSF.

Adverse effects
1. *Common:* bone pain, elevation of uric acid, lactate dehydrogenase, and alkaline phosphatase
2. *Uncommon:* fever, nausea, vomiting, rash, diarrhea, splenomegaly, erythema at injection site, hypotension, exacerbation of psoriasis, allergic reaction, acute respiratory distress syndrome, splenic rupture.

Recombinant Human GM-CSF

Indications
1. To accelerate myeloid recovery following stem cell transplantation
2. To accelerate myeloid recovery in a neutropenic patient with fungal infection, because it also accelerates macrophage recovery.

Contraindications
1. Excessive myeloid blasts in bone marrow or peripheral blood (>10%)
2. Juvenile chronic myeloid leukemia or monosomy 7 syndrome
3. Hypersensitivity to GM-CSF or yeast-derived proteins.

Dose and duration
1. The starting dose is 250 μg/m^2/day SC or IV over 2 hours.
2. When given to prevent engraftment delay, the first dose should be given 2–4 hours after stem cell transplant and continued for 21 days or until the ANC is greater than $10,000$ cells/mm^3.
3. Do not give within 24 hours of last chemotherapy or 12 hours of last radiation dose.

Adverse effects
1. *Common:* bone pain, reaction at injection site
2. *Uncommon:* fluid retention (peripheral edema, pleural effusion, pericardial effusion), leukocytosis, diarrhea, rash, malaise, fever, asthenia, headache, chills, arthralgias, chest pain, dyspnea, thrombocytopenia, thrombophlebitis, thrombosis, eosinophilia, weight gain, respiratory distress syndrome, bundle branch block, supraventricular arrhythmias. The first dose of GM-CSF may be followed within hours by a characteristic reaction involving skin flushing, tachycardia, hypotension, musculoskeletal pain, dyspnea, nausea and vomiting, and arterial oxygen desaturation.

Use of G-CSF or GM-CSF and risk of leukemia
1. Numerous clinical studies have not shown detectable adverse effects of G-CSF on stimulation of myeloid leukemic cell growth.
2. In aplastic anemia, the risk of myelodysplastic syndrome (MDS) or leukemia is increased in children treated with immunosuppressive therapy and G-CSF.
3. Seven percent of patients with severe chronic neutropenia treated for more than 8 years with G-CSF develop AML or myelodysplastic syndrome (MDS). Patients with cyclic neutropenia treated with G-CSF have not developed a secondary malignancy.

Recombinant Human Erythropoietin

When planning to use recombinant human erythropoietin (rHuEPO), the following points must be considered:

1. If the degree of anemia is disproportionate to the degree of thrombocytopenia and neutropenia, this may be due to other causes of low hemoglobin such as hemorrhage, iron deficiency, or hemolysis, and these will not be resolved by rHuEPO.
2. Not all patients respond to rHuEPO because of "end-organ" problems, such as myelodysplastic syndrome, and some anemias of chronic illness.
3. Patients on cisplatin-containing regimens who suffer renal damage may respond well to rHuEPO.

Indications
1. There are no proven indications in pediatric oncology.
2. Possible indications include:
   a. Anemia secondary to renal failure
   b. Anemia of chronic illness
   c. Anemia secondary to chemotherapy (to decrease the need for blood transfusions)
   d. Anemia associated with radiation therapy
   e. Anemia after allogeneic stem cell transplantation
   f. Anemia secondary to myelodysplastic syndromes when the serum erythropoietin is low.

Contraindications
1. Anemia secondary to nutritional deficiencies, hemorrhage, or hemolysis
2. Uncontrollable hypertension
3. Hypersensitivity to mammalian cell–derived products or to human albumin.

Dose and dose modification schedule
1. Obtain baseline serum erythropoietin and ferritin levels prior to starting therapy.
2. If ferritin is low, prescribe ferrous sulfate 6 mg elemental iron/kg/day divided into 3 daily doses.

3. Start rHuEPO at a dose of 150 Units/kg/day SC 3 times a week. Darbepoetin alpha is an analogue of erythropoietin with a longer plasma half-life and can be used once every 2–4 weeks. The starting dose is 2.25 µg/kg/dose.
4. If there is no response within 2–4 weeks, increase dose to 300 Units/kg/day 3 times a week or the darbepoetin dose to 4.5 µg/kg/week.
5. If the hemoglobin reaches 13 g/dL, discontinue rHuEPO until the hemoglobin is 12 g/dL; then resume at 25% dose.
6. If the hemoglobin increases very rapidly (>1 g/dL in 2 weeks) or hemoglobin reaches 12 g/dL, reduce the dose by 25%.
7. Give rHuEPO concurrently with chemotherapy.
8. Continue rHuEPO until the patient no longer requires red cell support.

Early initiation (prior to the need for transfusions), a low observed or predicted erythropoietin level (<0.825), and evidence of early response (more than 1 g/dL rise in hemoglobin within the first 4 weeks) are all associated with increased likelihood of response. Patients meeting all three of these criteria showed an 85% chance of significant response (more than 2 g/dL rise in hemoglobin).

Adverse reactions
1. *Common:* hypertension, pain at the injection site, headache, fever, diarrhea
2. *Uncommon:* nausea, malaise, seizures, thrombosis. There are reports of pure red cell aplasia due to neutralizing antibodies during erythropoietin treatment. Almost all of these patients have renal failure associated anemia and were treated with SC erythropoietin.

Interleukin-11

IL-11 acts synergistically with IL-3 and thrombopoietin (TPO) to stimulate various stages of megakaryocytopoiesis and thrombopoiesis. IL-11 has been evaluated in several human clinical trials. It is currently approved for the prevention of severe chemotherapy-induced thrombocytopenia in patients with nonmyeloid malignancies.

Indications
1. Prevention of severe thrombocytopenia after myelosuppressive chemotherapy.

Contraindications
1. Hypersensitivity
2. Children younger than 12 years of age
3. Myeloid malignancies
4. In patients with heart failure, atrial arrhythmias, thromboembolic disorders, major organ dysfunction, papilledema, or CNS tumors, IL-11 should be used with caution.

Dose and dose modification schedule
The dose is 50 µg/kg /day in adults. The dose in children may be 50–75 µg/kg/day, although efficacy studies have not been done in children.

Adverse reactions
1. *Common:* edema, tachycardia, headache, fatigue, dizziness, anorexia, nausea, conjunctivitis and papilledema in children, dyspnea, skin rashes, arthralgia, myalgia
2. *Uncommon:* atrial arrhythmia, thrombosis, cerebral infarction, syncope.

Prevention of Organ Toxicity

Prevention of Cardiac Toxicity

A baseline ECG and echocardiogram should be obtained before anthracycline treatment or thoracic radiotherapy.

During therapy, echocardiogram or radionuclide cardiac cineangiocardiography (RNA) should be performed regularly. If the planned cumulative dose of daunomycin/doxorubicin is less than 300 mg/m^2, testing is repeated after half the cumulative dose has been given. After the cumulative dose reaches more than 360 mg/m^2, testing is repeated before each cycle.

The following are criteria for progressive deteriorating cardiac function:

- A decrease in the fractional shortening (SF) by an absolute value of 10% from the previous test
- SF less than 29%
- A decrease in the RNA–left ventricular ejection fraction (RNA LVEF) by an absolute value of 10% from the previous test
- RNA LVEF less than 5%
- A decrease in the RNA LVEF with stress
- Development of arrhythmia.

If there is a documented infection or development of arrhythmia during therapy, anthracyclines should be discontinued and a cardiology consultation should be obtained.

Modification of Anthracycline Therapy

1. If both the SF and the RNA LVEF are abnormal, anthracycline therapy should be discontinued unless there is a recovery of SF and RNA LVEF to normal on two serial tests taken 1 month apart.
2. If one of the preceding test modalities is abnormal, while the other is normal, anthracyclines should be temporarily discontinued. Both tests should be repeated after 1 month.

If one remains normal and the other becomes normal or does not deteriorate further, therapy should be resumed. Therapy should be discontinued if further deterioration occurs in either tests. Patients who receive anthracyclines and/or thoracic radiotherapy should be evaluated by ECG and echocardiogram every year for 5 years.

Low-Dose Radiotherapy with Combination Chemotherapy

1. Appropriately lowered cumulative dose of anthracycline should be employed when radiotherapy is administered over the heart.
2. Use of less than 450 mg/m^2/cumulative dose for both doxorubicin and daunomycin and 125 mg/m^2 for idarubicin and 160 mg/m^2 for mitoxantrone. Patients who have received a cumulative dose of doxorubicin of more than 450 mg/m^2 should not receive mitoxantrone. The recommended cumulative dose of mitoxantrone for patients who have received prior treatment with doxorubicin is 120 mg/m^2.
3. Use of cardioprotective agents such as dexrazoxane (ICRF-187, Zinecard, DZR). The dose of dexrazoxane is 300 mg/m^2 (10 times the doxorubicin dose) IV bolus over 15 minutes followed by doxorubicin or daunomycin IV over 15 minutes, that is, before the elapsed time of 30 minutes (from the beginning of the dexrazoxane). Because of severe mucositis and increased risk of second malignancies it is not recommended.
4. Cardiac tissue damage serum marker (e.g., determination of cardiac troponin levels [cTnT], creatinine kinase [CK]-MB isozyme). cTnT is a thin-filament contractile protein that is released from damaged cardiomyocytes. Unlike CK-MB, cTnT is not found in the serum of a healthy person.

5. ECHO/MUGA surveillance studies as recommended.
6. Use of new anthracyclines with decreased potential for cardiotoxicity are being investigated.

See Chapter 27 for guidelines for long-term follow-up of patients who receive anthracyclines.

Prevention of Renal Toxicity

1. Maintain hydration at 125 mL/m²/h (i.e., twice maintenance) for a minimum of 2 hours prior to start of chemotherapy with agents such as high-dose methotrexate, moderate to high dose of cyclophosphamide, cisplatin, or ifosfamide to increase urine output to more than 3 mL/kg/h and decrease urinary specific gravity below 1.010.
2. During infusion of these agents, maintain hydration at 125 mL/m²/h and urinary output at ≥5 mL/kg/h.
3. After infusion, continue hydration at 90–125 mL/m²/h.
4. Maintain isovolemic fluid balance. When needed, use furosemide 0.5–1 mg/kg IV or mannitol 6 g/m² (200 mg/kg) in at least 25 mL of fluid over 15–60 minutes.
5. Use mesna for its uroprotective effect to prevent hemorrhagic cystitis caused by high-dose cyclophosphamide and ifosfamide. A total mesna dose equal to the total dose of cyclophosphamide (0.8 mg of mesna per 1 mg of cyclophosphamide) is recommended.
6. Adjust the doses of chemotherapy according to the glomerular filtration rate (GFR) (Table 26-14).
7. During infusion of cisplatin, add mannitol 15 g/m² (10–24 g/m²/L) and $MgSO_4$ in a dose of 20 mEq/L to the hydrating solution to prevent hypomagnesemia.
8. Continue postchemotherapy hydration with 5% dextrose/0.45% NaCl + 20 mEq/L KCl + 20 mEq/L $MgSO_4$ + 20 g/L mannitol.

Pain Management

Adequate pain management is crucial to the quality of life of a child with cancer. At diagnosis, pediatric oncology patients have tumor-related pain. As the treatment evolves, treatment-related pain predominates. The causes of pain in a child with cancer are:

1. *Cancer-related pain:* bone pain, compression of central or peripheral nervous system structures
2. *Procedure-related pain:* venipuncture, bone marrow aspiration and biopsy, lumbar puncture
3. *Treatment-related pain:*
   a. *Chemotherapy:* mucositis, peripheral neuropathy, aseptic necrosis of bone, steroid-induced myopathy
   b. *Radiation:* mucositis, radionecrosis, myelopathy, brachial/lumbar plexopathies
   c. *Postsurgical:* acute postoperative pain, phantom pain.

Pain management can be attained through an integration of drugs and other modalities. Pharmacologic analgesia is the mainstay of pain management. Nonpharmacologic methods of pain control are:

1. Preparation of the child prior to a procedure
2. Physical: massage, heat and cold, electrical nerve stimulation, acupuncture

Table 26-14. Suggested Percentage Dose of Chemotherapeutic Agents Adjusted for Glomerular Filtration Rate

>60 mL/min	30–60 mL/min (50–75% baseline)[a]			10–30 mL/min (25–49% baseline)		<10 mL/min (<25% baseline)	
100% dose	75%	50%	Omit	75%	Omit	50%	Omit
Adriamycin[b]	Bleomycin[c]	Cisplatin	Nitrosoureas	Carboplatin[d]	Cisplatin	Cyclophosphamide	Cisplatin
Bleomycin		Methotrexate	Bleomycin[a]	Ifosfamide[d]	Methotrexate		Methotrexate
Cisplatin			Cisplatin	Nitrosoureas	Nitrosoureas		
Cyclophosphamide							
Cytarabine[b]							
5-fluorouracil[b]							
Ifosfamide							
Melphalan[b]							
Methotrexate							
Nitrosoureas							
Vinblastine[b]							
Vincristine							

[a]Percentage of baseline may not be suitable if high urine output renal dysfunction present.

[b]No dose modification for decreased glomerular filtration rate.

[c]Recommendations vary per protocol.

[d]Reduce by 50%

[e]From Barnard DR, Friedman DL, Landier W, Larson-Tuttle C, Iacuone J. Monitoring and management of drug toxicity. In: Altman AJ, editor. Supportive care of children with cancer. Current therapy and guidelines from the Children's Oncology Group. 3rd ed. Baltimore: The Johns Hopkins University Press, 2004;100–48, with permission.

3. Behavioral: art and play therapy, exercise, relaxation, biofeedback, desensitization, operant conditioning
4. Cognitive: distraction, imagery, attention, hypnosis, music therapy, psychotherapy
5. Complementary and alternative medicine.

The recommended starting doses, route of administration, and schedules for analgesic medications are listed in Table 26-15.

The dosage and frequency of the analgesics are adjusted to the patient's pain, and are gradually increased as needed to maintain the patient free of pain. The next dose

Table 26-15. Recommended Starting Doses, Rate of Administration, and Schedules for Analgesic Medications

Medication	Dose (mg/kg)	Route	Schedule
Nonsteroidal anti-inflammatory drugs			
Acetaminophen	10–15	PO	q4h
	15–20	PR	q4h
Choline-magnesium salicylate	10–15	PO	q6–8h
Ibuprofen	5–10	PO	q6h
Rofecoxib	0.6 mg/kg (adult Dose 25 mg)	PO	qd
Ketorolac	0.5	IV	q6h
Opioids			
Codeine	0.5–1	PO	q4h
Fentanyl	0.001–0.002 (1–2 µg/kg)	IV	q1–2h
	0.002–0.004 (2–4 µg/kg)	IV	qh continuous infusion
Hydromorphone	0.02	IV	q3-4h
	0.1	PO	q4h
Methadone	0.1	IV	q4h × 2–3 doses; then q8–12h
	0.3–0.7/day	PO	Divide into 3 equal doses
Morphine	0.08–0.1	IV	q2-3h
	0.03–0.05	IV	qh continuous infusion
	0.2–0.3	PO	q4h
Morphine (MS Contin)	0.3–0.6	PO	q12h long acting
Oxycodone	0.15	PO	q4h
Oxycodone (OxyContin)	0.15	PO	q12h long acting
Adjuvants			
Amitriptyline	0.1–0.2	PO	qday at bedtime; advance to 0.5–2.0 mg/kg/day
Gabapentin	Initial 5 mg/kg or 300 mg	PO	qday at bedtime; advance dose to TID
Methylphenidate	0.1–0.2	PO	qdose; slowly advance dose as tolerated
Dextroamphetamine	0.1–0.2	PO	qdose; slowly advance dose as tolerated

Note: For all medications, dosages should be modified based on individual circumstances. Many of these agents have not yet received specific approval for infants and younger children. Certain doses are based on extrapolation from adult doses or from unpublished experience. For nonintubated infants age 4 months or less, reduce initial opioid doses to 1/3 to 1/4 of the recommended doses. Administer opioids with the patient in a location that permits close observation and immediate intervention. For the management of severe ongoing acute or chronic pain, increase opioid doses until comfort is achieved or until side effects prohibit further dose escalation.

From Sacks N, Ringwals-Smith K, Hale G. Nutritional support. In: Autumn AJ, editor. Supportive care of children with cancer. Current therapy and guidelines from the Children's Oncology Group. 3rd ed. Baltimore: The Johns Hopkins University Press, 2004; 243–61, with permission.

should be given before the previous dose has worn off fully to erase the memory and fear of pain. Analgesic medications include:

1. *Nonopioids:*
   a. Acetaminophen: Inhibits prostaglandin synthesis in the brain. The dose is 15 mg/kg/dose every 4 to 6 hours.
   b. Aspirin and nonsteroidal anti-inflammatory drugs (NSAIDs): Contraindicated in oncology patients because of adverse effects on platelet function. Choline magnesium salicylate has minimal effects on platelet function; however, its safety has not been established in severely thrombocytopenic patients. COX-2 inhibitors do not cause platelet dysfunction, but have not been tried in severely thrombocytopenic patients.
2. *Weak opioids:*
   a. *Codeine:* 0.5–1 mg/kg/dose orally every 4 hours.
   b. *Oxycodone:* 0.05–0.15 mg/kg/dose orally every 4–6 hours.
3. *Strong opioids.*

Table 26-16 lists the opioid analgesic initial dosage guidelines. With ongoing administration of narcotic analgesics, tolerance builds up, and increasing doses must be given to maintain the same level of analgesia. Combining a narcotic with tricyclic antidepressants, anticonvulsants, steroids, or topical agents may potentiate its analgesic activity. Guidelines for opioid therapy for persistent cancer pain are listed in Table 26-17, and Table 26-18 lists examples and dosages of adjuvant analgesics. Constipation, nausea, and somnolence are common side effects of opioid treatment. Management of these opioid side effects are listed in Table 26-19.

Patient-Controlled Analgesia

Patient-controlled analgesia (PCA) is a method of opioid administration using a computer-controlled pump that enables the patient to deliver small boluses as needed up to a preset maximum. It can be used with a baseline continuous infusion. The advantages of PCA are:

1. It permits titrated dosing to compensate for individual variation in pharmacokinetics and pain intensity.
2. It permits the patient to exercise control and diminishes anxiety.
3. It allows the patient to balance analgesia against its side effects such as sedation.

The usual starting dose is 0.01–0.02 mg/kg of morphine every 6–10 minutes with or without a basal infusion of 0.01–0.02 mg/kg/h.

Anesthesia for Painful Procedures

Painful or invasive procedures are a major source of anxiety for the child undergoing therapy for cancer. These procedures include insertion of intravenous lines, accessing of mediports, spinal taps, bone marrow aspirations, and pleural and peritoneal taps. Adequate local or general anesthesia, if indicated, can significantly reduce the child's fear.

Local Anesthesia

Local anesthesia is adequate for inserting intravenous lines, for accessing mediports, and for performing spinal taps and bone marrow aspirations on some children. Local anesthesia can be provided via:

1. EMLA (eutectic mixture of local anesthetics) cream (lidocaine 2.5% + prilocaine 2.5%) applied topically to the skin and covered with an occlusive dressing 1 hour prior to the procedure

Table 26-16. Opioid Analgesic Initial Dosage Guidelines

Drug	Equianalgesic doses		Usual starting IV or SC doses and intervals		Parenteral oral dose ratio	Usual starting oral doses and intervals	
	Parenteral	Oral	Child <50 kg	Child >50 kg		Child <50 kg	Child >50 kg
Codeine	120 mg	200 mg	NR	NR	1:2	0.5–1.0 mg/kg q3–4h	30–60 mg q3–4h
Morphine	10 mg	30 mg (chronic) 60 mg (single dose)	Bolus: 0.1 mg/kg q2–4h Infusion: 0.03 mg/kg/h	Bolus: 5–8 mg q2–4h Infusion: 1.5 mg/h	1:3 (chronic) 1:6 (single dose)	Immediate release 0.3 mg/kg q3–4h Sustained release: 20–35 kg: 10–15 mg q8–12h 35–50 kg: 15–30 mg q8–12h	Immediate release 15–20 mg q3–4h Sustained release 30–45 mg q8–12h
Oxycodone	NA	15–20 mg	NA	NA	NA	0.1–0.2 mg/kg q3–4h	5–10 mg q3–4h
Methadone[a]	10 mg	10–20 mg	0.1 mg/kg q4–8h	1:2	1:1.5–1.2	0.15–0.2 mg/kg q4–8h	7–10 mg q4–8h
Fentanyl	100 µg (0.1 mg)	NA	Bolus: 0.5–1.0 µg/kg q1–2h Infusion: 0.5–2.0 µg/kg/h	Bolus: 25–50 µg q1–2h Infusion: 25–100 µg/h	NA	NA	NA
Hydromorphone	1.5–2.0 mg	6–8 mg	Bolus: 0.02 mg q2–4h Infusion: 0.006 mg/kg/h	Bolus: 1 mg q2–4h Infusion: 0.3 mg/h	1:4	0.04–0.08 mg/kg q3–4h	2–4 mg q3–4h
Meperidine[b] (pethidine)	75–100 mg	300 mg	Bolus: 0.8–1.0 mg/kg q2–3h	Bolus: 50–75 mg q2–3h	1:4	2–3 mg/kg q3–4h	100–150 mg q3–4h

Note: Doses refer to patients older than 6 months. In infants younger than 6 months, initial doses per kilogram should begin at roughly 25% of the doses per kilogram recommended here. All doses are approximate and should be adjusted according to clinical circumstances.

Abbreviations: NA, not available; NR, not recommended.

[a]Methadone requires additional vigilance, because it can accumulate and produce delayed sedation. If sedation occurs, doses should be withheld until sedation resolves. Thereafter, doses should be substantially reduced or the dosing interval should be extended to 8 to 12 hours (or both).

[b]Meperidine should generally be avoided if other opioids are available, especially with chronic use, because its metabolite can cause seizures.

From Berde CB, Billett AL, Collins JJ. Symptom management in supportive care. In: Pizzo PA, Poplock DG, editors. Principles and Practice of Pediatric Oncology. 4th ed. Philadelphia: Lippincott, Williams & Wilkins. 2002; 1301–32, with permission.

Table 26-17. Guidelines for Opioid Therapy for Persistent Cancer Pain

Comprehensive assessment
- Define pain etiology, pathophysiology, and syndrome.
- Clarify status of disease.
- Determine impact of the pain and comorbid physical and psychosocial disturbances.

Drug selection
- Consider age and whether major organ failure is present, especially renal, hepatic, or respiratory.
- Consider drug-selective differences in side effect or toxicity profile.
- Consider the effects of concurrent drugs with possible pharmacokinetic and pharmacodynamic interactions.
- Consider individual differences (note prior treatment outcomes) and patient reference.
- Be aware of available preparations for route (e.g., oral, IV, subcutaneous injection, topical) and formulation (e.g., immediate or controlled-release).
- Be aware of cost differences.

Route selection
- Use least invasive route possible.
- Consider patient convenience and compliance.

Dosing
- Consider previous dosing requirements and relative analgesic potencies when initiating therapy.
- Start with low dose and increase until adequate analgesia occurs or dose-limiting side effects are encountered.
- Consider dosing schedule (e.g., around-the-clock or as needed) depending on the anticipated time course of pain.
- Consider "rescue medication" for breakthrough pain.
- Recognize that tolerance is rarely the driving force for dose escalation; consider disease progression when increasing dose requirements occur.

Treat side effects
- Give laxatives prophylactically.
- Be prepared to treat nausea, itch, and somnolence.
- Trial of alternative opioids.

Monitoring
- Monitor treatment efficacy and pain status over time and consider modification if necessary.

From Portenoy RK, Lesage P. Pain management—the series. Part 4: Cancer pain and end-of-life care. American Medical Association, with permission.

Table 26-18. Examples and Dosages of Adjuvant Analgesics

Dexamethasone	0.08–0.3 mg/kg/day PO, IV divided every 6–12 hours
Amitriptyline	0.1 mg/kg/dose PO at bedtime; increase as needed and tolerated to 0.5–2 mg/kg/dose
Gabapentin	300 mg PO three times a day (for children over 12 years old and adults)
Methylphenidate	0.3 mg/kg/dose before breakfast and lunch; may gradually increase to 1 mg/kg/day

Table 26-19. Approaches in the Management of Opioid Side Effects

Opioid side effect	Treatment
Constipation	General approach • Increase fluid intake and dietary fiber. • Encourage mobility and ambulation if appropriate. • Ensure comfort and convenience for defecation. • Rule out or treat impaction if present. Pharmacologic approach • Contact laxative plus stool softener (e.g., senna plus docusate). • Osmotic laxative (e.g., milk of magnesia). • Lavage agent (e.g., oral propylethylene glycol). • Prokinetic agent (metoclopramide). • Oral naloxone.
Nausea	General approach • Hydrate as appropriate. • Progressive alimentation. • Good mouth care. • Correct contributory factors. • Adjust medication. Pharmacological approach • If associated with vertiginous feelings, antihistamine (e.g., scopolamine, meclizine). • If associated with early satiety, prokinetic agent (e.g., metoclopramide). • In other cases, dopamine antagonist drugs (e.g., prochlorperazine, chlorpromazine, haloperidol, metoclopramide).
Somnolence or cognitive impairment	General approach • Reassurance. • Education. • Treatment of potential etiologies. Pharmacologic approach • If analgesia is satisfactory, reduce opioid dose by 25–50%. • If analgesia is satisfactory and the toxicity is somnolence, consider a trial of a psychostimulant (e.g., methylphenidate).

From Portenoy RK, Lesage P. Pain management—the series. Part 4: Cancer pain and end-of-life care. American Medical Association, with permission.

2. Lidocaine 2% injected superficially into the area of the procedure
3. Skin cooling with ice or fluorocarbon cooling sprays.

General Sedation/Anesthesia

General sedation/anesthesia is required for more painful procedures, such as bone marrow biopsies, and for lesser procedures in the young child who is extremely fearful. The following agents may used:

1. Propofol:
    a. Sedative hypnotic, not analgesic
    b. May produce respiratory depression and hypotension
    c. Supplied in an emulsion with egg lecithin; avoid use in patients with egg allergies

    d. Short-acting anesthetic; patients awaken when infusion is terminated

    e. Dosage: 2 mg/kg IV bolus followed by continuous infusion of 40–200 μg/kg/minute; reduce dose by half for patients with neurologic, cardiac, or respiratory disease

    f. Some patients develop tolerance and require higher doses.

2. Brevital (methohexital):
    a. Very short-acting anesthetic, barbiturate
    b. May produce respiratory depression, hypotension
    c. Dosage: 1–2 mg/kg/dose IV or 5–10 mg/kg/dose IM.

3. Ketamine:
    a. Rapid-acting anesthetic with profound analgesia
    b. Produces fuguelike state, disorientation, delirium, bizarre dreams
    c. Can be given along with midazolam dose to cause amnesia for the dreams
    d. Dosage: 2 mg/kg IV; increments of one half to the full dose may be repeated as needed.

4. DPT:
    a. Demerol 2 mg/kg IV, Phenergan 1 mg/kg IV, Thorazine 1 mg/kg IV
    b. Sedative, analgesic, and anesthetic
    c. Produces sedation for 3–4 hours.

If an anesthesiologist is available, propofol is preferred because it is extremely short acting, and the dose can be titrated as needed.

Management of Nausea and Vomiting

In most cases, nausea and vomiting can be prevented. Every effort should be made to provide adequate antiemetic coverage. The receptors for nausea and vomiting should be blocked before treatment starts and should continue as long as the effect is likely to occur. Scheduled doses should be administered regardless of symptoms.

Vomiting is mediated by the vomiting center located in the medullary lateral reticular formation. This center gets input from five sources:

1. Chemoreceptor trigger zone
2. Vagal and sympathetic afferents from viscera
3. Midbrain receptors that detect changes in intracranial pressure
4. Labyrinthine apparatus
5. Limbic system.

Chemotherapeutic agents may stimulate vomiting by direct effect on the vomiting center or through the chemoreceptor trigger zone. Serotonin (5-HT) receptors and substance P play a role in mediating emesis. The emetogenic potential of chemotherapeutic agents is listed in Table 26-20.

The etiology of vomiting should be identified before therapy is initiated. Unusual severity, timing, or duration should alert the physician to a diagnosis other than chemotherapy-induced nausea and vomiting. The three main categories of nausea and vomiting are:

1. Anticipatory nausea and vomiting occur before chemotherapy, arising from fear and anxiety about the treatment as well as the memory of previous episodes of emesis. The situation can be avoided most successfully if adequate antiemetic therapy is given with the first chemotherapy encounter.
2. Acute-onset nausea and vomiting occur within 24 hours of treatment (self-limiting).
3. Delayed-onset nausea and vomiting occur 24 hours or more after treatment (particularly with cisplatin therapy).

Table 26-20. Emetogenic Potential of Chemotherapeutic Agents[a]

Acute symptoms
  Highly emetogenic
    Actinomycin D
    Cisplatin ($\geq$40 mg/m^2)
    Cyclophosphamide ($\geq$1 g/m^2)
    Cytarabine ($\geq$1 g/m^2)
    Dacarbazine
    Ifosfamide
    Mechlorethamine
  Moderately emetogenic
    Anthracyclines (daunorubicin, doxorubicin, idarubicin)
    Carboplatin
    Cisplatin (<40 mg/m^2)
    Cyclophosphamide (<1 g/m^2)
    Cytarabine (IV <1 g/m^2, or IT)
    Mercaptopurine (IV)
    Methotrexate (IV >1 g/m^2)
    Nitrosoureas (carmustine, lomustine)
  Mildly emetogenic
    Bleomycin
    Epipodophyllotoxins (etoposide, teniposide)
    Paclitaxel
    Procarbazine
    Topotecan
    Vinblastine
  Nonemetogenic
    Asparaginase
    Mercaptopurine (PO)
    Methotrexate (low-dose IV, IM, PO, IT)
    Steroids
    Thioguanine
    Vincristine

Delayed symptoms
  Severe
    Cisplatin
  Moderate
    Cyclophosphamide

[a]Independent of route or dose unless specific route or dose is specified.

From Barnard DR, Friedman DL, Landier W, Larson-Tuttle C, Iacuone J. Monitoring and management of drug toxicity. In: Altman AJ, editor. Supportive care of children with cancer. Current therapy and guidelines from the Children's Oncology Group. 3rd ed. Baltimore: The Johns Hopkins University Press, 2004;100–48, with permission.

Table 26-21 lists the commonly used antiemetic agents, their doses, and side effects and Table 26-22 lists the antiemetic regimens used for the initial cycle of chemotherapy or radiotherapy.

Antiemetic agents can be given in combination to increase their efficacy. Commonly used effective regimens include:

1. Ondansetron alone or in combination with dexamethasone or with metoclopramide and Benadryl
2. Metoclopramide and Benadryl
3. Ativan and Compazine.

Table 26-21. Dosage and Side Effects of Commonly Utilized Antiemetic Agents

Medication	Dosage	Side effects	Comments
5-HT$_3$ (serotonin) antagonist Ondansetron (Zofran)	*Oral* Child 4–11 years: 4 mg before chemotherapy and every 4 hours for 2 doses Alternative therapy: single 12-mg dose before chemotherapy Child >11 years and adults: 8 mg before chemotherapy and every 4 hours for 2 doses Alternative therapy: single 24-mg dose before chemotherapy *Intravenous* Child >3 years: 0.15 mg/kg/dose before chemotherapy and every 4 hours for 2 doses Adult: 8–12 mg before chemotherapy and every 4 hours for 2 doses Alternative therapy: single 24–32 mg dose before chemotherapy	Headache, asthenia, light-headedness, dizziness, asymptomatic prolongation of electrocardiographic interval, constipation, diarrhea, abdominal pain, ataxia, fever, tremor, transient serum transaminase elevations, sedation, fatigue, warm sensation on IV administration	Oral therapy is considered as efficacious as IV therapy and less costly. Single-dose regimens preferred over multiple-dose regimens in adult patients. Antiemetic of choice for prophylactic therapy in pediatric and adult patients receiving chemotherapy with emetic potential of levels 3 through 5 (in combination with a corticosteroid). At equipotent doses, ondansetron, dolasetron, and granisetron are equally efficacious. Use in combination with corticosteroids for delayed emesis in adult and pediatric patients.

(Continues)

Table 26-21. (Continued)

Medication	Dosage	Side effects	Comments
Granisetron (Kytril)	*Oral* Adult: 2 mg before chemotherapy and every day or 1 mg twice daily *Intravenous* Child >2 years: 20–40 µg/kg before chemotherapy Adult: 10 µg/kg before chemotherapy		
Dolasetron (Anzemet)	*Oral* Child >2 years: 1.8 mg/kg before chemotherapy Adult: 100–200 mg before chemotherapy *Intravenous* Child >2 years: 1.8 mg/kg before chemotherapy Adult: 100 mg or 1.8 mg/kg before chemotherapy		
Corticosteroid Dexamethasone	*Oral/Intravenous* Child: 10 mg/m²/dose (maximum 20 mg) before chemotherapy and 5 mg/m²/dose (maximum 10 mg) every 6–12 hours as needed Adult: 20 mg before chemotherapy and 10–20 mg every 4–6 hours as needed	Anxiety, insomnia, dyspepsia, hyperglycemia, euphoria, behavioral changes, agitation, perineal burning after rapid IV infusion	Can be used as a single agent in prophylactic therapy for adult and pediatric patients receiving chemotherapy regimens with level 2 emetic potential. Should be added to 5-HT$_3$ receptor antagonist for adults and pediatric patients receiving chemotherapy with emetic potential of levels 3 through 5. Oral therapy as safe and effective as IV therapy.

Drug	Dose/Route	Toxicity	Comments
Methylprednisolone	*Oral/Intravenous* Child: 0.5–1 mg/kg/dose before chemotherapy and every 4 hours for 2 doses		Use for breakthrough nausea and vomiting in adult and pediatric patients. Use with metoclopramide or 5-HT$_3$ receptor antagonist for delayed emesis in adult patients. Use with lorazepam, 5-HT$_3$ receptor antagonist or chlorpromazine for delayed emesis in pediatric patients.
Benzodiazepine Lorazepam	*Oral/Intravenous* Child: 0.03 mg/kg/dose every 6–8 hours as needed. Maximum 2 mg/dose. Adult: 1–2 mg/dose every 6 hours as needed	Sedation, amnesia, behavior changes	May be effective to reduce anticipatory vomiting. Use for breakthrough nausea and vomiting in adult and pediatric patients. Use in combination with dexamethasone for delayed emesis in pediatric patients.
Phenothiazine Chlorpromazine	*Oral* Child >6 months: 0.5 mg/kg/dose every 4–6 hours as needed. Maximum dose 40 mg/day if <5 years; 75 mg/day if 5–12 years *Intravenous* Child: <6 months: 0.5 mg/kg/dose every 6–8 hours as needed. Maximum dose 40 mg/day if <5 years; 75 mg/day if 5–12 years	Sedation, extrapyramidal effects	Use for breakthrough nausea and vomiting in adult and pediatric patients. Use in combination with dexamethasone for delayed emesis in pediatric patients.

(Continues)

Table 26-21. (*Continued*)

Medication	Dosage	Side effects	Comments
Promethazine (Phenergan)	*Oral/Intravenous* Child: 0.25 mg–1 mg/kg/dose every 4–6 hours as needed. Maximum 25 mg/dose Adult: 12.5–25 mg/dose every 4 hours as needed	Sedation, extrapyramidal effects	Use for breakthrough nausea and vomiting in adult and pediatric patients. Use in combination with dexamethasone for delayed emesis in pediatric patients.
Benzamide Metoclopramide	*Oral/Intravenous* Adult: 2 mg/kg/dose IV every 2–4 hours for 2–5 doses. Delayed emesis: 0.5 mg/kg/dose or 30 mg IV every 4–6 hours for 3–5 days	Sedation, diarrhea, extrapyramidal effects	Use for breakthrough nausea and vomiting in adult patients. Use in combination with dexamethasone in delayed emesis in adult patients.
Butyrophenone Haloperidol	*Oral/Intravenous* Adult: 1–4 mg every 6 hours	Sedation, hypotension, tachycardia, extrapyramidal effects	Use for breakthrough nausea and vomiting in adult patients.
Cannabinoid Dronabinol	*Oral* Adult: 2.5–10 mg every 6 hours	Euphoria, dysphoria, drowsiness, dry mouth, anxiety, irritability, confusion	Use for breakthrough nausea and vomiting in adult patients.

Table 26-22. Antiemetic Algorithm for Initial Cycle of Chemotherapy or Radiotherapy[a]

Goal	Emetogenicity of the chemotherapy or radiotherapy	Treatment
Prophylaxis to prevent acute symptoms	High	5-HT$_3$ receptor antagonist, steroid
	Moderate	5-HT$_3$ receptor antagonist
	Mild	5-HT$_3$ receptor antagonist
Rescue (treatment of breakthrough of acute symptoms): advance up ladder, starting after agents already given for prophylaxis	Any	1. 5-HT$_3$ receptor antagonist 2. Steroid 3. Lorazepam 4. Dronabinol (if >6 yr old) 5. Metoclopramide (with diphenhydramine)
Prophylaxis to prevent delayed symptoms	High	Steroid (consider metoclopramide or 5-HT$_3$ receptor antagonist if breakthrough emesis in the first 24 h)
	Moderate	None (consider metoclopramide or 5-HT$_3$ receptor antagonist if breakthrough emesis in the first 24 h)
	Mild	None
Rescue (treatment of breakthrough delayed symptoms): advance up ladder, starting after agents already given for prophylaxis	Any	1. Dexamethasone 2. Metoclopramide 3. 5-HT$_3$ receptor antagonist 4. Lorazepam, dronabinol

Abbreviation: 5-HT$_3$, 5-hydroxytryptamine subtype 3.

[a]Data from the Dana-Farber Cancer Institute and Children's Hospital, Boston.

From Barnard DR, Friedman DL, Landier W, Larson-Tuttle C, Iacuone J. Monitoring and management of drug toxicity. In: Altman AJ, editor. Supportive care of children with cancer. Current therapy and guidelines from the Children's Oncology Group. 3rd ed. Baltimore: The Johns Hopkins University Press, 2004;100–48, with permission.

Nutritional Support

Progressive weight loss, protein energy malnutrition (PEM), and cachexia occur in advanced malignancies in children. Cachexia leads to decreased strength, impaired immune function, decreased pulmonary function, increased disability, and death. The clinical features of cachexia include:

- Wasting
- Anorexia
- Weakness
- Anemia
- Hypoalbuminemia
- Hypoglycemia
- Lactic acidosis
- Hyperlipidemia
- Impaired liver function
- Glucose intolerance
- Skeletal muscle atrophy
- Anergy.

The following factors interact to produce cachexia in pediatric oncology patients:

- Decreased intake secondary to mucositis
- Anorexia and altered taste perception (dysgeusia)
- Nausea and vomiting
- Decreased absorption secondary to the effects of chemotherapy, radiation therapy, or surgery
- Protein-losing nephropathy
- Steroid-induced diabetes
- Increased metabolic expenditure secondary to rapid tumor growth and metastases
- Endogenously produced cytokines such as TNF, IL-1, IL-6, and γ-interferon
- Hepatotoxicity with impaired liver synthetic capacity and altered protein, carbohydrate, and lipid metabolism
- Psychosocial factors such as depression and anticipatory vomiting.

The net result of the preceding factors is that intake fails to meet increased metabolic demands and tissue wasting occurs.

Treatment

It is crucial to increase nutritional intake both to improve quality of life and to increase survival from the underlying malignancy. Methods of nutritional support include:

1. Oral feeding with high-calorie supplements
2. Nasogastric tube feeding
3. Total parenteral nutrition (intravenous hyperalimentation).

Oral Feeding

If the child tolerates oral intake and can absorb nutrients, oral feeding is the treatment of choice. Supplemental diet formulas and elemental diets are helpful in these children (Table 26-23).

Tube Feeding

Oral feeding may not be adequate or may not be tolerated. Adequate nutrition may have to be supplied via nasogastric intubation if the patient has adequate blood counts and does not have mucositis. In cases where chronic tube feeding will be required, a gastrostomy tube may be placed. If bolus feeds are not tolerated, continuous low-volume infusions can be utilized to maximize caloric intake.

Intravenous Hyperalimentation or Total Parenteral Nutrition

Total parenteral nutrition (TPN) is indicated when enteral feeds cannot be tolerated. It is the most intensive modality of nutritional supplementation and requires a central intravenous device. Full nutritional requirements can usually be met. TPN should be continued until oral feedings can be resumed. Complications of TPN are hypoglycemia, hyperglycemia, fatty liver, and cholestatic jaundice.

Indwelling Intravenous Catheters

With ongoing therapy, it is difficult to find adequate peripheral venous access in pediatric oncology patients. In addition, chemotherapeutic agents produce venous sclerosis, further aggravating the problem of finding peripheral venous access.

Table 26-23. Characteristics of Enteral Products

Product description	1–10 Years of age		>10 Years of age	
	Tube feeding and/or oral	Tube feeding	Oral	

1. Standard or polymeric
Intact macronutrients intended as meal replacements
Requires normal digestive and absorptive capacity
Usually lactose free unless otherwise indicated
	PediaSure
	Kindercal
	Nutren Junior
	Resources Just for Kids TM
	Compleat Pediatric
		Isocal
		Osmolite
		Nutren
		Compleat
		Modified
		Promote
			Ensure
			Boost
			NuBasics
			Meritene
			
			Resource
			Fortashake
			Scandishake
			Carnation
			  Instant
			  Breakfast	

2. High nitrogen Intact macronutrients with >15% total calories as protein Useful for patients with increased protein need (i.e., poor wound healing, radiation)		Isocal HN Osmolite HN Criticare HN	Ensure HN Boost HN TwoCal HN	
3. Concentrated or high calorie Contains higher calorie per milliliter than standard formulas May be used with fluid restriction	Nutren 1.5 Nutren 2.0	Nutren 1.5 Nutren 2.0 TwoCal HN Deliver 2.0 Comply Isosource Jevity Plus	NuBasic Plus Ensure Plus Resource Plus Boost Plus TwoCal HN Jevity Plus	

(Continues)

743

Table 26-23. (Continued)

Product description	1–10 Years of age	>10 Years of age	
	Tube feeding and/or oral	Tube feeding	Oral
4. Predigested/elemental Predigested or partially hydrolyzed peptide-based diet that may be beneficial for child with impaired gastrointestinal function (diarrhea, mucositis, intestinal villous atrophy) Many contain medium-chain triglycerides to minimize fat tolerance Can have high osmolality	Peptamen Junior Neocate One Plus VivonexPeds TM PediaSure with Fiber EleCare L-Emental Pediatric	Peptamen Peptamen VHP Reabillin Tolerex Vivonex TEN Vivonex Plus Criticare HN Travasorb MCT	Vital HN
5. Fiber containing Containing fiber from natural sources or added soy polysaccharides to aid in bowel function	Kindercal PediaSure with Fiber Nutren Junior with Fiber	Jevity Ultracal Nutren 1.0 fiber FiberSource	Jevity Ultracal Nutren 1.0 with fiber
6. Disease specific Macro- and micronutrients modified for disease state		Diabetes: choice Dm, Glucerna Renal: Nepro, Suplena Pulmonary: Pulmocare, NutriVent Liver: NutriHep Metabolically stressed: Replete, Impact, Perative	Diabetes: choice DM, Glucerna Renal: Nepro, Suplena Pulmonary: Pulmocare NutriVent Metabolically stressed: Impact, Replete

7. Infant formulas (variety of formulas available for premature infants and for infants with poor tolerance). Many infants are lactose intolerant after chemotherapy and benefit from lactose-free formulas. Human breast milk should be used when possible (contains lactose and may not be tolerated well after chemotherapy).	Similac Enfamil Lactofree (lactose free) Gerber Carnation Good Start Similac PM 60/40	Isomil ProSobee	Pregestimil Alimentum Nutramigen
8. Modular components	Protein Casec Pro-mix ProMod Nutrisource Protein Elementra	Carbohydrate Polycose Moducal Liquid Carbohydrate (LC) Sumacal Nutrisource Carbohydrate Nutrisource (long- or medium-chain triglycerides)	Fat Vegetable oil (long-chain triglycerides) Microlipid (long-chain triglycerides) Medium-chain triglycerides
9. Oral electrolyte solutions Provides electrolytes, calories, and water during mild to moderate dehydration	Pedialyte Infalyte Equalyte		

From Sacks N, Ringwals-Smith K, Hale G. Nutritional support. In: Altman AJ, ed. Supportive care of children with cancer. Current therapy and guidelines from the Children's Oncology Group. 3rd ed. Baltimore: The Johns Hopkins University Press, 2004:243–261, with permission.

To alleviate this problem, permanently indwelling right atrial catheters are used. These catheters are recommended for:

- All young children and infants receiving chemotherapy
- Most older children and adults receiving chemotherapy if the protocol is prolonged and of moderate to high intensity
- Patients requiring TPN.

Types of Catheters and Methods of Insertion

Two major types of indwelling catheters are in use:

1. External tunneled catheters that lead to tubing that exits the skin. They can be single, double, and occasionally triple lumen. The most frequently used types are the Broviac catheter and the Hickman catheter.
2. Total implantable venous access devices or "ports" are right atrial catheters that lead to reservoirs totally embedded under the skin, replacing the external portion of the catheter. These are more cosmetically satisfactory to older children and adolescents.

Catheters are inserted via the subclavian, internal, or external jugular vein with a subcutaneous tunnel to the anterior or lateral chest wall. Alternatively, catheters can be placed via the femoral vein to the inferior vena cava with a tunnel to the abdominal wall.

Maintenance

1. Broviacs (or Hickmans) require daily or every-other-day heparin flushes, in addition to dressing changes three times a week.
2. Mediports require heparin flushes only once every 3–4 weeks and do not require dressing changes.
3. In both cases, completely sterile technique must be used in accessing the catheters.

Complications

The major complications are:

1. *Infection:* Episodes of catheter-related bacteremia occur and are most commonly due to coagulase-negative staphylococci. Management consists of appropriate intravenous antibiotic therapy. Antibiotic therapy without catheter removal is successful in approximately 75% of episodes. If the bacteremia fails to resolve, the patient develops uncontrolled clinical sepsis, or if there is infection overlying the subcutaneous tunnel, then the catheter must be removed. Occasionally, catheter-related fungal infection occurs and, in most of these cases, catheter removal is necessary.
2. *Thrombosis:* Thrombosis may be cleared by instilling tPA 0.5–1 mg and leaving it in for 30–60 minutes. If the catheter remains occluded after 2 doses, a continuous infusion of tPA is indicated. The dose is 0.01 mg/kg/hour for 6 hours. The dose may be increased to 0.02 mg/kg/hour for 6 hours, then to 0.03 mg/kg/hour for 6 hours if there is no resolution. The fibrinogen level should be monitored every 6 hours. If the line is still occluded, it should be removed.

Most patients develop the preceding complications from time to time. In the majority of cases, however, the morbidity associated with these complications is outweighed by the advantages of reliable, adequate venous access.

Psychosocial Support

Throughout the course of the disease, children with cancer and their families will face a number of psychological issues. In addition to the oncologist's skills in this area, specially trained psychologists, psychiatric social workers, and psychiatrists can be helpful in dealing with these matters as they arise. A detailed discussion of these issues is beyond the scope of this manual and the reader is referred to detailed review articles and books on this subject.

SUGGESTED READINGS

Alexander SW, Walsh TJ, Freifeld AG, Pizzo PA. Infectious complications in pediatric cancer patients. In: Pizzo PA, Poplack DG, editors. Principles and Practice of Pediatric Oncology. 4th ed. Philadelphia: Lippincott, Williams & Wilkins, 2002;1239–84.

Barnard DR, Friedman DL, Landier W, Larson-Tuttle C, Iacuone J. Monitoring and management of drug toxicity. In: Altman AJ, editor. Supportive Care of Children with Cancer. Current Therapy and Guidelines from the Children's Oncology Group. 3rd ed. Baltimore: The Johns Hopkins University Press, 2004;100–48.

Bechard LJ, Adiv OE, Jaksic T, Duggan C. Nutritional supportive care. In: Pizzo PA, Poplack DG, editors. Principles and Practice of Pediatric Oncology. 4th ed. Philadelphia: Lippincott, Williams & Wilkins, 2002;1285–300.

Berde CB, Billett AL, Collins JJ. Symptom management in supportive care. In: Pizzo PA, Poplack DG, editors. Principles and Practice of Pediatric Oncology. 4th ed. Philadelphia: Lippincott, Williams & Wilkins, 2002;1301–32.

Feusner J, Hastings C. Recombinant human erythropoietin in pediatric oncology: a review. Med Pediatr Oncol 2002;39:463–8.

Gorlin JB. Noninfectious complications of pediatric transfusion. In: Hillyer CD, Strauss RG, Luban NLC, editors. Handbook of Pediatric Transfusion Medicine. San Diego: Elsevier Academic Press, 2004;317–25.

Hughes WT, Armstrong D, Bodey GP, et al. 2002 guidelines for the use of antimicrobial agents in neutropenic patients with cancer. Clin Infect Dis 2002;34:730–51.

Jamali F, Ness PM. Infectious complications. In: Hillyer CD, Strauss RG, Luban NLC, editors. Handbook of Pediatric Transfusion Medicine. San Diego: Elsevier Academic Press, 2004;329–39.

Logdberg LE. Leukoreduced products: prevention of leukocyte-related transfusion-associated adverse effects. In: Hillyer CD, Strauss RG, Luban NLC, editors. Handbook of Pediatric Transfusion Medicine. San Diego: Elsevier Academic Press, 2004;85–90.

Orudjev E, Lange BJ. Evolving concepts of management of febrile neutropenic in children with cancer. Med Pediatr Oncol 2002;39:77–85.

Ozer H, Armitage JO, Bennett CL, et al. 2000 update of recommendations for the use of hematopoietic colony-stimulating factors: evidence-based, clinical practice guidelines. J Clin Oncol 2000;18(20):3558–85.

Pui CH, Mahmoud HH, Wiley JM, et al. Recombinant urate oxidase for the prophylaxis or treatment of hyperuricemias in patients with leukemia or lymphoma. J Clin Oncol 2001;19(3):697–704.

Rheingold SR, Lange BJ. Oncologic emergencies. In: Pizzo PA, Poplack DG, editors. Principles and Practice of Pediatric Oncology. 4th ed. Philadelphia: Lippincott, Williams & Wilkins, 2002;1177–1204.

Rizzo JD, Lichtin AE, Woolf SH, et al. Use of epoetin patients with cancer: evidence-based clinical practice guidelines of the American Society of Clinical Oncology and the American Society of Hematology. Blood 2002;100(7):2303–20.

Rogers ZR, Aquino VM, Buchana GR. Hematologic supportive care and hematopoietic cytokines. In: Pizzo PA, Poplack DG, editors. Principles and Practice of Pediatric Oncology. 4th ed. Philadelphia: Lippincott, Williams & Wilkins, 2002;1205–38.

Sacks N, Ringwals-Smith K, Hale G. Nutritional support. In: Altman AJ, editor. Supportive Care of Children with Cancer. Current Therapy and Guidelines from the Children's Oncology Group. 3rd ed. Baltimore: The Johns Hopkins University Press, 2004;243–61.

Wolff LJ, Altman AJ, Berkow RL, Johnson FL. The management of fever and neutropenia. In: Altman AJ, editor. Supportive Care of Children with Cancer. Current Therapy and Guidelines from the Children's Oncology Group. 3rd ed. Baltimore: The Johns Hopkins University Press, 2004;200–20.

Zempsky WT, Schechter NL, Altman AJ, Weisman SJ. The management of pain. In: Altman AJ, editor. Supportive Care of Children with Cancer. Current Therapy and Guidelines from the Children's Oncology Group. 3rd ed. Baltimore: The Johns Hopkins University Press, 2004;200–20.

27

EVALUATION, INVESTIGATIONS, AND MANAGEMENT OF LATE EFFECTS OF CHILDHOOD CANCER

Currently the overall 5-year survival rate in childhood cancer is 75%. The prevalence of U.S. childhood cancer survivors among young adults 15–45 years of age has been estimated to be 1 in 900 persons.

Late effects are defined as any physical or psychological outcome that develops or persists beyond 5 years from the diagnosis of cancer. Up to two thirds of childhood cancer survivors are likely to experience at least one late effect, with one fourth of survivors experiencing severe or life-threatening side effects. The most common late effects of childhood cancer are neurocognitive, psychological, cardiopulmonary, endocrine, musculoskeletal, and second malignancies.

Chemotherapy, radiation therapy, and surgery may all cause late effects involving any organ system. The three most common treatment-related causes of death are the development of a secondary cancer, cardiac toxicity, and pulmonary complications.

Some late effects of therapy are identified during childhood and adolescence and resolve without consequence. Other late effects become chronic and may progress to adult medical problems.

Information to be elicited in the follow-up of cancer survivors is listed in Table 27-1. Selected late effects associated with different childhood cancers are listed in Table 27-2, and the evaluation for suspected late effects can be seen in Table 27-3. Table 27-4 lists the radiosensitivity of various cell types, and Table 27-5 lists the radiation dose toxicity levels for subacute and late visceral effects.

MUSCULOSKELETAL SYSTEM

Radiation

Radiation has the following consequences:

- Scoliosis
- Atrophy or hypoplasia of muscles
- Avascular necrosis
- Osteoporosis
- Poor enamel and teeth formation with increased risk of cavities, malocclusion, and hypoplasia of mandible

Table 27-1. Information to be Elicited in Follow-Up of Survivors of Childhood Cancer

History of intercurrent illnesses
Review of systems
Development of any benign tumors or other cancers
Medications: prophylactic antibiotics
Educational status
   Grade completed; special education classes?
   Grade point average; results of intelligence quotient tests
   Areas of weakness
Employment status
Insurance coverage
   Individual policy, or coverage through parents?
   Difficulties in obtaining insurance?
Marital history
Menses, libido, sexual activity
Pregnancy outcome (patient or spouse)

From Pizzo PA, Poplock DG, editors. Principles and Practice of Pediatric Oncology. 4th ed. Philadelphia: Lippincott, Williams and Wilkins, 2002, with permission.

Table 27-2. Selected Potential Late Effects Associated with Childhood Cancer

Cancer	Potential late effects	
Leukemias	• Cognitive effects (e.g., learning disabilities) • Abnormal growth and maturation • Heart problems • Second cancers • Hepatitis C (effects of blood transfusion)	• Weakness, fatigue • Obesity • Osteoporosis • Avascular necrosis of bone • Dental problems
Brain cancer	• Neurologic and cognitive effects (e.g., learning disabilities) • Abnormal growth and maturation • Hearing loss	• Kidney damage • Hepatitis C • Infertility • Vision problems • Second cancers • Endocrinal abnormalities (craniopharyngioma)
Hodgkin disease	• Adhesions and intestinal obstruction (if spleen removed) • Decreased resistance to infection (potential for life-threatening sepsis) • Abnormal growth and maturation • Hypothyroidism (effects of neck radiation)	• Salivary gland malfunctioning (effect of jawbone irradiation) • Lung damage • Heart problems • Infertility • Hepatitis C • Second cancers (e.g., breast cancer in females)
Non-Hodgkin lymphoma	• Heart problems • Hepatitis C • Cognitive effects	• Infertility • Osteopenia/osteoporosis

(Continues)

Table 27-2. (*Continued*)

Bone tumor	• Amputation/disfigurement • Functional, activity limitations • Damage to soft tissues and underlying bones (radiation may cause scarring, swelling, or inhibit growth)	• Hearing loss • Heart problems • Kidney damage • Second cancers • Hepatitis C • Fertility problems
Wilms' tumor	• Heart problems • Kidney damage • Damage to soft tissues and underlying bones (radiation may cause scarring, swelling, or inhibit growth)	• Second cancers • Fertility problems • Scoliosis
Neuroblastoma	• Heart problems • Damage to soft tissues and underlying bones (radiation may cause scarring, swelling, or inhibit growth)	• Neurocognitive effects • Hearing loss • Hepatitis C • Second cancers • Kidney damage
Soft-tissue sarcoma	• Amputation/disfigurement • Functional activity limitations • Heart problems • Damage to soft tissues and underlying bones (radiation may cause scarring, swelling, or inhibit growth)	• Second cancers • Hepatitis C • Kidney damage • Cataracts • Infertility • Neurocognitive effects

From Hewitt M, Weiner SL, Simone JV, editors. Childhood cancer survivorship. Improving care and quality of life. Washington, DC: National Academies Press, 2003, with permission.

Table 27-3. Evaluation for Suspected Late Effects

Late effect	Screening test	Recommendations if screening results abnormal
Short stature	Growth curve	Bone-age, growth hormone test
	Sitting height	Thyroid function tests[a]
	Parental heights	Endocrine consultation
Obesity or weight loss	Growth curve	Thyroid function tests[a]
	Diet history	Nutritionist, endocrinologist, consultation
Scoliosis	Physical examination	Spine radiography; evaluate again during adolescent growth spurt Orthopedist consultation
Bone asymmetries (hypoplasia, atrophy)	Bone lengths, circumference	Orthopedist consultation; bone radiography; plastic surgeon consultation
Avascular necrosis or osteoporosis	History of pain, fractures Bone radiography	Bone scan Serum estradiol level; Ca, P Orthopedist consultation; physical therapist consultation
Soft-tissue hypoplasia, contractures, edema	Physical examination	Plastic surgeon consultation
Dental abnormalities	Physical examination	Dentist, oral surgeon consultation

(*Continues*)

Table 27-3. (*Continued*)

Late effect	Screening test	Recommendations if screening results abnormal
Learning disabilities	Communication with school, family; psychological testing	CT or MRI scan of head; special education classes
Leukoencephalopathy	CT or MRI (see also learning disabilities, above)	Cerebrospinal fluid basic myelin protein; neurologist consultation
Neuropathy	Physical examination	Neurologist consultation
Hearing loss	Audiogram	Otorhinolaryngologist consultation; audiologist consultation
Infertility	History (primary versus secondary dysfunction)	Endocrinologist consultation
	Gonadal function testing[b]	Obstetrician or gynecologist consultation
Thyroid dysfunction	Thyroid function testing[a]	Endocrinologist consultation
Cardiomyopathy or pericarditis	Electrocardiogram; echocardiogram; radionuclide angiography	Cardiologist consultation
Vaso-occlusive disease	Angiography; Doppler pulses	Vascular surgeon
Pneumonitis or pulmonary fibrosis	Chest radiography	Lung biopsy
	Pulmonary function tests	Pulmonologist consultation
Chronic enteritis	Growth curves	Serum folate, carotene
	Nutritional assessment	Small-bowel studies; barium enema; gastroenterologist consultation
Hepatitis or cirrhosis	Liver function tests	Liver biopsy, hepatitis screen; liver scan; gastroenterologist consultation
Nephritis, rickets (tubular defects)	Urinalysis; BUN, creatinine, serum electrolytes, CO_2, Ca, P, alkaline phosphatase; wrist radiographs	24-h creatinine clearance, glomerular filtration rate, intravenous urogram or sonogram; nephrologist consultation
Hemorrhagic cystitis	Urinalysis	Cytoscopy; urologist consultation
Thrombotic thrombocytopenic purpura	CBC/platelets, BUN, creatinine; peripheral blood smear	
Sepsis	Compliance with prophylactic antibiotics	
Second malignancy	Studies on an individual basis	Oncologist consultation

Abbreviations: BUN, blood urea nitrogen; CBC, complete blood cell count; CT, computed tomography; MRI, magnetic resonance imaging.

[a]Thyroid function tests include thyroxine (T_4), TSH.

[b]Gonadal function tests: Tanner staging for boys older than 14 years at the time of evaluation or girls not yet menstruating by age 12 years or if menses become irregular; follicle-stimulating hormone, luteinizing hormone, and testosterone (semen analysis) or estradiol, as appropriate.

From, Pizzo PA, Poplack DG, editors. Principles and Practice of Pediatric Oncology. 4th ed. Philadelphia: Lippincott, Williams and Wilkins, 2002, with permission.

Table 27-4. Cell Types in Order of Radiosensitivity

Radiosensitivity	Examples	Cell types
High	Hematopoietic stem cells; intestinal crypt cells; basal cells of the epidermis; lymphocytes[a]	Stem cells
Intermediate to high	Differentiating hematopoietic cells; spermatogonia and spermatocytes	Differentiating cells
Intermediate	Endothelial cells; fibroblasts	Connective tissue cells
Low to intermediate	Duct cells of the salivary glands, kidney cells, liver cells, epithelial cells; smooth muscle	Differentiated cells with some ability to divide cells
Low	Neurons; muscle cells; most mature hematopoietic cells	Differentiated, nondividing cells

[a]Differentiated, nondividing cells, but highly radiosensitive.

From Kun LE. General principles of radiation therapy. In: P.A. Pizzo and D.G. Poplack, editors. Principles and Practice of Pediatric Oncology. Philadelphia: Lippincott–Raven, 1997;289–321, with permission.

- Discrepancy in length of extremities
- Alteration in sitting to standing height ratio.

These late consequences are related to the dose, site, volume, and age of the child at the time of radiation. The higher the dose and the younger the child, the more pronounced the late effects.

Prevention

- Low-volume, low-dose radiation combined with effective systemic therapy (e.g., treatment for Hodgkin disease in children, treatment of early-stage Wilms' tumor with chemotherapy alone)
- Improvement in the delivery of radiation with advances in radiation technology
- Dental prophylaxis prior to radiotherapy in maxillofacial site.

Management

- *Length discrepancy:* contralateral epiphysiodesis, limb-shortening procedures
- *Pathologic fracture:* surgical repair of fracture; may require internal fixation
- *Osteonecrosis:* symptomatic care, joint replacement.

Chemotherapy

- Skin and tendon contracture following infiltration of vesicant drugs (e.g., nitrogen mustard, anthracycline, vincristine, actinomycin D)
- Steroid-induced avascular necrosis and osteoporosis. The increased use of dexamethasone in acute lymphocytic leukemia (ALL) therapy has resulted in an increased number of cases of avascular necrosis. Adolescents appear to be at higher risk. Recent Children's Oncology Group protocols have attempted to decrease this incidence by decreasing the number of continuous weeks of exposure to dexamethasone by the use of 1 week on and 1 week off when prolonged dexamethasone therapy is required after induction.

Investigators have found that bone mineral density is decreased in childhood cancer survivors and there is an increased incidence of osteopenia and osteoporosis. Use of bisphosphonates are being investigated in childhood cancer survivors to improve osteoporosis.

Table 27-5. Radiation Dose Toxicity Levels for Subacute and Late Visceral Effects

Organ	Toxicity	Whole organ irradiation			Partial organ irradiation				Chemotherapy effect
		5–10% incidence dose[a] (Gy)	RT±CTx	>25–50% incidence (Gy)	Volume	<5–10% incidence dose[a] (Gy)	RT±CTx	>25–50% incidence (Gy)	
Lung	Subacute pneumonitis or late fibrosis	18–20	(CTx−)	24–25	<30% of one lung	25–30	(CTx−)	45–50	++
		15–18	(CTx+)	21–24		<20	(CTx+)	>35	
Heart	Subacute pericarditis	35–40		>50	<50%	40–50		60–70	+/−
	Late cardiomyopathy	45–50	(CTx−)	>60	<25%	<40	(CTx−)	>70	+++
		30–40	(CTx+)	>50		30–40	(CTx+)	>50	
Liver	Subacute hepatopathy	25–30	(CTx−)	>40	<50%	30–40	NA	40	++
		20–25	(CTx+)	>35					
Kidney	Subacute nephropathy	18–20	(CTx−)	24–26	>50%	20–24	NA	>30	+
	Late nephropathy	16–18	(CTx+)	22–26					
	Late hypertension	Similar to subacute nephropathy			>50%	20–25	NA	>35	+/−
Small bowel	Subacute enteropathy	15–25	NA	>40	<50%	20–25	NA		+
Brain	Late necrosis	54–60	NA	>65	<50%	Equal to whole brain	NA	>60	+/−+++
Spinal cord	Subacute—late	40–45	NA	>50	<15%	45–50	NA	>55	−

Notes: (CTx−), without prior, concurrent, or subsequent chemotherapy; (CTx+), interaction with one or more chemotherapeutic agents; NA, not applicable.

[a]Dose assumes conventional fractionation (150–200 cGy once daily, 5 days per week). If ≥40% of liver excluded from dose ≥18 Gy, remainder of organ can receive doses up to 40+ Gy.

From Kun LE. General principles of radiation therapy. In: Pizzo PA, Poplack DG, editors. Principles and Practice of Pediatric Oncology. Philadelphia: Lippincott–Raven, 1997;289–321, with permission.

CARDIOVASCULAR SYSTEM

Chemotherapy, radiotherapy, or combined use of both have the potential to cause cardiac complications.

Anthracyclines

Anthracycline-induced myocyte death results in hypertrophy of existing myocytes, reduced thickness of the wall of the heart, and interstitial fibrosis. The heart is unable to compensate adequately to meet the demands of growth, pregnancy, or other cardiac stress, which results in late-onset anthracycline-induced cardiac failure.

The incidence of cardiomyopathy is related to the cumulative dose of anthracyclines. It occurs in 11% of cancer patients after a cumulative dose of less than 400 mg/m^2, 23% after 400–599 mg/m^2, 47% after 500–799 mg/m^2, and 100% after 800 mg/m^2.

Early-onset cardiotoxicity occurring during therapy or within 1 year of completion of therapy is the most significant risk factor for the development of late-onset cardiotoxicity (occurring longer than 1 year after completion of therapy). Female patients have an increased risk of cardiac dysfunction after anthracycline therapy. Mitoxantrone, idarubicin, and amacrine have also been associated with cardiotoxicity.

Late anthracycline-induced cardiomyopathy is a progressive disorder. It manifests with:

- Exercise intolerance
- Dyspnea
- Peripheral edema
- Pulmonary rales
- S3 and S4
- Hepatomegaly.

Rapid progression of symptoms may occur with pregnancy, anesthesia, isometric exercise, the use of illicit drugs (e.g., cocaine), prescription drugs (e.g., beta blockers), and alcohol. Factors that enhance the myocardial toxicity of anthracycline are:

- Mediastinal radiation
- Underlying cardiac abnormalities: involvement with tumor, uncontrolled hypertension, exposure to other chemotherapeutic agents (particularly cyclophosphamide, dactinomycin, mitomycin, dacarbazine [DTIC], vincristine, bleomycin, and methotrexate).

Appropriate Tests and Criteria for Deteriorating Cardiac Function

Electrocardiogram (ECG) findings include prolonged QT$_c$ ($\geq$0.45 or longer), second-degree atrioventricular (A-V) block, complete heart block, ventricular ectopy, ST elevation or depression, and T-wave changes. An association between prolongation of the QT$_c$ interval and an anthracycline dose greater than 300 mg/m^2 has been described in childhood cancer survivors.

Echocardiogram (ECHO) findings include fractional shortening (SF) and velocity of circumferential fiber shortening (VCF) for the measurement of left ventricular contractility. The normal SF value is 29% or more.

Radionuclide cardiac cineangiocardiography (RNA or MUGA) determines the ejection fraction and is useful for those patients in whom a good ECHO cannot be obtained. A left ventricular ejection fraction (LVEF) of 55% or more indicates normal systolic function.

The following are criteria for progressive deteriorating cardiac function:

- A decrease in the SF by an absolute value of 10% from the previous test
- SF less than 29%
- A decrease in the RNA LVEF by an absolute value of 10% from the previous test
- RNA LVEF less than 55%
- A decrease in the RNA LVEF with stress.

Therapy of Congestive Heart Failure

- Digoxin, to improve ventricular contractility
- Diuretics, to decrease sodium and water retention
- Angiotensin-converting enzyme-inhibiting agents (e.g., Captopril), to decrease sodium and water retention and decrease afterload
- Enalapril, to increase contractility and decrease afterload.

Patients with cardiomyopathy are at risk for ventricular arrhythmia. Such patients should undergo a 24-hour ECG monitoring on a regular basis. Arrhythmia will necessitate appropriate therapy.

Prognosis of late-onset heart failure is poor. Cardiac transplantation should be considered. The actuarial survival rate at 5 years after cardiac transplant is 77%.

Guidelines for Long-Term Follow-Up

The frequency of testing is determined by the cumulative anthracycline doses:

- Total cumulative dose less than 300 mg/m^2: Perform an ECHO before every other course of anthracyclines.
- Total cumulative dose greater than 300 mg/m^2 plus mediastinal radiation 1000 cGy or more: Perform an RNA (MUGA) in addition to an ECHO if indicated for better imaging and confirmation.
- Total cumulative dose greater than 400 mg/m^2 with or without mediastinal radiation: Perform an RNA in addition to an ECHO if indicated for better imaging and confirmation.

After completion of therapy all patients with any amount of anthracycline exposure or thoracic radiation therapy should have an EKG and ECHO ± RNA performed at 12 months after discontinuation of therapy. Patients with normal studies at the end of 1 year post-therapy may have an ECHO and ECG every 2–3 years. Patients with an abnormal study either at the end of therapy or at the time of initial long-term follow-up (5 years after diagnosis) should have more frequent follow-up.

Cyclophosphamide

Cyclophosphamide-induced cardiac effects occur primarily with high-dose preparatory regimens for stem cell transplantation. Cyclophosphamide causes intramyocardial edema and hemorrhage, often in association with serosanguineous pericardial effusion and fibrous pericarditis. This cardiotoxicity is usually reversible.

Cyclophosphamide may enhance anthracycline-induced cardiac toxicity.

Radiation

Cardiac doses of up to 25 Gy are generally safe. Chronic toxicity caused by radiotherapy usually involves pericardial effusion or constrictive pericarditis.

RESPIRATORY SYSTEM

Both chemotherapy and radiation therapy can cause acute and chronic lung injury. Younger children are at more risk than adolescents or adults for the development of chronic respiratory damage.

Radiation

Radiation therapy in children younger than 3 years of age results in increased toxicity. Radiation therapy to the lungs can cause impairment of the proliferation and maturation of alveoli, resulting in chronic respiratory insufficiency. This is thought to be consistent with a proportionate interference with the growth of both the lungs and chest wall. It also causes damage to the type II pneumocyte, which is responsible for the production of surfactant and the maintenance of patency of the alveoli. As a result of changes in surfactant production, there is a decrease in alveolar surface tension and compliance. These children exhibit decreased mean total lung volumes and DLCO (diffusion capacity of carbon monoxide) that is approximately 60% of predicted values.

The effects of direct radiation to the lungs also include damage to the endothelial cells of the capillaries, resulting in alterations of perfusion and permeability of the vessel wall. Currently, this complication is thought to be mediated by cytokine production that stimulates septal fibroblasts increasing collagen production and pulmonary fibrosis. The late radiation injury to the lung is characterized by the presence of progressive fibrosis of alveolar septa and obliteration of collapsed alveoli with connective tissue.

In adolescents treated for Hodgkin disease who are asymptomatic, chest radiographic findings or pulmonary function tests consistent with fibrosis have been found in 30–100% of patients. The changes have been detected months to years after radiation therapy. The incidence of radiation-induced fibrosis has decreased due to refinements in radiation therapy.

Children with malignant brain tumors receiving craniospinal radiation therapy have a significant risk of developing late restrictive lung disease.

Chemotherapy

The patterns of pulmonary toxicity include:

- Pneumonitis or fibrosis
- Acute hypersensitivity
- Noncardiogenic pulmonary edema.

Pneumonitis or Fibrosis

Etiologic agents include bleomycin, nitrosourea, cyclophosphamide, and methotrexate. The clinical manifestations usually occur months after a critical cumulative dose is reached or exceeded.

Bleomycin

- *Critical cumulative dose:* 400 units. At doses over 400 units of bleomycin, 10% of patients experience fibrosis.
- *Clinical manifestations:* dyspnea, dry cough, rales.
- *Radiographic findings:* interstitial pneumonitis with reticular or nodular pattern.
- *Pulmonary function tests:* restrictive ventilatory defect with hypoxia, hypercapnia, and chronic hyperventilation (diffusion capacity of carbon monoxide is considered to be the most sensitive test).

- *Aggravating factors:* radiation therapy, renal insufficiency, cisplatin, cyclophosphamide, exposure to high levels of oxygen, pulmonary infections.

Nitrosourea

- *Critical cumulative dose:* >1500 mg/m^2 in adults; >750 mg/m^2 in children.
- *Clinical manifestations:* same as bleomycin.

Pulmonary fibrosis is more commonly associated with BCNU.

Acute Hypersensitivity Reaction

- Agents associated with this reaction: methotrexate, 6-mercaptopurine, procarbazine, bleomycin
- *Pathology:* desquamative interstitial pneumonitis or an eosinophilic pneumonitis.

Noncardiogenic Pulmonary Edema

Etiologic agents include cytosine arabinoside, methotrexate, ifosfamide, and cyclophosphamide. This complication occurs within days of the beginning of treatment. Children under 8 years of age who develop methotrexate-induced lung toxicity may reveal abnormalities in pulmonary function on long-term follow-up studies.

Other factors contributing to chronic pulmonary toxicity include asthma, infection, smoking, and having had a history of assisted ventilation.

Detection and Screening for Lung Toxicity

Clinical

Table 27-6 shows a scoring system for shortness of breath.

Nuclear Medicine Studies

- Perfusion and ventilation scan (V/Q scan)
- Gallium scan
- Quantitative ventilation-perfusion scintigraphy consists of three different studies: (1) ventilation per unit volume, (2) blood flow to ventilated alveoli, and (3) blood flow per unit ventilated lung volume.

Table 27-6. Shortness of Breath Scoring System

Grade	Description
0	No shortness of breath with normal activity. Shortness of breath with exertion, comparable to a well person of the same age, height, and sex
1	More shortness of breath than a person of the same age while walking quietly on the level or on climbing an incline or two flights of stairs
2	More shortness of breath and unable to keep up with persons of the same age and sex while walking on the level
3	Shortness of breath while walking on the level and while performing everyday tasks at work
4	Shortness of breath while carrying out personal activities (e.g., dressing, talking, walking from one room to another)

From McDonald S, Rubin P, Schwartz CL. Pulmonary effects of antineoplastic therapy. In: Schwartz CL, Hobbie WL, Constine LS, Ruccione KS, editors. Survivors of Childhood Cancer: Assessment and Management. St. Louis: Mosby, 1994;177–95, with permission.

Blood flow to ventilated alveoli has proved most useful in quantifying radiation injury to the lungs.

Radiography

- Chest films
- Computed tomography (CT) scan of the chest
- Quantitative CT scan of the chest, which provides the following information: total aerated lung volume, total opacified lung volume, and percentage of opacified lung volume.

Management of Pulmonary Toxicity

- Chest radiograph, pulmonary function studies every 2–5 years in asymptomatic patients
- Lung biopsy to differentiate chronic fibrosis from lung metastasis
- Awareness of the risks of general anesthesia in patients with pulmonary toxicity
- Corticosteroids for symptomatic relief
- Bronchodilators, expectorants, antibiotics, and oxygen, when indicated.

CENTRAL NERVOUS SYSTEM
Pathogenesis of Central Nervous System Toxicity

Radiation

- Altered capillary wall permeability, resulting in alterations in cerebral blood flow
- Primary damage to glial cells, especially oligodendroglia
- Demyelination of glial tissue
- Focal white matter destruction
- Impaired neuronal differentiation, including dendritic formation and synaptogenesis.

Chemotherapy

The pathogenesis of chemotherapy-induced central nervous system (CNS) toxicity is not well understood. In addition to damage to the glial and capillary tissue, the neurotransmitter function of the brain may also be impaired.

With current trends in the use of higher doses of methotrexate, as well as the increased frequency with which methotrexate is used in intrathecal therapy, induced neurologic sequelae have been on the rise.

The four pathologic effects of prophylactic CNS therapy in leukemia are:

1. Leukoencephalopathy
2. Mineralizing microangiopathy
3. Subacute necrotizing leukomyelopathy
4. Brain tumors (second malignant neoplasm).

Leukoencephalopathy

- *Clinical manifestations:* seizure, ataxia, lethargy, slurred speech, spasticity, dysphagia, lowered IQ scores, memory impairment, and confusion
- *Onset of symptoms:* usually 4 months after cranial radiation

- *Radioimaging findings:* dilatation of the ventricles and subarachnoid space, indicative of cerebral atrophy; white matter hypodensity by CT scan and hyperdensity on magnetic resonance imaging (MRI) indicative of leukoencephalopathy
- *Correlation with treatment:* 20-Gy cranial RT and use of both intratheal (IT) methotrexate (MTX) and systemic MTX (>40 mg/m² weekly). This combination of therapy is most neurotoxic.

With the use of current treatments, this severe form of leukoencephalopathy is seen infrequently. The subclinical form of leukoencephaly is more common, characterized by radiologic abnormalities on CT scan and MRI without clinical symptoms. It occurs in approximately 55–60% of patients receiving CNS prophylaxis. Nonirradiated patients generally do not show both white matter changes (i.e., low-density areas) and gray matter changes (widening of sulci and ventricles). This combination of findings is seen more often in patients treated with cranial radiation, IT MTX, and systemic MTX.

Mineralizing Microangiopathy

- *Clinical manifestations:* seizures, electroencephalogram (EEG) abnormalities, inco-ordination, gait abnormalities, memory deficits, learning disabilities, decrease in IQ scores, behavioral problems
- *Onset of symptoms:* 10 months to several years after CNS prophylaxis (the risk of these complications increases proportionately with higher doses of IT MTX and irradiation combined with systemic chemotherapy. Irradiation is the main cause of this complication).
- *Radioimaging findings:* changes primarily in the gray matter of the brain mainly in the region of basal ganglia and less frequently in the cerebellar gray matter.

Histologically, there is deposition of calcium in the small blood vessels, causing lumen occlusion by mineralized debris. There may be dystrophic calcification of the surrounding neural tissue.

Subacute Necrotizing Leukomyelopathy

This unusual complication occurs after the use of cranial or craniospinal irradiation combined with IT MTX. Histologically, it shows focal myelin necrosis on the posterior and/or lateral columns of the spinal cord.

Brain Tumors (Second Malignant Neoplasm)

Patients with ALL who are younger than 5 years of age at the time of cranial irradiation are at a 1% risk to develop brain tumors within the first 10 years after therapy. Children treated under 6 years of age have an increased risk of developing high-grade gliomas. They are at risk for developing meningioma 10–20 years after cranial irradiation.

Children treated before 5–6 years of age, especially those treated before 3 years of age, are at a higher risk for developing cognitive impairments than those treated after the age of 8–10 years. Table 27-7 lists the clinical manifestations of neurotoxicity associated with irradiation therapy, and Table 27-8 lists the neurologic complications secondary to chemotherapy.

Detection of Neurotoxic Sequelae

In addition to history and physical examination, neurocognitive evaluation is essential to detect learning disability. It should be performed in all children under 10 years

Table 27-7. Radiation-Related Neurotoxicity

Type	Timing	Etiology	Syndrome	Signs and symptoms
Acute	During or immediately after RT	Peritumoral edema	Increased intracranial pressure	Worsening focal signs; headache, vomiting; nausea
Subacute	Weeks to 3 months	Transient demyelina-tion (? oligo-dendroglial dysfunction)	Somnolence	Somnolence lasting days to weeks; anorexia
			Myelitis	Paresthesia down spine
			Endocrinologic	Growth failure; hypothy-roidism; hypogonadism
			Neurocognitive	School difficulties; memory loss; retardation
Chronic	Months to years after RT	Vasculitis; oligoden-droglial dysfunction; autoimmune etiology	Radionecrosis	Focal deficits; seizures; symptoms of increased intracranial pressure
			Large vessel occlusion	Focal deficits; seizures
			Mineralizing micro-angiopathy	Focal deficits; seizures; headaches
			Myelopathy	Paraparesis; quadripare-sis; bowel and bladder dysfunction
			Peripheral neuropathy	Cranial nerve palsies; autonomic dysfunction weakness

From Moore IM, Packer RJ, Karl D, Bleyer WA. Adverse effects of cancer treatment on the central nervous system. In: Schwartz CL, Hobbie WL, Constine LS, Ruccione KS, editors. Survivors of Childhood Cancer: Assessment and Management. St. Louis: Mosby, 1994;81–95, with permission.

of age who have received extensive cranial irradiation, intrathecal chemotherapy, and high-dose systemic MTX therapy. Baseline evaluation should be done during the initial phase of illness or 8–12 weeks after the start of cranial irradiation. Follow-up neuropsychological evaluations should be performed twice a year. In ALL patients, neuropsychological evaluations have revealed decreases in attention capacities and nonverbal cognitive processing skills.

Neuroradiologic studies should include either CT or MRI. MRI, however, is preferred because of its greater sensitivity in delineating white matter damage. The degree of white matter changes is mild, moderate, or severe. Mild change is represented by occasional punctate areas of signal abnormality, moderate is large or multiple areas of damage, and severe is confluent areas of white matter damage. Patients with severe white matter damage manifest impairment in mentation, motor deficits, and seizures.

EEG abnormalities are relatively nonspecific. A positron emission tomography (PET) scan may help in differentiating radiation-induced necrosis from recurrence of malignant tumor, the former being characterized by decreased metabolism and the latter by increased metabolism.

Learning Disabilities

Neuropsychological screening should be performed routinely in children treated for ALL and brain tumors. An age-standardized battery of tests should be used that

Table 27-8. More Common Neurologic Complications Secondary to Chemotherapy (Excluding Methotrexate)

Drug	Acute and subacute	Chronic
Cytosine arabinoside		
Intrathecal	Meningitis; seizures; radiculitis; myelitis; brain necrosis following intraparenchymal infusion	Leukoencephalopathy myelitis; peripheral neuropathy
IV high-dose	Cerebellar ataxia; encephalopathy	Cerebellar ataxia; ? demyelinating polyneuropathy
5-Fluorouracil	Cerebellar syndrome; encephalopathy	Reversible encephalopathy
Ifosfamide	Encephalopathy; cerebellar ataxia; weakness; cranial nerve dysfunction; seizures	? Encephalopathy
BCNU		
Intra-arterial	Focal brain necrosis; blindness; seizures; encephalopathy	Blindness; seizures; encephalopathy; brain necrosis
Cisplatin		
Intra-arterial	Encephalopathy; blindness	Blindness; progressive brain necrosis
IV	Increased intracranial pressure; seizures; retrobulbar neuritis	Peripheral neuropathy; ototoxicity[a]
Vincristine	Muscle cramps; paresthesias; jaw pain; cranial neuropathy (sensory and motor); autonomic neuropathy; constipation; reversible	Peripheral neuropathy
L-Asparaginase	Metabolic encephalopathy; cerebral vascular accidents due to thrombosis or hemorrhage	Sequelae of cerebral vascular accidents
Procarbazine	Encephalopathy; peripheral neuropathy; ataxia; autonomic neuropathy; psychosis with high dosages	

[a]Enhanced by radiotherapy.
From Moore IM, Packer RJ, Karl D, Bleyer WA: Adverse effects of cancer treatment on the central nervous system. In: Schwartz CL, Hobbie WL, Constine LS, Ruccione KS, editors. Survivors of Childhood Cancer: Assessment and Management. St. Louis: Mosby, 1994:81–95, with permission.

measures intellectual ability, visual and somatosensory perception, visual motor and motor skills, language memory and learning behavior, and academic and social functioning. Repeat testing should be performed every 2–3 years until early adulthood.

Management

Educational intervention may be required to minimize problems with school performance.

ENDOCRINE SYSTEM

The hypothalamic–pituitary axis plays a central role in translating neurologic and chemical signals from the brain into endocrine responses through its neuronal circuitry with the brain involving afferent and efferent pathways. It also produces peptide hormones and biogenic amines that serve as regulators of anterior pituitary hormones. These hypothalamic factors are supplied to the anterior pituitary gland by way of the portal venous system.

Table 27-9 shows the anterior pituitary hormones, their physiologic functions, and their hypothalamic regulatory hormones.

Table 27-10 describes the neuroendocrine complications, their clinical manifestations, standard fractionated radiation dose limits responsible for brain damage, diagnostic studies, and treatment.

Management

Growth Hormone Deficiency

If growth failure is due to documented growth hormone (GH) deficiency, then growth hormone is appropriate treatment. Growth failure can occur due to the systemic effects of cancer or cancer treatment and not necessarily due to GH deficiency, in which case GH should not be administered. The following are clinical considerations in the use of GH:

- It does not increase the incidence, but does worsen the degree of scoliosis.
- It may cause benign intracranial hypertension (pseudotumor cerebri), which resolves with medical management (i.e., acetazolamide and dexamethasone) and discontinuation of GH therapy.
- Children with prior neoplastic disease may develop a second cancer following GH therapy, but the incidence does not appear to be greater than expected.

GH treatment is useful for children with a history of previous cancer who have GH deficiency. They should be cancer free for 1–2 years following cessation of chemotherapy. Patients should understand the benefits of GH therapy in terms of

Table 27-9. Anterior Pituitary Hormones, Their Physiologic Functions, and Their Hypothalamic Regulatory Factors

Pituitary hormone	Functions of pituitary hormone	Hypothalamic regulatory factor
Growth hormone (GH)	Bone and soft-tissue growth through insulinlike growth hormones (ISF-1)	Growth-hormone-releasing hormones (GHRH) (+) Somatostatin (−)
Prolactin (PRL)	Induction of lactation and interruption of ovulation and menstruation during postpartum period	Dopamine (−)
Gonadotropins Luteinizing hormone (LH)	In males, LH stimulates Leydig cells to produce testosterone; in females, LH is responsible for normal steroidogenesis and ovulation	Gonadotropin-releasing hormone (GnRH) (+)
Follicle-stimulating hormone (FSH)	In males, FSH stimulates spermatogenesis; in females, FSH is responsible for normal steroidogenesis and ovulation	Gonadotropin-releasing hormone (GnRH) (+)
Thyroid-stimulating hormone (TSH)	TSH regulates thyroid hormone production for thyroid gland	Thyrotropin-releasing hormone (+)
Adrenocorticotropin (ACTH)	ACTH regulates adrenal steroidogenesis	Corticotropin-relasing Hormone (+)

Notes. (+), stimulating effect; (−), inhibitory effect.
From Sklar CA. Neuroendocrine complications of cancer therapy. In: Schwartz CL, Hobbie WL, Constine LS, Ruccione KS, editors. Survivors of childhood cancer: assessment and management. St. Louis: Mosby, 1994:97–110, with permission.

Table 27-10. Summary of Neuroendocrine Complications, Their Clinical Manifestations, Standard Fractionated Radiation Dose Limits to Brain Responsible for Damage, Diagnostic Studies, and Treatment

Disorder	Clinical presentation	Radiation dose (Gy)	Diagnostic studies	Treatment
GH deficiency	Short stature	≥18–20	Plotting growth on growth velocity chart; GH stimulation test; Bone age; Frequent sampling for 12–24 hours GH	Recombinant GH[a]
Gonadotropin deficiency	In young child, failure to enter puberty and primary amenorrhea; in adults, infertility, sexual dysfunction, and decreased libido	>30	Basal serum concentration of LH, FSH, estradiol, or testosterone; GnRH stimulation test	Estrogen/progestin (women); Depot testosterone (men)
Precocious puberty	Female 8 years of age or younger with appearance of breast and genital development and male 9 years of age or younger with testicular development; Accelerated skeletal growth and premature epiphyseal fusion	>10 (?)	GnRH stimulation test; Estradiol or testosterone concentration; Bone age; Pelvic ultrasound (women); GH stimulation tests	GnRH agonists plus recombinant GH (if GH deficient)
TSH deficiency	Often subclinical	>30	Basal serum T_3 uptake, T_4, and TSH; TRH stimulation test	L-Thyroxine
ACTH deficiency	Decreased stamina, lethargy, fasting hypoglycemia, dilutional hyponatremia	>30	Basal serum cortisol concentration; Adrenal stimulation test (e.g., insulin, ACTH)	Hydrocortisone

Abbreviations: GH, growth hormone; TSH, thyroid-stimulating hormone; ACTH, adrenocorticotropin; LH, luteinizing hormone; FSH, follicle-stimulating hormone; GnRH, gonadotropin-releasing hormone; TRH, thyrotropin-releasing hormone.

[a]See text discussion on use of growth hormone.

Modified from Sklar CA. Neuroendocrine complications of cancer therapy. In: Schwartz CL, Hobbis WL, Constine LS, Ruccione KS, editors. Survivors of Childhood Cancer: Assessment and Management. St. Louis: Mosby, 1994;97–110, with permission.

greater adult height versus the potential mitogenic risks, which have not been established.

Luteinizing and Follicle-Stimulating Hormone Deficiency

- Estrogen and progestin therapy in females
- Androgen therapy in males.

Precocious Puberty

- Gonadotropin-releasing hormone (GnRH) analogues to suppress puberty
- GnRH plus GH for patients with coexistent GH deficiency.

Thyroid-Stimulating Hormone Deficiency

- Daily thyroxine therapy.

Adrenocorticotropin Deficiency

- Low-dose hydrocortisone therapy daily
- Stress doses of hydrocortisone during febrile illness or under anesthesia.

Hyperprolactinemia

Bromocriptine or related dopamine agonists are used to reduce prolactin levels in young women with amenorrhea and infertility as a result of hyperprolactinemia.

Thyroid Deficiency

Hypothyroidism is the most common sequela following radiotherapy to the neck. Elevated thyroid-stimulating hormone (TSH) levels with normal T_3, T_4, indicative of subclinical hypothyroidism, is detected in up to two thirds of patients treated with mantle field (greater than 2600 cGy) in Hodgkin disease. However, in Hodgkin disease treated with low-dose radiotherapy, the incidence of hypothyroidism is 10–28%.

Patients with subclinical hypothyroidism (i.e., elevated levels of TSH with normal thyroxin level) are treated with thyroxine. Patients with a palpable thyroid abnormality should be evaluated with ultrasound and ^{99m}TC scanning. Ultrasound detects the location, number, and density of the nodules, and ^{99m}TC scan detects the functional status of the nodules. Detection of a nodule warrants biopsy. Papillary thyroid carcinoma is treated with total thyroidectomy, radioactive iodine, and TSH suppression with thyroxine.

Ovarian Dysfunction

Radiation

Elevated follicle-stimulating hormone (FSH) and luteinizing hormone (LH) values occur in 95% of patients receiving craniospinal plus abdominal radiation (RT) including ovaries.

Chemotherapy

Prepubertal ovaries are more resistant than postpubertal ovaries to damage by alkylating agents. Females treated between the ages of 3 and 17 years with 2.8–9.0 g/m² cyclophosphamide for Burkitt lymphoma have about a 1-year delay in menarche and 94% of these have unimpaired fertility. Females treated with MOPP for Hodgkin disease during their teens retain regular menses compared with females older than 30 years of age who have a high chance of developing amenorrhea after 5–6 cycles of MOPP.

Females treated for malignant germ cell tumors who have an intact ovary and uterus retain fertility. This applies only to patients treated with chemotherapy alone for germ cell tumors. Radiotherapy to the ovaries should be avoided.

Laboratory investigations of primary or secondary amenorrhea consist of:

- *Radioimaging studies:* bone age, ultrasound of ovaries
- *Blood tests:* T_3, T_4, TSH, dehydroepiandrosterone sulfate (DHEAS), testosterone, prolactin, FSH, LH, estradiol.

A complex hormonal regimen (estrogen, Premarin, gonadotropins, growth hormones) may be required to manage amenorrhea.

Pregnancy and Delivery

1. The rate of birth defects is the same as in the general population.
2. The rate of perinatal mortality is higher than in the general population.
3. There is a fourfold increase for low-birth-weight infants in women who received abdominal RT for the treatment of Wilms' tumor during their childhood. These women also are at risk for premature labor and fetal malposition.

Factors responsible for high-risk pregnancy and delivery after RT to the abdomen during childhood:

- Damage to elastic properties of the uterine musculature
- Damage to the vasculature of the uterus.

Testicular Dysfunction

The incidence of impaired fertility is higher in males than in females following cancer treatment. Spermatogenesis is affected more frequently than testosterone production by Leydig cells. Thus, male patients are at significant risk of infertility; however, progression through normal puberty and maintenance of male sexual phenotype are affected less often.

Prior to beginning therapy that could adversely impact fertility, sexually mature males should be informed and offered the option of preserving sperm prior to treatment. Table 27-11 shows the effects of fractionated testicular irradiation on spermatogenesis and Leydig cell function.

Cyclophosphamide

Total doses of 300–350 mg/kg cyclophosphamide cause sterility in adults, and in pubertal and prepubertal boys these doses cause oligospermia and azoospermia without effecting normal progression of puberty.

MOPP

In prepubertal and adult males, there is an 80–100% incidence of azoospermia after 5–6 cycles of MOPP. Twenty percent of these patients recover spermatogenesis 7 years after therapy. A 50% incidence of sterility occurs after 3 cycles of MOPP. Leydig cell damage due to the use of MOPP in boys (ages 11–16 years) results in gynecomastia, reduced testosterone level, and elevated levels of FSH and LH.

Table 27-11. Effect of Fractionated Testicular Irradiation on Spermatogenesis and Leydig Cell Function

Testicular dose in Gy (100 rad)	Effect on spermatogenesis	Effect on Leydig cell function
<0.1	No effect	No effect
0.1–0.3	Temporary oligospermia Complete recovery by 12 months	No effect
0.3–0.5	Temporary azoospermia at 4–12 months following irradiation 100% recovery by 48 months	
0.5–1.0	100% temporary azoospermia for 3–17 months from irradiation Recovery beginning at 8–26 months	Transient rise in FSH with eventual normalization
1–2	100% azoospermia from 2 months to at least 9 months Recovery beginning at 11–20 months with return of sperm counts at 30 months	Transient rise in FSH and LH No change in testosterone
2–3	100% azoospermia beginning at 1–2 months Some will suffer permanent azoospermia; others show recovery starting at 12–14 months Reduced testicular volume	Prolonged rise in FSH with some recovery Slight increase in LH No change in testosterone
3–4	100% azoospermia No recovery observed up to 40 months All have reduced testicular volume	Permanent elevation in FSH Transient rise in LH Reduced testosterone response to hCG stimulation
12	Permanent azoospermia Reduced testicular volume	Elevated FSH and LH Low testosterone Decreased or absent testosterone response to hCG stimulation Testosterone replacement may be needed to ensure pubertal changes
>24	Permanent azoospermia Reduced testicular volume	Effects more severe and profound than at 12 Gy Prepubertal testes appear more sensitive to the effects of radiation Replacement hormone treatment probably needed in all prepubertal cases

Notes. FSH, follicle-stimulating hormone; LH, luteinizing hormone; HCG, human chorionic gonadotropin.
From Leventhal BG, Halperin EC, Torano AE. The testes. In: Schwartz CL, Hobbie WL, Constine LS, Ruccione KS, editors. Survivors of Childhood Cancer: Assessment and Management. St. Louis: Mosby, 1994:225–44, with permission.

ABVD

Adult patients treated with ABVD develop azoospermia in 33% of cases. Recovery of spermatogenesis occurred in 67% of these patients. Abnormalities in Leydig cell function do not occur.

Retroperitoneal Lymph Node Dissection

Damage to the thoracolumbar sympathetic plexus during retroperitoneal lymph node dissection results in ejaculatory failure. Evidence of testicular damage can be determined clinically or by laboratory assessment.

Clinical Assessment

- Tanner score for the stages of development of secondary sexual characteristics
- Presence of gynecomastia.

Laboratory Assessment

- Spermatogenesis. If the patient is old enough, semen can be analyzed for sperm count, morphology, and motility
- Bone age
- Hormonal studies.

Table 27-12 presents an evaluation of the hypothalamic–pituitary axis using an analysis of pertinent hormonal assays.

GENITOURINARY SYSTEM

Ifosfamide, carboplatin, and cisplatin can cause renal complications, including acute tubular dysfunction manifested by increased excretion of potassium, phosphorus, and magnesium. Carboplatin is less nephrotoxic than cisplatin. Ifosfamide can cause hypophosphatemic rickets. Risk factors for ifosfamide nephrotoxicity include:

- Younger age group
- Hydronephrosis
- Prior administration of cisplatin
- Cumulative dose of ifosfamide greater than 72 g/m^2.

Indicators of significant Fanconi syndrome are serum glucose less than 150 mg/dL and a ratio of urine protein to urine creatinine of less than 0.2. Serum phosphate, <3.5 mg/dL; K$^+$, <3 mEq/L; bicarbonate, <17 mEq/L; and 1+ glycosuria.

Hemorrhagic cystitis and fibrosis of the bladder can occur often after treatment with cyclophosphamide and ifosfamide, especially when the bladder is included in the radiation field. Hypoplastic kidney and renal arteriosclerosis can occur after the use of a combination of radiation therapy in a dose of 10–15 Gy with chemotherapy

Table 27-12. Evaluation of Hypothalamic–Pituitary Axis

	Testosterone	FSH	LH	Response to GnRH	Response to hCG
Primary Leydig cell disease	nl/lo	hi	hi	—	lo
Primary disease of germinal epithelium	nl	hi	nl	—	—
Hypothalamic disease	nl/lo	nl/lo	nl/lo	nl	—
Pituitary disease	nl/lo	nl/lo	nl/lo	lo	—

Abbreviations: nl, normal; lo, low; hi, high; GnRH, gonadotropin-releasing hormone, hCG, human chorionic gonadotropin.

From Leventhal BG, Halperin EC, Torano AE. The testes. In: Schwartz CL, Hobbie WL, Constine LS, Ruccione KS, editors. Survivors of Childhood Cancer: Assessment and Management. St. Louis: Mosby, 1994; 225–44, with permission.

or radiation therapy alone in a dose of 20–30 Gy. Nephrotic syndrome can occur after radiation therapy in a dose of 20–30 Gy of RT.

Abnormal bladder function is seen in children with pelvic rhabdomyosarcoma in whom radiation has been used. Twenty-seven to 100% of these children experience dribbling and nocturnal enuresis.

Adenovirus is a well-known cause of hemorrhagic cystitis. This infection compounded with high doses of cyclophosphamide can cause significant morbidity.

OCULAR COMPLICATIONS

- *Lacrimal glands:* decreased tearing or fibrosis following radiation therapy (RT) of more than 50 Gy
- *Cornea:* ulceration, neovascularization, keratinization, edema following RT of more than 40–50 Gy
- *Lens:* cataract following steroids or RT of more than 10–15 Gy
- *Iris:* neovascularization, glaucoma, atrophy following RT of more than 50 Gy
- *Retina:* infarction, exudates, hemorrhage, telangiectasia, neovascularization, macular edema following RT of more than 50 Gy
- *Optic nerve:* optic neuropathy following RT of more than 50 Gy.

AUDITORY COMPLICATIONS

- Chronic otitis following RT of more than 40–50 Gy.
- Sensorineural hearing loss following cisplatin and/or RT of more than 40–50 Gy.
- Amifostine has been shown to not protect hearing loss associated with cisplatin therapy.
- Aminoglycoside therapy can also contribute to hearing loss.

GASTROINTESTINAL SYSTEM

- *Enteritis:* Occurs following the use of RT greater than 40 Gy. Actinomycin D or doxorubicin enhances RT effect.
- *Fibrosis:* Occurs anywhere from esophagus to colon following the use of RT greater than 40–50 Gy.
- *Hepatitic fibrosis/cirrhosis:* Occurs following the use of chemotherapy agents, such as methotrexate, actinomycin D, 6-mercaptopurine (6-MP), and 6-thioguanine (6-TG) and/or RT greater than 40-Gy dose.

Patients treated with blood transfusion prior to adequate blood donor screening for hepatitis C are at risk for chronic liver disease secondary to hepatitis C.

Recent studies using 6-TG in ALL have shown an increased risk of veno-occlusive disease of the liver associated with the use of 6-TG.

Guidelines for Modification of Chemotherapeutic Agents That Produce Liver Toxicity

6-Mercaptopurine and 6-Thioguanine

Discontinue the drugs if liver enzymes are 5.0–20.0 times the normal values and/or bilirubin is 1.5–3 times the normal value, or if the drugs are the cause of liver function abnormalities (exclude viral hepatitis, Gilbert disease, or tumor effect).

Restart at 50% dose, when liver enzyme values decrease to 2.5–5.0 times normal values and bilirubin is less than 1.5 times the normal value. If toxicity persists, a liver biopsy should be performed to determine the histologic findings to assess the extent of liver damage.

Methotrexate

Methotrexate can cause fibrosis and cirrhosis. Follow the same guidelines as above for management of liver toxicity.

IMMUNOLOGIC SYSTEM

In children with continuous complete remission of ALL, defects in both normal and cellular immunity resolve within 6 months to 1 year after cessation of chemotherapy. However, the intensity of chemotherapy for ALL may determine the degree and duration of immune deficiency. Evaluation of children treated with the BFM-ALL protocol at our institution revealed that in some patients immune deficiency persisted for more than 2 years after completion of therapy. More than half of the children had no protective antibodies to one or more previously administered vaccines or related infections. Although most of them were able to produce antibodies after reimmunization, some patients repeatedly were unable to make protective antibodies after reimmunization or despite natural disease.

Additional studies of larger numbers of long-term cancer survivors are necessary to determine the incidence, duration, and severity of immune defects.

OBESITY

Adult survivors of childhood ALL have been found to be at a marked increased risk for obesity. They are at 2–3 times the risk for obesity relative to sibling controls (the odds ratio was 2.59 for females and 1.86 for males). Adult leukemia survivors were found to be more physically inactive and to have reduced exercise capacity, which further increased their risk for obesity.

Interventions to prevent obesity and promote physical activity should decrease cardiovascular morbidity and improve the quality of life in this population. Follow-up with assessment of weight and physical activity is important in the evaluation of childhood cancer survivors.

SECOND MALIGNANT NEOPLASMS

The incidence of secondary neoplasms is 3–12% within the first 20 years from diagnosis. Childhood cancer survivors have 10–20 times the lifetime risk of second malignant neoplasms compared to age-matched controls. Second malignant neoplasms are the most common cause of death in longtime survivors after recurrence of the primary cancer.

Patients with retinoblastoma, Hodgkin disease, and Ewing sarcoma are at the greatest risk for developing second malignant neoplasms. An estimated 10% of children with ALL have a defect in the drug metabolizing enzyme (thiopurine methyl transferase), which places them at increased risk for the development of a second cancer. Long-term survivors who have an underlying inherited susceptibility to cancer have a second malignant neoplasm rate that approaches 50%. Neurofibromatosis also increases the risk of additional neoplasms. Li–Fraumeni syndrome can be associated with breast cancer and sarcomas at an early age. Because hepatoblastoma has been associated with familial polyposis, children with hepatoblastoma should be examined for the polyposis gene and then screened for colon cancer if needed.

Table 27-13 lists the second malignant neoplasms, their predisposing factors, signs and symptoms, and recommendations for follow-up.

Leukemia Secondary to Alkylating Agents

- Most commonly acute AML; usually preceded by a myelodysplastic phase
- Correlation with total dose of alkylating agents
- Cytogenetic abnormalities: aberrations in the long arm of chromosome 5, 7, or both
- Latency period: 3.5–5.5 years
- Cumulative risk: 1% at 20 years.

Acute Myelocytic Leukemia Secondary to MOPP Treatment

- Risk increases with increase in the number of courses.
- Risk increases with splenectomy.
- Radiotherapy does not add to the leukemia risk from chemotherapy.

Acute Promyelocytic Leukemia Secondary to Chemotherapy in Hodgkin Disease

This has a relatively good prognosis, similar to *de novo* acute promyelocytic leukemia.

Leukemias Associated with Epipodophyllotoxins

- Type of leukemia: monoblastic
- Correlation with dose and schedule
- Cytogenetic abnormalities: aberrations involving chromosomes 11q23 and 21q22
- Latency period: 2–6 years
- Cumulative risk: 3.8–44%, depending on intensity of dose and schedule.

Intercalating topoisomerase II inhibitors (such as doxorubicin and dactinomycin), when combined with alkylating agents, may also cause secondary acute myelocytic leukemia (AML).

The prognosis for patients with secondary acute leukemia is poor. Very few long-term survivors have been reported. Allogeneic hematopoietic stem cell transplantation is the treatment of choice. Radiotherapy does not contribute significantly to the development of secondary leukemias. At St. Jude Children's Research Hospital, Memphis, TN, analysis of a study of subsequent malignancies in children and adolescents after treatment for Hodgkin disease revealed the estimated cumulative risk of second malignancies was 1.5% at 5 years and 7.7% at 15 years. Patients 10 years of age or older at initial diagnosis appeared to be at greater risk for developing second malignant neoplasms. Also, adolescent females treated for recurrent Hodgkin disease appeared to be at greater risk for second malignant neoplasms.

Second Solid Tumors

The most common second solid tumor type is bone sarcoma. The median time to the development of a second malignant neoplasm is 7 years (range 1 year 11 months to 15 years 9 months). The 10-year cumulative incidence is 1.7%. Genetic abnormalities such as neurofibromatosis or family histories suggestive of Li–Fraumeni

Table 27-13. Predisposing Factors, Signs and Symptoms, and Follow-Up in Second Malignant Neoplasms

Second malignant neoplasm	Predisposing factor	Other	Signs and symptoms	Recommended follow-up
Bone or soft-tissue sarcomas	Radiotherapy (RT)	Doses >3000 cGy; adolescents	Pain or mass in irradiated area	Radiograph, other imaging, baseline every 5 years or if symptoms arise
	Ratinoblastoma	Familial and bilateral cases		
	Li-Fraumeni syndrome	Family history may be revealing; constitutional p53 mutation (?)		
	Neurofibromatosis (NF)	Diagnosis based on clinical findings; influence of RT not established		
Pineoblastoma	Retinoblastoma	Bilateral and familial cases		
Brain tumor	RT	Younger children at greater risk	Change in sleep pattern Seizures, headaches, altered mental status	Neuroimaging baseline, then if symptoms
	NF			
	Nevoid basal cell carcinoma syndrome	Ionizing RT increases risk and shortens latiant period		
Thyroid	RT	Younger children at greater risk	Enlarged thyroid, nodules	Ultrasound, baseline, then if symptoms, ^{131}I scan
Breast	RT	Preadolescent females; interaction with family history (?)	Breast mass	Mammography at age 25, every 2 years to age 40, then every year; biopsy pm mass
Skin	RT	Ionizing RT increases risk and shortens latent period	New lesion or change in skin color or texture	Biopsy
	Nevoid basal cell carcinoma syndrome Xeroderma pigmentosa	Risk associated with ultraviolet light		
Leukemia	Alkylating agents	Dose response, melphalan>nitrogen mustard>cyclophosphamide; associated with chromosome 5 and 7 abnormalities	Pallor, bruising, fatigue, petechiae	Complete blood count annually
	Epipodophyllotoxins	Associated with 11q23 abnormality; schedule or dose dependent (?)		
	NF	Juvenile chronic myslogenous leukemia (JCML) most common; xanthomas; may develop monosomy 7		Bone marrow evaluation for symptoms

From Meadows AT, Fenton JG. Follow up care of patients at risk for the development of second malignant neoplasms. In: Schwartz CI, Hobble WL, Constine LS, Ruccione HS, editors. Survivors of Childhood Cancer: Assessment and Management. St. Louis: Mosby, 1994, 3 19–28, with permission.

syndrome appear to predispose these patients to the development of second solid neoplasms.

In a study of the role of radiation and genetic factors in the development of second neoplasms after a first cancer in childhood, it was found that both genetic factors (p53 mutation and neurofibromatosis) and exposure to radiation have independent effects on the risk of development of second primary neoplasms.

Analysis of second malignant neoplasms occurring in survivors of osteosarcoma at St. Jude Children's Research Hospital showed that the overall 10-year cumulative incidence of second malignancies was 2±1% for localized osteosarcoma and 8±5% for those who presented with metastatic disease at initial diagnosis of osteosarcoma. The study concluded that, with the increased success of chemotherapy, more patients with osteosarcoma are surviving and, therefore, the number of patients with osteosarcoma who develop second malignant neoplasms is also expected to increase. A review of late mortality in long-term survivors of childhood cancer from St. Jude Children's Research Hospital reported the following results. The study included 2053 patients who survived 5 years or longer. They were grouped by treatment eras that reflected increased intensity of therapy and significantly improved survival, namely: early era, 1962–1970; recent era, 1971–1983. There were 258 deaths in 2053 cancer survivors; 169 occurred 5–10 years postdiagnosis and 89 occurred 10 years postdiagnosis. Deaths were attributed to the recurrence of malignancies in 61% of cases, second malignancies in 20%, nonneoplastic complications in 5%, and unintentional injury/suicide in 8%. Comparison of the two eras showed that late death from recurrent disease decreased significantly for survivors treated in the recent era, whereas the risk of death from second malignancies increased, although not statistically significantly.

The National Wilms' Tumor Study (NWTS) reported 43 second malignant neoplasms following treatment of Wilms' tumor in 5278 patients. The various types of second tumors included hematologic malignancies, various bone and/or soft-tissue sarcomas, hepatocellular carcinoma, and other carcinomas. It was concluded that abdominal irradiation (35 Gy) received as part of the initial therapy increased the risk of a second malignant neoplasm. The radiation effect was potentiated by doxorubicin. Treatment of relapses further increased the risk for second malignant neoplasm by a factor of 4 or 5.

Women who were treated with mantle irradiation for childhood Hodgkin disease face a significant increased risk for the development of breast cancer with a cumulative incidence of about 35% at 20–25 years post-therapy. Onset of breast cancer has been noted as early as 8 years postradiation with a median age at diagnosis of 31.5 years and a median interval from radiation of 15.7 years.

There is an increased risk of basal cell carcinomas and squamous cell carcinoma in young children with Hodgkin disease, non-Hodgkin lymphoma, soft-tissue sarcomas, and Wilms' tumor who were treated with radiation therapy.

In general, it appears that both genetic susceptibility and exposure to cytotoxic therapy, especially alkylating agents, topoisomerase inhibitors, and radiotherapy, play important roles in the development of second malignant neoplasms in childhood.

SUGGESTED READINGS

Beaty O, Hudson MM, Greenwald C, Luo X, Fang L, Wilmas JA, Thompson EI, Kun LE, Pratt CB. Subsequent malignancies in children and adolescents after treatment for Hodgkin's disease. J Clin Oncol 1995;13:603–9.

Bhatia S. Late effects among survivors of leukemia during childhood and adolescence. Blood Cells Mol Dis 2003;31:84–92.

Breslow NE, Takashina JR, Whitton JA, D'Angio GJ, Green DM. Second malignant neoplasms following treatment of Wilms' tumor: a report from the National Wilms' Tumor Study Group. J Clin Oncol 1995;13:1851–9.

Dreyer ZE, Blatt J, Bleyer A. Late effects of childhood cancer and its treatment. In: Pizzo PA, Poplack DG, editors. Principles and Practice of Pediatric Oncology. 4th ed. Philadelphia: Lippincott, Williams and Wilkins, 2002.

Friedman DL, Meadows AT. Late effects of childhood cancer therapy. Pediatr Clin North Am 2002;49:1063–81.

Hewitt M, Weiner SL, Simone JV, editors. Childhood Cancer Survivorship Improving Care and Quality of Life. Washington, DC: National Academic Press, 2003.

Heym R, Hoeberlen V, Newton WA, Ragab AH, Raney RB, Teft M, Wharam M, Ensign LG, Mauera H. Second malignant neoplasm in children treated for rhabdomyosarcoma. J Clin Oncol 1993;11:262–70.

Hudson MH, Jones D, Boyelt J, Sharp GB, Pui CH. Late mortality of long term survivors of childhood cancer. J Clin Oncol 1997;15:2205–13.

Hudson MH, Mertens AC, Yasui Y, Hobbie W, Chen H, Gurney JG, Yeazel M, Rechlites CJ, Marina N, Robinson LR, Oeffinger KC. Health status of adult long term survivors of childhood cancer. A report from the Childhood Cancer Survivor Study. JAMA 2003;290:1583–92.

Iacuone JL, Steinherz L, Oblender MG, Bernard DR, Ablin AR. Modifications for toxicity. In: Ablin AR, editor. Supportive Care of Children with Cancer: Current Therapy and Guidelines from the Children's Cancer Group. 2nd ed. Baltimore: Johns Hopkins University Press, 1997.

Kong SJ, de Vathaire F, Chompret A, Shumsaldim A, Grimaud E, Raguin MA, Oberlin O, Borugleres L, Feunteun Eschwege J, Lemerle J, Bonaiti-Peuie C. Radiation and genetic factors in the risk of second malignant neoplasms after a first cancer in childhood. Lancet 1997;350:91–5.

Lipshultz SE, Colon SD. Cardiovascular trials in long term survivors of childhood cancer. J Clin Oncol 2004;22:769–73.

Moshang T. Use of growth hormone in children surviving cancer. Med Pediatr Oncol 1998;31:170–2.

Pratt CB, Meyer WH, Luo X, Cain AM, Kaste SC, Pappo AS, Rao BN, Flemming ID, Jenkins JJ. Second malignant neoplasms occurring in survivors of osteosarcoma. Cancer 1997;80:960–5.

Pui CH, Cheng C, Leung W, Rai SN, Rivera GK, Sandlund JJ, Ribiero RC, Rolling MV, Kien LE, Evans WE, Hudson MH. Extended follow-up of long term survivors of childhood acute lymphoblastic leukemia. N Engl J Med 2003;349(7):640–9.

Robinson LL, Bhatia S. Late effects among survivors of leukemia and lymphoma during childhood and adolescence. Br J Haematol 2003;122:345–59.

Ross L, Johansen C, Dalton SO, Mellemkjaer L, Thomassen LH, Martensen PB, Olsen JH. Psychiatric hospitalization among survivors of cancer in childhood and adolescence. N Engl J Med 2003;349(7):650–7.

Sandoval C, Pui CH, Bowman LC, Heaton D, Hurwitz C, Raimondi SL, Behm FG, Head DR. Secondary acute myeloid leukemia in children previously treated with alkylating agents, intercalating topoisomerase II inhibitors and irradiation. J Clin Oncol 1993;11:1039–45.

Schwartz CL, Hobbie WL, Constine LS, Ruccione KS. Survivors of Childhood Cancer: Assessment and Management. St. Louis: Mosby, 1994.

Smith S, Schiffman G, Karayalcin G, Bonagura V. Immune deficiency in long-term survivors of acute lymphoblastic leukemia treated with Berlin–Frankfurt–Munster therapy. J Pediatr 1995;127:68–75.

Walter AW, Hancock ML, Pui CH, Hudson MM, Ochs JS, Rivera GK, Pratt CB, Bayett JM, Kuh LE. Secondary brain tumors in children treated for acute lymphoblastic leukemia at St. Jude Children's Research Hospital. J Clin Oncol 1998;16:3761.

APPENDIX 1

HEMATOLOGIC REFERENCE VALUES

The normal range for most hematologic parameters in infancy and childhood is different from that in adults. Dramatic changes occur during the first few weeks of life. The recognition of variables in the pediatric age group prevents unnecessary medical and laboratory investigations.

RED CELL VALUES AND RELATED SERUM VALUES

Table A1-1. Hemoglobin Concentrations (g/dL) for Iron-Sufficient Preterm Infants[a]

Age	Number	Birth weight (g)	
		1000–1500	1501–2000
2 weeks	17, 39	16.3 (11.7–18.4)	14.8 (11.8–19.6)
1 month	15, 42	10.9 (8.7–15.2)	11.5 (8.2–15.0)
2 months	17, 47	8.8 (7.1–11.5)	9.4 (8.0–11.4)
3 months	16, 41	9.8 (8.9–11.2)	10.2 (9.3–11.8)
4 months	13, 37	11.3 (9.1–13.1)	11.3 (9.1–13.1)
5 months	8, 21	11.6 (10.2–14.3)	11.8 (10.4–13.0)
6 months	9, 21	12.0 (9.4–13.8)	11.8 (10.7–12.6)

[a]These infants were admitted to the Helsinki Children's Hospital during a 15-month period. None had a complicated course during the first 2 weeks of life or had undergone an exchange transfusion. All infants were iron sufficient, as indicated by a serum ferritin greater than 10 ng/mL.

From Lundstrom U, Siimes MA, Dallman PR. At what age does iron supplementation become necessary in low-birth-weight infants J Pediatr 1997;91:878, with permission.

Table A1-2. Red Cell Values on First Postnatal Day

	Gestational age (weeks)							
	24-25 (7)[a]	26-27 (11)	28-29 (7)	30-31 (25)	32-33 (23)	34-35 (23)	36-37 (20)	Term (19)
RBC × 10^6	4.65[b]	4.73 ± 0.45	4.62 ± 0.75	4.79 ± 0.74	5.0 ± 0.76	5.09 ± 0.5	5.27 ± 0.68	5.14 ± 0.7
Hb (g/dL)	19.4 ± 1.5	19.0 ± 2.5	19.3 ± 1.8	19.1 ± 2.2	18.5 ± 2.0	19.6 ± 2.1	19.2 ± 1.7	19.3 ± 2.2
Hematocrit (%)	63 ± 4	62 ± 8	60 ± 7	60 ± 8	60 ± 8	61 ± 7	64 ± 7	61 ± 7.4
MCV (L)	135 ± 0.2	132 ± 14.4	131 ± 13.5	127 ± 12.7	123 ± 15.7	122 ± 10.0	121 ± 12.5	119 ± 9.4
Reticulocytes (%)	6.0 ± 0.5	9.6 ± 3.2	7.5 ± 2.5	5.8 ± 2.0	5.0 ± 1.9	3.9 ± 1.6	4.2 ± 1.8	3.2 ± 1.4
Weight (g)	725 ± 185	993 ± 194	1174 ± 128	1450 ± 232	1816 ± 192	1957 ± 291	2245 ± 213	

[a]Number of infants.
[b]Mean values ± SD.
From Zaizov R, Matoth Y. Red cell values on the first postnatal day during the last 16 weeks of gestation. Am J Hematol 1976;1:276, with permission.

Table A1-3. Mean Hematologic Values in the First 2 Weeks of Life in the Term Infant

Hematologic value	Cord blood	Day 1	Day 3	Day 7	Day 14
Hb (g/dL)	16.8	18.4	17.8	17.0	16.8
Hematocrit	0.53	0.58	0.55	0.54	0.52
Red cells (×10^{12}/L)	5.25	5.8	5.6	5.2	5.1
MCV (fL)	107	108	99.0	98.0	96.0
MCH (pg)	34	35	33	32.5	31.5
MCHC (%)	31.7	32.5	33	33	33
Reticulocytes (%)	3-7	3-7	1-3	0-1	0-1
Nucleated RBC (mm^3)	500	200	0-5	0	0
Platelets (×10^9/L)	290	192	213	248	252

From Oski FA, Naiman JL. Hematologic Problems in the Newborn. 3rd ed. Philadelphia: Saunders, 1982, with permission.

Table A1-4. Red Cell Values at Various Ages: Mean and Lower Limit of Normal (–2 SD)[a]

Age	Hemoglobin (g/dL)		Hematocrit (%)		Red cell count (10¹²/L)		MCV (fl)		MCH (pg)		MCHC (g/dL)		Reticulocytes	
	Mean	–2 SD	Mean	–2 SD	Mean	–2 SD	Mean	–2 SD	Mean	–2 SD	Mean	–2 SD	Mean	–2 SD
Birth (cord blood)	16.5	13.5	51	42	4.7	3.9	108	98	34	31	33	30	3.2	1.8
1–3 days (capillary)	18.5	14.5	56	45	5.3	4.0	108	95	34	31	33	29	3.0	1.5
1 week	17.5	13.5	54	42	5.1	3.9	107	88	34	28	33	28	0.5	0.1
2 weeks	16.5	12.5	51	39	4.9	3.6	105	86	34	28	33	28	0.5	0.2
1 month	14.0	10.0	43	31	4.2	3.0	104	85	34	28	33	29	0.8	0.4
2 months	11.5	9.0	35	28	3.8	2.7	96	77	30	26	33	29	1.6	0.9
3–6 months	11.5	9.5	35	29	3.8	3.1	91	74	30	25	33	30	0.7	0.4
0.5–2 years	12.0	10.5	36	33	4.5	3.7	78	70	27	23	33	30	1.0	0.2
2–6 years	12.5	11.5	37	34	4.6	3.9	81	75	27	24	34	31	1.0	0.2
6–12 years	13.5	11.5	40	35	4.6	4.0	86	77	29	25	34	31	1.0	0.2
12–18 years														
Female	14.0	12.0	41	36	4.6	4.1	90	78	30	25	34	31	1.0	0.2
Male	14.5	13.0	43	37	4.9	4.5	88	78	30	25	34	31	1.0	0.2
18–49 years														
Female	14.0	12.0	41	36	4.6	4.0	90	80	30	26	34	31	1.0	0.2
Male	15.5	13.5	47	41	5.2	4.5	90	80	30	26	34	31	1.0	0.2

[a]These data have been compiled from several sources. Emphasis is given to recent studies employing electronic counters and to the selection of populations that are likely to exclude individuals with iron deficiency. The mean ±2 SD can be expected to include 95% of the observations in a normal population.

From Dallman PR. Blood and blood-forming tissue. In: Rudolph A, editor. Pediatrics. 16th ed. E. Norwalk, CT: Appleton-Century-Crofts, 1977, with permission.

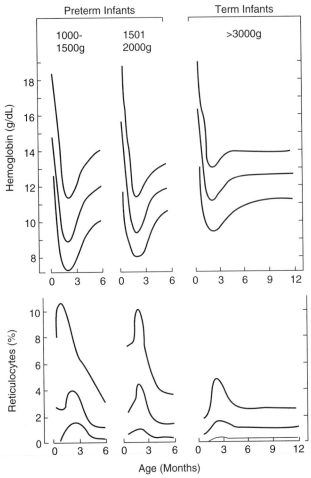

Fig. A1-1. Physiologic nadir for term and preterm infants. The mean and range of normal hemoglobin and reticulocyte values for term and preterm infants are shown. Premature infants reach nadir of erythrocyte production sooner and require longer to recover than their term infant counterparts. (From Dallman PR: Anemia of prematurity. Ann Rev Med 1981; 32:143, reproduced with permission.)

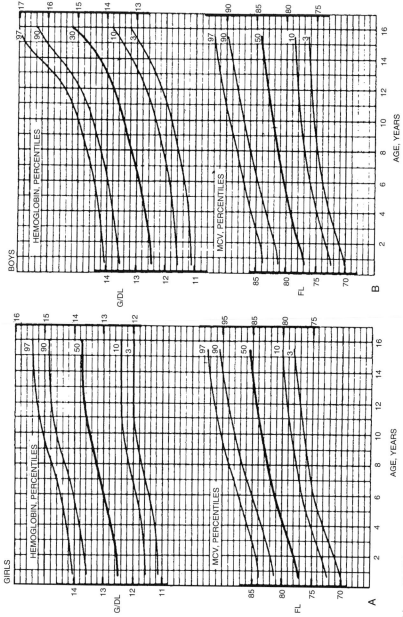

Fig. A1-2. (A) Hemoglobin and MCV percentile curves for girls. (B) Hemoglobin and MCV percentile curves for boys. (From Dallman PR, Siimes MA. Percentile curves for hemoglobin and red cell volume in infancy and childhood. J Pediatr 1979;94:28, with permission.)

Table A1-5. Serum Ferritin Values

Age	ng/ml
Newborn	25–200
1 month	200–600
2–5 months	50–200
6 months–15 years	7–140
Adult:	
Male	15–200
Female	12–150

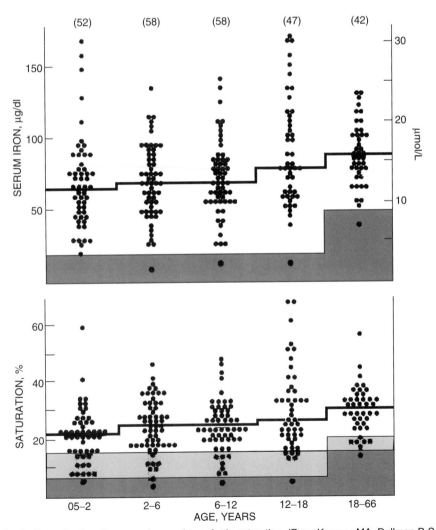

Fig. A1-3. Normal values for serum iron and transferrin saturation. (From Koerper MA, Dallman P. Serum iron concentration and transferrin saturation in the diagnosis of iron deficiency in children: normal developmental changes. J Pediatr 1977;91:870, with permission.)

Table A1-6. Values of Serum Iron (SI), Total Iron-Binding Capacity (TIBC), and Transferrin Saturation (S%) from Infants during the First Year of Life

		Age (months)						
		0.5	1	2	4	6	9	12
SI								
Median	μmol/L	22	22	16	15	14	15	14
95% range		11–36	10–31	3–29	3–29	5–24	6–24	6–28
	μg/dL	120	125	87	84	77	84	78
		63–201	58–172	15–159	18–164	28–135	34–135	35–155
TIBC (mean ± SD)	μmol/L	34 ± 8	36 ± 8	44 ± 10	54 ± 7	58 ± 9	61 ± 7	64 ± 7
	μg/dL	191 ± 43	199 ± 43	246 ± 55	300 ± 39	321 ± 51	341 ± 42	358 ± 38
S%								
Median		68	63	34	27	23	25	23
96% range		30–99	35–94	21–63	7–53	10–43	10–39	10–47

Notes: These data were obtained from a group of heathly, full-term infants who were born at the Helsinki University Central Hospital. Infants received iron supplementation in formula and cereal throughout the 12-month period. Infants with hemoglobin below 10 g/dL, mean corpuscular volume of red blood cells below 71 fL, or serum ferritin below 10 ng/mL were excluded from the study. The 95% range of the transferrin saturation values indicates that the lower limit of normal is about 10% after 4 months of age.

From Saarinen UM, Siimes MA. Serum iron and transferrin in iron deficiency. J Pediatr 1977;91:876, with permission.

Table A1-7. Mean Serum Iron and Iron Saturation Percentage

Age (years)	Serum iron (μg/dL)	Saturation (%)
0.5–2	68 ± 3.6 (16–120)	22 ± 1.1 (6–38)
2–6	72 ± 3.4 (20–124)	25 ± 1.2 (7–43)
6–12	73 ± 3.4 (23–123)	25 ± 1.2 (7–43)
18+	92 ± 3.8 (48–136)	30 ± 1.1 (18–46)

From Koerper MA, Dallman PR. Serum iron concentration and transferrin saturation are lower in normal children than in adults. J Pediatr Res 1977;11:473, with permission.

Table A1-8. Normal Serum Folic Acid Levels (ng/ml)

Folate	Age	Range	Mean±SD
	Normal premature infants		
Serum folate	1–4 days	7.17–52.00	29.54 ± 0.98
	2–3 weeks	4.12–15.62	8.61 ± 0.55
	1–2 months	2.81–11.25	5.84 ± 0.35
	2–3 months	3.56–11.82	6.95 ± 0.50
	3–5 months	3.85–16.50	8.92 ± 0.86
	5–7 months	6.00–12.25	9.02 ± 0.74
	Normal children		
	1 year	3.0–35	9.3
	1–6 years	4.12–21.15	11.37 ± 0.82
	1–10 years	6.5–16.5	10.3
	Normal adults		
	20–45 years	4.50–28.00	10.29 ± 1.14
Red cell folate	Infants <1 year	74–995	277
	Children 1–11 years	96–364	215
	Adults	160–640	316
Whole blood folate	Infants <1 year	20–160	87
	Infants 1 year	31–400	86
	Infants 2–24 months	34–160	96
	Children 1–11 years	52–164	97
	Adults	50–400	195

From Shojania A, Gross S. Folic acid deficiency and prematurity. J Pediatr 1964;64:323, with permission.

Table A1-9. Percentage of Hemoglobin F in the First Year of Life[a]

Age	Number tested	Mean	2 SD	Range
1–7 days	10	74.7	5.4	61–79.6
2 weeks	13	74.9	5.7	66–88.5
1 month	11	60.2	6.3	45.7–67.3
2 months	10	45.6	10.1	29.4–60.8
3 months	10	26.6	14.5	14.8–55.9
4 months	10	17.7	6.1	9.4–28.5
5 months	10	10.4	6.7	2.3–22.4
6 months	15	6.5	3.0	2.7–13.0
8 months	11	5.1	3.6	2.3–11.9
10 months	10	2.1	0.7	1.5–3.5
12 months	10	2.6	1.5	1.3–5.0
1–14 years and adults	100	0.6	0.4	—

[a]HbF measured by alkali denaturation.

Data from Schröter W, Nafz C. Diagnostic significance of hemoglobin F and A2 levels in homo- and heterozygous beta-thalassemia during infancy. Helv Paediatr Acta 1981;36:519.

Table A1-10. Percentage of Hemoglobin F and A_2 in Newborn and Adult

	Hemoglobin F (%)	Hemoglobin A_2 (%)
Newborn	60–90	<1.0
Adult	<1.0	1.6–3.5

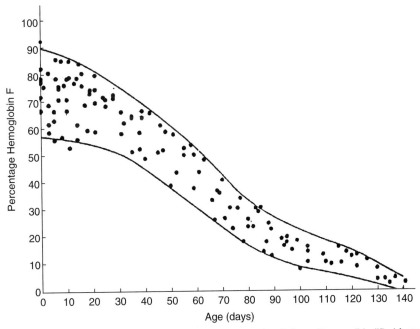

Fig. A1-4. Relative concentration of hemoglobin F in infants and variation with age. (Modified from Garby L, Sjolin S, Vuille JC. Studies on erythro-kinetics in infancy. II The relative rate of synthesis of haemoglobin F and haemoglobin A during the first months of life. Acta Paediatr 1962;51:245, with permission.)

Table A1-11. Estimated Blood Volumes

Age	Plasma volume (PV) (ml/kg)	Red cell mass (RCM) (ml/kg)	Total blood volume (ml/kg) (From PV)	(From RCM)
Newborn	43.6	43.1	80.0	85.4
1–7 days	51–54	37.9	82–86	77.8
1–12 months	46.1	25.5	78.1	72.8
1–3 years	45.8	24.9	77.8	69.1
4–6 years	49.0	25.5	82.8	67.5
7–9 years	50.6	24.3	86.8	67.5
10–12 years	49.0	26.3	85.4	67.4
13–15 years	51.2		88.3	
16–18 years	50.1		90.2	
Adult	39–44	25–30	68–88	55–75

Modified from Price DC, Ries C: In Handmaker H, Lowenstein JM (eds): Nuclear Medicine in Clinical Pediatrics. New York, Society of Nuclear Medicine, 1975, p 279.

Table A1-12. Methemoglobin Levels in Normal Children[a]

	Number of cases	Number of determinations	Methemoglobin (g/dL)			Number of cases	Number of determinations	Methemoglobin as percentage of total hemoglobin		
			Mean	Range	SD			Mean	Range	SD
Prematures (birth–7 days)	29	34	0.43	(0.02–0.83)	±0.07	24	28	2.3	(0.08–4.4)	±1.26
Prematures (7–72 days)	21	29	0.31	(0.02–0.78)	±0.19	18	23	2.2	(0.02–4.7)	±1.07
Prematures (total)	50	63	0.38	(0.02–0.83)	±0.10	42	51	2.2	(0.08–4.7)	±1.10
Cook County Hospital prematures (1–14 days)	8	8	0.52	(0.18–0.83)	±0.08	—	—	—	—	—
Newborns (1–10 days)	39	39	0.22	(0.00–0.58)	±0.17	25	30	1.5	(0.00–2.8)	±0.81
Infants (1 month–1 year)	8	8	0.14	(0.02–0.29)	±0.09	8	8	1.2	(0.17–2.4)	±0.78
Children (1–14 years)	35	35	0.11	(0.00–0.33)	±0.09	35	35	0.79	(0.00–2.4)	±0.62
Adults (14–78 years)	30	30	0.11	(0.00–0.28)	±0.09	27	27	0.82	(0.00–1.9)	±0.63

[a]The premature and full-term infants were free of known disease. None had respiratory distress or cyanosis. Analysis of milk and water ingested by these infants revealed the nitrate level to be less than 0.027 ppm. The premature infants routinely received vitamin C orally each day from the seventh day of life.

From Kravitz H, Elegant LD, et al. Methemoglobin values in premature and mature infants and children. Am J Dis Child 1956;91:2, with permission.

Table A1-13. Serum Erythropoietin Levels

RIA method	<5–20 mU/mL
Hemagglutination method	25–125
Bioassay method	5–18

Table A1-14. Comparison of Enzyme Activities and Glutathione Content in Newborn and Adult Red Blood Cells

Enzyme	Activity in normal adult RBC in IU/g Hb (mean±1 SD at 37°C)	Mean activity in newborn RBC as percentage of mean (100%) activity in normal adult RBC
Aldolase	3.19 ± 0.86	140
Enolase	5.39 ± 0.83	250
Glucose phosphate isomerase	60.8 ± 11.0	162
Glucose-6-phosphate dehydrogenase	8.34 ± 1.59	
WHO method	12.1 ± 2.09	174
Glutathione peroxidase	30.82 ± 4.65	56
Glyceraldehyde phosphate dehydrogenase	226 ± 41.9	170
Hexokinase	1.78 ± 0.38	239
Lactate dehydrogenase	200 ± 26.5	132
NADH-methemoglobin reductase	19.2 ± 3.85 (at 30 ~C)	Increased
Phosphofructokinase	11.01 ± 2.33	97
Phosphoglycerate kinase	320 ± 36.1	165
Pyruvate kinase	15.0 ± 1.99	160
6-Phosphogluconate dehydrogenase	8.78 ± 0.78	150
Triose phosphate isomerase	211 ± 397	101
Glutathione	6570 ± 1040 nmol/g Hb	156

Note: The percentage activity in newborn RBC compared to mean adult (100%) values is presented with quantitative data from studies on adult RBC. Newborn data from Konrad et al., 1972; quantitative data from Beutler, 1984.

From Hinchliffe RF, Lilleyman JS, editors. Practical Paediatric Haematology: A Laboratory Worker's Guide to Blood Disorders in Children. New York: Wiley, 1987, with permission.

Table A1-16. Polymorphonuclear Leukocyte and Band Counts in the Newborn during the First 2 Days of Life[a]

Age	Absolute neutrophil count (mm³)	Absolute band count (mm³)	B/N ratio
0	3,500–6,000	1300	0.14
12	8,000–15,000	1300	0.14
24	7,000–13,000	1300	0.14
36	5,000–9,000	700	0.11
48	3,500–5,200	700	0.11

[a]Normal values were obtained from the assessment of 3100 separate white blood cell counts obtained from 965 infants; 513 counts were from infants considered to be completely normal at the time the count was obtained and for the preceding and subsequent 48 hours. There was no difference in the normal ranges when infants were compared by either birth weight (~2500 g) or gestational age.

From Manroe BL, Browne R, et al. Normal leukocyte (WBC) values in neonates. Pediatr Res 1976;10:428, with permission.

WHITE CELL VALUES

Table A1-15. Normal Leukocyte Counts[a]

Age	Total leukocytes Mean	(Range)	Neutrophils Mean	(Range)	%	Lymphocytes Mean	(Range)	%	Monocytes Mean	%	Eosinophils Mean	%
Birth	18.1	(9.0–30.0)	11.0	(6.0–26.0)	61	5.5	(2.0–11.0)	31	1.1	6	0.4	2
12 hours	22.8	(13.0–38.0)	15.5	(6.0–28.0)	68	5.5	(2.0–11.0)	24	1.2	5	0.5	2
24 hours	18.9	(9.4–34.0)	11.5	(5.0–21.0)	61	5.8	(2.0–11.5)	31	1.1	6	0.5	2
1 week	12.2	(5.0–21.0)	5.5	(1.5–10.0)	45	5.0	(2.0–17.0)	41	1.1	9	0.5	4
2 weeks	11.4	(5.0–20.0)	4.5	(1.0–9.5)	40	5.5	(2.0–17.0)	48	1.0	9	0.4	3
1 month	10.8	(5.0–19.5)	3.8	(1.0–9.0)	35	6.0	(2.5–16.5)	56	0.7	7	0.3	3
6 months	11.9	(6.0–17.5)	3.8	(1.0–8.5)	32	7.3	(4.0–13.5)	61	0.6	5	0.3	3
1 year	11.4	(6.0–17.5)	3.5	(1.5–8.5)	31	7.0	(4.0–10.5)	61	0.6	5	0.3	3
2 years	10.6	(6.0–17.0)	3.5	(1.5–8.5)	33	6.3	(3.0–9.5)	59	0.5	5	0.3	3
4 years	9.1	(5.5–15.5)	3.8	(1.5–8.5)	42	4.5	(2.0–8.0)	50	0.5	5	0.3	3
6 years	8.5	(5.0–14.5)	4.3	(1.5–8.0)	51	3.5	(1.5–7.0)	42	0.4	5	0.2	3
8 years	8.3	(4.5–13.5)	4.4	(1.5–8.0)	53	3.3	(1.5–6.8)	39	0.4	4	0.2	2
10 years	8.1	(4.5–13.5)	4.4	(1.8–8.0)	54	3.1	(1.5–6.5)	38	0.4	4	0.2	2
16 years	7.8	(4.5–13.0)	4.4	(1.8–8.0)	57	2.8	(1.2–5.2)	35	0.4	5	0.2	3
21 years	7.4	(4.5–11.0)	4.4	(1.8–7.7)	59	2.5	(1.0–4.8)	34	0.3	4	0.2	3

[a]Numbers of leukocytes are in thousands per cubic millimeter, ranges are estimates of 95% confidence limits, and percentages refer to differential counts. Neutrophils include band cells at all ages and a small number of metamyelocytes and myelocytes in the first few days of life.

From Dallman PR. Blood and blood-forming tissues. In: Rudolph AM, editors. Pediatrics. 16th ed. E. Norwalk, CT: Appleton-Century-Crofts, 1977, with permission.

Table A1-17. Lymphocyte Subsets (25th, 50th, and 75th Percentiles) in Children and Adults

Subset	Percentage T cells				Percentage B cells			Percentage natural killer (NK) cells		
CD numbers	CD3				CD19			CD16+/CD56+, CD3−,		
Reagent	Leu 4				Leu12			Leu 11+ / 19+, Leu 4−		
Percentile		P_{25}	P_{50}	P_{75}	P_{25}	P_{50}	P_{75}	P_{25}	P_{50}	P_{75}
Age group	Number									
Cord blood	24	49	55	62	14	20	23	14	19.5	30
1 day–11 months	31	55	60	67	19	25	29	11	15	19
1–6 years	54	62	64	69	21	25	28	8	11	15
7–17 years	31	64	70	74	12	16	23	8.5	11	15.5
18–70 years	300	67	72	76	11	13	16	10	14	19

Subset	Percentage T helper cells				Percentage T suppressor cells			Helper/suppressor (CD4/CD8) ratio		
CD number	CD4				CD8			CD4,	CD8	
Reagent	Leu 3				Leu 2			Leu 3	Leu 2	
Percentile		P_{25}	P_{50}	P_{75}	P_{25}	P_{50}	P_{75}	P_{25}	P_{50}	P_{75}
Age group	Number									
Cord blood	24	28	35	42	26	29	33	0.80	1.15	1.75
1 day–11 months	31	35	41	48	18	23	28	1.35	1.80	2.25
1–6 years	54	32	37	40	25	32	36	1.00	1.20	1.60
7–17 years	31	33	36	40	28	31	36	1.05	1.20	1.40
18–70 years	300	38	42	46	31	35	40	1.00	1.20	1.50

Data obtained using flow cytometry. Kindly supplied by Dr. F. Hulstaert, Becton Dickinson Immunocytometry Systems Medical Department, Cockeysville, MD.

PLATELET VALUES

Table A1-18. Normal Platelet Counts

Subject	Platelet count/mm³ (mean±1 SD)
Preterm, 27–31 weeks	275,000 ± 60,000
Preterm, 32–36 weeks	290,000 ± 70,000
Term infants	310,000 ± 68,000
Normal adult or child	300,000 ± 50,000

From Oski FA, Naiman JL. Normal blood values in the newborn period. In: Hematologic Problems in the Newborn. Philadelphia: Saunders, 1982, with permission.

COAGULATION VALUES

Table A1-19. Reference Values for Coagulation Tests in Healthy Full-Term Infants during First 6 Months of Life

	Day 1		Day 5		Day 30		Day 90		Day 180		Adult	
	M	B	M	B	M	B	M	B	M	B	M	B
PT (s)	13.0	(10.1–15.9)[a]	12.4	(10.0–15.3)[a]	11.8	(10.0–14.3)[a]	11.9	(10.0–14.2)[a]	12.3	(10.7–13.9)[a]	12.4	(10.8–13.9)
INR	1.00	(0.53–1.62)	0.89	(0.53–1.48)	0.79	(0.53–1.26)	0.81	(0.53–1.26)	0.88	(0.61–1.17)	0.89	(0.64–1.17)
APTT (s)	42.9	(31.3–54.5)	42.6	(25.4–59.8)	40.4	(32.0–55.2)	37.1	(29.0–50.1)[a]	35.5	(28.1–42.9)[a]	33.5	(26.6–10.3)
TCT (s)	23.5	(19.0–28.3)[a]	23.1	(18.0–29.2)	24.3	(19.4–29.2)[a]	25.1	(20.5–29.7)[a]	25.5	(19.8–31.2)[a]	25.0	(19.7–30.3)
Fibrinogen (g/dL)	2.83	(1.67–3.99)[a]	3.12	(1.62–4.62)[a]	2.70	(1.62–3.78)[a]	2.43	(1.50–3.79)[a]	2.51	(1.50–3.87)[a]	2.78	(1.56–4.00)
II (units/mL)	0.48	(0.26–0.70)	0.63	(0.33–0.93)	0.68	(0.34–1.02)	0.75	(0.45–1.05)	0.88	(0.60–1.16)	1.08	(0.70–1.46)
V (units/mL)	0.72	(0.34–1.08)	0.95	(0.45–1.45)	0.98	(0.62–1.34)	0.90	(0.48–1.32)	0.91	(0.55–1.27)	1.06	(0.62–1.50)
VII (units/mL)	0.66	(0.28–1.04)	0.89	(0.35–1.43)	0.90	(0.42–1.38)	0.91	(0.39–1.43)	0.87	(0.47–1.27)	1.05	(0.67–1.43)
VIII (units/mL)	1.00	(0.50–1.78)[a]	0.88	(0.50–1.54)[a]	0.91	(0.50–1.57)[a]	0.79	(0.50–1.25)[a]	0.73	(0.50–1.09)	0.99	(0.50–1.49)
vWF (units/mL)	1.53	(0.50–2.87)	1.40	(0.50–2.54)	1.28	(0.50–2.46)	1.18	(0.50–2.06)	1.07	(0.50–1.97)	0.92	(0.50–1.58)
IX (units/mL)	0.53	(0.15–0.91)	0.53	(0.15–0.91)	0.51	(0.21–0.81)	0.67	(0.21–1.13)	0.86	(0.36–1.36)	1.09	(0.55–1.63)
X (units/mL)	0.40	(0.12–0.68)	0.49	(0.19–0.79)	0.59	(0.31–0.87)	0.71	(0.35–1.07)	0.78	(0.38–1.18)	1.06	(0.70–1.52)
XI (units/mL)	0.38	(0.10–0.66)	0.55	(0.23–0.87)	0.53	(0.27–0.79)	0.69	(0.41–0.97)	0.86	(0.49–1.34)	0.97	(0.67–1.27)
XII (units/mL)	0.53	(0.13–0.93)	0.47	(0.11–0.83)	0.49	(0.17–0.81)	0.67	(0.25–1.09)	0.77	(0.39–1.15)	1.08	(0.52–1.64)
PK (units/mL)	0.37	(0.18–0.69)	0.48	(0.20–0.76)	0.57	(0.23–0.91)	0.73	(0.41–1.05)	0.86	(0.56–1.16)	1.12	(0.62–1.62)
HMW-K (units/mL)	0.54	(0.06–1.02)	0.74	(0.16–1.32)	0.77	(0.33–1.21)	0.82	(0.30–1.46)[a]	0.82	(0.36–1.28)[a]	0.92	(0.50–1.36)
XIII[a] (units/mL)	0.79	(0.27–1.31)	0.94	(0.44–1.44)[a]	0.93	(0.39–1.47)[a]	1.04	(0.36–1.72)[a]	1.04	(0.46–1.62)[a]	1.05	(0.55–1.55)
XIII[b] (units/mL)	0.76	(0.30–1.22)	1.06	(0.32–1.80)	1.11	(0.39–1.73)[a]	1.16	(0.48–1.84)[a]	1.10	(0.50–1.70)[a]	0.97	(0.57–1.37)

Abbreviations: PT, prothrombin time; APTT, activated partial thromboplastin time; TCT, thrombin clotting time; VII, factor VIII procoagulant; vWF, von Willebrand's factor; PK, prekallikrein; HMW-K, high molecular weight kininogen; INR, international normalized ratio.

All factors except fibrinogen are expressed as units per milliliter (units/mL) where pooled plasma contains 1.0 unit/mL. All values are expressed as mean (M) followed by the lower and upper boundary (B) encompassing 95% of the population. Between 40 and 77 samples were assayed for each value for the newborn. Some measurements were skewed due to a disproportionate number of high values. The lower limit, which excludes the lower 2.5% of the population, has been given.

From Andrew M. Bailliere's Clin Hematol 1991;4:251, with permission.

[a]Values are indistinguishable from the adult.

Table A1-20. Reference Values for Coagulation Tests in Healthy Premature Infants (30–36 Weeks' Gestation) during First 6 Months of Life[a]

	Day 1		Day 5		Day 30		Day 90		Day 180		Adult	
	M	B	M	B	M	B	M	B	M	B	M	B
PT (s)	13.0	(10.6–16.2)[b]	12.5	(10.0–15.3)[b,c]	11.8	(10.0–13.6)[b]	12.3	(10.0–14.6)[b]	12.5	(10.0–15.0)[b]	12.4	(10.8–13.9)
APTT (s)	53.6	(27.5–79.4)[c]	50.5	(26.9–74.1)[c]	44.7	(26.9–62.5)	39.5	(28.3–50.7)	37.5	(21.7–53.3)[b]	33.5	(26.6–40.3)
TCT (s)	24.8	(19.2–30.4)[b]	24.1	(18.8–29.4)[b]	24.4	(18.8–29.9)[b]	25.1	(19.4–30.8)[b]	25.2	(18.9–31.5)[b]	25.0	(19.7–30.3)
Fibrinogen (g/L)	2.43	(1.50–3.73)[b,c,d]	2.80	(1.60–4.18)[b,c,d]	2.54	(1.50–4.14)[b,c]	2.46	(1.50–3.52)[b,c]	2.28	(1.50–3.60)[d]	2.78	(1.56–4.00)
II (units/mL)	0.45	(0.20–0.77)[c]	0.57	(0.29–0.85)[c]	0.57	(0.36–0.95)[c,d]	0.68	(0.30–1.06)	0.87	(0.51–1.23)	1.08	(0.70–1.46)
V (units/mL)	0.88	(0.41–1.44)[b,c,d]	1.00	(0.46–1.54)	1.02	(0.48–1.56)	0.99	(0.59–1.39)	1.02	(0.58–1.46)	1.06	(0.62–1.50)
VII (units/mL)	0.67	(0.21–1.13)	0.84	(0.30–1.38)	0.83	(0.21–1.45)	0.87	(0.31–1.43)	0.99	(0.47–1.51)[b]	1.05	(0.67–1.43)
VIII (units/mL)	1.11	(0.50–2.13)[b,c]	1.15	(0.53–2.05)[b,c,d]	1.11	(0.50–1.99)[b,c,d]	1.06	(0.58–1.88)[b,c,d]	0.99	(0.50–1.87)[b,c,d]	0.99	(0.50–1.49)
vWF (units/mL)	1.36	(0.78–2.10)[b]	1.33	(0.72–2.19)[c]	1.36	(0.66–2.16)[c]	1.12	(0.75–1.84)[b,c]	0.98	(0.54–1.58)[b,c]	0.92	(0.50–1.58)
IX (units/mL)	0.35	(0.19–0.65)[b,d]	0.42	(0.14–0.74)[c,d]	0.44	(0.13–0.80)[c]	0.59	(0.25–0.93)	0.81	(0.50–1.20)[c]	1.09	(0.55–1.63)
X (units/mL)	0.41	(0.11–0.71)	0.51	(0.19–0.83)	0.56	(0.20–0.92)	0.67	(0.35–0.99)	0.77	(0.35–1.19)	1.06	(0.70–1.52)
XI (units/mL)	0.30	(0.08–0.52)[c,d]	0.41	(0.13–0.69)[d]	0.43	(0.15–0.71)[d]	0.59	(0.25–0.93)[d]	0.78	(0.46–1.10)	0.97	(0.67–1.27)
XII (units/mL)	0.38	(0.10–0.66)[d]	0.39	(0.09–0.69)[d]	0.43	(0.11–0.75)	0.61	(0.15–1.07)	0.82	(0.22–1.42)	1.08	(0.52–1.64)
PK (units/mL)	0.33	(0.09–0.57)	0.45	(0.28–0.75)[c]	0.59	(0.31–0.87)	0.79	(0.37–1.21)	0.78	(0.40–1.16)	1.12	(0.62–1.62)
HMWK (units/mL)	0.49	(0.09–0.89)	0.62	(0.24–1.00)[d]	0.64	(0.16–1.12)[d]	0.78	(0.32–1.24)	0.83	(0.41–1.25)[b]	0.92	(0.50–1.36)
XIII[a] (units/mL)	0.70	(0.32–1.08)	1.01	(0.57–1.45)[b]	0.99	(0.51–1.47)[b]	1.13	(0.71–1.55)[b]	1.13	(0.65–1.61)[b]	1.05	(0.55–1.55)
XIII[b] (units/mL)	0.81	(0.35–1.27)	1.10	(0.68–1.58)[b]	1.07	(0.57–1.57)[b]	1.21	(0.75–1.67)	1.15	(0.67–1.63)	0.97	(0.57–1.37)
Plasminogen (CTA, units/mL)	1.70	(1.12–2.48)[c,d]	1.91	(1.21–2.61)[d]	1.81	(1.09–2.53)	2.38	(1.58–3.18)	2.75	(1.91–3.59)[d]	3.36	(2.48–4.24)

[a]All values are given as a mean (M) followed by the lower and upper boundaries (B) encompassing 95% of the population. Between 40 and 96 samples were assayed for each value for newborns.

[b]Values indistinguishable from the adult.

[c]Measurements are skewed owing to a disproportionate number of high values. Lower limit that excludes the lower 2.5% of the population is given (B).

[d]Values differ from those of full-term infants.

From Andrew M, Paes B, Milner R, et al. Development of the human coagulation system in the healthy premature infant. Blood 1988;72:1651, with permission.

Table A1-21. Reference Values for Inhibitors of Coagulation in the Healthy Full-Term Infant during the First 6 Months of Life[a]

Inhibitors	Day 1 (n)	Day 5 (n)	Day 30 (n)	Day 90 (n)	Day 180 (n)	Adult (n)
AT-III (units/mL)	0.63 ± 0.12 (58)	0.67 ± 0.13 (74)	0.78 ± 0.15 (66)	0.97 ± 0.12 (60)[b]	1.04 ± 0.10 (56)[b]	1.05 ± 0.13 (28)
α_2-M (units/mL)	1.39 ± 0.22 (54)	1.48 ± 0.25 (73)	1.50 ± 0.22 (61)	1.76 ± 0.25 (55)	1.91 ± 0.21 (55)	0.86 ± 0.17 (29)
α_2-AP (units/mL)	0.85 ± 0.15 (55)	1.00 ± 0.15 (75)[b]	1.00 ± 0.12 (62)[b]	1.08 ± 0.16 (55)[b]	1.11 ± 0.14 (53)	1.02 ± 0.17 (29)
C_1E-INH (units/mL)	0.72 ± 0.18 (59)	0.90 ± 0.15 (76)[b]	0.89 ± 0.21 (63)	1.15 ± 0.22 (55)	1.41 ± 0.26 (55)[b]	1.01 ± 0.15 (29)
α_1-AT (units/mL)	0.93 ± 0.22 (57)[b]	0.89 ±0.20 (75)[b]	0.62 ± 0.13 (61)	0.72 ± 0.15 (56)	0.77 ± 0.15 (55)	0.93 ± 0.19 (29)
HCII (units/mL)	0.43 ± 0.25 (56)	0.48 ± 0.24 (72)	0.47 ± 0.20 (58)	0.72 ± 0.37 (58)	1.20 ± 0.35 (55)	0.96 ± 0.15 (29)
Protein C (units/mL)	0.35 ± 0.09 (41)	0.42 ± 0.11 (44)	0.43 ± 0.11 (43)	0.54 ± 0.13 (44)	0.59 ± 0.11 (52)	0.96 ± 0.16 (28)
Protein S (units/mL)	0.36 ± 0.12 (40)	0.59 ± 0.14 (48)	0.63 ± 0.15 (41)	0.86 ± 0.16 (46)[b]	0.87 ± 0.16 (49)[b]	0.92 ± 0.16 (29)

Abbreviations: AT-III, antithrombin III; α_2-M, alpha$_2$-macroglobulin; α_2-AP, alpha$_2$-antiplasmin; C_1E-INH, C_1-esterase inhibitor; α_1-AT, alpha$_1$-antitrypsin; HCII, heparin cofactor II.

[a]All values expressed in units/mL as mean ± 1 SD; *n*, numbers studied.

[b]Values indistinguishable from those of adults.

From Andrew M, Paes B, Milner R, et al. Development of the human coagulation system in the healthy premature infant. Blood 1988;72:1651, with permission.

Table A1-22. Reference Values for the Inhibitors of Coagulation in Healthy Premature Infants during the First 6 Months of Life[a]

	Day 1		Day 5		Day 30		Day 90		Day 180		Adult	
	M	B	M	B	M	B	M	B	M	B	M	B
AT-III (units/mL)	0.38	(0.14–0.62)[d]	0.56	(0.30–0.82)[b]	0.59	(0.37–0.81)[d]	0.83	(0.45–1.21)[d]	0.90	(0.52–1.28)[d]	1.05	(0.79–1.31)
α_2-M (units/mL)	1.10	(0.56–1.82)[c,d]	1.25	(0.71–1.77)[b]	1.38	(0.72–2.04)	1.80	(1.20–2.66)[c]	2.09	(1.10–3.21)[c]	0.86	(0.52–1.20)
α_2-AP (units/mL)	0.78	(0.40–1.16)	0.81	(0.49–1.13)[b]	0.89	(0.55–1.23)[d]	1.06	(0.64–1.48)[b]	1.15	(0.77–1.53)	1.02	(0.68–1.36)
C_1E-INH (units/mL)	0.65	(0.31–0.99)	0.83	(0.45–1.21)	0.74	(0.40–1.24)[c,d]	1.14	(0.60–1.68)[b]	1.40	(0.96–2.04)[c]	1.01	(0.71–1.31)
α_1-AT (units/mL)	0.90	(0.36–1.44)[d]	0.94	(0.42–1.46)[d]	0.76	(0.38–1.12)[d]	0.81	(0.49–1.13)[b,d]	0.82	(0.48–1.16)[b]	0.93	(0.55–1.31)
HCII (units/mL)	0.32	(0.00–0.80)[d]	0.34	(0.00–0.69)	0.43	(0.15–0.71)	0.61	(0.20–1.11)[c]	0.89	(0.45–1.40)[b,c,d]	0.96	(0.66–1.26)
Protein C (units/mL)	0.28	(0.12–0.44)[c]	0.31	(0.11–0.51)	0.37	(0.15–0.59)[d]	0.45	(0.23–0.67)[d]	0.57	(0.31–0.83)	0.96	(0.64–1.28)
Protein S (units/mL)	0.26	(0.14–0.38)[d]	0.37	(0.13–0.61)	0.56	(0.22–0.90)	0.76	(0.40–1.12)[d]	0.82	(0.44–1.20)	0.92	(0.60–1.24)

[a]All values expressed in units/mL where pooled plasma contains 1.0 unit/mL. All values are given a mean (M) followed by the lower and upper boundaries (B) encompassing 95% of the population. Between 40 and 75 samples were assayed for each value for the newborn.

[b]Values are indistinguishable from the adults.

[c]Measurements are skewed owing to a disproportionate number of high values. Lower limit which excludes the lower 2.5% of the population is given (B).

[d]Values differ from those of full-term infants.

From Andrew M, Paes B, Milner R, et al. Development of the human coagulation system in the healthy premature infant. Blood 1988;72:1651, with permission.

Table A1-22a. Reference Values for the Components of the Fibrinolytic System in the Healthy Full-Term Infant and the Healthy Premature Infant During the First 6 Months of Life

Fibrinolytic system	Day 1 M	Day 1 B	Day 5 M	Day 5 B	Day 30 M	Day 30 B	Day 90 M	Day 90 B	Day 180 M	Day 180 B	Adult M	Adult B
Healthy full-term infant												
Plasminogen (units/mL)	1.95	(1.25–2.65)	2.17	(1.41–2.93)	1.98	(1.26–2.70)	2.48	(1.74–3.22)	3.01	(2.21–3.81)	3.36	(2.48–4.24)
t-PA (ng/mL)	9.60	(5.00–18.9)	5.60	(4.00–10.0)[a]	4.10	(1.00–6.00)[a]	2.10	(1.00–5.00)[a]	2.80	(1.00–6.00)[a]	4.90	(1.40–8.40)
α_2 AP (units/mL)	0.85	(0.55–1.15)	1.00	(0.70–1.30)[a]	1.00	(0.76–1.24)[a]	1.08	(0.76–1.40)[a]	1.11	(0.83–1.39)[a]	1.02	(0.68–1.36)
PAI (units/mL)	6.40	(2.00–15.1)	2.30	(0.00–8.10)[a]	3.4	(0.00–8.80)[a]	7.20	(1.00–15.3)	8.10	(6.00–13.0)	3.6	(0.00–11.0)
Healthy premature infant												
Plasminogen (units/mL)	1.70	(1.12–2.48)[b]	1.91	(1.21–2.61)[b]	1.81	(1.09–2.53)	2.38	(1.58–3.18)	2.75	(1.91–3.59)[b]	3.36	(2.48–4.24)
t-PA (ng/mL)	8.48	(3.00–16.70)	3.97	(2.00–6.93)[a]	4.13	(2.00–7.79)[a]	3.31	(2.00–5.07)[a]	3.48	(2.00–5.85)[a]	4.96	(1.46–8.46)
α_2 AP (units/mL)	0.78	(0.40–1.16)	0.81	(0.49–1.13)[b]	0.89	(0.55–1.23)[b]	1.06	(0.64–1.48)[a]	1.15	(0.77–1.53)	1.02	(0.68–1.36)
PAI (units/mL)	5.40	(0.00–12.2)[a,b]	2.50	(0.00–7.10)[a]	4.30	(0.00–11.8)[a]	4.80	(1.00–10.2)[a,b]	4.90	(1.00–10.2)[a,b]	3.60	(0.00–11.0)

Abbreviations: t-PA, tissue plasminogen activator; α_2AP, α_1 antiplasmin; PAI, plasminogen activator inhibitor. For α_2 AP, values are expressed as units per milliliter (units/mL) where pooled plasma contains 1.0 unit/mL. Plasminogen units are those recommended by the Committee on Thrombolytic Agents. Values for t-PA are given as nanograms per milliliter. Values for PAI are given as units per milliliter; one unit of PAI-I activity is defined as the amount of PAI-I that inhibits one international unit of human single-chain TA. All values are given a mean (M) followed by the lower and upper boundary encompassing 95% of the population (B).

[a]Values that are indistinguishable from those of the adult.

[b]Values that are different from those of the full-term infant.

From Andrew M, Paes B, Johnston M, et al. Development of the hemostatic system in the neonate and young infant. Am J Pediatr Hematol Oncol 1990;12:95–104.

Table A1-23. Bleeding Time (min) in Children and Adults[a]

Subjects	Number tested	Mean	SD	Range
Children	36	4.6	1.4	2.5–8.5
Adults	48	4.6	1.2	2.5–6.5

[a]Bleeding time performed using a template technique, with incision 6 mm long and 1 mm deep and sphygmomanometer pressure 40 mmHg. Using this technique, bleeding times up to 11.5 min have been observed in apparently healthy children tested in the author's laboratory.

From Buchanan GR, Holtkamp CA. Prolonged bleeding time in children and young adults with hemophilia. Pediatrics 1980;66:951.

Table A1-24. Bleeding Time (min) in Newborns and Children[a]

Subjects	Number tested	Sphygmomanometer pressure (mmHg)	Mean	Range
Term newborn	30	30	3.4	1.9–5.8
Preterm newborn:				
<1000 g	6	20	3.3	2.6–4.0
1000–2000 g	15	25	3.9	2.0–5.6
>2000 g	5	30	3.2	2.3–5.0
Children	17	30	3.4	1.0–5.5
Adults	20	30	2.8	0.5–5.5

[a]Bleeding time performed using a template technique, with incision 5 mm long and 0.5 mm deep. All subjects had normal platelet counts.

From Feusner JH. Normal and abnormal bleeding times in neonates and young children utilizing a fully standardized template technique. Am J Clin Pathol 1980;74:73.

Table A1-25. Coagulation Factor Assays (Mean±1 SD) and Screening Tests in the Fetus and Neonate[a]

Assays of coagulation factors	Normal adult values	28–31 weeks' gestation	32–36 weeks' gestation	Term	Time at which values attain adult norms
Fibrinogen (mg/dL)	150–400	215 ± 28 (SE)	226 ± 23 (SE)	246 ± 18 (SE)	b
		270 ± 85	244 ± 55	246 ± 55	
II (%)	100	30 ± 10	35 ± 12	45 ± 15	2–12 months
V (%)	100	76 ± 7 (SE)	84 ± 9 (SE)	100 ± 5 (SE)	b
		90 ± 26	72 ± 23	98 ± 40	
VII and X (%)	100	38 ± 14	40 ± 15	56 ± 16	2–12 months
VIII (%)	100	90 ± 15 (SE)	140 ± 10 (SE)	168 ± 12 (SE)	b
		70 ± 30	98 ± 40	105 ± 34	
IX (%)	100	27 ± 10	NA	28 ± 8	3–9 months
XI (%)	100	5–18	NA	29–70	1–2 months
XII (%)	100	NA	30±	51 (25–70)	9–14 days
XIII (%)	100	100	100	100	b
Bioassay (%)					
Quantitative (units/mL)	21 ± 5.6	5 ± 3.5	NA	11 ± 3.4	3 weeks
Prothrombin time (s)[c]	12–14	23±	17 (12–21)	16 (13–20)	1 week
Activated partial thromboplastin time (s)[c]	44	NA	70±	55 ± 10	2–9 months
Thrombin time (s)[c]	10	16–28	14 (11–17)	12 (10–16)	Few days

[a]Assays quoted are biologic unless otherwise specified. SE, standard error; NA, not available.

[b]Adult levels attained prenatally.

[c]Values vary among laboratories, depending on reagents employed.

From Hathaway WE. The bleeding newborn. Semin Hematol 1975;12:175, and from Gross SJ, Stuart MJ. Hemostasis in the premature infant. Clin Perinatal 1977;4:260, with permission.

Table A1-26. Vascular-Platelet Interactions in the Fetus and Neonate

Vascular-platelet interactions	Normal adult values	27–31 weeks' gestation	32–36 weeks' gestation	Term	Term infant >1–2 months
Capillary fragility	N	Increased	N	N	N
Platelet count (10^3/mm^3)	300±50	275±60	290±70	310±68	280±56
Platelet retention (%)	N	NA	NA	N or decreased	N
Platelet aggregation with ADP, epinephrine collagen	N	Abn	Abn	Abn	
Platelet aggregation with ristocetin	N	NA	NA	N or increased	N
Platelet release I (adenide nucleotides)	N	Abn	Abn	Abn	
Platelet factor 3	N	Abn	Abn	Abn	
Platelet factor 4	N	NA	NA	N	N
Bleeding time (min)	4.0±1.5		4±1.5	4 ±1.5	N

Abbreviations: N, normal; Abn, abnormal; NA, not available.

From Hathaway WE. The bleeding newborn. Semin Hematol 1975;12:175, and from Gross SJ, Stuart MJ. Hemostasis in the premature infant. Clin Perinatol 1977;4:260, with permission.

BONE MARROW CELLS

Table A1-27. Bone Marrow Cell

Cell type	Month				
	0 (n = 57)[b]	1 (n = 71)	2 (n = 48)	3 (n = 24)	4 (n = 19)
Small lymphocytes	14.42 ± 5.54	47.05 ± 9.24	42.68 ± 7.90	43.63 ± 11.83	47.06 ± 8.77
Transitional cells	1.18 ± 1.13	1.95 ± 0.94	2.38 ± 1.35	2.17 ± 1.64	1.64 ± 1.01
Proerythroblasts	0.02 ± 0.06	0.10 ± 0.14	0.13 ± 0.19	0.10 ± 0.13	0.05 ± 0.10
Basophilic erythroblasts	0.24 ± 0.25	0.34 ± 0.33	0.57 ± 0.41	0.40 ± 0.33	0.24 ± 0.24
Early erythroblasts	0.27 ± 0.26	0.44 ± 0.42	0.71 ± 0.51	0.50 ± 0.38	0.28 ± 0.30
Polychromatic erythroblasts	13.06 ± 6.78	6.90 ± 4.45	13.06 ± 3.48	10.51 ± 3.39	6.84 ± 2.58
Orthochromatic erythroblasts	0.69 ± 0.73	0.54 ± 1.88	0.66 ± 0.82	0.70 ± 0.87	0.34 ± 0.30
Extruded nuclei	0.47 ± 0.46	0.16 ± 0.17	0.26 ± 0.22	0.19 ± 0.12	0.16 ± 0.17
Late erythroblasts	14.22 ± 7.14	7.60 ± 4.84	13.99 ± 3.82	11.40 ± 3.43	7.34 ± 2.54
Early/late erythroblast ratio[c]	1 : 50	1 : 15	1 : 18	1 : 22	1 : 23
Fetal erythroblasts	14.48 ± 7.24	8.04 ± 5.00	14.70 ± 3.86	11.90 ± 3.52	7.62 ± 2.56
Blood reticulocytes	4.18 ± 1.46	1.06 ± 1.13	3.39 ± 1.22	2.90 ± 0.91	1.65 ± 0.73
Neutrophils					
Promyelocytes	0.79 ± 0.91	0.76 ± 0.65	0.78 ± 0.68	0.76 ± 0.80	0.59 ± 0.51
Myelocytes	3.95 ± 2.93	2.50 ± 1.48	2.03 ± 1.14	2.24 ± 1.70	2.32 ± 1.59
Early neutrophils	4.74 ± 3.43	3.27 ± 1.94	2.81 ± 1.62	3.00 ± 2.18	2.91 ± 2.01
Metamyelocytes	19.37 ± 4.84	11.34 ± 3.59	11.27 ± 3.38	11.93 ± 13.09	6.04 ± 3.63
Bands	28.89 ± 7.56	14.10 ± 4.63	13.15 ± 4.71	14.60 ± 7.54	13.93 ± 6.13
Mature neutrophils	7.37 ± 4.64	3.64 ± 2.97	3.07 ± 2.45	3.48 ± 1.62	4.27 ± 2.69
Late neutrophils	55.63 ± 7.98	29.08 ± 6.79	27.50 ± 6.88	31.00 ± 11.17	31.30 ± 7.80
Early/late neutrophil ratio	1 : 12	1 : 9	1 : 9	1 : 9	1 : 11
Total neutrophils	60.37 ± 8.66	32.35 ± 7.68	30.31 ± 7.27	34.01 ± 11.95	34.21 ± 8.61
Total eosinophils	2.70 ± 1.27	2.61 ± 1.40	2.50 ± 1.22	2.54 ± 1.46	2.37 ± 4.13
Total basophils	0.12 ± 0.20	0.07 ± 0.16	0.08 ± 0.10	0.09 ± 0.09	0.11 ± 0.14
Total myeloid cells	63.19 ± 9.10	35.03 ± 8.09	32.90 ± 7.85	36.64 ± 2.26	36.69 ± 8.91
Monocytes	0.88 ± 0.85	1.01 ± 0.89	0.91 ± 0.83	0.68 ± 0.56	0.75 ± 0.75
Miscellaneous					
Megakaryocytes	0.06 ± 0.15	0.05 ± 0.09	0.10 ± 0.13	0.06 ± 0.09	0.06 ± 0.06
Plasma cells	0.00 ± 0.02	0.02 ± 0.06	0.02 ± 0.05	0.00 ± 0.02	0.01 ± 0.03
Unknown blasts	0.31 ± 0.31	0.62 ± 0.50	0.58 ± 0.50	0.63 ± 0.60	0.56 ± 0.53
Unknown cells	0.22 ± 0.34	0.21 ± 0.25	0.16 ± 0.24	0.19 ± 0.21	0.23 ± 0.25
Damaged cells	5.79 ± 2.78	5.50 ± 2.46	5.09 ± 1.78	4.75 ± 2.30	4.80 ± 2.29
Total	6.38 ± 2.84	6.39 ± 2.63	5.94 ± 1.94	5.63 ± 2.36	5.66 ± 2.30

[a]Percentages of cell types (means ± standard deviation) in tibial bone marrow of infants from birth to 18 months of age. Data were obtained from normal American infants of black, white, and Asian racial origin. The changes in the marrow during the first 18 months of postnatal life are based on differential counts of 1000 cells classified on stained smears on each of 10 serial marrow samples aspirated from the same population of infants. Criteria for including bone marrow data in this study consisted of the absence of any clinical evidence of disease, normal rate of growth, and normal serum proteins and transferrin saturations.

Populations of Normal Infants[a]

Month					
5 (*n* = 22)	6 (*n* = 22)	9 (*n* = 16)	12 (*n* = 18)	15 (*n* = 12)	18 (*n* = 19)
47.19 ± 9.93	47.55 ± 7.88	48.76 ± 8.11	47.11 ± 11.32	42.77 ± 8.94	43.55 ± 8.56
1.83 ± 0.89	2.31 ± 1.16	1.92 ± 1.39	2.32 ± 1.90	1.70 ± 0.82	1.99 ± 1.00
0.07 ± 0.10	0.09 ± 0.12	0.07 ± 0.09	0.02 ± 0.04	0.07 ± 0.12	0.08 ± 0.13
0.47 ± 0.33	0.32 ± 0.24	0.31 ± 0.24	0.30 ± 0.25	0.38 ± 0.37	0.50 ± 0.34
0.55 ± 0.36	0.41 ± 0.30	0.39 ± 0.28	0.39 ± 0.27	0.46 ± 0.36	0.59 ± 0.34
7.55 ± 2.35	7.30 ± 3.60	7.73 ± 3.39	6.83 ± 3.75	6.04 ± 1.56	6.97 ± 3.56
0.46 ± 0.51	0.38 ± 0.56	0.39 ± 0.48	0.37 ± 0.51	0.50 ± 0.65	0.44 ± 0.49
0.14 ± 0.11	0.16 ± 0.22	0.22 ± 0.25	0.23 ± 0.25	0.17 ± 0.12	0.21 ± 0.19
8.16 ± 2.58	7.85 ± 4.11	8.34 ± 3.31	7.42 ± 4.11	6.72 ± 1.80	7.62 ± 3.63
1 : 15	1 : 17	1 : 19	1 : 17	1 : 15	1 : 10
8.70 ± 2.69	8.25 ± 4.31	8.72 ± 3.34	7.81 ± 4.26	7.18 ± 1.95	8.21 ± 37.1
1.38 ± 0.65	1.74 ± 0.80	1.67 ± 0.52	1.79 ± 0.79	2.10 ± 0.91	1.84 ± 0.46
0.87 ± 0.80	0.67 ± 0.66	0.41 ± 0.34	0.69 ± 0.71	0.67 ± 0.58	0.64 ± 0.59
2.73 ± 1.82	2.22 ± 1.25	2.07 ± 1.20	2.32 ± 1.14	2.48 ± 0.94	2.49 ± 1.39
3.60 ± 2.50	2.89 ± 1.71	2.48 ± 1.46	3.02 ± 1.52	3.16 ± 1.19	3.14 ± 1.75
11.89 ± 3.24	11.02 ± 3.12	11.80 ± 3.90	11.10 ± 3.82	12.48 ± 7.45	12.42 ± 4.15
14.07 ± 5.48	14.00 ± 4.58	14.08 ± 4.53	14.02 ± 4.88	15.17 ± 4.20	14.20 ± 5.23
3.77 ± 2.44	4.85 ± 2.69	3.97 ± 2.29	5.65 ± 3.92	6.94 ± 3.88	6.31 ± 3.91
29.73 ± 7.19	29.86 ± 6.74	29.86 ± 7.36	30.77 ± 8.69	34.60 ± 7.35	32.93 ± 7.01
1 : 8	1 : 10	1 : 12	1 : 10	1 : 10	1 : 10
33.12 ± 8.34	32.75 ± 7.03	32.33 ± 7.75	33.79 ± 8.76	37.76 ± 7.32	36.06 ± 7.40
1.98 ± 0.86	2.08 ± 1.16	1.74 ± 1.08	1.92 ± 1.09	3.39 ± 1.93	2.70 ± 2.16
0.09 ± 0.13	0.10 ± 0.13	0.11 ± 0.13	0.13 ± 0.15	0.27 ± 0.37	0.10 ± 0.12
35.40 ± 8.54	34.93 ± 7.52	34.18 ± 8.13	35.83 ± 8.84	41.42 ± 7.43	38.86 ± 7.92
1.29 ± 1.06	1.21 ± 1.01	1.17 ± 0.97	1.46 ± 1.52	1.68 ± 1.09	2.12 ± 1.59
0.08 ± 0.09	0.04 ± 0.07	0.09 ± 0.12	0.05 ± 0.08	0.00 ± 0.00	0.07 ± 0.12
0.05 ± 0.11	0.03 ± 0.07	0.01 ± 0.03	0.03 ± 0.07	0.07 ± 0.12	0.06 ± 0.08
0.50 ± 0.37	0.56 ± 0.48	0.42 ± 0.50	0.37 ± 0.33	0.46 ± 0.32	0.43 ± 0.45
0.17 ± 0.22	0.10 ± 0.15	0.14 ± 0.17	0.11 ± 0.14	0.13 ± 0.18	0.20 ± 0.23
4.86 ± 1.25	5.04 ± 1.08	4.89 ± 1.60	5.34 ± 2.19	4.99 ± 1.96	5.05 ± 2.15
5.66 ± 1.41	5.78 ± 1.16	5.55 ± 1.74	5.90 ± 2.03	5.65 ± 2.02	5.81 ± 2.16

[b]*n*, number of infants studied at each stage.

[c]Expressed in round figures for facilitating comparison. Means ± SD were calculated from values obtained in individual infants, and statistical comparisons were performed.

From Rosse C, Kraemer MJ, et al. Bone marrow cell populations of normal infants: the predominance of lymphocytes. J Lab Clin Med 1977;89:1228, with permission.

Table A1-28. Normal Serum Vitamin E Levels (mg/dL) in Newborns[a]

Weeks	1	2	3	4	5	6	7	8	9	10
<1500 g 28–32 weeks	0.40 [0.05][a]	0.30 [0.04]	0.25 [0.03]	0.25 [0.03]	0.25 [0.03]	0.25 [0.03]	0.25 [0.03]	0.25 [0.03]	0.35 [0.04]	0.45 [0.05]
1500–2000 g 32–36 weeks	0.45 [0.05]	0.40 [0.05]	0.40 [0.05]	0.45 [0.05]	0.45 [0.05]	0.45 [0.05]	0.50 [0.05]	0.50 [0.05]	0.60 [0.06]	0.70 [0.06]
2000–2500 g 36–40 weeks	0.50 [0.05]	0.45 [0.05]	0.50 [0.05]	0.60 [0.06]	0.70 [0.06]	0.75 [0.06]	0.75 [0.60]	0.75 [0.60]	0.75 [0.60]	0.80 [0.70]
>2500 g term	0.55 [0.60]	0.55 [0.60]	0.55 [0.60]	0.60 [0.60]	0.75 [0.70]	0.80 [0.70]	0.85 [0.80]	0.85 [0.80]	0.85 [0.80]	0.85 [0.80]

[a]Mean±1 SD.

From Klaus M, Fanaroff A. Care of the High Risk Neonate. 3rd ed. Philadelphia: Saunders, 1986, with permission.

Table A1-29. Homovanillic Acid and Vanillylmandelic Acid in Different Age Groups in normal infants and children

Age	HVA (μg/mg urinary creatinine)		VMA (μg/mg urinary creatinine)	
	Range	Mean ± SD	Range	Mean ± SD
0–3 months	11.3–35.0	22.3 ± 7.5	5.0–37.0	19.5 ± 10.3
3–12 months	8.4–44.9	27.8 ± 9.6	8.4–43.8	22.8 ± 10.6
1–2 years	12.2–31.8	19.7 ± 6.0	7.9–23.0	14.9 ± 3.9
2–5 years	3.4–32.0	15.3 ± 7.7	2.9–23.0	11.3 ± 7.6
5–10 years	6.8–23.7	12.8 ± 5.1	5.8–18.7	9.3 ± 3.7
10–15 years	3.2–13.6	8.1 ± 3.9	1.6–10.6	5.2 ± 2.5
>15 years	3.2–9.6	5.7 ± 1.9	2.8–8.3	4.5 ± 1.8

Abbreviations: HVA, homovanillylic acid; VMA, vanillylmandelic acid.

From Tuchman M, Moriss CI, Rammaraine ML, et al. Value of urinary homovanillic acid and vanillylmandelic acid levels in the diagnosis and management of patients with neuroblastoma: comparison with 24-hour urine collections. Pediatrics 1985;75:324, with permission.

Table A1-30. Values for Soluble Interleukin-2R (SIL-2R)

Cord blood	267–799 units/mL
2.5–9 months	580–1712 units/mL
9.5–19.5 months	341–2337 units/mL
20–60 months	322–1207 units/mL
10+ years	80–600 units/mL
Adults	71–477 units/mL

Table A1-31. Thyroid Values

TSH, μIU/mL	0.3–5.0	Immunoradiometric assay
Total T-3, ng/dL	50–190	Radioimmunoassay
Total T-4, μg/dL	4.0–13.0	Radioimmunoassay

APPENDIX 2

CD ANTIGEN DESIGNATIONS

The following summary table provides an up-to-date list of all presently accepted CD designations and some basic information concerning the molecules defined by these antibodies.

CD designation	Common name	Workshop section
CD1a, b, c		T cell/B cell/Dendritic
CD2	E rosette/LFA-2 receptor	T cell
CD3	Tcr T cell receptor complex	T cell
CD4	mature helper T cell	T cell
CD5	Association with TCR	T cell/some B cell
CD6		T cells/some B cell
CD7	Earliest precursor T cell	T cell
CD8	mature cytotoxic T cells	T cell
CD9		Platelet, early B cell
CD10	neutral endopeptidase CALLA	Pre B
CD11a, b, c	leukocyte integrin	Leukocytes
CDw12		Monocyte, neutrophil, platelet
CD13	Aminopeptidase	Leukocyte
CD14	receptor for LPS	Monocyte, macrophages
CD15	Selectin ligand	Myeloid
CD16		NK macrophages, neutrophils
CD17		Neutrophils
CD18	Integrin beta 2	Leukocyte
CD19		B cells
CD20		B cells
CD21		Mature B cells
CD22		B cells
CD23	Fc epsilon R11 IgE receptor	B cells, IL4 activated T cells
CD24		B cells/myeloid
CD25	IL-2R	Active T cells, B cells
CD26	cell surface protease	Active T cells
CD27		T cells
CD28		T cells
CD29	Beta 1 integrin/platelet GPIIa	Leukocyte
CD30	Ki-1	T cells/B cells
CD31	Platelet endothelial cells adhesion molecule	Platelet, monocyte granulocytes, endothelial
CD32	Fc gamma R 11	NK monocyte, granulocytes, B cell
CD33		Myeloid
CD34		Immature hematopoietic cells
CD35		Granulocyte, monocyte, B cell

(Continues)

CD designation	Common name	Workshop section
CD36		Platelets, monocytes
CD40		Mature B active T cells
CD41	integrin alpha 11b/platelet adhesion	Platelets
CD42a		Platelet
CD43		Leukocytes
CD44		Leukocytes
CD45RC	Restricted epitope of CD45	Nonlineage
CD52	CDw52	Nonlineage
CD65	CDw65	Myeloid
CD65s	Sialylated form of CD65	Myeloid
CD66f	PMG-1	Myeloid
CD84	CDw84	B cell
CD90	CDw90, Thy-1	Adhesion
CD101	CDw101	Myeloid
CD114	G-CSFR	Myeloid
CD109	CDw109	Endothelial
CD116	CDw116, GM-CSFR	Cytokine
CD121a	CDw121a, IL-1R; type 1	Cytokine
CDw123	IL-3Rα	Cytokine
CD124	CDw124, IL-4R	Cytokine
CDw125	IL-5Rα	Cytokine
CD127	CDw127, IL-7R	Cytokine
CD130	CDw130, IL-6R-gp130 signal transducer	Cytokine
CDw131	Commonβ	Cytokine
CD132	Commonγ	Cytokine
CD134	OX40	Cytokine
CD135	Flt3, Flk2	Cytokine
CDw136	MSP-R, macrophage-stimulating protein receptor	Cytokine
CDw137	4–1BB	Cytokine
CD138	Syndecan-1	B cell
CD139		B cell
CD140a	PDGFRα, platelet-derived growth factor receptor	Endothelial
CD140b	PDGFRβ, platelet-derived growth factor receptor	Endothelial
CD141	Thrombomodulin	Endothelial
CD142	Tissue factor	Endothelial
CD143	ACE, angiotensin-converting enzyme	Endothelial
CD144	VE-cadherin	Endothelial
CDw145		Endothelial
CD146	MUC18, S-endo	Endothelial
CD147	Neurothelin, basigin	Endothelial
CD148	HPTP-eta, p260 phosphatase	Nonlineage
CDw149	MEM-133	Nonlineage
CDw150	SLAM, IPO-3	Nonlineage
CD151	PETA-3	Platelet
CD152	CTLA-4	T cell
CD153	CD30L, CD30 ligand	T cell
CD154	CD40L, CD40 ligand, T-BAM	T cell
CD155	PVR, polio virus receptor	Myeloid

(Continues)

CD designation	Common name	Workshop section
CD156	ADAM8, MS2 (mouse homologue)	Myeloid
CD157	BST-1, MO-5	Myeloid
CD158a	p58.1, MHC class I specific NK receptors	NK cell
CD158b	p58.2 MHC class I specific NK receptors	NK cell
CD161	NKRP-1	NK cell
CD162	PSGL-1	Adhesion
CD163	M130	Myeloid
CD164	MGC-24	Adhesion
CD165	GP37/AD2	Adhesion
CD166	ALCAM	Adhesion

From Kishimoto T, et al. CD antigens. Blood 1996;89:3502, with permission.

APPENDIX 3

BIOLOGICAL TUMOR MARKERS

Tumor marker	Diagnostic significance	Normal values
Oncofetal proteins		
α-fetoprotein in serum	Hepatoblastoma Hepatocellular carcinoma Endodermal sinus tumor Embryonal carcinoma Pancreatoblastoma	Table 24-4, average normal serum α-fetoprotein of infants at various ages
Carcinoembryonic antigen (CEA) in serum	Adenocarcinoma of colon	2.5 ng/mL
Hormones		
Beta-human chorionic go-nadotropin (beta-hCG) in serum	Choriocarcinoma Hepatoblastoma	5 mIU/mL
Catecholamines urinary VMA/HVA	Neuroblastoma	Appendix 1
Plasma and urinary cate-cholamines and urinary metanephrine and VMA	Pheochromocytoma	
Testosterone serum	Leydig cell tumor (testis) Sertoli–Leydig cell (ovary)	D.O.M.
Estrogen serum	Granulosa cell tumor (ovary) Sertoli cell tumor (testis)	D.O.M.
Cortisol, aldosterone, testosterone, and estrogen serum	Adrenal hyperplasia Adrenal adenoma Adrenal carcinoma Ectopic adrenal rests (liver, testis, ovary)	D.O.M.
Thyrocalcitonin serum	Medullary (C-cell) thyroid carcinoma	D.O.M.
T_3, T_4 serum	Hyperthyroidism Thyroid adenoma Thyroid carcinoma	Appendix 1
Parathormone serum	Parathyroid hyperplasia Parathyroid adenoma Parathyroid carcinoma Hepatoblastoma	D.O.M.
Vasoactive intestinal peptide (VIP)	Neuroblastoma Vipoma	<75 pg/mL
Renin serum	Wilms' tumor	D.O.M.

(Continues)

Tumor marker	Diagnostic significance	Normal values
Erythropoietin serum	Wilms' tumor Adrenal carcinoma Renal carcinoma Hepatoma	Appendix 1
Enzymes		
Neurone-specific enolase in serum	Neuroblastoma Primitive neuroectodermal tumors Medulloblastoma	15 ng/mL
Lactic dehydrogenase (LDH) in serum	Acute leukemias Non-Hodgkin lymphoma Neuroblastoma Ewing sarcoma Osteosarcoma Germ cell tumor	297–537 units/L (depending on laboratory)
Specific proteins		
Immunoglobulins	Multiple myeloma and other gammopathies	See reference values
Cytokines		
Soluble interleukin-2 receptor (SIL-2R) in serum	Acute lymphoblastic leukemia Non-Hodgkin lymphoma Hodgkin disease Hemophagocytic histiocytic syndrome	Appendix 1
Mucins and other glycoproteins		
CA 125	Ovarian cancer	<35 units/mL
CA 19–9	Colon cancer, pancreatic cancer	~37 units/mL (for investigation use only)
CA 15–3	Breast cancer	<31 units/mL
Other tumor markers		
5-Hydroxyindoleacetic acid in urine (5-HIAA)	Carcinoid tumor	24-hour urine: 2–8 mg/dL
Neopterins in urine	Non-Hodgkin lymphoma Hemophagocytic lymphohistiocytosis	7–150 µg/L
Ferritin	Neuroblastoma Hodgkin disease Hepatocellular carcinoma Germ cell tumor	6 months–15 years: 12–113 ng/mL; 15–49 years: 12–156 ng/mL

Notes: D.O.M., dependent on method. The reader should consult reference laboratory or standard textbook for normal values.

APPENDIX 4

PHARMACOLOGIC PROPERTIES OF COMMONLY USED CHEMOTHERAPY AGENTS

Drug	Synonyms	Route	Dose/m²	Schedule	Toxicities
Alkylating agents					
Mechlorethamine	Mustargen, HN$_2$, nitrogen mustard	IV	6 mg	Weekly × 2, q 28 days	M, N and V, A, phlebitis, vesicant, mucositis; NT (HD)
Cyclophosphamide	Cytoxan, CTX	IV / PO	250–1800 mg / 100–300 mg	Daily × 1–4, q 21–28 days / Daily	M, N and V, A, cystitis, water retention; cardiac (HD)
Ifosfamide	IFOS, IFEX	IV	1800 mg	Daily × 5, q 21–28 days	M, N and V, A, cystitis, NT, renal
Melphalan	Alkeran, L-PAM	IV	16 mg / 140–200 mg	Every 2 weeks × 4 then every 4 weeks / Single dose (ABMT)	M, N and V; mucositis and diarrhea (HD)
Lomustine	CeeNU, CCNU	PO	100–150 mg	Single dose, q 4–6 weeks	M, N and V, renal and pulmonary
Carmustine	BiCNU, BCNU	IV	200–250 mg	Single dose, q 4–6 weeks	M, N and V, renal and pulmonary
Cisplatin	Platinol, CDDP	IV	50–200 mg / 20 mg	Over 4–6 hours, q 21–28 days / Daily × 5, q 21–28 days	M (mild), N and V, A, renal, NT, ototoxicity, allergic
Carboplatin	CBDCA, Paraplatin	IV	560 mg / 175 mg	q 28 days / Weekly × 4, q 6 weeks	M (Plt), N and V, A, hepatic (mild)
Dacarbazine	DTIC	IV	250 mg	Daily × 5, q 21–28 days	M (mild), N and V, flulike syndrome, hepatic
Procarbazine	Matulan	PO	100 mg	Daily for 10–14 days	M, N and V, NT, rash, mucositis
Busulfan	Myleran	PO	1.8 mg	Daily	M, A, pulmonary; N and V, mucositis, NT, hepatic (HD)
Antimetabolites					
Methotrexate	MTX	PO, IM / IV	7.5–30 mg	Weekly or biweekly / Bolus or CI (6–42 hours)	M (mild), mucositis, rash, hepatic; renal, NT (HD)
6-Mercaptopurine	Purinethal, 6-MP	PO	75–100 mg	Daily	M, hepatic, mucositis
6-Thioguanine	6-TG	PO	40 mg	Daily or 2 × day	M, N and V, mucositis, hepatic
Hydroxyurea	Hydrea	PO	500 mg	Daily titrated to effect	M, N and V, diarrhea, A, renal toxicity
Cytarabine	Cytosine arabinoside, Cytosar, Ara-C	IV, SC / IV	100–200 mg / 3000 mg	q12 h or CI for 5–7 days / q12 h for 4–6 doses	M, N and V, mucositis, GI, hepatic; NT, ocular, skin (HD)

Drug	Other names	Route	Dose	Schedule	Toxicity
5-Fluorouracil	5-FU	IV	500 mg; 800–1200 mg	Single or daily × 5; CI (24–120 hours)	M (bolus), mucositis, N and V, diarrhea, skin, NT, ocular
Antibiotics					
Adriamycin	Doxorubicin, ADR	IV	45–75 mg; 20–30 mg	Single, q 21 days; Weekly × 2 every 4 weeks	M, mucositis, N and V, A, vesicant, cardiac (acute and chronic)
Daunomycin	Daunorubicin, DNR, Cerubidine	IV	30–45 mg	Daily × 3 or weekly	Same as Adriamycin
Bleomycin	Blenoxane, BLEO	IV, IM, SC	10–20 units	Weekly	Lung, skin, hypersensitivity, Raynaud disease
Dactinomycin	Cosmegen, ACT-D, actinomycin D	IV	0.45 mg (max 0.5 mg)	Daily × 5, q3–6 weeks	M, N and V, A, mucositis, vesicant, hepatic
Idarubicin	IDA	IV	10–12 mg	Daily or weekly × 3	M, mucositis, N and V, diarrhea, A, vesicant, cardiac (acute and chronic)
Mitoxantrone	Novantrone	IV	10 mg	Daily × 3	M, mucositis, N and V, A, cardiac, cough
Plant alkaloids					
Vincristine	Oncovin, VCR	IV	1.0–2.0 mg (max 2.0 mg)	Weekly × 3–6	NT, A, SIADH, hypotension, vesicant
Vinblastine	Velban, VLB	IV	3.5–6.0 mg	Weekly × 3–6	M, A, mucositis, mild NT, vesicant
Etoposide	VePesid, VP16	IV	60–120 mg	Daily × 3–5, q 3–6 weeks	M, A, N and V, mucositis, mild NT, hypotension, allergic
Teneposide	VM-26, Vumon	IV	165 mg	Twice weekly for 8–9 doses	Same as etoposide
Miscellaneous					
Prednisone	Deltasone, PRED	PO	40 mg	Daily	Multiple
Prednisolone		PO, IV	40 mg	Daily	Multiple
Dexamethasone	Decadron, DEX	PO, IV	6 mg	Daily	Multiple
L-Asparaginase	Elspar, L-ASP	IV, IM	6000 IU	3 times per week	Allergic, coagulopathy, pancreatitis, hepatic, NT

Abbreviations: IV, intravenous; PO, oral; IM, intramuscular; SC, subcutaneous; CI, continuous infusion; ABMT, autologous bone marrow transplant; M, myelosuppression; N and V, nausea and vomiting; A, alopecia; NT, neurotoxicity; GI, gastrointestinal toxicity; HD, high dose.

INDEX

Page numbers followed by an *f* indicate figures, and those followed by a *t* indicate tables

A

Abdominal crisis and acute abdomen, differentiation between, 161*t*

Abdominal emergencies, 701–702

ABO isoimmunization, 24–26, 25*t*

Abscess, perirectal, 702

Absolute neutrophil count (ANC), 213

Abt-Letterer-Siwe disease, 608

Acanthocytes (spur cells), abnormalities in anemia, 5*t*

Acanthocytosis, hereditary, 150

Acetylsalicylic acid (ASA), impaired platelet aggregation, 288

Acquired immunodeficiency syndrome (AIDS), 82–83, 82*t*. *See also* Human immunodeficiency virus (HIV)

Activated prothrombin complex concentrate (aPCC), treatment in hemophilia, 318–319, 318*t*

Addison disease, hematologic manifestations, 75

Adenopathy, mediastinal. *See* Lymphadenopathy

Adenosylcobalamin and methylcobalamin deficiencies, 55*f*, 57–58

Adenosylcobalamin deficiency, 55*f*, 56

Adenotonsillar hypertrophy, in SCD, 167

Adrenal gland disease, hematologic manifestations, 75

Adrenocorticotropin deficiency, late effects of childhood cancer, 763*t*, 764, 765*t*

Agammaglobulinemia, 219, 220. *See also* Neutropenia

Agnogenic myeloid metaplasia, with myelofibrosis (AMM), 412

AIDS, 79–83, 82*t*

AILD-type lymphoma, 371–372, 382*t*

Airway management with large mediastinal mass, 467

Alkylating agents, leukemia secondary to, 771

Alport syndrome, 287*t*

ALPS. *See* Autoimmune lymphoproliferative syndrome (ALPS)

Amegakaryocytic purpura. *See* TAR syndrome

Analgesia, 730–735, 730*t*

   adjuvant analgesics, examples and dosages, 733*t*

   anesthesia for painful procedures, 731, 734–735

   opioid

      initial dosage, 732*t*

      side effects, management of, 734*t*

      therapy for persistent pain, 733*t*

   patient-controlled analgesia, 731

Anaphylactoid purpura, 293

Anemia

   aplastic (*See* Aplastic anemia)

   congenital dyserythropoietic (*See* Congenital dyserythropoietic anemias (CDAs))

   defined, 1

   diagnosis of, 1–11

      blood smear, 1, 4*f*

      bone marrow examination, 1, 9*t*

      mean corpuscular volume (MCV), 1, 8*f*, 29*f*

      red cell distribution width (RDW), 9*t*

      reticulocyte count, 1, 8*f*, 9

   Diamond-Blackfan anemia (*See* Diamond-Blackfan anemia (DBA))

   due to hemorrhage, 12–15

   etiologic classification and diagnostic features, 2–4*t*

   hemolytic (*See* Hemolytic anemia)

   infections, 78

   iron deficiency (*See* Iron-deficiency anemia)

   in liver disease, 73

   macrocytic, 4*f*

   megaloblastic (*See* Megaloblastic anemia)

   microcytic, 4*f*

   during the neonatal period, 12–30

      causes of, 13–14*t*

      clinical and laboratory evaluation of, 30*t*

      diagnostic approach to, 28, 29*f*

      hemorrhage, 12–15

   normocytic, 4*f*

   pernicious, 51*t*

   physiologic, 27

   refractory, 396

      with excess blasts in transformation (RAEB-T), 396

      with excess blasts (RAEB), 396

   sideroblastic (*See* Sideroblastic anemia)

   steps in the investigation of, 2–4*t*, 4*f*, 5–7*t*, 8*f*, 9–11

   X-linked, 276

Anemia of prematurity, 27, 28*t*

Angiocentric immunolymphoproliferative disorders, 372–373

Angiofollicular lymph node hyperplasia, 373–374, 374*t*

Angioimmunoblastic lymphadenopathy with dysproteinemia (AILD), 371–372, 382*t*

Angiomatous lymphoid harmartoma, 373–374, 374*t*

Aniridia, in Wilms' tumor, 548, 549*t*

Anorexia nervosa, hematologic manifestations, 85–86

Anthracyclines
  late effects of childhood cancer, 755
  therapy, cardiotoxicity, 726–728
Antibiotics
  prophylactic, 716–717
  therapy for fever and neutropenia, 707–708,
    707*t*, 708*f*, 709–710*t*, 712–713*t*
Anticardiolipin antibodies (ACLAs), 341–343, 342*t*
  treatment, 344*t*
Anti-D therapy, immune thrombocytopenia, 260–261
Antiemetic agents, dosage and side effects,
    737–740*t*
Antifibrinolytic therapy, 317
Antifungal therapy, 709, 714*t*, 715*t*, 717
Antiphospholipid syndrome, 338–343
  anticardiolipin antibodies (ACLAs), 341–343, 344*t*
  diagnosis, 340*t*
  effects of, 339
  histopathological features of, 339
  lupus anticoagulant and thrombosis, 340–341
  manifestations of, 339
  prevalence, 338–339
  promotion of thrombosis, 339
  syndromes of thrombosis associated with
    antiphospholipid antibodies, 342*t*
  thrombocytopenia, 264, 336
Antiplatelet therapy, 357–358
Antithrombin (AT) deficiency, 345
Antithrombotic agents
  antiplatelet therapy, 357–358
  heparin therapy, 351–353
  heparin-induced thrombocytopenia, 354–355
  low-molecular-weight heparin, 353–354
  special conditions for use of, 360–362
  thrombolytic therapy, 358–360
  warfarin therapy, 355–357, 358*t*
Antiviral therapy, 716*t*
Aplastic anemia, 1
  acquired
    causes, 115–116*t*
    clinical features, 117
    etiologic classification, 115*t*
    laboratory investigations, 117–118
    pathophysiology, 114–116
    prognostic factors, 119*t*
    severity, 118
    treatment, 118*t*
      choices and long-term follow-up, 123
      hematopoietic stem cell transplantation,
        120–121, 120*t*
      high-dose cyclophosphamide therapy, 124,
        124*t*
      immunosuppressive therapy, 121–123, 121*t*
      long-term sequelae following treatment,
        124–125, 125*t*
      moderate aplastic anemia, 125–126
      salvage therapy, 123–124
      supportive care, 118–120
  congenital
    anemias with constitutional chromosomal
      abnormalities, 114
    dyskeratosis congenita, 112–114
    Fanconi anemia, 105–112

paroxysmal nocturnal hemoglobinuria (PNH),
    131*t*
  prognostic factors, 119*t*
Arteriosclerosis, renal, late effects of childhood
    cancer, 768
Arthritis, rheumatoid, hematologic manifestations
    of, 77
Askin tumor, 599
Astrocytomas, 519–521
  high-grade, 521
  histologic subtypes, 519–520
  low-grade, 520–521, 520*t*
Atypical lymphocytes, causes, 247*t*
Auditory complications, late effects of childhood
    cancer, 769
Autoimmune disorders, thrombocytopenia in, 264
Autoimmune lymphoproliferative syndrome
    (ALPS)
  characteristics, 384
  hematologic findings, 384–385
  immunologic findings, 385
  mechanism of autoimmunity, 386
  origin of α/β-DNT cells, 386
  pathophysiology, 385–386
  prognosis, 387
  thrombocytopenia, 264
  treatment, 386–387
Avascular necrosis (AVN), SCD, 166

B

Babesiosis, hematologic manifestations, 84
Barth syndrome, 223
Bartonellosis, hematologic manifestations, 84
Basophilia, causes, 211*t*
Basophilic stippling, abnormalities in anemia, 7*t*,
    153
Beckwith-Wiedemann syndrome, in Wilms' tumor,
    549–550, 553
Bernard-Soulier syndrome, 252*t*, 283*t*, 284*t*, 285, 329*t*
Biological tumor markers, 803–804
Birbeck granules, 604
Bladder, late effects of childhood cancer, 768, 769
Blalock-Taussig shunts, 335
  antithrombotic therapy, 361
Bleeding time
  children and adults, 793*t*
  evaluation of platelets and platelet function, 292
  newborns and children, 793*t*
Bleomycin, late effects of childhood cancer,
    757–758, 768, 769
Blister cells, abnormalities in anemia, 7*t*
Blood component therapy
  indications for small-volume RBC transfusion in
    preterm infants, 27, 28*t*
  intrauterine intravascular transfusion (IUIVT), 23
  in iron-deficiency anemia
    packed red cell transfusion, 45
    partial exchange transfusion, 45–46
  maternofetal transfusion, polycythemia due to,
    200–201
  oncologic emergencies, 717–722
    alloimmunization and refractoriness, 718

Blood component therapy (*Continued*)
  benefits of leukoreduced blood products, 718*t*
  general guidelines, 719
  graft *versus* host disease, 719
  granulocyte transfusions, 721–722
  platelet transfusions, 720–721, 721*t*
  red cell transfusions, 719–720
  risk estimates of viral transmission, 719*t*
  risks of transfusion complications per unit, 717*t*
  transfusion reactions, 717–718
  transmission of infectious agents, 718–719
  thrombocytopenia associated with
      erythroblastosis fetalis or exchange
      transfusion, 274
  twin-to-twin transfusion, and prenatal blood
      loss, 15
Blood loss. *See* Hemorrhage
Blood smear
  diagnosis of anemia, 1, 4*f*
  evaluation of platelets and platelet function, 292
  in iron deficiency anemia, 38
Blood volumes, estimated, 783*t*
Bone disease, in Hodgkin disease, 462
Bone marrow
  disorders
      with neonatal thrombocytopenia, 280
      with neutropenia, 223
  erythroid series, 10*f*
  examination, 1, 9*t*
  failure, 94–135
      of all cell lines, 3*t*
      causes of, 95*t*
      infiltration, 3*t*
      inherited syndromes, 96*t*
      of single cell line, 2*t*
  foam cells in, 91
  infiltration, 86–93, 86*t*, 87*f*, 88*t*, 89*t*, 90*t*
  involvement in Hodgkin disease, 463
  megaloblastic, 10*f*
  normoblastic, 10*f*
  sideroblastic, 10*f*
  transplantation (*See* Hematopoietic stem cell
      transplantation (HSCT))
Bone marrow aspiration, central nervous system
    malignancies, 517
Bone marrow cells, reference values, 796–797*t*
Bone marrow transplantation *See* Hematopoietic
    stem cell transplantation
Bone tumors, malignant, 585–602. *See also* Central
    nervous system (CNS) malignancies
  incidence, 585
      age-specific incidence rate, 586*f*
  secondary, late effects of childhood cancer, 771,
      772*t*, 773
Bones, in SCD, 165–166
Bordetella pertussis, hematologic manifestations, 83
Brain stem tumors, 524–525
Brain tumors. *See* Central nervous system (CNS)
    malignancies
Budd-Chiari syndrome, 132, 341
Burkitt lymphoma. *See* Lymphoma, non-Hodgkin
    (NHL)
Burr cells, 6*t*

C

Cabot's Ring bodies, abnormalities in anemia, 7*t*,
    66
Cachexia, in pediatric oncology patients, 741–745
  clinical features of, 741
  treatment, 742, 743–745*t*
Ca^{2+} mobilization, defects in, 288
Canale-Smith syndrome. *See* Autoimmune
    lymphoproliferative syndrome (ALPS)
Cancer
  childhood, late effects, 749–773
      defined, 749
      evaluation for suspected late effects, 751–752*t*
      information from follow-up of survivors, 750*t*
      potential late effects, 750–751*t*
      radiation dose toxicity levels, 754*t*
      radiosensitivity of cell types, 753*t*
      second malignant neoplasms, 770–773, 772*t*
  in children with HIV infection, 80–83, 81*t*
Carcinoma
  embryonal
      ovarian, 660
      testicular, 659–660
  renal cell, 559–560
Cardiac catheterization, arterial thromboic event
    and, 334–335
Cardiac toxicity, prevention of, 726–728
Cardiovascular system
  late effects of childhood cancer, 755–756
  SCD, 163–164
  tissue effects of iron-deficiency anemia, 37*t*
Carney traid, 563
Castleman disease, 365*t*, 373–374
  histologic types and clinical features, 374*t*
Catheters, indwelling, intravenous, nutritional
    support, cancer patients, 745–746
CD antigen designations, 800–802
CDAs. *See* Congenital dyserythropoietic anemias
    (CDAs)
Central nervous system (CNS)
  late effects of childhood cancer, 759–762, 761*t*,
      762*t*
  malignancies, 512–529
      clinical manifestations
          intracranial tumors, 513–514
          spinal tumors, 515, 515*t*
      children less than 3 years, 528–529
      conditions associated with, 512
      diagnostic evaluation
          bone marrow aspiration and bone scan, 517
          cerebrospinal fluid examination, 517
          computed tomography (CT), 515
          magnetic resonance angiography, 516
          magnetic resonance imaging, 516
          magnetic resonance spectroscopy, 516
          positron emission tomography (PET),
              516–517
          of spinal cord, 517
      frequency of childhood brain tumors, 512,
          513*t*
      management of specific tumors, 519–529
          astrocytomas, 519–521, 520*t*
          brain stem tumors, 524–525

in children and infants less than 3 years of age, 528–529
craniopharyngiomas, 527
ependymomas, 525
intracranial germ cell tumors, 527–528
medulloblastoma, 521–524
optic gliomas, 526–527
pathology, 512–513
cytogenic abnormalities identified in brain tumors, 513*t*
molecular pathology of CNS neoplasms, 513
treatment
chemotherapy, 518–519
radiotherapy, 518
surgery, 517
SCD, 161–163
tissue effects of iron-deficiency anemia, 36*t*
Chédiak—Higashi syndrome, 230–231, 286, 329*t*, 620
Chelation therapy, β-thalassemia, 186–187, 188
Chemotherapeutic agents
emetogenic potential of, 736*t*
pharmacologic properties of, 804–805
Chemotherapy
cardiovascular system, late effects of childhood cancer, 755, 756
central nervous system, late effects of childhood cancer, 759–760, 762*t*
endocrine system, late effects of childhood cancer, 762–768
Ewing sarcoma, 601–602
gastrointestinal system, late effects of childhood cancer, 769–770
genitourinary system, late effects of childhood cancer, 768–769
germ cell tumors, 653*t*, 654*t*, 660*t*
hepatoma, 666, 666*t*
high-dose followed by autologous stem cell transplant, 660*t*
Hodgkin disease, 470–471, 471*t*, 472–473*t*, 473, 481–482*t*, 482–483, 483*t*
immune system, late effects of childhood cancer, 770
musculoskeletal system, late effects of childhood cancer, 753
neuroblastoma, 538, 541*t*, 543, 546
osteosarcoma (OS), 590–595
ovarian dysgerminoma, 653, 653*t*, 654*t*
post-transplant LPDs, 379, 382*t*
recurrent soft-tissue sarcomas, 582*t*
regimens for initial cycle of, 741*t*
respiratory system, late effects of childhood cancer, 757–759, 758*t*
retinoblastoma, 637, 637*t*, 638–639
rhabdomyosarcoma, 571, 572–573*t*, 574*f*
second malignant neoplasms, late effects of childhood cancer, 773
teratoma, 653*t*, 656
Cholesterol, coronary artery disease and, 337–338
Chronic granulomatous disease (CGD), 231–233
reactions of the respiratory burst pathway, 231, 232*t*

Chronic illness, hematologic manifestations of, 76–85
Chuvashian polycythemia (CP), clinical manifestations of, 205, 206*t*
Cigarette smoking, coronary artery disease and, 337
Closure time, evaluation of platelets and platelet function, 292
CNS. *See* Central nervous system (CNS)
Coagulation factors, 296*t*
assays and screening tests in fetus and neonate, 794*t*
commercially available concentrates, 313*t*
disorders
acquired, 304–309
inherited, 309–328
in liver disease, 73–74
natural inhibitors of coagulation, 299–301, 300*t*
reference values
healthy infant, first 6 months of life, 790*t*
healthy premature infant, first 6 months of life, 791*t*
treatment of rare coagulation deficiencies, 328*t*
Coagulation tests
hemostasis, 304*t*
reference values
healthy infants, first 6 months of life, 788*t*
healthy premature infants, first 6 months of life, 789*t*
vitamin K deficiency, 305*f*
Coagulopathy, in cyanotic heart disease, 72
Cobalamin *See* Vitamin in B$_{12}$
Cognitive impairments, late effects of childhood cancer, 760–762
Common variable immunodeficiency (CVID), 220
Congenital dyserythropoietic anemias (CDAs)
clinical manifestations
types I-III, 100–102*t*
types IV-VI, 102*t*
diagnostic tests, 103*t*
erythroblasts showing dysplastic changes, 103*t*
treatment, 101, 103–104
Congenital leukemia, 450
Congenital pure red cell aplasia. *See* Diamond-Blackfan anemia (DBA)
Conjunctiva, small lymphotic infiltrates of, 372
Connective tissue disorders, 291
hematologic manifestations of, 77–78
Coombs' test, 19, 28, 30*t*
Corticosteroid therapy, Diamond-Blackfan anemia, 99
Cow's milk, hypersensitivity to, iron-deficiency anemia and, 34, 35*t*
Craniopharyngiomas, 527
C-reactive protein (CRP), 337
Cryoablation, retinoblastoma, 638
Cutaneous manifestation, in Hodgkin disease, 463–464
Cyclooxygenase synthetase deficiency, 287
Cyclophosphamide, late effects of childhood cancer, 756, 766

Cyclosporine
    prophylaxis, graft versus host disease (GVHD),
        679
    treatment
        Diamond-Blackfan anemia, 99
        paroxysmal nocturnal hemoglobinuria, 133
Cystic fibrosis, hematologic manifestations, 73
Cystinosis, 91–92, 365*t*
Cystitis, hemorrhagic, late effects of childhood
    cancer, 768–769
Cytokines
    in Hodgkin disease tumors, 467*t*
    treatment of thrombocytopenia, 280
Cytomegalovirus (CMV) infection, complication of
    stem cell transplantation, 684–685
Cytopenia, refractory, 396

D

Dactylitis, SCD, 165
DDAVP-(1-deamino-8-D-arginine vasopressin)
    therapy, 314
Denys-Drash syndrome, 548, 553
Dermatitis herpetiformis, hematologic
    manifestations, 76
Desferrioxamine (Desferal) in thallasemia, 186–187
Diabetes, coronary artery disease and, 338
Diamond-Blackfan anemia (DBA)
    clinical features, 97
    diagnosis, 97, 98*t*
    differentiating from transient
        erythroblastopenia, 97–99, 98*t*
    genetics
        dominant inheritance, 94–95
        recessive inheritance, 97
    pathophysiology, 94
    prognosis, 99–100
    treatment, 99
Dianzani autoimmune lymphoproliferative
    disease (DALD), 387
DIDMOAD (Wolfram) syndrome, 48*t*, 64–65, 126*t*
Diencephalic syndrome, 514
Diet, prevention of iron-deficiency anemia, 31
Disseminated intravascular coagulation (DIC),
    306*t*, 307–309
    disease states associated with, 308*t*
    low-grade DIC, 308
    thrombocytopenia in, 78, 265, 270*t*, 275
    treatment, 307*t*
Döhle bodies, 209
Donath-Landsteiner cold hemolysin, 143*t*, 195
Down syndrome, myelodysplastic syndrome,
    396–397
Drug-induced thrombocytopenia, 265
Drugs, implicated in platelet dysfunction, 290*t*
Dubowitz syndrome, 221
Dysfibrinogenemia, 347
Dysgerminoma, ovarian
    chemotherapy, 653, 653*t*, 654*t*
    prognosis, 654
    radiotherapy, 653–654
    signs and symptoms, 652
    surgery, 653

Dyskeratosis congenita, 112–114
    clinical course, 113
    genetics, 113
    hematologic manifestations, 76
    pathophysiology, 112–113
    therapy, 113–114
Dysplasminogenemia, 348

E

Ears, in SCD, 167
Epstein-Barr Virus, 79, 246*f*, 453–454
Echinocytes (burr cells), abnormalities in
    anemia, 5*t*
Eczema, hematologic manifestations, 76
Ehlers-Danlos syndrome, 255*t*, 291
    hematologic manifestations, 76
ELISA technique, 40
Elliptocytes, abnormalities in anemia, 6*t*
Elliptocytosis, hereditary, 147–148
Embden-Meyerhof anaerobic pathway, 151*f*
Embryonal Carcinoma, 659–660
Endocrine emergencies, 695–700
Endocrine glands, hematologic manifestations, 75
Endocrine manifestations, in Hodgkin disease,
    464–465
Endocrine system, late effects of childhood cancer,
    762–768, 763*t*, 765*t*, 767*t*, 768*t*
Endodermal sinus tumor (yolk sac tumor)
    ovarian, 659
    pathology 645–646
    testicular, 658
Endovascular stents, 335
Enteritis, late effects of childhood cancer, 769
Enterocyte cobalamin malabsorption, 50, 51*t*, 52,
    56*t*
Enteropathy, exudative, 32*t*, 35*t*
Enucleation of the eye, retinoblastoma, 639
Enzyme activities and glutathione content in
    newborn and adult red blood cells, 785*t*
Enzyme defects, 151–157
Enzyme-linked immunosorbent assay (ELISA)
    technique, 40
Eosinophilia, 235–242
    causes of, 235–236*t*, 237*f*
    diagnostic studies for evaluation of, 243*f*
    familial, 242
    grading of severity, 236
    hypereosinophilic syndrome (HES), idiopathic,
        236, 239–240
        treatment, 241*t*
    mechanism of eosinophil production in bone
        marrow, release in circulation, and
        migration in tissue, 238*f*
    during the newborn period, 241–242
    nonidiopathic
        non eosinophilic clonic disorders, 240–241
        primary clonal eosinophilic disorders, 240
        secondary clonal eosinophilic disorders, 240
    normal mean eosinophil count in circulating
        blood, 236
    treatment, 241*t*
Eosinophilic granuloma, 607

Ependymomas, 525

Epipodophyllotoxins, leukemia associated with, 771

Epstein syndrome, 287t

Epstein-Barr virus (EBV)
-associated LPD, 375–376
cellular responses in control of EBV infection, 375–376
EBV antigens associated with the lytic cycle, 375
functions of EBV latent antigens, 375
patterns of EBV gene expression, 376f
associated with Hodgkin disease, 453–454
hematologic manifestations, 79

Erythroblastopenia, transient, 98t, 104–105, 145, 159–160

Erythroblastosis fetalis, 20–21
thrombocytopenia with, 274

Erythrocyte protoporphyrin, free, in iron deficiency anemia, 38, 39t

Erythrocytes, abnormal. *See also* Red blood cells
acquired erythrocyte defects, 17–27
ABO isoimmunization, 24–26
late-onset anemia in immune hemolytic anemia, 26
nonimmune hemolytic anemia, 14t, 26
prevention of hemolytic disease, 24
Rh isoimmunization
clinical features, 17–18t, 19
laboratory findings, 19
management, 19–24, 21f
congenital erythrocyte defects,
Rh isoimmunization
clinical features, 17, 19
laboratory findings, 19
management, 19–23, 21f

Erythrocytosis, 205

Erythropoietin, recombinant human
benefits of 75t
contraindications, 725
dose and schedule, 725–726
indications, 725
treatment in prematures, 27
treatment in renal disease, 74–75, 75t

Erythropoietin serum levels, 784t

European Bone Marrow Transplantation Working Party, 125

Evans syndrome, thrombocytopenia, 264

Ewing sarcoma, 596–602
atypical Ewing Sarcoma, 596
clinical features, 598–599
diagnostic evaluation, 599–600
differential diagnosis, pathology, 597t, 598t
differentiation from other small blue-cell tumors, 598t
differentiation from typical, atypical Ewing sarcoma and PPNET, 597t
DNA ploidy and proliferative indices, 597
epidemiology, 596
molecular genetics, 597–598, 598t
pathology, 596–597
primary sites of origin, 599t
prognosis, 602
radiographic findings, 600t

treatment
chemotherapy, 601
high-risk and metatastic at presentation, 601
radiation, 601
relapse, 601–602
surgery, 600–601

Eyes, in SCD, 166

F

Factor IX inhibitors, treatment of, 320–321, 321

Factor V Leiden mutation, 343–345

Factor V Quebec, 286–287

Factor VIII concentrate replacement therapy, 317–318, 318t, 321
porcine, 318t, 319

Fanconi anemia, 105–112
clinical features, 106–108
complementation groups, 107t
complications, 108t
diagnostic investigations, 111t
differential diagnosis, 108–109, 109t
indications for screening studies, 110t
laboratory studies, 110t
malignancy and liver disease in, 108t
management, 109–112
pathophysiology, 106
prognosis, 112
screening studies, 110t
thrombocytopenia, 271f

Fanconi syndrome, indicators of, 768

Farnesyl protein transferase (FPTase) inhibitor, 401

Favism, 155

Fechtner syndrome, 287t

Felty's syndrome, hematologic manifestations, 77

FEP, 38, 39t

Ferritin, serum
in iron deficiency anemia, 38–39, 40f
values, 780t

α-fetoprotein, normal values, 550, 651t, 646–648t, 650–651, 655, 657, 664

Fever management, in the oncology patient, 704–711
antibiotic therapy for fever and neutropenia, 707–708, 707t, 708f, 709–710t
febrile neutropenic patients, 706, 709–710t
febrile nonneutropenic patients, 705
fever of unknown origin, 708–711
in patients with indwelling venous catheters, 705–706

Fibrin degradation products (D-Dimers), 337

Fibrinogen, 337

Fibrinolysis, 298–299, 299f, 300t

Fibrinolytic system, reference values, healthy full-term and healthy premature infants, first 6 months of life, 792t

Fibrosarcoma, 562t

Fibrosis, late effects of childhood cancer, 757–758, 769

FIGLU, 64

Foam cells, in bone marrow, 91

Folic acid, normal serum folic acid levels, 782t

Folic acid deficiency
  acquired, 59, 60
  cause of megaloblastosis, 48*t*
  causes of, 59–60*t*
  clinical features of, 65–66
  diagnosis, 66–68
  inborn errors of folate transport and
      metabolism, 60, 61–62*t*, 63–64
    functional methionine synthase
        deficiency, 64
    glutamate formiminotransferase deficiency, 64
    hereditary folate malabsorption, 60, 63
    methylene-tetrahydofolate reductase
        deficiency, 63–64
  treatment, 69
Follicle-stimulating hormone deficiency, late
    effects of childhood cancer, 763*t*, 764
Fontan procedure, 335, 360–361
Food
  cobalamin malabsorption, 50, 56*t*
  iron content of, 32–33, 33*t*
Formimiglutamic (FIGLU) acid excretion, 64
"Founder effect," 105
FPTase inhibitor, 401
Functional methionine synthase deficiency, 64

G

Gammaglobulin, intravenous, immune
    thrombocytopenia, 260
Gardner syndrome, 662*t*
Gastrointestinal system, late effects of childhood
    cancer, 769–770
Gastrointestinal tract
  hematologic manifestations, 72–73
  tissue effects of iron-deficiency anemia, 36*t*
Gaucher disease, 86–90
  cellular pathophysiology, 87*f*
  clinical classification, 88*t*
  diagnosis and evaluation, 87–88
  monitoring, 89*t*
  pathogenesis, 86–87
  treatment, 88, 89*t*, 90
  Type I disease, 87, 88*t*
G-CSF
  receptor, congenital neutropenia, 218
  recombinant human, 724
G-6 PD, *See* glucose-6-phosphate dehydrogenase
    deficiency
Gene therapy, β-thalassemia, 189
Genitourinary system, late effects of childhood
    cancer, 768–769
Genitourinary-priapism, SCD, 167
Germ cell tumors, 645–667
  clinical association of histologic variants, 650*t*
  clinical features, 646, 649*t*
  diagnostic features, 646, 647
  histogenesis, 646*f*
  incidence, 645
  intracranial, 527–528
  pathology, 645–646, 647–648*t*
  staging systems, 652*t*
  treatment, 651–660, 653*t*, 654*t*

  relapsed and resistant germ cell tumors, 660,
      660*t*
  tumor markers, 650–651
    deviation of normal serum AFP in infants, 651*t*
Germinoma, 651–652
  extragonadal, 653*t*, 654–655
Giant lymph node hyperplasia, 373–374, 374*t*
Glanzmann thrombasthenia, 283*t*, 285, 329*t*
Gleich syndrome, 241
Glucose-6-phosphate dehydrogenase deficiency,
    153–156
  agents inducing hemolysis in G6PD-deficient
      subjects, 155*t*
  clinical features, 154–156
  drugs causing hemolysis, 155*t*
  genetics, 153–154
  in leukocytes, 234
  pathogenesis, 154
  treatment, 156
  WHO classification of G6PD variants, 154
Glutamate formiminotransferase deficiency, 64
Glutamyl cysteine synthetase disorder, 156
Glutathione peroxidase deficiency, 157
Glutathione reductase deficiency, 156, 234
Glutathione synthetase deficiency, 156, 233–234
Glycoprotein GP Ib deficiency, 283*t*, 285
GM-CSF, recombinant human, 724, 725
Gonadotropin deficiency, late effects of childhood
    cancer, 764, 765*t*
Gorlin syndrome, 512
Graft versus host disease (GVHD), 685–691
  acute
    clinical manifestations, 686, 687*t*
    histologic grades of, 688*t*
    treatment
      prophylaxis, 688, 689*t*
      therapy, 688–689
  causes of, 686
  chronic
    classification, 690*t*
      extensive tissue involvement, 690
      limited tissue involvement, 689
    incidence, 689
    predictors, 689
    prognosis, 690
    treatment, 690–691
  comparison of acute and chronic GVHD, 688*t*
  incidence, 685–686
  prophylaxis, 689*t*
    cyclosporin, 679
    methotrexate, 679
    methylprednisone, 680, 690–691
    thalidomide, 691
  veno-occlusive disease, 691–692
Graft versus leukemia effect (GVL), 409–411
Granulomas, in Hodgkin disease, 465
Gray platelet, 283*t*, 286, 329*t*
Griscelli syndrome, 620
Growth and development, in SCD, 168–169
Growth factors, treatment, cytopenia, 133, 722–726
Growth hormone deficiency, late effects of
    childhood cancer, 763–764, 763*t*, 765*t*
Guaiac test, for occult bleeding, 42

H

Ham test, 101–102*t*
Hand-Schuller-Christian disease, 607–608
Haptocorrin deficiency, 52, 53*t*, 56*t*
Hashimoto-Pritzker syndrome, 608
β-hcG, 650–651, 664
Heart disease
  cyanotic congenital, thrombocytopenia in, 268–269
  hematologic complications of, 71–73
Heinz bodies
  abnormalities in anemia, 7*t*
  formation of in hemolytic anemia, 16–17, 180
Hemangioma, giant, thrombocytopenia
    (Kasabach-Merritt syndrome), 275
Hematolgic values
  first 2 weeks of life, 776*t*
  at various ages, 777*t*, 779*t*
Hematologic manifestations, in Hodgkin disease,
    464
Hematoma, 18*t*
Hematopoietic growth factors, oncologic
    emergencies
  basic biology of growth factors, 722, 723*f*, 723*t*
  use of G-CSF, GM-CSF erythropoietin, and
    IL-11, 724–726
Hematopoietic stem cell transplantation (HSCT),
    401, 669–693
  allogenic transplantation
    advantages/disadvantages of, 672*t*
    blood bank support in bone marrow
      transplantation, 673*t*
    bone marrow harvesting and transplantation,
      674–678
      preconditioning regimens
        aplastic anemia, 677
        hemoglobinopathies and inherited
          disorders, 677
        leukemia, 676–677
        nonmyeloablative regimens, 677–678
      pretransplantation investigations, 676*t*
      sources of hematopoietic stem cells for
        transplantation, 671*t*
      stem cell transplantation preparative
        regimens, 676, 676*t*
    donor selection, 673–674
    evidence of engraftment, 678
    graft versus host disease prophylaxis, 679–680
    histocompatibility testing, 674
    indications for, 670*t*
    late sequelae of in children, 693*t*
    results, 679*t*
  autologous transplantation
    acute lymphocytic leukemia, 681
    advantages/disadvantages of, 672*t*
    conditioning regimen for, 523*t*
    disease-free survival, 680*t*
    high-risk solid tumors, response to HSCT, 681*t*
    Hodgkin disease, 483–484
    indications for, 671*t*, 680–681
    β-thalassemia, 189
  characteristics in post-solid organ
    transplantation and post-hematopoietic
    stem cell transplantation, 380*t*

complications, 682–693
  effects of conditioning regimens, 683
  immunodeficiency, 682
  infections, 682, 683–685, 684*t*, 686*t*
  interstitial pneumonitis, 685
  pancytopenia, 685
  prophylaxis and supportive care, 683*t*
  reimmunization schedule after
    transplantation, 682–683, 682*t*
  veno-occlusive disease, 691–692
in Aplastic anemia, 677
in Diamond-Blackfan anemia, 99
in leukemia patients
  high-risk group, 672
  standard-risk group, 672
graft versus host disease (*See* Graft versus host
    disease (GVHD))
paroxysmal nocturnal hemoglobinuria, 133
post-stem cell transplantation therapy, 692–693
in SCD, 177–188
in solid tumors, 681
Hemihypertrophy and Wilms' tumor, 549
Hemoglobin
  concentrations for iron-sufficient preterm
    infants, 775*t*
  in iron deficiency anemia, 38
  and MCV percentile curves, 779*f*
  and reticulocyte values for term and preterm
    infants, 778*f*
  values in first 2 weeks of life, 776*t*
Hemoglobin Barts, 183
Hemoglobin C, 179
Hemoglobin C disease (homozygous CC), 179
Hemoglobin C trait, 179
Hemoglobin Chesapeake, 180, 204*t*
Hemoglobin Constant Spring, 182
Hemoglobin D and E disease, 180, 180*t*, 181*t*
Hemoglobin defects, 157–181
Hemoglobin F
  and A$_2$, percentage in newborn and adult, 782*t*
  percentage in first year of life, 782*t*, 783*f*
  relative concentration according to age, 783*t*
Hemoglobin H, 182, 183*t*
Hemogobin Köln, 13*t*, 41*t*, 180–180*t*
Hemoglobin Lepore, 41*t*, 182
Hemoglobin M, 180
Hemoglobin SC disease, 179–180
Hemoglobin S/thalassemia, 180
Hemoglobin Zurich, 13*t*, 16, 180–180*t*
Hemoglobinopathies, unstable, 180, 180*t*, 181*t*
Hemoglobinuria
  causes of in hemolytic anemia, 141*t*
  paroxysmal (PNH)
    clinical manifestations, 131*t*
    complications, 132
    course of the disease, 132
    diagnosis
      flow cytometric analysis of GPI-linked
        molecules, 132–133
      laboratory findings, 133*t*
      treatment, 133–134
    mechanism of defective hematopoiesis, 131
    mechanism of hemolysis and hemoglobinuria,
      131

Hemoglobinuria (*Continued*)
    mechanism of hypercoagulable state, 131
    pathogenesis, 129–131
    surface proteins missing on blood cells, 130*t*
Hemolysis, in heart disease, 71–72
Hemolytic anemia, 13–14*t*, 16–27, 136–196
    approach to diagnosis, 136
    cause of unconjugated hyperbilirubinemia, 17–18*t*
    causes of
        acquired erythrocyte defects
            ABO isoimmunization, 24–26
            late-onset anemia in immune hemolytic
                anemia, 26
            nonimmune hemolytic anemia, 14*t*, 26
            prevention of hemolytic disease, 24
            Rh and ABO incompatibility, 25*t*
            Rh isoimmunization
                clinical features, 17–18*t*, 19
                laboratory findings, 19
                management, 19–24, 21*f*
                vitamin E deficiency, 26–27
        congenital erythrocyte defects, 16–17
        corpuscular defects, 137*t*
        extracorpuscular defects, 138*t*
        hemoglobinuria, 141*t*
        tests, 142*t*, 143*t*
    classification, 3–4*t*
    clinical features, 136
    corpuscular
        enzyme defects, 151–157
        membrane defects, 142–151
    extracorpuscular
        immune, 191–195
            cold autoimmune, 194–195
                Donath-Landsteiner cold hemolysin, 195
            warm autoimmune, 191–194
                giant cell hepatitis and Coombs-positive
                    AIHA, 194
        nonimmune, 195–196
            hypersplenism, 196
            microangiopathic, 195–196, 196*t*
    hemoglobin defects, 157–181
    laboratory findings
        extravascular hemoglobin catabolism, 139*f*,
            141
        increased erythropoiesis, 141–142
        intravascular hemoglobin catabolism, 140*f*,
            141
        tests to demonstrate, 142–143*t*
    microangiopathic, 195–196, 196*t*, 265
    thalassemias, 181–191
Hemolytic uremic syndrome (HUS),
    thrombocytopenia, 265–266, 339
Hemophagocytic lymphohistiocytosis, 620–623,
    621*t*
Hemophilia, 309–322
    ancillary therapy
        antifibrinolytic, 317
        DDAVP, 314
        management of inhibitors, 317–321, 318*t*, 320*t*
    ancillary therapy, spontaneously acquired
        inhibitory antibodies to coagulation factors,
        318*t*, 321–322
    clinical course, 310

    commercial coagulation factor concentrates, 313*t*
    common sites of hemorrhage, 312*t*
    hemophilia A carrier detection, 310
    hemophilia B carrier detection, 310
    incidence, 309–310
    incidence of severity and clinical manifestations,
        312*t*
    prenatal diagnosis, 310
    severity of clinical manifestations and factor
        levels, 311*t*
    treatment (factor replacement therapy), 311–312,
        314
    treatment of bleeding episodes, 315–316*t*
    treatment of rare coagulation factor deficiencies,
        310*t*
Hemorrhage
    as cause of anemia in the newborn
        intranatal blood loss, 15
            15,13*t*, 12
        postnatal blood loss, 13*t*, 15
        prenatal blood loss
            intraplacental and retroplacental, 12
            transplancental fetomaternal, 12
            twin-to-twin transfusion, 15
    as cause of iron-deficiency anemia, 32*t*, 34
    characteristics of acute and chronic blood loss in
        the newborn, 14*t*
    intracranial, in immune thrombocytopenia, 259*t*
    treatment of children with life-threatening
        hemorrhage, 263
Hemorrhagic telangiectasia, 73, 76, 255*t*, 291
Hemostasis
    coagulation tests and normal values, 304*t*
    fibrinolysis, 298–299, 299*f*, 300*t*
    natural inhibitors of coagulation, 299, 300*f*, 300*t*,
        301
    in the newborn, 301–302, 301*t*
    physiology of
        fibrin thrombus formation, 296–297, 298*t*
        half-life and plasma levels of coagulation
            factors, 296*t*
        primary hemostatic mechanism (platelet
            phase), 296, 297*f*
        relevant components, 295–296
    preoperative evaluation of, 304
Hemostatic defects, detection of, 302–304, 304*t*
Henoch-Schönlein purpura, 255*t*, 293
    hematologic manifestations, 78
Heparin Cofactor II deficiency, 348
Heparin therapy, 351–353
    low-molecular-weight heparin, 353–354
Heparin-induced thrombocytopenia (HIT), 264,
    354–355
Hepatic artery thrombosis, 335–336
Hepatic dysfunction, vitamin K deficiency,
    305–306
Hepatoblastoma. *See* Hepatoma
Hepatocellular carcinoma. *See* Hepatoma
Hepatoma
    clinical features, 662, 663*t*
    demographic features of tumors in children,
        660, 661*t*
    diagnostic evaluation, 662, 664–665
    disorders with increased risk of, 661, 662*t*

epidemiology, 661
frequency of signs and symptoms, 664*t*
incidence, 660
malignant and benign liver tumors in children,
661*t*
pathology, 661–662
prognosis, 667
staging, 665, 665*t*
treatment
chemotherapy, 666, 666*t*
liver transplantation, 667
radiation, 666
recommendations, 666–667
surgery, 665
Hepatosplenomegaly, 17
Hereditary folate malabsorption, 60, 63
Hereditary hemorrhagic telangiectasia, 73, 76,
255*t*, 291
Hereditary spherocytosis. *See* Spherocytosis,
hereditary
Hermansky-Pudlak syndrome, 286, 327, 329*t*
Hexose monophosphate shunt, 151*f*
Histiocytes
identifying features of cells, 605*t*
ontogeny of, 605*f*
Histiocytomas, solitary, with dendritic cell
phenotypes, 620
Histiocytosis syndromes, 604–628
classification of histiocytosis syndromes in
children, 606*t*
classification of histocyte disorders, 606*t*
hemophagocytic lymphohistiocytosis
familial, 620–623, 621*t*
infection-associated, 623–625, 623*t*, 624*t*
nonfamilial, 623
identifying features of cells of the histocyte
system, 605*t*
macrophage activation syndrome, 624–625,
625*t*
malignancy-associated hemophagocytic syndrome, 623–624, 624*t*
juvenile xanthogranuloma, 620
Langerhans cell histiocytosis (LCH), 604–619
clinical and laboratory evaluation, 613–614,
614*t*, 615*t*
clinical features, 607–613
complications, 619
diagnosis, 607*t*
incidence, 604
involvement by site of disease
bone, 608, 609*t*
central nervous system, 610–613
cerebellar syndrome/neurologic
degeneration, 613
classification of CNS lesions according to
MRI morphology, 611*t*
clinical characteristics of patients with
LCH who develop CNS disease, 611*t*
hypothalamic pituitary involvement, 612
space-occupying CNS lesions, 612–613
endocrine system, 610
gastrointestinal system, 610
hematopoietic dysfunction, 609–610
liver, 609

lymph nodes, 610
skin, 609
long-term complications, 619
pathology, 604–607, 607*t*
prognosis, 618
recurrent or refactory disease, 616–618
risk factors for developing residual disabilities, 618
staging system, 619*t*
treatment
recurrent or refractory disease, 616–618
risk groups, Histiocyte Society ICH-III trial,
617*t*
solitary bone lesion, 614, 616
specific site, 616
systemic therapy for LCH, 617*t*
malignant histiocytic disorders, 626–628, 627*t*
classification, 627*f*
criteria for, 628*t*
ontogeny of histiocytes, 605*f*
secondary dendritic cell processes, 619–620
sinus histiocytosis with massive
lymphadenopathy, 626
solitary histiocytomas with dendritic cell
phenotypes, 620
HIV. *See* Human immunodeficiency virus (HIV)
Hodgkin disease (HD), 453–489
classification
by age group, 457*t*
revised European-American and Rye
classifications compared, 456*t*
clinical features, 458–465
bone disease, 462
bone marrow involvement, 463
cutaneous manifestation, 463–464
endocrine and metabolic manifestations,
464–465
frequency of initial sites of involvement, 460*t*
granulomas, 465
hematologic manifestations, 464
liver disease, 463
lymph node regions, 459*f*
lymphadenopathy, 458, 459*f*
mediastinal adenopathy, 458–459
neurologic manifestations, 461–462
paraneoplastic manifestations, 462
polymyositis, 465
pulmonary disease, 461
renal manifestations, 464
scleroderma, 465
splenomegaly, 460
systemic symptoms, 461
complication from therapy, 486–488
dental evaluation and care, 489
Epstein-Barr virus associated with, 453–454
etiology and epidemiology, 453
familial, 454
follow-up evaluations, 488–489
immunophenotypic features, 456*t*, 457*t*
investigations in, 469*t*
laboratory features
biochemical findings, 465–466
clinical and pathologic presentation with
detection of cytokines in HD tumors, 467*t*

Hodgkin disease (HD) (*Continued*)
  hematologic features, 465
  immune profiles in HD, 466*t*
  immunologic features, 466–467*t*
  late effects of childhood cancer, 771, 773
  mediastinal masses, airway management,
    467–468
  pathology
    cytogenics of HD, 458
    histologic variants of, 455–456*t*
    histopathology, 454–456*t*, 457*t*
    immunophenotypic features, 456–458, 457*t*,
      458*t*
    lymphocyte depletion, 456*t*
    lymphocyte predominance (LP), 455*t*
    lymphocyte-rich classical HD, 456*t*
    macroscopic features, 454
    mixed cellularity (MC), 455*t*
    nodular sclerosis (NS), 455*t*
  prognosis, 477
    treatment results in advanced-stage HD, 480*t*
    treatment results in early-stage HD, 478–479*t*
  prognostic factors, 484–486
  relapsed disease, 481–484
    alternative salvage combination
      chemotherapy regimens, 481–482*t*
    autologous stem cell transplantation, 483–484,
      510*t*
    ifosfamide and vinorelbine regimen, 482–483,
      483*t*
    molecular targeted therapies, 484
    vinorelbine and gemcitabine regimen, 483*t*
  staging, 468–470
    Ann Arbor classification of HD, 468*t*
    investigation in HD, 469*t*
    radionuclide scanning, 470
    staging laparotomy, 470
  treatment, 470–486
    chemotherapy regimens, 470–471, 471*t*,
      472–473*t*, 473–477
    dose-intensive response-based treatment for
      intermediate-risk children and
      adolescents, 476*t*
    lymphocyte-predominant HD, 477
    radiation therapy, 470, 471*t*, 474
    relapsed disease, 481–484
    risk-adapted therapy, 475–477
    stage and response-adapted therapy, 474–475,
      474*t*
Homocysteine, 336
Hookworm, hematologic manifestations, 85
Howell-Jolly bodies, abnormalities in anemia, 7*t*, 66
HSCT. *See* Hematopoietic stem cell transplantation
  (HSCT)
Human immunodeficiency virus (HIV)
  anemia, 79
  cancers in children with HIV infection, 80–83,
    81*t*
  coagulation abnormalities, 80
  hematologic manifestations, 79–83
  neutropenia, 79
  pathogenesis of hematologic disorders, 80
  thrombocytopenia, 79, 263–264
HVA, normal values, 798*t*

Hydroxyurea therapy, SCD, 176–178
Hyperbilirubinemia, unconjugated. *See also*
  Jaundice, neonatal
  causes of, 17–18*t*
  investigation of, 19*f*
Hypercalcemia, in tumor lysis syndrome, 698–699
Hypercoagulable states, 131, 330*t*, 331*t*
Hypereosinophilic syndrome (HES), idiopathic,
  236, 239–240
  treatment, 241*t*
Hyperglycinemia with ketosis, thrombocytopenia,
  280
Hyperhomocysteinemia, 55, 336
Hyperimmunoglobulin M syndrome, 222–223
Hyperkalemia, in tumor lysis syndrome, 698
Hyperleukocytosis, 695–696, 696*t*
Hyperphosphatemia, in tumor lysis syndrome,
  698
Hyperprolactinemia, late effects of childhood
  cancer, 764
Hypersplenism
  neutropenia, 226
  nonimmune, hemolytic anemia, 196
  thrombocytopenia, 269
Hypertension, coronary artery disease and, 338
Hyperthyroidism, in mothers, and neonatal
  thrombocytopenia, 280
Hyperuricemia, in tumor lysis syndrome, 697
Hypocalcemia, in tumor lysis syndrome, 698
Hypochromic anemia, 40–41
  disorders associated with, 41*t*
Hyposplenism, functional, SCD, 169
Hypothalamic-pituitary axis, evaluation of, 768*t*
Hypoxia, intrauterine, polycythemia due to, 202

I

Idiopathic pulmonary hemosiderosis, 75, 76
Imerslund-Gräsbeck syndrome, 48*t*, 50, 51*t*, 52,
  56*t*
Immune system
  late effects of childhood cancer, 770
  tissue effects of iron-deficiency anemia, 37*t*
Immune-tolerance induction (ITI), 319–320, 320*t*
Immunodeficiencies associated with development
  of LPDs, 376–377
Immunoneutropenia, 223–225
Inappropriate antidiuretic hormone secretion
  syndrome, in tumor lysis syndrome, 699–700
Infantile pyknocytosis, 6*t*, 16
Infarct, arterial, antithrombotic therapy, 361
Infections
  bacterial, management of, 707*t*, 709–710*t*, 711
  fungal, management of, 711, 714*t*, 715*t*, 717
  hematologic manifestations, 78
  in oncology patients, management of, 704–717
    susceptibility of oncology patients to infec-
      tions, 704
  protozoan, 713, 715
  viral, management of, 711, 716, 716*t*
Infectious lymphocytosis, 84
Infectious mononucleosis
  chronic, 247–248
  complications, 247*t*

differential diagnosis, 242, 244
EBV-specific antibody responses, 246*f*
frequency of signs and symptoms, 244–245*t*
laboratory findings, 245–246*t*
treatment, 245
α-Interferon, treatment, congenital
dyserythropoietic anemia, 103–104
Interleukin-ll, 726
Interleukin-2R, soluble (SIL-2R), reference values,
799*t*
Intestinal absorption, impaired, cause of iron-
deficiency anemia, 34, 35*t*
Intranatal blood loss, 15
Intraplacental and retroplacental blood loss, 12
Intrauterine intravascular transfusion (IUIVT), 23
Intrinsic factor, deficiency (S-binder), 50, 56*t*
Iron
content of infant foods, 33*t*
iron-containing compounds, 36*t*
oral iron medications, 44
serum
iron, total iron-binding capacity, and transferrin saturation during first year of life,
781*t*
iron and iron saturation percentage, 781*t*
iron and transferrin saturation values, 780*f*
Iron deficiency
gastrointestinal tract, 72–73
infants at high risk for, 33*t*
tissue effects of, 36–38*t*
Iron (III) hydroxide sucrose complex, for iron-
deficiency anemia, 44–45
Iron-deficiency anemia
causes, 32*t*
classification, 35*t*
cow's milk and, 34, 35*t*
diagnosis
blood findings, 38–40, 39*t*, 41*t*
FEP levels, 38, 39*t*
serum ferritin, 38–39, 40*f*
serum iron, 39
therapeutic trial, 39
differential diagnosis
hypochromic anemia, 40–41, 41*t*
microcytic anemia, 41, 43*f*, 43*t*
etiologic factors
blood loss, 32*t*, 34
dietary requirements, 31
food iron content, 32–33, 33*t*
growth, 33
impaired absorption, 34, 35*t*
nonhematologic manifestations, 34, 36–38*t*
exudative enteropathy in, 32*t*, 35*t*
infants at high risk for, 33*t*
iron-containing compounds, 36*t*
prevalence, 31
prevention, 31
tissue effects of iron deficiency, 36–38*t*
treatment
blood transfusion, 45
nutritional counseling, 42, 44
oral iron medication, 44
parenteral therapy
intramuscular, 44–45

intravenous, 45
partial exchange transfusion, 45–46
Iron-dextran, for iron-deficiency anemia, 44–45
Isovaleric acidemia, thrombocytopenia, 280
ITP. *See* Thrombocytopenic purpura: immune,
idiopathic

J

Jacobsen syndrome, 277
Jaundice, neonatal, 156
causes of unconjugated hyperbiliruminemia,
17–18*t*
clinical features, 17
investigation of, 19–21*f*
Job syndrome, 230

K

Kaposi sarcoma, in children with AIDS, 83
Kasabach-Merritt syndrome, 251*t*, 275
Kawasaki disease, 336
hematologic manifestations, 77–78
Kearns-Sayre syndrome, 126*t*, 129
Kelly-Paterson syndrome, 36*t*
Kernicterus, 17
Ki-1+ anaplastic large-cell lymphoma, 506–507*t*,
508, 508*f*
Kidney, in SCD, 164–165
Kidney disease. *See* Renal disease
Kikuchi-Fujimoto disease, 366*t*
Kleihaver-Betke Smear, 11, 12, 143*t*
Knudson, A.G., two-hit hypothesis of
carcinogenesis, 631
Kostmann disease, 215, 216–217*t*

L

Langerhans cell histiocytosis (LCH). *See*
Histiocytosis syndromes
Laparotomy, staging, Hodgkin disease, 470
Lazy-leukocyte syndrome, 229–230
Lead intoxication, hematologic manifestations, 41*t*,
85
Learning disabilities, late effects of childhood
cancer, 762
Leg ulcers, in SCD, 166–167
Leiomyoma, 83
Leiomyosarcoma, 563*t*
and leiomyomas, in children with HIV
infection, 83
Leishmaniasis, hematologic manifestations, 84
Leptospirosis, hematologic manifestations, 84
Lesch-Nyhan syndrome, 48*t*, 65
Leukemia, acute, 415–450
acute lymphoblastic (ALL), 416–439
bone and joint involvement, 418
cardiac involvement, 419
classification
B-cell and T-cell ontogeny, 422*f*
of bone marrow remission status in ALL,
427*t*
cytochemical features of acute leukemias,
421*t*

Leukemia, acute (*Continued*)
    cytochemical features of morphologic
        types, 420*t*
    cytogenetics and molecular characteristics,
        425*t*
    frequency of specific genotypes of ALL
        children, 423*f*
    future directions, 426–427
    immunology, 424
    immunophenotype distribution of ALL,
        424–425
    molecular genetics, 425
    morphologic characteristics, 420*t*
    morphology, 424
    nonrandom chromosomal translocations in
        childhood ALL, 423*t*, 425–426
    prognostic factors, 426
    proposed risk classification system, 427*t*
    clinical features, 416–419
    clinical and laboratory features, 417*t*
    clinical manifestations from lymphoid system
        invasion, 417
    clinical manifestations of extramedullary
        invasion, 417–418
    cytochemistry, 424
    diagnosis, 419
    etiology, 415–416
    incidence, 415
    gastrointestinal involvement, 418
    general systemic effects, 416
    genitourinary tract involvement, 418
    hematologic effects from bone marrow
        invasion, 416
    Immunology, 424
    laboratory studies, 419–420
    lung involvement, 419
    prognostic factors, 426
    skin involvement, 419
    treatment
        bone marrow relapse, 431, 436
            Memorial Sloan-Kettering protocol for
                ALL in bone marrow relapse, 438*t*
        central nervous system relapse, 436
        Comprehensive Cancer Network
            recommendations for ALL relapse, 437*f*
        general, 427–428
        minimal residual disease (MRD), 429, 430*t*
        newly diagnosed ALL, 429–430
        protocol for B-cell ALL and B-cell NHL,
            434–435*t*
        protocol for high-risk pre-B-cell ALL,
            432–433*t*
        protocol for ALL in bone marrow relapse,
            438*t*
        protocol for recurrent ALL, 439*t*
        protocol for T-cell ALL, 435*t*
        schema for ALL with CNS relapse, 439*t*
        testicular relapse, 436
        therapy for standard-risk pre-B-cell ALL,
            430–431*t*
acute mixed-lineage leukemia (AMLL),
    449–450
acute myeloblastic leukemia (AML)
    age incidence, 439

    bone marrow criteria for diagnosis of AML
        subtypes, 441*t*
    classification, 440–441
    clinical features, 420*t*, 421*t*, 440
    cytogenic abnormalities, 443–444*t*
    familial platelet deficiency/AML, 277
    immunophenotype of AML, 441, 442*t*
    inherited disorders predisposing to AML, 440
    molecular genetics, 442, 443–444*t*, 445*f*
    monoclonal antibody targeted therapy for
        AML, 449
    patients with refractory or recurrent AML, 448*t*
    prognosis, 445
    reinduction protocol for relapsed AML, 449*t*
    treatment of newly diagnosed AML, 442, 445
        AML-protocol, 446*t*
        DCTER regimen, 446*t*
    treatment of refractory or recurrent AML, 448,
        448*t*, 449*t*
acute promyelocytic leukemia (type M3) with
    trans-retinoic acid (ATRA)
    assessment of MRD, 448
    management of, 448
    treatment
        dose of ATRA, 447
        leukocytosis following the use of ATRA,
            447–448
        side effects, 447
acute undifferentiated leukemia (AUL)
    subtypes, 449
in children with AIDS, 83
chronic myelogenous (*See* Leukemia, chronic
    myelogenous (CML))
congenital, 450
etiology, 415–416
features of, 212*t*
incidence, 415
juvenile myelomonocytic (JMML) (*See*
    Leukemia, juvenile myelomonocytic
    (JMML))
late effects of childhood cancer, 770–771, 772*t*
pathogenesis, 415–416
types, 415
Leukemia, chronic myelogenous (CML),
    401–411
allogenic stem cell transplantation for CML, 409,
    410*f*, 411
biology, 404–405
blast crisis, 403
    WHO criteria for diagnosis, 403*t*
clinical phases
    accelerated phase, 402–403
    blast phase, 403
    chronic phase, 402
incidence, 401
minimal residual disease, 408
monitoring response to therapy, 408
novel therapies, 411
treatment
    allogeneic stem cell transplantation, 409, 410*f*,
        411
    of advanced stages, 409
    of chronic phase, 405–408, 407*t*
    with IFN-α, 407–408

with IFN-α and Ara-C, 408
  with imatinib mesylate, 405–407
    drug interactions, 406–407
    management of side effects, 406
  metabolic problems, 405
Leukemia, juvenile myelomonocytic (JMML),
    397–401
  biology, 399, 400*f*
  clinical features, 397–398
  diagnostic guidelines, 398*t*
  differential diagnosis, 398–399
  epidemiology, 397
  incidence, 397
  laboratory features, 398
  molecular events, 399
  natural history, 399–400
  prognosis, 400
  treatment, 400–401
Leukemoid reaction, features of, 212*t*
Leukocytes (white blood cells)
  alterations in, with chronic infections, 78
  disorders of, 209–235
  disorders of function, 226–235, 228*t*
    Chédiak–Higashi syndrome, 230–231
    chronic granulomatous disease (CGD), 231–233
      reactions of the respiratory burst pathway,
        231, 232*t*
    classification and investigations, 228*t*
    glucose-6-phosphate dehydrogenase
      deficiency in leukocytes, 234
    glutathione reductase deficiency, 234
    glutathione synthetase deficiency, 233–234
    lazy-leukocyte syndrome, 229–230
    leukocyte adhesion deficiencies, 226, 229
    localized juvenile periodontitis (LJP), 230
    neutrophil production and destruction in
      newborns, 234–235
    syndrome of elevated immunoglobulin E,
      Eczema, and recurrent infection (Job
      syndrome), 230
  normal leukocyte counts, 786*t*
  polymorphonuclear leukocytes and band count
    in first 2 days of life, 785*t*
  white cell values, at various ages, 786*t*
Leukocytosis, causes, 210*t*
Leukopenia, 209, 213
Leydig cell function, late effects of childhood
    cancer, late effects of childhood cancer, 766,
    767*t*
Lhermitte Syndrome, 462
Li-Fraumeni Syndrome, 512, 565, 586, 662*t*
Lipoprotein, venous thrombosis and, 336–337
Liposarcoma, 563*t*
Liver and biliary system in SCD, 164
Liver disease
  hematologic manifestations, 73–74
  in Hodgkin disease, 463
  late effects of childhood cancer, 769–770
  platelet disorders and, 289
  SCD, 165
Liver tumors. *See* Hepatoma
Livido reticularis, 342
Loeffler Syndrome, 235t, 241
LPDs. *See* Lymphoproliferative disorders (LPDs)

Lungs
  involvement, in ALL, 419
  late effects of childhood cancer, 759
  in SCD, 163–164
Lupus anticoagulant antibody (LA), 340–341
Lupus erythematosus, systemic, hematologic
    manifestations, 77
Luteinizing-stimulating hormone deficiency, late
    effects of childhood cancer, 763*t*, 764
Lymphadenopathy, 363–367
  biopsy, precautions and studies, 366
  causes, 363, 365*t*
  character, 364
  differential diagnosis, 364*t*
  history, 364
  in Hodgkin disease, 458–459
  investigations to elucidate cause, 366
  location, 364
  massive, with sinus histiocytosis with, 626
  size, 364
Lymphocyte depletion (LD), Hodgkin disease,
    456*t*
Lymphocyte predominance (LP), nodular,
    Hodgkin disease, 455*t*
Lymphocyte-rich classical Hodgkin disease, 456*t*
Lymphocytes subsets in children and adults, 787*t*
Lymphocytic and/or histiocytic (L&H) cells, 457
Lymphocytic infiltrates of the orbit and
    conjunctiva, 372
Lymphocytosis
  acute infectious, 84, 242
    causes of, 244*t*
  atypical, causes of, 247*t*
Lymphohistiocytosis, hemophagocytic
  familial, 620–623, 621*t*
  infection-associated hemophagocytic, 623–625,
    623*t*, 624*t*
  nonfamilial, 623
Lymphoma, Non-Hodgkin (NHL), 491–511
  Burkitt, 494–495*t*, 496*t*
  in children with HIV infection, 81
  classification
    histologic classification for NHL, 494*t*
    synonyms in various classifications, 495
    WHO classification for NHL, 492–493*t*
  clinical features
    abdomen, 493, 496
    constitutional symptoms, 497
    head and neck, 496
    mediastinum, 496–497
    other primary sites, 497
  diagnosis, 497–498, 497*t*
  epidemiology, 491–492, 496*t*
  incidence, 491
  prognosis, 508–509*t*
  staging, 498, 498*t*
  treatment
    complications in children with NHL, 499
    gastrointestinal complications, 499–500
    intrathoracic lesions, 499
    pericardial effusion, 499
    relapse, 509
    BEAM regimen for stem cell transplantation
      in NHL, 510*t*

Lymphoma, Non-Hodgkin (NHL) (*Continued*)
    CBV regimen for stem cell transplantation in
        NHL, 510*t*
    relapsed ALCL, 510*t*
    relapsed NHL, 510*t*
    tumor lysis syndrome, 696*t*, 697–700
    prognosis, 509*t*
    radiation therapy, 508
    surgical therapy, 508
    treatment categories
        advanced-stage BL, BLL, and DLCL including
            B-cell ALL and B-cell NHL, 503–504,
            505–506*t*
        intermediate-risk BL, BLL, and DLCL, 503,
            504*t*
        Ki-1+ anaplastic large-cell lymphoma,
            506–507*t*, 508, 508*f*
        localized BL, BLL, and DLCL, 502–503
        localized lymphoblastic lymphoma, 500–501*t*,
            502, 502*f*
        stage III and IV lymphoblastic NHL, 502
Lymphomas, central nervous system, in children
    with HIV infection, 81–82
Lymphomatoid papulosis (LyP) in children,
    387–388, 389*t*
Lymphopenia, causes of, 244*t*
Lymphoproliferative disorders (LPDs), 371–388
    angiocentric immunolymphoproliferative
        disorders, 372–373
    angioimmunoblastic lymphadenopathy with
        dysproteinemia (AILD), 371–372, 382*t*
    autoimmune lymphoproliferative syndrome
        (ALPS)(Canale-Smith syndrome)
        characteristics, 384
        Dianzani ALP disease, 387
        hematologic findings, 384–385
        immunologic findings, 385
        mechanism of autoimmunity, 386
        origin of α/β-DNT cells, 386
        pathophysiology, 385–386
        prognosis, 387
        treatment, 386–387
    Castleman disease, 373–374
        histologic types and clinical features, 374*t*
    Epstein-Barr virus-associated LPD, 375–376
        cellular responses in control of EBV infection,
            375–376
        EBV antigens associated with the lytic cycle,
            375
        functions of EBV latent antigens, 375
        patterns of EBV gene expression, 376*f*
    immunodeficiencies associated with
        development of LPDs, 376–377
    lymphocytic infiltrates of the orbit and
        conjunctiva, 372
    lymphomatoid papulosis (LyP) in children,
        387–388, 389*t*
    post-transplant LPDs
        characteristics in post-solid organ
            transplantation and post-hematopoietic
            stem cell transplantation, 380*t*
        classification of, 378*t*
        common sites of involvement in B-cell PTLDs,
            379*t*

diagnosis of, 377–378
treatment
    of B-cell LPD in immunosuppressed
        patients, 379, 381–382
    chemotherapy, 379, 382*t*
    WHO classification of, 378*t*
X-linked lymphoproliferative syndrome
    clinical manifestations, 383
    diagnostic criteria for, 384*t*
    pathophysiology, 382–383
    prognosis, 384
    treatment, 383–384

M

Macrophage activation syndrome, 624–625, 625*t*
Magnetic resonance angiography, central nervous
    system malignancies, 516
Magnetic resonance imaging, central nervous
    system malignancies, 516
Magnetic resonance spectroscopy, central nervous
    system malignancies, 516
Malabsorption syndrome, iron-deficiency anemia
    and, 34
Malaria, hematologic manifestations, 84, 157
Malignancy-associated hemophagocytic syndrome
    (MAHS), 623–624, 624*t*
Malnutrition, hematologic manifestations, 85
Marble bone disease, 92
Marfan syndrome, 291
Mast cell disease, hematologic manifestations,
    76
May Hegglin anomaly, 252*t*, 270, 277, 278*t*, 287
McLeod Syndrome, 232
MDS. *See* Myelodysplastic syndrome (MDS)
Mean corpuscular hemoglobin concentration
    (MCHC), 1
Mean corpuscular hemoglobin (MCH), 1
Mean corpuscular volume (MCV)
    classification of nature of the anemia, 9*t*
    diagnosis of anemia, 1, 8*f*, 29*f*
    hemoglobin and MCV percentile curves, 779*f*
    at various ages, 779*t*
Meckel's diverticulum, 34
Medulloblastoma, 521–524
    Chang staging system for PNET, 522*t*
    prognosis, 523–524
    relapsed medulloblastoma, 524
    risk categories, 522*t*
    therapy, 522–523
        conditioning regimen for autologous stem cell
            transplantation, 523*t*
Megaloblastic anemia, 47–69. *See also* Folic acid
    deficiency; Vitamin B$_{12}$ deficiency
    age at presentation, 53–54*t*, 67*t*
    causes of, 48*t*
    diagnosis, 66–68
    disorders giving rise to, 67*t*
    Lesch-Nyhan syndrome, 65
    orotic aciduria, 65
    thiamine-responsive anemia in DIDMOAD
        (Wolfram) syndrome, 64–65
Megaloblastic bone marrow morphology, 10*f*
Mesoblastic, nephroma, congenital, 558–559

Metabolic diseases, in neutropenia, 212*t*, 223
Metabolic emergencies, 695–700
Metabolic manifestations, in Hodgkin disease, 464–465
Metabolism disorders, vitamin B$_{12}$ deficiency
 acquired, 49*t*, 58
 congenital, 49*t*, 52, 53–54*t*, 55–58, 56*t*
Methemoglobin levels in normal children, 784*t*
Methemoglobinopathies, 180
Methionine synthase deficiency, functional, 64
Methylcobalamin synthesis deficiency, 55*f*, 57
Methylene-tetrahydofolate reductase deficiency, 63–64
5,10-Methylenetetrahydrofolate reductase mutation, 346
Methylmalonic acidemia, 55
 thrombocytopenia, 280
Methylmalonyl-CoA mutase deficiency, 55*f*, 56–57
Microangiopathic hemolytic anemia, 195–196, 196*t*
Microcytic anemia, 41–42
 diagnosis of, 42*t*
 diagnosis using MCV and RDW, 43*f*
 studies in, 43*t*
Mitochondrial diseases with bone marrow failure syndromes, 126–129
 classification, 126–127*t*
Mixed cellularity (MC), Hodgkin disease, 455*t*
Monocytopenia, causes of, 210*t*
Monocytosis, causes of, 210*t*
Mononucleosis. *See* Infectious mononucleosis
Monosomy 7 abnormality in childhood MDS, 394
Moschowitz syndrome, 266–268, 266*t*
Mucosa-associated lymphoid tissue (MALT), proliferative lesions of in children with AIDS, 82–83, 82*t*
Musculoskeletal system
 late effects of childhood cancer, 749, 753
 tissue effects of iron-deficiency anemia, 37*t*
Myelodysplastic syndrome (MDS), 388–397
 abnormalities associated with JMML and MDS, 393*t*
 in children with Down syndrome, 396–397
 classification
  French-American-British, 391*t*
  World Health Organization, 392*t*
 clinical features, 394
 cytogenics, 394
 diagnostic categories of MDS and myeloproliferative diseases in children, 393*t*
 diagnostic criteria, 390*t*
 differential diagnosis, 395*t*, 396*t*
 incidence, 392–393
 investigations for diagnosis and pertinent differential diagnosis, 390*t*
 issues, 388, 392
 minimal diagnostic criteria, 390*t*
 pathophysiology, 394
 prognosis, 395, 395*t*
 therapy-related MDS, 393–394
 treatment, 396
Myeloid metaplasia, agnogenic, with myelofibrosis (AMM), 412

Myelokathexis and WHIM syndrome, 220–221
Myeloperoxidase deficiency, 233
Myelopoiesis, ineffective, 226
Myeloproliferative disorders
 agnogenic myeloid metaplasia, with myelofibrosis (AMM), 412
 chronic myelogenous leukemia (CML), 401–411
MYH9-related disease, 287
Myoclonus, 532–533

N

Nausea and vomiting, management of, 735–741
 antiemetic agents, dosage and side effects, 737–740*t*
 categories, 735
 emetogenic potential of chemotherapeutic agents, 736*t*
 regimens for initial cycle of chemotherapy or radiotherapy, 741*t*
 vomiting center, 735
Neonatal jaundice. *See* Jaundice, neonatal
Neonatal thrombocytopenia. *See* Thrombocytopenia: neonatal
Neonate. *See* Newborn
Neoplasms. *See also* Cancer
 secondary, late effects of childhood cancer, 770–773, 772*t*
Neoplastic disease, hematologic manifestations, 92–93
Nephroblastoma. *See* Wilms' tumor
Nephroblastomatosis, 558
Nephroma, mesoblastic, congenital, 558–559
Neuroblastoma, 530–546
 anatomic site, 531–532
 clinical features, 530–532
 conditions associated with, 531*t*
 constitutional symptoms, 532
 diagnosis
  criteria from INSS Conference, 534*t*
  screening program for early diagnosis, 534
  studies for assessment of extent of disease, 535
 histopathologic classifications of Shimada and Joshi, 531*t*
 immunocytochemistry, 598*t*
 incidence, 530
 laboratory studies for disease status, 545*t*
 modified International Neuroblastoma (INRC) definitions of response to treatment, 536*t*
 neonatal, 533
 nonspecific constitutional symptoms, 532
 paraneoplastic syndromes
  manifestations
   acute myoclonic encephalopathy: syndrome of opsoclonus and myoclonus (OM), 532–533
   excessive catecholamine secretion, 532
   vasoactive intestinal peptide (VIP), 532
  pathophysiology of OM, 533
  treatment of OM, 533
 pathology, 531*t*
 prognosis, 531*t*, 537*t*, 546

Neuroblastoma (*Continued*)
  risk factors for specific relapse at a specific site, 544
  staging systems (INSS and COG), 535–536*t*
  treatment
    chemotherapy, 539, 546
    consolidation therapy, 543, 544*t*
    dumbbell neuroblastoma and spinal cord compression, 545–546
    follow-up laboratory studies to determine disease status, 545*t*
    induction chemotherapy and response rates, 541*t*, 543
    minimal residual disease therapy, 544
    radiation, 538, 546
    risk group assignment, 538*t*
      high-risk, 542–545
      intermediate-risk, 540–542
      low-risk, 539–540
    surgery, 538, 546
  in young adult and adults, 546
Neuroectodermal tumor, primitive peripheral (PPNET), 596, 597*t*. *See also* Ewing sarcoma
Neurofibromatosis, with optic nerve tumors, 526–527, with rhabomyosarcoma, 565
Neurologic emergencies, 703–704
Neurologic manifestations, in Hodgkin disease, 461–462
Neutropenia, 17
  abnormal cellular immunity in cartilage-hair hypoplasia, 220
  alloimmune neonatal, 224
  antibiotic therapy for, 707–708, 707*t*, 708*f*, 709–710*t*
  autoimmune, 224–225
  autosomal recessive agammaglobulinemia, 220
  benign ethnic neutropenia, 214
  bone marrow disease, 223
  causes, 212–213*t*
  chronic benign, 218
  clinical features, 214
  common variable immunodeficiency (CVID), 220
  cyclic, 218–219
  defined, 213
  diagnosis, 214*f*
  drug-induced, 223–224
  familial benign, 216–217*t*
    Dubowitz syndrome, 221
  hyperimmunoglobulin M syndrome, 222–223
  hypersplenism, 226
  ineffective myelopoiesis, 226
  infections, 226
  investigations in, 227*t*
  management of, 228*t*
  metabolic diseases, 223
  myelokathexis and WHIM syndrome, 220–221
  neonatal, 224
  neonatal preeclampsia-associated neutropenia, 235
  nonimmune, 225–226
  pancreatic insufficiency (Shwachman–Diamond syndrome), 221–222
  selective IgA deficiency and, 221

  severe congenital neutropenia (SCN)and Kostmann disease
    clinical and hematologic features, 216–217*t*
    clinical manifestations, 215
    cytogenic evaluation, 215, 218
    epidemiology, 215
    G-CSF receptor, 218
    incidence, 215
    treatment, 218
  severity of, according to ANC, 213
  X-linked agammaglobulinemia, 219
Neutrophil production and destruction in newborn infants, 234–235
Neutrophilia, causes, 211*t*
Nevus Sabaceous of Jadassohn, 565
Newborn
  causes of anemia in, 13–14*t*
    anemia of prematurity, 27
    blood loss, 12, 13t, 15
    failure of red cell production, 27
    hemolytic anemia, 16–27
    intranatal blood loss, 15
    physiologic anemia, 27
    postnatal blood loss, 15
    prenatal blood loss
      intraplacental and retroplacental, 12
      transplancental fetomaternal, 12
      twin-to-twin transfusion, 15
  characteristics of acute and chronic blood loss in the newborn, 14*t*
  clinical and laboratory evaluation of anemia in, 30*t*
  diagnostic approach to anemia in, 28, 29*f*
  eosinophilia during the newborn period, 241–242
  hemostasis in the, 301–302, 301*t*
  neutrophil function in, 234–235
  polycythemia in, 199–202
  stroke, 350*t*
  thrombotic disorders in, 348–351
NHL. *See* Lymphoma, Non-Hodgkin (NHL)
Niemann-Pick disease, 90–91, 90*t*, 365*t*
Nitrosoureas, late effects of childhood cancer, 758
Non-Hodgkin lymphoma. *See* Lymphoma, non-Hodgkin (NHL)
Nonneuroblastoma levels, random HVA and VMA, in different age groups, 798*t*
Nonrhabdomyosarcoma soft-tissue sarcomas (NRSTS), 561, 562–563*t*
Nonthrombocytopenic purpura, 293–294
Noonan syndrome, 397
Normoblastic bone marrow morphology, 10*f*
Nuclear medicine studies, respiratory system, late effects of childhood cancer, 758–759
Nucleated red blood cells, abnormalities in anemia, 7*t*
Nutrition
  counseling, iron-deficiency anemia, 42, 44
  support, oncology, 741–746, 743–745*t*
  Vitamin B$_{12}$ deficiency, 49–50
Nutritional disorders, hematologic manifestations, 85–86

O

Obesity
  cardiovascular disease and, 338
  late effects of childhood cancer, 770
Ocular complications, late effects of childhood
    cancer, 769
Omenn Syndrome, 235t
OMIM, 50
Oncologic emergencies
  by anatomic regions
    abdominal, 701–702
    neurologic, 703–704
    thoracic, 700–701
  infectious complications, 704–717
  supportive care and management, 695–747
Ophthalmic therapies, retinoblastoma, 638
Opsoclonus and myoclonus (OM), syndrome of,
    532–533
Optic gliomas, 526–527
Orbit, small lymphotic infiltrates of, 372
Orotic aciduria, 48t, 65
Oroya fever, 84
Osler-Weber-Rendu disease, 76, 255t, 291
  hematologic manifestations, 73
Osteogenesis imperfecta, 291
Osteomyelitis, and bone infarction, differentiation
    between, 160t
Osteopetrosis, infantile malignant, 92
Osteosarcoma (OS), 585–596
  classification, 587t
  clinical manifestations, 587
  diagnostic evaluation, 587–589
  epidemiology
    bone growth, 585
    environmental factors, 586–587
    genetic factors, 585–586
  follow-up studies, 595
  pathology, 587
  primary sites of origin, 588f
  prognosis, 595–596
  second malignant neoplasms, late effects of
      childhood cancer, 773
  treatment
    chemotherapy, 590–595
      event-free survival (EFS), 590, 591f
      histologic response to preoperative
        chemotherapy, 590t
      metatastic disease, 593, 594f, 595f
      recurrent disease, 593–594
      Pediatric Oncology Group POG-8651
        protocol, 590, 592f
      Rizzoli's 4th protocol, 591, 593, 593f
    surgery, 589–590
Ovarian dysfunction, late effects of childhood
    cancer, 764.766

P

Packed red cell transfusion
  in Diamond–Blackfan anemia, 99
  in iron deficiency anemia, 45
Pain management
  in childhood cancer, 728–735
    analgesic medications, dosage and frequency,
      730–735, 730t
      adjuvant analgesics, examples and dosages,
        733t
      anesthesia for painful procedures, 731,
        734–735
      opioid analgesic initial dosage, 732t
      opioid side effects, management of, 734t
      opioid therapy for persistent pain, 733t
      patient-controlled analgesia, 731
    causes of, 728
    chemotherapeutic agents, percentage dose of,
      729t
    nonpharmacologic methods, 728, 730
  sickle cell disease, 172–174, 173t
Pancreatic insufficiency (Shwachman–Diamond
    syndrome), in neutropenia, 73, 221–222
Pancreatitis, hemorrhagic, 73
Pancytopenia
  complication of stem cell transplantation, 685
  differential diagnosis of, 105f
  investigations in patients with, 106t
Parasitic illnesses with marked hematologic
    sequelae, 84–85
Parenteral therapy, iron-deficiency anemia,
    intravenous, 45
Parinaud Syndrome, 514
Paris-Trousseau syndrome, 252t, 277
Paroxysmal nocturnal hemoglobinuria (PNH)
  clinical manifestations, 131–132, 131t
  complications, 132
  course of the disease, 132
  diagnosis
    flow cytometric analysis of GPI-linked
      molecules, 132–133
    laboratory findings, 133t
  mechanism of defective hematopoiesis, 131
  mechanism of hemolysis and hemoglobinuria,
    131
  mechanism of hypercoagulable state, 131
  pathogenesis, 129–131
  treatment, 133–134
  surface proteins missing on blood cells, 130t
Parvovirus B19, 78–79
Pathogens, in children with cancer, 705t
Pearson syndrome, 126t, 128–129
  hematologic manifestations, 73
Pediatric Oncology Group POG-8651 protocol for
    osteosarcoma, 590, 592f
Periodontitis, juvenile, 230
Pernicious anemia, congenital and acquired
    defects of vitamin B_{12} absorption, 50, 51t, 52
Petechiae, 17, 254, 255t
Peutz–Jeghers syndrome, colon cancer, 73
Phlebotomy, prophylactic, congenital
    dyserythropoietic anemia, 101
Phosphofructokinase deficiency, 153
Phosphoglycerate Kinase deficiency, 153
Photoablation, retinoblastoma, 638
Physical inactivity, cardiovascular disease and,
    338
Pica, 36t
Plasma VFW deficiency, 283t, 285
Plasmapheresis, immune thrombocytopenia, 262

Plasmapheresis with immunoadsorption, 319

Plasminogen activator Inhibitor 1, 337

Plasminogen activator inhibitor deficiency, 348

Platelet aggregation

  defects

    acetylsalicylic acid (ASA) and, 288

    disorders causing, 289*t*

  evaluation of platelets and platelet function

    in platelet-rich plasma, 292–293

    in whole blood, 293

Platelet arachidonic acid pathways, abnormalities in, 287

Platelet count

  in iron deficiency anemia, 38

  normal values, 787*t*

Platelet disorders, 250–294

  associated with cardiac disease, 72

  hereditary disorders of platelet function, 328–329, 329*t*

  laboratory evaluation of platelets and platelet function, 292–293

  platelet size, diseases based on, 251*t*

  qualitative

    acquired, 288–289, 289*t*

    congenital, 282–288

      classification, 283*t*

      laboratory findings, 284*t*

      drugs implicated in platelet dysfunction, 290*t*

      management of defects in platelet function, 289–290

Platelet procoagulant activity, deficiency of, 283*t*, 288

Platelet receptor-agonist interaction, 283, 285

Platelet secretion disorders, 286–287, 287*t*

Platelet transfusions, immune thrombocytopenia, 262, 720–721*t*

Platelet vessel-wall interaction, 285

Platelet-platelet interaction, 285

Platelets

  characteristics of, 250

  α-granule in, 286, 322

  gray platelets, 286

Pneumocystis carinii, prophylactic antibiotics for, 716

Pneumonia, and pulmonary infarction, differentiation between, 161*t*

Pneumonitis

  interstitial, complication of stem cell transplantation, 685

  late effects of childhood cancer, 757–758

Polyarteritis nodosa, hematologic manifestations, 77

Polycythemia

  cause of unconjugated hyperbilirubinemia, 18*t*

  in childhood

    causes, 204*t*

      combined characteristics, 205

      primary polycythemia, 202

      secondary polycythemia, 202, 205

    pathogenesis of, 203*f*

    treatment, 205–207

  Chuvashian polycythemia (CP), clinical manifestations of, 205, 206*t*

in heart disease, 72

in the newborn, 199–202

  causes of, 200*t*

  definition of, 199

  factors increasing viscosity, 200*t*

  incidence, 199

  laboratory findings

    polycythemia due to intrauterine hypoxia, 202

    polycythemia due to maternofetal transfusion, 200–201

  symptoms, signs, and complications, 201*t*

  treatment, 202

primary familial and congenital polycythemia (PFCP), clinical manifestations of, 206*t*

Von Hippel-Lindau mutations in, 205

Polycythemia vera

  clinical manifestations, 206*t*

  criteria for diagnosis of, 207*t*

  in high-risk patients, 206–207

  intermediate-risk patients, 207

  in low-risk patients, 206

Polymyositis, in Hodgkin disease, 465

"Popcorn cells," 457

Porcine factor VIII concentrate, 318*t*, 319

Positron emission tomography (PET), central nervous system malignancies, 516–517

Posterior fossa PNET. *See* Medulloblastoma

Post-splenectomy infection, 711

Post-transplant LPDs

  characteristics in post-solid organ transplantation and post-hematopoietic stem cell transplantation, 380*t*

  classification of, 378*t*

  common sites of involvement in B-cell PTLDs, 379*t*

  diagnosis of, 377–378

  treatment

    of B-cell LPD in immunosuppressed patients, 379, 381–382

    chemotherapy, 379, 382*t*

  WHO classification of, 378*t*

PPNET, 596, 597*t*

Prednisone treatment

  Diamond-Blackfan anemia, 99

  infectious mononucleosis, 245

Pregnancy

  late effects of childhood cancer, 766

  venous thrombosis and, 338

Priapism in SCD, 167–168

Primary familial and congenital polycythemia (PFCP), clinical manifestations of, 206*t*

Primitive neuroectodermal tumor (PNET), 596, 597*t*

Proliferating cell nuclear antigen (PCNA), 597

Protein C deficiency, 346

Protein deficiency, hematologic manifestations, 85

Protein S deficiency, 346–347

Prothrombin complex concentrate (PCC), treatment in hemophilia, 318, 318*t*

Prothrombin G20210A mutation, 345

Pseudolymphoma, orbit and conjunctiva, 372

Pseudoneutropenia, 225–226

Pseudoxanthoma elasticum, 291

Psoriasis, hematologic manifestations, 76

Psychosocial support, in cancer patients, 747

Puberty, precocious, late effects of childhood cancer, 764, 765t

Pulmonary disease
  hematologic manifestations, 75–76
  with Hodgkin disease, 461

Pulmonary embolism, diagnosis of, 333t

Pulmonary infarction and pneumonia, differentiation between, 161t

Pulmonary syndrome, 608

Purpura factitia, 255t, 294

Purpura fulminans, 255t, 307t

Pyknocytosis, infantile, 6t, 16

Pyropoikilocytosis, hereditary, 148–149

Pyruvate kinase deficiency, 152

Q

Quebec platelet disorder (QPD), 286–287

R

Radionuclide scanning, Hodgkin disease, 470

Radiotherapy
  cardiovascular system, late effects of childhood cancer, 756
  central nervous system, late effects of childhood cancer, 759–762, 761t
  endocrine system, late effects of childhood cancer, 764–766, 765t, 767t
  hepatoma, 666
  musculoskeletal system, late effects of childhood cancer, 749, 753, 753t
  Non-Hodgkin lymphoma, 508
  ovarian dysgerminoma, 653–654
  regimens for initial cycle of, 741t
  respiratory system, late effects of childhood cancer, 757
  retinoblastoma
    episcleral plaque, 638
    external beam, 637–638
  rhabdomyosarcoma, 570–571, 571t

RB1 gene mutations. *See* Retinoblastoma
  in osteosarcoma, 586

R-binder deficiency, 52, 53t, 56t

Recombinant factor VII (rFVIIª), treatment in hemophilia, 318t, 319

Red blood cells. *See also* Erythrocytes, abnormal
  failure of production
    acquired, viral diseases, 27
    congenital, 14t, 27
  impaired red cell formation, 2t
  indications for small-volume RBC transfusion in preterm infants, 27, 28t
  in iron-deficiency anemia, 37–38t
  morphologic abnormalities in anemia, 5–7t
  nucleated, 7t
  zinc protoporphyrin/heme ratio, in iron deficiency, 40

Red cell distribution width (RDW), 9t

Red cell values and related serum values, 775–785
  blood volumes, estimated, 783t

enzyme activities and glutathione content in newborn and adult red blood cells, 785t
  on first postnatal day, 776t
  hemoglobin and MCV percentile curves, 779f
  hemoglobin and reticulocyte values for term and preterm infants, 778f
  hemoglobin concentrations for iron-sufficient preterm infants, 775t
  hemoglobin F
    and A$_2$, percentage in newborn and adult, 782t
    percentage in first year of life, 782t
    relative concentration according to age, 783t
  hemoglobin values in first 2 weeks of life, 776t
  methemoglobin levels in normal children, 784t
  normal serum folic acid levels, 782t
  serum erythropoietin levels, 784t
  serum ferritin values, 780t
  serum iron, total iron-binding capacity, and transferrin saturation during first year of life, 781t
  serum iron and iron saturation percentage, 781t
  serum iron and transferrin saturation values, 780f
  at various ages: mean and lower limit of normal, 777t

Reed-Sternberg cells, 456–458, 457t

Renal artery thrombosis, 335

Renal disease
  benefits of recombinant human erythropoietin in children with, 75t
  clear cell sarcoma, 559
  hematologic manifestations, 74–75
  hypoplastic kidney, late effects of childhood cancer, 768–769
  late effects of childhood cancer, 768–769
  renal cell carcinoma, 559–560
  rhabdoid tumor of, 559

Renal failure, platelet disorders and, 289

Renal manifestations, with Hodgkin disease, 464

Renal toxicity, prevention of, 728

Respiratory burst oxidase, 231

Respiratory burst pathway, reactions, 231, 232t

Respiratory system, late effects of childhood cancer, 757–759, 758t

Reticular dysgenesis, 216–217t

Reticulocyte count
  in anemia, 1, 8f, 9
  in iron deficiency anemia, 38

Reticulocyte index, 9

Retinoblastoma, 630–643
  classification
    focality, 631
    genetics, 631–633
      genetic counseling, 632
      hereditary retinoblastoma, 631–632
      nonhereditary retinoblastoma, 632
      prenatal diagnosis, 632
      RB1 gene, 631
      two-hit hypothesis (Knudson), 631
    international classification system for intraocular retinoblastoma, 637t
    laterality, 631

Retinoblastoma (*Continued*)
  clinical features
    patterns of spread, 634
    presenting signs and symptoms, 634
    trilateral retinoblastoma, 634–635
  diagnostic procedures, 635, 636*t*
  epidemiological data, 632–633
  future perspectives, 642–643, 643*t*
  incidence, 630
  pathology
    retinoblastoma, 633–634
    retinocytoma, 634
  post-treatment management
    disease-related follow-up, 640–641
    toxicity-related follow-up, 641, 642*t*
  Reese–Ellsworth staging for intraocular
      retinoblastoma, 635, 636*t*
  second malignant neoplasms, risk for, 633
  staging, 635–636*t*
  treatment
    of extraocular retinoblastoma, 639–640, 640*t*
    of intraocular retinoblastoma, 637–639, 637*t*
    of recurrent retinoblastoma, 640
Retinocytoma, 634
Retinopathy, in SCD, 166–167
Rh isoimmunization
  clinical features, 17–18*t*, 19
  laboratory findings, 19
  management
    antenatal, 19–23, 21*f*, 22*f*
    postnatal, 24
  prevention, 24
Rhabdoid tumor, of kidney, 551*t*, 559
Rhabdomyosarcoma (RMS), 561–583
  assays used in the differential diagnosis of,
      564
  clinical features
    primary sites, 565, 566*t*
    signs and symptoms, 565, 566–567*t*, 567
  diagnostic evaluation, 567–568
  epidemiology, 561
  examinations in special sites, 568
  genetics of
    clinical genetic factors, 565
    molecular genetics, 565
  histologic subtypes, 564*t*
  nonrhabdomyosarcoma soft-tissue sarcomas
      (NRSTS), 561, 562–563*t*
  pathologic classification, 564
    histologic subtypes, 564*t*
  prognosis
    age, 580
    cellular DNA (ploidy), 581
    extent of disease, 579
    failure-free survival at 3 years
      according to histologic subtype, 580*t*
      by stage and group on IRS-IV, 580*t*
    histologic and cytologic type, 580*t*
    primary tumor site, 580
    recurrent disease, 581–583, 582*t*
    recurrent soft-tissue sarcomas, 582*t*
    response to therapy, 581
    risk stratification and survival data fro IRS-III
        and IRS-IV, 581*t*

  sites of metastases, 581*t*
  tumor burden at diagnosis, 580
  staging, 568–569
    Intergroup Rhabdomyosarcoma Study (IRS),
        569*t*
    TNM staging system, 569*t*
  treatment
    chemotherapy, 571, 572–573*t*, 574*f*, 575*f*,
        576*f*,
    follow-up after completion of therapy,
        578–579
    future perspectives for, 583
    radiotherapy, 570–571, 571*t*
    for specific anatomic sites
      bladder neck/trigone and prostate, 578
      extremities, 571*t*, 573*t*, 577
      genitourinary tract, 572–573*t*, 578
      head and neck (extraorbital), 571, 572*t*,
          574, 575*f*, 576*f*
      orbit and eyelid, 572*t*, 574, 574*f*
      paratesticular lesions, 571*f*, 574, 576–577,
          572*t*,
      retroperitoneal area, 573*t*, 577–578
      vagina, uterus, and bladder dome, 578, 572*t*
    surgery, 570
Rituximab, immune thrombocytopenia, 261–262
Rizzoli's 4th protocol for osteosarcoma, 591, 593,
    593*f*
RMS. *See* Rhabdomyosarcoma (RMS)
Rosai–Dorfman disease, 608, 626

S

Sacrococcygeal teratoma. *See* Teratoma
Sarcoma. *See also* Rhabdomyosarcoma
  clear cell, of kidney, 551*t*, 559
Sarcoma botryoides, 564*t*, 567
SCD. *See* Sickle cell disease (SCD)
Schilling test, 51*t*, 67
Schistocytes, abnormalities in anemia, 6*t*
Schulman Syndrome, 241
Scleroderma, with Hodgkin disease, 465
Sclerosis, nodular, Hodgkin disease, 455*t*
Scurvy, hematologic manifestations, 85
Sebastian syndrome, 287*t*
Serum iron and iron saturation percentage, in iron
    deficiency anemia, 39
Serum transferrin receptor levels (STR), measure
    of iron deficiency, 39–40
Shwachman–Diamond syndrome, 221–222
  hematologic manifestations, 73
Sickle cell disease (SCD), 157–181
  clinical features by age, 159*f*, 161–169
  crises, 159*f*, 159–161*t*
    aplastic crisis, 159–160
    differentiation between bone infarction and
        osteomyelitis, 160*t*
    differentiation between painful abdominal
        crisis and acute abdomen, 161*t*
    differentiation between pneumonia and pul-
        monary infarction, 161*t*
    erythroblastopenic crisis, 159–160
    hyperhemolytic crisis, 161
    painful crisis, 172–173

splenic sequestration crisis, 160, 172, 174*t*
vaso-occlusive crisis, 160*t*, 161*t*
diagnosis, 170, 171*t*
genetics, 157
health maintenance-related laboratory studies,
175*t*
hematology findings, 158
hemostatic changes, 169
incidence, 157
management, 172–176
acute chest syndrome, 175*t*
hematopoietic stem cell transplantation,
177–188
hydroxyurea therapy, 176
new treatment modalities, 176
pain crisis
dose and interval of analgesics for adequate
pain control, 173*t*
serum α-hydroxybutyric dehydrogenase,
173*t*
in pregnancy, 175–176
prognosis, 170
protocol, patients under 5 years of age, with
fever, 172*t*
psychological support, 176
sickle cell trait, 178–179
splenic sequestration crisis, 160, 172, 174*t*
transfusion therapy, 174
neurologic deficit, 162*t*
organ dysfunction, 161–169
pathophysiology, 157–158, 158*f*
Sickle cell trait (heterozygous form, AS),
178–179
Sideroblastic anemia, 126–129
classification, 126–127*t*
iron and heme metabolism: distinct features in
erythroid cells, 128*t*
pathophysiology, 127–128
treatment, 128–129
Sideroblastic bone marrow morphology, 10*f*
Sinovenous thrombosis, therapy, 361
Skin, in SCD, 167
Skin disease, hematologic manifestations, 76
Sodium ferric glutonate, for iron-deficiency
anemia, 45
Soft-tissue sarcomas. *See also* Rhabdomyosarcoma
(RMS)
nonrhabdomyosarcoma soft-tissue sarcomas
(NRSTS), 561, 562–563*t*
Spermatogenesis, late effects of childhood cancer,
766, 767*t*
Spherocytes, abnormalities in anemia, 5*t*
Spherocytosis, hereditary, 143–147
biochemistry, 145
classification of and indications for splenectomy,
146*t*
clinical features, 145
complications, 145
diagnosis, 145
genetics, 143
hematology, 144
pathogenesis, 143
treatment, 147
Spinal cord compression, 703–704

Spinal tumors. *See* Central nervous system (CNS):
malignancies
Splenic index in Hodgkin disease, 460
Splenectomy
β-thalassemia, 187
in congenital dyserythropoietic anemia, 101
immune thrombocytopenia, 262–263
indications for, hereditary spherocytosis, 146*t*
Splenomegaly, 367–370
causes, 368*t*
diagnostic approach
detailed history, 367
laboratory investigations, 369–370
physical examination, 369
with Hodgkin disease, 460
visceroptosis of spleen, 367
Stem cell transplantation. *See* Hematopoietic stem
cell transplantation (HSCT)
Steroid treatment, immune thrombocytopenia,
258–259
Stomatocytes, abnormalities in anemia, 6–7*t*
Stomatocytosis, hereditary, 149–150
Storage pool deficiencies, 286
Streptokinase, 359
Stroke, antithrombotic therapy, 361

T

Tapeworm, hematologic manifestations, 85
TAR syndrome, 109*t*, 270*t*, 277, 279
Target cells, abnormalities in anemia, 5*t*
Tear drop cells, abnormalities in anemia, 6*t*
Telangiectasia, hereditary hemorrhagic, 255*t*, 291
hematologic manifestations, 76
Teratoma
anatomic and histologic grading, 656*t*
chemotherapy, 653*t*, 656
groups, 655
mediastinal, 653*t*, 657–658
ovarian, 657
prognosis, 656–657
radiotherapy, 656
surgery, 655–656
Testicular dysfunction, late effects of childhood
cancer, 766–768, 767*t*
Thalassemias, 181–191
α-thalassemia, 157, 182, 183*t*, 191
basic features, 181–182, 181*f*
β-thalassemia, 181–182, 182*t*
biochemistry, 184
causes of death, 185–189
clinical features, 184–185
complications, 185
hematology, 184
heterozygous states, 182*t*
homozygous or doubly heterozygous states,
182*t*
management
of the acutely ill patient, 189–190
chelation therapy, 186–187, 188
gene therapy, 189
hematopoietic stem cell transplantation,
189
hypertransfusion protocol, 185–186

Thalassemias (*Continued*)
    pharmacologic upgrading of fetal
        hemoglobin synthesis, 188–189
    splenectomy, 187
    supportive care, 187–188
  pathogenesis, 182
  sequelae, 184
  β-thalassemia intermedia, 190
  β-thalassemia minor or trait, 190–191
  differential diagnosis, 42*t*
Theophylline, treatment for erythrocytosis, 205
Therapeutic trial, criterion in iron-deficiency
    anemia, 39
Thiamine-responsive anemia in DIDMOAD
    (Wolfram) syndrome, 48*t*, 64–65
Thoracic emergencies, 700–701
Thrombocythemia, essential (ET), 281–282
  conditions associated with, 281*t*
  diagnostic criteria, 281
  differentiation from reactive thrombocytosis,
    282*t*
  treatment, 282
Thrombocytopenia
  cytokines in treatment of, 280
  heparin-induced, 264, 354–355
  hyporegenerative, 17
  neonatal, 269–280
    amegakaryocytic, 277, 278*t*, 279–280
    autoimmune, 271–272
    alloimmune, 272–274
      congenital
        with bilateral absence of radii (TAR
          syndrome), 277, 279
        hypoplastic thrombocytopenia with
          microcephaly, 279
        without anomalies, 277
      with radio-ulnar synostosis (ATRUS), 279
      thrombocytopenia agenesis of corpus
        callosum syndrome, 279
      thrombocytopenia associated with trisomy
        syndrome, 280
      thrombocytopenia in rubella syndrome, 279
    bone marrow disorders, 280
    causes, 269–270*t*
    diagnostic approach to, 271*f*
    incidence, 269
    inherited thrombocytopenia
      autosomal, 276–277
      sex-linked, 276
    megakaryocytic, 271–276
      associated with erythroblastosis fetalis,
        274
      causes, 269–270*t*
      disseminated intravascular coagulation,
        270*t*, 275
      drug-induced thrombocytopenia in the
        mother, 257–258*t*, 275
      giant hemangioma, 275–276
      idiopathic (autoimmune) purpura in
        passive transfer of platelet antibody
        from mother, 271–272
      infection, 274–275
      isoimmune (alloimmune) purpura,
        272–274

Thrombocytopenic purpura
  amegakaryocytic (TAR syndrome)
    causes, 270*t*
    differentiating from Fanconi anemia, 109*t*
  immune, idiopathic (ITP), 250–263
    causes of
      based on pathophysiology, 251–253*t*
      based on platelet size, 251*t*
    characteristics of, 250
    clinical features of acute and chronic ITP, 253*f*,
      254
    diagnostic criteria, 257
    drug causes, 257–258*t*
    incidence, 253
    intracranial hemorrhage in ITP, 259*t*
    investigations in patients with purpura,
      256–257
    laboratory findings, 256
    pathogenesis
      platelet antibodies, 253
      platelet survival, 254
    prognosis, 263
    signs, 256
    symptoms
      clinical approach to, 255*f*
      internal organs, 255
      mucous membranes, 255
      skin, 254–255
    treatment, 258–263, 259*t*
      anti-D therapy, 260–261
      of children with life-threatening
        hemorrhage, 263
      gammaglobulin, intravenous, 260
      plasmapheresis, 262
      platelet transfusions, 262
      rituximab, 261–262
      splenectomy, 262–263
      steroid, 258–259
  secondary, 263–269
    autoimmune disorders, 264
    cyanotic congenital heart disease, 268–269
    disseminated intravascular coagulation, 265
    drug-induced, 265
    hemolytic uremic syndrome, 265–266
    heparin-induced, 264
    HIV-1 infection, 263–264
    hypersplenism, 269
    microangiopathic hemolytic anemia, 265
    thrombopoietin deficiency, 269
    thrombotic thrombocytopenic purpura
      syndrome, 266–268, 266*t*
Thrombocytosis, 280–290
  essential thrombocythemia (ET), 281–282
    conditions associated with, 281*t*
    diagnostic criteria, 281
    differentiation from reactive thrombocytosis,
      282*t*
    treatment, 282
Thrombolytic therapy, 358–360
Thrombophilia, 328–330, 348
Thrombosis. *See also* Antithrombotic agents
  antiphospholipid syndrome, 338–343
  antithrombotic therapy in special conditions,
    360–362

arterial, predisposing causes of, 333, 334–335*t*, 335–338
clinical manifestations of hypercoagulable states, 330*t*
laboratory findings in hypercoagulable states, 331*t*
mechanisms of, in inherited thrombophilia, 329–330
venous, 330, 332
  detection of, 333*t*
  diagnosis of pulmonary embolism, 333*t*
  predisposing factors, 331–332*t*
  treatment, 333*t*
Thrombotic disorders. *See also* Thrombosis
hereditary, 343–348
in newborns, 348–351
  acquired, 349–350
  congenital, 348–349
  diagnosis and treatment of neonatal thromboembolism, 351*t*
  risk factors for perinatal stroke, 350–351*t*
Thrombotic thrombocytopenic purpura syndrome, 266–268, 266*t*, 339
Thromboxane synthetase deficiency, 287
Thyroid gland
deficiency, late effects of childhood cancer, 764
hematologic manifestations of disease, 75
hyperthyroidism, in mothers, and neonatal thrombocytopenia, 280
values, 799*t*
Thyroid-stimulating hormone deficiency, late effects of childhood cancer, 763*t*, 764, 765*t*
Tissue plasminogen activator (t-PA), 337, 348, 358
Tissues, cellular changes in iron-deficiency anemia, 38*t*
Torch infections, hematologic manifestations, 83
Transcobalamin I, (R-binder) partial deficiency, 52, 53*t*, 56*t*
Transcobalamin II, abnormalities, vitamin B$_{12}$ deficiency, 52, 53*t*, 56*t*
Transfusions. *See* Blood component therapy
Transient erythroblastopenia, differentiating from Diamond-Blackfan anemia (DBA), 97–99, 98*t*, 104
clinical features, 104
Transient ischemic attacks, antithrombotic therapy, 361
Transplancental fetomaternal blood loss, 12
Triosephosphate isomerase deficiency, 153
Trisomy 21 abnormality in childhood MDS, 394
Trisomy 8 abnormality in childhood MDS and JMML, 397
Trypanosomiasis, hematologic manifestations, 85
Tuberculosis, hematologic manifestations, 84
Tumor lysis syndrome, 696*t*, 697–700
Tumor markers, 650–651, 803–804
deviation of normal serum AFP in infants, 651*t*
staging systems, 652*t*
Tumor necrosis factor alpha (TNF-α), 399
Turcot Syndrome, 512
Twin-to-twin transfusion, and prenatal blood loss, 15
Typhlitis, 701–702

U

Umbilical artery catheterization, 335
Unstable hemoglobins, 180, 180*t*, 181*t*
Urokinase, 358–359

V

Valve replacement, antithrombotic therapy, 360
Varicella exposure, prophylactic antibiotics for, 717
Vascular-platelet interactions, in fetus and neonate, 795*t*
Vasoactive intestinal peptide (VIP), 532
Vaso-occlusive crisis *See* Sickle cell disease
Veno-occlusive disease (VOD), complication of stem cell transplantation, 691–692
Viral illnesses with marked hematologic sequelae, 78–84
Visceroptosis of spleen, 367
Vitamin B$_{12}$ deficiency
absorption of dietary vitamin B$_{12}$, 47
cause of megaloblastosis, 48*t*
causes of, 48–49*t*
  defective absorption, 50, 51*t*, 52
  defective transport, 52, 54–55*t*
  disorders of metabolism, 52–58, 53*f*, 54–55*t*
  nutritional deficiency, 49–50
clinical features, 65–66
clinical manifestations, 49
diagnosis, 66–68, 67*t*
treatment, 68–69
Vitamin E, normal serum levels, newborns, 798*t*
Vitamin E deficiency, 26–27
Vitamin K deficiency, 304–309
coagulation tests and interpretation, 305*f*
conditions associated with, 306*t*
disseminated intravascular coagulation, 307–309
  disease states associated with, 308*t*
  treatment, 307*t*
hepatic dysfunction, 305–306
laboratory findings, 306*t*
VMA, normal values, 798*t*
Vomiting. *See* Nausea and vomiting, management of
von Hippel-Lindau mutations, causing polycythemia, 205, 512
von Willebrand disease (vWD), 322–328
acquired vWD, 327, 550–551*t*, 555
classification of, 324*t*
comparison with Hemophilia A, 323*t*
defective platelet function, 283*t*, 285
platelet-type pseudo-vWD, 324*t*, 327
protein structure, 325*f*
treatment, 326*t*, 555
type 1, 322, 324*t*
type 2A, 322–323, 324*t*
type 2B, 323, 324*t*
type 2M, 324*t*, 325
type 2N, 323, 324*t*, 325
type 3, 325, 327
von Willebrand factor (vWF), 322

W

WAGR syndrome, 548, 553
Warfarin therapy, 355–357
  effects of drugs on warfarin response, 358*t*
Wegener granulomatosis, hematologic
    manifestations, 77
Weibel-Palade body in epithelial cells, 322
Weil disease, hematologic manifestations, 84
Well syndrome, 241
WHIM syndrome, 220–221
White blood cells. *See* Leukocytes
Wilms' tumor, 548–560
  anaplastic, 552–553
  associated congenital anomalies
      aniridia, 548, 549*t*
      Beckwith-Wiedemann syndrome, 549–550
      follow-up of patients with, 550
      hemihypertrophy, 549
      incidence, 549*t*
  bilateral, 557–558
      prognostic factors, 557, 557*t*
      treatment, 558
  clinicopathologic staging system, 552*t*
  cytogenic and molecular features, 553
  incidence, 548
  laboratory studies, 551, 551*t*
  pathology, 551–553
  prognosis, 557, 557*t*
  second malignant neoplasms, late effects of
      childhood cancer, 773
  signs and symptoms, 550, 550*t*
  staging system, 551, 552*t*
  treatment

  of acquired von Willebrand disease, 555
  NWTS recommendations for Wilms' tumor,
      554*t*
  post-therapy follow-up, 555–556
  radiation therapy, 554–555
  of relapse, 556–557
  surgery, 553–554
  tumors inoperable because of size, 555
Wiskott-Aldrich syndrome, 252*t*, 276, 327, 329*t*
Wolfram syndrome, 64–65, 129

X

Xanthogranuloma, juvenile, 620
Xerocytosis, hereditary, 150–151
X-linked anemia, 276
X-linked lymphoproliferative syndrome
  clinical manifestations, 383
  diagnostic criteria for, 384*t*
  pathophysiology, 382–383
  prognosis, 384
  treatment, 383–384

Y

Yolk sac tumor
  ovarian, 659
  testicular, 658

Z

Zinc protoporphyrin/heme ratio, in iron
    deficiency, 40
Zollinger-Ellison syndrome, iron deficiency in, 72